Rudolph's
PEDIATRICS
22ND EDITION
SELF-ASSESSMENT
AND BOARD REVIEW

Rudolph's
PEDIATRICS
22ND EDITION
SELF-ASSESSMENT
AND BOARD REVIEW

Editor

Michael D. Cabana, MD, MPH

Professor of Pediatrics, Epidemiology, and Biostatistics
Chief, Division of General Pediatrics
Department of Pediatrics
University of California, San Francisco
UCSF Benioff Children's Hospital
Philip R. Lee Institute for Health Policy Studies
San Francisco, California

Consulting Editors

Hilary M. Haftel, MD, MHPE

Professor of Pediatrics
Department of Pediatrics and Communicable Diseases
University of Michigan
Ann Arbor, Michigan

Sunitha V. Kaiser, MD

Assistant Professor of Pediatrics
Department of Pediatrics
University of California, San Francisco
San Francisco, California

Julie Stein O'Brien, MD

Assistant Professor of Pediatrics
Department of Pediatrics
University of California, San Francisco
San Francisco, California

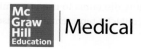

New York   Chicago   San Francisco   Athens   London   Madrid
Mexico City   Milan   New Delhi   Singapore   Sydney   Toronto

1 2 3 4 5 6 7 8 9 0   CTP/CTP   18 17 16 15 14 13

ISBN 978-0-07-178109-1
MHID 0-07-178109-9

The book was set in Minion Pro by Thomson Digital.
The editors were Alyssa K. Fried and Peter J. Boyle.
The production supervisor was Catherine H. Saggese.
Project management was provided by Ritu Joon, Thomson Digital.
The designer was Alan Barnett.
China Translation & Printing Services, Ltd., was printer and binder.

This book was printed on acid-free paper.

Library of Congress Cataloging-in-Publication Data

Rudolph's pediatrics self-assessment and board review / editor, Michael Cabana.
   p. ; cm.
 Pediatrics self-assessment and board review
 Complemented by: Rudolph's pediatrics / editor-in-chief, Colin D. Rudolph; editors,
Abraham M. Rudolph ... [et al.]. 22nd ed. c2011.
 Includes index.
 ISBN-13: 978-0-07-178109-1 (paperback : alk. paper)
 ISBN-10: 0-07-178109-9 (paperback : alk. paper)
 ISBN-13: 978-0-07-178110-7 (ebook)
 I. Cabana, Michael D., editor of compilation. II. Rudolph's pediatrics. Complemented by (work):
III. Title: Pediatrics self-assessment and board review.
 [DNLM: 1. Pediatrics—Examination Questions. WS 18.2]
 RJ45
 618.92—dc23
                                                                          2013025619

International Edition ISBN 978-1-25-909516-0; MHID 1-25-909516-9.
Copyright © 2014. Exclusive rights by McGraw-Hill Education, for manufacture and export. This book cannot be re-exported from the country to which it is consigned by McGraw-Hill Education. The International Edition is not available in North America.

McGraw-Hill Education books are available at special quantity discounts to use as premiums and sales promotions, or for use in corporate training programs. To contact a representative please visit the Contact Us pages at www.mhprofessional.com.

To Cewin, Alexandra, Abigail, Annie, and Binko
—*MDC*

To Mindy, Gene, George, and Georgia
—*JSO*

To Dan, Lirit, and Shoshana
—*HMH*

To Rao, Vasu, Scott, and Varun
—*SVK*

CONTENTS

CONTENTS

CONTRIBUTORS

Ayesha Ahmad, MBBS
Assistant Professor of Pediatrics
Division of Genetics
University of Michigan
Ann Arbor, Michigan
Chapter 11

Duha Al-Zubeidi, MD
Pediatric Infectious Diseases Fellos
Department of Pediatrics
Washington University School of Medicine
St. Louis, Missouri
Chapter 17

Alan P. Baptist, MD, MPH
Assistant Professor of Medicine
Department of Medicine
Division of Allergy and Clinical Immunology
University of Michigan School of Medicine
Ann Arbor, Michigan
Chapter 14

Sara M. Buckelew, MD, MPH
Associate Professor of Pediatrics
Department of Pediatrics
University of California, San Francisco
San Francisco, California
Chapter 6

Kristin L. Van Buren, MD
Assistant Professor of Pediatrics
Department of Pediatrics
Baylor College of Medicine
Houston, Texas
Chapter 21

Natalie J. Burman, DO, MA
Instructor of Pediatrics
Department of Pediatrics
University of California, San Francisco
San Francisco, California
Chapter 1

Michael D. Cabana, MD, MPH
Professor of Pediatrics, Epidemiology, and Biostatistics
Chief, Division of General Pediatrics
Department of Pediatrics
University of California, San Francisco
UCSF Benioff Children's Hospital
Philip R. Lee Institute for Health Policy Studies
San Francisco, California
Chapters 3, 17, and 20

Diana Camarillo, MD
Pediatric Dermatology Fellow
Department of Dermatology
University of California, San Francisco
San Francisco, California
Chapter 18

Cewin Chao, MS, RD, MBA
Director, CTSI Bionutrition Core
Department of Medicine
University of California, San Francisco
San Francisco, California
Chapter 3

Eric H. Chiou, MD
Assistant Professor of Pediatrics
Department of Pediatrics
Baylor College of Medicine
Houston, Texas
Chapter 21

Christine S. Cho, MD, MPH, MEd
Assistant Professor of Pediatrics and Emergency Medicine
Departments of Pediatrics and Emergency Medicine
University of California, San Francisco
San Francisco, California
Chapter 8

Elizabeth A. Cristofalo, MD, MPH
Assistant Professor of Pediatrics
Department of Pediatrics
Johns Hopkins University School of Medicine
Baltimore, Maryland
Chapter 5

Colleen Hughes Driscoll, MD
Assistant Professor of Pediatrics
Department of Pediatrics
University of Maryland School of Medicine
Baltimore, Maryland
Chapter 5

Ada M. Fenick, MD
Assistant Professor of Pediatrics
Department of Pediatrics
Yale School of Medicine
New Haven, Connecticut
Chapter 2

Amy G. Filbrun, MD, MS
Clinical Assistant Professor of Pediatrics
Department of Pediatrics and Communicable Diseases
University of Michigan
Ann Arbor, Michigan
Chapter 27

Susan Fisher-Owens, MD, MPH
Associate Professor of Pediatrics
Department of Pediatrics
University of California, San Francisco
San Francisco, California
Chapter 20

Amy A. Gelfand, MD
Clinical Instructor
Departments of Pediatrics and Neurology
University of California, San Francisco
San Francisco, California
Chapter 29

Danielle M. Goetz, MD
Assistant Professor of Pediatrics
Department of Pediatrics
University of Buffalo
Buffalo, New York
Chapter 27

W. Christopher Golden, MD
Assistant Professor of Pediatrics
Department of Pediatrics
Johns Hopkins University School of Medicine
Baltimore, Maryland
Chapter 5

Robert Goldsby, MD
Professor of Pediatrics
Department of Pediatrics
University of California, San Francisco
San Francisco, California
Chapter 24

Andrea K. Goldyn, MD
Pediatric Endocrinology and Diabetology Fellow
Department of Pediatrics
Indiana University School of Medicine
Indianapolis, Indiana
Chapter 28

Deepti Gupta, MD
Pediatric Dermatology Fellow
Department of Dermatology
University of California, San Francisco
San Francisco, California
Chapter 18

Hilary M. Haftel, MD, MHPE
Professor of Pediatrics
Department of Pediatrics and Communicable Diseases
University of Michigan
Ann Arbor, Michigan
Chapters 13, 15, and 16

Lauren B. Hartman, MD
Instructor of Pediatrics
Department of Pediatrics
University of California, San Francisco
San Francisco, California
Chapter 6

D. Micah Hester, PhD
Professor of Medical Humanities and Pediatrics
Division of Medical Humanities
University of Arkansas for Medical Sciences
Little Rock, Arkansas
Chapter 1

Bernadette A. Hillman, MD
Clinical Instructor of Pediatrics
Department of Pediatrics
Yale-New Haven Hospital
New Haven, Connecticut
The Hospital of Central Connecticut
New Britain, Connecticut
Chapter 5

James Huang, MD
Professor of Pediatrics
Department of Pediatrics
University of California, San Francisco
San Francisco, California
Chapter 23

Tannie Huang, MD
Clinical Instructor
Department of Pediatrics
University of California, San Francisco
San Francisco, California
Chapter 23

Sunitha V. Kaiser, MD
Assistant Professor of Pediatrics
Department of Pediatrics
University of California, San Francisco
San Francisco, California
Chapters 9 and 17

Dylan C. Kann, MD
Assistant Professor
Department of Pediatrics
University of California, San Francisco
San Francisco, California
Chapter 17

David B. Kershaw, MD
Associate Professor of Pediatrics
Department of Pediatrics and Communicable Diseases
University of Michigan
Ann Arbor, Michigan
Chapter 10

Alaina K. Kipps, MD
Assistant Professor of Pediatrics
Department of Pediatrics
Stanford Medical School
Palo Alto, California
Chapter 26

Cornelia Latronica, MD
Attending Physician
Department of Pediatric Emergency Medicine
Children's Hospital and Research Center Oakland
Oakland, California
Chapter 8

Sarah Shrager Lusman, MD
Assistant Professor of Pediatrics
Department of Pediatrics
Columbia University Medical Center
New York, New York
Chapter 22

Ann L. Marqueling, MD
Assistant Clinical Professor
Departments of Dermatology and Pediatrics
Stanford University School of Medicine
Palo Alto, California
Chapter 18

Erin F.D. Mathes, MD
Assistant Professor of Dermatology
Department of Dermatology
University of California, San Francisco
San Francisco, California
Chapter 18

Anna K. Meyer, MD
Assistant Professor of Otolaryngology
Department of Otolaryngology
University of California, San Francisco
San Francisco, California
Chapter 19

Kendall B. Nash, MD
Assistant Professor of Pediatrics and Neurology
Departments of Pediatrics and Neurology
University of California, San Francisco
San Francisco, California
Chapter 29

Todd D. Nebesio, MD
Associate Professor of Clinical Pediatrics
Department of Pediatrics
Indiana University School of Medicine
Indianapolis, Indiana
Chapter 28

Haley C. Neef, MD
Assistant Professor of Pediatrics
Department of Pediatrics and Communicable Diseases
University of Michigan
Ann Arbor, Michigan
Chapters 21 and 22

Julie Stein O'Brien, MD
Assistant Professor of Pediatrics
Department of Pediatrics
University of California, San Francisco
San Francisco, California
Chapter 7

Vikash Oza, MD
Pediatric Dermatology Fellow
Department of Dermatology
University of California, San Francisco
San Francisco, California
Chapter 18

Erica Pan, MD, MPH
Associate Clinical Professor of Pediatrics
Department of Pediatrics
University of California, San Francisco
San Francisco, California
Director
Alameda County Public Health Department
Division of Communicable Disease Control and Prevention
Oakland, California
Chapter 17

Jerusha Pearson-Lev, MD
Attending Physician
Denver Emergency Center for Children
Denver Health
Denver, Colorado
Chapter 8

Julie C. Philp, MD
Pediatric Dermatology Fellow
Department of Dermatology
University of California, San Francisco
San Francisco, California
Chapter 18

Kartik Pillutla, MD
Attending Pediatric Nephrologist
Dell Children's Medical Center of Central Texas
Austin, Texas
Chapter 25

Laura A. Robertson, MD
Associate Professor of Pediatrics
Department of Pediatrics
University of California, San Francisco
San Francisco, California
Chapter 26

Kristina W. Rosbe, MD
Professor of Clinical Otolaryngology
Department of Otolaryngology
University of California, San Francisco
San Francisco, California
Chapter 19

Tina Rutar, MD
Assistant Professor of Pediatrics and Ophthalmology
Departments of Pediatrics and Ophthalmology
University of California, San Francisco
San Francisco, California
Chapter 30

Angela Scheuerle, MD
Clinical Assistant Professor
McDermott Center for Human Genetics
University of Texas (UT) Southwestern
Medical Director
Texas Birth Defects Research Center
UT Houston School of Public Health
Dallas, Texas
Chapter 12

Lance M. Siegel, MD
Associate Clinical Professor
Department of Ophthalmology
University of California, Los Angeles (UCLA)
Los Angeles, California
Director
Children's Eye Institute
Upland, California
Chapter 30

Laura L. Sisterhen, MD, MPH
Associate Professor
Department of Pediatrics
University of Arkansas for Medical Sciences
Little Rock, Arkansas
Chapter 1

Aimee Leyton Speck, MD
Fellow
Department of Medicine
Division of Allergy and Clinical Immunology
University of Michigan School of Medicine
Ann Arbor, Michigan
Chapter 14

Martin T. Stein, MD
Professor of Pediatrics
Department of Pediatrics
University of California, San Diego (UCSD)
San Diego, California
Chapter 7

Christopher C. Stewart, MD
Associate Professor of Pediatrics
Department of Pediatrics
University of California, San Francisco
San Francisco, California
Chapter 4

John I. Takayama, MD, MPH
Professor of Clinical Pediatrics
Department of Pediatrics
University of California, San Francisco
San Francisco, California
Chapter 9

Marie H. Tanzer, MD
Attending Pediatric Nephrologist
Department of Pediatrics
Maine Medical Partners Pediatric Specialty Care
Portland, Maine
Chapter 10

Ashley Ward, MD
Assistant Professor of Pediatrics
Department of Pediatrics
University of California, San Francisco
San Francisco, California
Chapter 24

Erica Winnicki, MD
Assistant Professor
Department of Pediatrics
University of California, Davis
Sacramento, California
Chapter 25

Nanci Yuan, MD
Clinical Associate Professor of Pediatrics
Department of Pediatrics
Stanford University School of Medicine
Palo Alto, California
Chapter 27

Barrett J. Zlotoff, MD
Associate Professor
Department of Dermatology
University of New Mexico
Albuquerque, New Mexico
Chapter 18

FOREWORD

True knowledge exists in knowing that you know nothing.

Socrates

In the 22nd edition of *Rudolph's Pediatrics*, we provided a comprehensive review of the development of the normal infant and child and of the disorders and diseases that may affect them. A prime objective was the consideration of the biologic basis for normal and abnormal development and for the changes associated with the disease. With this vast amount of background information, it may be difficult to define the role of etiological factors and the significance of various clinical observations in differential diagnosis and management.

In this *Self-Assessment and Board Review*, Dr. Cabana and his colleagues follow the tradition of the great teacher Socrates by providing a series of questions designed to assist the reader in analyzing the importance of abnormal physiologic, biochemical, genetic, and other features in pediatric disorders and to highlight clinical features that aid in differential diagnosis. Stimulating questions allow the student to assess the extent of their own knowledge. Brief explanations illustrate key points, and readers are conveniently referred to the core textbook for in-depth learning. We congratulate the authors for creating this valuable resource to help all of us evaluate our knowledge of pediatrics, and thereby assure we provide children with the best care possible.

Colin D. Rudolph, MD, PhD
Clinical Professor
Department of Pediatrics
University of California, San Francisco

Abraham M. Rudolph, MD
Professor Emeritus
Department of Pediatrics
University of California, San Francisco

PREFACE

It is much simpler to buy books than to read them, and easier to read them than to absorb their contents.

William Osler, MD
1848–1919

Rudolph's Pediatrics 22nd Edition Self-Assessment and Board Review builds upon the 22nd edition of the textbook, *Rudolph's Pediatrics*. Although *Rudolph's Pediatrics* is already a key resource and reference, our goal was to create a companion book that would allow readers to more easily and quickly absorb the contents presented in *Rudolph's Pediatrics*.

As a result, this book contains over 1500 questions that place the content in *Rudolph's Pediatrics* in a clinical context. While the textbook presents a general overview of different pediatric topics, this *Self-Assessment and Board Review* book actively questions the reader about the clinical application of such material in terms of the epidemiology, pathophysiology, presenting symptoms, clinical decision making, therapeutics, and prognosis of different pediatric disorders. This book is designed for practicing pediatricians who need to quickly assess their knowledge of pediatrics, by topic. This book then gives the reader a quick reference to the pertinent sections in *Rudolph's Pediatrics* to reinforce the reader's knowledge about the topic.

We have been able to enlist an outstanding group of pediatric clinician educators who have provided a collection of challenging questions for each chapter. These questions highlight the key clinical issues from *Rudolph's Pediatrics*. In addition, the thirty topics presented in this book parallel the thirty topics and chapters in *Rudolph's Pediatrics*. This feature allows readers the opportunity to focus on any one specific topic, based on their own learning needs.

We are sure that you will find this review book both comprehensive and challenging. We hope you find this book indispensable as part of your preparation and review for the Pediatric Board examination.

Michael D. Cabana, MD, MPH
San Francisco, California

ACKNOWLEDGMENTS

We would like to thank the team at McGraw-Hill who have helped us throughout this process, including Dominik Pucek, Christine Barcellona, and Alyssa Fried. A special thanks to Abraham Rudolph, MD, who introduced us to the McGraw-Hill team and entrusted us with developing this project. In addition, thanks to Nancy Tran, from the University of Vermont, who helped us edit and prepare this text.

We would also like to thank our respective Chairs, Donna Ferriero, MD, at the University of California, San Francisco (UCSF), and Valerie Castle, MD, at the University of Michigan for their support and leadership. We acknowledge our medical students, residents, and trainees who keep us sharp with their questions and excited about our work with their enthusiasm. UCSF Benioff Children's Hospital and C.S. Mott Children's Hospital are very special places to work. Every single day, outstanding patient care, clinical education, new discoveries, and advocacy for children are applied to provide the best possible care for children, families, and communities.

CHAPTER 1 | Fundamentals of Pediatrics

Laura L. Sisterhen, Natalie J. Burman, and D. Micah Hester

1-1. You are working in a community clinic setting and the clinic is implementing an electronic medical record system for the first time. You have been asked to give input on behalf of the other pediatricians in your clinic that will allow the system to better serve your patients and facilitate communication between providers caring for your patients. Which of the following recommendations will best serve your patient population well into the 21st century?

   a. A diagnosis list that is reduced to contain pediatric-specific diagnoses only

   b. An automated system that selects the best empiric antibiotic for specific infectious diseases

   c. An electronic reminder system that notifies you when labs are abnormal and contains family contact information to relay the results

   d. A system that can be highly individualized to allow each provider to routinely choose the asthma treatment approach that works best for each individual provider

   e. The ability to generate a lab requisition printout for a patient to carry with him or her to the laboratory

1-2. You are a hospitalist at a community hospital. The respiratory therapists have asked that you give a talk on aerosolized treatments for bronchiolitis. Specifically, they have asked the following question: "In infants hospitalized with bronchiolitis, does 3% hypertonic saline compared with 0.9% saline result in decreased length of stay?" Which of the following study titles is most likely to best answer the clinical question?

   a. Nebulized hypertonic saline without adjunctive bronchodilators for children with bronchiolitis: a retrospective cohort study

   b. Nebulized 3% hypertonic saline solution treatment in hospitalized infants with viral bronchiolitis: a randomized, double-blind, controlled trial

   c. Hypertonic saline in the treatment of acute bronchiolitis in the emergency department: a case series

   d. Nebulized hypertonic saline and recombinant human DNAse in the treatment of pulmonary atelectasis in newborns

   e. Inhaled hypertonic saline in infants and toddlers with bronchiolitis: short-term tolerability, adherence, and safety

1-3. You are reviewing a new study for journal club. The authors enrolled 50 infants admitted to the hospital with bronchiolitis and randomized them to receive either treatment with a nasal decongestant or placebo. Following administration of the nasal drops, a research assistant measured the change in oxygen saturation. One parent withdrew consent; thus, 49 of the 50 patients completed the study. The results showed that there was no statistical difference in change in oxygen saturation between groups ($P > .05$). As part of your discussion, you critically appraise the evidence. Which of the following is the most accurate statement?

   a. The results of the study could have been affected by a small sample size.

   b. The results demonstrate that topical nasal decongestants are not effective in reducing length of stay for infants with bronchiolitis.

   c. Infants who were randomized to the treatment group, but did not receive the drug due to tachycardia, should not have been included in the treatment group during analysis.

   d. This is a cohort study that is able to equalize study groups for known, but not unknown, confounding factors.

   e. The number of patients lost to follow-up was unacceptable.

1-4. You receive a daily e-mail summarizing the latest pediatric research on your handheld device. One study on bullying behaviors catches your attention. On further reading, you learn that the study was based on an analysis of a nationally representative, cross-sectional survey of 15,000 students in grades 6 to 10. Involvement in bullying and self-reported physical symptoms such as headaches, stomachaches, backaches, dizziness, and sleeping difficulties were measured. The results showed that 15% of the students were involved in bullying as a victim and/or as a bully at least once a week. Students who reported at least 1 or more physical symptoms, which occur several times a week, were 3 times more likely to be involved in frequent bullying incidents, as compared with students who did not experience frequent symptoms. What is the most accurate conclusion you can determine from the results of this study?

a. Involvement in bullying causes stress in school-aged children resulting in physical symptoms of headaches, stomachaches, and backaches.

b. Physical symptoms of headaches, stomachaches, and backaches in children cause them to engage in more frequent bullying.

c. In preadolescent and adolescent students in grades 6 to 10, the incidence of bullying behaviors is 15%.

d. There is an association between bullying behaviors and somatic complaints that merits further investigation with a stronger observational study.

e. Physical symptoms of headaches, stomachaches, and backaches in children are the result of being a victim of frequent bullying.

1-5. You are a clinician who is approached by a researcher to collaborate in a study. The researcher would like to examine the effect of a new prethickened formula on gastroesophageal reflux disease in infants. As a clinician, you are most interested in patient-centered outcomes as opposed to disease-oriented outcomes. Which of the following study designs will you recommend as the most clinically useful study?

a. A double-blind, randomized trial of prethickened versus standard formula in infants with symptomatic reflux comparing the reduction of pain symptoms and weight gain in the 2 groups

b. An observational study of infants measuring their symptom severity score before and after initiating the new prethickened formula

c. A double-blind, randomized trial examining the effect of the prethickened formula on gastroesophageal reflux using scintigraphic measurement of gastric emptying time

d. A placebo-controlled crossover study examining the effects of the thickened formula on gastroesophageal reflux using intraluminal impedance

e. A placebo-controlled, randomized trial of the thickened formula using direct laryngoscopy to examine for the presence of reflux-related extraesophageal tissue injury

1-6. A mother comes in with her newborn son and her 3-year-old daughter to establish care for the infant. She is concerned about the baby's slow weight gain. As you begin to discuss breast-feeding with the mother, the 3-year-old sister begins telling you about her new doll that she brought to the visit and she wants you to examine the abrasion on her knee from a fall this morning. While you find the 3-year-old compelling and adorable, it is difficult to focus the encounter on the new baby and his mother's concerns. What is the most effective way to redirect this patient encounter?

a. Ask the mother if the toddler can go out into the waiting room with her grandmother, since the grandmother is visiting to help with the new adjustment.

b. Ask the toddler if she helps her mother to take care of the new baby and then ask her to hold onto the pacifier while the baby breast-feeds so you can evaluate the latch.

c. Discuss with the mother that this is typical sibling rivalry behavior and give her several strategies on how to assist the toddler with the adjustment.

d. Excuse yourself from the mother and baby to examine the toddler's abrasion and give her appropriate reassurance.

e. Speak directly to the toddler and tell her she needs to be quiet because today it is her brother's turn and she will get her turn at her appointment.

1-7. A 5-year-old girl is here with her mother to see you for her kindergarten entrance physical. When you walk into the room, the 5-year-old begins crying and says, "No, I don't want a shot." As you begin to engage the family, which of the following statements is the best choice for promoting relationship building with the child and her mother?

a. As you enter the room, you take a few minutes to read the electronic medical record and begin reviewing her past medical history and previous clinic notes.

b. As you walk into the room, you make direct eye contact with the mother and introduce yourself to her, making sure you learn the mother's first name and then introduce yourself to the patient.

c. You efficiently go through any new concerns, review the past medical history, and begin your physical examination so you can stay on schedule.

d. You introduce yourself to the child first and say, "Wow, you are already to start kindergarten! You must be so excited. Did you get any new school supplies yet?"

e. You sit down on the examination table right next to the girl and say, "Don't worry, we don't do any shots in this room. The nurse will take you to the shot room when we are all done here."

1-8. You are seeing a 2-year-old child in your clinic. Her parents state she has been refusing to walk the past couple of days. One week ago she had a febrile illness. They do not report any trauma. On observation, you see that she is in no respiratory distress. She cries as you approach her for examination. While auscultating her chest, she leans down to bite your arm. As part of your assessment, you want to assess her reflexes and motor strength. What is the most appropriate next step to complete your examination?

a. Defer the examination until she is more cooperative with your neurological examination.

b. Explain to the child that she must do what the doctor says or we cannot help her feel better.

c. Enlist the family to make her follow your directions and hold her head if necessary.

d. Ask for a physical therapy consult for a more comprehensive evaluation.

e. Use toys to encourage her to stand while blowing bubbles that she can reach for and pop.

1-9. Mrs Johnson brings her 6-year-old daughter in for a scheduled asthma recheck. You scheduled a 10-minute visit and are behind in your schedule. She is very chatty about her recent divorce, and her daughter's sleep disturbances, bedwetting, and itchy rash on her arms that seems to be getting worse with the over-the-counter cream they are using. You note that since the last visit, she has made 2 emergency department visits for wheezing. Today, you want to obtain spirometry and manage her asthma, which is not well controlled. What is the best response in order to plan the visit with the patient, and prioritize the asthma?

a. "Let's make sure we talk about her asthma and eczema. It sounds like you also want to make sure we cover her bedwetting. If we can't get to the other concerns, let's schedule another visit to discuss her adjustment to the divorce."

b. "When a visit is scheduled for an asthma recheck, the only diagnosis I have time to address today is your daughter's asthma. The bedwetting will probably get better once she has adjusted to the divorce."

c. "You are concerned about issues that are not related to your daughter's asthma, which is the most important diagnosis for us to discuss. I'll refer your daughter to a counselor to help her adjust to the recent divorce."

d. "Next time you call for an appointment, let them know that you need an hour with me, so I can address all of your concerns at once."

e. "Your divorce seems to be having an effect on your daughter, given all of her symptoms. How were you hoping I could help?"

1-10. You are caring for a girl who was diagnosed with obesity 4 years ago based on her BMI percentile at her 6-year-old well visit. She comes in today with her mother for her 10-year-old well visit and continues to have an elevated BMI. When you ask the patient how confident she is on a scale of 1 (not at all confident) to 10 (very confident) that she can cut soda out of her diet, she tells you "6." Choose the best response to her answer based on your knowledge of motivational interviewing.

a. "Six, which is really great. I am really glad you chose a higher number today than you did at your last visit."

b. "That is excellent; I can tell you are ready to make a change."

c. "Okay, why not lower?"

d. "Do you think you are ready to make a change?"

e. "How confident are you that you can cut out fast food?"

1-11. A 15-year-old girl is accompanied by her father for a sport's physical. As you walk into the examination room, you sense there is some tension between the adolescent and her father. After completing the past medical history with most of the answers from her father and a few mumbled answers from the adolescent, you politely ask the father to wait in the waiting room so that you can complete the physical examination. You explain to him this procedure is routine for all patients over age 12. Once he leaves the room, you begin the HEADSS examination. During this assessment, she says, "My father and I don't really get along. He always wants to be in my business." Which of the following questions would be the best response to her statement?

   a. "Does he invade your privacy?"

   b. "Don't you think he is just concerned for your safety?"

   c. "Do you feel overly restricted by his concerns for you?"

   d. "When was the last time he got into your business?"

   e. "Why do you think he is concerned about your business?"

1-12. You are seeing a 2-year-old with reactive airway disease in your office. She comes in today with her mother who is frustrated by the frequency of her cough. While taking the history, you ask if anyone in the household smokes tobacco. She responds, "I'm tired of being asked about my smoking every time I bring my daughter to the doctor." What is the best reflective statement in response to her statement during the encounter?

   a. "You do know that the best thing you can do for your health is to quit smoking, don't you?"

   b. "I'm sorry, I apologize. I won't ask you about your smoking anymore."

   c. "May I give you some information about secondhand smoke exposure?"

   d. "Do you know how harmful smoking in the home is to your daughter's health?"

   e. "It sounds like you are frustrated by health care providers asking if you smoke."

1-13. A 2-year-old boy comes in for his annual well visit accompanied by his mother. Early into the visit, she discloses to you that there is marital discord in the home and she is struggling with the behavior that is exhibited by her son. As you review the *Bright Futures* checklist of items to discuss at this visit, you realize that you cannot address all of the guidelines recommended for a 2-year-old well visit during the 20-minute appointment. Which clinic system would be most important to have in place so that you can best meet the needs of this child and his mother?

   a. A handout discussing multiple safety concerns appropriate for 2-year-olds

   b. A list of community resources that support families coping with stress

   c. An established referral network that includes developmental pediatricians

   d. Developmental surveillance questions included on your well visit encounter form

   e. Reach Out and Read volunteers to enhance early literacy in the waiting room

1-14. You are seeing a 13-year-old girl with cystic fibrosis today for a follow-up visit from her recent admission. You have been following her since her abnormal newborn screen for elevated trypsinogen. She initially had surgery as an infant for bowel obstruction and was closely followed for poor weight gain until age 2. Over the past year, she has become colonized with a mucoid strain of *Pseudomonas* and was admitted for the first time for intravenous and inhaled antibiotics to attempt to eradicate her colonization and treat pneumonia. As you are starting to feel overwhelmed by her changing medical condition and the stress the admission has put on the family, you stop to think about your role in her care as a general pediatrician. Within the larger system of care for this patient's disease, which of the following is your responsibility?

   a. Coordinating her follow-up bronchial aspiration procedure through the pediatric anesthesia department

   b. Ensuring she is on the clinic registry as a high-risk patient to receive the annual influenza immunization once it becomes available

   c. Optimizing her outpatient antibiotic and pulmonary treatment regimen for her current respiratory status

   d. Organizing multidisciplinary clinics to address all of her cystic fibrosis needs

   e. Selecting appropriate educational materials and providing cystic fibrosis education to teach her about the progression of her condition

1-15. A 7-week male infant is brought into your afternoon clinic by his father for a concern of fever. The infant has been feeding well, but a little fussier than usual. His father became concerned and obtained a rectal temperature this morning at 101.3°F (38.5°C) and brought the baby in for an evaluation. Using a systems-based approach, which of the following is the best choice in proceeding to care for this infant?

   a. Conferring with your colleague down the hall, to see what she thinks you should do for this infant

   b. Discussing with the father if he feels comfortable taking the infant home with a follow-up appointment in 24 hours

   c. Referring to your institutional clinical practice guideline on fevers that was last updated 10 years ago

   d. Requesting your nurse recheck the temperature to ensure the infant is currently febrile

   e. Using the online source for National Guideline Clearinghouse to find the most recent guideline for fever in an infant

1-16. As you are finishing up your charting after a long and busy summer day, you check your inbox to find 5 patient phone calls to address before you can leave for the day. Three of the 5 calls are regarding difficulty scheduling appointments with you for well and follow-up visits. These 3 families have been in your practice for quite a while. This problem has become a routine issue and you contemplate what can be done to fix this. Which of the following changes would be most effective in improving access for your established patients?

   a. Ask your front desk staff to complete all registration paperwork and insurance verification in the waiting room so that any problems can be addressed before the patient is in the examination room.

   b. Begin charting patient demand for appointments to determine which patient needs are and aren't being met by your current appointment templates.

   c. Confirm that your supply storage room is fully stocked so you can go to a central place to obtain all necessary supplies during patient encounters.

   d. Increase the length of your appointments from 20 to 30 minutes so you can accomplish more at each visit, reducing the need for follow-up visits.

   e. Increase the number of acute appointments in your summer templates so that families who need same-day care are appointed more quickly, leaving more available appointments in the future for routine care.

1-17. Graduate medical education has shifted its focus from structure- and process-based experience to competency-based training. Six core competencies have been embraced by multiple medical education organizations and many accrediting bodies. These competencies consist of medical knowledge, patient care, interpersonal and communication skills, professionalism, practice-based learning and improvement, and systems-based practice. Which of the following statements best describes the reason for this new emphasis on competency-based training and physician performance?

   a. A report put out by the Institute of Medicine that outlined this new structure for medical education.

   b. The Accreditation Council for Graduate Medical Education (ACGME) developed these to address the need for improved quality of care.

   c. The Flexner report issued by the Carnegie Foundation set forth this approach to medical education.

   d. The Joint Commission requests to see these 6 competencies evaluated for each physician within a health care organization.

   e. The need for teaching hospitals to be more financially solvent in an increasingly competitive medical marketplace.

1-18. The Accreditation Council for Graduate Medical Education (ACGME) has outlined 6 core competencies to guide assessment of all residents within a residency program. Which of the following is the correct competency–description pair?

   a. Interpersonal and communication skills—Residents must be able to provide compassionate, appropriate, and effective patient care for the treatment of health problems and the promotion of health.

   b. Medical knowledge—Residents must demonstrate knowledge of established and evolving biomedical, clinical, epidemiological, and social–behavioral sciences and demonstrate the ability to apply this knowledge to patient care.

   c. Patient care—Residents must demonstrate interpersonal and communication skills that result in the effective exchange of information and collaboration with patients, their families, and health professionals.

   d. Practice-based learning and improvement—Residents must demonstrate an awareness of and a responsiveness to the larger context and system of health care, as well as the ability to call effectively on other resources in the system to provide optimal health care.

   e. Systems-based practice—Residents must demonstrate the ability to investigate and evaluate their care of patients, to appraise and assimilate scientific evidence, and to continuously improve patient care based on constant self-evaluation and lifelong learning.

1-19. You are a hospitalist in an academic center. This morning you conducted bedside work rounds with your medical team. Your medical team consists of medical students, interns, residents, a bedside nurse, a respiratory therapy coordinator (R.T.), dietician, and social worker. Your first patient was a 9-year-old admitted for an asthma exacerbation and oxygen requirement. After the intern completes his presentation, you examine the patient, elicit concerns of the family, and discuss discharge criteria. The R.T. reports the patient's response to treatment and suggests that the team prescribe the inhaled corticosteroid that is the preferred medication on the patient's insurance formulary. The nurse reports that the patient's father is interested in quitting smoking and the team refers him to the free, statewide tobacco dependence treatment program. During this discussion, the intern updates a discharge instruction summary that will be faxed to the patient's primary care provider. The residency program director asks you to identify the competencies of the Accreditation Council for Graduate Medical Education (ACGME) that you incorporated during rounds this morning. The rounding encounter described above best describes which ACGME competency?

a. Medical knowledge

b. Practice-based learning and improvement

c. Systems-based practice

d. Interpersonal and communication skills

e. Professionalism

1-20. A 5-year-old child presents to ambulatory surgery for an elective procedure. The father informs the anesthesiologist that his child is deaf and the child becomes very upset when he cannot read lips. The father explains that last time his son had surgery, he became very combative when he was taken from his parents for induction of anesthesia. Because he reads lips, and all the staff members were wearing surgical masks over their mouths, he became very anxious. Which response by the anesthesiologist best expresses the principles of patient- and family-centered care?

a. "We all have to wear surgical masks for infection control and your son is getting older, so he should be able to handle his fears better than the last time."

b. "You know that we will be very nice to Johnny and he has nothing to be afraid of. We will take very good care of him."

c. "Would it help your son if you accompany him to induction of anesthesia and if we wait to place our surgical masks on until he is comfortable?"

d. "I'm sorry the last operation was such an unpleasant experience; we'll make sure that your son receives the best care this time."

e. "It's alright, you don't have anything to worry about; it won't take us long to induce sedation and he won't remember anything."

1-21. You are asked to give a lecture to medical students about patient- and family-centered care. You describe the key principles of family-centered care including respect, information sharing, participation, collaboration, and flexibility. Which of the following organizational processes best supports the philosophy of family-centered care?

a. The emergency department encourages family members to be present for resuscitations even if they do not wish to witness the resuscitation.

b. Family members are allowed in the intensive care unit at all hours except during work rounds and nursing change of shift.

c. A multidisciplinary committee develops educational materials about the dangers of secondhand smoke for parents who smoke tobacco.

d. Two patient and family advisors serve as nonvoting members on the Patient Care Committee and the Bioethics Committee.

e. Two patient and family advisors are invited to join a working group that is beginning an improvement project to improve medication reconciliation.

1-22. You are the attending on an inpatient ward team. As part of your team orientation with the new students, you discuss the process for conducting family-centered rounds. Which of the following best reflects family-centered care principles?

a. You instruct the students and/or bedside nurses to make sure parents are awake between 10 and noon, when your team will be conducting walk rounds on all patients.

b. Your team will conduct bedside rounds on all patients with 1 exception: when the patient is admitted for the evaluation of child maltreatment syndrome.

c. The students present the vital signs, physical examination, and laboratory findings outside the patients' rooms. Following the hallway presentation, the team enters the room to give the family the plan and answer any questions they may have.

d. You ask the students to obtain permission from the patients and families to round in the patient's room. When the team enters the room, they knock on the door, introduce themselves, and invite the caregivers to participate in the discussion of their child.

e. During rounds at the bedside, you teach families how to take care of their child with special health care needs and model this family teaching for the students.

1-23. You have recently signed an employment contract with a pediatric clinic in Galveston, Texas. Because this town is located on the Gulf of Mexico, it has an increased risk of being impacted by a devastating hurricane. As a part of your new role, you have been asked to be the disaster preparedness representative from the clinic to work directly with a local hospital committee to plan for disaster response. Your role also includes dissemination of information to your partners on their role in disaster preparedness. Which of the following is the responsibility of every pediatrician in disaster preparedness?

a. Ensure all of your patients have been vaccinated against hepatitis A because the last disaster in your area rendered all drinking water unsafe and there was a hepatitis A epidemic.

b. Become a member of the Incident Command System, which facilitates the efficient coordination and mobilization of resources necessary in a disaster response.

c. Discuss the development of a disaster plan with the families of patients with special health care needs because of their dependence on specialized medications and equipment.

d. Focus all of your preparedness on hurricanes since this is the natural disaster threat to your population and other disasters are much more rare.

e. Take a continuing medical education course on diagnosis and treatment of posttraumatic stress disorder in children to increase your proficiency in its management.

1-24. You are asked to give the medical students a pediatric lecture on disaster preparedness as a part of their section on disaster medicine. Which of the key points is most accurate about the role of the pediatrician and the effects of disasters on pediatric patients?

a. Because of the rapid growth and development of infants, they are less susceptible to toxins than older children.

b. Children are very resilient to disasters and, therefore, should not be diagnosed with posttraumatic stress disorder.

c. Children inhale and ingest larger quantities of contaminated air, food, and water for their weight than adults do.

d. Discussion in the household about violence, death, and disaster increases fear of disasters and decreases the resilience of children.

e. Pediatricians are not skilled to address the community on disaster preparedness; this should be left to the local health authorities.

1-25. Ms B brings her infant, Anna, to see you for her 2-month checkup. After doing a thorough examination, you state, "Now, it is time to start Anna on her immunizations. Would you like that in 1 shot that contains many vaccines, or we can give multiple shots with 1 vaccine in each?" Ms B states that she does not wish to get any vaccinations. She has read that they may lead to autism and other health-related problems.

You should respond to Ms B accordingly:

a. "I'm sorry that you feel that way, but I will not be able to continue as your child's pediatrician."

b. "I'm concerned that the media may have distorted your understanding of vaccinations."

c. "I would like to talk to you more about the scientific basis of this, and in the meantime we can wait on starting the immunizations."

d. "You are putting your child and the society at serious risk, and I will need to call in Child Protective Services if you do not agree to the immunizations right now."

e. "I will have to have a social worker come evaluate this situation to determine if you are fit to continue to care for your child."

1-26. Julie is 15 years old and has been brought into the emergency department after fainting during volleyball practice. You are the ED physician seeing Julie, and during the examination you ask whether Julie has been sexually active and would like to get a pregnancy test. Julie hesitates to disclose information and asks whether she can rely on you to not tell her mother.

You should respond to Julie accordingly:

a. "What you say to me I take to be confidential. However, there are some things I must report to others."

b. "I'm sorry, but as a minor, I have to tell your parents everything that we talk about."

c. "Are you afraid of your parents for some reason? Should I call in Child Protective Services?"

d. "The confidentiality of our discussion is safe with me. In fact, no one else need know what we talk about in here."

e. "You are too young to be sexually active. Abstinence is the best way to avoid unwanted pregnancy and sexually transmitted diseases."

1-27. Billy has severe scoliosis and needs corrective surgery because breathing is becoming increasingly difficult. He is 12 years old and his parents are members of the Jehovah's Witness faith. If the surgery is not performed, Billy will eventually require a ventilator, tracheostomy, and may lose lung function altogether. The surgeon is unwilling to do the surgery without consent to use blood products if necessary, but Billy's parents refuse to consent for blood products.

The surgeon should:

a. Do the surgery anyway, and just not use blood even if Billy's medical condition warrants it.

b. Before performing the surgery, get a court order to allow blood products during the surgery, but only use them if necessary.

c. Perform the surgery as an "emergent" issue without parental consent for blood products.

d. Ask Billy what he would want and follow Billy's wishes as a mature minor.

e. Get a social worker to evaluate whether the parents are fit to continue to care for Billy.

1-28. You are working in the emergency department when Justin is brought in by his babysitter, who is on summer break from college. Justin, who is 6 years old, was riding his bike when he lost control and fell. He was not wearing his helmet, but the babysitter insists that he was "not going too fast." You notice that Justin has a cut that looks to need stitches, and his head has a large bump on it. The babysitter says that she cannot get hold of Justin's parents on their cell phones; she has no other phone numbers for the parents or family members. A nurse attempts to contact the parents as well, but is not successful, either.

The nurse asks you what you will do next. You decide to:

a. Wait until the parents can be contacted to do anything other than keeping Justin comfortable as possible.

b. Track down phone numbers of Justin's grandparents in order to gain their consent for any medical treatments.

c. Find a hospital administrator to consent to treatments for Justin.

d. Get consent from the babysitter to admit Justin so that he can be properly monitored until his parents can be found.

e. Close Justin's wounds and get any tests and scans necessary to be sure that his injuries are properly diagnosed. Debrief the parents once they are located.

1-29. Bobby is 16 years old and has been diagnosed with Hodgkin disease. While undergoing his first round of chemotherapy, he begins to look on the Internet for alternative therapies because the current medications make him sick and tired all the time. Once the first phase is over, he decides that he will instead take vitamins he has read about online. His parents are not sure what is best for Bobby, but they homeschooled him precisely because they wanted their son to learn to be independent and make decisions for himself. So, even though they would like to see him continue his current therapy, they do not want to go against their son's wishes.

Bobby's health care team should:

a. Stop all treatments and allow Bobby to pursue the alternative therapies he desires.

b. Convince Bobby's parents that he is wrong, and gain their consent to continue chemotherapy.

c. Talk further with Bobby in order to address his concerns and possibly develop a plan that can provide both chemotherapy and adjuncts that meet his interests.

d. Get a court order to force Bobby to have chemotherapy.

e. Stop chemotherapy, but provide the alternative therapies to Bobby so as to maintain the patient–professional relationship.

1-30. Nicole is 17 years old and just married her high school boyfriend. He is in the military and is out of the country. Nicole lives with her parents while he is away. One night, on her way home from an evening class her car is hit by another vehicle. She ends up in the intensive care unit on a ventilator. She has spinal cord and brain injuries, but the physician believes she is making neurological progress and should recover decision-making capacity, though she may not walk again. Her parents have been at her bedside throughout. Now, 2 weeks into her hospital stay, the physicians want to talk about a tracheostomy to secure Nicole's airway long-term. The need for a tracheostomy is not emergent, at this point in time.

The physician should:

a. Try to contact Nicole's husband abroad to get his consent for the procedure.

b. Since Nicole is a minor, obtain consent for the procedure from Nicole's parents.

c. Since Nicole cannot speak for herself, have a judge appoint a guardian ad litem who can objectively evaluate whether the procedure is in Nicole's best interest.

d. Wait a few more weeks to see if Nicole recovers decisional capacity, giving her the chance to decide for herself.

e. Get a court to declare Nicole incompetent and appoint one of her family members as surrogate.

ANSWERS

Answer 1-1. c

The emphasis of patient care has changed from the 20th century to the 21st century to become more patient- and family-focused. Patients and their families desire increased access to information, more timely information, and quality care that is evidence-based. By incorporating an alert system that notifies a provider of an abnormal result with easy access to the family's contact information allows a physician to readily respond to abnormal results and notify the family of the result and the intended next step. This system change also facilitates a timely and reliable method of alerting physicians of potentially concerning information.

A diagnosis list limited to pediatric diagnoses may facilitate easier billing on a routine basis, but it can be overly limiting. As more children are being diagnosed with what were traditionally considered adult diseases, it is important to allow for the flexibility of changing epidemiology.

While a system that automatically determines empiric antibiotics for specific infectious diseases might be helpful, it would be very difficult for this to be reflective of local antibiotic-resistant patterns and may not address other factors associated with infectious diseases that could require other empiric treatment (eg, a child who is diagnosed with lymphadenitis may have a young kitten at home leading to a diagnosis of *Bartonella*, rather than Group A *Streptococcus*, and would require different antibiotic coverage).

Flexibility in electronic medical records is helpful to allow physicians to document in a way that works efficiently for each provider. However, with medicine moving toward an emphasis on quality care, approaches to treatment should be based on evidence in research rather than individual physician preferences.

Lastly, the generation of a lab requisition through an electronic medical record saves time for a physician, but there is still a chance of the requisition getting lost before a patient arrives at the lab. Ideally the lab order should be electronically delivered to the lab through a secure network to avoid human error in transporting the order.

(Page 1-2, Section 1: Fundamentals of Pediatrics, Chapter 1: Role of the Pediatrician)

Answer 1-2. b

The respiratory therapists have developed a complete and answerable clinical question in the PICO (patient or problem, intervention, comparison, outcome) format. Framing the question in this format allows one to conduct a practical and focused search of the literature. Well-done systematic reviews, such as in the *Cochrane Database of Systematic Reviews*, may be sufficient to answer the question. However, a physician wanting to keep up with the most up-to-date information would want to search for original studies published since the review was conducted.

A prospective, blinded comparison trial is the most useful to determine the efficacy of an intervention. Randomization is an effective strategy to minimize known, as well as unknown, allocation bias. Therefore, a study using a randomized, double-blind, controlled trial design would be the most appropriate publication to retrieve and critically appraise in order to answer the question.

Cohort studies are limited by the possibility of confounders that may influence the association being studied. For example, consider a cohort study that examined the medical records for length of stay among infants hospitalized for bronchiolitis. The study would be limited by the fact that there may have been an unmeasured difference (such as educational level of the caregivers or the initial severity of illness) between the groups of infants who received 3% saline and those who did not receive saline. Unmeasured differences may have affected their length of stay and biased the results. A case series would not be useful to assess efficacy, because of the small sample size, lack of randomization, and lack of a comparison group. The other titles address safety of hypertonic saline and treatment of pulmonary atelectasis, but do not include the outcome of interest (length of stay).

(Page 3-4, Section 1: Fundamentals of Pediatrics, Chapter 2: Decision Making: Use of Evidence-based Medicine)

Answer 1-3. a

In this "negative" study that shows no statistically significant difference between groups, it is possible that a real difference in change of oxygen saturation between study groups was missed. There are 2 possible errors that can occur with any study (see the display table below). In a "positive" study, the study results may suggest a difference exists between therapies, when a difference does not actually exist. This situation is a Type I error and is mitigated by assessing the P value (the chance of a Type I error). However, in the case above, the study is a "negative" study. In this situation, there is the risk of a Type II error: the authors suggest that no difference exists and it is possible that a difference may actually exist. In this situation, it is important to assess if the study had an adequate sample size (or power) to avoid this error. In general, a sample size calculation and justification should be included in the text of the published study to allow the reader to critically appraise this possibility.

	Actual Truth	
Study Results	**No Difference Exists**	**Difference Exists**
Difference exists	Type I error	(Correct)
No difference exists	(Correct)	Type II error

Answer b is incorrect because the length of stay was not the primary outcome measure of this study. This study was a randomized controlled trial that permitted the authors to limit the effects of both known and unknown confounding factors. In a randomized trial, patients should be analyzed in the groups to which they were randomized, allowing investigators to determine how the potential treatment performs in the real world. Thus, answers c and d are incorrect. A high dropout rate or withdrawal rate can compromise the validity of any study. In this case, only

1 of the patients withdrew from the study; however, the 98% follow-up and completion rate was reasonable for this study.

(Page 4, Section 1: Fundamentals of Pediatrics, Chapter 2: Decision Making: Use of Evidence-based Medicine)

Answer 1-4. d

Answer d is correct because a cross-sectional study can only determine associations between an exposure and a disease. A cross-sectional study cannot establish causation because it measures both the prevalence of disease and exposure at the same time. Thus, answers a, b, and e are incorrect. Incidence of disease is defined as the number of new cases of a disease that occur during a specified period of time in a population at risk. A cross-sectional study cannot determine incidence of disease because the population is surveyed at one moment in time, not over time. For this reason, answer c is incorrect.

(Page 4, Section 1: Fundamentals of Pediatrics, Chapter 2: Decision Making: Use of Evidence-based Medicine)

Answer 1-5. a

Answer a is the most clinically useful study. A double-blind, placebo-controlled, randomized trial is most appropriate to examine the efficacy of a therapeutic intervention, such as a prethickened formula. Patient-centered outcomes focus on measures that can be identified by the patient such as hospitalization rate, pain severity, or length of stay. Disease-oriented outcomes include improvement in laboratory values, or other physical measurements such as intraluminal impedance or pH probe monitoring of gastric reflux. Direct laryngoscopy would be invasive to the patient and the effect of reflux on laryngeal tissue injury is another disease-oriented outcome measure. Therefore, answers c, d, and e are incorrect. Answer b is incorrect because it is an observational, before-and-after study without a control group. Without a control group, the investigators cannot attribute the improved symptoms to the prethickened formula. Another confounding factor could have influenced the desired outcome.

(Page 3, Section 1: Fundamentals of Pediatrics, Chapter 2: Decision Making: Use of Evidence-based Medicine)

Answer 1-6. b

Communication with families in the pediatric clinic can be challenging when there are siblings present during an encounter. In addition, time of family transitions such as the birth of a new baby can compound the situation. In this case, it is essential to give the mother–infant dyad appropriate attention to address their interaction and not be overly distracted by the older sibling. Because the older sibling is accustomed to seeing a pediatrician in the context of being the patient, she is feeling left out. She may also be experiencing some jealousy of the new baby. According to Miller's habit of humanism, a physician must identify multiple perspectives in each encounter, reflect on possible conflicts that could help or hinder forming a relationship with the patient, and choose to act altruistically.

Answer b is the best choice because this allows you to validate the importance of the big sister's new role in an age-appropriate manner, but also redirect the visit toward the mother's weight concern. Answer a will not validate the sibling and may create more delays in the visit if she becomes upset and refuses to go to the waiting room. Answer c may be helpful, but detracts from the focus of the visit, the newborn. This may be helpful to address at the end of the visit if there is additional time and especially if it is a concern for the mother. Answer d may appease the sibling's desire for your attention, but also detracts from the visit. Answer e may be viewed as scolding the child and can hinder the relationship you are establishing with the mother. In addition, the sibling is not being validated and will likely continue to compete for attention.

(Page 6, Section 1: Fundamentals of Pediatrics, Chapter 3: Communication)

Answer 1-7. d

Building a relationship with a scared child can be very difficult, especially when his or her fears, such as getting an immunization, are well founded. There are several verbal and nonverbal communication skills that can be used to assist in this process. Answer d is the best choice because you are directly engaging the patient by acknowledging her on an age-appropriate level that relates to the purpose of the visit. Answers a and c are incorrect because you are avoiding establishing rapport with the mother or the child by immediately delving into the purpose of the visit without showing any interest in the 2 other people in the room. Answer b is an appropriate way to address the parent, but it would be better to address the patient, followed by the parent, to better establish rapport with the patient and encourage her participation in her own medical care on an age-appropriate level. Answer e is unlikely to be effective because the child is already scared of what might happen when you enter the room and this can be further exacerbated by quickly approaching her personal space and then discussing the impending immunizations that she is so worried about.

(Page 9, Table 3-4, Section 1: Fundamentals of Pediatrics, Chapter 3: Communication)

Answer 1-8. e

The examination of a 2-year-old requires physician flexibility and ability to adjust the physical examination techniques as needed in order to engage the child. It is developmentally normal for a willful and anxious toddler to refuse being examined and appear uncooperative. Appropriate developmentally based communication during the 2-year-old examination includes play. By providing toys and using bubbles as a distraction technique, the physician will be more likely to assess whether or not a toddler can bear weight or pull to stand than simply asking her to stand up and walk.

It is not appropriate to defer the examination as it is important to identify whether or not the child is weak and to exclude neurological causes of her refusal to walk. A 2-year-old is too young to engage in discussions about cooperating with your examination, so answers a and c are incorrect. A physical therapy consult may be appropriate depending on the diagnosis but not in the initial assessment during a clinic visit.

(Page 6, Section 1: Fundamentals of Pediatrics, Chapter 3: Communication)

Answer 1-9. a

Applying the Four Habits Model of communication will help to build and sustain this relationship with Mrs Johnson and her daughter. The first habit in this model is termed "invest in the beginning." Investing in the beginning of the encounter includes skills such as creating rapport quickly, eliciting the patient's (or parent's) concerns, and planning the visit. Planning the visit with Mrs Johnson includes prioritizing her asthma, which is not well controlled. By negotiating the agenda for the encounter, you can acknowledge her concerns while making it clear that you have limited time for the visit. Answers b and c do not acknowledge mother's concerns, while answer d is unrealistic in a busy practice. Answer e acknowledges the stress on the family and is an appropriate way to explore the impact the divorce has had on the family; however, it does not prioritize the asthma for this visit.

(Page 6-8, Section 1: Fundamentals of Pediatrics, Chapter 3: Communication)

Answer 1-10. c

Based on the motivational interviewing technique using readiness rulers, following her rating with a question of "why not lower?" helps you to address her strengths in her perceived ability to make this change. A further response can be followed up by another question of "why not higher?" to determine what her perceived barriers in addressing this change might be. Answer a is a positive answer but doesn't really address her readiness to make a change. Answer b is incorrect because it makes the assumption she is ready to make a change without addressing any barriers she may face. Answer d doesn't take into account the principle of using the readiness ruler, but does attempt to address readiness to change. However, this question is not open-ended and may elicit a socially desired response rather than the truth. Answer e changes the subject and avoids more in-depth knowledge about whether the patient is ready to address her soda intake.

(Page 14, Section 1: Fundamentals of Pediatrics, Chapter 4: Interviewing Techniques)

Answer 1-11. e

Communicating with adolescents can feel more difficult than communicating with a parent of a young child, but similar interviewing techniques can be used. Open-ended answers require engagement between the patient and provider. When discussing behavior, it is recommended that 4 open-ended questions be used for every closed-ended question. Answer e is the best response because it is the only question that is open-ended and will allow you to explore what the adolescent meant by her statement. Her answer will be richer in content and will help you to determine if this is just a concerned father, an overly controlling father, or an adolescent who might be engaging in some problematic behavior.

Answer a is a closed-ended question and will not produce much information. Answer b is a leading question and implies you are taking the side of her father that may compromise your rapport with the patient. Answer c may be a useful question as you learn more about what she meant by the initial statement, but this question may best be used as a follow-up to more open-ended questions. Answer d is another closed-ended question that will be unlikely to yield any useful information.

(Page 13, Section 1: Fundamentals of Pediatrics, Chapter 4: Interviewing Techniques)

Answer 1-12. e

A motivational tool that can be used in brief clinical encounters is the reflective statement. The reflective statement is a restatement of the content or feeling expressed by the patient or caregiver. It is especially helpful in response to meeting resistance from a patient or caregiver. The ability to phrase statements that stimulate a conversational response is a crucial skill in reflective listening.

The other responses are not reflective statements. Answer b prevents the opportunity of the physician to conduct motivational interviewing or assist the parent in quitting smoking in the future. Answer a has a concluding tone that is designed to elicit a confirmatory "yes" response. It prevents the physician from eliciting any thoughts from the parent about her smoking. Answer c is an appropriate response to a parent who is not ready to quit smoking, but is open to discussion about his or her smoking; however, it is not a reflective statement.

(Page 14, Section 1: Fundamentals of Pediatrics, Chapter 4: Interviewing Techniques)

Answer 1-13. b

Office systems to support clinical care assist a pediatrician in providing quality care that meets parents' needs. Because all of the recommended topics for each well visit cannot be addressed in the usual 20-minute appointment, the focus of the appointment must elicit parents' concerns, identify psychosocial risk factors, incorporate appropriate anticipatory guidance regarding development, and be tailored to the family's needs. Systems can be designed to assist the pediatrician in both accomplishing some of the preventive care guidelines before the child is seen and improving the efficiency of time spent with the patient. Answer b is correct because it is specific to this family's needs, which addresses the mother's concerns, and will

help to further identify psychosocial risk factors that cannot be addressed by the pediatrician during the well-child visit.

Answer a is helpful in addressing appropriate anticipatory guidance but is not directed specifically to the concerns that are addressed by the mother. Answer c is incorrect because there is no evidence that this child has developmental delay. Answer d is incorrect because the recommended practice is to do targeted developmental screening rather than superficial developmental surveillance. In addition, this can be accomplished prior to the encounter with a designated developmental screening tool. Answer e is not specific to this family's need, but is an evidence-based intervention that promotes early literacy.

(Page 15, Section 1: Fundamentals of Pediatrics, Chapter 5: Systems of Practice and Office Management)

Answer 1-14. b

Pediatricians are increasingly caring for patients with chronic diseases. While these patients often have multiple providers to care for their highly specialized needs, the general pediatrician still plays a valuable role. The chronic care model (Figure 5-1) shows how the community, the health system, the patient, and the physician all have a role in improving patient outcomes. Answer b is the best answer. This answer is a good example of using clinical information systems to facilitate prompt patient care to implement clinical guidelines and track patients who do not receive timely follow-up. Preventive medicine, such as the administration of an annual influenza immunization, is well within the purview of a primary care pediatrician. Answers a and c may be necessary to optimize her therapy, but the coordination of care is best managed by the specialist who is most skilled at performing the necessary procedure and most experienced at determining the optimal therapy for this specific condition. Answer d is another example of a benefit to the patient that incorporates a proactive team, but would best be coordinated by the pulmonologist who directly partners with the involved subspecialists. Answer e again is an important part of informing the patient how to be an active participant in his or her care, but this role would be better filled in the setting of a specialized clinical center for cystic fibrosis.

(Page 15-16, Section 1: Fundamentals of Pediatrics, Chapter 5: Systems of Practice and Office Management)

Answer 1-15. e

Approaching common clinical problems with a systems approach that is evidence-based links to higher-quality and cost-effective care. Fever in an infant is a common clinical problem for which practice guidelines exist. Guidelines for common clinical problems, such as fever in an infant, can be found through the National Guideline Clearinghouse, American Academy of Pediatrics, and many children's hospital Web sites. In addition, many hospitals and practices often develop their own specific clinical pathways, standing order sets, references to national guidelines, parent or patient information sheets, and discharge goals. Answer e is the best answer because it is an efficient way to find up-to-date clinical guidelines that are original sources.

Answer a may be helpful if your colleague is well versed in this particular guideline, but it bypasses a systems approach and doesn't ensure the most evidence-based answer to the clinical question. Answer b does not incorporate a systems approach and is not supported by fever guidelines for this age patient. Answer c is a systems approach, but a guideline that is over 10 years old is unlikely to contain the most current evidence-based approach and should be verified with another online source. If this older guideline contains a reference to the parent guideline, that can be used to guide an online search for the most current recommendation. Answer d is incorrect because it does not apply a systems approach and could potentially distract a provider for properly caring for a young febrile infant.

(Page 16-17, Section 1: Fundamentals of Pediatrics, Chapter 5: Systems of Practice and Office Management)

Answer 1-16. b

Clinic access and efficiency have become more evidence-based with a trend toward *open* or *advanced access*. The goal for *open access* is to predict the demand and respond to it effectively by matching supply with demand, while reducing inefficiency. This can be enabled by having same-day availability not only for acute visits but also for well-child care and follow-up care. This decreases waits in the system and allows patients increased access to their own physician, improving patient satisfaction and quality of care. According to Table 5-2 (Principles of Advanced Access), answer b is correct because it lays the groundwork for transitioning to an open access approach to office management. By determining the specific demand of your patient population over a period of time, this can be used to predict the demand so that the supply can be adjusted accordingly.

Answer a is incorrect because this strategy may decrease efficiency. Ideally registration and insurance can be completed prior to the appointment by mailings and phone verification so that the patient can be seen by the provider on arrival to the waiting room. Delays in registration and insurance verification lead to delays in physician schedules that are difficult to overcome once the schedule becomes delayed. Answer c is incorrect because the supplies should be readily accessible and stocked in the examination rooms, not a central storage room. Well-stocked examination rooms help to avoid inefficiencies in direct patient care. Answer d is incorrect because longer appointments mean a decreased number of total appointments in a day. The need for follow-up is rarely averted by increased length of appointments. Answer e is incorrect because the demand for appointments in the summer is typically shifted more toward well care, rather than acute. The winter time may need to be adjusted to include more acute visits and less well visits.

(Page 17, Table 5-2, Section 1: Fundamentals of Pediatrics, Chapter 5: Systems of Practice and Office Management)

Answer 1-17. b

Answer b is correct because the 6 core competencies initially described by the ACGME were a response to the Institute of Medicine report *To Err Is Human*. This report highlighted the significant gaps in the quality of care for patients within the United States. The medical education community felt that there was a need to ensure that physicians were competent in a variety of areas. It was no longer sufficient to expect physicians to be competent based on a specific quantity of time in various training experiences, which were often evaluated by global assessments.

Answer a is incorrect because the Institute of Medicine report did not recommend a specific approach to medical education; it just highlighted the problems that contributed to poor quality of care and proposed that leaders in medical education have a role in addressing the quality of care issue. Answer c is incorrect because Flexner report was completed in 1910 and changed medical education significantly at that time to standardize the student's educational experience. Medical education did not change significantly again until the Institute of Medicine report that was followed by the ACGME's move to focus on outcomes-based training. This emphasis became highlighted during the last decade of the 20th century and the beginning of the 21st century. Answer d is incorrect because the Joint Commission does not evaluate these competencies in physicians. It does ask health care organizations to use role-specific competency assessment for all clinical staff in the organization. Answer e is incorrect because there is no direct financial incentive for implementing these 6 competencies into resident or physician assessment, despite the need for financial solvency to keep an organization in existence.

(Page 17-18, Section 1: Fundamentals of Pediatrics, Chapter 6: Core Competencies)

Answer 1-18. b

Answer b is correct according to Table 6-1 as the description of the competency of medical knowledge. Answer a is incorrect because the description belongs to patient care. Answer c is incorrect because the description belongs to interpersonal and communication skills. Answer d is incorrect because the description belongs to systems-based practice. Answer e is incorrect because that is the description for practice-based learning and improvement.

(Page 18, Table 6-1, Section 1: Fundamentals of Pediatrics, Chapter 6: Core Competencies)

Answer 1-19. c

Answer c is correct because although multiple competencies may be assessed in 1 patient encounter, the rounds described above best fit with systems-based practice evaluation. To show achievement in systems-based practice, residents must demonstrate an interdisciplinary approach to patient care. In the scenario above, the respiratory therapist and the patient's nurse were effectively part of the health care team and addressed important issues that may impact the patient's asthma control. If the patient's medication is not covered by insurance, adherence to prescribed therapy may be diminished. The patient will also have more difficulty controlling her symptoms if she is exposed to tobacco smoke. By referring the patient's caregiver to a statewide tobacco dependence treatment program, the team demonstrated the ability to access other resources in the health care system to provide optimal chronic disease management.

Lastly, the team recognized the importance of continuity of care by communicating the discharge instructions to the patient's medical home. Medical knowledge is not demonstrated by the residents in this scenario as they did not express understanding of scientific knowledge and its application to patient care. Practice-based learning and improvement is not correct because there is no evidence during rounds that the residents conducted self-evaluation of their patient care. Interpersonal and communication skills may have been demonstrated during the encounter, but the effective exchange of information is not described above. Professionalism and adherence to ethical principles is also not addressed in the scenario.

(Page 18, Section 1: Fundamentals of Pediatrics, Chapter 6: Core Competencies)

Answer 1-20. c

Patient- and family-centered care is best described by the principles of respect, information sharing, participation, collaboration, and flexibility. Fundamental to the model of patient- and family-centered care is the concept that partnership with the family will result in improved patient care outcomes. Of all the response options, proposing that the parent accompany the child to induction of anesthesia and being flexible about when to wear the surgical masks is the most patient- and family-centered response.

Reassuring the parent that the medical team will be kind, efficient, or provide the best care is one approach when a family member voices a concern about his or her child; however, it does not demonstrate a partnership with the parent. Another family-centered approach would be to ask the family what has worked well in the past and negotiate a plan with the family to reduce their child's anxiety about not being able to communicate with the health care team.

(Page 19, Section 1: Fundamentals of Pediatrics, Chapter 7: Patient and Family-centered Care)

Answer 1-21. e

By inviting patient and family members to participate in a working group focused on improving an organizational process, the hospital is demonstrating an awareness of the importance of collaboration with families to improve the health care system. Pediatric hospital systems have shown the benefits of collaboration with families including improved patient and satisfaction scores and decreased cost.

Answer a is incorrect because families are not given an option to be present and, thus, the department is not demonstrating flexibility to meet the individual needs of the families. Answer b is incorrect because the unit is excluding family members during important transitions of care and medical team interactions that would potentially benefit from family participation. Answer c does not describe active participation of patients or family members in the development of materials. Answer d is incorrect because although the family advisors are members of the hospital committees, they are not actively involved as full participants with voting privileges.

(Page 19, Section 1: Fundamentals of Pediatrics, Chapter 7: Patient and Family-centered Care)

Answer 1-22. d

By asking for permission to round in the patients' rooms, the team is demonstrating respect for the individual preferences of each patient and his or her family. The team introductions help to facilitate communication with families during rounds. Inviting caregivers to participate in the care planning for their child demonstrates a willingness to partner with families. Respect, information sharing, participation, and collaboration are key principles of family-centered care.

Answer b excludes some families from communicating with the medical team during team rounds as provided to other families of hospitalized children. Families of children admitted for evaluation of child maltreatment still need medical information from the team, unless they lose custody or rights to visitation from a state agency. Answer c is incorrect because the families are excluded from decision making by the team and there is no evidence of collaboration with families to determine a care plan. Answer e does not describe a collaborative approach to managing a child's chronic disease, and does not demonstrate the physician's willingness to partner with the family or provide choices in medical decision making.

(Page 19, Section 1: Fundamentals of Pediatrics, Chapter 7: Patient and Family-centered Care)

Answer 1-23. c

Disaster preparedness consists of 4 phases that include preparedness (advanced planning), response (direct actions during the disaster), recovery (return to normalcy after acute event), and mitigation (actions to decrease the vulnerability of a disaster and reduce the need to respond in a disaster). Pediatricians have a role in each of these components whether they are key players or community members. Answer c is correct and is included in the preparedness phase. Children with special health care needs have increased vulnerabilities because they require more rare medications and specialized equipment, and can be dependent on an electrical source for life-maintaining equipment such as ventilators. Having a conversation with their caregivers in advance of a disaster and addressing all aspects of care and backup systems can prevent additional casualties caused by short supply of medications or electricity failures. A written disaster plan allows for all participants in the care of these children to ensure necessary supplies and equipment are available.

Answer a is not the best answer because vaccination prophylaxis should not be limited to just hepatitis A. While it is important to respond to lessons learned from prior disasters, it would not be prudent to focus vaccination only on hepatitis A. Ideal mitigation of vaccine-preventable infectious diseases would include proper immunization of all vaccine-preventable diseases to minimize the population susceptibility from increased herd immunity. Answer b is incorrect because the Incident Command System is a mechanism for collaborative management. This system allows for coordination of both public and private emergency management agencies and uses best practices to coordinate all resources and facilities. Local community leadership and stakeholders designate representatives to participate in the Incident Command System. This system does not include every pediatrician but does benefit from having a pediatric representative to address the unique health care needs of children.

Answer d is incorrect because disaster preparedness requires physicians to be prepared to care for patients in a wide variety of disaster situations to include natural, biological, traumatic, nuclear, chemical, and humanitarian disasters (Table 8-1). In this instance, hurricane disaster preparedness is essential because of the increased likelihood, but this community is also susceptible to disasters such as plane crashes, terrorist attacks, pandemic infections, and others. Answer e is not the best answer because it is a very limited approach to the recovery phase of disaster preparedness. Posttraumatic stress disorder is not an infrequent result of any disaster. Pediatricians should have a heightened suspicion for this in children who have survived disasters, but the general pediatrician is not expected to be able to diagnose and treat these patients. The essential role of a pediatrician is to recognize the signs and assist families with accessing mental health services.

(Page 21-23, Section 1: Fundamentals of Pediatrics, Chapter 8: Disaster Preparedness)

Answer 1-24. c

Disaster is "a sudden calamitous event bringing great damage, loss, or destruction," which can include any event in which the needs of a population exceed the local capacity to meet them. Children are uniquely affected because of their growth rate, developmental level, and dependence on adults. Answer c is correct because the smaller the child, the larger the relative quantity of contamination he or she is exposed to. Children have increased respiratory and increased metabolic rates in relation to their weight when compared with adults.

Answer a is incorrect and the opposite is true. Young children and fetuses are more susceptible to toxins because of their rapid growth and early stages of development. They also have a greater potential time to live after the exposure, allowing for larger cumulative effects and time to demonstrate long-term effects of toxins. Answer b is incorrect because children are susceptible to developing posttraumatic stress disorder after a disaster. It is important for pediatricians to be aware of this, address it early, and assist families with access to mental health services if it is suspected. Answer d is incorrect. By helping parents learn

to talk with their children about violence, death, and disaster that occurs in our daily environment and addressing children's fears, pediatricians can increase the resiliency of children to disasters. Answer e is also incorrect because pediatricians are a valuable resource for disaster preparedness and recognize the unique challenges that families with children face. Together, pediatricians and local health authorities can address a larger population regarding disaster preparedness than public health authorities alone. Pediatricians are valuable and trusted liaisons to the public for many issues that impact families.

(Page 21-23, Section 1: Fundamentals of Pediatrics, Chapter 8: Disaster Preparedness)

Answer 1-25. c

While you may believe that Ms B is choosing a poor course of action for her child, and even though there are implications for schooling and pandemic quarantines when a child is not immunized, all states recognize that the scope of parental authority is quite broad with regard to many issues, including immunizations. In fact, parental authority is trumped only when parents are abusive or medically negligent. All 50 states allow medical exemptions for immunizations, and thus such refusals are not considered medical negligence. As a result, answers d and e are incorrect. Forty-eight of the 50 also allow religious and/or philosophical exemptions. Answer a is incorrect, as excusing this family from your practice may increase the chance that they will never be willing to get immunizations. As a pediatrician, care and trustworthiness are paramount values to maintain. Listening carefully to Ms B's reasons, providing education, and maintaining a working relationship are your best hope of changing Ms B's mind. A response similar to answer b, without understanding the parent's source of information or perspective on this issue, may be off-putting. One potential advantage of a primary care relationship and continuity of care is the potential opportunity to revisit the issue of childhood immunizations at a future visit. It might be possible to get her to agree to some immunizations, even if she does not agree to all of them. As a result, answer c is the best response.

(Page 24-25, Section 1: Fundamentals of Pediatrics, Chapter 9: Law, Ethics, and Clinical Judgment)

Answer 1-26. a

Confidentiality is a paramount obligation for all health care providers. Ethically, confidentiality demonstrates trustworthiness and protects patient privacy. Legally, most states have statutory protections for confidentiality of minor patients with regard to their sexual health (making answer b incorrect), although statutes vary on what the exact protections are and whether/when a minor's confidentiality can be broken. However, strict confidentiality between physician and patient cannot be guaranteed (ruling out answer d). For example, if the patient uses her parents' insurance to pay for the visit and treatment, that information will be reported to the insurance company and, thus, will be available to her parents. Also, certain transmittable diseases must be disclosed to state health officials, who themselves—depending on the state and the disease—may be required to disclose the patient's condition to specific individuals. Further, as "mandated reporters" in cases of suspected abuse, all pediatricians may have to tell state authorities when they have suspicions that a patient has been abused. Finally, some mental health conditions, such as suicidality, may require involuntary confinement and evaluation. Answer c is incorrect because state intervention is not considered before it is warranted, and answer e is incorrect because the response does not address the patient's concern for privacy. It is best to both acknowledge the importance of confidentiality and inform the patient of possible limits that she should be aware of before she discloses anything to you.

(Page 26, Section 1: Fundamentals of Pediatrics, Chapter 9: Law, Ethics, and Clinical Judgment)

Answer 1-27. b

This scenario demonstrates a tension between respecting parental values as they raise their children and providing necessary medical treatments to protect the patient from undue harms. Answer c is incorrect because the surgery, while important, even necessary, for Billy's well-being, is not emergent. Further, Billy's parents do not want harm to come to Billy, and they do not object to the surgery, only the use of blood (so answer e is incorrect). However, there is a conflict because there is a strong likelihood that due to the extensive surgery, Billy will require blood, and without the administration of these blood products, Billy may die. If Billy were an adult with decisional capacity, he would have the right to refuse medical interventions of any sort at any time. As a 12-year-old, Billy may be a bright, insightful boy, but few would argue that he has reached a level of developmental maturity to be covered by spirit of the mature minor doctrine. Thus, his wishes, while important to know, cannot be the determining factor in this scenario (ruling out answer d).

In response to answer a, in the 1944 US Supreme Court case *Prince v. Massachusetts*, Justice Rutledge stated the now famous legal principle that parents are entitled to make martyrs of themselves, but not of their children. The case itself was not strictly about parental health care decisions, but as Justice Rutledge notes, "The right to practice religion freely does not include liberty to expose the community or the child to communicable disease or the latter to ill health or death." Obtaining an ethics consult can allow the parents to air their concerns more carefully, but if they continue both to want surgery and to refuse blood products, the court order will be necessary.

(Page 24-25, Section 1: Fundamentals of Pediatrics, Chapter 9: Law, Ethics, and Clinical Judgment)

Answer 1-28. e

While respect for parental decision-making authority is important to maintain, under emergent conditions providing necessary medical treatment for a child is paramount (making answers a and b incorrect). Justin's cut is large enough to require skillful closure, and since head trauma can have significant consequences if not diagnosed, both the closure and tests should be performed during the current visit. In many states grandparents, and even babysitters, can give legally authorized consent for the treatment of a minor; however, neither is necessary in this case. Further, it places a significant moral burden on the babysitter who may be in no better position to make the decision than the physician, and the time and effort to find the grandparents places an undue burden on the hospital staff, the grandparents, and the patient himself (answer d is incorrect as well). Also, although some hospitals have policies allowing for "administrative" consent, this is rarely a type of consent recognized in the law (thus, answer c is incorrect). And again, emergent situations require physicians to act to stabilize the patient's condition whenever there is no one otherwise authorized to make medical decisions for the patient.

(Page 24, Section 1: Fundamentals of Pediatrics, Chapter 9: Law, Ethics, and Clinical Judgment)

Answer 1-29. c

Given that Bobby is 16 years old, it is possible that he can demonstrate the maturity and decisional capacity necessary to make important health care decisions. And yet, as a minor, the burden of proof for his maturity in this regard lies with him. In the face of the fact that the efficacy of treatments in Hodgkin disease is quite good (70%-80% remission rates), it is reasonable to withhold final judgment on whether Bobby should be granted full decisional authority. His parents, too, are not entirely convinced that Bobby is making the best choice. Therefore, answers a and e are incorrect. It is their desire to maintain a loyal and supportive relationship with their son that moves them not to oppose his position. None of this speaks to initializing state intervention, but instead to strive for greater communication and the development of creative solutions. Therefore, answer c is correct.

(Page 25-26, Section 1: Fundamentals of Pediatrics, Chapter 9: Law, Ethics, and Clinical Judgment)

Answer 1-30. d

By being married, Nicole is an emancipated minor entitled to make her own medical decisions, as long as she has decisional capacity. Thus, answer b is incorrect. The question, then, is does this decision need to be made now? If so, her husband would be next of kin, and have decisional authority (this situation makes answers c and e incorrect, regardless). However, while decisions like these cannot be put off indefinitely, and while maintaining the airway will be more complicated without a tracheostomy, the decision to have surgery is not so emergent. More time can be given to see whether Nicole reaches a cognitive state where she can make the decision for herself.

(Page 25, Section 1: Fundamentals of Pediatrics, Chapter 9: Law, Ethics, and Clinical Judgment)

CHAPTER 2 | Health Promotion and Disease Prevention

| Ada M. Fenick

2-1. A "medical home" is:

a. The health parameters of the entire community where a child lives and learns

b. A location for children with special health care needs to live when their medical issues overwhelm their parents

c. A psychological construct that describes the place that children most feel at home discussing their medical problems

d. The location in the house where the family does most of their medical care, for example, bandaging and distribution of medications

e. The place where health supervision occurs, which optimally promotes health and builds on the recognized strengths of the child and family

2-2. Which of the following does not appear as a specific area of importance in each *Bright Futures* age-based visit?

a. Context (brief overview of developmental tasks and milestones usually achieved at specific age levels)

b. Evidence (background papers and specific data from randomized controlled trials regarding utility of the recommendations)

c. Priorities for the visit (the concerns of the parents and 5 additional topics for discussion in the visit)

d. Health supervision (special details of history, observation, developmental surveillance, physical examination, screening, and immunizations)

e. Anticipatory guidance (more detail for the visit priorities for the provider, specific health promotion questions, and information for the parent and child)

2-3. The most important priority topics in *Bright Futures* are:

a. Parental concerns

b. Nutrition and activity

c. Mental health issues of child and family

d. Injury prevention and health promotion

e. Developmental milestones

2-4. An 18-month-old toddler is in your office for a well-child visit. In the last few visits, he has grown more apprehensive when you enter the room. Which of the following techniques is most likely to calm him so that you can complete the physical examination?

a. Attempt to meet his gaze directly as soon as possible.

b. Allow his mother to hold him on her lap.

c. Perform the examination as soon as you enter the room.

d. Examine him in the usual head-to-toe approach.

e. Have his father firmly position him while you examine his ears.

2-5. A 12-month-old breastfed female arrives in your office for well-child care. After your nurse is done weighing the child, you review the growth chart. What is your next step?

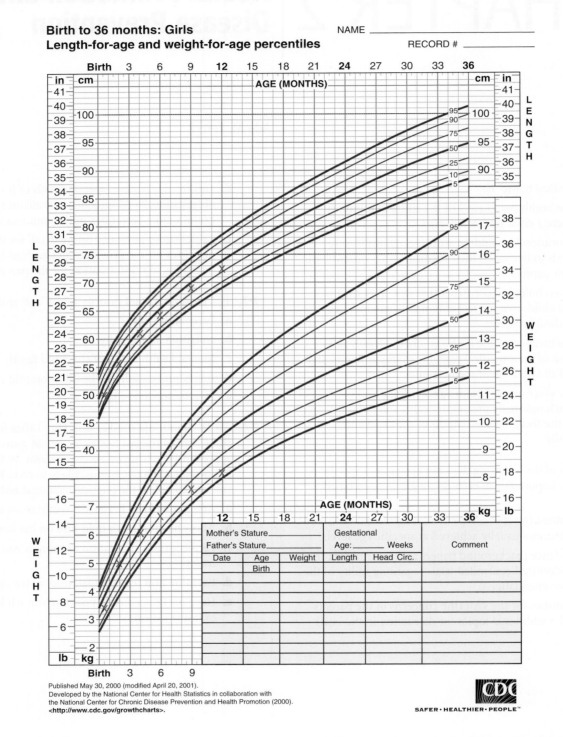

Birth to 36 months: Girls
Length-for-age and weight-for-age percentiles

NAME _____

RECORD # _____

Published May 30, 2000 (modified April 20, 2001).
Developed by the National Center for Health Statistics in collaboration with
the National Center for Chronic Disease Prevention and Health Promotion (2000).
<http://www.cdc.gov/growthcharts>.

CDC

SAFER · HEALTHIER · PEOPLE™

a. Obtain a bone age.

b. Obtain blood and urine for preliminary failure to thrive tests.

c. Obtain an extensive dietary history.

d. Replot these growth points on the World Health Organization (WHO) growth charts.

e. Reassure the parents that this growth pattern is normal.

2-6. Visit closure would be unlikely to include:

   a. Reviewing high-priority areas that were discussed in the visit

   b. Handing out pamphlets and tip sheets

   c. Modeling positive reinforcement techniques

   d. Creating the plan for the next visit

   e. Giving a Reach Out and Read book

2-7. You wish to improve identification of obesity in your practice. You convene a team of physicians, nurses, and front desk staff, and discover through baseline data collection that you are identifying the weight status of 40% of your patients. You decide that the nurses will place a sticky note on all charts where the child's growth points fall at greater than the 95th percentile, prompting you to enter a diagnosis in the problem list. After 1 week, you review the charts again and note that you are now up to 60% identification. You note the improvement, but want a higher level of fidelity, and you decide to alter your plan to having the nurses flag children when they are at greater than the 85th percentile. Which part of your described activities comprised the "study" segment of the plan–do–study–act (PDSA) cycle?

   a. Discover through baseline data that you are identifying the weight status of 40% of patients.

   b. Decide that the nurses will place a sticky note on all charts where the growth is greater than the 95th percentile.

   c. Review the charts again and note that you are now up to 60% identification.

   d. Note the improvement, and decide to alter your plan.

   e. Have the nurses flag children when they are at greater than the 85th percentile.

2-8. You are giving a presentation about child development to a parent–teacher organization. You are asked about the concept of "resilience" in relation to development. Resilience is:

   a. Any external, environmental factor that promotes child development

   b. A physical characteristic; specifically, the ability for a child to withstand corporal punishment or physical abuse

   c. A characteristic that is inherent and present in equal amounts in all children

   d. A relative resistance to environmental risk experiences, or overcoming stress or adversity

   e. A characteristic not associated with optimism

2-9. A 30-month-old arrives for well-child care. His medical history includes intermittent asthma. His mother is concerned about slow motor development; she says that he can't jump or walk up stairs one foot at a time. Which of the following would be a risk factor for poor motor development?

   a. The bedtime routine includes nightly reading by a parent.

   b. You observe that child is checking back with the mother frequently during his exploration of the room.

   c. You recall that the mother and an older sibling of this child have a strong relationship.

   d. You review the chart and note a history of prematurity, with birth at 31 weeks EGA.

   e. The child scores in the gray area on the Ages and Stages Questionnaire for gross motor skills.

2-10. The motherhood constellation is:

   a. The people around a new mother who provide emotional and physical assistance

   b. A mental state of a mother in which she prioritizes the infant and her relationship with the infant

   c. A group of symptoms and signs of pregnancy, including amenorrhea, morning nausea, breast enlargement, and mild weight gain

   d. The people with whom a mother interacts on a regular basis, whether or not they provide support

   e. A group of early symptoms of postpartum depression, such as insomnia, poor appetite, and mild sadness

2-11. Which of the following is unnecessary to secure attachment between a child and her parent?

   a. Parents' provision of age-appropriate toys

   b. Parents' emotional availability

   c. Ability of parents to manage their own state of arousal

   d. High parental sensitivity

   e. Appreciation of the infant's needs as independent of the parents' own

2-12. During a well-child visit, you learn that 4-year-old Mimi is very proud of her newly found abilities to pick out her own clothing and put it on. Her parents describe a relatively calm drop-off at preschool, when she very briefly clings and then joins in with activities. However, at school she will frequently grab toys from others instead of waiting calmly or asking to share. When she is challenged by the teachers on this behavior, she sometimes has a temper tantrum that reminds her parents of the "terrible 2s." Unlike the tantrum at the age of 2, she now will recover much more quickly than in the past.

Which area of development is Mimi having trouble mastering at this point?

- **a.** Autonomy
- **b.** Separation
- **c.** Mastery
- **d.** Self-regulation
- **e.** Individuation

2-13. A 2-month-old comes in with his mother, who is a neurobiologist. She tells you that he is beginning to smile and coo when he sees her. You tell her that this behavior is occurring because neurodevelopmentally he is beginning to make connections to his:

- **a.** Right hemisphere
- **b.** Amygdala
- **c.** Anterior cingulate
- **d.** Right orbitofrontal cortex
- **e.** Right hippocampus

2-14. You have successfully implemented developmental screening in your practice. One of your nurses has a friend who recently completed a child life program specializing in development, who has been trained for Healthy Steps. She is looking for a job, and you are looking for a way to enhance development while spending all that reimbursement you *did* receive for the developmental screening using the Common Procedural Terminology (CPT) Evaluation and Management (E&M) code, 96110. Should you hire her?

- **a.** No, because Healthy Steps has not been shown to give an advantage to children in the practices tested.
- **b.** Yes, because parents in Healthy Steps practices reported enhanced parenting abilities related to sleep position, feeding, and infant development.
- **c.** Yes, even though parents had worse satisfaction with care in Healthy Steps practices.

- **d.** No, although depressed mothers were more likely to discuss their mood with someone in the practice, they were more likely to leave the Healthy Steps practices.
- **e.** No, because parents in Healthy Steps practices were more likely to use harsh or severe discipline.

2-15. Group well-child care:

- **a.** Eliminates all ability to have individual discussion between the family and provider
- **b.** Limits the amount of time available to discuss anticipatory guidance topics
- **c.** Limits the ability of the provider to observe parent–child interaction and child behavior and development
- **d.** Decreases the family's ability to obtain information about their child's care and development
- **e.** Is associated with increased patient and provider satisfaction

2-16. You are asked to consult on a pediatric advisory panel for the health department. The health department is deciding whether or not to include a new screening test for a disease ("Fictionuria") in the newborn screening panel. You learn that "Fictionuria" is not rare (1 case for every 1000 births), and is a serious disease that is potentially lethal by the second decade of life. Early intervention can mitigate the symptoms of "Fictionuria" and dramatically improve life expectancy by several decades. The screening test has an extremely high sensitivity (only 1 false-negative for every 1,000,000 cases) and an equally high specificity (estimated to be only 1 false-positive for every 1,000,000 children without the disease). Although family history does not seem to be predictive of the disease, in utero tobacco exposure is associated with an increase in the likelihood of disease by a factor of 45.

Which consideration is *least* influential in determining whether the newborn screening test for "Fictionuria" should be added?

- **a.** "Fictionuria" is serious if untreated.
- **b.** "Fictionuria" can be treated with minimal side effects.
- **c.** A sensitive and specific screening test for "Fictionuria" is available.
- **d.** Early diagnosis will favorably influence the outcome of infants diagnosed with "Fictionuria."
- **e.** A specific characteristic (eg, in utero tobacco exposure) has been identified that is associated with a 45 times increase in the risk of "Fictionuria."

2-17. A 4-day-old newborn was born at full term in a birthing center, to a 26-year-old mother who had negative screening tests for HIV, hepatitis B, and syphilis. The dyad was discharged from the birthing center at 10 hours of age. The infant passed the hearing screening test, received the hepatitis B vaccine, and underwent blood screening for the newborn panel. She now comes to you for her first office visit. The mother is taking no medications; she is breast-feeding. The infant has lost 8% of her birth weight.

a. You recommend a repeat newborn screen, due to the risk of false-negatives.

b. You recommend repeat hearing test, due to the risk of false-negatives.

c. You recommend a second hepatitis B vaccination, due to poor immunogenicity in the first 24 hours of life.

d. You recommend that the mother supplement with formula due to the weight loss.

e. You recommend that the mother be tested for group B Strep (GBS).

2-18. Which of the following children does *not* need a referral to an eye specialist as a result of your vision screening?

a. A 6-month-old whose red reflex is brighter in the left eye

b. An 8-month-old whose mother says he is crossing eyes when tired

c. A 4-year-old who does not manage the visual acuity test using the tumbling E

d. A 4-year-old who can read the 20/40 line correctly, but fails the 20/30 line

e. A 7-year-old who can read the 20/20 line with left eye, and 20/40 line with right eye

2-19. An 18-month-old male presents to your office for establishment of care, and a well-child care visit. He is a pleasant, happy-appearing child who seems to be developing normally. His mother states that he was a full-term infant, was hospitalized in the newborn intensive care unit for 10 days for respiratory issues and a rule-out sepsis, and has since been healthy. The examination is normal. There is no family history of any medical problems. Outside of normal testing for this age, what screening test or referral should you request?

a. Hearing evaluation, audiology

b. Vision screening, ophthalmology

c. Dental evaluation, dentistry

d. Renal function testing, nephrology

e. Echocardiogram, cardiology

2-20. A 6-month-old female presents to your office for a well-child care visit. She is developing normally, and the nurse has obtained growth parameters, which show a child on the 10th percentile for height, weight, and head circumference. The examination is normal. You review the chart and thus remind yourself that this infant was the result of a 32-week gestation and was in the newborn intensive care unit for 4 weeks, first with transient NEC, and then as a "feeder and grower." She is just about to get her vaccines, but you remember that you should obtain a specific vital sign before she gets upset.

a. Temperature

b. Blood oxygenation

c. Respirations

d. Pulse

e. Blood pressure

2-21. Which child is at highest risk for coronary artery disease?

a. A 4-year-old with a history of Kawasaki disease with normal coronary arteries

b. A 7-year-old with congenital cardiac disease

c. A 10-year-old with type 1 diabetes mellitus

d. A 13-year-old with obesity (BMI z-score of 4.5)

e. A 16-year-old with type 2 diabetes mellitus

2-22. The primary source of lead contamination in children in the United States at this time is:

a. Factories producing lead-containing products

b. Paint chips and dust in older homes

c. Water from the pipes in older homes

d. Lead-containing products such as medications or makeup

e. Aviation fuel for aircraft with piston engines

2-23. Which child below does *not* need to be screened for iron-deficiency anemia?

a. A 4-month-old female born at 32 weeks estimated gestational age

b. An 18-month-old male living in poverty

c. A 5-year-old female with hemochromatosis

d. A 9-year-old male who eats a vegetarian diet

e. A 14-year-old female who appears generally healthy

2-24. A family of a 6-month-old presents to your office for a well-child visit. The infant (who was born at term) has recently stopped breast-feeding and has begun to take formula. You begin your usual talk about starting foods, and the mother tells you she is particularly worried about iron-deficiency anemia because she herself is anemic and because the family is vegetarian. You tell her:

  a. He is not at risk because he was not premature.

  b. Drinking regular-iron formula will take care of any risk he has.

  c. He will not be at risk if she gives him 3 servings of iron-fortified cereal a day.

  d. Vegetables with a higher iron content should keep him from becoming anemic.

  e. You will be checking him for anemia regularly.

2-25. A 3-year-old child presents to your office for well-child care. You screen him for tuberculosis and find that he had had no family members with tuberculosis or a positive tuberculin skin test, but he was born in a country identified by WHO as a high-incidence area for tuberculosis and received a BCG vaccine. A tuberculin skin test (TST) is placed in the right forearm, and 2 days later he returns for reading. Your nurse uses the "ballpoint method" and measures the induration at 12 mm perpendicularly to the long axis of the arm. Your appropriate next step is:

  a. Do nothing, as this is a negative TST.

  b. Repeat the measurement, as one must measure with the long axis of the arm.

  c. Repeat the skin test, as this is an equivocal TST.

  d. Obtain radiographs of the chest, as this is a positive TST.

  e. Refer the patient to an infectious disease specialist.

2-26. The most common dental problem is:

  a. Caries

  b. Malocclusion

  c. Erosion

  d. Fluorosis

  e. Odontodysplasia

2-27. Which of the following children is at lowest risk of early childhood caries?

  a. A 6-month-old male whose mother has moderate dental caries

  b. A 1-year-old female whose family is on the Supplemental Nutrition Assistance Program

  c. A 6-year-old with cerebral palsy and oromotor dyskinesia

  d. A 12-year-old who has been wearing braces for 8 months

  e. A 15-year-old who drinks regular cola daily, at lunch and dinner only and water at other times

2-28. Which of the following children is experiencing unusual tooth eruption?

  a. A 6-month-old male, primary mandibular central incisor

  b. A 1-year-old female, primary maxillary first molar

  c. An 18-month-old female, primary mandibular canine

  d. A 6-year-old male, permanent second premolar

  e. A 12-year-old male, permanent second molar

2-29. Which of the following statements concerning oral health anticipatory guidance for infants is correct?

  a. For infants without teeth, the parent should clean the infant's gums with a clean damp cloth at least once per day until the first tooth erupts.

  b. Upper molar teeth are the first to erupt at approximately 13 months of age.

  c. Teething pain is quite common and topical benzocaine gels are recommended as an initial treatment.

  d. Infants less than 12 months of age do not require fluoride supplementation.

  e. Parents can be reassured that infant consumption of beverages high in sugar content via a sippy cup does not increase the risk of dental caries, as long as a bottle is not used.

2-30. A family you know well comes in for well-child care. The 3-, 6-, and 12-year-old children all see the same pediatric dentist. After stating that teeth should be brushed twice per day, you also add:

  a. The 3-year-old can start to brush his or her own teeth.

  b. The 12-year-old should transition to an adult dentist.

  c. All 3 children should be encouraged to chew gum.

  d. All 3 children should be taking fluoride supplements.

  e. All 3 children should be avoiding foods high in sugar and sticky carbohydrates.

2-31. What statement about complementary and alternative medicine (CAM) is true?

    a. CAM use in adults is uncommon.

    b. CAM use among parents does not predict CAM use in their children.

    c. CAM use in children is more common for minor ailments.

    d. Most pediatricians ask about CAM.

    e. Most pediatricians are concerned about side effects of CAM.

2-32. "Like cures like" is a basic tenet of which of the following complementary and alternative medicine (CAM) therapies?

    a. Chiropractic

    b. Ayurveda

    c. Homeopathy

    d. Naturopathy

    e. Acupuncture

2-33. Your 17-year-old vegan patient arrives for an urgent care visit. She has a history of asthma, but today she complains of palpitations that she has been feeling intermittently for a few weeks, not instigated by increased activity. She has not had any asthma symptoms lately, so has not used her inhaler. She denies tobacco use. While her examination is unrevealing, you note vital signs of a pulse rate of 80, blood pressure 140/85, respirations 14, and oxygen saturation of 99%. Which herbal remedy may be causing her symptoms?

    a. *Echinacea*

    b. *Ginkgo biloba*

    c. Lavender

    d. Licorice

    e. St. John's wort

2-34. A 7-year-old with a history of behavioral issues arrives for his well-child checkup. Which strategy will best elicit a history of CAM use?

    a. Allow the family to bring up CAM treatment without your specific questioning.

    b. Ask about "any other medications" the family has used for treatment.

    c. Ask about "alternative medicines" the family has used for treatment.

    d. Ask about "any herbal or dietary therapies" the family has used for treatment.

    e. Ask about "any other doctors" the family sees for his treatment.

2-35. A family from Ecuador comes in for an assessment of Gustavo's behavior. He is 7, and has always been very active, but is now having trouble in school, as he is unable to sit still and pay attention to the teacher. Which question is most likely to elicit explanation about this family's understanding of their child's behavior?

    a. Tell me what happens at home. How does Gustavo act lately?

    b. What do you think causes Gustavo to behave how he does?

    c. What does Gustavo's teacher think about his behavior?

    d. What has the teacher tried at school that helps Gustavo?

    e. Is Gustavo managing to sit and finish his homework after school?

2-36. You are seeing a family from Guatemala for their son's 2-month well-child care appointment. You are aware that there is a higher incidence of bed sharing in their home country. How can you sensitively open this issue?

    a. "Tell me where your son sleeps."

    b. "Does your son sleep with you?"

    c. "Is your son sleeping in a crib as we discussed last time?"

    d. "He's in a crib, right?"

    e. "Tell me how he spends his day."

2-37. You are seeing a 6-year-old, Marta, for her well-child care appointment. She and her mother have recently arrived from Colombia, and Marta has been learning English rapidly in school. However, they have brought along Marta's uncle, who has been living in the country for several years, to interpret. You remember some of your high school Spanish. Your office medical assistant is also from Colombia. Which of the following is true?

    a. Since Marta is learning English so well, you don't need an interpreter.

    b. The uncle can serve as an interpreter.

    c. The medical assistant can serve as an interpreter.

    d. You don't need an interpreter, because you remember your high school Spanish.

    e. A trained interpreter is necessary.

2-38. Which of the following statements regarding children of gay fathers or lesbian mothers, compared with children of heterosexual parents, is correct?

   a. Behavioral problems are more likely to be related to sexual orientation of the parents than to issues of parental stress and conflict.

   b. Children of nonheterosexual couples are more likely to report being teased and being concerned about being harassed.

   c. Children of heterosexual parents score higher on cognitive tests.

   d. Children of lesbian parents are more emotionally well adjusted and have better motor skills.

   e. Children of heterosexual parents score higher on tests of psychological adjustment.

2-39. Which of the following practices will not support a safe and inclusive environment for same-gender parents and their children?

   a. Health care office staff attitudes are addressed with interventions, for example, diversity training.

   b. Ensure that all office staff learn the precise details of each family member's situation.

   c. Medical power of attorney designation forms are available in the practice.

   d. Standard office forms are modified to include gender-neutral terms, for example, "parent" instead of "mother."

   e. Posting a nondiscrimination policy for the office.

2-40. A 7-year-old presents to your office with malaise, nausea, headache, and dizziness. Which of the following environmental toxins do you suspect?

   a. Carbon monoxide

   b. Lead

   c. Mercury

   d. Nitrates

   e. Pesticides

2-41. A 3-month-old is admitted for cyanosis. Her oxygenation is poor, but cardiac and respiratory disease is ruled out. In putting together a broad differential, you consider potential environmental etiologies. You suspect that she could potentially have been exposed to:

   a. An improperly ventilated fireplace

   b. Paint chips from the windows in her bedroom

   c. A button battery

   d. Formula made with well water

   e. The ant poison that was put in the kitchen near where her formula was made

2-42. Acute radiation sickness includes which of the following:

   a. Headache, conjunctivitis, palmar rash, fever

   b. Photophobia, headache, abdominal pain

   c. Anxiety, sadness, insomnia

   d. Periorbital edema, weight gain, poor appetite

   e. Nausea, vomiting, diarrhea, leukopenia, thrombocytopenia

2-43. A family moves from a town near Lake Michigan to your practice. They describe their main hobbies by Lake Michigan as sport fishing (salmon), ice hockey, and reading. The mother has been breast-feeding. You are concerned about the 6-month-old's exposure to:

   a. Air pollution

   b. Ionizing radiation

   c. Nitrates

   d. Pesticides

   e. Polychlorinated biphenyls

2-44. Below are pollutants and cancers that have been associated with them. Which pair is correct?

   a. Nitrates—thyroid cancer

   b. Ionizing radiation—non-Hodgkin lymphoma

   c. Solar radiation—melanoma

   d. Mercury—astroglioma

   e. Pesticides—neuroblastoma

2-45. Which of the below comprises an exposure to organic mercury?

   a. Amalgam used in dental fillings

   b. Calomel teething powders

   c. Phenylmercuric acetate found in latex paint

   d. Quicksilver used in blood pressure cuffs

   e. Thimerosal used in vaccine preservation

2-46. A 4-year-old with asthma presents to your office with an exacerbation in the afternoon. She had been at her favorite area of a local playground, which was next to a parking lot where a car rally was being organized. Which of the following air pollutants is most likely responsible?

   a. Aflatoxins

   b. Mycotoxins

   c. Nitrogen oxide

   d. Sulfur compounds

   e. Radon

2-47. The family of your 4-year-old patient with asthma and cerebral palsy who uses a wheelchair due to severe lower extremity paresis arrives for a pretravel consultation. They are planning on going to Thailand for 3 weeks. Your best advice is that:

a. The airline will automatically know what accommodations he needs.

b. He should receive his set of booster vaccines now (MMR, VZV, DTaP, IPV).

c. He should receive the yellow fever vaccine.

d. They should take his albuterol, but don't need to worry about taking a course of steroids as medications will be readily available.

e. They should not worry about diarrhea.

2-48. The best source for medical information regarding planned travel to a particular country is:

a. AAP *Red Book*

b. CDC *Yellow Book*

c. US Department of State Travel Warnings

d. *Rudolph's Pediatrics*

e. The Web site of the country's health department

2-49. Which pathogen must pilgrims to Mecca be vaccinated against?

a. Hepatitis A

b. Japanese B encephalitis

c. Meningococcus

d. Rabies

e. Typhoid

2-50. Which of the following is true about traveler's diarrhea?

a. It is the second most common travel-related illness in children and adults.

b. China is in a high-risk area for development of traveler's diarrhea.

c. Electrolyte imbalance is the primary risk in children with traveler's diarrhea.

d. Oral rehydration packets, bismuth subsalicylate, and loperamide can be used in children over 8 years.

e. Presumptive treatment with antibiotics is not recommended in children.

2-51. You see a family in the well newborn nursery. They are planning to take the new baby to see her grandmother in Scotland, but are worried about air travel. Which is not a risk of air travel?

a. Infection from recirculated air

b. Mild decrease in oxygen saturation

c. Expansion of gases in body cavities, for example, the middle ear

d. Injury during turbulence if held on the lap of an adult

e. Limited ability for the caregiver to clean his or her hands

2-52. You receive a call from Greece. The healthiest patient in your practice, a 17-year-old, has gone on a summer cruise and is now feeling poorly. Besides some mild chest pain and shortness of breath, he is describing numbness and tingling in his extremities, fatigue, dizziness, and mild weakness. You suspect:

a. Asthma exacerbation

b. Traveler's diarrhea

c. Motion sickness

d. Altitude sickness

e. Decompression illness

2-53. A family and its functioning has been likened to:

a. Hanging mobile

b. Yo-yo

c. Stacking blocks

d. Rubik's cube

e. Interlocking puzzle

2-54. All of the following entail changes to the family constellation except:

a. Birth of a child

b. Adult returning from incarceration

c. Death of a sibling

d. Chronic illness of a parent

e. Move to a new home

2-55. Your 2-year-old patient, Mary, and her parents come in for her well-child visit. The mother tells you that she is 7 months pregnant, and that the infant is almost sure to have trisomy 21. Which of the following should you advise them to?

a. Not worry about it until the baby is born, at which time they will all work it out.

b. When the diagnosis is sure, give Mary detailed information about exactly what is wrong with the new baby.

c. Expose Mary to their emotions about the new baby so that she will continue to feel a part of the family.

d. When the baby is born, make sure to take time with Mary to play with her as they do now, even though it will by necessity be less.

e. Begin reducing the time they spend with Mary now, so that she won't feel it as much when the new baby comes.

2-56. Which of the following is true regarding foster care?

    a. In recent years, the majority of children are placed in foster care due to illness or death of parents or extreme poverty.

    b. Foster care is meant to be a stepping stone on the way to adoption; thus, efforts are made to match the child with a family similar to his or her birth family.

    c. Foster children who have experienced abuse and/or neglect tend to respond to foster parents with dysfunctional patterns.

    d. The incidence of child maltreatment in foster homes is less than 5%, and is limited to nonphysical abuse.

    e. Younger children who blame themselves for the placement in foster care are more likely to easily accept the foster parent.

2-57. The mother of one of your patients brings in a 6-year-old whom she is now taking care of through the foster system. You take a full medical history, and recall that:

    a. Most children in foster care with medical problems are over the age of 5.

    b. Children in foster care have 4 times the rate of mental health problems as do children in the general population.

    c. The incidence of developmental delay in children in foster care does not differ from that in the general population.

    d. The foster mother can make all medical decisions for the child.

    e. Most children in foster care remain in the child welfare system for several years.

2-58. Internationally adopted children do *not* have an increased incidence of:

    a. Allergies

    b. Learning disabilities

    c. Tuberculosis

    d. Attention-deficit hyperactivity disorder

    e. Substance abuse

2-59. A family comes to you for their well-child care. You ask the mother of the 10-, 7-, 4-, and 2-year-olds if there are problems in her marriage or relationship, and she tearfully tells you that she and their father are going to be divorced. She is worried about their reaction, and their long-term outcomes. You tell her to expect:

    a. The 2-year-old to be most resilient and not be easily rattled by the emotional state of caregivers

    b. The 4-year-old to be able to understand the long-term ramifications of the divorce

    c. The 7-year-old to wonder if the divorce would have happened if he had been "better" and wish his parents to reunite

    d. The 10-year-old to act out, and become quite aggressive and perhaps hypersexual

    e. That an older teenager would feel guilty, but in the end be most accepting

2-60. Special assessment for children experiencing moderate or severe marital stress will likely not include:

    a. Evaluating the parents' ability to understand the child's needs

    b. Assessing the child's functioning in school and home

    c. Evaluating the parent's modeling of eating, sleep, and exercise habits

    d. Assessing the child's mood state, friendships, and activities

    e. Reviewing the child's view of the stress or divorce and his or her relationships with parents

2-61. An approach that most helps a child and family who are grieving is to say:

    a. "I'm sure you will feel better soon."

    b. "At least your father is no longer in pain."

    c. "You are the man of the house now that your father has died."

    d. "You must be very sad."

    e. "I'm very sorry to hear that your father died."

2-62. Concepts about death that a child must come to understand include all but:

    a. All living things eventually die.

    b. Death is irreversible.

    c. Other people in his or her family also feel sad about death.

    d. All life functions end completely at the time of death.

    e. A realistic understanding of the cause of death.

2-63. The mother of a 5-year-old contacts you to ask about whether her child should go to the funeral of her father-in-law. He is a normally developing child who was quite attached to the grandfather who has passed away. You respond that:

   a. She should take him with her and make sure he participates in all aspects so he understands that death is final.

   b. She should explain to him what the funeral entails and find a way to involve him.

   c. Whether he goes to the funeral or not, he will have the equal support of family and friends.

   d. Whether he goes to the funeral or not, he will be able to understand and accept what has occurred.

   e. He is too young to go to a funeral; she should make sure she keeps him home and that someone cares for him there.

2-64. The members of the local school district are concerned about high ozone levels and their association with lung disease. You are asked by the local school district to participate as a child health expert on ways to reduce ozone levels. You learn that school buses idle outside the schools when they wait for students at the end of the day. You suggest an anti-idling program for school buses. You use the following to explain the rationale:

   a. School buses directly produce ozone, especially after the buses have been running for long periods of time.

   b. Motor vehicle exhaust, such as that from idling school buses, provides precursor compounds that later become ozone.

   c. School bus use is more common in the winter, which is when ozone levels are highest.

   d. School bus use is highest in the morning, which is when ozone levels are highest.

   e. School buses and cars are the only source of ozone or precursor compounds.

2-65. You are treating a 7-year-old child in your practice for lead exposure. Which of the following statements about lead exposure treatment is correct?

   a. A normal lead level is <10 µg/dL.

   b. Chelation therapy is initiated at lead levels >25 µg/dL.

   c. Inpatient chelation therapy is initiated at lead levels >45 µg/dL or for those children with symptoms of encephalopathy.

   d. A health department inspection is initiated for children with lead levels >45 µg/dL.

   e. 2,3-Dimercaptosuccinic acid (DMSA) and CaNa2EDTA are preferred treatment over penicillamine.

ANSWERS

Answer 2-1. e

The medical home is the setting where health supervision occurs, which includes health promotion, prevention, surveillance and management, and the coordination of care for children and youth with special health care needs. The medical home is the setting for diagnosing, managing, and treating health-related problems, but it is also a place for promoting health and building on the strengths of the child and family. The health care professional can coordinate the complex care of children with chronic illness, disability, and other special needs, and can advocate for appropriate services and facilitate communication among the specialists involved.

(Page 27, Section 2: Health Promotion and Disease Prevention/ Well-child Care)

Answer 2-2. b

The third edition of *Bright Futures* was revised following a careful examination of available evidence supporting each recommendation. However, this evidence is not explicitly reviewed in the detailed section covering each age-based visit. For each age-based visit, *Bright Futures* outlines the health supervision visit using 4 areas of importance: context, priorities, health supervision, and anticipatory guidance. *Bright Futures* can be found online at http://brightfutures.aap.org/3rd_Edition _Guidelines_and_Pocket_Guide.html.

Although *Bright Futures* is theory-driven and evidence-driven, in many cases, there are few, if any, randomized controlled trials that have been conducted for the specific recommendations at each age-based visit. The *Bright Futures* recommendations are based on evidence from clinical trials, observational studies, existing clinical practice guidelines, consensus recommendations, and expert opinion.

(Page 29, Section 2: Health Promotion and Disease Prevention/ Well-child Care)

Answer 2-3. a

Prioritizing the concerns of the family will accomplish several goals. Besides helping the parents to see the well-child visit as a partnership instead of a provider-directed or school-ordered task and emphasizing their participation, it will allow them to later focus on any additional priorities for the visit that the provider may bring to light instead of worrying or becoming frustrated at not having these concerns addressed. Additionally, it will allow the provider to understand at what intellectual level the family members are functioning and bring some insight into family function, thus allowing the provider to better tailor information and advice.

(Page 29, Section 2: Health Promotion and Disease Prevention/ Well-child Care)

Answer 2-4. b

Children at this age can be quite apprehensive about medical providers. A parent holding the child can reassure the child both verbally and physically most effectively. Other techniques commonly used fall in the categories of distraction (again both verbally using constant banter and physically by allowing the child to hold interesting objects), demonstration (eg, listening to a doll's heart before the child's), and recruitment (eg, allowing the child to "help" by holding a tongue depressor).

Additionally, the provider should avoid causing further fear. Approaching the child slowly and avoiding gaze initially, delaying the examination until the child is used to the provider's presence, and modifying the examination to begin with noninvasive examinations all may help to ameliorate the anxiety that prior visits with their attendant invasive and perhaps painful procedures have engendered.

While it is helpful for a parent to be the one holding a child in position for a particular examination element, this is unlikely to calm the infant.

(Page 31, Section 2: Health Promotion and Disease Prevention/ Well-child Care)

Answer 2-5. d

The WHO growth charts are based on an international set of samples of healthy breastfed children, and are thus a growth *standard*. The CDC growth charts (such as the one shown here) are based on several US datasets including breastfed or formula-fed and healthy or unhealthy children, and are a growth *reference*. The 2 charts differ slightly, and current recommendations by the CDC are to use the WHO growth charts for children from birth to age 2. Replotting these growth points on that chart would show a child growing resolutely on the 25th percentile.

If the chart were to show true failure to thrive, often defined as a crossing of 2 percentile lines on the chart, a thorough history and examination would be in order, and one would consider preliminary laboratory examination if the history and examination did not point in any specific direction.

The bone age might be considered if this child was showing signs of short stature.

(Page 31, Section 2: Health Promotion and Disease Prevention/ Well-child Care [also Page 110, Section 3: Nutrition/ Assessment of Nutritional Adequacy])

Answer 2-6. e

Reach Out and Read books should be given to families at the beginning of an encounter. They are not a reward for a good visit. Observing a parent and child with a developmentally and culturally appropriate book is an opportunity to not only discuss reading and language but also assess the child's interaction with the book and the parents' interactions with the child. It is also an opportunity to provide anticipatory guidance regarding child development (Zuckerman, 2010).

Visit closure should include a review of high-priority areas, giving the family further sources of information, and creation of a plan for follow-up. It is also an opportunity for the provider to model positive reinforcement techniques by praising the child for maintaining good health habits.

Zuckerman B, Khandekar A. Reach out and read: evidence-based approach to promoting early child development. *Curr Opin Pediatr.* 2010;22:539–544.

(Page 32, Section 2: Health Promotion and Disease Prevention/ Well-child Care)

Answer 2-7. c

The PDSA cycle provides a rough template for quality improvement activities. After identifying the aim of the improvement, the "plan" step involves understanding the background and devising a strategy, or method, for improvement. In the "do" stage, this strategy is implemented, and in the "study" stage, data are collected, analyzed, and interpreted. In "action," conclusions are drawn and decisions about next steps are taken, leading to yet another PDSA cycle. The aim is multiple rapid cycles, leading inexorably toward improvement.

(Page 33, Section 2: Health Promotion and Disease Prevention/ Well-child Care)

Answer 2-8. d

Resilience is defined as "an interactive concept that refers to a relative resistance to environmental risk experiences, or overcoming stress or adversity." Resilience refers to neither an external factor nor a physical factor. It is an innate quality, which is different in each individual and allows that individual to overcome adversity. Examples include behavioral, emotional, and cognitive self-regulation, as well as an optimistic attitude about life. A high level of resilience is one important factor that helps children overcome developmental risk factors (eg, poverty, poor access to health care or education) and increase the likelihood of achievement in life.

(Page 35, Section 2: Health Promotion and Disease Prevention/ Child Development)

Answer 2-9. d

Multiple risk factors exist for developmental delay. While prematurity falls into the category of a biological risk, one must also consider psychosocial risks such as family poverty or an unresponsive caring environment.

On the other hand, attachment theory states that a stable, responsive, nurturing environment may serve to ameliorate some of these risks. The child's exploration behavior, development of bedtime routines (especially those that include language learning), and a known strong family relationship all bode well for this child's future developmental ability.

While the gray area of the Ages and Stages Questionnaire does serve as a caution, this scale does not indicate a risk for future development as much as indicate that motor skills might be an area of concern at the time of administration.

(Page 35, Section 2: Health Promotion and Disease Prevention/ Child Development)

Answer 2-10. b

The motherhood constellation is a psychological construct that explains the mental state of a mother, beginning in pregnancy and lasting for several years afterwards, which enables her to bond with her own baby (making it *her* baby and not just any baby), and leads to her desire to protect and nurture it. An additional portion of this construct is the "holding environment," which is a psychologically enabling environment where the mother gathers supportive persons who will empower her in her new role.

(Page 35, Section 2: Health Promotion and Disease Prevention/ Child Development)

Answer 2-11. a

The provision of age-appropriate toys is important and may enhance developmental outcome; however, without the interaction of the parent, the toys are de facto unable to promote attachment. Children need their parents' engagement in play and other interactions to promote their ability to form relationships. An infant as young as 2 months old can read a range of affective states of the parent. The infant can also respond to these states in a way that promotes ongoing connection. Parents may face multiple challenges, but their ability to calm themselves and respond to the child's overtures will improve the bond. This ability will allow the child to use the parent as an external organizer of his or her state until the child forms his or her own ability to mitigate environmental stressors.

(Page 39, Section 2: Health Promotion and Disease Prevention/ Child Development)

Answer 2-12. d

Self-regulation is the ability of an individual to respond to his or her own emotions in a way that allows for a reduction in negative feelings without becoming overwhelmed or experiencing severe, unmanageable psychological distress. Grabbing toys instead of asking for them and displaying a tantrum instead of using words to describe wants or emotional states demonstrate a diminished capacity for self-regulation. Lack of regulatory capacities predicts higher frequencies of behavior problems in the future, lower levels of social competence, and poor school readiness.

In contrast, Mimi does demonstrate some achievement of behavioral independence (autonomy) in her ability to recover from the tantrum. She has begun to individuate, as can be seen by her choice of clothing, and mastered new skills, as evidenced by her ability to independently dress. Her parents describe a child who is skilled at separating from her parents in safe locations.

(Page 39-40, Section 2: Health Promotion and Disease Prevention/Child Development)

Answer 2-13. b

At birth, the infant is able to respond to external stimuli and produce autonomic and arousal responses due to the function of the amygdala.

By 8 weeks, the limbic system is maturing, including the anterior cingulate, allowing them to process more complex emotions and facial expressions, and better modulate the autonomic nervous system.

The right orbitofrontal cortex matures by the end of the first year of life until the middle of the second year, exerting a regulating effect on material processed through the amygdala and allowing the infant to manage emotional responses with greater complexity and more thought, and to modulate strong urges.

Overall, the right hemisphere, responsible for decoding emotional meaning conveyed through emotional tone of voice, gestures, and images, and for conscious and nonconscious reception, expression, and regulation of emotions, dominates in size and function in the first 3 years of life. The left hemisphere, with its more "cognitive" skills, becomes dominant after the age of 3.

(Page 40, Section 2: Health Promotion and Disease Prevention/ Child Development)

Answer 2-14. b

Healthy Steps for Young Children (found online at www. healthysteps.org) is a model of care that uses additional personnel trained in specific communication skills and in development to enhance the capacity and effectiveness of the practice. During the visit, the developmental specialist meets with parents and children and looks for opportunities to address parents' questions and concerns about child development and behavior using "teachable moments," with the goal to promote positive parent–child interactions based on observed behavior during the visit.

The evaluation of this program demonstrated that parents reported enhanced parenting practices related to sleep position, feeding, and infant development, discussed more anticipatory guidance topics, and were less likely to use harsh or severe discipline. Parents reported greater satisfaction with care, as well. Depressed mothers were more likely to discuss their mood. Families reported greater satisfaction with care and were more likely to stay in the practice. Sustainability may be an issue; in the past, reimbursement was not available for screening and thus additional study is needed.

(Page 41, Section 2: Health Promotion and Disease Prevention/ Child Development)

Answer 2-15. e

Group well-child care has been shown to increase both patient and provider satisfaction.

Usually the group well-child care appointments are much longer than appointments for individual visits, being made up of time slots for multiple children put together. Thus, there is ample time for the provider and families to discuss anticipatory guidance topics, including general care of children and development, as well as for the provider to observe the children and families in action.

Typically, there is a brief time for the child's physical examination during which the family can ask a quick question. While matters of interest to all the families are deferred to the whole group, individual concerns can be either quickly addressed or deferred to an individual contact, either in person (another appointment) or by telephone.

(Page 41, Section 2: Health Promotion and Disease Prevention/ Child Development)

Answer 2-16. e

Global screening tests are useful for common and serious conditions that have both a good (sensitive/specific) test available for them and an acceptable treatment that favorably influences the outcome. Thus, the decision whether to implement a screening test weighs these factors against the costs of the screening, including not only the direct costs of the screening but also the subsequent diagnostic, therapeutic, and supportive services that will be required and the psychological impact on individuals identified as false-positives.

In some cases, it may be necessary to identify patients at high risk of an illness. Clinically, the positive predictive value (PPV) of a screening tool may provide the most valuable information. As the population prevalence of a condition being sought diminishes, the PPV decreases as it directly reflects the proportion of true-positive to false-positive results. Thus, in

some cases, it may make the most sense to screen high-risk subgroups if they are the ones most at risk of the condition, as a positive result will be most dependable in this group. However, in this case, although the disease is not particularly common, the screening test characteristics (an extremely high specificity and high sensitivity) suggest that general screening may be reasonable. In general, if the 4 conditions listed above (eg, a serious disease if untreated, an available treatment, a highly sensitive and specific test, and a highly improved prognosis with early intervention) are met, then screening of the general population (as opposed to subgroup screening) can be an appropriate approach.

(Page 42, Section 2: Health Promotion and Disease Prevention/ Screening)

Answer 2-17. a

Newborn screening for certain disorders, for example, phenylketonuria, requires time for buildup of the metabolite for which the state is testing. Testing done earlier than 24 hours of life may be inaccurate, and thus repeat testing is recommended. Blood transfusions, dialysis, parenteral feeding, use of antibiotics, and prematurity all may interfere with accurate testing and thereby necessitate repeat testing.

The risk of false-negatives for the hearing test is not altered by time of discharge, and is relatively low. However, if there are signs of hearing loss, or other risk factors for hearing loss, retesting would then be recommended.

The US Advisory Committee on Immunization Practices recommends that hepatitis B immunization be given in the birth hospitalization; the ideal is to give this dose at less than 12 hours of life.

The weight loss seen is not excessive for 4 days of life, and supplementation is not necessarily indicated.

GBS documentation is lacking in this mother, but the opportunity for prophylaxis has passed, as the highest risk for early disease is in the first 48 hours of life. Thus, testing this mother is not indicated.

(Page 43, Section 2: Health Promotion and Disease Prevention/ Screening)

Answer 2-18. c

There are multiple picture tests available to enable screening preschool children for visual acuity issues, among them the Allen and the Lea; most of these systems can be taught to preschoolers even if not immediately understood by the child. Thus, the 4-year-old can be trained to recognize the various shapes, or to indicate the direction of the legs of the tumbling E.

An asymmetric red reflex can indicate simple disconjugate gaze, but can also indicate more severe pathology, and thus a child with this finding should be referred to an ophthalmologist. By 4 months of age, all children should have conjugate vision thus, a child over this age who is repeatedly crossing his eyes or whose examination indicates disconjugacy (eg, by abnormal corneal light reflex or by asymmetric red reflex) should be referred as well. The visual acuity testing should be better than 20/40 for a preschooler, better than 20/30 for a child over 6 years of age. Any child with a discrepancy of more than 1 line in acuity should be referred as well.

(Page 44, Section 2: Health Promotion and Disease Prevention/Screening)

Answer 2-19. a

Multiple risk indicators (see Table 12-1) are associated with hearing loss, including receipt of neonatal intensive care for more than 5 days. Additionally, this child presumably received

TABLE 12-1. Risk Indicators Associated with Hearing Loss

Caregiver concern[a] regarding hearing, speech, language, or developmental delay
Family history[a] of permanent childhood hearing loss
Neonatal intensive care of more than 5 days or any of the following regardless of length of stay: extracorporeal membrane oxygen,[a] assisted ventilation, exposure to ototoxic medications (gentamicin and tobramycin) or loop diuretics (furosemide/Lasix), and hyperbilirubinemia that requires exchange transfusion
In utero infections, such as cytomegalovirus,[a] herpes, rubella, syphilis, and toxoplasmosis
Craniofacial anomalies, including those that involve the pinna, ear canal, ear tags, ear pits, and temporal bone anomalies
Physical findings, such as white forelock, associated with a syndrome known to include a sensorineural or permanent conductive hearing loss
Syndromes associated with hearing loss or progressive or late-onset hearing loss,[a] such as neurofibromatosis, osteopetrosis, and Usher syndrome; other frequently identified syndromes include Waardenburg, Alport, Pendred, and Jervell and Lange-Nielsen
Neurodegenerative disorders,[a] such as Hunter syndrome, or sensory motor neuropathies, such as Friedreich ataxia and Charcot-Marie-Tooth syndrome
Culture-positive postnatal infections associated with sensorineural hearing loss,[a] including confirmed bacterial and viral (especially herpes viruses and varicella) meningitis
Head trauma, especially basal skull/temporal bone fracture[a] that requires hospitalization
Chemotherapy[a]

[a]These risk indicators are of greater concern for delayed-onset hearing loss.

Source: Reproduced, with permission, from Joint Committee on Infant Hearing. Year 2007 position statement: principles and guidelines for early hearing detection and intervention programs. *Pediatrics*. 2007;120:898–921.

an ototoxic antibiotic, gentamicin, for at least a few days during his stay to manage his presumptive infection. Thus, referral to audiology to rule out any hearing loss would be warranted.

Most infants in the United States do receive audiologic testing before departing the nursery, but a passed test at this stage does not imply that the child will be able to hear later. The newborn nursery screening can have false-negatives. Additionally, children can develop hearing difficulties later in infancy or childhood.

There is no specific indication in this case for vision, dental, renal, or cardiac screening, although the American Association of Pediatric Dentistry recommends establishment of a dental home by age 1 for all children.

(Page 44, Section 2: Health Promotion and Disease Prevention/Screening)

Answer 2-20. e

All children who have a history of prematurity, especially those who have had umbilical catheterization, are at risk of hypertension and should have blood pressure screening even before the standard age of 3 years. This applies also to children who have congenital heart disease; renal disease including urologic malformations, recurrent urinary tract infections, hematuria, or proteinuria *or* a family history of congenital renal disease; a history of malignancy or transplantation (both solid organ and bone marrow); evidence of elevated intracranial pressure; and systemic illness or medications associated with hypertension. It is probably a good idea, overall, to obtain any vital signs in children before submitting them to potentially painful procedures such as vaccination.

There is no indication in a well-appearing infant for obtaining temperature readings before immunization. One may wish to check respirations or blood oxygenation if the child had a history of respiratory issues during a stay in the newborn intensive care unit, especially if the child were on diuretic medications, but this infant had no such history. If there were a history of cardiac disease, obtaining blood pressure, pulse rate, and oxygenation might be of interest if these were questionable in the past.

(Page 44-45, Section 2: Health Promotion and Disease Prevention/Screening)

Answer 2-21. c

While all the children listed do have higher risk than the norm for heart disease, the highest risk for coronary artery disease at less than 30 years of age accrues to children with type 1 diabetes, as well as those with homozygous familial hypercholesterolemia, chronic renal disease, Kawasaki disease with coronary aneurysms, and history of orthotopic heart transplantation.

For children with Kawasaki disease, risk increases with degree of coronary artery involvement. Thus, children with normal coronary arteries are at lowest risk (although still at higher than the general population), those with regressed coronary aneurysms are at moderate risk, and those with current coronary aneurysms are at highest risk. Children with congenital heart disease are thought to be at higher risk than the general population and fall into the same "at-risk" category as children with Kawasaki disease with no coronary artery involvement.

Both type 1 and type 2 diabetes mellitus confer risk of atherosclerosis, but the risk is higher for children with type 1 than with type 2.

Obesity is associated with the "metabolic syndrome," a constellation of findings including hyperlipidemia, hypertension, insulin resistance, and central adiposity, which put the patient at higher-than-normal risk of coronary artery disease.

(Page 45, Section 2: Health Promotion and Disease Prevention/ Screening)

Answer 2-22. b

While lead-based paint for homes was banned for sale in the 1970s, many older homes will have layers of paint on walls or windows. Thus, renovation of older homes, or even frequent movement of the windows, may create chips or dust that expose children, and in fact this is the most frequent source of lead contamination that affects children.

Adults are most often exposed occupationally, at workplaces that produce lead-containing products, such as ammunition, aviation fuel for piston engine aircraft, soldering, or ceramic glazes.

Pediatric providers should be aware that lead might be an ingredient in makeup (eg, kohl), in medications (eg, certain ayurvedic medicines), or imported products (eg, some ceramics, candies, and toys). The New York City Department of Health Web site at http://www.nyc.gov/html/doh/html/lead/ lead-herbalmed.shtml is one source for detailed information about some of these risks.

(Page 45, Section 2: Health Promotion and Disease Prevention/ Screening)

Answer 2-23. c

The patient with hemochromatosis is least likely to have anemia; she is more likely to be suffering from iron overload if not treated. Thus, iron studies would be indicated in this child, but not because of anemia risk.

All children should be screened once between 9 and 12 months of age for iron-deficiency anemia. Additionally, children should be screened at 4 months of age if premature, of low birth weight, or drinking low-iron formula or cow's milk. Screening frequently in the preschool age (at 18 months and 2, 3, 4, and 5 years of age) is recommended for children living in poverty or having limited access to iron-containing food, and for children with special health needs that limit their iron intake. Lastly, any child on a strict vegetarian diet who does not receive iron supplementation and any woman of childbearing age (including adolescent females) should be screened as well.

(Page 46, Section 2: Health Promotion and Disease Prevention/ Screening)

Answer 2-24. e

Infants at higher risk for iron-deficiency anemia, including those who are vegetarian and have a diet low in iron, as well as those who live in poverty, have limited access to food, or have certain special health needs, should be screened for anemia more frequently.

Prematurity does give a risk for iron-deficiency anemia, but as there are other risks, it would be inappropriate to reassure the mother on this basis. While drinking regular formula (as opposed to low-iron), eating iron-fortified cereal, and being aware of vegetables with increased iron will be helpful, iron from nonheme sources is less well absorbed, and this does not obviate the need for testing.

(Page 46, Section 2: Health Promotion and Disease Prevention/ Screening)

Answer 2-25. d

For children younger than 4 years of age, any induration of greater than or equal to 10 mm is considered a positive tuberculin skin test; this is also true for children who are born in other countries. The definitions of positivity apply regardless of BCG vaccination. Appropriate next steps are to obtain chest radiography and subsequently to begin appropriate therapy (dictated by the results of the chest radiography).

A tuberculin skin test should be measured between 48 and 72 hours after placement. Measurement should identify the amount of induration perpendicular to the long axis of the arm. The amount of induration identified as positive depends on any other history or physical findings (see Table 12-5 for identification of categories).

If the radiograph were to show findings consistent with tuberculosis (ie, lymphadenopathy out of proportion to parenchymal disease), referral to an infectious disease specialist might be warranted, although often a primary care provider in a medical home can oversee treatment of primary tuberculosis. However, children with latent TB (those with positive TST but negative radiographs) can be well managed by a medical home. Some states require notification of positive TSTs.

(Page 46, Section 2: Health Promotion and Disease Prevention/ Screening)

Answer 2-26. a

Caries are the most common dental problem in children and adults. The incidence is high; in the United States, primary dentition is affected in 42% of children aged 2 to 11, and secondary dentition is affected in 21% of children from ages 6 to 11. It is 5 times more common than asthma. Risk can be ameliorated by behavioral strategies, and thus it is incumbent on the pediatric care provider to be aware of this risk, to learn to evaluate a child's dental status from an early age, and to provide anticipatory guidance to families that can prevent or slow the onset of caries.

(Page 47, Section 2: Health Promotion and Disease Prevention/ Oral Health Supervision)

TABLE 12-5. Questions for Determining Risk of Latent Tuberculosis Infection

Has a family member or contact had tuberculosis disease?

Has a family member had a positive tuberculin skin test?

Was your child born in a high-risk country (countries other than the United States, Canada, Australia, New Zealand, or Western European countries)?

Has your child traveled (had contact with resident populations) to a high-risk country for more than 1 week?

Definitions of positive tuberculin skin test results in infants, children, and adolescents[a]

Induration ≥5 mm

Children in close contact with known or suspected contagious people with tuberculosis disease

Children suspected to have tuberculosis disease:

    Findings on chest radiograph consistent with active or previous tuberculosis disease

    Clinical evidence of tuberculosis disease[b]

Children receiving immunosuppressive therapy[c] or with immunosuppressive conditions, including HIV infection

Induration ≥10 mm

Children at increased risk of disseminated tuberculosis disease:

    Children younger than 4 years of age

    Children with other medical conditions, including Hodgkin disease, lymphoma, diabetes mellitus, chronic renal failure, or malnutrition

Children with increased exposure to tuberculosis disease:

    Children born in high-prevalence regions of the world

    Children frequently exposed to adults who are HIV infected, homeless, users of illicit drugs, residents of nursing homes, incarcerated or institutionalized, or migrant farm workers

    Children who travel to high-prevalence regions of the world

Induration ≥15 mm

Children 4 years of age or older without any risk factors

[a]These definitions apply regardless of previous bacille Calmette-Guérjn immunization; erythema at tuberculin skin test site does not indicate a positive test result. Tests should be read at 48-72 hours after placement.

[b]Evidence by physical examination or laboratory assessment that would include tuberculosis in the working differential diagnosis (eg, meningitis).

[c]Including immunosuppressive doses of corticosteroids.

Source: Reproduced, with permission, from American Academy of Pediatrics. Tuberculosis. In: Pickering LK, Baker CJ, Long SS, McMillan J, eds. *Red Book: 2006 Report of the Committee on Infectious Diseases.* 27th ed. Elk Grove Village, IL: American Academy of Pediatrics; 2006:678–698.

Answer 2-27. e

While it is understood that sodas may not be the drink of choice for other health reasons, for the purposes of oral health, keeping sugared drinks to mealtimes only is much better than consuming them throughout the day. Constant exposure to the sugar allows growth of bacteria; salivary action between episodes of intake may help to retard this growth.

Parents frequently attempt to limit juice by watering it down, but for the above reason a better way to limit juice is to allow it only during meals and use water in between.

Dental decay in a parent or sibling is a risk factor for early caries (see Table 13-1) as there is vertical transmission of pathogenic *Streptococcus mutans* bacteria; families should be cautioned to attempt to delay this transmission as long as possible by not sharing utensils or "cleaning" pacifiers that have fallen by placing them in their mouths. Children whose families are of low socioeconomic status are also at higher risk of caries, as are those who do not have regular dental visits. Other children at risk include those with any situation that decreases salivary flow, or any situation that impairs the cleaning of teeth, such as orthodonture or illness that impairs the ability to open the mouth or use a toothbrush.

(Page 48, Section 2: Health Promotion and Disease Prevention/ Oral Health Supervision)

Answer 2-28. d

Formation, eruption, and exfoliation/replacement of teeth follow a generally predictable pattern, and the pediatric provider should be aware of this and be able to assess the timing, both as a measure of physical maturity and as a cause for dental referral. Eruption of primary teeth is typically symmetric, with mandibular teeth usually, but not always, presenting before maxillary teeth. Eruption of permanent dentition, with associated preceding exfoliation of the primary teeth, usually follows a similar pattern.

See Figure 13-1 for more detail.

(Page 49, Section 2: Health Promotion and Disease Prevention/ Oral Health Supervision)

Answer 2-29. a

Cleaning the infant's gums with a clean, damp cloth will decrease the levels of *Streptococcus mutans*, which is associated with the early development of childhood caries. When the tooth erupts, the caregiver can use a soft toothbrush and plain water.

The first teeth to erupt are the lower central incisors at 6 to 10 months of age (see Figure 13-1). The upper first molars and lower first molars erupt at 13 to 19 months of age. Teething can cause pain, which can be reduced with sucking on a wet washcloth, chewing on a chilled teething ring, or using a clean finger to massage the gum. Benzocaine gels are not recommended as they can be ingested and are associated with aspiration and methemoglobinemia. Consumption of

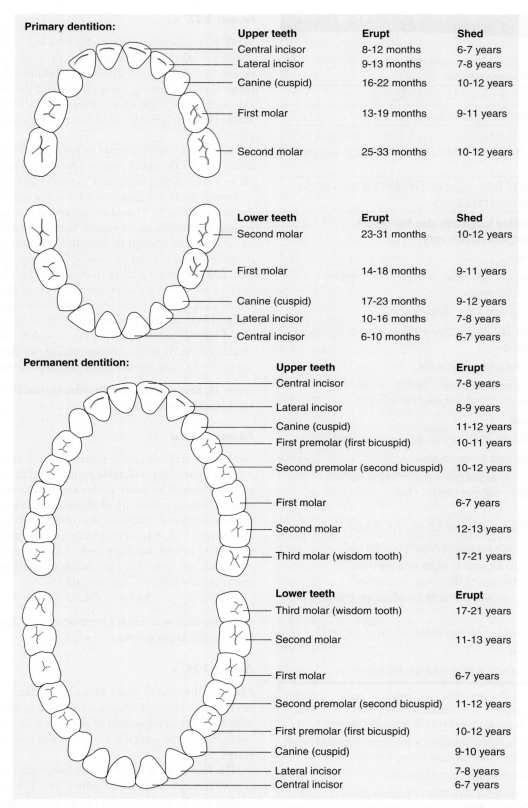

Primary dentition:

Upper teeth	Erupt	Shed
Central incisor	8-12 months	6-7 years
Lateral incisor	9-13 months	7-8 years
Canine (cuspid)	16-22 months	10-12 years
First molar	13-19 months	9-11 years
Second molar	25-33 months	10-12 years

Lower teeth	Erupt	Shed
Second molar	23-31 months	10-12 years
First molar	14-18 months	9-11 years
Canine (cuspid)	17-23 months	9-12 years
Lateral incisor	10-16 months	7-8 years
Central incisor	6-10 months	6-7 years

Permanent dentition:

Upper teeth	Erupt
Central incisor	7-8 years
Lateral incisor	8-9 years
Canine (cuspid)	11-12 years
First premolar (first bicuspid)	10-11 years
Second premolar (second bicuspid)	10-12 years
First molar	6-7 years
Second molar	12-13 years
Third molar (wisdom tooth)	17-21 years

Lower teeth	Erupt
Third molar (wisdom tooth)	17-21 years
Second molar	11-13 years
First molar	6-7 years
Second premolar (second bicuspid)	11-12 years
First premolar (first bicuspid)	10-12 years
Canine (cuspid)	9-10 years
Lateral incisor	7-8 years
Central incisor	6-7 years

FIGURE 13-1. Dental growth and development. (Reproduced, with permission, from American Dental Association. Oral health topics, A-Z, tooth eruption charts. Available at: http://www.ada.org/public/topics/tooth_eruption.asp. Accessed January 29, 2008.)

sugar-sweetened beverages will increase the risk of caries regardless of the mode of ingestion. Fluoride supplementation should begin at 6 months of age.

(Page 50, Section 2: Health Promotion and Disease Prevention/ Oral Health Supervision)

Answer 2-30. e

All persons who wish to maintain good dentition should be avoiding foods high in sugar, for example, juice, soda, candy, and sticky carbohydrates, for example, dried fruits and rolled dried fruits, as these can increase the growth of *Streptococcus mutans* and lead to increased caries. Some gums contain sugar, and thus should be avoided, and gum chewing by young children can be a choking hazard. However, for older children, gums containing xylitol have been shown to reduce dental caries by lowering plaque index scores.

Children should not brush their own teeth until they have sufficient fine motor dexterity and cognitive capacity to methodically do so, usually when they reach school age. A child who cannot tie shoelaces probably does not have sufficient capacity to adequately address all tooth surfaces.

Fluoride supplementation has been shown to decrease caries formation, but is based on the drinking water content as oversupplementation can lead to fluorosis, a disturbance of the tooth enamel. Thus, it would be inappropriate to supplement fluoride without assessing other sources. Pediatric providers should be aware of the availability of public water and of fluoridation programs in their communities.

Transition to an adult dentist typically should not happen until late adolescence.

(Page 50-51, Section 2: Health Promotion and Disease Prevention/Oral Health Supervision)

Answer 2-31. e

The 2002 National Health Interview Survey of adults found that 62% had used some form of CAM in the last 12 months. Use in parents is the number one predictor of use in children. CAM use in children with special health care needs is more common than that in the general pediatric population. Despite this high prevalence, in surveys, less than 40% of pediatricians asked about CAM in their routine pediatric history. Most pediatricians in this survey were concerned about side effects and were concerned that CAM use might delay mainstream care.

(Page 52, Section 2: Health Promotion and Disease Prevention/ Complementary and Alternative Medicine [CAM])

Answer 2-32. c

Homeopathy is a whole medical system founded in the late 18th century with 2 principles—the law of similar ("like cures like") and the law of dilutions. Homeopathic remedies, made from plant, animal, and mineral substances that are diluted to extremely small doses, are prescribed by practitioners based on the symptomatology of the patient, with the more dilute preparations thought to have increased power. Homeopathic remedies are easily available without a prescription.

Chiropractic therapies consist of musculoskeletal manipulations. Spinal manipulation may have serious adverse events in children and may have limited effect.

Ayurveda is a natural healing system developed in India, putting an equal emphasis on body, mind, and spirit. Primary treatments include diet, exercise, meditation, herbs, massage, exposure to sunlight, and controlled breathing. Some ayurvedic medicines contain lead.

Naturopathy is a medical system with a central belief that nature has a healing power, and that living organisms have the power to maintain a state of balance and health, and to heal themselves. Practitioners use treatment approaches that they consider to be most natural and least invasive, such as diet modification and nutritional supplements as well as herbal medicine, acupuncture and Chinese medicine, hydrotherapy, massage, and lifestyle counseling.

Naturopaths are trained in a 4-year, graduate-level, accredited program and receive a degree entitled "Doctor of Naturopathic Medicine," or ND. Some naturopaths recommend avoiding vaccinations. Studies of naturopathic medicine have mixed results.

Acupuncture is intended to remove blockages in the flow of vital energy (qi), and consists of stimulation of specific points on the body using needles, heat, laser, or massage along "energy meridians." It may have benefit in treatment of pain, headaches, nausea, and allergy.

(Page 54, Section 2: Health Promotion and Disease Prevention/ Complementary and Alternative Medicine [CAM])

Answer 2-33. d

Licorice is often used for respiratory symptoms, including asthma and URI, as well as some digestive disturbances. Long-term use may lead to a mineralocorticoid effect, hypertension, potassium wasting, and arrhythmias.

While herbal remedies can sound "natural," it is important to be cautious with their use as many of them do have side effects that are not well advertised and may develop only after some prolonged use. In addition, the preparations sold can vary widely in amount of the herb per dose.

Echinacea is often used internally to prevent or treat URIs, but its effectiveness even there is in doubt.

G. biloba has many claimed uses, including improvements in circulatory, arthritic, neurological, and respiratory problems. Its most important side effect is to interfere with the coagulation system.

Lavender is used topically as a sedative, for headaches, and as insect repellent. Generally, it is considered safe to use.

St. John wort is typically used for depression and anxiety. Its side effects include gastrointestinal symptoms, sedation, dizziness, confusion, and rarely a severe photosensitivity.

(Page 56-59, Section 2: Health Promotion and Disease Prevention/Complementary and Alternative Medicine [CAM])

Answer 2-34. d

Studies show that 12% to 21% of healthy children have some CAM use, and more widespread use among children with special health care needs. Asking about specific therapies, such as herbal or dietary therapies, is most likely to elicit report of use of these treatments. One can also name other therapies commonly used for the specific condition that the child comes in for, or ask if the family brings the child to "any other health professionals."

Waiting for families to bring it up on their own or asking in a judgmental fashion, or using potentially pejorative terms such as "alternative," "unproved," or "unconventional," is less likely to be productive. As only certain types of CAM practitioners are titled doctor, asking about other doctors is more likely to elicit visits to allopathic specialists, as opposed to any providers of homeopathy, chiropractic, or other types of CAM.

(Page 60, Section 2: Health Promotion and Disease Prevention/ Complementary and Alternative Medicine [CAM])

Answer 2-35. b

The relevance of culture to medicine is much more than quantifying beliefs and cataloging practices of groups of people; it is about understanding how culture shapes the ways that individual patients make sense of disease. Thus, people's explanatory models provide insight into how they are making sense of their experience, using ideas and beliefs that may have origin in their ancestry but also may have come from other sources of experience.

The second question is the only one of this grouping that asks for specific ideas of the family as to source or motivation; the others all ask for examples of behavior or therapy. Other questions that may be useful to elicit the meaning of the issue to the family are those such as "How severe is Gustavo's problem?," "What are the most important results that you hope to obtain for Gustavo through treatment?," or "What do you fear most about Gustavo's problem?"

(Page 61, Section 2: Health Promotion and Disease Prevention/ Culture and Pediatric Practice)

Answer 2-36. a

Issues of culture involve uncertainty, and thus may often be avoided. However, this important cause of infant death should be addressed with parents regardless.

Beginning with an open-ended question about the topic at hand holds best promise for a truthful and textured answer. It can be followed up with a question about motivation ("So he sleeps in the bed with you. Can you tell me how you decided to have him do that?") that can then best help the provider use a patient-centered method, arriving at an agreement that best matches the family's goals and priorities with the physician's.

Asking a question that directs the family to the provider's desired response as in the third or fourth questions may help the provider move along and check off a box, but may not get at the truth; additionally it may diminish rapport. Likewise,

presupposing, as in the second question, that the patient is not behaving safely with the child may diminish rapport or cause confusion on the part of the family—"No doc, last time we talked about this, and you told me that the back is safest, so I listened to you! Why, can he sleep with me now?"

The fifth is too general and may not elicit response about sleeping location.

(Page 62, Section 2: Health Promotion and Disease Prevention/ Culture and Pediatric Practice)

Answer 2-37. e

There is no substitute for a trained interpreter. These professionals know medical terminology, are trained to keep information private, and can help the provider to understand the patient's culture. They further can use their knowledge of the language and culture of a patient to make the information shared maximally understood by both sides. Not using an interpreter can lead to misunderstandings that can affect patient care negatively.

A child is not a sufficient interpreter, as there may be information that is inappropriate to share through her, either from you to the mother or vice versa. Additionally, she will not know much medical terminology.

While the uncle was brought in as an interpreter, he is likewise not ideal. Although his grasp on both languages is sure to be better than Marta's, there may still be privacy and terminology issues that interfere with his ability to provider full understanding.

While your check-in assistant is linguistically and culturally adept and may even know the medical terminology you wish to share, she may not be trained adequately in clear provision of information. Furthermore, for cultures that have small or close-knit communities in the United States, sharing of medical information with non–health care staff may lead to issues of privacy.

Your Spanish, while it may be excellent, may still not be sufficient. Not only must you make yourself clearly understood, but your language skills must also make the family feel confident that you understand their questions—or they will not ask them.

(Page 63, Section 2: Health Promotion and Disease Prevention/ Culture and Pediatric Practice)

Answer 2-38. b

While adult children of lesbian families recall an overall amount of teasing and bullying that is similar to that experienced by adults who grew up in heterosexual single-parent homes, in 1 study, children from nonheterosexual couples did report being more likely than those of heterosexual couples to be teased and to be concerned about being harassed.

A study that compared lesbian couples and heterosexual couples whose children were conceived via donor insemination found that child behavior problems were unrelated to family structural variables such as maternal sexual orientation, but rather were associated with higher levels of parental stress and interparental conflict.

In contrast, every study that has compared children with heterosexual parents with children of lesbian mothers has concluded that there is no difference in terms of psychological health, social relationships, or cognitive functioning. Motor skills have not been well evaluated.

(Page 64, Section 2: Health Promotion and Disease Prevention/ Gay and Lesbian Parents)

Answer 2-39. b

The challenge for the medical staff that cares for children lies in creating an environment in which individuals feel comfortable enough to disclose and discuss their sexual orientation and family constellation. While attitudes of office staff should be addressed with interventions as needed, there must be strict guidelines regarding confidentiality, as otherwise family privacy will be compromised. Thus, the family structure, like all such information, should be shared on a need-to-know basis.

The other practices are more supportive of families with same-gender parents, or any families with members who may be in family structures that are nonnormative compared with the local community.

(Page 65, Section 2: Health Promotion and Disease Prevention/ Gay and Lesbian Parents)

Answer 2-40. a

Carbon monoxide is an odorless gas produced by incomplete combustion of carbon-containing material. Mild-to-moderate exposures present with general symptoms similar to influenza or gastroenteritis: malaise, nausea, vomiting, dyspnea, headache, dizziness, and confusion. More severe poisoning is characterized by syncope, seizures, coma, cardiorespiratory depression, and death. Besides house fires, common sources include improperly ventilated water heaters, stoves, furnaces, fireplaces, and space heaters.

Lead poisoning is more insidious, and can present with neurobehavioral abnormalities including decreased intelligence quotients and developmental delay, or when very severe, encephalopathy and cerebral edema.

Mercury poisoning can be acute, presenting with rash, vomiting, muscle pain, and tachycardia, or chronic, initially presenting with insomnia, forgetfulness, loss of appetite, and mild tremor.

Nitrate-contaminated water can lead to methemoglobinemia, which should be suspected in a cyanotic patient with no respiratory or cardiac disease. Long-term exposure to nitrate in drinking water may increase the risk of certain cancers, hyperthyroidism, and diabetes.

Organophosphate or carbamate pesticides can acutely result in cholinergic excess, manifesting in signs such as bronchorrhea, bronchospasm, weakness, muscular incoordination, and fasciculations.

(Page 66-68, Section 2: Health Promotion and Disease Prevention/Environmental Pediatrics)

Answer 2-41. d

Nitrate-contaminated water can lead to methemoglobinemia, which should be suspected in a cyanotic patient with no respiratory or cardiac disease. Infants less than 4 months of age are particularly susceptible, because of the lower acidity of their intestines, which allows flourishing of the bacteria that metabolize nitrates to nitrite, because of the higher concentration of fetal hemoglobin, and because of the functional immaturity of the NADH-dependent methemoglobin reductase enzyme.

An improperly ventilated fireplace can result in exposure to carbon monoxide (CO), an odorless gas produced by incomplete combustion of carbon-containing material. Symptoms can be as mild as generalized malaise, nausea, and emesis, and as serious as syncope, seizures, coma, cardiopulmonary depression, and death.

Paint chips that are scraped off of windows with lead paint can be a source of lead exposure. However, this exposure will typically result in an older child's mouthing of toys that have lead-containing dust on them, not exposure to a nonmobile infant. Lead poisoning is insidious, and can present with neurobehavioral abnormalities including decreased intelligence quotients and developmental delay, or when very severe, encephalopathy and cerebral edema.

While most button batteries contain nickel and cadmium, some contain mercury. However, most ingestions happen in mobile children. Mercury poisoning can be acute, presenting with rash, vomiting, muscle pain, and tachycardia, or chronic, initially presenting with insomnia, forgetfulness, loss of appetite, and mild tremor.

Pesticides, typically organophosphate or carbamate, can acutely result in cholinergic excess, manifesting in signs such as bronchorrhea, bronchospasm, weakness, muscular incoordination, and fasciculations. It is unlikely that a nonmobile infant would be in danger of an ingestion.

(Page 69, Section 2: Health Promotion and Disease Prevention/ Environmental Pediatrics)

Answer 2-42. e

Acute radiation sickness consists of nausea, vomiting, diarrhea, declining white blood cell count, and thrombocytopenia.

The other descriptions may provide diagnoses of partial Kawasaki syndrome (headache, conjunctivitis, palmar rash, fever), migraine (photophobia, headache, abdominal pain), depression (anxiety, sadness, insomnia), and minimal change disease (periorbital edema, weight gain, poor appetite).

(Page 69, Section 2: Health Promotion and Disease Prevention/ Environmental Pediatrics)

Answer 2-43. e

Polychlorinated biphenyls (PCBs) are clear, nonvolatile, hydrophobic oils that resist metabolism and persist in the environment. Chronic exposure is associated with lower developmental and intelligence test scores, including lower psychomotor scores, defects in short-term memory, and lowered IQ.

The main source of exposure for most people is contaminated food, and the most concentrated source is sport fish from contaminated waters since the residues bioconcentrate, with fish typically the food at the highest part of this food chain that is consumed by humans. For young children, the major dietary source is human milk. Since the chemicals are not well metabolized or excreted, even very small doses accumulate over years. Fish advisories for Lake Michigan recommend that individuals not eat more than 1 meal per month of salmon.

Exposure to the other environmental pathogens named should not be any higher than those of other families in your practice based on the history proposed.

(Page 68-69, Section 2: Health Promotion and Disease Prevention/Environmental Pediatrics)

Answer 2-44. c

Skin cancers may be induced by ultraviolet light, although they rarely occur in childhood unless there is markedly heightened sensitivity. Children who experience repeated sunburns are at risk. Prevention includes avoidance of solar radiation at peak times and use of sunblock or protective clothing.

Exposure to nitrates has been associated with increased risk of non-Hodgkin lymphoma, gastric cancer, and bladder cancer. Japanese children exposed to the atomic bomb experienced an excess of thyroid cancer. Exposure to pesticides seems to be associated with childhood leukemia, brain cancers, and non-Hodgkin lymphoma. There are no documented increases in cancer incidence resulting from exposure to mercury; its main effects are related to the nervous system.

(Page 68-69, Section 2: Health Promotion and Disease Prevention/Environmental Pediatrics)

Answer 2-45. e

Of the substances mentioned above, all of which contain mercury in some form, only thimerosal contains an organic form, ethylmercury.

Mercurous chloride (in calomel teething powders) and phenylmercuric acetate (in some latex paints) are forms of inorganic mercury, while some dental fillings and blood pressure cuffs have used elemental mercury.

Symptoms of all 3 types of mercury poisoning are primarily neurological in nature, but the symptom constellations are somewhat different. Organic mercury toxicity progresses from paresthesias to ataxia, to generalized weakness, visual and hearing impairment, tremor and muscle spasticity, and then coma and death. Guidelines for maximum mercury exposure differ by issuing agency, but range from 0.1 to 0.4 $\mu g/kg/day$.

(Page 67-68, Section 2: Health Promotion and Disease Prevention/Environmental Pediatrics)

Answer 2-46. c

Although nitrogen oxides typically are more concentrated indoors than outside, one source of outdoor nitrogen oxides is motor vehicle emissions. Nitrogen oxides are associated with wheezing, cough, and shortness of breath in children.

Aflatoxins are not associated with air pollution. They are associated with peanuts, maize, soybeans, and cassava. The typical presentation includes vomiting, fever, abdominal pain, dizziness, and diarrhea, as opposed to respiratory symptoms.

Sulfur-containing compounds are usually found as products of burning coal plants, smelters, and paper mills.

Mycotoxins are typically found indoors after exposure to water damage. They are definitely associated with upper and lower respiratory tract symptoms.

Radon is not an air pollutant, and concentrates in homes, particularly in basements. It is associated with lung cancer and acute myeloid leukemia (AML).

(Page 70, Section 2: Health Promotion and Disease Prevention/Environmental Pediatrics)

Answer 2-47. b

A child's risk of vaccine-preventable diseases is higher in many countries outside the United States, especially developing countries. Thus, children should be fully immunized with all routine childhood vaccines prior to traveling out of the country. Specific travel vaccinations will depend on the area to which the family is traveling, and sometimes whether they plan to stay in cities or in rural areas.

It is important for families of children and youth with special health care needs to plan ahead for accommodations. Airlines do not routinely track the needs of passengers, particularly child passengers, and thus the family will need to call the airline to describe their child's needs. The family should also take medications that may be needed with them, as the medications available may differ in composition or dosage from those that the child usually takes, and thus may have different effects.

Traveler's diarrhea is the most common travel-related illness. High-risk areas include developing countries in Latin America, Africa, the Middle East, and Asia.

(Page 72, Section 2: Health Promotion and Disease Prevention/Travel Medicine)

Answer 2-48. b

The Centers for Disease Control and Prevention (CDC) maintains the travel Web site at http://wwwnc.cdc.gov/travel, with information available for any particular country. The same site hosts an online version of the *Yellow Book*, which is an excellent resource for the primary care provider, giving thoughtful and concise information that can be passed to the traveler. The table of contents can be found at http://wwwnc.cdc.gov/travel/yellowbook/2012/table-of-contents.htm.

The AAP *Red Book* gives specific information on many infectious diseases, as does *Rudolph's Pediatrics*. Web sites of national health departments are not often designed for the traveler, and thus may not carry the information needed and may not be in a language that the provider or traveler understands.

The US Department of State Web site lists travel warnings; however, these warnings refer to protracted conditions that make a country politically unstable or dangerous due to violence, kidnapping, or terrorist activity.

(Page 72, Section 2: Health Promotion and Disease Prevention/ Travel Medicine)

Answer 2-49. c

Because of epidemics that have occurred in Saudi Arabia among pilgrims making Hajj, this country requires all pilgrims to have been vaccinated between 10 days and 3 years before arrival. Epidemics have also occurred in the Indian subcontinent, but most cases overall occur in the "meningitis belt" of sub-Saharan Africa.

Typhoid vaccine is also recommended by the CDC for travel to Saudi Arabia, as is hepatitis A (although the latter is on the standard schedule for childhood vaccination published by the US Advisory Committee on Immunization Practices).

Japanese B encephalitis is typically found in rural areas of Asia. Rabies is endemic in many countries in Africa, Asia, and Central and South America; however, the primary method of vaccination takes place after exposure.

(Page 73, Section 2: Health Promotion and Disease Prevention/ Travel Medicine)

Answer 2-50. d

Traveler's diarrhea is the most common travel-related illness in children and adults, and can be bacterial, protozoal, or viral in origin. High-risk areas include developing countries of Latin America, Africa, the Middle East, and Asia. China is in the intermediate-risk area, which also includes the Mediterranean and Israel. Low-risk areas include North America, Northern Europe, Australia, and New Zealand.

Dehydration is the primary risk in children with traveler's diarrhea. Families should be aware that oral rehydration packets are commonly found in most developing countries, and should be used with bottled or boiled water. Bismuth subsalicylate can decrease the rate of stooling, as can loperamide, which should be avoided in children less than 8 years, or in older children with fever or bloody stools. Presumptive treatment is recommended in children and adults, and azithromycin and ciprofloxacin are the drugs of choice.

(Page 74, Section 2: Health Promotion and Disease Prevention/ Travel Medicine)

Answer 2-51. a

Air exchange in an aircraft is not associated with an increased risk of bacterial and viral infection. The infant is more at risk from nearby passengers who may be ill, or from the decreased availability of hand-hygiene measures aboard an aircraft.

The difference in pressures can lower oxygen saturation; while typically healthy children will likely not experience any ill effect from this, a child with sickle cell or cardiopulmonary disease may. However, the decrease in pressure can definitely cause discomfort in body cavities, including the middle ear, sinus, and gastrointestinal tract. Ear pain during changes in pressure can be partly ameliorated for infants by breast-feeding or sucking on a bottle, and for older children by chewing gum or using the Valsalva maneuver to open the Eustachian tubes.

Children who are sitting on the lap of an adult can be hurt during turbulence and nonfatal crashes, and the AAP recommends the use of a child-safety seat.

(Page 75, Section 2: Health Promotion and Disease Prevention/ Travel Medicine)

Answer 2-52. e

Decompression illness is a result of rapid ascent from deep scuba diving to the surface, causing overexpansion of air in the lungs and nitrogen bubbling in the bloodstream and tissues. Symptoms include the above as well as arthralgias, mottling or marbling of skin, itching, and neurological changes from personality change, to tremors or paralysis, to unconsciousness. Treatment consists of hyperbaric oxygen chamber therapy.

While an asthma exacerbation may cause the symptoms listed, these symptoms are unlikely to suddenly arise in an otherwise healthy patient.

The sine qua non of traveler's diarrhea is diarrhea itself, not listed in this young man's symptoms.

While motion sickness often strikes people traveling on smaller boats, those on cruise ships are less likely to be affected. Additionally, symptoms typically include nausea, vomiting, pallor, sweating, and vertigo, and none of the above.

Altitude sickness, also known as acute mountain sickness, occurs with rapid ascension to higher altitudes, strenuous exercise, and insufficient acclimatization. Common symptoms include headache, fatigue, irritability, nausea, vomiting, dizziness, and sleep disturbance.

(Page 76, Section 2: Health Promotion and Disease Prevention/ Travel Medicine)

Answer 2-53. a

The hanging mobile is an apt metaphor for the family for a host of reasons. Each level corresponds to a different generation; family members are interconnected and depend on each other. A force that disturbs the family will change the balance, but eventually the family will return to its original configuration. Changing the role of a member, for example, through illness or loss of a job, can change the balance points but, again, the family will come back to an equilibrium, even though it may not be identical to the starting point.

(Page 77, Section 2: Health Promotion and Disease Prevention/ Family Function and Birth of a Child)

Answer 2-54. e

The family constellation can be altered by additions to the family or losses to the family. Additions can be new children, whether by birth, adoption, or marriage; new adults, such as grandparents or new partners for the primary caregiver; or adults who have left and then return, such as adult children returning home or a return of a partner from separation, or from distant employment, the military, or incarceration. Losses typically entail death, permanent separation, or a temporary loss (for employment, military service, or incarceration). A loss of function, whether through injury or acute or chronic illness, will also mean adjustment of family roles.

While a move to a new home is an adjustment, it typically does not alter the family roles.

(Page 77, Section 2: Health Promotion and Disease Prevention/Family Function and Birth of a Child)

Answer 2-55. d

The birth of a child is a shock to any younger sibling, who will inevitably feel the reduction in attention due to the parent's need to care for a new infant. Any family should plan to make time with older siblings to focus on their interests and desires. In the case of a child with special health care needs, it is important to tailor the information and messaging to the older sibling's developmental level. A 2-year-old will certainly not understand the technicalities of her brother's problem, but should rather be told about the situation in more general terms—"the baby is born, and we love him, but he is sick and needs help from the doctors to make sure he stays healthy." Likewise, young children will not benefit from sharing the brunt of their parents' distress in the face of medical problems; instead they should be shielded as much as possible, with parents being aware of all the nonverbal cues that the child is exposed to.

(Page 78-79, Section 2: Health Promotion and Disease Prevention/Family Function and Birth of a Child)

Answer 2-56. c

Children who have experienced abuse and neglect are less likely to have a secure attachment with biological parents, are less likely to view caregivers as consistently available and nurturing, and thus may respond to foster parents with dysfunctional patterns. This may lead to foster parents withdrawing at times from the relationship or inflicting further abuse or maltreatment—one estimate is that 12% to 25% of children are maltreated in their foster homes. Younger children who blame themselves for the separation may resist developing a relationship with the foster parents out of a sense of loyalty to the biological parent.

While in the past most children in foster care were placed there due to parental illness or death, or extreme family poverty, in recent years approximately 70% of children are placed because of parental abuse and/or neglect. Foster care

is intended to be a temporary legal arrangement, enabling the child to be nurtured and protected while the biological parents receive supportive services with the aim of providing reunification.

(Page 79-81, Section 2: Health Promotion and Disease Prevention/Foster Care and Adoption)

Answer 2-57. b

Children in foster care suffer high rates of medical, developmental, and mental health problems that have typically developed before their placement in foster care. Between 44% and 82% of children in foster care are believed to have a chronic medical condition, with children under 2 with highest prevalence. At least 60% of preschool children in foster care have some type of developmental delay, in contrast with approximately 15% in the general population, and up to 80% of children entering foster care have a significant mental health problem, compared with 16% to 22% in the general population.

Only about 10% of children in foster care remain in the child welfare system for years, while about 50% return to their biological families within 6 months of placement. Typically, when the child is in foster care, the state agency serves as guardian.

(Page 79-81, Section 2: Health Promotion and Disease Prevention/Foster Care and Adoption)

Answer 2-58. a

Studies have documented an increased incidence of acute and chronic medical problems in internationally adopted children, including infectious diseases such as HIV, hepatitis, and tuberculosis, but not allergies. These children also have increased risk of developmental delays and speech and language disorders, as well as disrupted emotional development and behavior, including abnormal stress responses and attachment disorders. Adopted children in general have a higher risk of learning disabilities, externalizing behaviors, reactive attachment disorders, and attention-deficit hyperactivity disorder, and substance abuse.

(Page 82-83, Section 2: Health Promotion and Disease Prevention/Foster Care and Adoption)

Answer 2-59. c

While there are ongoing themes about how children react to divorce, the reactions do differ by developmental ability. Infants and toddlers may actually be most affected, as they are in constant contact with caregivers who are at an emotionally difficult point. Four- and 5-year-olds will not be able to grasp the longer time frame and finality of a divorce. Typically, children of this age have a rich fantasy life and thus may feel responsible for what is happening in the family. Children of school age can more realistically understand the cause of the divorce, and often feel caught in loyalty conflicts. They may also still wonder about their own contribution to the divorce, particularly if they have been, as is often the case, a central figure in a parental argument. Older school-age children and adolescents may react oppositionally, but may be more likely to react less directly, for example, with increasing complaints of psychosomatic disorders. The acceptance of divorce ultimately depends on the individual resilience of the family member and the parents' abilities to maintain relationships with the children despite their feelings about each other.

(Page 84-85, Section 2: Health Promotion and Disease Prevention/Family Discord and Divorce)

Answer 2-60. c

While the pediatric provider will often routinely be assessing the child's eating, sleep, and exercise habits, in times of family stress, the specific modeling of the parents in these habits will likely not be a primary point of concern.

Understanding the child's view of the divorce and the relationships with his or her parents is critical and will likely happen at multiple time points as the child grows. A trusted pediatric provider may ask at each major developmental stage whether the child's view of the divorce has changed, whether he or she might want any information or have new questions, and what he or she senses are any ongoing effects of the divorce. Providing an opportunity for children to discuss these feelings over time and helping them develop a better understanding and acceptance of the divorce is an invaluable service.

There are referral sources available to help families with some of the other issues mentioned. For example, children having trouble with school function or showing signs of altered mood state can be referred for mental health evaluation. Children whose parents are having trouble understanding their children's needs in the divorce situation may benefit from a family mental health evaluation, or may even need a guardian ad litem to take their side in a court of law.

(Page 85-86, Section 2: Health Promotion and Disease Prevention/Family Discord and Divorce)

Answer 2-61. e

It is most important to create an environment where the patient feels it is safe and welcome to discuss his or her thoughts and feelings related to the death. Thus, an empathic sentence that opens the conversation and allows the child or adolescent to state *his or her* emotions about the event may be most helpful. It is less helpful to try to cheer up those who are actively grieving, to encourage them to be strong or to hide or minimize their distress, or to tell them how they should be feeling. A willingness to be with the individual who is actively grieving, the time to actively listen, and an offer of help now or in the future are most beneficial.

(Page 86-87, Section 2: Health Promotion and Disease Prevention/Supporting the Grieving Child and Family)

Answer 2-62. c

Do not presume that sadness is the predominant feeling for either the child or his or her family. Children have difficulty sustaining strong emotions for extended periods of time, and thus may have spurts of emotion, delay or limit their engagement in the process overall, or use play or behavior to communicate and process their feelings. Young children often feel guilty about the death, feeling that if they had thought or acted a different way, the death would not have happened.

However, for the adjustment ultimately to take place, the child must understand 4 basic concepts—the irreversibility of death (their loved one will not return), the finality of death (life functions are over, so there is no physical suffering), the inevitability of death (neither the child nor the deceased did something special to bring it on), and the cause of the particular death. Most children learn these concepts by the age of 5 to 7 years, but personal experience and education can accelerate comprehension.

(Page 86-87, Section 2: Health Promotion and Disease Prevention/Supporting the Grieving Child and Family)

Answer 2-63. b

In order to have an understanding about death, a child who loses a loved one must learn about the irreversibility, inevitability, and finality of death, and about what caused the death of this loved one. However, it does not follow that he should be pushed to participate in events that he may be uncomfortable with. Each child has a different threshold for involvement in a funeral, and while some may feel comfortable witnessing the entire event, some may prefer to be present for only part of it or on the periphery. If the child does not attend the funeral at all, he will miss out on the support of family and friends who are present to celebrate the life of a person he loves. Thus, the death of the grandfather should be discussed with the 5-year-old and a description of the funeral process provided, and he can participate to the extent that he desires. If he chooses not to attend the funeral, it would be beneficial for him to be with someone who is familiar with the family structure and is able to answer questions about the grandfather's passing in a truthful and caring way.

(Page 87-88, Section 2: Health Promotion and Disease Prevention/Supporting the Grieving Child and Family)

Answer 2-64. b

Ozone is a pervasive outdoor air pollutant and the principal component of urban summer smog. It is produced in the atmosphere when volatile organic compounds and nitrogen oxides react in the presence of sunlight. Motor vehicle exhaust, chemical factories, and refineries provide precursor compounds for these reactions.

Generally, levels are highest on hot summer days and are highest in the late afternoon. Levels of other air pollutants, particularly particulates and acid aerosols, may also increase concomitantly.

(Page 70, Section 2: Health Promotion and Disease Prevention/ Environmental Pediatrics)

Answer 2-65. e

Lead has no physiologic function. As a result, a "normal" lead level is zero. Health department inspection should be initiated for any level over the action level, which is currently 5 μg/dL. Chelation therapy is reserved for children with a blood lead level greater than 45 μg/dL. Inpatient chelation therapy is initiated at lead levels >70 μg/dL or for those children with symptoms of encephalopathy. DMSA and CaNa2EDTA are preferred treatments over penicillamine due to toxicity associated with penicillamine.

(Page 67, Section 2: Health Promotion and Disease Prevention/ Environmental Pediatrics)

CHAPTER 3 | Nutrition

Michael D. Cabana and Cewin Chao

3-1. A 4-year-old presents with a 2-day history of fever, conjunctivitis, hacking cough, and congestion. According to the mother, there is no "bark" and there is no "whoop" with his cough. Examination of his mouth is notable for pinpoint white dots on a red base. The patient moved 3 years ago from Australia at 1 year of age. His parents have refused immunizations.

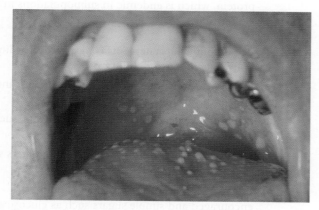

(Reproduced, with permission, from Rudolph CD, Lister A, Gershon A, Rudolph A, First L. *Rudolph's Pediatrics.* 22nd ed. New York: McGraw-Hill, 2011.)

Which vitamin supplement would you include in your treatment plan?

a. Vitamin D

b. Vitamin A

c. Vitamin E

d. Vitamin B$_{12}$

e. Vitamin K

3-2. A 17-year-old girl presents after being recently diagnosed a week ago with anorexia nervosa. The diagnosis was based on a >30-kg weight loss over the last 8 months. She had been restricting herself to less than 1000 kcal/day. Although hospitalization was recommended last week, the family refused inpatient treatment. She now presents with a recent onset of confusion, ataxia, and nystagmus for 2 days. On further questioning, she admits to a recent eating binge 3 days ago to avoid hospitalization. She consumed foods high in carbohydrates. On examination, she has a BMI of 15.9. Eye examination reveals both vertical and horizontal nystagmus. Mini-mental state examination reveals a score of 21 out of 30. She has gait ataxia. Urine toxicology screen is negative. CT scan shows diffuse cortical atrophy consistent with restrictive dietary intake.

Which vitamin deficiency is suspected in this patient?

a. Thiamin (B$_1$)

b. Riboflavin (B$_2$)

c. Niacin (B$_3$)

d. Vitamin A

e. Vitamin E

3-3. While working at an underserved health clinic in Southeastern Asia, an 11-month-old baby boy presents with shortness of breath. The parents note that he also has a hoarse, weak cry with poor feeding. One month prior to presentation, the child was treated for a viral gastroenteritis and diarrhea. During the visit 1 month ago, the mother was advised to stop feeding infant formula temporarily and give rice water. The diarrhea was quickly controlled; however, during your diet history, you learn that the mother never restarted infant formula and has instead continued with rice water for the last month. On examination, the infant has a heart rate of 152 beats/min. There is an S3 gallop. Liver is noted 3 cm below the left costal margin. There is sacral and pedal edema.

Given the dietary history and examination findings, which vitamin deficiency is suspected in this patient?

a. Vitamin A

b. Thiamin (B$_1$)

c. Niacin (B$_3$)

d. Vitamin D

e. Vitamin E

3-4. You are asked for an inpatient consult on a 16-year-old girl who has just been admitted with a diagnosis of anorexia nervosa. She was admitted with a 40% weight loss over the past 6 months. During that time she had placed herself on a calorie-restricted diet (about 400 kcal/day). One month prior to admission, she had become irritable and had a depressed mood. Over the past week she has also developed diarrhea (not related to laxative abuse) and an erythematous rash that is exacerbated by sunlight exposure. Over the past week, the skin in the erythematous area has become rough, cracked, and thick. In addition, the diarrhea has also persisted along with continued irritability and confusion.

Given the dietary history and examination findings, which vitamin deficiency is suspected in this patient?

a. Vitamin A

b. Thiamin (B_1)

c. Niacin (B_3)

d. Vitamin D

e. Vitamin E

3-5. You are asked to interpret dietary reference ranges for a vitamin provided by the National Academy of Science and the Food and Nutrition Board. The data available include the intake that would be associated with a tolerable upper limit (UL) for a vitamin, the estimated average requirement (EAR) for a vitamin, and the recommended dietary allowance (RDA) for a vitamin. You need to provide a range that not only could ensure that deficiency will not occur but would also avoid vitamin toxicity. What would you recommend?

a. Select an intake level above the EAR, but below the RDA.

b. Select an intake level above the EAR, but below the UL.

c. Select an intake level above the RDA, but below the UL.

d. Select an intake level above the RDA, but below the EAR.

e. None of the above.

3-6. Total body water composition changes with age. Which statement accurately describes the changes in total body water composition of children?

a. Water accounts for almost all 85% to 90% of body weight for infants and decreases over time (to 60%) in adolescents and young adults.

b. Water accounts for 70% to 75% of body weight for infants and decreases over time (to 50%-60%) in adolescents and young adults.

c. Water accounts for less than half (40%-50%) of body weight for infants and decreases over time (to 35%) in adolescents and young adults.

d. Water accounts for 40% to 50% of body weight for infants and increases over time (to 50%-60%) in adolescents and young adults.

e. Water accounts for 60% of body weight for infants and increases over time (to 85%) in adolescents and young adults.

3-7. Which of following statements is *correct* regarding protein intake for children?

a. Compared with carbohydrates and fats, children can derive more kilocalories (kcal) per gram from protein.

b. Unlike carbohydrates, both fat and protein are sufficient dietary sources of nitrogen.

c. Dietary protein requirements beyond infancy are easily obtained in the typical Western diet.

d. Protein needs are approximately 2.0 g/kg/day in infancy and linearly increase over time until they triple by late adolescence.

e. Kwashiorkor refers to excessive intake of dietary protein, which is endemic in subpopulations in the United States.

3-8. Which of following statements is *incorrect* regarding carbohydrate intake for children?

a. Dietary carbohydrate provides between 35% and 60% of the average American diet.

b. Fruits and vegetables contain simple sugars, such as glucose, fructose, and sucrose.

c. Soda, sweets, and candy contain simple sugars such as fructose.

d. Intake of complex carbohydrates should be encouraged and simple sugars such as glucose and fructose should be eliminated.

e. Glucose is the preferred energy substrate for the brain.

3-9. A 1-year-old girl is noted to have failure to thrive and persistent diarrhea with foul-smelling stool for several months. The mother describes the stool as "greasy." On examination, you note that the child has a scaly, diffuse dermatitis and hair loss. As you prepare to work up the underlying condition, you are also concerned about the possibility of a nutritional deficiency. Which of the following is the most likely nutritional deficiency present in this child?

a. Linoleic acid deficiency

b. Vitamin C deficiency

c. Vitamin B_{12} deficiency

d. Protein deficiency (kwashiorkor)

e. Protein and caloric deficiency (marasmus)

3-10. Which of following statements is *incorrect* regarding fat intake for children?

    a. Essential fatty acids include linoleic acid and linolenic acid.

    b. Hair loss, diarrhea, and poor wound healing are all symptoms of essential fatty acid deficiency.

    c. Prematurity and fat malabsorption are risk factors for essential fatty acid deficiency.

    d. Linoleic acids comprise a smaller percentage of total calories in human milk compared with typical commercial infant formulas.

    e. Linoleic deficiency can be diagnosed by low plasma linoleic acid levels, as well as a high buildup of serum levels of arachidonic acid.

3-11. Which of the following nutritional factors is least helpful in preventing later bone loss?

    a. A high peak bone density in the third decade of life

    b. High green vegetable intake

    c. High cow's milk intake

    d. High intake of phosphates (eg, cola drinks)

    e. High levels of human milk intake during infancy

3-12. Which of the following situations is not a contraindication for breast-feeding?

    a. A 22-year-old mother with human immunodeficiency virus infection in the United States

    b. A 32-year-old mother with active tuberculosis who has been treated for 1 week

    c. A 21-year-old mother with a history of cocaine use with a positive urine screen for cocaine and marijuana

    d. A 29-year-old mother currently on therapeutic doses of chemotherapy

    e. A 19-year-old mother with hepatitis B infection

3-13. Which of the following has the lowest potential renal solute load (PRSL)?

    a. Skim milk

    b. Whole milk

    c. Raw cow whole milk

    d. Soy-based infant formula

    e. Cow's milk–based infant formula

3-14. According to the World Health Organization, which of the following hospital-based nursery interventions is associated with increased newborn breast-feeding rates?

    a. Initiation of breast-feeding for all babies within the first hour after birth

    b. Separation of babies and mothers from other siblings

    c. Screening for galactosemia in the newborn period

    d. A strict breast-feeding schedule of feeding every 3 hours

    e. All of the above

3-15. You are counseling the mother of a newborn about breast-feeding. Which recommendations will help increase prolactin and breast milk production?

    a. Establishment of a breast-feeding routine

    b. The touch, sight, or smell of an infant

    c. Emptying the breast of milk with each feed

    d. Infant sucking of the breast

    e. All of the above

3-16. A 10-day-old former 3.02-kg full-term infant presents for a routine follow-up visit. The infant is breast-feeding. He was discharged at 2 days of age from the nursery. His discharge weight was 2.85 kg. At 4 days of age, his weight reached a nadir of 2.79 kg. Parents report that stools transitioned from meconium to yellow/mustard-colored by 3 days of age. He is now 3.03 kg today at his 10-day-old visit. He has several wet diapers per day. All of the following are signs of the adequacy of breast-feeding *except*:

    a. Regaining birth weight by 10 days of age

    b. Loss of less than 10% of birth weight

    c. Transition to mustard-colored stools by 5 days of age

    d. Presence of several wet diapers per day

    e. None of the above

3-17. A 3-day-old infant presents after discharge from the nursery for routine follow-up. The mother has been breast-feeding, but complains of breast tenderness. Since discharge, the infant has been slowly establishing a routine of feeding every 3 hours. Both breasts are warm and throbbing. She denies fever, chills, or aches. There is no specific area of tenderness. The areola and nipple appear normal with no shiny or flaky skin. What do you recommend to the mother?

    a. Miconazole or nystatin cream applied to the mother's nipples

    b. A 10- to 14-day course of antibiotics to cover *Staphylococcus aureus* for a mastitis

    c. Warm compresses to treat a plugged duct

    d. Increase feedings to 10 to 12 times per day; hand expression and application of cold compresses for engorgement

    e. Discontinuation of breast-feeding

3-18. A breast-feeding mother complains of breast pain. The following factors are associated with candidal infection of the nipple of a breast-feeding mother *except*:

a. Recent antibiotic use by the mother.

b. History of diabetes.

c. Maternal fever.

d. Mother is sleeping with milk-soaked breast pads.

e. History of maternal vaginal candidiasis.

3-19. You are asked by a parent about infant nutrition for her 3-month-old child. The mother plans to stop breast-feeding over the next week. She notes that infants can be fed a cow's milk–based infant formula; however, unmodified whole cow's milk is not recommended for infants less than 1 year of age. She asks why infants can't be fed the same whole cow's milk that she feeds to her 19-month-old child. Which of the following reasons supports the recommendation not to feed infants (less than 1 year of age) unmodified cow's milk?

a. Unmodified cow's milk has unacceptable low protein content.

b. Unmodified cow's milk has a high renal solute load that is not appropriate for infants.

c. Unmodified cow's milk has excessive iron content that increases the risk for constipation.

d. Unmodified cow's milk increases the risk of development of allergic disease.

e. Unmodified cow's milk has an increased whey protein to casein protein ratio, compared with human milk.

3-20. Place the following steps in the introduction of complementary foods in appropriate order by age:

Age	Complementary Food Introduced
4-6 months	
6-8 months	
8-10 months	
10-12 months	
12-24 months	

a. Mashed table food, plain yogurt, cooked scrambled eggs

b. Iron-fortified infant cereal

c. Wheat cereal, strained chicken, mashed cooked beans

d. Mixed table food (avoiding grapes, nuts, hot dogs, raisins, peanut butter)

e. Strained fruited and vegetables

3-21. You are seeing a 4-week-old infant for the first time. She is the product of a 33-week gestation. The infant currently weighs 2.84 kg. She was recently discharged from the nursery on 22 kcal/oz preterm discharge formula. The parents ask you when she can transition to a routine newborn formula. What are the general recommendations for when to transition a former premature infant to a routine newborn formula?

a. When the infant is greater than 3 kg

b. When the infant is 6 months of age

c. When the infant has achieved catch-up growth to the 10th percentile for adjusted age

d. A and B

e. A and C

3-22. During a well-child visit for an 18-month-old, you learn that your patient consumes over 32 oz of whole milk per day. Which of the following recommendations would you include in your counseling?

a. Immediately eliminate all whole milk intake.

b. Encourage increased intake of red meat, but decreased intake of fish and poultry.

c. Encourage consumption of foods high in vitamin C.

d. Suggest replacement of whole cow's milk with soy milk.

e. No recommendations are necessary.

3-23. You are caring for an exclusively breastfed 2-month-old infant. The mother is a strict vegetarian or vegan and does not eat any animal products. What specific dietary supplementation would you recommend for the mother?

a. Vitamin D.

b. Vitamin A.

c. Vitamin B_{12}.

d. Vitamin E.

e. No supplementation is necessary.

3-24. You are a consultant on a medical relief mission and are asked to help manage a child with a severely malnourished 7-year-old boy. All of the following recommendations would be appropriate *except*:

a. Check baseline potassium, phosphorus, calcium, and magnesium. If baseline levels are low, correct and continue supplementation.

b. Administer thiamin before refeeding.

c. Monitor for signs of cardiac and respiratory distress.

d. Start aggressive caloric replacement and gradually taper to full routine feeds when at 10% of ideal body weight.

e. Do not exceed maintenance fluid needs.

3-25. A 10-year-old boy presents for a well-child examination. Height is 130 cm. Weight is 35.5 kg. Head circumference is not obtained.

Based on the child's body mass index, what would be the appropriate description of this child?

a. There is not enough information provided to determine a BMI.

b. This child would be considered underweight.

c. This child is neither overweight nor obese.

d. This child would be considered overweight.

e. This child would be considered obese.

Boys, 2-20 years

Name _____

BODY MASS INDEX FOR AGE PERCENTILES

Record # _____

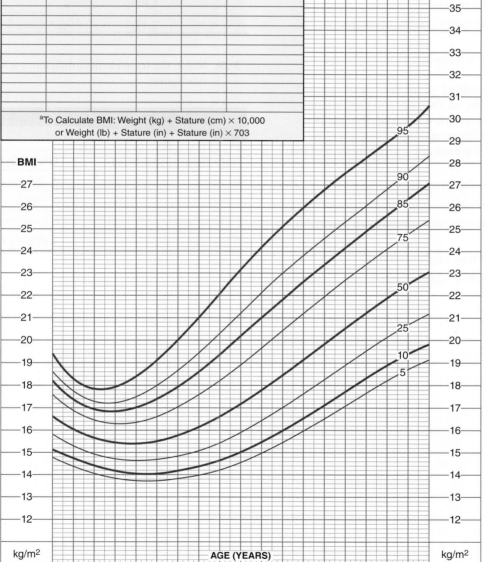

(Reproduced from Centers for Disease Control and Prevention.)

3-26. Match the symptom or sign with the condition associated with obesity:

1. Polyuria and polydipsia
2. Cranial nerve VI palsy
3. Knee pain
4. Oligomenorrhea or amenorrhea
5. Undescended testicle
6. Red hair

a. Pseudotumor cerebri
b. Slipped capital femoral epiphyses
c. Prader-Willi syndrome
d. Type 2 diabetes mellitus
e. Proopiomelanocortin (POMC) deficiency syndromes
f. Polycystic ovary disease

3-27. You are asked to consult on for the care of a patient who is unable to be fed enterally and requires long-term nutritional support. A hematocrit suggests iron-deficiency anemia, and iron replacement is needed. What is the most appropriate method of iron replacement?

a. Intravenous bolus infusion
b. Prolonged intravenous iron administration
c. Addition of iron to routine prolonged parenteral nutrition
d. Subcutaneous iron administration
e. Intramuscular iron administration

3-28. Match the vitamin deficiency with the clinical syndrome:

Vitamin	Clinical Syndrome
1. Vitamin A	a. Megaloblastic anemia
2. Vitamin D	b. Rickets
3. Vitamin K	c. Night blindness, poor growth, photophobia
4. Folate	d. Scurvy
5. Vitamin B$_{12}$	e. Dermatitis, dementia, diarrhea
6. Niacin	f. Pernicious anemia
7. Vitamin C	g. Hemorrhagic disease during the newborn period

3-29. Match the trace element deficiency with the clinical syndrome:

Trace Element Deficiency	Clinical Syndrome
1. Zinc	a. Glucose intolerance
2. Fluoride	b. Growth failure
3. Chromium	c. Cardiomyopathy
4. Selenium	d. Dental caries

ANSWERS

Answer 3-1. b

The child in this vignette has measles. The lesions in the mouth are Koplik spots, which are pathognomonic for measles. Although measles usually presents with a rash, the rash usually appears after the fever, cough, coryza, and conjunctivitis. Vitamin A deficiency is associated with decreased resistance of infection. In addition, although vitamin A deficiency is rare in the United States, there is an association between measles infection and vitamin A deficiency. As a result, the American Academy of Pediatrics recommends consideration of treatment with vitamin A for all children hospitalized for measles.

(Page 1172, Infectious Diseases/Page 92, Nutrition)

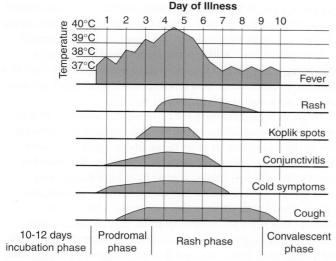

Clinical features of measles. (Reproduced from Expanded Programme on Immunization Team. *Manual for the Laboratory Diagnosis of Measles and Rubella Virus Infection.* 2nd ed. Geneva, Switzerland: WHO Document Production Services; 2007.)

Answer 3-2. a

This patient has a triad of symptoms (confusion, ataxia, and nystagmus) classic for Wernicke encephalopathy. If untreated, the condition can lead to psychosis, coma, and death. Classically, Wernicke encephalopathy occurs in the setting of thiamin (vitamin B_1) deficiency with acute administration of glucose. In this case, the patient has long-standing malnutrition and most likely low thiamin intake. In this setting, the body can deplete thiamin stores in weeks. In addition, prior to the onset of symptoms, the patient had engaged in a carbohydrate eating binge. If Wernicke encephalopathy is suspected, treatment consists of thiamin replacement. Although there is some overlap of these patient's symptoms and other manifestations of other vitamin deficiencies listed above, thiamin deficiency is the best response.

Riboflavin and vitamin A deficiency are also associated with visual symptoms. Riboflavin deficiency presents with photophobia and loss of visual acuity, and vitamin A deficiency classically presents with night blindness. Niacin deficiency is associated with pellagra that includes dermatitis, diarrhea, and dementia. Vitamin E deficiency is associated with hemolytic anemia in premature infants, as well as loss of neural integrity, but not necessarily ataxia.

(Page 113, Malnutrition and Feeding; Page 393, Hypoglycemia/ Acute Neurological Dysfunction)

Answer 3-3. b

This infant has beriberi, which is a deficiency of thiamin (vitamin B_1). Thiamin is critical for carbohydrate metabolism, voluntary muscle action, and nerve impulse conduction. Sources of thiamin include legumes, pork, yeast, and whole grain brown rice. Milled white rice is a poor source of thiamin. Deficiency of thiamin can manifest as Wernicke encephalopathy or beriberi. There are 2 forms of beriberi, which may overlap slightly. "Wet" beriberi is characterized by congestive heart failure and may be preceded by aphonia, including a weak or hoarse dry. "Dry" beriberi is associated with peripheral neuropathy and is characterized by muscle wasting, ataxia, paresthesias, neuritis, and loss of deep tendon reflexes.

Beriberi is rare in the United States. Populations at risk include patients with anorexia nervosa, patients with chronic gastrointestinal disease with poor nutritional supplementation, children in families who practice food faddism, and adolescents after bariatric surgery. In this case, the child's baseline poor nutritional status was exacerbated by 1 month of poor nutrition from rice water. This child has signs of wet beriberi and congestive heart failure. Treatment includes parenteral thiamin replacement.

Vitamin A deficiency may manifest with impaired resistance to infection or poor growth, but classically presents with night blindness. Niacin deficiency is associated with pellagra that includes dermatitis, diarrhea, and dementia, but not congestive heart failure. Vitamin E deficiency is associated with hemolytic anemia in premature infants, which may predispose to congestive heart failure; however, this is less likely given the age of the patient. Vitamin D in infants presents as rickets, which includes skeletal findings, including a rachitic rosary and frontal bossing.

(Page 93, Vitamins, Nutrition)

Answer 3-4. c

This patient has an underlying malnutrition and a classic triad of symptoms (diarrhea, dementia, and dermatitis) that is associated with pellagra or niacin deficiency. There is no specific order in which the symptoms present. The dermatitis tends to be symmetrical and erupts in sun-exposed areas. After the initial erythematous appearance, the skin develops a rough texture.

The term pellagra is derived from the Italian words meaning "rough skin." If not treated, pellagra is associated with multiorgan system failure and death. Treatment is niacin supplementation.

The other vitamin deficiencies listed do not have dermatologic findings. Vitamin A deficiency may manifest with impaired resistance to infection or poor growth, but classically presents with night blindness. Thiamin deficiency is associated with beriberi and Wernicke encephalopathy. Vitamin E deficiency is associated with hemolytic anemia in premature infants. Vitamin D in infants presents as rickets, which includes skeletal findings, including a rachitic rosary and frontal bossing.

(Page 93, Nutrition)

Answer 3-5. c

The EAR is the "estimated nutrient intake value that meets the requirements of half the healthy individuals in a group or population according to accepted scientific research." The RDA is "the average daily dietary intake level that is sufficient to meet the nutrient requirements of virtually all (97%-98%) healthy individuals in a group or population." The UL is "the highest level of daily nutrient intake found to pose no risks of adverse effects in individuals of a healthy population. The risk of adverse effects and toxicities increases with an increase in consumption above these limits." To avoid deficiency, the level about the RDA should be selected. To avoid toxicity, a level below the UL should be selected. Sometimes an "adequate intake (AI)" value is listed. If EAR is not known due to lack of data, an AI is provided.

(Page 89, Nutrition)

Answer 3-6. b

Total body water, as a percentage of weight, decreases with age. For infants, 70% to 75% of weight is composed of water. Adults have 50% to 60% of body weight in the form of water. They also have a greater relative percentage of fat in their body composition. Free water should not be provided to infants; however, providing nutrition without adequate amounts of fluid increases the risk for dehydration. Infants are at greater risk for dehydration due to the increased relative surface area and an inability for infant kidneys to concentrate urine.

(Page 90, Nutrition/Normal Nutritional Requirements)

Answer 3-7. c

Typical Western diets easily meet dietary protein requirements. Kwashiorkor refers to insufficient intake of protein of high quality and is rare in the United States. Unlike carbohydrates and fats, protein provides a source of nitrogen for growth. Fat is more efficient in storing energy, as it can provide 9 kcal/g, compared with only 4 kcal/g provided by carbohydrates and protein. Protein needs stay relatively constant at around 2 to 2.4 kcal/kg/day. This dips slightly to 1.5 kcal/kg/day at 6 months of age before increasing again during childhood and adolescence to approximately 2.2 kcal/kg/day.

(Page 91, Nutrition/Normal Nutritional Requirements)

Answer 3-8. d

Complex carbohydrate intake should be encouraged and simple sugar intake should be *minimized*. It is impossible to avoid all simple sugars. For example, fruits and vegetables contain simple sugars, such as glucose, fructose, and sucrose; however, fruits and vegetables also contain dietary fiber.

(Page 91, Nutrition/Normal Nutritional Requirements)

Answer 3-9. a

This child has steatorrhea, which is associated with malabsorption of fat-soluble vitamins (eg, vitamins D, E, A, and K), as well as fatty acids. This child has a history suggestive of linoleic acid deficiency. Linolenic acid and linoleic acid are considered essential fatty acids. Children at greatest risk for fatty acid deficiency include premature infants who do not receive adequate linoleic acid, children on long-term parenteral nutrition without intravenous lipid, and children with fat malabsorption. In this case, long-standing fat malabsorption led to low levels of linoleic acid and an essential fatty acid deficiency. Linoleic acid is an essential fatty acid and can be lengthened to form arachidonic acid. For the diagnosis of linoleic acid deficiency, there are low serum levels of linoleic acid, as well as a decrease in arachidonic acid levels. Linoleic acid deficiency also presents with a scaly dermatitis and hair loss.

Vitamin B_{12} is necessary for erythrocyte development and presents with pernicious anemia and neurological symptoms due to demyelination of large nerve fibers. Typical Western diets easily meet dietary protein requirements. Kwashiorkor refers to insufficient intake of protein of high quality and is rare in the United States. Marasmus includes protein and caloric insufficiency that is also rare in the United States. Vitamin C is not a fat-soluble vitamin. It is found in citrus fruits, tomatoes, green vegetables, and human milk. Although both vitamin C deficiency and linoleic deficiency present with poor wound healing, deficiency of vitamin C leads to scurvy that presents with diffuse tissue bleeding and hemorrhage, as well as loose teeth and easy bone fractures.

(Page 93, Nutrition)

Answer 3-10. e

Linoleic acid is an essential fatty acid and can be lengthened to form arachidonic acid. For the diagnosis of linoleic acid deficiency, there are low serum levels of linoleic acid, as well as a decrease in arachidonic acid levels.

(Page 91-93, Nutrition/Normal Nutritional Requirements)

Answer 3-11. d

A high peak bone density is inversely related to the risk of later osteoporosis. Foods with high calcium to phosphorus ratio prevent bone loss. As a result, green vegetables, human milk, and cow's milk have a high Ca:P ratio and prevent later bone loss. Foods high in phosphates are associated with bone loss.

(Page 93, Nutrition/Normal Nutritional Requirements)

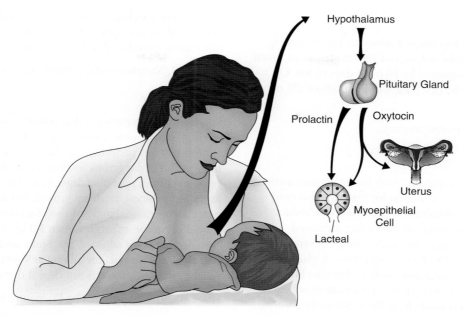

FIGURE 24-1. The physiology of lactation. Suckling stimulates proprioceptors in the aerola and nipple, transmitting impulses to the hypothalamus, which in turn stimulates the release of oxytocin by the posterior pituitary and prolactin by the anterior pituitary. Oxytocin stimulates smooth muscle contraction and milk ejection by the alveolus in the breast. Prolactin stimulates milk production. Emptying the breast stimulates milk production. (Reproduced, with permission, from Rudolph CD, Lister A, Gershon A, Rudolph A, First L. *Rudolph's Pediatrics.* 22nd ed. New York: McGraw-Hill, 2011.)

Answer 3-12. e

With few contraindications, all infants should be breastfed. In the United States, maternal HIV, HTLV I, or HTLV 2 infection is a contraindication to breast-feeding. Active tuberculosis is a contraindication unless there is at least 2 weeks of treatment. Hepatitis B infection is not a contraindication to breast-feeding.

(Page 95, Nutrition/Breast-feeding)

Answer 3-13. e

PRSL is measured in terms of milliosmole per liter (mOsm/L). The infant kidney is not capable of handling high-concentration fluids. Skim, whole, or goat milk is not recommended in infants less than 12 months. Raw milk is not recommended as it increases the risk of *E. coli* or *Salmonella* infection, which can be found in raw beverages.

PRSL for varying fluids are listed as follows:

Skim milk	326 mOsm/L
Whole milk	308 mOsm/L
Soy-based infant formula	160 mOsm/L
Cow's milk–based formula	135 mOsm/L

(Page 90, Nutrition/Normal Nutritional Requirements)

Answer 3-14. a

The World Health Organization and the American Academy of Pediatrics have promoted several interventions to improve breast-feeding rates. These include initiation of breast-feeding for all babies within the first hour after birth, as well as encouragement of on-demand feeding. Galactosemia is a contraindication to breast-feeding.

(Page 96, Nutrition/Breast-feeding)

Answer 3-15. e

The "let-down reflex" is also known as the "ejection reflex" for breast-feeding (Figure 24-1). Stress or anxiety can inhibit the let-down reflex. Infant sucking of the breast stimulates proprioceptors in the areola and nipple. A signal is sent to the hypothalamus that triggers the release of prolactin from the anterior pituitary gland and oxytocin from the posterior pituitary gland. Oxytocin stimulates smooth muscle (myoepithelial) cells in the breast to contract and eject milk. Prolactin stimulates milk production. In addition, the emptying of breast milk will also stimulate milk production. The sight, touch, or cry of an infant will stimulate oxytocin production, which stimulates myoepithelial cells in the breast to contract and improve milk ejection. The establishment of a regular breast-feeding routine is necessary to ensure continued breast milk production.

(Page 96, Nutrition/Breast-feeding)

Answer 3-16. e

All of the following options suggest adequate breast-feeding. Average weight loss should not exceed 10% for the term infant. This weight should be regained by 10 to 14 days of life. On average, weight loss in the first 3 days of life is about 7% of birth weight.

(Page 96-97, Nutrition/Breast-feeding)

Answer 3-17. d

The symptoms are most consistent with breast engorgement. During the first 4 days, it is common for breasts to become engorged as the child establishes a breast-feeding schedule. Warm compresses in this situation may cause increased swelling. Increasing feedings, hand expression, or even pumping may help drain the breasts to relieve symptoms. A plugged duct can also present with soreness and swelling, but also lumpiness of the breast. A warm compress or hand massage may help move the plug. Mastitis is unlikely, as there is usually a warm, tender, pie-shaped area on the breast, accompanied by flu-like symptoms, fevers, and/or chills. Candidal infection is usually noted on the nipple and areola. Mothers with diabetes or recent antibiotic use are at greater risk.

(Page 97, Nutrition/Breast-feeding)

Answer 3-18. c

Pain and fever are most associated with mastitis. Candidal infection is usually noted on the nipple and areola. Mothers with diabetes, vaginal candidiasis, or recent antibiotic use have increased risk. There may also be nonstabbing or stabbing breast pain. Sleeping with milk-soaked breast pads also increases candidal risk.

(Page 97-98, Nutrition/Breast-feeding)

Answer 3-19. b

Unmodified cow's milk has high levels of protein, sodium, chloride, and phosphorous. Together, these components create a high renal solute load that is not appropriate for infants. Unmodified cow's milk should not be introduced until after 12 months of age. Unmodified cow's milk also has inadequate amounts of iron, vitamin C, zinc, and essential fatty acids. In addition, human milk has a whey to casein ratio of 60% to 40%, compared with 18% to 82% in unmodified cow's milk. The development of allergic disease is multifactorial. Both delayed and late introduction of foods have been associated with the development of food allergy.

(Page 99, Nutrition/Infant Formula and Complementary Food)

Answer 3-20. b, e, c, a, d

Please refer to Table 25-2. Guidelines for the introduction of complementary food suggest introducing foods that are developmentally appropriate. At 4 to 6 months, infants should be able to sit with support and hold their head steady. By 8 months of age, infants can bite into foods and use the finger and thumb to manipulate food. Gradually, a mixed food table diet can be introduced at 12 months of age.

(Page 105, Nutrition/Infant Formula and Complementary Food)

Answer 3-21. e

Specialized "preterm formulas" contain increased protein, calcium, phosphorous, and vitamins. However, it is not appropriate for "preterm formulas" to be used postdischarge, due to ingestion of dangerous levels of nutrients when fed ad lib at greater volumes post discharge. As a result, "preterm discharge formulas" promote catch-up growth, but decrease the risk of potential nutritional toxicity. Use of a preterm discharge formula should occur for infants less than 3.0 kg or until infants are at the 10th percentile for adjusted age. Some studies have shown that postdischarge formula for as long as 9 months leads to better weight gain; however, it is not clear if this effect is sustained.

(Page 106-107, Nutrition/The Premature Infant After Discharge)

Answer 3-22. c

Increased intake of whole cow's milk increases the risk of iron deficiency. Recommended milk intake is between 16 and 24 oz/day. It is not necessary to eliminate all whole milk intake. Red meat, as well as fish and poultry, is an iron-rich food and can be encouraged. Vitamin C helps increase iron absorption. As a result, it is important to also encourage consumption of foods high in vitamin C.

(Page 108, Nutrition/Table 27-1: Dietary Subgroups at Risk for Nutrient Deficiencies)

Answer 3-23. c

Vitamin B_{12} is found in only animal products. As a result, vegans must obtain vitamin B_{12} supplementation through fortified foods or supplements. Vegan mothers may have baseline low levels of B_{12}. It is recommended that supplementation should occur throughout pregnancy and lactation. Infants breastfed by mothers who are deficient in B_{12} are at high risk for B_{12} deficiency, as well. All infants who are exclusively breastfed will require vitamin D, which is given directly to the infant, not the mother.

(Page 109-110, Nutritional Issues)

Answer 3-24. d

Refeeding syndrome is characterized by electrolyte and fluid shifts during the refeeding of severely malnourished patients. With refeeding, increased glucose intake leads to increased insulin levels and increased production of fat and protein. There is a resulting hypophosphatemia, hypokalemia, and hypomagnesemia. The low phosphate levels lead to cardiac arrhythmias. Low magnesium leads to weakness and tremor. Thiamin deficiency is associated with malnutrition. Quick replenishment of glucose in the setting of thiamin deficiency can lead to Wernicke encephalopathy.

(Page 113, Nutrition/Malnutrition and Refeeding)

Answer 3-25. d

$$\text{Body mass index (BMI)} = \frac{\text{weight [kg]}}{(\text{height})^2 \text{ [m]}}$$

The child's BMI is 21.0, which places the child between the 90th and 95th percentiles for BMI.

A BMI greater than the 85th percentile is considered overweight; a BMI greater than the 95th percentile is considered obese.

(Page 123-124, Nutrition/The Overweight or Obese Child)

Answer 3-26. 1—d, 2—a, 3—b, 4—f, 5—c, 6—e

POMC deficiency syndromes are associated with severe early onset obesity, adrenal insufficiency, and red hair due to a complete loss of function mutation of the human *POMC* gene.

(Page 123-124, Tables 32-1, 32-3)

Answer 3-27. a

Ideally, iron should be provided enterally; however, in this case, intravenous bolus infusion is the best choice. Prolonged intravenous administration is associated with iron overload, oxidant injury, and gram-negative septicemia. Intramuscular administration is associated with pain and staining of skin. Subcutaneous administration is not effective. Finally, adding iron to parenteral nutrition is not compatible with a lipid preparation.

(Page 132, Nutrition/Specialized Nutrition Support)

Answer 3-28. 1—c, 2—b, 3—g, 4—a, 5—f, 6—e, 7—d

Answer: 1—c. Vitamin A plays a crucial role in vision, reproduction, growth, and bone development. It is a component of retinal pigments. A metabolite of vitamin A, retinal, is necessary for vision in dim light, as well as color vision. Vitamin A is also necessary as retinoic acid for epithelial cell growth and wound healing.

Answer: 2—b. Vitamin D is involved in calcium and phosphorous metabolism, and vitamin D deficiency leads to rickets. In adults, vitamin D deficiency manifests as osteomalacia. Vitamin D is unique, as it can be synthesized during sun exposure or ingested (as vitamin D_2 or vitamin D_3).

Answer: 3—g. Vitamin K deficiency bleeding (VKDB), previously labeled as hemorrhagic disease of the newborn (HDN). VKDB occurs due to the fact that specific clotting factors (factors II, VII, IX, and X) are vitamin K–dependent. Neonates may have inadequate levels of vitamin K. Without vitamin K prophylaxis in the nursery, the incidence of VKDB is reportedly as high as 1.7%.

Answer: 4—a. Both folate and cobalamin (vitamin B_{12}) are necessary for DNA synthesis. There is a high rate of cell division in the bone marrow to replenish red blood cells. The anemia associated with folate deficiency is megaloblastic.

TABLE 32-3. History, Symptoms, and Signs of Conditions Caused by or Associated With Overweight and Obesity

History and Symptoms	
Polyuria, polydipsia, weight loss anxiety, school avoidance, social isolation	Depression Type 2 diabetes mellitus
Headaches	Pseudotumor cerebri
Nighttime breathing difficulties	Sleep apnea, hypoventilation syndrome, asthma
Daytime sleepiness	Sleep apnea, depression
Abdominal pain, regurgitation	Gastroesophageal reflux, cholelithiasis, constipation
Hip or knee pain	Slipped capital epiphysis, Blount disease
Oligomenorrhea or amenorrhea	Polycystic ovary syndrome
Hyperphagia	History of hypothalamic malformation or injury
Pharmacotherapy (if any)	Glucocorticoids, appetite stimulants, antidepressants, antipsychotics, oral hypoglycemic agents
Signs	
Poor linear growth	Hypothyroidism, Cushing disease, genetic syndromes
Enlarged thyroid gland	Hypothyroidism
Dysmorphic features (or red hair)	Genetic syndromes
Acanthosis nigricans	Type 2 diabetes mellitus, insulin resistance
Hirsutism and excessive acne	Polycystic ovary syndrome, Cushing disease
Violaceous striae	Cushing disease
Papilledema, cranial nerve VI palsy	Pseudotumor cerebri
Tonsillar hypertrophy	Sleep apnea
Abdominal tenderness	Gastroesophageal reflux, cholelithiasis
Hepatomegaly	Nonalcoholic fatty liver disease
Undescended testicle	Prader-Willi syndrome
Limited hip range of motion	Slipped capital femoral epiphysis
Lower leg bowing	Blount disease

Reproduced, with permission, from Rudolph CD, Lister A, Gershon A, Rudolph A, First L. *Rudolph's Pediatrics.* 22nd ed. New York: McGraw-Hill, 2011.

Answer: 5—f (and a). Vitamin B$_{12}$ (also called cobalamin) deficiency is also associated with megaloblastic anemia (answer a). In addition, vitamin B$_{12}$ absorption in the ilium requires intrinsic factor, which is produced in the stomach. Pernicious anemia, which is rare in childhood, occurs due to the improper absorption of vitamin B$_{12}$ (eg, autoimmune disease, gastritis, surgical resection), which then leads to the associated megaloblastic anemia.

Answer: 6—e. Niacin deficiency leads to pellagra, which has a classic triad of symptoms (diarrhea, dementia, and dermatitis). There is no specific order in which the symptoms present. Niacin is necessary for glycogen synthesis and fatty acid breakdown, which explains a variety of effects including dermatitis, neuropathy, encephalopathy, and atrophy of mucosal tissue, which is associated with diarrhea.

Answer: 7—d. Vitamin C (or ascorbic acid) is necessary for collagen synthesis. Vitamin C deficiency is associated with scurvy, which manifests as diffuse tissue bleeding, poor wound healing, and friable gingiva.

(Page 92, Nutrition/Normal Nutritional Requirements)

Answer 3-29. 1—b, 2—d, 3—a, 4—c

Answer: 1—b. Zinc deficiency has been recognized in association with growth failure. As a cofactor for over 100 different enzymes, it is involved in a variety of metabolic processes. In addition, it is needed for protein synthesis and nucleic acid metabolism.

Answer: 2—d. Fluoride deficiency is associated with dental caries and increased tooth decay. Over half of the US water supply is supplemented with fluoride. Other sources of fluoride include oral supplements and fluoridated toothpaste.

Answer: 3—a. Chromium is necessary for glucose metabolism. It improves the efficiency of insulin in glucose uptake as a cofactor for insulin receptor binding. Chromium deficiency is associated with glucose intolerance.

Answer: 4—c. Selenium deficiency is a rare condition that is associated with cardiomyopathy. Selenium is a cofactor for glutathione peroxidase, as well as other enzymes. The association with pediatric cardiomyopathy was first reported in Keshan, a region in China with low selenium intake.

(Page 94-95, Nutrition/Normal Nutritional Requirements)

CHAPTER 4 | Abuse, Neglect, and Violence

Christopher C. Stewart

4-1. Which of the following statements is correct, based on epidemiologic data collected about child abuse?

a. Most child maltreatment occurs outside the home.

b. Females are equally likely as males to be perpetrators of sexual abuse.

c. Of substantiated child abuse cases, neglect is the most common type.

d. If all types of child abuse are included, males are the most likely perpetrators of child abuse.

e. Females are more commonly perpetrators in child abuse death cases.

4-2. A single mother brings a developmentally normal 16-month-old child to the emergency department for an upper respiratory illness and a laceration. The child has a healing laceration on his forehead above the left eyebrow that is open and healing and will likely leave a scar. It is too late to stitch or glue the laceration closed. The mother states the child sustained this laceration when he fell while running in the house 4 days ago. She states that it was hard to stop the bleeding. When asked by the nurse when alone whether somebody hit him, the child replies "no."

Which of the following factors makes this injury most suspicious for child abuse?

a. The mother is single and thus is at increased risk for abusing her child.

b. The history of falling while running is not within a 16-month-old child's developmental abilities.

c. The mother delayed seeking care for the child soon after the injury.

d. The child's response when asked by the nurse when alone whether somebody hit him.

e. The child appears very fearful and cries when even experienced pediatricians try to examine him.

4-3. A 3-month-old boy is brought to the hospital with a history of falling off a couch onto a carpeted floor. He has been having seizures, and on CT scan of the head he is noted to have subdural hemorrhages and swelling of the brain. He has bilateral posterior rib fractures and extensive retinal hemorrhages.

In reviewing the parents' background, which of the following factors that are identified is *not* associated with an increased risk of abusing their child?

a. The mother is a teenager.

b. Both the parents are strongly religious.

c. The father has a substance abuse problem.

d. There is a history of intimate partner violence in the family.

e. The mother was maltreated as a child.

4-4. A 2-year-old boy is brought to your clinic by child protective services for a clearance examination. The child is noted to have a bruise on the glans of his penis with some swelling. The child can urinate. Urinalysis reveals no blood. There are no other injuries to the child's genitals or anus noted. The child is also noted to have multiple bruises on the abdomen and buttocks and cheeks. Nucleic amplification tests of the urine for chlamydia and gonorrhea, and complete blood count, PT, PTT, INR, and blood tests for HIV, syphilis, and hepatitis B and C are also negative.

This child's findings would be best classified as which of the following types of maltreatment?

a. Exploitation

b. Emotional abuse

c. Neglect

d. Physical abuse

e. Sexual abuse

4-5. A 14-month-old child comes into your clinic for hot water burns. There are scalding water burns on both the infant's feet. The second-degree burns cover the feet and the lower part of the legs. On each leg, there are straight, well-demarcated burn lines approximately 2 cm above the ankles.

The child is developmentally normal, and was born full-term. He has no past medical history, and his immunizations are up to date. His parents have missed 2 appointments since birth that had to be rescheduled. The father reports that the bathtub was running with hot water as he prepared the bath for the child. He went into another room to clean up the child's soiled underwear. He also reports he and the child's mother have been trying to potty train their child. He reports when he came back into the bathroom, the child had climbed into the bathtub, and was found crying in the water. The father did not bring the child in for care until he noticed blistering of the burn site later in the evening.

The factor that most makes this burn suspicious for abuse is:

a. The delay in bringing in the child for care

b. The unlikely ability of the 14-month-child to climb into the bath

c. The fact that the child was potty training and soiled his underwear

d. The history of missed appointments

e. Sharply demarcated lines of the burn

4-6. A 2-year-old child is brought in for buttock bruising noticed by a day care worker when changing their diaper. In clinic, the child is acting developmentally normally for their age, and they do not seem fearful or in pain.

After complete history and physical, the best workup for this patient would be which of the following?

a. Complete blood and platelet count, prothrombin, and partial thromboplastin time

b. Skeletal survey

c. Bleeding time and a von Willebrand factor (vWF)

d. Computed tomography scan of the head and neck without contrast

e. Ophthalmology examination with dilated pupils

4-7. An accurate statement about violence exposure is that:

a. A child's exposure to intimate partner violence (IPV) increases the likelihood of being abused.

b. Peer violence is more likely to be chronic than sibling violence.

c. Over 95% of victims of IPV are women.

d. Teen pregnancy is a protective factor for IPV.

e. A child's exposure to violence affects mental, but not physical, health.

4-8. You are referred a 3-month-old nonambulatory child from a day care center staff who noticed bruising on the infant's buttocks during a diaper change. The parents and other caretakers deny any history of trauma. The child appears well on examination, and is interactive and playful. Although you are concerned about abusive injuries given the location of the bruising, you create a differential diagnosis.

Your differential diagnosis would most likely *not* include which of the following?

a. Henoch-Schonlein purpura

b. Idiopathic thrombocytopenic purpura

c. Acute lymphocytic leukemia

d. Dermal melanocytosis

e. Vitamin A deficiency

4-9. You see a 3-year-old girl brought in for possible sexual abuse. The mother says the girl has made statements about being touched by her father's brother, who lives in the house with the family. The girl is well appearing. The mother denies any bleeding, itching, dysuria, and frequency. The girl has otherwise been acting her normal self per the mother's report. You perform a physical examination, including a genital examination. Laboratory testing is done for sexually transmitted infections, including HIV, syphilis, gonorrhea, and chlamydia.

The finding most indicative of sexual abuse in this case would be which of the following?

a. A confirmed genital human papilloma virus (HPV) wart on the child's labia majora

b. A crescentic hymen through which the vaginal mucosa can be seen

c. A 1-cm circular bruise on the inner thigh

d. A confirmed case of *Neisseria gonorrhoeae* vulvovaginitis

e. The child's statement that the uncle touched her "down there"

4-10. A 30-month-old developmentally normal boy presents to your clinic with a chief complaint of not walking and inability to bear weight on his right leg. The parents noted this yesterday, and are bringing the child in today because the apparent pain with weight bearing has not resolved. The parents give no history of falls or trauma. The child has not had any other complaints. On contacting their primary pediatrician, you learn that there have been no previous fractures or other significant past medical history concerning for abuse.

On physical examination of the entire body, there is no evidence of bruising or other concerning findings, and neurologic and mental status examinations are normal. You are not able to obtain an adequate retinal examination. In examining the right leg, there are no obvious bruises. There is full range of motion, with a question of some point tenderness over the distal tibial plateau on the right side. The child is reluctant to walk, and cries when prompted to do so, with a noticeable limp on the right leg. There are no other significant physical examination findings. A radiograph reveals a nondisplaced spiral fracture of the distal right tibia.

The next best diagnostic procedure for this child is:

a. Check levels of calcium, phosphorus, alkaline phosphatase, and 25-hydroxyvitamin D.

b. No further workup is indicated given the information at this point.

c. Obtain a CT scan of the head looking for subdural hemorrhages.

d. Get an ophthalmology consult to look for retinal hemorrhages.

e. Perform a full skeletal survey, looking for unsymptomatic abusive fractures.

4-11. A 6-month-old developmentally normal infant is referred to the ED for radiographs. The baby presented at the primary pediatrician's office with a swollen left thigh. There was pain on examination when the left lower extremity was moved. There are no bruises, and the leg is distally neurovascularly intact. There are no other concerning signs on the baby's body on physical examination, and the baby appears to be neurologically normal.

The baby was at home with a baby sitter, and mother noted the baby being fussy that evening after the sitter went home. The mother decided to bring the infant in the next day when the fussiness continued, and she noticed the left thigh swelling. The radiograph shows an oblique/spiral nondisplaced fracture through the left femoral diaphysis, with associated soft tissue swelling noted. The baby sitter reports no history of falls or trauma, and the mother reports none either.

Which of the following is the most accurate statement concerning the likelihood of abuse associated with this fracture?

a. Oblique/spiral fractures without a trauma history in 6-month-old children are concerning for abuse.

b. Over 50% of fractures in children less than 3 years of age are from abuse.

c. Undiagnosed osteogenesis imperfecta accounts for 1% of unexplained fractures in infants.

d. The mother should have noticed the fracture right away and brought in her child earlier.

e. A skeletal survey is not indicated as the child is asymptomatic in other parts of the body.

4-12. A 3-month-old baby is admitted for suspicion of abusive head trauma. The caretaker gives a history of the baby falling off a couch. The baby cried immediately, but then became lethargic and unresponsive. The baby was rushed to a nearby hospital, where they were stabilized. A CT scan of the head shows a thin layer subdural hemorrhage over the right hemisphere. A chest radiograph reveals a number of posterior rib fractures that appear acute. On ophthalmology examination, retinal hemorrhages are noted.

The most accurate statement regarding retinal hemorrhages would be which of the following?

a. Retinal hemorrhages can be from birth, and these usually persist for months.

b. Only 1 type of retinal hemorrhage is associated with abusive head trauma.

c. Retinal hemorrhages usually cause irreversible blindness for the child.

d. Retinal hemorrhages only occur near the macula due to presence of retinal blood vessels.

e. Retinal hemorrhages can result from certain types of infections.

4-13. A 14-month-old developmentally normal boy is brought into the hospital with concerns for abuse by his mother. The mother states she has noticed marks on the child over the past several days when picking him up from day care. At first she thought these were normal bruises from the child playing, but she has been more concerned recently given the number and type. The child also seems to be crying and scared when dropped off at day care, which is a new phenomenon. On physical examination the child is noted to have a number of cutaneous findings.

Which of the following findings would be most concerning for abusive injuries?

a. Bruises on the shins

b. Red and green color bruises indicating different ages

c. Bruises on the forearms

d. Bruises on the lower back

e. A bruise on the right forehead, just above the eye

4-14. A 17-month-old boy is admitted for suspicions of abuse. The boy was noted to have multiple bruises on the buttocks, upper arms, trunk, and ears. On physical examination, the child is interactive and otherwise well appearing. A complete blood count revealed normal platelets, and coagulation factors are normal as well. A skeletal survey is done to evaluate for possible fractures.

Which of the following statements about a skeletal survey is most accurate?

a. Is a series of x-rays of the long bones, chest, and spine, but not the skull

b. Usually shows evidence of any fractures within the last year

c. Should be obtained for every child with suspicious fractures less than 7 years old

d. Is sometimes repeated in 2 weeks to look for additional fractures not initially observed

e. Can rule out abuse if it is found to be negative

4-15. A 15-year-old girl is brought in for possible sexual assault by an adult man. She met the man on the Internet, and eventually agreed to go to his apartment to meet him. She became intoxicated while drinking alcohol with him, and eventually "blacked out." She does not recall anything else, except waking up in a park, where police officers found her and brought her into the hospital. Her blood alcohol level was 0.02 on arrival at the ER. Examination was otherwise unremarkable, except for some abrasions over her knees and right shoulder, and several 1 to 2 cm circular bruises on her left arm. The girl complains of pain in the genital area. A sexual assault examination is performed. The examination is found to be normal. The girl tests positive for chlamydia on the urine test and culture performed on the day of the possible sexual assault.

Which of the following statements is correct?

a. The normal genital examination does not rule out a sexual assault.

b. The positive chlamydia test is proof that the girl was raped.

c. The bruises suggest that the girl was assaulted.

d. The girl would not benefit from postexposure prophylaxis.

e. The blood alcohol level suggests the girl was raped.

4-16. A previously full-term 4-month-old girl presents to the ED with an apparent life-threatening event (ALTE). The baby was sleeping with mother and was noted to turn blue and stop breathing for over 1 minute. Mother reports starting CPR before the baby responded. The baby was brought in by ambulance with the mother. EMTs reported a well-appearing baby when they got to the house. In the ED, physical examination was normal, and a history and review of symptoms was unremarkable. The baby was observed in the hospital over the next several days, and had 6 more "events" of stopping breathing over the next several days, and continues to be observed in the hospital. Workup for infections including blood and urine cultures, RSV, and pertussis was negative. An EKG was normal, as was a pH probe, and the events do not seem to be associated with feeding. There is no reported seizure activity, and an EEG is normal. Head CT scan is unremarkable.

Before further workup is initiated, one of the members of your team points out that the only time the events occur are when mother is with the baby alone in her room. You suspect medical child abuse (Munchausen syndrome by proxy).

Which statement about medical child abuse is most accurate?

a. Medical child abuse rarely is fatal.

b. Medical child abuse is usually straightforward to diagnose.

c. ALTEs are most likely to be from medical child abuse.

d. Perpetrators of medical child abuse are often nonparent caretakers.

e. Fever is a common presentation of medical child abuse.

4-17. A recently turned 3-year-old boy is being evaluated for poor weight gain. The child has crossed 2 percentile lines for weight in the last 6 months, going from 50th percentile at 32 lb to between 5th and 10th percentiles at 27 lb. Height and head circumference have not crossed percentile lines. There are multiple family stressors, including a recent divorce, and the primary caregiver has been struggling with finances and employment. The child also has had multiple URIs over the past several months, though has never been hospitalized.

On physical examination, the child seems thin and is active and cooperative, although he has a flat affect. He has multiple bruises over his left and right shins, has 2 café au lait spots on his trunk, and is noted to have a faint 1/6 systolic ejection murmur at the left sternal border, which mother says was noted in previous visits since the age of 18 months, and she was told it was a "Still's murmur." His examination is otherwise unremarkable. You are concerned about neglect, but realize you must also evaluate the child for other possible causes of poor weight gain.

The most appropriate next step is which of the following?

a. Obtain an EKG and 4 limb blood pressures.

b. Get baseline electrolytes prior to feeding.

c. Obtain a skeletal survey.

d. Obtain a careful feeding history.

e. Obtain a head CT scan.

4-18. A 5-month-old baby fell onto a hard wood floor from a 4 ft high changing table when mother's boyfriend was reaching to get the diapers. The boyfriend brings the child immediately into the emergency department as the mother is working. The baby is noted to have slight superficial soft tissue swelling with erythema noted over the right parietal area. Otherwise, the child's examination is normal. The ED doctor decides to get a skeletal survey, because they "don't have a good feeling about the boyfriend."

Of these possible acute fractures found on the survey, the most specific for abuse is:

a. A linear skull fracture of the right parietal bone

b. A classic metaphyseal lesion of the right distal radius

c. An oblique fracture of the right femoral diaphysis

d. A buckle fracture of the left distal tibial metaphysis

e. A mid-diaphyseal transverse fracture of the right clavicle

4-19. A 3-month-old baby presents with apnea and unresponsiveness at home under the care of a babysitter. The sitter says they went to get a bottle for the baby, and when they returned, the baby was blue and not breathing. CPR was performed by the sitter while waiting for EMTs to arrive, and the baby responded and became alert. On arrival by EMTs, the baby appeared alert and responsive, but began to have seizure activity in the ambulance on the way to the hospital. In the ER, the baby was stabilized, and apparent seizures resolved with medication. On chest x-ray, several acute posterior rib fractures were noted. A head CT scan showed a right subdural hemorrhage layering over the hemisphere and into the convexity. Otherwise the baby appeared to have an unremarkable physical examination, with no bruising or other signs of head trauma.

The next step that would be most helpful in supporting the diagnosis of abusive head trauma would be to obtain which of the following?

a. Liver function tests

b. Coagulation studies and a complete blood count

c. A dilated retinal examination by ophthalmology

d. Serum Ca^{2+}, PO_4^-, and alkaline phosphatase

e. Serum amino acids

4-20. A 2-year-old girl is brought in when her divorced mother gets concerned after picking her up from a weekend visit with father. The mother noted blood in the girl's underwear, and called the father to ask if he had noticed this as well. The father says the girl fell and banged her perineal area while straddling a toy horse while playing in the house. She reportedly cried when this occurred, but settled down and consoled easily. The father reports he did not notice any bleeding, and did not think anything more of it, as the girl continued to play without problems.

On genital examination of the girl, the most concerning finding for sexual abuse would be which of the following?

a. Bruise and laceration on the labia majora

b. Urine test positive for chlamydia

c. Prolapsed urethra with bleeding

d. Thinning of the skin with subepidermal hemorrhages of the vulva

e. Perianal group A streptococcal infection with bleeding

ANSWERS

Answer 4-1. c

Among the types of maltreatment, neglect makes up almost two thirds of substantiated cases. National data suggest that women make up more than half of the perpetrators of child abuse, although perpetrators of sexual abuse are overwhelmingly male. In addition, more than two thirds of child abuse deaths are perpetrated by males. National survey data also suggest that most child abuse occurs in the child's home.

(Page 137-138, Chapter 35: Child Maltreatment: Neglect to Abuse)

Answer 4-2. c

Five types of history should raise the suspicion of child abuse. These include a child with a serious injury and no history of trauma offered; a history that is not consistent with the mechanism, severity, or timing of an injury; a delay in seeking care for a significant injury; a history that changes during the course of evaluation; and a history of recurrent injuries.

In this case the fact that the laceration would likely leave a scar and the fact that it was difficult to contain the bleeding make this history concerning. However, there may be many reasons for a delay in, or an absence of, seeking care in a case like this that are not related to trying to hide abuse. These reasons include, but are not limited to, a lack of understanding about laceration healing, a lack of understanding of the importance of cleaning and possible closure to prevent scarring, or limited access to medical care issues due to socioeconomic factors.

Although single parenting is a risk factor for child abuse, in this case it is not the most concerning factor. In addition, the majority of single parents do not abuse their children. A 16-month-old child described as developmentally normal would be expected to be able to run and fall. As a result, from a developmental standpoint, the injury is not suspicious. A developmentally normal 16-month-old child's reply to a question of whether they were hit or not is probably not helpful in determining a cause of the injury. A 16-month-old child would also be considered developmentally normal if they were fearful and crying when strangers tried to examine them, regardless of abuse history.

(Page 138-139, Chapter 35: Child Maltreatment: Neglect to Abuse)

Answer 4-3. b

There are a number of factors associated with abuse or neglect of children, including those associated with the child, the parents, the family unit, and the social setting. Parental risk factors for child abuse include young maternal age, and abuse of alcohol or drugs. There is also a strong association between a history of abuse as a child and abusing one's own child

(the "intergenerational transmission of abuse"), although the majority of parents who were abused as children do not abuse their own children. Intrafamilial violence such as intimate partner or domestic violence is an independent risk factor for child maltreatment. Being strongly religious has not been associated with child abuse.

(Page 138, Chapter 35: Child Maltreatment: Neglect to Abuse)

Answer 4-4. d

Maltreatment includes physical abuse, neglect, sexual abuse, exploitation, and emotional maltreatment. Physical abuse is an act of commission toward the child by a parent or other caregiver that results in harm or intended harm to the child. Neglect is an act of omission, such as failure to provide adequate nutrition, shelter, or health care, among other needs. Sexual abuse is the involvement of children or adolescents in sexual activities that they do not fully understand, to which they cannot give informed consent because of their developmental understanding, and that break societal or family taboos. Exploitation is the use of a child in work or other activities for the benefit of others, such as child labor, commercial sexual exploitation of children, and child trafficking. Emotional maltreatment is the most difficult form of maltreatment to define and can include repeated verbal denigration.

In the case presented, the bruise is associated with other bruises that suggest physical abuse. Although one might argue the bruise to the penis is sexual in nature, bruising of the penis is commonly a result of punishment (such as for potty training accidents when the penis is pinched, or shut in the toilet seat). In addition, the lack of other suggestion of sexual abuse in this case, as well as the associated bruising in areas concerning for physical abuse, makes physical abuse the most likely classification for this case.

(Page 137, Chapter 35: Child Maltreatment: Neglect to Abuse)

Answer 4-5. e

Demarcated lines are associated with abusive scald injuries, whereas nonabusive scalds tend to be asymmetric from one extremity to the other, and have less sharply demarcated borders. Nonabusive scalding should reveal splash marks that indicate the child tried to avoid the injury. In this case, if the child climbed into a tub himself, one would expect splash marks as the child tried to avoid the pain of the hot water.

Delay in bringing a child into care is certainly a concerning factor in abuse. However, burns may not appear immediately concerning to a lay person. In addition, delay in seeking care is not as specific for abuse as the physical findings in this case. In this case, it may be part of an overall concern and suspicion, but not as clearly suspicious as the absence of splash marks and the sharply demarcated lines of the burn. Although it may seem implausible that a 14-month-old child could get into a bathtub by themselves, a 2005 study in *Pediatrics* revealed that of 176 children between 10 and 18 months of age, 35% were able to climb into a standard bath tub on their own.

Providers need to be careful in their assumptions about the developmental abilities of young children. The fact that the child was potty training may indeed have been a trigger for frustration in a caregiver, but in itself is not as clearly suspicious as the physical examination in this case. The history of missed appointments, though potentially indicating a pattern of avoidance of medical care or neglect, is also quite nonspecific as a concern. The developmental ability of a child needs to be matched with the history offered for an injury; inconsistencies raise serious concerns and suspicion.

(Page 139, Chapter 35: Child Maltreatment: Neglect to Abuse)

Answer 4-6. a

In every case of suspected abuse, a complete history and physical examination is indicated. Often, health care providers neglect to perform a full examination of the skin, including the perigenital and anal areas. Providers should pay close attention to the ears, and the mouth, as injuries are missed. With bruising, in general a complete blood count, platelet count, prothrombin, and partial thromboplastin time are indicated as a first set of laboratory tests to be sure there is not an obvious bleeding disorder (eg, ITP, leukemia). Further coagulation or platelet studies such as a von Willebrand panel (which includes von Willebrand factor) may be indicated, depending on the presentation. Although any of the tests listed may be indicated with further history and physical examination, the initial labs should be obtained given the bruising noted, as unsuspected medical conditions could obviate the need for further testing.

A skeletal survey is generally indicated in a child less than 2 years of age who presents with a history or physical examination suspicious for sexual or physical abuse. In children 2 years of age or older, there may be some yield to a skeletal survey, but this should usually be considered after the blood cell, platelet, and coagulation studies, and in consultation with a child abuse expert.

A CT scan of the head may be indicated when there is suspected physical abuse in a young child with concern for head injury, particularly in a child younger than 1 year with history or physical examination suggesting physical abuse. In the absence of acute neurologic symptoms, an MRI of the head is a more revealing study, without the radiation exposure risks. An MRI is a more expensive study that often requires sedation. Similarly, ophthalmology examinations are useful in cases of suspected abusive head trauma to evaluate the presence of retinal hemorrhages.

(Page 142, Chapter 35: Child Maltreatment: Neglect to Abuse)

Answer 4-7. a

The risk of child maltreatment increases as the level of violence in the household increases. Children exposed to IPV are 6 to 15 times more likely to be abused. Overall, sibling violence tends to result in fewer serious injuries than peer violence and involves the use of fewer potentially injurious weapons; however, sibling violence is more likely to be chronic and therefore may hold greater potential for trauma symptoms. Although IPV is present in relationships across class, culture, race/ethnicity, and sexual orientation, this phenomenon is characterized by a gender disparity; in 2001, the US Bureau of Justice Statistics reported that 85% of victims of IPV are women. Pregnant teens also experience a sharply elevated risk of violence in intimate relationships. An estimated 7% to 26% of adolescent females report violence during pregnancy inflicted by a partner or family member. There are overwhelming data that exposure to violence affects mental health, and more and more data to support that long-term physical health is also affected.

(Pages 144-147, Chapter 36: Family and Community Violence)

Answer 4-8. e

Buttock bruises are concerning for child abuse in many cases. The differential diagnosis for bruises can include a number of acute or chronic medical conditions. Henoch-Schonlein purpura is a disease that can cause abdominal and joint pain, as well as purpura, often on the buttocks, which may be mistaken for bruising. Abnormalities affecting the coagulation process such as idiopathic thrombocytopenic purpura, an autoimmune disorder leading to platelet destruction resulting in decreased platelet counts, can increase the propensity to bruise easily. Similarly, a bone marrow infiltrative process such as acute lymphocytic leukemia can present with easy bruising. Birthmarks such as dermal melanocytosis (previously called Mongolian spots) are often located in the buttocks area, and can easily be mistaken for bruises. Bruising may be associated with malnutrition, such as deficiencies of vitamins B_{12}, C, K, or folic acid. However, vitamin A is not likely to be a cause of easy bruising by itself.

(Page 142, Chapter 35: Child Maltreatment: Neglect to Abuse)

Answer 4-9. d

A confirmed vaginal infection with *Neisseria gonorrhoeae* is considered diagnostic of sexual abuse if it is not perinatally acquired. It is important to confirm this diagnosis, particularly if the test is done with a urine sample using nucleic acid amplification technology, or other nonculture tests. Other vaginal infections considered diagnostic of sexual abuse in a prepubertal child include chlamydia, syphilis, and HIV, assuming no blood transfusion, perinatal or other obvious means of acquisition. Herpes simplex type 2 can be concerning for sexual abuse and requires a full investigation, but is not diagnostic.

HPV is not diagnostic of sexual abuse, and can result from nonsexual autoinoculation. Like HSV, genital warts in a prepubertal child should trigger an evaluation for possible sexual abuse. Normal prepubertal girls may have any of a variety of hymen shapes including crescentic, annular, and fimbriated or redundant. Vaginal mucosa can be seen through such a normal hymen. There is a myth that the hymen covers the vaginal opening, and that it can be "popped" or broken. However, in normal prepubertal girls there is generally a hymenal opening through which one may see the vaginal mucosa on routine examination. Lack of a hymenal opening is called hymenocolpos, and can present at puberty when menstrual blood cannot exit the vagina. A small bruise on the inner thigh of a 3-year-old girl could raise concerns; however, it is not diagnostic of sexual abuse. A 3-year-old's statement that an uncle touched her down there, though perhaps concerning, could mean a variety of things, including that the uncle was helping with normal potty training. The statement, by itself, would not be diagnostic of sexual abuse.

(Page 141, Chapter 35: Child Maltreatment: Neglect to Abuse)

Answer 4-10. b

Spiral fractures in themselves are not diagnostic of physical abuse. Careful consideration of the nature and severity of the injury, the proposed mechanism of injury, and the developmental abilities of the child should be undertaken when spiral fractures are diagnosed. In a nonambulatory child, spiral fractures certainly raise suspicion for abuse. In an ambulatory 2- or 3-year-old child, spiral fractures can occur accidentally. The term "toddler's fracture" refers to a nondisplaced spiral fracture, usually of the distal tibia. Although one cannot rule out abuse, such fractures can occur with a twisting or planting motion in an ambulatory child as they are running or walking. It would be expected that the parents may not witness or be aware of the actual injury.

Given the overall lack of other findings or social concerns, this would be a reasonable diagnosis to make for this child. When there are fractures that are not consistent with the developmental age of a child or mechanism or history provided, obtaining laboratory tests to rule out some underlying disease that could affect bone strength, such as rickets, may be helpful. Checking levels of calcium, phosphorus, alkaline phosphatase, and 25-hydroxyvitamin D would be a reasonable first step. Other labs might include a workup for osteogenesis imperfecta, or other rare disorders that might affect bone fragility such as Menkes disease. If there is suspicion of head trauma in a young child, then a workup might include a retinal examination to evaluate for retinal hemorrhages, and a CT or MRI scan of the head to evaluate for intracranial bleeding. In this case, with a normal mental status examination and no findings concerning for head trauma, these diagnostic studies would not be indicated. A skeletal survey is a series of radiographs examining all the long bones as well as the skull, chest, and spine. A skeletal survey is a helpful screening tool when suspicion of abuse is present in children less than 2 years old. A skeletal survey can be helpful in up to 5-year-olds in certain clinical situations.

(Page 140, 142, Chapter 35: Child Maltreatment: Neglect to Abuse)

Answer 4-11. a

About 25% of fractures in children under 3 years old are believed to be from abuse. Whereas an oblique/spiral femur fracture in an ambulatory child could be accidental from a planting and twisting motion during running or walking, a similar femur fracture in a nonambulatory infant without any history of trauma is very concerning for abuse.

Underlying bone diseases such as osteogenesis imperfecta must be considered, but most of these are rare, and can be excluded by a thorough physical examination, laboratory testing, and careful review of the radiographs. Osteogenesis imperfecta is a very rare spectrum of diseases that affect collagen and bone strength, sometimes associated with clinical findings such as blue sclerae, dental abnormalities, hyperflexibility, and short stature. Radiographs may reveal wormian bones (extra sutures) in the skull. Some cases may not have any findings, but these are likely less than 1 per 10,000 to 20,000 live births. Fractures of the femur may not be readily apparent, and a delay by a mother of 1 night to bring in her child in this case would not be overly concerning, although in general delay in care for obvious injuries is a red flag. One study reported femur fractures in newborns were not recognized by medical personnel often for days, and sometimes weeks. In this case, as in all cases of children less than 2 years old who have injuries suspicious for abuse, a skeletal survey would be indicated to look for non–clinically evident fractures.

(Page 140, 142, Chapter 35: Child Maltreatment: Neglect to Abuse)

Answer 4-12. e

Retinal hemorrhages can occur from a number of causes, including infections causing meningitis, sepsis, or coagulation disturbances, from birth, and abusive head injury. Retinal hemorrhages from birth usually resolve within 2 weeks, although hemorrhages have been documented lasting almost 2 months. There are a number of types of retinal hemorrhages including preretinal and intraretinal hemorrhages, and hemorrhages may have descriptions such as "splinter" hemorrhages and "blot and dot" hemorrhages. All of these types of hemorrhages have been associated with abusive head trauma.

Retinal hemorrhages usually resolve without any effect on vision, although severe hemorrhages can affect vision. Retinal hemorrhages can occur anywhere in the retina, and are not found only near the macula. Greater numbers of retinal hemorrhages distributed throughout the retina are more specific for abusive head trauma than a few scattered hemorrhages around the macula. In general, it is important to document the number, type, and location of retinal hemorrhages.

(Page 139-140, Chapter 35: Child Maltreatment: Neglect to Abuse)

Answer 4-13. d

Bruises on the trunk are more concerning for abuse, as they are less likely to occur accidentally, and bruising on the posterior surface of the body is highly suspicious at any age. Accidental bruises on the front of the developmentally normal 1-year-old boy would not be unexpected. Bruises over bony prominences such as shins, elbows/forearms, and the face are not unusual, especially when children are learning to walk and might fall forward. Multiple bruises in these areas, especially the shins, are common. The color of bruises can vary, and dating bruises is inexact.

(Page 139-140, Chapter 35: Child Maltreatment: Neglect to Abuse)

Answer 4-14. d

The skeletal survey is a series of radiographs that includes the skull, spine, chest, pelvis, and long bones. A skeletal survey is generally used as a screening tool when there is suspicion of abuse or neglect in children less than 2 years old. In specific cases, skeletal surveys may be indicated for children up to 5 years of age. The skeletal survey can detect unsuspected recent or old fractures that may be clinically undetectable. However, many fractures will heal within 6 months or less, and so the survey does not detect all previous fractures in a child. Repeating skeletal surveys in 10 to 14 days can sometimes reveal fractures not obvious initially, due to callous formation that makes them more apparent.

(Page 140, 142, Chapter 35: Child Maltreatment: Neglect to Abuse)

Answer 4-15. a

A normal genital examination does not rule out sexual abuse or assault. A study of pregnant adolescents found 2/36 had definitive findings of vaginal penetration. Only 5% of children referred for sexual abuse have positive findings on their genital examinations. Among those cases in which a perpetrator was convicted, only 23% of the genital examinations were considered suspicious. A chlamydia test being positive on the day of a sexual contact in a postpubertal girl would more likely be the result of a previously existing infection, particularly in a sexually active person. In this case, a positive chlamydia test would not be proof of rape. In cases of suspected or known sexual assault, postexposure prophylaxis for pregnancy, syphilis, chlamydia, gonorrhea, and HIV may be indicated, depending on the situation. State laws around age of consent and ability to provide these medications vary, but in this case such prophylaxis may benefit the girl. In general, for HIV and pregnancy prophylaxis, the earlier the medications are taken, the more effective they are. Beyond 72 hours the benefit is greatly diminished.

For syphilis, chlamydia, and gonorrhea, the decision is often made, to treat before results of diagnostic tests, especially due to poor follow-up rates. There is no treatment to prevent hepatitis C, although immunization against hepatitis B should be ensured. A blood alcohol level that is elevated only suggests alcohol ingestion, and does not suggest rape in itself.

(Page 141, Chapter 35: Child Maltreatment: Neglect to Abuse)

Answer 4-16. e

Medical child abuse includes a spectrum of abuse types (often referred to as Munchausen syndrome by proxy, factitious disorder by proxy, pediatric falsification syndrome, pediatric condition falsehood, and other names), in which a parent exaggerates or fabricates symptoms of an illness or causes a child to be ill. It has a high fatality rate because it is often difficult to recognize or diagnose, as often focus is on the child's symptoms rather than the possibility that they could be caused by a parent. The most common presentations of medical child abuse are seizures, apnea, diarrhea, and fever. Although the etiology of ALTEs is unknown as often as half the time, studies suggest up to 2% to 3% of ALTEs may be from medical child abuse.

(Page 140, Chapter 35: Child Maltreatment: Neglect to Abuse)

Answer 4-17. d

Neglected children commonly present with poor growth due to inadequate nutrition. Weight usually is the first parameter affected, then height, and then head circumference. Often there is accompanying developmental delay, particularly in language and social interactions. Although there are a myriad of possible causes of poor weight gain (or failure to thrive), whether evaluating for organic or nonorganic causes, a careful feeding history is critical in order to estimate the caloric intake of the child as well as evaluate the potential social and environmental contributions to the weight loss. Evaluation might focus on questions such as how food is prepared, and how the child responds to it, past feeding problems, and parental concerns.

Prior to other medical tests, obtaining a complete developmental history would also be an important next step, including the child's developmental milestones, temperament, and interactions with family and others. Although one might suspect neglect, which is the most common form of abuse, in the absence of other concerning signs a skeletal survey in a 3-year-old would not be indicated, nor would a CT scan of the head. The murmur may require further workup, but would not be as important as a feeding history in this situation. Assessment of serum electrolyte levels would not be useful, given the child does not have other signs to suggest that he is severely malnourished at this point.

(Page 140, 142, Chapter 35: Child Maltreatment: Neglect to Abuse)

Answer 4-18. b

Two types of fractures that are specific for abuse are classic metaphyseal fractures (also called bucket handle or corner fractures related to their appearance depending on the angle of the x-ray) and posterior (or lateral) rib fractures. Linear skull fractures would be consistent with a simple fall onto a hard surface, and an underlying epidural (and even localized subdural) hematoma could be consistent with this mechanism of injury, assuming no other suspicious findings.

An oblique fracture of the femur, though concerning, could potentially be caused by a fall onto a hard surface. A transverse clavicle fracture could be associated with birth trauma in an infant, although a fall could cause this. Birth fractures would usually be healed, and certainly would not be acute appearing (without callus formation) at 5 months of age. A buckle (sometimes called torus) fracture implies longitudinal forces, which could occur from a fall directly onto the foot. Buckle fractures occur in the metaphyseal region of the bone, but are different than the type of classic metaphyseal lesion with strong specificity for abuse.

(Page 140, Chapter 35: Child Maltreatment: Neglect to Abuse)

Answer 4-19. c

Head injuries are the most common cause of death from abuse in children. Abusive head trauma is a spectrum of presentations resulting from inflicted injuries to the head, with or without injuries to other parts of the body. There is often no clear history to direct health care providers to a trauma as the mechanism for the presentation. Infants with abusive head trauma can be asymptomatic, or present with severe findings, and even coma or death. Seizures are not uncommon. Often there are no other signs of abuse, including no external signs of head trauma such as bruises or swelling.

Abusive head trauma often is accompanied by retinal hemorrhages, which can involve various layers of the retina and can be extensive, out the periphery of the retina. Studies suggest that other professionals are reasonably good at identifying retinal hemorrhages on clinical examination; however, a retinal examination by an experienced ophthalmologist is important to obtain when there is suspicion of abusive head trauma. Important labs to rule out potential mimics of abusive head trauma would include coagulation studies with a complete blood count to evaluate for coagulation abnormalities. It should be noted that head trauma, particularly severe trauma, can cause coagulation disorders as a secondary response to injury. Some rare disorders, such as glutaric acidemia type 1, can present with retinal hemorrhages and

subdural hemorrhages, and tests for these might include serum amino acids. LFTs can screen for occult abdominal injuries in young infants and children with suspicious injuries, but would not directly support the diagnosis of abusive head trauma in the same manner as retinal hemorrhages. Serum calcium, phosphorus, and alkaline phosphatase would be labs to obtain to work up fractures.

(Page 139-140, 142, Chapter 35: Child Maltreatment: Neglect to Abuse)

Answer 4-20. b

A positive urine test for chlamydia would be the most concerning finding for sexual abuse. Given the low prevalence of chlamydia in the 2-year-old female population, a confirmatory test by culture or by repeat urine testing using a different probe (nucleic acid amplification or PCR) would be necessary to rule out a false-positive test. Treating children in these cases should be deferred until a positive culture or repeated positive test allows confirmation of infection.

A bruise and/or laceration to the external female genitalia such as the labia majora would be consistent with a straddle injury as described by the father. Prolapsed urethra often presents with bleeding, occurs more often in obese African American girls, and is often mistaken for sexual abuse on examination by an inexperienced provider. Treatment is usually with topical steroids. Lichen sclerosis presents with hypopigmented thinning of the skin often in the perianal or genital area. These lesions are from an unclear cause, and can also present with bleeding and/or pain, and are also sometimes mistaken for sexual abuse. Treatment is usually with topical steroids. Perianal streptococcal dermatitis is sharply demarcated bright red rash caused by group A β-hemolytic streptococci. Symptoms can include blood-streaked stools in one third of patients, and it primarily occurs in children between 6 months and 10 years of age. A rapid streptococcal test of the area can make the diagnosis, and treatment is similar to strep throat, with amoxicillin or penicillin being effective.

(Page 141, 143, Chapter 35: Child Maltreatment: Neglect to Abuse)

CHAPTER 5 | Newborn

W. Christopher Golden, Elizabeth A. Cristofalo,
Bernadette A. Hillman, and Colleen Hughes Driscoll

5-1. Which of the following statements regarding vitamin K administration in the newborn period is correct?

a. Two 1-mg doses of intramuscular vitamin K are required in the first 48 hours of age.

b. Vitamin K cannot be given safely to neonates as an oral preparation.

c. Neonates receiving a 2-mg dose of oral vitamin K require no additional dosing in infancy.

d. Oral vitamin K administration dosing has been standardized with internationally accepted guidelines.

e. Parental nonadherence with additional doses of oral vitamin K is a major factor in oral vitamin K failures.

5-2. A 4130-g male infant is born via vaginal delivery after 40 6/7 weeks' gestation. The mother recently migrated from Ecuador and received no prenatal care. In the delivery room, the baby developed mild tachypnea and intercostal retractions. Pulse oximetry from the infant's left foot registers 95% saturation in room air. Physical examination findings include a flat abdomen and audible bowel sounds over the left side of the infant's chest. Clear breath sounds are noted over the right side of the chest. Heart sounds are best auscultated at the left sternal border.

The most appropriate *initial* step in management of this neonate is:

a. Needle decompression of the right hemithorax

b. Positive pressure ventilation using a bag and mask

c. Decompression of the stomach with a nasogastric tube

d. Positive pressure ventilation with a T-piece resuscitator

e. Transillumination of the right hemithorax

5-3. A 4550-g male neonate is delivered vaginally after a 37 6/7 weeks' gestation complicated by gestational diabetes. One application of a vacuum extractor to the neonate's head was required to facilitate delivery. On examination at 12 hours of age, the baby has a well-circumscribed, fluctuant mass over the parietal skull that does not cross suture lines. The overlying skin is erythematous but intact. He is active and alert, and the rest of his examination is unremarkable. His hematocrit (measured from a capillary sample) is 45%.

Which of the following steps is next indicated in the management of this neonate?

a. Administration of intravenous ampicillin and cefotaxime

b. Monitoring serum and/or transcutaneous bilirubin levels

c. Careful aspiration of the mass with a tuberculin syringe

d. Application of topical bacitracin zinc ointment to the mass

e. Transfusion of packed red blood cells

5-4. An obstetric colleague asks you to provide prenatal counseling for a new patient to his practice. The woman, currently at 34 3/7 weeks' gestation, transferred her medical care from an out-of-state obstetrical group. Her past medical history is notable for poorly controlled type 1 diabetes. The mother asks about fetal growth and neonatal body habitus in pregnancies complicated by diabetes.

Which of the following statements regarding growth in fetuses and infants of diabetic mothers (IDMs) is true?

a. Growth hormone (GH) is the primary anabolic growth factor in the fetus.

b. If a mother has advanced diabetes-related vascular disease (ie, diabetic retinopathy), fetal growth is not affected.

c. IDMs have excess fat distribution in the extremities

d. Hypertrophic cardiomyopathy (HCM) in IDMs may result in ventricular outflow tract obstruction.

e. IDMs have equally increased weight, length, and head circumference percentiles at birth.

5-5. A 3840-g female infant is delivered by cesarean section after a 39 5/7 weeks' gestation. In the delivery room, she develops tachypnea and cyanosis when quiet. Physical examination reveals clear bilateral breath sounds when the infant is crying. However, the nurse is unable to pass a 5 French suction catheter through the nares into the posterior pharynx.

The most appropriate initial step in management of this neonate is:

a. Oral airway placement

b. Intranasal dexamethasone instillation

c. Nasal cannula oxygen administration

d. Supine positioning

e. Nasal continuous positive airway pressure (CPAP)

5-6. A 9-week-old female infant is seen for a follow-up appointment with her pediatrician. The baby weighed 4330 g at birth, and was delivered vaginally (from the breech presentation) at 40 weeks' gestation. In the nursery, hip examination was unremarkable bilaterally on Ortolani and Barlow maneuvers. Physical examination at this visit shows normal movement of the lower extremities.

The appropriate screening strategy for developmental dysplasia of the hip (DDH) in this infant at this time is:

a. Repeat Ortolani and Barlow maneuvers only

b. Measurement and comparison of the lower extremity length (from the anterior superior iliac crest to the heel)

c. Ultrasonography of both hips

d. Radiographs of both hips

e. Magnetic resonance imaging of both hips

5-7. A 1200-g male infant is delivered vaginally after a 28 3/7 weeks' gestation complicated by preterm rupture of membranes and preterm labor. On arrival to the delivery room table, the neonate receives positive pressure ventilation (PPV) after the neonatal nurse dries the skin and suctions the oropharynx.

After 3 minutes of PPV, the nurse notes the baby has a heart rate of 110 beats/min with cyanosis and intercostal retractions. The pediatric resident decides to intubate the infant. Brief visual inspection of the mouth, mandible, and tongue reveals no abnormalities.

Which of the following combinations of laryngoscope blade and endotracheal tube is indicated for intubating this patient?

a. Number 0 blade, 3.0 mm endotracheal tube

b. Number 00 blade, 4.0 mm endotracheal tube

c. Number 1 blade, 3.5 mm endotracheal tube

d. Number 00 blade, 3.5 mm endotracheal tube

e. Number 0 blade, 4.0 mm endotracheal tube

5-8. An infant born at 26 weeks' gestation with a birth weight of 900 g is now 42 weeks postmenstrual age (PMA). He had respiratory distress syndrome (RDS) in his early neonatal intensive care unit (NICU) course and continues to have a supplemental oxygen requirement.

Which of the following characteristics of his past or current neonatal course would support the diagnosis of bronchopulmonary dysplasia (BPD) in this infant?

a. He was born due to maternal chorioamnionitis and was mechanically ventilated for 21 days.

b. He was mechanically ventilated for 2 weeks, and now requires an FiO_2 of 0.5 via CPAP (+5 cm H_2O) to keep his saturations >97%.

c. He requires 2 liters per minute (LPM) of nasal cannula oxygen with an FiO_2 of 0.6 to maintain oxygen saturations of 98% to 100%.

d. He developed *Bacteroides fragilis* sepsis at 2 weeks of age and required mechanical ventilation until 34 weeks PMA.

e. He requires 1 LPM nasal cannula oxygen with an FiO_2 of 0.45 to maintain oxygen saturations of 91% to 93%.

5-9. A 600-g male infant was born at 24 1/7 weeks' gestation to a 26-year-old, gravida 2, para 0020 woman with a history of cervical incompetence. His hospital course was complicated by cholestatic jaundice, feeding intolerance, and chronic respiratory failure requiring intubation from birth until his death from *E. coli* pneumonia and bacteremia at 105 days of age. The family has requested a complete autopsy to better understand his lung disease.

Which of the following features would you expect to see on pathologic examination of this infant's lungs?

a. Lung development consistent with his postmenstrual age

b. Uniform lung tissue with no evidence of emphysematous changes

c. Localized elastin fibers at the branch points of the alveoli

d. Increased alveolar diameter with decreased number of alveoli

e. Normal pulmonary vasculature with evidence of pulmonary edema

5-10. A 30-year-old, gravida 1 woman presents to the Labor and Delivery unit at 26 6/7 weeks' gestation. She reports uterine contractions every 5 minutes and leakage of clear amniotic fluid 1 hour prior to her arrival. Physical examination confirms rupture of her amniotic membranes as well as 9.5 cm of cervical dilation. She is afebrile and has a normal heart rate and blood pressure. The obstetricians page the neonatal intensive care unit (NICU) team to the Labor and Delivery unit, anticipating an imminent delivery.

After delivery, which of the following management strategies in the NICU would decrease the risk of this infant developing bronchopulmonary dysplasia (BPD)?

a. Initiation of parenteral erythromycin within 24 hours of birth

b. Application of positive pressure ventilation in the delivery room, using high inspiratory pressures of 40 to 60 cm water after the first 5 infant breaths

c. Initiation of high-dose corticosteroids if the neonate requires more than 7 days of mechanical ventilation.

d. Supplementation with enteral ascorbic acid (vitamin C) when the infant is on full-volume gastric feeds

e. Use of supplemental oxygen to keep saturations within gestational-age-specific target parameters while in the NICU

5-11. A 26-year-old, gravida 3 female presents to your office at 25 4/7 weeks' gestation for a prenatal consult. She tells you that the fetus, a female, has a "rectal mass." The prenatal ultrasound report notes the mass to be most consistent with a sacrococcygeal teratoma (SCT). The mother asks about the possibility of resecting the mass prior to delivery.

Which of the following statements regarding fetal surgery for a SCT is correct?

a. The primary goal of fetal surgery is prevention of fetal hydrops.

b. The removal of pelvic components of the teratoma is accomplished prenatally.

c. The development of hydrops fetalis is an insignificant concern in this case.

d. The anorectal sphincter complex should be removed during fetal surgery.

e. The surgical intervention should occur only after complete hydrops fetalis occurs.

5-12. Which of the following pathophysiologic mechanisms is associated with neonatal hypoxic-ischemic brain injury?

a. Loss of high-energy phosphorylated compounds

b. Reduction in cellular oxidative stress

c. Accelerated reuptake of glutamate at the synaptic cleft

d. Decrease in intracellular calcium levels

e. Sustained inhibition of neuronal apoptosis

5-13. A 3210-g female neonate was delivered by emergent cesarean section due to a maternal seizure and cardiorespiratory arrest after a 37 6/7 weeks' gestation. The infant required mechanical ventilation and chest compressions in the delivery room. Her Apgars were 1, 2, and 4 at 1, 5, and 10 minutes of age, respectively. Her initial arterial blood gas at 45 minutes of age showed a pH of 6.78 and a base deficit of −20mmol/L. On admission to the NICU, the radiant warmer was not turned on in anticipation of hypothermia therapy to prevent hypoxic ischemic encephalopathy (HIE). Her rectal temperature was 35.1°C at 60 minutes of age.

Which of the following statements regarding therapeutic hypothermia in this infant is correct?

a. If the infant had severe abnormalities on amplitude-integrated electroencephalography (aEEG) on NICU admission, selective head cooling would provide the most neuroprotection.

b. The minimum length of therapeutic hypothermia for prevention of HIE in this infant is 12 hours.

c. Therapeutic hypothermia would accelerate free radical production in this patient.

d. Based on clinical trial data, whole body hypothermia would reduce the risk of death or moderate to severe disability in this infant at 12 to 18 months of age.

e. Hypothermia will preserve executive functioning and psychosocial development in this infant at 15 years of age.

5-14. Which of the following statements regarding neonatal venous strokes is correct?

a. Based on randomized clinical trials, low-molecular-weight heparin is the anticoagulant of choice for treatment of venous thromboses.

b. Venous infarctions may be associated with neonatal group B *Streptococcus* sepsis.

c. Venous infarctions are 3 times as likely as arterial strokes in neonates.

d. Hemorrhagic venous infarcts in neonates usually spare the deep gray matter.

e. Trials of supratherapeutic doses of erythropoietin in humans have demonstrated benefit in treating neonatal strokes.

5-15. A 4-day-old male infant born at 37 2/7 weeks' gestation presents for his first well-child care visit. He weighed 4000 g at birth and his length was 55.5 cm (both greater than the 90th percentile for gestational age). His newborn course was notable for episodes of "low sugar," per the mother; the nursery pediatrician suggested the mother feed the infant every 2 hours because he was a "large baby." The mother had a normal oral glucose tolerance test during pregnancy.

On physical examination, the infant has a prominent tongue and bilateral ear creases. Abdominal examination is notable for slight separation of the rectus abdominis muscles but without herniation of intestinal contents. He is alert and interactive. A serum glucose taken in the office is 39 mg/dL. He takes 30 cm³ of formula in the office in 15 minutes without respiratory distress or diaphoresis.

The etiology of hypoglycemia in this infant is related to:

a. Congestive heart failure

b. Impaired fatty acid oxidation

c. Pancreatic hypertrophy

d. Swallowing dysfunction

e. Impaired glycogenolysis

5-16. You meet a 23-year-old primigravida female student, who presents for a routine fetal ultrasound at 20 2/7 weeks' gestation. She is a postbaccalaureate student who will be applying to graduate school. She has an interest in fetal circulation, particularly the oxygen concentration in the heart and blood vessels. She asks you, "Which of the following sites has the highest oxygen concentration in the fetus?" What is the best answer?

a. Inferior vena cava

b. Umbilical vein

c. Umbilical artery

d. Right ventricle

e. Ductus arteriosus

5-17. A 1200-g white male infant is born (at 29 1/7 weeks' gestation) to a 25-year-old, gravida 2, para 1001 woman who presented to the hospital in preterm labor. The infant has an uncomplicated delivery and requires only routine drying, warming, and tactile stimulation. He is admitted to the NICU secondary to prematurity. He requires no respiratory support initially, but at 3 hours of life, he is started on nasal continuous positive airway pressure (CPAP) due to tachypnea, grunting, nasal flaring, and sternal retractions.

What is the *most likely* cause of his symptoms?

a. Persistent pulmonary hypertension of the newborn

b. Transient tachypnea of the newborn

c. Respiratory distress syndrome (RDS)

d. Meconium aspiration syndrome

e. Congenital heart disease

5-18. A 2100-g infant was born at 33 1/7 weeks' gestation by repeat cesarean section to a 28-year-old primigravida woman. At delivery, the male infant was noted to have respiratory distress characterized by grunting, retractions, and hypoxia. The infant is intubated and given a dose of surfactant. The father, a graduate student in biochemistry, asks you about the properties of surfactant and its production and role in the normal lung.

Which of the following statements about surfactant is correct?

a. Surfactant lipids and proteins are synthesized in the alveolar epithelial type II cells.

b. Phosphatidylglycerol (PG) is the major component responsible for decreasing alveolar surface tension.

c. Congenital surfactant protein A (SP-A) deficiency causes fatal respiratory distress in affected full-term infants.

d. Surfactant synthesis and storage begins at 28 to 38 weeks' gestation.

e. Antenatal testing of amniotic fluid after 34 weeks' gestation will show a lecithin–sphingomyelin (L/S) ratio of 1:1 in infants with mature lungs.

5-19. A 2500-g female infant was born at 34 3/7 weeks' gestation to a 30-year-old, gravida 3, para 1102 woman. Shortly after birth, the infant developed tachypnea (respiratory rate of 60 breaths/min), and increased work in breathing (manifested by intercostal retractions). She is brought to the special care nursery for evaluation and management of her respiratory distress. Physical examination shows coarse bilateral breath sounds, no cardiac murmur, and strong, equal peripheral pulses. She is alert and active.

What is the *most appropriate initial* management strategy for this infant?

a. Intubate the infant; immediately begin high-frequency oscillatory ventilation (HFOV).

b. Begin continuous positive airway pressure (CPAP) with supplemental oxygen and nitric oxide (iNO).

c. Intubate the infant and begin intermittent mechanical ventilation (IMV).

d. Support the infant with CPAP and supplemental oxygen to maintain appropriate oxygen saturations for gestational age.

e. Place the infant under a hood and titrate nitrogen (N_2) and oxygen (O_2) into the hood to generate an FiO_2 of 0.16.

5-20. A 36 2/7–week, 1800-g male infant is born to a 32-year-old, gravida 1 woman with pregnancy-induced hypertension. At 30 seconds of age, he is spontaneously crying on the delivery room table, and has a heart rate of 110 beats/min.

Which of the following steps is most important in the *initial management* of this infant?

a. Administer positive pressure ventilation (PPV) via a self-inflating bag.

b. Provide continuous positive airway pressure (CPAP) using a T-piece resuscitator.

c. Administer a 10 cm³/kg intravenous bolus of normal saline via an umbilical venous catheter.

d. Dry the infant with warm towels and suction his mouth and nose.

e. Deliver a 2 cm³/kg intravenous bolus of 10% dextrose via an umbilical venous catheter.

5-21. A 2200-g infant was born at 39 6/7 weeks' gestation (via spontaneous vaginal delivery) to a 34-year-old woman with a history of chronic hypertension. In the nursery at 2 hours of age, the baby's blood glucose was 24 mg/dL before feeding. After taking 20 mL of age-appropriate formula, the blood glucose increased to 50 mg/dL.

What is the *most likely* cause for the initial hypoglycemia in this infant?

a. Increased gluconeogenesis

b. Decreased neonatal insulin sensitivity

c. Increased placental transport of maternal insulin in utero

d. Increased serum epinephrine levels

e. Decreased glycogen stores

5-22. A 1500-g female infant is born at 34 weeks' gestation to a 40-year-old, gravida 4, para 3003 woman by cesarean section due to reverse end-diastolic flow noted on fetal sonography. The pregnancy was complicated by intrauterine growth restriction (IUGR) and pregnancy-induced hypertension. Due to respiratory distress in the delivery room, the baby is transferred to the NICU for intravenous nutrition and respiratory support.

The infant is at high risk for developing which of the following?

a. Low plasma concentrations of fatty acid and triglycerides if she receives intravenous lipids

b. Low basal oxygen consumption and total energy expenditure (relative to an appropriate-for-gestational-age [AGA] infant)

c. Increased intestinal protein losses with enteral nutrition

d. Higher serum insulin levels in the neonatal period

e. High immunoglobulin levels during infancy

5-23. Which of the following statements regarding neonatal glucose metabolism is correct?

a. Postnatal increases in catecholamines and glucagon modulate neonatal glucose concentrations shortly after birth.

b. Neonatal hepatic glycogen content may remain elevated up to 72 hours after birth without exogenous glucose delivery.

c. Neonatal insulin levels surge immediately after delivery.

d. Basal glucose production in a neonate is approximately 10% to 15% the basal rate of an adult.

e. Inhibition of long-chain fatty acid oxidation increases circulating glucose concentrations.

5-24. A 4050-g male neonate was delivered by emergent cesarean section due to fetal bradycardia after a 39 2/7 weeks' gestation. He required mechanical ventilation, chest compressions, and intravenous epinephrine in the delivery room. The baby's Apgars were 1, 1, and 6 at 1, 5, and 10 minutes of age, respectively. His initial arterial blood gas at 45 minutes of age showed a pH of 6.97 and a base deficit of −17 mmol/L. He developed seizures at 30 minutes of age, and was placed on whole-body hypothermia (for prevention of hypoxic ischemic encephalopathy) at 75 minutes of age. He also was placed on a high-frequency oscillator and started on maintenance intravenous fluids of 85 cm³/kg/day containing 10% dextrose via an umbilical venous catheter.

At 24 hours of age, the baby's total urine output for the day is 0.2 cm³/kg/h. He has 2-second capillary refill and strong peripheral pulses. A set of serum chemistries at that time demonstrates the following:

Sodium	122 mEq/L
Potassium	6.2 mEq/L
Chloride	89 mEq/L
CO_2	14 mEq/L
Blood urea nitrogen (BUN)	45 mg/dL
Creatinine	2.6 mg/dL
Calcium	6.9 mg/dL
Glucose	67 mg/dL

Which of the following steps is appropriate in the management of this infant?

a. Administration of furosemide, 0.5 mg/kg intravenous

b. Administration of normal saline, 10 cm³/kg intravenous, over 30 minutes

c. Administration of bumetanide, 0.1 mg/kg intravenous

d. Reduction of intravenous fluids to 30 cm³/kg/day

e. Increase of dextrose in the intravenous fluids to 15%

5-25. A 3700-g male infant, born vaginally at 39 2/7 weeks' gestation, required intubation in the delivery room for apnea. The mother is a 31-year-old, gravida 3, para 2002 woman with no significant medical history. She received routine prenatal care during this uncomplicated pregnancy. She developed more frequent uterine contractions at home (4 hours prior to birth) and, subsequently, her amniotic membranes ruptured

(1 hour prior to birth). On arrival to Labor and Delivery, her cervix was fully dilated, and she delivered the baby shortly thereafter.

The pediatric resuscitation team arrived at 3 minutes of life to find a limp, cyanotic infant under the radiant warmer receiving stimulation and blow-by oxygen. The baby's heart rate was greater than 100 beats/min, but he demonstrated little respiratory effort. He was intubated easily by the pediatric intern and brought to the NICU. Apgars were 4 and 4 (2 points each for color and heart rate) at 5 and 10 minutes, respectively. Cord blood was not sent for blood gas measurement, but the infant's initial arterial blood gas in the NICU at 30 minutes of age revealed a pH of 6.98 and base deficit of −14 mmol/L.

At 45 minutes of age, he continues to be hypotonic and apneic (despite stimulation from NICU caregivers), with pupils that are nonreactive to light.

Which of the following statements is correct, and should be considered in the management of this infant?

a. There is no report of a prenatal or antenatal event that would cause hypoxia–ischemia, making this infant's presentation most consistent with an inborn error of metabolism.

b. Administration of prophylactic phenobarbital is indicated for seizure prophylaxis in this infant for a minimum of 72 hours after birth.

c. If the neurologic examination does not improve, this infant will be a candidate for whole-body hypothermia, which should begin at 12 hours of life.

d. Results of MRI imaging and electroencephalogram will be useful for discussing long-term prognosis.

e. Tracking degree of clinical encephalopathy is useful for predicting duration of hospitalization, but does not contribute additional information when predicting later prognosis.

5-26. A 34-year-old, gravida 1 woman presents at 18 weeks for a level 2 screening ultrasound. The fetus is noted to have a hypoplastic nasal bone, increased nuchal fold, and short humeri and femora.

What profile of α-fetoprotein (α-FP), human chorionic gonadotropin (hCG), and unconjugated estriol (uE) would have been *most likely* seen on the woman's triple screen prior to the ultrasound?

a. Low α-FP, low hCG, low uE

b. Low α-FP, high hCG, low uE

c. Low α-FP, low hCG, high uE

d. High α-FP, high hCG, high uE

e. High α-FP, high hCG, low uE

5-27. A 25-year-old, gravida 2, para 1001 woman presents at 38 6/7 weeks' gestation in labor. She is placed on a tocodynamometer. The following tracing is obtained:

Which of the following is the *most likely* cause of the above findings?

a. Low fetal oxygen tension

b. Intermittent umbilical cord compression

c. Fetal hiccups (singultus)

d. Fetal head compression

e. Normal fetal movement

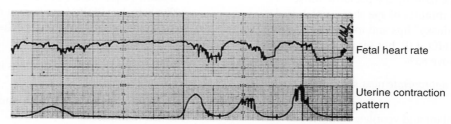

Fetal heart rate

Uterine contraction pattern

(Reproduced, with permission, from Parer JT. Fetal heart rate. In: Creasy R, Resnick R, eds. *Maternal-Fetal Medicine: Principles and Practice*. 3rd ed. Philadelphia: Saunders; 1994.)

5-28. A 29-year-old, gravida 4, para 1203 woman presents to her obstetrician for a routine appointment at 27 6/7 weeks' gestation. Her urine dipstick demonstrates 4+ protein, and her blood pressure is 170/100 mm Hg. Her baseline (prepregnancy) blood pressure is 116/70 mm Hg, and her blood pressure at 24 2/7 weeks' gestation was 140/88 mm Hg. She denies headache, visual changes, or abdominal pain, and has no facial or extremity edema on physical examination. She has normal urine output and a serum creatinine of 1.1 mg/dL. Her obstetrician admits his patients to a tertiary care obstetrical center.

Which is the *most appropriate initial* step in management of this patient?

a. Admission to Labor and Delivery for an emergent cesarean section delivery

b. Admission to Labor and Delivery for hemodialysis and delivery within the next 48 hours

c. Admission to Labor and Delivery and intravenous magnesium sulfate administration only

d. Admission to Labor and Delivery for intravenous magnesium sulfate and corticosteroid administration

e. Admission to Labor and Delivery for corticosteroid administration therapy only

5-29. A 10-day-old male infant born at 28 1/7 weeks' gestation develops hypotension, tachypnea, and an increasing number of desaturation and bradycardia episodes. The infant was born vaginally after the mother presented to the hospital with a 4-day history of ruptured amniotic membranes. She received a course of antenatal betamethasone. He was intubated in the delivery room, given 3 doses of surfactant over his initial NICU course for respiratory distress syndrome, and extubated at 4 days of age to CPAP (FiO$_2$ 0.3). The infant also received 48 hours of antibiotics (beginning at birth) for presumed sepsis. Enteral feeds were initiated at 5 days of age. Physical examination is notable for a holosystolic murmur. An echocardiogram demonstrates a large patent ductus arteriosus (PDA) with left-to-right flow. His complete blood count shows a white blood cell count of 4000/mm^3 with 20% band forms.

The *most likely* reason for presentation of this symptomatic PDA at this time is:

a. Extubation on day 4, which decreased pulmonary vascular resistance.

b. Failure to receive indomethacin prophylaxis for intraventricular hemorrhage in the first 48 hours of life.

c. Inadequate antibiotic treatment for presumed sepsis, resulting in prostaglandin release.

d. Failure of the mother to receive antenatal steroids due to precipitous delivery.

e. Advances in enteral feeding caused shunting to mesenteric circulation.

5-30. How many grams per deciliter of hemoglobin is deoxygenated when cyanosis becomes apparent in a neonate?

a. 0.5 to 1.0

b. 3 to 5

c. 9 to 11

d. 15 to 20

e. 25 to 30

5-31. A 27-year-old woman presented to the emergency department of a local community hospital in active labor. She has had no prenatal care and does not remember her last menstrual period. She was transferred to the Labor and Delivery suite, where a bedside ultrasound dated the fetus at approximately 40 weeks' gestation. Three hours later, the woman vaginally delivered a 4700-g male infant. Physical examination of the baby by the pediatric nurse practitioner at 15 minutes of age shows unlabored respirations but "dusky" lips and tongue. He is given blow-by oxygen (FiO$_2$ 1.0), but his oxygen saturations never increase above 85%.

What is the *most appropriate* next step in management of this neonate?

a. Intubate the infant and ventilate him with an anesthesia bag.

b. Administer a bolus of 10% dextrose intravenously.

c. Admit infant to full-term nursery.

d. Obtain a computerized tomogram (CT) of the chest.

e. Consult a cardiologist at a tertiary care children's hospital.

5-32. A 3800-g male infant was born at 41 3/7 weeks' gestation to a 26-year-old woman. She had unremarkable cultures and serologies except for a positive vaginal group B *Streptococcus* culture (at 36 3/7 weeks' gestation), for which she received intrapartum antibiotics. Amniotic membranes were ruptured at delivery, and the amniotic fluid was noted to be meconium stained. At birth, the infant was initially apneic and hypotonic with a heart rate of 90 beats/min. He was intubated easily on the first attempt, and a moderate amount of meconium was aspirated from the trachea. He began to breathe when the endotracheal tube was removed, but subsequently developed tachypnea and intercostal retractions. He was admitted to the NICU and placed on supplemental oxygen (FiO$_2$ 1.0) via an oxygen hood.

Which of the following conditions is the *most likely* cause of the baby's respiratory distress?

a. Mechanical obstruction of the airways

b. Bacterial pneumonia

c. Decreased surfactant production

d. Pulmonary vasodilation

e. Tracheal edema

5-33. A 4500-g female infant was born at 37 6/7 weeks' gestation to a 30-year-old woman with poorly controlled gestational diabetes. The delivery occurred vaginally (with forceps assistance) and was complicated by shoulder dystocia. Three hours after birth, the infant develops respiratory distress and needs supplemental oxygen (FiO$_2$ 0.35) to keep her saturations greater than 95%. Physical examination of the infant is notable for shallow respirations but clear bilateral breath sounds. The baby has limited movement of the left arm on elicitation of the Moro reflex. The intern orders a chest radiograph.

Which of the following findings is *most likely* to be seen on the radiograph?

a. Herniation of the stomach and small bowel into the left hemithorax

b. A decrease in pulmonary vascular markings bilaterally

c. Elevation of the left hemidiaphragm by 3 intercostal spaces (relative to the right hemidiaphragm)

d. A left pleural fluid density compressing the lung

e. Multiple cystic lesions in the upper lobe of the left lung

5-34. A 2700-g female infant is admitted to the NICU after delivery by cesarean section at 36 0/7 weeks' gestation. The mother is a 25-year-old, gravida 1 who developed severe preeclampsia (after an uncomplicated pregnancy) and was treated with a magnesium sulfate drip.

Which of the following findings on initial physical examination is normal given the clinical scenario?

a. Bursts of 8 to 10 sucks on a pacifier within 5 seconds, followed by pauses lasting 5 to 10 seconds

b. Visual fixation on a bull's eye with sustained tracking

c. Strong flexor tone in the upper extremities and semiflexion in the lower extremities

d. Absence of the Moro and palmar grasp reflexes

e. Movement of the right elbow to the left shoulder when the right arm is pulled across the chest to the left

5-35. The Pediatrics team was called to a delivery by the Obstetrics team due to fetal bradycardia. On arrival to the delivery room, the Labor and Delivery nurse told the pediatricians that the mother was a 27-year-old, gravida 4, para 2103 woman at 39 0/7 weeks' gestation. The mother had regular prenatal care, and her labor was progressing normally. Rupture of membranes occurred 5 hours ago (clear amniotic fluid).

At delivery, the baby was cyanotic, hypotonic, and apneic, but had an appropriate response to stimulation and positive pressure ventilation delivered by the pediatric respiratory therapist. The pediatric resident performed the initial newborn examination 30 minutes after birth.

Which of the following findings on physical examination of this baby would raise suspicion for central nervous system injury?

a. An intermittent disconjugate gaze when he is not fixating or tracking an object

b. Unsustained clonus when his ankle jerk reflex is elicited

c. Changes in the upper and lower extremity tones with rotation of his head from left to right

d. Truncal extensor tone that exceeds his flexor tone

e. Rapid grasp when the palm of his hand is pressed

5-36. A 2700-g female infant was born vaginally (with vacuum assistance) after induction of labor at 36 6/7 weeks' gestation (due to maternal preeclampsia). Apgar scores were 8 (−1 color, −1 tone) and 9 (−1 color) at 1 and 5 minutes, respectively. The baby was permitted to stay with mother and receive couplet care. While holding her at 48 hours of age, the mother felt the baby moving but "not breathing" and called the postpartum nurse. The baby recovered quickly but was transferred from couplet care to the NICU for monitoring. During the workup, a noncontrast CT scan of the brain is performed. Before you can review the CT results, the radiology technologist mentions to the baby's nurse that the scan "... looks like a stroke."

Which of the following statements regarding the brain injury in this infant is correct?

a. The timing of the seizure indicates that the insult occurred after delivery, and mother should be questioned about having dropped the baby.

b. The timing of the seizure indicates that the insult occurred after delivery, and the baby most likely has a congenital cardiac mixing lesion.

c. The stroke is most likely venous in origin, and evaluation for a hypercoagulable state is a high priority.

d. Anticoagulation is effective therapy for neonatal thrombotic stroke regardless of the origin (arterial vs venous).

e. This baby's perinatal risk factors for stroke include maternal preeclampsia and vacuum-assisted delivery.

5-37. A 2600-g male infant, born to a 16-year-old, gravida 1 female who did not receive prenatal care, was admitted to the neonatal intensive care unit with mild tachypnea. At 3 days of age, his respiratory distress has resolved, and a developmental pediatrician is asked to help determine his gestational age. On his examination, the baby has very weak, intermittent finger flexion when his palm is pressed, and no arm flexion when traction is placed on his arms. He has interest in a pacifier, and will suck on it 4 to 5 times before requiring a 10-second pause.

These findings are most consistent with an infant of what gestational age?

a. Less than 30 weeks' gestation

b. 30 to 31 weeks' gestation

c. 32 to 33 weeks' gestation

d. 34 to 35 weeks' gestation

e. Greater than 36 weeks' gestation

5-38. A 7-day-old female infant was born at 30 weeks' gestation by cesarean section for maternal preeclampsia. She required CPAP for 3 days for respiratory distress syndrome, and received 48 hours of antibiotics before blood cultures were negative. Today, the pediatric intern noted the baby is tachypneic with an active precordium. On examination, he hears a continuous cardiac murmur and palpates full peripheral pulses. Echocardiogram reveals a large patent ductus arteriosus with left-to-right flow.

Which of the following factors could have contributed to the infant's clinical status?

a. Elevated cortisol concentrations due to antenatal betamethasone administration

b. Decreased sensitivity of premature ductal tissue to prostaglandins

c. Antenatal treatment of maternal headache with ibuprofen

d. Elevated serum concentration of prostaglandin E_2 (PGE_2)

e. Omission of surfactant administration after delivery

5-39. Which of the following statements about necrotizing enterocolitis (NEC) in near-term and term infants is true?

  a. NEC in near-term and term infants is usually preceded by a perinatal infectious risk factor such as maternal chorioamnionitis or prolonged rupture of membranes.

  b. NEC in near-term and term infants typically involves the proximal small bowel, rather than the colon.

  c. NEC typically occurs sooner after birth in near-term and term infants when compared with premature infants.

  d. Near-term and term infants with NEC are more likely to require surgical intervention than premature infants.

  e. Near-term and term infants rarely develop a spontaneous intestinal perforation (SIP) if there are no risk factors for intestinal hypoperfusion, such as indomethacin exposure.

5-40. Which of the following statements is correct based on the studies currently available about prevention of necrotizing enterocolitis?

  a. Exposure to antenatal steroids is associated with a decreased risk of necrotizing enterocolitis in premature infants.

  b. Intermittent increases in metabolic demand from bolus feeding put very-low-birth-weight infants at risk for necrotizing enterocolitis.

  c. When compared with formula, feeding with maternal breast milk protects against necrotizing enterocolitis, but feeding with donor breast milk confers a risk similar to feeding with formula.

  d. Rapid advancement of enteral feeding in premature, very-low-birth-weight infants increases the risk of necrotizing enterocolitis.

  e. Dosing of probiotic strains for the prevention of NEC has been standardized internationally and requires a minimum of 1.0×10^{10} colony-forming units/day.

5-41. Which of the following interventions decreases an infant's risk of developing germinal matrix/intraventricular hemorrhage (IVH)?

  a. Antenatal administration of phenobarbital

  b. Postnatal administration of glucocorticoids

  c. Postnatal infusion of fresh frozen plasma

  d. Treatment of maternal chorioamnionitis with antibiotics

  e. Rapid correction of hypotension with fluid boluses

5-42. A newborn female presents for a weight check a few days after discharge from the neonatal intensive care unit. She was born at 35 4/7 weeks' gestation, weighing 2570 g. The mother, a 27-year-old unemployed woman, had good prenatal care. She developed preterm labor on the day of her daughter's birth, and delivered vaginally shortly after rupture of membranes. She was admitted to the neonatal intensive care unit for transient tachypnea of the newborn, which resolved by 12 hours of life. Antibiotics were started on admission, but discontinued after 48 hours when blood cultures were negative. She was initially slow with oral feeding, but took an adequate amount prior to discharge.

The mother has been reading about prematurity and neurodevelopment on the Internet, and she asks the general pediatrician what to expect for her daughter.

Which of the following statements is accurate regarding outcomes of premature infants later in life?

  a. Since her infant was almost 36 weeks' gestation at delivery, she does not need to worry about neurodevelopmental problems.

  b. Determination of her daughter's need for special assistance in school (due to intellectual disability) will be evident by her daughter's third birthday.

  c. Her daughter is at risk for risk-taking behavior as a teenager due to her prematurity.

  d. If the baby's birth weight had been less than 1500 g, she would have been extremely unlikely to graduate from high school.

  e. Preterm children are more likely to have language disorders, reading disability, and difficulty with arithmetic.

5-43. The Obstetrics attending asks the Neonatology attending to counsel a 36-year-old female who presented to the Labor and Delivery (L&D) suite in active labor. The patient reported to the L&D nurse that she is "at full term." The patient received prenatal care in a community clinic, including a dating ultrasound at 10 weeks' gestation. After a normal ultrasound at 20 weeks' gestation, she was told that she didn't require additional follow-up. The patient reports that she has been taking her prenatal vitamins and that her fetus has remained active. The obstetrician is concerned that the patient's fundal height is only 33 cm and the fetus must be more premature than 36 weeks' gestation or significantly growth restricted.

Which of the following statements is correct and should be included in the consultation with the mother?

a. For a low-birth-weight infant, the likelihood of developing serious neonatal complications is primarily related to size at delivery, not gestational age.

b. If there has been growth restriction in utero that has affected the body, but has spared the head, her child's cognitive outcome should not be adversely affected.

c. If there has been growth restriction due to uteroplacental insufficiency, her child will have a greater risk for developing hypertension and diabetes as an adult.

d. Since third-trimester intrauterine growth restriction (IUGR) stimulates a response that interferes with fetal lung maturation, her baby must be intubated in the delivery room.

e. If sent to a pathologist within 6 hours of delivery, the placenta, on gross examination, will provide definitive information about the reason for IUGR.

5-44. A 4325-g term infant born with meconium aspiration syndrome has severe hypoxic respiratory failure. Despite aggressive management with high-frequency ventilation, inhaled nitric oxide, and phosphodiesterase inhibitors, stable oxygenation cannot be achieved. The NICU team decides to utilize extracorporeal membrane oxygenation (ECMO) for this infant.

Which of the following statements regarding the outcomes of neonates treated with ECMO is correct?

a. The increased frequency of treatment of neonatal hypoxic respiratory failure with ECMO has resulted in a decrease in ECMO complications and better survival.

b. Neonates who require treatment with ECMO for neonatal hypoxic respiratory failure have a risk of neurodevelopmental impairment that is significantly greater than neonates who respond to conventional therapy (including high-frequency ventilation) and inhaled nitric oxide.

c. The most common cause of mortality in infants treated with ECMO for hypoxic respiratory failure is hemorrhage.

d. The risk of hearing impairment in extremely premature infants is significantly greater than in term infants with respiratory and other organ failure.

e. Survival rate for infants treated with ECMO in the United States is less than 50%.

5-45. Which of the following statements is correct about neurodevelopmental impairment in premature infants?

a. It is possible to diagnose a major neurodevelopmental impairment prior to NICU discharge based on brain MRI and abnormalities on serial neurologic examinations.

b. Detection of abnormalities on magnetic resonance imaging (MRI) of the brain is the "gold standard" for predicting major neurodevelopmental disabilities.

c. More than half of the premature survivors who were born at the limit of viability, prior to 26 weeks' gestation, develop intellectual disability, cerebral palsy, or both.

d. Complications of prematurity including chronic lung disease, sepsis, and necrotizing enterocolitis confer additional risk for problems with neurodevelopment above the risk of prematurity.

e. The most common type of cerebral palsy in premature survivors born at the limit of viability is spastic hemiplegia.

5-46. Which of the following statements regarding the cardiorespiratory transition from intrauterine to extrauterine life is correct?

a. Compliance in the neonatal lung decreases due to fluid shifts.

b. Surfactant is released into the alveolar space via lung inflation and increased blood catecholamine levels.

c. Pulmonary vascular resistance increases in response to increased arterial oxygen tension.

d. Clearance of fetal lung fluid occurs primarily through egress via the trachea.

e. Neonatal blood flow pattern is unchanged from the fetal blood flow pattern.

5-47. A premature male infant born at 26 1/7 weeks' gestation has a cranial ultrasound performed at 4 days of age. The study shows a hemorrhage limited to the right germinal matrix.

Which of the following statements is correct regarding this patient's management/outcome?

a. Since the hemorrhage is limited to the germinal matrix/subependymal area, additional brain imaging is not necessary for several weeks.

b. Male infants with germinal matrix/intraventricular hemorrhages are less likely to have neurologic sequelae than female infants.

c. Since the hemorrhage is limited to the germinal matrix/subependymal area, the infant's development should be normal.

d. Cranial ultrasound should be repeated within the first week of life due to an increased risk of a primary hemorrhage into the left germinal matrix.

e. Cranial ultrasound should be repeated within the first week of life, as the hemorrhage in the right germinal matrix may extend into the ventricles.

5-48. Which of the following infants is at *highest risk* of developing a germinal matrix–intraventricular hemorrhage (GM-IVH)?

a. A term male infant born by vacuum-assisted vaginal delivery who required intubation, positive pressure ventilation, and chest compressions in the delivery room

b. A 20-day-old male infant born at 24 weeks' gestation who develops hypotension from a patent ductus arteriosus

c. A female infant born at 26 weeks' gestation by precipitous vaginal delivery who develops hyperoxia and hypocarbia after intubation and surfactant administration in the delivery room

d. A male infant born by cesarean section at 34 weeks' gestation who required positive pressure ventilation in the delivery room

e. A female infant born at 28 weeks' gestation (due to maternal chorioamnionitis) who develops a right-sided tension pneumothorax after reintubation at 17 days of age

5-49. A male infant born at 25 2/7 weeks' gestation (birth weight 800 g) develops tachycardia and abdominal distension prior to passing a blood-tinged stool. His physical examination reveals decreased tone and activity, tenderness on palpation of the abdomen, and a paucity of bowel sounds. His abdominal x-ray shows diffuse pneumatosis without pneumoperitoneum or portal venous air. His parents arrive during initial stabilization of their infant and ask to speak to the attending neonatologist.

Which of the following statement regarding this infant's condition is correct?

a. Because of his abdominal findings, the infant likely has hypersensitivity to mother's breast milk, and she should stop pumping.

b. Unless intestinal perforation occurs, their infant's risk for growth failure is not significantly increased as a result of this condition.

c. Their infant is unlikely to develop an intestinal stricture if there is no bowel perforation.

d. This condition puts their infant at increased risk for neurodevelopmental impairment.

e. The incidence of this condition is inversely related to gestational age and birth weight, but these characteristics do not increase the risk of mortality.

5-50. A 1460-g male infant is delivered by cesarean section after a 30 1/7 weeks' gestation to a 29-year-old woman with acute lymphoblastic leukemia. The infant is placed on the delivery room table. Drying the skin and suctioning the oropharynx is initiated, followed by positive pressure ventilation (PPV). After 20 seconds of PPV, the neonatal nurse notes that the infant has a heart rate of 40 beats/min and no chest wall movement.

Which of the following interventions is indicated at this time in the resuscitation?

a. Flexion of the head and neck

b. Confirmation of an appropriate seal of the face mask

c. Intravenous infusion of 10 cm³/kg of normal saline

d. External cardioversion

e. Intravenous infusion of 0.1 mg/kg of 1:10,000 epinephrine solution

5-51. A 3690-g male infant was born vaginally after a 38 6/7 weeks' gestation. The pregnancy was notable for polyhydramnios. He required only suctioning, drying, and stimulation in the delivery room. He passed meconium on the delivery room table. Apgar scores were 8 and 9 at 1 and 5 minutes, respectively.

At 6 hours of age, the mother tells the postpartum nurse that the baby is "spitty" with feeding. The nurse notes the infant has copious clear secretions from the mouth. The nasopharynx and oropharynx appear normal on physical examination. A large-bore nasogastric tube is placed; a subsequent chest x-ray shows the tube ending at the level of the sixth cervical vertebrae.

The most appropriate initial step in management of this neonate is:

a. Intravenous antibiotics

b. Barium enema

c. Oral airway placement

d. Suction applied to the nasogastric tube

e. Contrast study of the upper gastrointestinal tract

5-52. Which of the following statements regarding fetal cortisol is correct?

    a. Steroidogenic enzymes present in the adult adrenal gland are absent in the fetal adrenal gland.

    b. Fetal cortisol is necessary for normal intrauterine development.

    c. Circulating fetal cortisol peaks during the middle of the first trimester of development.

    d. Most of the circulating fetal cortisol is derived from the maternal adrenal gland.

    e. Elevated fetal cortisol levels in the third trimester assist in neonatal respiratory adaptation.

5-53. A 4950-g female neonate is delivered vaginally after a 38 6/7 weeks' gestation complicated by poorly controlled type 2 diabetes. The obstetrician reported shoulder dystocia during the delivery. On examination at 4 hours of age, the baby's left arm is internally rotated, and the forearm is extended and pronated. The baby does not move her left arm when the examiner assesses the Moro reflex.

Which of the following physical examination findings is most associated with the findings in the arm?

    a. An absent left thumb

    b. A hyperpigmented patch on the left chest

    c. A 2-vessel umbilical cord

    d. A constricted left pupil

    e. An enlarged left fifth finger

5-54. Which of the following neonates should receive hepatitis B immune globulin within 12 hours after birth?

    a. A 38 weeks' gestation neonate (birth weight 3600 g) whose mother is hepatitis B surface antigen (HBsAg) negative

    b. A 39 weeks' gestation neonate (birth weight 3750 g) whose mother has HBsAg serology that is unknown, but will be confirmed within 24 hours after delivery

    c. A 37 weeks' gestation neonate (birth weight 3550 g) whose mother is positive for hepatitis C antibody only

    d. A 34 weeks' gestation neonate (birth weight 2500 g) whose mother is HBsAg negative but developed chorioamnionitis in labor

    e. A 36 weeks' gestation neonate (birth weight 1850 g) whose mother has HBsAg serology that cannot be resulted until 36 hours after delivery

5-55. A 4885-g female infant was delivered via cesarean section due to cephalopelvic disproportion after a 40 3/7 weeks' gestation. Maternal serologies were unremarkable, and cultures (including a cervical culture

for group B *Streptococcus* at 36 weeks' gestation) were negative. The mother has a 10-year history of poorly controlled type 2 diabetes mellitus.

The baby only required brief blow-by oxygen in the delivery suite. The infant's Apgar scores were 8 and 9 at 1 and 5 minutes, respectively. Her initial newborn examination was normal.

The neonate fed well in the term nursery after birth. At 60 hours of age, she developed rhythmic, generalized jerking of her head and extremities. After the ictal event, vital signs and the physical examination were unremarkable, and a capillary glucose was 69 mg/dL.

Which of the following tests should be ordered to evaluate this infant?

    a. Serum calcium level

    b. Serum sodium level

    c. Serum C-reactive protein

    d. Computerized tomography (CT) scan of the head

    e. Magnetic resonance imaging (MRI) of the head

5-56. A 3440-g male neonate is delivered vaginally after a 39 6/7 weeks' gestation complicated by fetal bradycardia. On arrival at the delivery room table, the baby has no respiratory effort or spontaneous movement. He is covered in particulate meconium. The nurse palpates the pulse in the umbilical cord stump and detects 5 beats in 6 seconds.

Which of the following steps is next indicated in resuscitation of this neonate?

    a. Initiation of chest compressions

    b. Placement of a 5 French nasogastric tube

    c. Suctioning of the mouth and nose with a bulb syringe

    d. Catheterization of the umbilical vein

    e. Intubation and suctioning the trachea

5-57. A 2-day-old term female neonate is undergoing her discharge physical examination in the nursery. On exam, you note the liver edge 1 cm below the right costal margin and the spleen tip is not palpable. The umbilical stump is dry. Bowel sounds are audible in the abdomen. When the infant cries, you note that there is a slight distention of the abdominal space between the rectus abdominis muscles.

Which of the following steps is indicated for this infant?

    a. Order a liver and gallbladder ultrasound

    b. Discharge the baby home with her parents

    c. Obtain a peripheral blood smear

    d. Order a voiding cystourethrogram

    e. Consult a pediatric surgeon

5-58. A 27-year-old woman brings her 3-year-old son into your office for a well-child care visit. The child had documented intrauterine growth restriction (IUGR), and weighed 1990 g at birth (at 39 1/7 weeks' gestation). The mother is currently 8 weeks pregnant and wants to decrease the risk of fetal growth restriction during her current gestation. She has no acute or chronic medical problems. She smokes 0.5 pack of cigarettes per week.

Which of the following interventions would reduce the likelihood of fetal growth restriction during this pregnancy?

  a. Consumption of 4 oz of red wine daily

  b. Avoiding food rich in β-carotene

  c. Initiation of a strict vegan diet

  d. Dietary supplementation with folic acid

  e. Cessation of cigarette smoking

5-59. Which of the following statements regarding neonatal and infant mortality is correct?

  a. Infant mortality rates are higher for infants of pregnancies where prenatal care commences in the first trimester.

  b. Asian or Pacific Islander ethnicity is a risk factor for infant mortality.

  c. The introduction of surfactant therapy and antenatal steroids has reduced neonatal mortality.

  d. Female sex is a risk factor for neonatal mortality.

  e. Neonatal mortality for low-birth-weight infants is reduced in high-care-level, low-volume neonatal intensive care units (NICUs).

5-60. Which of the following neonates is most likely to experience a normal anion gap metabolic acidosis?

  a. A 2-day-old term male with weak femoral pulses (relative to brachial pulses) and a serum lactate of 5.9 mmol/L

  b. A 3-day-old female born at 24 4/7 weeks' gestation with bounding palmar pulses and a serum creatinine of 1.8 mg/dL

  c. A 1-day-old male born at 28 1/7 weeks' gestation with mild respiratory distress syndrome and an initial urine pH of 7.5

  d. A 4-day-old term female male with lethargy and a serum lactate of 1.2 mmol/L

  e. A 5-day-old infant born at 32 2/7 weeks' gestation with hypotension and a blood culture positive for gram-negative rods

5-61. A 28-day-old male presents to his pediatrician's office with a 1-week history of intermittent vomiting and alternating irritability and lethargy. He was delivered vaginally (with assistance of forceps) after a 40 4/7 weeks' gestation complicated by fetal bradycardia. His discharge physical was notable for marked bruising. On examination, he is afebrile with a normal cardiorespiratory examination. He has well-circumscribed, indurated nodules over the cheeks at the site of forceps placement.

Which of the following laboratory values is most associated with this infant's presentation?

  a. A serum glucose of 29 mg/dL

  b. A serum ammonia of 135 μmol/L

  c. A serum lactate of 5.0 mmol/L

  d. A serum calcium of 13.1 mg/dL

  e. A serum urea nitrogen of 1.8 mg/dL

5-62. A 28 3/7–week male was born by cesarean section due to worsening maternal preeclampsia. Due to respiratory distress in the delivery room, he is intubated and placed on mechanical ventilation.

At 6 hours of age, the infant develops mottling of the skin, tachycardia, and desaturations (measured by bedside pulse oximetry). A stat echocardiogram shows a structurally normal heart with a patent ductus arteriosus.

Which of the following interventions would improve the infant's blood pressure?

  a. Initiation of an intravenous prostaglandin E1 (PGE1) infusion

  b. Increase in the infant's peak end-expiratory pressure (PEEP) on the ventilator

  c. Increase in the infant's peak inspiratory pressure (PIP) on the ventilator

  d. Initiation of an intravenous immune globulin infusion

  e. Initiation of an intravenous dopamine infusion

5-63. A 1900-g male infant is delivered by C-section after a 29 1/7 weeks' gestation secondary to fetal supraventricular tachycardia (SVT) and progressive hydrops fetalis. The infant is placed on the delivery room table, and positive pressure ventilation (PPV) begins after drying the skin and suctioning the oropharynx. Physical examination is notable for diffuse anasarca. After 4 minutes of PPV, the nurse notes the neonate has a heart rate of 190 beats/min, central cyanosis, and intercostal retractions.

Which of the following steps is indicated at this point in the resuscitation?

  a. Infusion of 0.3 mg/kg of 1:10,000 epinephrine solution via an umbilical venous catheter

  b. Endotracheal intubation and ventilation using a T-piece resuscitator

  c. Weaning the infant to blow-by oxygen

  d. Infusion of 0.1 mg/kg of adenosine via an umbilical venous catheter

  e. Weaning the infant to nasal cannula

5-64. Which of the following statements regarding thermoregulation in neonate is correct?

  a. Heat production in the neonate (controlling for body weight) is greater than heat production in the adult.

  b. Heat production in the neonate (relative to body weight) must be lower in the neonate to maintain a normal body temperature.

  c. The capacity for neonatal adaptation to cold stress is similar to that of an adult.

  d. Brown fat stores are less abundant in the neonate than in the adult.

  e. Circulating free fatty acids serve as an acute source of energy during cold stress in the neonate.

5-65. You are asked by the obstetrical service to counsel a 25-year-old primigravida woman who is experiencing preterm labor. Her pregnancy is notable for a twin gestation.

  Which of the following statements is true regarding multiple births?

  a. Twin–twin transfusion syndrome usually occurs in dizygotic pregnancies as compared with monozygotic pregnancies.

  b. Most infants born following multifetal gestations are premature.

  c. The rate of multiple births has remained stable over recent decades.

  d. Fetuses of twin pregnancies are more likely to be born in a vertex position as compared with fetuses of singleton pregnancies.

  e. Monozygotic twins account for two thirds of all spontaneous twin births.

5-66. A newborn infant is born at 26 6/7 weeks' gestation following a spontaneous vaginal delivery. Resuscitative efforts include warming, and drying the infant followed by clearing and positioning the airway. The infant developed spontaneous respiratory effort within 1 minute of life. However, he develops intercostal retractions, minimal air entry on auscultation, grunting, and decreased tone. He then develops apnea, cyanosis, and bradycardia (heart rate of 80 beats/min). Positive pressure ventilation is given via self-inflating bag and face mask, but the infant remains apneic.

  Which is the most appropriate next step in the management of this infant?

  a. Administration of continuous positive airway pressure (CPAP) via nasal prongs

  b. Needle decompression of the right hemithorax

  c. Provision of supplemental oxygen via nasal cannula

  d. Endotracheal intubation for mechanical ventilation and surfactant administration

  e. Administration of inhaled nitric oxide

5-67. A 30-day-old infant was born at 24 4/7 weeks' gestation. Until today, she had been intubated and ventilated using the synchronized intermittent mandatory ventilation (SIMV) mode. Based on improved blood gases, she was extubated 12 hours ago to room air. In the last 20 minutes, she has developed nasal flaring and intermittent subcostal retractions. Her current blood gas shows a pH of 7.34 and a pco_2 of 56 mm Hg. Her pulse oxygen saturations have decreased to 82%. Her chest radiograph reveals a normal cardiothymic silhouette, decreased lung expansion, and air bronchograms.

  What is the most appropriate next step in the management of this patient?

  a. Endotracheal intubation and synchronized intermittent mandatory ventilation (SIMV)

  b. Provision of supplemental oxygen via nasal cannula

  c. Administration of continuous positive airway pressure (CPAP) via nasal prongs

  d. Endotracheal intubation and high-frequency ventilation (HFV)

  e. Repeat blood gas sampling in 1 hour

5-68. A 4-day-old term neonate with congenital pneumonia is being mechanically ventilated for respiratory failure. He is ventilated using the synchronized intermittent mandatory ventilation (SIMV) mode. His settings are:

  Positive inspiratory pressure—19 mm Hg

  Positive end-expiratory pressure—5 mm Hg

  Rate—25 breaths/min

  For the past several hours you notice that the ventilator is displaying wide variability in measured tidal volumes. His most recent arterial blood gas shows a pH of 7.5 and pco_2 of 30 mm Hg. On the same ventilator settings, the previous arterial blood gas had a pH of 7.3 and pco_2 of 51 mm Hg.

  What is the most appropriate next step in the management of this patient?

  a. Change the mode to intermittent mandatory ventilation.

  b. Add pressure support of 10 mm Hg to his current ventilator settings.

  c. Change the mode to assist control ventilation.

  d. Change the mode to high-frequency oscillation ventilation.

  e. Change the mode to volume-targeted ventilation.

5-69. A term 3-day-old infant was born through meconium-stained amniotic fluid. Following aspiration of meconium, the infant developed respiratory failure. On current examination, he has a systolic murmur and a loud second heart sound. His chest radiograph reveals a hyperlucent background in addition to patchy areas of opacity. Despite the use of high-frequency oscillation and an inspired oxygen fraction of 1.0, the postductal pulse oximeter does not read above 90%.

Which of the following treatment options is most likely to be effective in addressing the underlying pathophysiology?

a. Permissive hypercarbia

b. Diuretic therapy

c. Inhaled nitric oxide

d. Opiate therapy

e. Albuterol

5-70. A 1-week-old infant born at 23 6/7 weeks' gestation has developed sudden onset of hypotension and tachycardia. She is mechanically ventilated, has been NPO since birth, and recently completed a course of antibiotics and hydrocortisone for septic shock. Prenatal history is notable for intrauterine growth restriction and perinatal indomethacin exposure for preterm labor. On examination, she has abdominal distention and guarding, lethargy, and hypoperfusion. Chest and abdominal x-rays reveal pulmonary edema and a pneumoperitoneum. There is no pneumatosis intestinalis or portal venous gas noted.

Which of the following is the most likely etiology of the infant's acute decompensation?

a. Necrotizing enterocolitis (NEC)

b. Cow's milk protein allergy

c. Spontaneous intestinal perforation (SIP)

d. Volvulus

e. Duodenal atresia

5-71. A term infant was born to a 26-year-old, gravida 7 woman at home following a precipitous delivery. When the emergency medical team arrived, the infant was vigorous but still attached to the placenta. The infant was transported to a local hospital where his physical examination was normal. Several hours later, the infant develops irritability and poor feeding. On examination, he is tachypneic and lethargic. The remainder of the examination is within normal limits.

Which of the following tests should be ordered first in evaluating this infant?

a. Hematocrit

b. Cranial sonogram

c. Thyroid-stimulating hormone level

d. Stool occult blood test

e. Chest radiograph

5-72. You are seeing a 3-day-old Korean male infant in your clinic for the first time since his hospital discharge. He was born by spontaneous vaginal delivery at 36 2/7 weeks' gestation to a 25-year-old woman with negative prenatal serologies. The pregnancy, delivery, and postpartum admission were uncomplicated. He has been breast-feeding every 1 to 2 hours, but his weight on your examination has decreased 12% from birth weight. The remainder of his examination is unremarkable.

Which screening test is most important to perform at this visit?

a. Hemoglobin level

b. Vitamin D level

c. C-reactive protein

d. Serum lead level

e. Total serum bilirubin level

5-73. A 2-day-old infant born at 35 1/7 weeks' gestation to a diabetic mother presents to your office with jaundice. She is breast-feeding every 2 hours, has wet diapers with every feed, and has passed at least 1 meconium stool. Vital signs include weight decreased 2% from birth weight, a rectal temperature of 37.4°C, heart rate of 147 beats/min, respirations of 50 breaths/min, and blood pressure of 45/28 mm Hg. Her anterior fontanelle is soft and flat. She is alert with appropriate tone, and is icteric to her mid-calf. Her total serum bilirubin (TSB) level is 14.0 mg/dL, and direct bilirubin level is 0.4 mg/dL at 48 hours of life.

Which of the following is the appropriate management of this infant's hyperbilirubinemia?

a. Administer intravenous immunoglobulin (IV Ig).

b. Initiate phototherapy, continue breast-feeding, and recheck TSB level in 4 hours.

c. Initiate phototherapy, replace breast-feeding with formula feeding, and recheck TSB in 4 hours.

d. Initiate phototherapy, discontinue breast-feeding, initiate IV hydration, and recheck TSB in 4 hours.

e. Place central arterial and venous catheters for exchange transfusion.

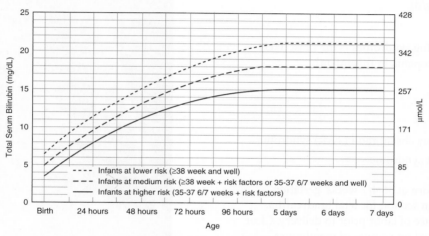

- Use total bilirubin. Do not subtract direct-reacting or conjugated blirubin.
- Risk factors : isoimmune hemolytic disease, G6PD deficiency, asphyxia, significant lethargy, temperature instability, sepsis, acidosis, or albumin <3.0 g/dL (if measured).
- For well infants 35-37 6/7 weeks can adjust TSB levels for intervention around the medium-risk line. It is an option to intervene at lower TSB levels for infants closer to 35 weeks and at higher TSB levels for those closer to 37 6/7 weeks.
- It is an option to provide conventional phototherapy in hospital or at home at TSB levels 2-3 mg/dL (35-50 mmol/L) below those shown, but home phototherapy should not be used in any infant with risk factors.

(Reproduced, with permission, from Subcommittee on Hyperbilirubinemia. Management of hyperbilirubinemia in the newborn infant 35 or more weeks of gestation. *Pediatrics.* 2004;114:297–316.)

5-74. A 24-year-old, gravida 2, para 1 Hispanic woman is being seen for the first time for prenatal care. Her previous delivery occurred in El Salvador, and she has recently immigrated to the United Stated for this delivery. Based on her last menstrual period, the pregnancy is dated at 34 0/7 weeks' gestation. Ultrasound examination of the fetus reveals thickened subcutaneous tissue and fluid in the pleural cavity. Sampling of the amniotic fluid is significant for bile pigment, and percutaneous umbilical blood sampling shows fetal anemia.

Which of the following is the most likely cause of this infant's presentation?

a. Human parvovirus B19

b. Cytomegalovirus

c. Rh antibody exposure

d. Complex congenital heart disease

e. Supraventricular tachycardia

5-75. A 2-week-old infant presents to the pediatrician with a large reddish blue mass under the lower middle aspect of the abdomen, measuring 3 cm × 4 cm. According to her mother, the lesion was noticed after discharge home from the nursery, but has enlarged over the past 2 weeks. The mass is nontender and warm, and a bruit is heard on auscultation of the overlying skin. The infant is vigorous with normal vital signs and strong lower extremity pulses. There is no hepatosplenomegaly, pallor, or petechiae. The results of her complete blood count are:

White blood cells—15,000/μL

Hemoglobin—11.5 g/dL

Platelets—19,000/μL

Which of the following syndromes is the most likely cause of thrombocytopenia in this infant?

a. Trisomy 13

b. Trisomy 18

c. Fanconi anemia

d. Thrombocytopenia absent radii (TAR) syndrome

e. Kasabach-Merritt syndrome

5-76. A male infant was born at 36 4/7 weeks' gestation by emergent cesarean section for fetal bradycardia. There was no evidence of labor prior to delivery. Clear amniotic fluid is noted on rupture of membranes during the operative delivery. The infant's Apgars were 9 and 9 at 1 and 5 minutes, respectively. However, he developed grunting and tachypnea approximately 30 minutes after birth. On current examination, his respiratory rate is 70 breaths/min and the preductal and postductal pulse oximeters read 97% while he is breathing room air. His physical examination is otherwise normal. A chest radiograph demonstrates prominent vascular markings, an opacity in the transverse fissure, and flattening of the diaphragms. An arterial blood gas reveals:

pH—7.46

pco$_2$—34 mm Hg

Pao$_2$—89 mm Hg

HCO$_3$—24 mEq/L

Which of the following mechanisms is most likely responsible for this infant's respiratory distress?

a. Evolving chemical pneumonitis

b. Delayed sodium transport across the alveolar apical and basolateral cell membranes

c. Ascending infection through the birth canal

d. Increased pulmonary vascular tone

e. Increased alveolar surface tension

5-77. A 2-week-old female infant was born at 24 1/7 weeks' gestation. She has significant respiratory insufficiency secondary to surfactant deficiency and is currently intubated and on high-frequency mechanical ventilation. Chest x-rays have persistently demonstrated diffuse pulmonary interstitial emphysema. Early this morning, she abruptly became tachypneic and agitated. On examination, she is tachycardic and hypotensive, and the cardiac impulse (PMI) is shifted to the right, with diminished breath sounds over the left chest. Her chest x-ray is shown below:

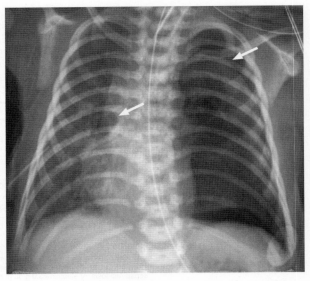

(Reproduced, with permission, from Rudolph CD, Rudolph A, Lister G, First L, Gershon A. *Rudolph's Pediatrics.* 22nd ed. New York: McGraw-Hill, 2011.)

Which of the following is the most appropriate next step in the management of this patient?

a. Decompressing the left hemithorax with an angiocatheter, followed by chest tube placement

b. Repositioning the endotracheal tube

c. Inserting a nasogastric tube and aspirating gastric air and fluid

d. Increasing mean airway pressure on the ventilator

e. Performing an emergent pericardiocentesis

5-78. A 23-year-old primigravida woman presented to Labor and Delivery today for decreased fetal movement. Her pregnancy history was significant for chronic ibuprofen use to treat low back pain in the third trimester. Nonstress testing revealed nonreassuring fetal heart tones, and the woman underwent an emergent cesarean section. Thirty minutes following delivery, the baby has tachypnea, nasal flaring, and grunting. His preductal and postductal pulse oximeter readings are 97% and 86%, respectively. His chest x-ray shows hyperlucent lung fields and an enlarged cardiothymic silhouette. A postductal arterial blood gas on room air demonstrates the following values:

pH—7.30

pco_2—37 mm Hg

Pao_2—55 mm Hg

HCO_3—19 mEq/L

Which of the following tests is the preferred method to confirm this patient's diagnosis?

   a. Echocardiography with Doppler studies

   b. Serial blood gas sampling

   c. Pulse oximetry

   d. Tracheal aspirate for bacterial culture

   e. Arterial blood sample for bacterial culture

5-79. In which of the following scenarios is pulmonary hemorrhage most frequently associated?

   a. A term 2-day-old born following maternal cocaine use

   b. A term 2-day-old with sepsis

   c. A term 2-day-old born with perinatal depression

   d. A preterm 2-day-old with a patent ductus arteriosis

   e. A term 1-month-old with congenital heart disease

5-80. A 3-day-old infant born at 25 weeks' gestation is undergoing high-frequency oscillatory ventilation for respiratory insufficiency. Her x-rays since birth have demonstrated a diffuse reticulogranular pattern with low lung volumes. Approximately 2 hours after administration of exogenous surfactant, she developed pallor, bradycardia, and a bloody nasal discharge. A chest x-ray now reveals patchy infiltrates throughout the lung fields. Abruptly, her pulse oximeter saturations decline.

What is the first step in the management of this patient?

   a. Suction and secure the airway.

   b. Transfuse packed red blood cells.

   c. Transfuse platelets.

   d. Increase the mean airway pressure.

   e. Administer indomethacin.

ANSWERS

Answer 5-1. e

Early vitamin K deficiency bleeding (VKDB), previously known as hemorrhagic disease of the newborn (HDN), is caused by inadequate levels of active vitamin K–dependent clotting factors (factors II, VII, IX, and X) and has an incidence that has been reported as high as 1.7% (AAP, 2003). VKDB can result in intracranial, gastrointestinal, or generalized bleeding in the neonate. Due to limited neonatal stores at birth and supplies from enteral sources (including breast milk), vitamin K supplementation is necessary to prevent neonatal hemorrhage.

A single 1-mg dose of intramuscular vitamin K in the first few hours of life will prevent VKDB. Some parents request oral vitamin K administration (in lieu of an intramuscular injection). Oral administration of the intramuscular formulation by mouth is safe. However, although a single 2-mg oral dose of vitamin K will prevent VKDB for a few days, the effect will be transient and the dose must be repeated in early infancy. Guidelines for sequential oral dosing of vitamin K vary. Some physicians recommend a second dose at 6 to 8 months of age; others recommend weekly dosing while breast-feeding. Failure of vitamin K therapy to prevent VKDB has been reported, and is associated with noncompliance with therapy (Srehle, 2010; Doran, 1995). In addition, newborns receiving incomplete oral prophylaxis have a higher risk of developing VKDB.

In 1993, the Vitamin K Ad Hoc Task Force of the American Academy of Pediatrics (AAP) reviewed concerns about the association of intramuscular vitamin K injection and the incidence of childhood leukemia. The committee concluded that there was no association between the intramuscular administration of vitamin K and childhood leukemia or other cancers. This conclusion has been supported by several subsequent case–control studies (AAP, 2003).

(Page 186, Section 5: Newborn)

American Academy of Pediatrics Committee on the Fetus and the Newborn. Controversies concerning vitamin K and the newborn. *Pediatrics.* 2003;112:191–192.

Doran O, Austin NC, Taylor BJ. Vitamin K administration in neonates: survey of compliance with recommended practices in the Dunedin area. *N Z Med J.* 1995;108:337–339.

Srehle EM, Howey C, Jones R. Evaluation of the acceptability of a new oral vitamin K prophylaxis for breastfed infants. *Acta Paediatr.* 2010;99:379–383.

Answer 5-2. c

The neonate in this vignette has physical examination findings consistent with a congenital diaphragmatic hernia (CDH). This is a rare condition with an overall incidence of 1 in 2500 births. The large majority of cases are detected by routine prenatal ultrasound. The majority of CDHs (roughly 85%) occur on the left side through a posteriolateral defect (Bochdalek hernia).

Infants with CDH develop respiratory failure due to pulmonary hypoplasia (decreased lung volume on the affected side) and pulmonary hypertension (due to abnormal pulmonary vascular development). Other examination findings include a scaphoid abdomen (due to displacement of the peritoneal contents into the thorax) and displacement of the heart to the midline.

Initial management involves decompression of the stomach with a nasogastric tube (to reduce gastric distention impacting thoracic and mediastinal contents [heart and great vessels]). Subsequent respiratory management should include endotracheal intubation. Positive pressure ventilation with a T-piece resuscitator (a flow-controlled resuscitation device with adjustable peak inspiratory and positive end-expiratory pressures) or a bag and mask will insufflate the stomach and may impair respiratory function. Transillumination or needle decompression of a normal right hemithorax is not indicated in this case.

(Page 257, Section 5: Newborn)

Answer 5-3. b

The infant in this vignette has a cephalohematoma, which is a subperiostial hemorrhage often associated with trauma during labor (see figure). The hemorrhage presents hours after delivery as a fluctuant mass over the affected skull bone (often the parietal or occipital bone). The hemorrhage is limited by the periosteum of the skull bone and, as a result, does not extend beyond the suture lines. Blood loss is minimal, and affected infants usually do not require transfusion of blood products. The most common neonatal complication is hyperbilirubinemia due to the breakdown of the extravasated blood. In the absence of localized or systemic infection, antibiotics should not be administered. Needle aspiration of the hematoma is not indicated and may introduce skin flora into the hematoma, resulting in infection of the mass and surrounding skin.

A cephalohematoma should be distinguished from 2 other entities (see figure). A caput succedaneum is edema of the scalp and tends to cross suture lines. A subgaleal hemorrhage is bleeding between the galea aponeurotica and the skull. This condition can lead to extensive hemorrhage and shock. As a result, this is an emergency situation requiring close monitoring, as well as potential replacement of blood and clotting products.

(Page 177, Chapter 5: The Newborn)

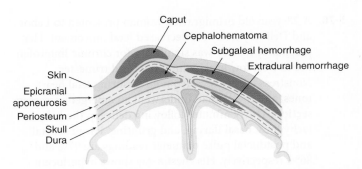

(Reproduced, with permission, from Hay W, Levin M, Deterding R, Abzug M. *Current Diagnosis & Treatment Pediatrics*. 21st ed. New York: McGraw-Hill, 2012.)

Answer 5-4. d

Most IDMs are macrosomic, which is defined as a birth weight greater than the 90th percentile for gestational age or over 4000 g. This increased body weight is a result of deposition of fuel sources, resulting in increased body fat and mass of visceral organs, including the heart.

HCM involves overgrowth of the intraventricular septum and 1 or both ventricular walls, leading to ventricular outflow tract obstruction. Due to this ventricular outflow tract obstruction coupled with decreased myocardial function, the neonate with HCM has decreased cardiac output and may develop congestive heart failure.

Insulin, not GH, represents the primary anabolic fetal growth factor. Excess glycogen and fat deposition occurs in the presence of insulin and high glucose levels, and this fat is primarily deposited in the abdomen and subscapular areas, putting these infants at risk for shoulder dystocia. However, this excess growth does not affect skeletal muscle, leading IDMs to have higher weight percentiles at birth relative to length and head circumference.

Interestingly, not all IDMs are macrosomic. In women with pregestational diabetes and associated nephropathy, retinopathy, or chronic hypertension, placental insufficiency may occur. The placental insufficiency limits nutrient and oxygen delivery, which can result in a small-for-gestational-age (SGA) infant.

(Page 196-197, Section 5: Newborn)

Answer 5-5. a

The neonate in this vignette has examination findings consistent with bilateral choanal atresia. The etiology is due to a persistence of a bony septum (90%) or a soft tissue membrane (10%) (see figure below).

This condition is an emergency situation in neonates (who are obligate nose breathers). Placement of an oral airway and/or putting the baby in a prone position at the time of clinical presentation will bypass the nasal obstruction and allow for air exchange.

Neither supplemental oxygen and pressure (via nasal cannula or CPAP) nor intranasal steroids will overcome the anatomic obstruction. While unilateral atresia can generally be delayed until the child is 1 to 2 years of age, bilateral choanal atresia requires prompt repair.

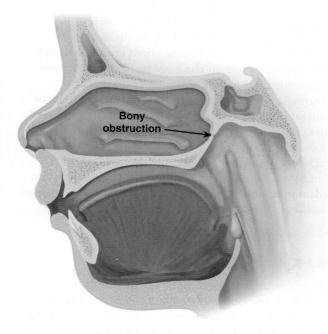

(Page 256, Section 5: Newborn)

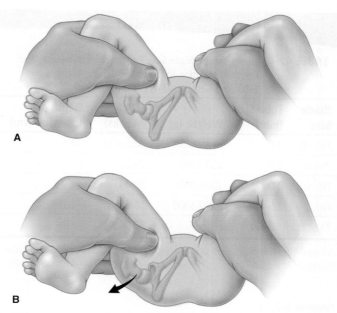

FIGURE 215-1. The Barlow test for developmental dislocation of the hip in a neonate. (**A**) With the infant supine, the examiner holds both of the child's knees and gently adducts 1 hip and pushes posteriorly. (**B**) When the examination is positive, the examiner will feel the femoral head make a small jump (arrow) out of the acetabulum (Barlow sign). When the pressure is released, the head is felt to slip back into place. (Reprinted with permission from Herring JA, ed. *Tachdjian's Pediatric Orthopaedics.* 4th ed. Philadelphia: Saunders; 2007.)

Answer 5-6. c

Although her physical examination findings at birth were unremarkable, the infant presented in this vignette is at risk for DDH due to a history of breech presentation. As DDH can develop any time in the first year of life, the Ortolani and Barlow maneuvers (see Figures 215-1 and 215-2) may initially be negative. Risk factors increasing the incidence of this condition in infants include female sex and birth from the breech position. In this infant with 2 risk factors, current guidelines for DDH screening recommend hip ultrasonography at 6 weeks of age. Radiographs are not reliable until 4 to 6 months of age, when there is greater ossification of the femoral head (AAP, 2000).

Leg length discrepancy or gluteal/leg fold asymmetry may be significant in infants with DDH, but these findings are not diagnostic. Magnetic resonance imaging is not the recommended imaging modality for diagnosis of DDH. Reexamination of the hips should be performed at every well-child care visit during the first year of life but should not replace screening hip imaging in at-risk infants.

American Academy of Pediatrics. Committee on Quality Improvement, Subcommittee on Developmental Dysplasia of the Hip. Clinical practice guideline: early detection of developmental dysplasia of the hip. *Pediatrics.* 2000;105:896.

(Page 188, Section 5: Newborn)

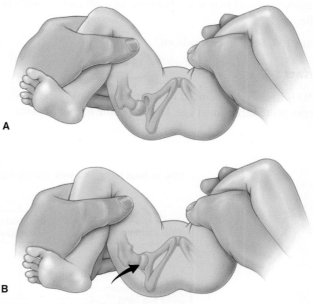

FIGURE 215-2. The Ortolani test for developmental dislocation of the hip in a neonate. (**A**) The examiner holds the infant's knees and gently abducts the hip while lifting up on the greater trochanter with 2 fingers. (**B**) When the test is positive, the dislocated femoral head will fall back into the acetabulum (arrow) with a palpable (but not audible) "clunk" as the hip is abducted (Ortolani sign). When the hip is adducted, the examiner will feel the head redislocate posteriorly. (Reprinted with permission from Herring JA, ed. *Tachdjian's Pediatric Orthopaedics.* 4th ed. Philadelphia: Saunders; 2007.)

TABLE 42-4. Laryngoscope Blade Size, Endotracheal Tube Size, and Depth of Insertion for Babies of Various Weights and Estimated Gestational Age (EGA)

Blade Size	Tube Size (mm)	Weight (g)	EGA (Weeks)	Depth of Insertion (cm)
No. 00	2.5	Below 750	Below 27	~6.5
No. 0	2.5	750-1000	27-28	~7.0
No. 0	3.0	1000-2000	28-34	~7.0-8.0
No. 1	3.5	2000-3000	34-38	~8.0-9.0
No. 1	3.5-4.0	>3000	>38	~9.0-10.0

Adapted from Kattwinkel J. *Textbook of Neonatal Resuscitation.* 5th ed. Elk Grove Village, IL: American Academy of Pediatrics and American Heart Association; 2006.

Answer 5-7. a

Endotracheal intubation may be performed at any point during neonatal resuscitation. The infant in this vignette requires intubation based on worsening respiratory distress despite prolonged PPV.

Using data in Table 42-4, an infant weighing 1200 g should be intubated with a 3.0 mm endotracheal tube, and the airway should be visualized using a number 0 laryngoscope blade. The presence of anatomic variations in the trachea (ie, airway masses, stenosis) may necessitate use of a smaller endotracheal tube.

(Page 168, Section 5: Newborn)

Answer 5-8. e

BPD is defined as the need for supplemental oxygen at 36 weeks postconceptional age. However, due to inconsistent practice among clinicians, supplemental oxygen use and target saturations vary widely in clinical practice. Walsh and colleagues developed an oxygen-need test to make the diagnosis of BPD more uniform. The infant in this vignette would meet the "Walsh criteria" for BPD if he met the conditions of choice e (saturations between 90% and 96% while receiving an FiO_2 of over 0.3). If maintained on an FiO_2 of greater than 0.3 to keep saturations greater than 96%, he would require a room air challenge (with demonstration of oxygen saturations of 90% or less) to be diagnosed with BPD. During a room air challenge, those infants who cannot maintain saturations >90% during weaning and in room air for over 30 minutes were also diagnosed with BPD.

The diagnostic definition of BPD as oxygen need at 36 weeks does not require antecedent exposures (eg, RDS, mechanical ventilation), abnormalities on a chest radiograph, antecedent infectious exposures (antenatal chorioamnionitis or postnatal sepsis), or any laboratory test.

(Page 253, Section 5: Newborn)

Answer 5-9. d

Bronchopulmonary dysplasia (BPD) is a disease due to immature lung development (see Figure 59-1). Infants who die from BPD show pathologic changes consistent with arrest of lung development. The lungs have an emphysematous appearance due to decreased alveolarization. In addition, alveoli present in these lungs have large diameters and contain dysplastic type II cells.

Other pathologic findings include decreased pulmonary microvasculature, an interrupted collagen network, and abnormal elastin localization (ie, distribution away from fibers where alveolar septations should later occur). The lungs may also demonstrate acute inflammatory changes due to the bacterial infection at the time of the infant's demise.

(Page 254, Section 5: Newborn)

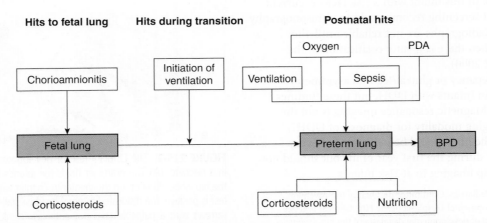

FIGURE 59-1. Risk factors for bronchopulmonary dysplasia, a disease with a single root cause: a very immature lung. Multiple factors then contribute to injury and interfere with lung development. Fetal exposures to chorioamnionitis and corticosteroids, preterm birth with lung injury during resuscitation, and postnatal care (ventilatory and oxygen) and diseases such as sepsis and patent ductus arteriosus represent a series of "hits" to the preterm lung. (Reproduced, with permission, from Rudolph CD, Rudolph A, Lister G, First L, Gershon A. *Rudolph's Pediatrics.* 22nd ed. New York: McGraw-Hill, 2011. <http://www.accesspediatrics.com>.)

Answer 5-10. e

BPD has a multifactorial etiology, and no single intervention has been demonstrated to reduce its incidence. Lung immaturity is a major factor in the pathogenesis of BPD; therefore, preventing preterm delivery would have the most substantial impact on decreasing the incidence of BPD. However, as in this vignette, interruption of progressive preterm labor (and, ultimately, preterm delivery) is not always possible. Therefore, treatment strategies should be implemented in preterm neonates to reduce BPD. Supplemental oxygen use (based on gestation-specific guidelines) and low ventilatory pressures during resuscitation and mechanical ventilation can reduce the initiation and progression of BPD. Postnatal, high-dose corticosteroids may facilitate extubation of ventilator-dependent infants, but do not decrease the incidence of BPD. Furthermore, antioxidant therapy (with drugs such as vitamin C) and reducing *Ureaplasma* colonization from birth (with parenteral erythromycin) have not been shown to decrease the incidence or prevent BPD.

(Page 254-255, Section 5: Newborn)

Answer 5-11. a

Antenatal removal of a SCT is one of the few indications for open fetal surgery. This tumor, thought to be a remnant of the primitive streak in early development, affects only 1 in 25,000 live births. However, the consequences of a rapidly expanding teratoma (preterm labor, polyhydramnios, hydrops, fetal congestive heart failure) are significant to the mother and fetus.

The primary goal of fetal surgery for SCT is interruption of the large vascular connections between the tumor and the fetus that result in nonimmune hydrops. Successful fetal surgery for SCT is accomplished at the time of initial onset of hydrops, not late in the course. Preservation of the anorectal sphincter complex, if possible, is attempted, and removal of pelvic components is deferred until after the infant delivers.

(Page 159, Section 5: Newborn)

Answer 5-12. a

The cellular processes associated with neonatal hypoxic ischemic encephalopathy can be divided into 2 separate pathophysiologic phases. Primary energy failure occurs secondary to decreases in cerebral blood flow, resulting in reduced substrate (ie, glucose) and oxygen delivery to brain tissue. Cellular derangements include loss of high-energy compounds (such as adenosine triphosphate [ATP] and phosphocreatine), excessive release or failure of reuptake of excitatory neurotransmitters (such as glutamate), disturbed ionic homeostasis (including increases in intracellular calcium), and decreased cellular protein synthesis. Secondary energy failure, whose severity is related to the degree of primary energy failure, results in a constellation of neurodegenerative processes (including oxidative injury, neuronal apoptosis, accumulation of excitatory neurotransmitters, and inflammation).

(Page 222, Chapter 5: The Newborn)

Answer 5-13. d

Hypothermia (defined as a reduction in core temperature by 1°C-6°C) has been demonstrated to reduce the deleterious cellular effects of brain ischemia in experimental animal models, including excitatory neurotransmitter release, microglial activation, and free radical production. Data from 2 large randomized control trials and 1 large pilot trial of therapeutic hypothermia in neonates were published in 2005. In all of these studies, hypothermia was initiated within 6 hours of birth and maintained for 48 to 72 hours.

Both the NICHD randomized trial and the pilot trial by Eicher et al used whole-body hypothermia; newborns with HIE receiving this therapy had decreased death or moderate-to-severe disability at 12 months (Eicher) or 18 months (NICHD) relative to HIE infants who were kept normothermic. The CoolCap Trial, which provided selective head cooling to infants with moderate-to-severe encephalopathy, demonstrated protective effects (decreased death or disability in survivors at 18 months) in infants with HIE who demonstrated less severe aEEG abnormalities at admission to the study. Recent data from subsequent studies (the European Network study, the UK Total Body Hypothermia [TOBY] trial, and the Australasian Infant Cooling Evaluation [ICE] study) have further advanced the understanding of the benefits of hypothermia. However, data on neurodevelopmental outcomes in adolescents treated with hypothermia as neonates have not been ascertained.

(Page 223-224, Chapter 5: The Newborn)

Answer 5-14. b

Venous cranial infarcts are less common than arterial strokes in neonates. Factors that may predispose neonates to venous strokes include hypovolemia, polycythemia, decreased blood flow (in the setting of preeclampsia), and infection. Magnetic resonance imaging (MRI) may demonstrate injury to the deep gray matter and thalamus. Additionally, concomitant magnetic venography may show occlusion or recanulation of the affected vessel as well as development of collateral circulation. At present, there are no definite anticoagulant therapies available for management of neonatal stoke based on data from large randomized clinical trials. Additionally, trials of erythropoietin in the prevention of neonatal strokes in humans are in progress and have not demonstrated clinical benefit in reducing effects of stroke.

(Page 225-226, Chapter 5: The Newborn)

Answer 5-15. c

The neonate in this vignette has findings consistent with Beckwith-Wiedemann syndrome (BWS), an overgrowth disorder associated with neonatal hypoglycemia. Visceromegaly, including pancreatic hypertrophy, occurs in these infants, which is associated with hyperinsulinemia and hypoglycemia; however, other factors may be involved.

Symptoms may extend beyond the immediate neonatal period. Hypoglycemia in these infants may improve with more frequent feedings or supplemental glucose administration. Fatty acid oxidation defects and impaired glycogenolysis can result in neonatal hypoglycemia but are not associated with BWS. The infant's feeding trial in the office does not indicate congestive heart failure or swallowing dysfunction as a cause of increased caloric demand or impaired calorie intake.

(Page 212-213, Section 5: Newborn; also see Chapter 545: Endocrine Causes of Hypoglycemia > Hyperinsulinism > Congenital Hyperinsulinism)

Answer 5-16. b

Umbilical venous blood, which is delivered from the placenta, has the highest oxygen concentration in fetal blood (see figure). This blood is streamed across the right atrium, through the foramen ovale, and into the left atrium, where this well-oxygenated blood is delivered to the head and upper extremities. Less-oxygenated blood from the vena cava is streamed through the right atrium and ventricle, and then through the ductus arteriosus to the descending aorta and the umbilical arteries.

(Page 242-243, Section 5: Newborn)

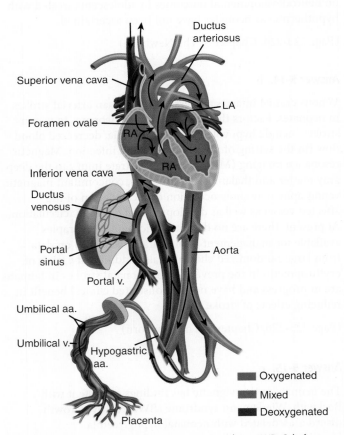

(Reproduced, with permission, from Strange GR, Ahrens WR, Schafermeyer RW, Wiebe RA, eds. *Pediatric Emergency Medicine*. 3rd ed. New York: McGraw-Hill, 2009.)

Answer 5-17. c

Neonatal RDS or hyaline membrane disease (HMD) is the most common cause of respiratory failure in the first days after birth, occurring in 1% to 2% of newborn infants. Until about 25 years ago, approximately 50% of infants with this condition died. However, improved methods of treatment over the past 3 decades have markedly reduced mortality from this condition. RDS occurs mainly in premature infants and is more common in white infants than in black infants. The characteristic clinical features of infants with RDS are expiratory grunting, tachypnea, retractions (involving the intercostal and sternal muscles), and central cyanosis.

Persistent pulmonary hypertension of the newborn and transient tachypnea of the newborn are more common causes of respiratory distress in near-term (born at 34 0/7-36 6/7 weeks' gestation) and term (born at 37 0/7 weeks' gestation or later) infants. Meconium passage in utero before 32 weeks' gestation is rare, making meconium aspiration syndrome less likely in this infant. Congenital heart disease could present at 6 hours of life, but is less common than RDS in an infant of this gestational age.

(Page 233-234, Section 5: Newborn)

Answer 5-18. a

Pulmonary surfactant, a mixture of proteins and phospholipids, is synthesized in alveolar epithelial type II cells. The phospholipid dipalmitoylphosphatidylcholine makes up about 45% to 50% of the mass of surfactant and is the main surfactant component that lowers surface tension. The ratio of amniotic fluid concentrations of surfactant phospholipids (lecithin ([L] and sphingomyelin [S]) has been used to determine fetal lung maturity.

An L:S ratio of 2:1 suggests a lower risk of the fetus developing respiratory distress syndrome after birth. Of the 4 surfactant apoproteins (surfactant proteins A, B, C, and D), a congenital deficiency in surfactant protein B production has been associated with fatal respiratory failure in term neonates. Synthesis and storage of surfactant begin around 16 weeks' gestation, but it is not secreted into the amniotic fluid until 28 to 38 weeks' gestation, at approximately the same time alveolar development begins.

(Page 236, Section 5: Newborn)

Answer 5-19. d

Neonates with respiratory distress should receive the least invasive therapy that supports their pulmonary needs. The infant in this vignette is a late preterm infant with clinical evidence of respiratory distress syndrome (RDS). Physiologically, the infant has atelectasis and hypoxia, which can be reversed with positive pressure and oxygen support. Since she is not apneic, the baby should receive respiratory support with CPAP and supplemental oxygen to maintain age-appropriate oxygen saturations. Intubation and mechanical ventilation (either IMV or HFOV) should be started only if she develops worsening respiratory distress (with respiratory acidosis apnea, or hypoxia) while on CPAP. Nitric oxide is a pulmonary vasodilator used for conditions causing respiratory failure in term newborns (such as meconium aspiration syndrome) but is not indicated for routine use in premature infants with RDS. Titrating nitrogen into the oxyhood would decrease the FiO_2 and potentially worsen the infant's respiratory distress.

(Page 237, Section 5: Newborn)

Answer 5-20. d

Small-for-gestational-age (SGA) infants lose heat rapidly because of their large surface area relative to body weight and their scant subcutaneous fat stores. To prevent hypothermia, this infant should be dried quickly and completely, placed under a radiant warmer, and protected from drafts with warmed blankets. He is crying and has a heart rate above 100 beats/min; therefore, administering PPV, CPAP, or intravenous volume would not be appropriate for his resuscitation in the delivery room. Although SGA infants are at risk for hypoglycemia, administration of dextrose in the delivery room is not indicated.

(Page 193, Section 5: Newborn)

Answer 5-21. e

Hypoglycemia is common in small-for-gestational-age (SGA) infants, including the infant in this vignette. Of note, hypoglycemia increases with the severity of intrauterine growth restriction. The risk of hypoglycemia is greatest during the first 3 postnatal days, but fasting hypoglycemia may occur repetitively for several days after birth. This early hypoglycemia usually results from insufficient hepatic and skeletal muscle glycogen content and is exacerbated by the lack of alternative energy sources (because of scant adipose tissue and decreased lactate concentrations). Early enteral feeding usually can prevent hypoglycemia. Less commonly, hyperinsulinemia and/or increased sensitivity to insulin may also contribute to hypoglycemia. This insulin is fetally/neonatally derived, as maternal insulin does not cross the placenta. Finally, deficient catecholamine responses to low blood sugar levels (seen in SGA infants) may also result in persistent hypoglycemia.

Increased gluconeogenesis would decrease, not increase, the incidence of hypoglycemia in this infant.

(Page 194, Section 5: Newborn)

Answer 5-22. c

Small-for-gestational-age (SGA) infants have multiple metabolic abnormalities in the neonatal period. Protein digestion and absorption is impaired in these infants due to decreased intestinal size and function. SGA infants have lower muscle masses relative to AGA infants, and although muscle accretion is a priority in these babies, their tolerance of high protein/amino acid administration may be limited.

SGA babies also have increased plasma triglyceride concentrations due to deficient cellular uptake. Additionally,

these infants have higher oxygen consumption and higher resting energy expenditure due to increased heat loss. Finally, SGA infants have impaired insulin secretion (leading to poor anabolic growth) and impaired immunologic function during infancy and childhood (resulting in subtherapeutic response to vaccinations).

(Page 195, Section 5: Newborn)

Answer 5-23. a

Establishment of glucose homeostasis in the newborn occurs via a series of hormonal and enzymatic changes initiated with clamping of the umbilical cord. Basal glucose production in a neonate is approximately 2- to 3-fold greater than adult production, which is related to the large consumption of glucose by the neonatal brain. Hepatic glycogen stores are converted to glucose in response to increases in circulating catecholamines and glucagon at delivery as well as decreases in serum insulin levels. The glycogen stores rapidly decline in the term infant and are nearly exhausted by 12 hours of age, requiring gluconeogenesis or delivery of exogenous glucose to achieve acceptable glucose levels.

Gluconeogenesis is regulated by increases in cytosolic phosphoenylpyruvate kinase (triggered by delivery) and the oxidation of free fatty acids (in particular, medium-chain triglycerides).

(Page 173, Chapter 5: The Newborn)

Answer 5-24. d

The infant in this vignette has developed hyponatremia secondary to inappropriate antidiuretic hormone secretion and renal failure after perinatal depression. Of the choices listed, reduction in intravenous fluid infusion (as well as serial monitoring of electrolytes) is the correct choice for management of this infant. Administration of additional fluid (a normal saline bolus) is not indicated in a well-perfused infant with intrinsic renal failure (oliguria with a BUN/creatinine ratio of 10-20). Diuretic administration (either furosemide or bumetanide) is not indicated in infants with intrinsic renal failure; furthermore, diuretics increase renal sodium losses and may worsen hyponatremia. Increasing the dextrose in maintenance fluids of a normoglycemic infant may cause hyperglycemia, which introduces free water into the vascular space and may worsen hyponatremia.

(Page 219, Chapter 5: The Newborn)

Answer 5-25. d

This infant's presentation is most consistent with neonatal encephalopathy (probably hypoxic ischemic encephalopathy [HIE]). There is no history of a prenatal or intrapartum event that would compromise fetal blood flow, but in many cases of neonatal encephalopathy, such an event cannot be identified. Information that can be useful in the first hours of life to assist in management of these infants includes serial neurodevelopmental assessments, neuroimaging, and electroencephalography. Based on this infant's initial presentation (moderate-to-severe encephalopathy with metabolic acidosis), strong consideration should be given to initiating hypothermia.

This therapy has shown efficacy if initiated within the first 6 hours of life (not 12 hours of life), and can be initiated before obtaining neuroimaging or an electroencephalogram, especially if transport to another hospital is required. Neonatal seizures can occur as a result of HIE, and may exacerbate the brain injury. Empiric phenobarbital therapy has been considered for neonates with HIE; however, this strategy has not been demonstrated to reduce cerebral palsy or mental retardation in these infants. Clinicians cannot predict definitively neurologic outcomes for infants with HIE. However, certain neonatal MRI findings (as described on page 225), in addition to clinical and electroencephalographic evidence of ongoing encephalopathy (over the first week of life), are poor prognostic signs for neurodevelopment in these neonates.

(Page 222-225, Section 5: Newborn)

Answer 5-26. b

The features of the ultrasound are suggestive of Down syndrome. The risk of Down syndrome increases with maternal age. Women at high risk of having a fetus with Down syndrome will have low serum α-FP, high hCG, and low uE levels adjusted for gestational age. If the maternal plasma tests indicate increased risk, a level 2 ultrasound can identify structural findings in the fetus frequently associated with Down syndrome (increased nuchal fold, nasal bone hypoplasia, and decreased fetal extremity length). The diagnosis can be confirmed by karyotype of fetal cells from amniotic fluid.

(Page 156, Section 5: Newborn)

Answer 5-27. a

Fetal heart rate and uterine contraction monitoring are used routinely throughout labor to assess fetal status and the labor pattern. While fetal monitoring is not highly predictive of outcomes, some fetuses at high risk for birth depression can be identified. The above tocodynamometer tracing shows a fall in fetal heart rate after the onset of uterine contractions, with a gradual return to baseline after the contractions have ceased. This pattern is consistent with late decelerations and suggests decreased fetal oxygenation due to reduced placental perfusion (which occurs with uterine contractions). With intermittent cord compression, variable decelerations may occur, which present as abrupt dips in the fetal heart rate (usually a brief acceleration followed by a deceleration).

Vagal stimulation due to fetal head compression would cause an early deceleration (as opposed to a late deceleration). An early deceleration is manifested as a decrease in fetal heart rate associated with the contraction. Normal fetal movement would result in an acceleration of the fetal heart rate. Fetal hiccups (singultus) do not decrease the fetal heart rate.

(Page 156, Section 5: Newborn)

Answer 5-28. d

A complication of 7% to 10% of all pregnancies, preeclampsia results from vasoregulatory abnormalities in the placenta and the gravid woman. Mild preeclampsia is diagnosed by an increase in blood pressure (greater than 140/90 mm Hg) and proteinuria. The woman in this vignette, however, has evidence of severe preeclampsia (with blood pressure of greater than 160/90 mm Hg and 3+-4+ proteinuria).

Emergent cesarean section is not indicated presently, as more data should be collected regarding maternal and fetal status. Medical management of the pregnancy at this time includes hospital admission, intravenous magnesium sulfate administration (to decrease the risk of seizures and provide fetal neuroprotection), antihypertensive therapy (β-blockers, calcium channel blockers) to control blood pressure, and monitoring maternal blood pressure, urine output, and end-organ (renal, hepatic, hematologic, and neurologic) function. Fetal well-being, amniotic fluid index, and estimated fetal weight should also be assessed.

Ultimately, however, if the preeclampsia worsens, delivery of the fetus would be indicated. If preeclampsia occurs at a gestational age earlier than 34 weeks, maternal corticosteroid therapy should be given, with delay of delivery for 48 hours (if possible). Antenatal steroids decrease the risk and severity of certain conditions seen in premature infants, including respiratory distress syndrome and necrotizing enterocolitis. Hemodialysis is not an appropriate therapy in this patient.

(Page 157, Section 5: Newborn)

Answer 5-29. c

During fetal development, the ductus arteriosus diverts blood away from the fetal lungs to the descending aorta and placenta (see Figure 494-3). Postnatally, the ductus arteriosus closes through vasoconstriction and remodeling. The risk of PDA is inversely associated with gestational age.

Multiple interacting factors, including increased sensitivity to prostaglandins, influence patency of the ductus arteriosus in premature infants. During episodes of sepsis or necrotizing enterocolitis, circulating prostaglandin E_2 concentrations can reach pharmacologic levels in premature infants, causing vasodilation of the ductus. Under these circumstances, responsiveness of ductal tissue to inhibitors of prostaglandin synthesis (indomethacin or ibuprofen) is limited. Levels of indomethacin on day 8, following early administration of intraventricular hemorrhage prophylaxis, would not be adequate to promote PDA closure.

Antenatal steroid therapy is associated with a decreased (not increased) risk of PDA. Decreased peak end-expiratory pressure after extubation is unlikely to play a major role in the maintenance of ductal patency. Enteral feeding results in shunting of blood to the mesenteric circulation. This could decrease the degree of left-to-right shunting, which could result in less pulmonary overcirculation but not increase the risk of prolonged PDA patency.

(Page 240, Section 5: Newborn)

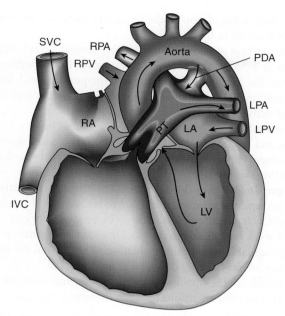

FIGURE 494-3. Patent ductus arteriosus. (Reproduced, with permission, from Rudolph CD, Rudolph A, Lister G, First L, Gershon A. *Rudolph's Pediatrics*. 22nd ed. New York: McGraw-Hill, 2011. <http://www.accesspediatrics.com>.)

Answer 5-30. b

Cyanosis is due to the presence of deoxygenated hemoglobin in vessels visible on the skin surface and mucosa. Cyanosis in the neonate tends to become apparent when there is about 3 to 5 g/dL of deoxygenated hemoglobin, but detection varies widely depending on lighting, observer differences, and pigmentation of the skin, among other factors. The oxygen binding capacity of fetal hemoglobin in the newborn (which is higher than the capacity in an adult) also decreases the degree of desaturation at a given Pao_2.

(Page 198, Section 5: Newborn)

Answer 5-31. e

The infant in this vignette has central cyanosis with no respiratory distress and a minimal response to supplemental oxygen. These findings suggest cyanotic congenital heart disease in this neonate. At this point, the caregiver should seek advice from a cardiologist and transfer the baby to a tertiary care center for an echocardiogram and careful monitoring in a neonatal intensive care unit (NICU). It is important to remember that oxygen may promote ductus arteriosus closure and increase pulmonary vasodilation, which may exacerbate the hypoxia in children with left-sided obstructive lesions (eg, hypoplastic left heart syndrome). Thus, titration of oxygen (to an FiO_2 0.4-0.6) in this infant is appropriate until his cardiac lesion can be defined.

Admitting a cyanotic infant to a full-term nursery at any hospital is not appropriate. Additionally, in the absence of respiratory distress, intubation and ventilation is not necessary in this infant. A chest CT may be useful in pulmonary and/or

cardiac anomalies in this infant but is not the most appropriate initial management step. Finally, administering dextrose may be necessary if this large-for-gestational-age (LGA) infant is hypoglycemic but is not the most important intervention for this infant at this time.

(Page 201, Section 5: Newborn)

Answer 5-32. a

Approximately 10% to 15% of all live births are associated with meconium-stained amniotic fluid, although only 4% to 5% of these infants will develop meconium aspiration syndrome. Meconium represents the contents of the fetal intestine and consists of a variety of substances, including bile-containing intestinal secretions, blood, and amniotic fluid. Meconium can injure the lung through multiple mechanisms, including mechanical obstruction of the airways, chemical pneumonitis, inactivation of endogenous surfactant, and vasoconstriction of pulmonary vessels, all of which prevent adequate ventilation and oxygenation in the immediate postnatal period. The ease of intubation of the baby in the vignette would make in airway edema a less likely answer. Bacterial pneumonia or primary surfactant deficiency also would be a less likely cause of this neonate's respiratory distress.

(Page 200, Section 5: Newborn)

Answer 5-33. c

This infant with a history of shoulder dystocia and a left-sided Erb's palsy likely has a brachial plexus injury. In addition to left arm weakness, the injury in this infant will result in limited left diaphragm movement (due to phrenic nerve injury). A chest radiograph would demonstrate the left hemidiaphragm higher than the right hemidiaphragm. Based on the physical examination findings, this infant is less likely to have a congenital diaphragmatic hernia (indicated radiographically by peritoneal contents in the left hemithorax), right-sided heart congenital disease or pulmonary hypertension (evidenced by decreased pulmonary vascular markings), a cystic congenital adenomatoid malformation (CCAM, with cystic lesions in the lung), or a pleural effusion (fluid in the pleural space creating mass effect).

(Page 200, Section 5: Newborn)

Answer 5-34. a

Fetal neuromaturation prior to term typically progresses in a standard manner with some individual variation. The late preterm infant in this vignette is likely to have a coordinated pattern of sucking with discrete pauses for breathing, although her suck may be weaker than the suck of a term infant. Additionally, she should fixate on a bull's eye (ability present at 34 weeks' gestation) with minimal, unsustained tracking that will develop over subsequent weeks.

In the third trimester of pregnancy, flexor tone increases initially in the lower extremities and progresses in a cephalad direction. Therefore, this infant should not have good flexor tone in the upper extremities in the absence of full flexion of the lower extremities. Some tone in the shoulders and upper extremities, however, exists by 36 weeks' gestation, and would prevent the infant from stretching her right elbow to the contralateral shoulder (the anterior scarf sign). The degree of upper extremity tone will increase over subsequent weeks, keeping the elbow from reaching the midline when this maneuver is attempted at term.

Antenatal magnesium exposure can temporarily alter the neurologic examination, and cause decreased tone. However, despite magnesium exposure, the primitive reflexes should be present in this neonate.

(Page 180-182, Chapter 5: The Newborn)

Answer 5-35. d

The resuscitation scenario above raises concern for perinatal depression in the baby, which can result in hypoxic-ischemic injury to the brain. The baby's rapid response to positive pressure ventilation, however, suggests minimal perinatal depression. However, in this situation, the infant's initial examination is important for assessment of his baseline neurologic function. One component of the neurologic examination is assessment of primitive reflexes, which are normal findings on the newborn examination. Examples of these reflexes include the palmar grasp (rapid grasp of the examiner's finger with pressure on the palm of the baby's hand) and the asymmetric tonic neck reflex (lateralized changes in the baby's extremity tone with rotation of his head). Other normal findings on the examination include very responsive and brisk deep tendon reflexes (that can produce a few beats of clonus) and intermittent disconjugate gaze if the infant is not focused on an object. As the cerebral cortex matures over the first 6 to 9 months of age, the primitive reflexes and periods of dysconjugate gaze should diminish and disappear, and then deep tendon reflexes should relax. Newborns can exhibit brief periods of pronounced active trunk extension (when crying, eg), but in the normal newborn, trunk extensor is not stronger than trunk flexor tone. When evaluated in the quiet, alert state, extensor tone should be minimal to absent, and flexor tone should be present.

(Page 182, Section 5: Newborn)

Answer 5-36. e

Signs and symptoms of a neonatal stroke can present shortly after birth, or later in the neonatal period. When presenting symptoms occur days after delivery, perinatal causes should still be considered, especially when there are noted risk factors. Instrumented vaginal delivery using forceps or vacuum is associated with increased risk of birth trauma. Because this baby in this vignette required vacuum assistance for delivery, she has an increased risk of traumatic bleeding that could result in an intracranial hemorrhage. A perinatal hemorrhage may evolve and progress in size hours to days after delivery, increasing pressure on adjacent normal brain tissue. The resultant ischemia may result in later clinical evidence of a stroke (ie, seizures). Preeclampsia, which can result in

compromised blood flow to the fetus, also increases the risk of perinatal stroke in this case.

Investigation of neonatal brain injury should always include trauma as a part of the differential diagnosis. In this scenario, however, the timing of the seizure and the perinatal risk factors are most consistent with trauma having occurred around the time of delivery, not due to a postnatal injury.

Postnatal strokes can be related to congenital heart lesions and repair, as blood flow can bypass the pulmonary vasculature. However, postnatal seizure is unlikely to be the presenting symptom.

Approximately two thirds of neonatal strokes are arterial in origin, and the remainder are due to sinovenous thrombus. This injury is, therefore, less likely to be venous in origin. Recent work has raised questions of the value of a workup for a hypercoagulable state in the evaluation of a neonatal stroke.

There are no large randomized clinical trials of anticoagulation therapy for neonatal strokes, and there are no definitive recommendations for such therapy in this case.

(Page 225-226, Section 5: The Newborn)

Answer 5-37. d

Neurologic development of the fetus over the third trimester of pregnancy progresses in a sequence that is generally predictable, allowing for estimation of gestational age. The assessment gives the more accurate results after the first few days of life, allowing the neonate to recover from perinatal complications or exposures, and the effect of in utero positioning.

The infant described in the scenario has weak finger grasp (also referred to as palmar grasp), which typically emerges at 34 to 35 weeks' gestation. Coordinated breathing and sucking typically begins to organize around 32 weeks' gestation with slow sucks, little negative pressure, and brief sucking bursts (fewer than 3 sucks) alternating with 15- to 20-second periods of breathing. This infant demonstrates a sucking pattern more consistent with an infant born at 34 to 35 weeks' gestation, with longer bursts, a greater number of more rapid strong sucks, and shorter pauses for breathing. Finally, the baby has no flexor tone elicited in the upper extremities with traction, which is typically present by 36 weeks' gestation.

(Page 181, Examination of the Newborn Infant)

Answer 5-38. d

Closure of the ductus arteriosus in infants is regulated by several factors that change during in utero development. In the term infant, factors promoting closure of the ductus arteriosus include an increase in arterial blood oxygen tension (Pao_2), a decrease in ductal luminal blood pressure, a decrease in circulating PGE_2, and a decrease in PGE_2 receptors.

In contrast, factors that facilitate ductal patency in premature infants include:

1. Continued synthesis of the dominant PGE_2 receptor (E_4), rendering the ductus sensitive to the vasodilatory effects of PGE_2.

2. Higher prostaglandin levels due to less efficient metabolism and clearance of circulating prostaglandins and increased PGE_2 production due to increased expression of the COX-2 isoform.

3. The production of increased amounts of other vasodilators (such as nitric oxide and interleukin-6).

4. Absence of the normal fetal cortisol surge, which occurs in the third trimester and initiates physiologic changes that are necessary for survival in the extrauterine environment (including ductus closure). Preterm infants whose mothers receive antenatal betamethasone have a decreased risk of prolonged ductal patency.

As pulmonary vascular resistance decreases in premature infants, increased left-to-right shunting and resultant pulmonary edema can exacerbate respiratory compromise. Intermittent hypoxemia and additional respiratory support that may be needed for management will contribute to lung injury and the risk of chronic lung disease. In this scenario, early administration of surfactant would have improved lung compliance, and the PDA may have become symptomatic sooner. Surfactant administration, however, does not decrease the likelihood of having a PDA.

Maternal use of ibuprofen (or other nonsteroidal anti-inflammatory drugs) is associated with intrauterine closure of the ductus arteriosus.

(Page 239-240, Section 5: The Newborn)

Answer 5-39. c

Characteristics of NEC are different in near-term and term neonates than in premature neonates. An episode of NEC in a term or near-term newborn commonly involves the presence of a risk factor such as congenital heart disease, gastroschisis, intrauterine growth restriction, perinatal depression, or polycythemia. Additionally, NEC typically presents earlier in these babies (first week of life) than in more premature infants (second or third week of life). In addition, the area of intestine affected is different in more mature infants when compared with premature infants. NEC is more likely to affect the colon in near-term and term neonates. In premature infants, NEC occurs primarily in the jejunum and ileum; the most common site is the distal ileum. Finally, near-term and term infants with NEC have a lower risk of requiring surgery than premature infants.

SIPs are more likely to occur in premature neonates. However, when present in a more mature neonate, a SIP occurs earlier (typically 0-3 days of age), and is not usually accompanied by 1 of the typical risk factors (ie, indomethacin therapy) associated with a SIP in a more premature neonate.

(Page 246-247, Section 5: The Neonate)

Answer 5-40. a

Although it has been difficult to elucidate the specific pathophysiology leading to necrotizing enterocolitis in premature infants, multiple studies have aimed to identify risk factors and test potential prophylactic measures/therapies.

At present, the following factors and strategies have been identified as protective in premature infants:

1. Antenatal corticosteroids (protective mechanism unclear).
2. Feeding with human milk (maternal or donor breast milk) when compared with feeding with formula.
3. Fluid restriction.
4. Administration of enteral antibiotics (not recommended due to concern for the development of resistant organisms).
5. Treatment with specific probiotic strains (in infants with birth weight less than 1000 g) based on the results of a variety of clinical trials. However, there has been no consistency in strain, dose, or regimen in any of the reported studies, to date.

Other strategies studied (ie, different enteral feeding styles, administration of immunoglobulins or amino acid supplements) have not changed the incidence of necrotizing enterocolitis.

(Page 249, Section 5: The Newborn)

Answer 5-41. d

The most effective prophylaxis against IVH is prolongation of pregnancy, as the risk of IVH decreases with increased birth weight and gestational age. In addition, timely interventions to treat complications that can lead to preterm delivery are associated with lower risk of IVH including administration of antibiotics to women in preterm labor. Although premature delivery may occur, antenatal antibiotic therapy may result in a less severe inflammatory response (a hypothesized component of the pathophysiologic pathway of IVH), and better hemodynamic stability.

Although hypotension is an important risk factor for intraventricular hemorrhage, rapid correction with intravenous fluid boluses may compound the risk (due to germinal matrix reperfusion injury). Antenatal administration of betamethasone is associated with decreased incidence of intraventricular hemorrhage. In contrast, postnatal glucocorticoid administration does not influence the risk of intraventricular hemorrhage and can have a detrimental effect on neurodevelopment. Studies that have evaluated other potential prophylactic therapies such as phenobarbital or fresh frozen plasma have not shown any benefit in these agents preventing IVH.

(Page 253, Chapter 5: The Newborn)

Answer 5-42. e

Extremely premature and very-low-birth-weight infants have a significant risk of neurodevelopmental impairment, including intellectual disability and cerebral palsy. Studies following very-low-birth-weight survivors into adolescence and adulthood have revealed more functional limitations in this group. These problems include lower academic achievement scores (relative to peers born at term), an increased risk of emotional, behavioral, and attention problems, and neurosensory impairment. However, parents of low-birth-weight neonates report less risk-taking behavior and the majority of children (74%-82%) graduate from high school and pursue productive lives.

In general, major neurodevelopmental impairments such as cerebral palsy and intellectual disability can be diagnosed by 3 years of age. However, more subtle problems with cognition and motor function may not present until school age, when more complex functioning is necessary. Preterm children with no neurologic problems or intellectual disability are more likely to have language disorders, reading disability, and difficulty with arithmetic than their peers who were born at term. In addition, they have a greater prevalence of visual perceptual problems, executive dysfunction, and behavior problems than children born at term. Finally, children born to parents with lower socioeconomic status are more likely to have cognitive impairments as opposed to cerebral palsy.

Recent studies have better elucidated the risks of neurodevelopmental impairment for late preterm infants (who may not be low birth weight). For example, infants born at 33 to 36 weeks' gestation have a significantly greater risk for reading and spelling problems than infants born at 39 to 40 weeks' gestation. Thus, the absence of risk factors such as extreme prematurity or low birth weight does not guarantee a normal outcome.

(Page 261-263, Section 5: The Newborn)

Answer 5-43. c

IUGR can occur at different times in pregnancy. Timing and etiology of growth restriction can affect the intrauterine growth pattern, often manifested in the anthropometric measures of the newborn. The relative sparing of head growth in a growth-restricted fetus ("head-sparing IUGR") is thought to be a fetal adaptation to uteroplacental insufficiency; as nutritional supply is limited, somatic growth is sacrificed to allow for brain growth. If nutrient supply is further decreased relative to fetal needs, accelerated pulmonary and neurologic maturation prepare the fetus for extrauterine survival. However, sparing of head growth does not completely protect the brain from inadequate intrauterine nutrition and subsequent neurodevelopmental sequelae in childhood. Children who had evidence of head-sparing IUGR at delivery have demonstrated lower cognitive scores on testing when compared with controls who were born at a size appropriate for gestational age. Furthermore, the acceleration of lung maturity may not prevent respiratory complications in this infant, including respiratory distress syndrome (RDS).

Low birth weight at delivery has been identified as a risk factor for various health outcomes in infancy, childhood, and later life, including the risk of hypertension, diabetes, and cardiovascular disease in adulthood. However, gestational age, which represents the degree of physiologic maturity, is predictive neonatal mortality and morbidity. In fact, prior to 30 to 32 weeks' gestation, an infant born small for gestational age does not have a greater risk for mortality, morbidity, or later neurodevelopmental disability above that conferred by degree of prematurity.

The inability to identify the cause of IUGR may lead to a presumptive diagnosis of uteroplacental insufficiency. Certain findings on placental pathology, such as an infarct noted on gross examination, or an inflammatory response seen on microscopic examination may provide additional information. However, despite data from placental pathology, the definitive cause(s) of IUGR may not be determined.

(Page 263, Chapter 5: The Neonate)

Answer 5-44. c

ECMO is a therapy with significant risks that is reserved for infants with the most profound respiratory or cardiorespiratory failure. The overall survival rate for infants who are treated with ECMO is 80% in the United States. The most common cause of death for infants treated with ECMO is hemorrhage. The risk of neurodevelopmental problems, including cognitive and motor impairment and sensorineural hearing loss, is not considered to be greater with ECMO than the risk conferred by the underlying illness and conventional therapies. Hearing impairment is more common in term infants with respiratory and other organ failure than in extremely premature infants. Because less invasive therapies are being used more effectively for neonatal respiratory failure, the use of ECMO has decreased in recent years.

(Page 261 and 263, Chapter 5: The Newborn)

Answer 5-45. d

Infants born prematurely have a significantly increased risk of mortality when compared with infants born at term, and premature survivors have a significantly increased risk of neurodevelopmental problems. In addition, the risk of major neurodevelopmental impairments (intellectual disability, cerebral palsy, visual impairment, hearing impairment) increases with decreasing birth weight and gestational age at delivery.

High rates of neurodevelopmental impairment occur primarily in the survivors born at the limit of viability (prior to 25 completed weeks' gestation). Data currently available show that as many as half of these infants have intellectual disability, and up to one quarter of survivors develop cerebral palsy (most commonly, spastic diplegia). These infants also are at the highest risk for complications of prematurity (such as chronic lung disease, necrotizing enterocolitis, retinopathy of prematurity, and bacterial sepsis), which represent additional risk factors for abnormal neurodevelopment. It is important to focus on risk factors in discussing outcomes of premature infants with parents, since diagnosis or exclusion of neurodevelopmental impairments is not possible prior to NICU discharge. The impact of abnormal radiographic or physical findings in the NICU on neurologic function is typically not apparent until after infancy. Furthermore, although MRI of the brain can be helpful for identifying abnormalities that predict neurodevelopmental impairments, no single neuroimaging study has been recognized as a clinical practice standard.

(Page 262-263, Chapter 5: The Neonate)

Answer 5-46. b

Surfactant production increases in the fetal lung during the later stages of intrauterine development. Stimulated by the catecholamine surge that accompanies birth and inflation of the lungs, surfactant is released into the alveolar space, decreasing surface tension and preventing collapse of the distal air spaces with expiration. Additionally, neonatal lung compliance is increased due to sustained, regular respirations at birth and resorption of fetal lung fluid across the pulmonary epithelium via transcellular sodium movement. Circulatory adaptations at birth include a reduction in pulmonary vascular resistance and a change in neonatal blood flow from a fetal pattern (pulmonary and systemic circulations in parallel) to an adult pattern (pulmonary and systemic circulations in series).

(Page 170-171, Chapter 5: Newborn)

Answer 5-47. e

Premature infants in whom a germinal matrix hemorrhage has occurred require close evaluation, especially during the days following the primary bleed (when the hemorrhage is most likely to extend into the ventricle and cause additional complications). Serial evaluations should include daily measurement of head circumference, and repeat cranial ultrasound at the end of the first week of life, or sooner if there is clinical suspicion of more bleeding (ie, rapid increase in head circumference, drop in hematocrit, seizure).

After the first few days of age, their risk of bleeding on the contralateral side does not increase. In the absence of profound coagulopathy, hemodynamic instability, and/or mass effect from the initial bleed, the risk of a primary bleed on the contralateral side should decrease.

Although bleeding that is limited to the germinal matrix has not been associated with an increased risk of major developmental problems, at this stage, it is possible that this infant's bleed will progress into the ventricles, resulting in posthemorrhagic hydrocephalus, and various related complications, including a greater risk of neurodevelopmental impairment. In addition, male infants are more likely to have neurologic sequelae from intraventricular hemorrhage.

(Page 249-252, Section 5: Newborn)

Answer 5-48. c

There are many factors that can contribute to the development of a GM-IVH as outlined in Figure 58-1. The final common pathway is their relationship to, or effect on, the delicate germinal matrix, the site of origin of this type of intracranial hemorrhage. Perinatal asphyxia and vigorous resuscitation are risk factors for intraventricular hemorrhage in a premature baby, as cerebral hemodynamics are influenced by the respiratory condition of an infant. Establishing a stable respiratory status in a premature infant can result in hyperoxia and hypocarbia, which can cause a decrease in cerebral blood flow (ischemia) through the germinal matrix vessels.

When cerebral blood flow subsequently increases, additional reperfusion injury can result in rupture of the germinal matrix vessels, causing a GM-IVH. In premature infants, germinal matrix hemorrhages primarily occur within the first few days of life, which may be due to a later adaptation to extrauterine life that provides stability to this vascular structure. Despite risk factors such as hemodynamic and respiratory instability that are present in choices b and e, it is less likely for a premature infant to have a primary GM-IVH after 5 days of age. The infant in choice d had respiratory distress in the delivery room, but his gestational age (greater than 32 weeks' gestation) decreases his risk for a GM-IVH. Furthermore, the germinal matrix has involuted completely in the majority of term infants, making putting the infant in choice a at low risk for GM-IVH but at higher risk for another form of intracranial hemorrhage (ie, subgaleal hemorrhage).

(Page 250-251, Section 5: Newborn)

Answer 5-49. d

Necrotizing enterocolitis (NEC) occurs most commonly in premature infants. The incidence of NEC is inversely related to 2 important risk factors: birth weight and gestational age. In addition, the risk of mortality from NEC is higher for the smallest infants born at lower gestational ages. Mortality is also related to the need for surgical intervention, and the extent of bowel involvement, with survival directly related to the length of remaining bowel after surgical resection. Even in the absence of surgical intervention, NEC increases the incidence of other prematurity-related complications, including chronic lung disease, growth failure, neurodevelopmental delays, and hospital-acquired infections. Additionally, infants with NEC who require surgery have a greater risk of neurodevelopmental impairment (2-3 times greater risk than infants managed with medical therapy alone). There is no evidence to suggest that hypersensitivity to breast milk is involved in NEC pathophysiology. Strictures may occur weeks to months after an episode of NEC, even in the absence of bowel perforation.

(Page 246-249, Section 5: The Neonate)

Answer 5-50. b

The infant in this vignette has received inadequate PPV during the initial steps of resuscitation, resulting in bradycardia. Inadequate airway positioning and poor seal with the neonatal face mask are the most common causes of a lack of a response to PPV (which include chest rise and a rise in the neonatal heart rate). The first steps in evaluating a poor response to PPV are repositioning the airway (with mild extension of the head and neck) and ensuring an appropriate seal between the mask and the infant's face (see Table 42-3).

Of note, the mask should rest snugly around the mouth and be supported by the chin and the bridge of the nose. Volume infusion and epinephrine administration may be necessary (to treat hypovolemia and bradycardia, respectively) but are not indicated at this point in the resuscitation. Cardioversion

TABLE 42-3. Strategies to Achieve Chest Rise During Bag–Mask Ventilation (MR SOPII)

M (mask)	Check the seal of your mask
R (reposition)	Make sure the infant is truly in the open airway (mild extension) position
S (suction)	Remove obstructing secretions
O (open the mouth)	Sometimes in an effort to get a good seal, the mouth is accidentally closed. The higher resistance of the nasal passages will limit effective ventilation
P (pressure)	Try increasing the inflation pressure if possible
I (inflation time)	Increase I_T to 1-2 seconds for 2-3 breaths in an effort to insure a functional residual capacity is established
I (intubate)	If all previous steps have failed to achieve chest rise, it is time to intubate!

Reproduced, with permission, from Rudolph CD, Rudolph A, Lister G, First L, Gershon A. *Rudolph's Pediatrics*. 22nd ed. New York: McGraw-Hill, 2011.

to correct a neonatal arrhythmia is not performed during the initial neonatal resuscitation.

(Page 167-168, Section 5: Newborn)

Answer 5-51. d

The neonate in this vignette has findings consistent with isolated esophageal atresia, which can present prenatally with polyhydramnios (due to inability of the fetus to swallow amniotic fluid). Postnatal findings include excessive oral secretions and respiratory distress. Radiographic findings include failure of a nasoenteric tube to pass to the stomach,

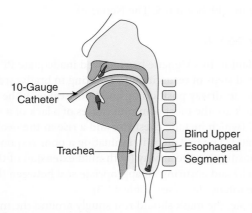

FIGURE 392-2. Diagnosis of esophageal atresia is confirmed by inability to pass a 10 French orogastric tube beyond 10 cm from the gums. (Reproduced from Beasley SW. Esophageal atresia and tracheoesophageal fistula. In: Oldham KT, Colombani PM, Foglia RP, et al, eds. *Principles and Practice of Pediatric Surgery*. Philadelphia: Lippincott Williams & Wilkins; 2005:1040.)

with curling of the tube in the proximal esophageal pouch. Initial management involves decompression of the proximal pouch by suctioning the nasogastric tube (to prevent pooling of oral secretions).

Subsequent steps in management may include contrast imaging of the proximal pouch and esophagus (to delineate anatomy) and intravenous antibiotics (if pneumonia is suspected due to aspiration of secretions). A barium enema is not indicated for isolated esophageal atresia. An oral airway is not needed in this infant with normal pharyngeal findings.

(Page 257, Section 5: Newborn)

Answer 5-52. e

Fetal cortisol concentrations increase during development, beginning at the end of the first trimester and rapidly increasing during the final weeks of the third trimester. This increase in cortisol facilitates the development of molecular pathways in several organs, including mechanisms for lung fluid clearance at birth and surfactant production. The majority of fetal cortisol is derived from the fetal adrenal gland, and the synthetic capacity of the fetal adrenal gland equals the capacity of the adult adrenal gland. However, placental and/or maternal steroids may allow for normal development in situations where fetal steroidogenesis is insufficient.

(Page 172, Chapter 5: The Newborn)

Answer 5-53. d

The infant in this vignette has evidence of an Erb's palsy, an acquired injury of the upper portion (cervical roots 5 and 6) of the brachial plexus secondary to avulsion or lateral traction during delivery. This phenomenon often occurs in infants during deliveries associated with shoulder dystocia (ie, deliveries of macrosomic babies). The injury leads to paralysis of the deltoid, biceps, and brachialis muscles of the affected arm and shoulder, resulting in positioning of the affected arm as described in the question. Associated findings include ptosis, miosis, and enophthalmos of the ipsilateral eye due to cervical sympathetic nerve injury (Horner syndrome) and diaphragmatic paralysis (due to ipsilateral phrenic nerve injury). The other physical findings are congenital anomalies not associated with Erb's palsy.

(Page 177-178, Chapter 5: The Newborn)

Answer 5-54. e

Vertical transmission of hepatitis B infection can be prevented with appropriate antenatal serologic screening of pregnant women. For infants born to HBsAg seropositive mothers, appropriate immunoprophylaxis includes administration of hepatitis B vaccine and hepatitis B immune globulin.

For a variety of reasons, including inability to access maternal records, maternal hepatitis B serostatus may be unknown at the time of delivery. In these cases, HBsAg serology on the mother should be drawn immediately on admission for delivery, and the hepatitis B vaccine should be administered to the neonate within 12 hours of age. Guidelines for administration of hepatitis B immune globulin are based on infant weight (using a weight cutoff of 2000 g) as well as the timing of determination of maternal serology status.

Because of the variable immune response to the hepatitis B vaccine in neonates born under 2000 g, hepatitis B immune globulin should be given to these infants if maternal serology status cannot be determined within 12 hours. For infants with a birth weight over 2000 g, immune globulin administration may be delayed if the maternal serology status can be determined within 7 days. Infants born to mothers who are HBsAg negative should only receive the hepatitis B vaccine. Maternal chorioamnionitis and hepatitis C seropositive status are not indications for administration of hepatitis B immune globulin.

(Page 186, Section 5: Newborn)

Answer 5-55. a

The infant of a diabetic mother in this vignette most likely is experiencing seizures due to hypocalcemia. Calcium is actively transported across the placenta from the mother to the fetus, with a corresponding decrease in fetal parathyroid hormone (PTH). At birth, neonatal PTH levels surge to account for the decreased transplacental calcium delivery. However, relative to normal infants, infants of diabetic mothers have reduced PTH levels as well as decreased end-organ sensitivity to PTH. The resultant hypocalcemia manifests clinically at 48 to 72 hours of age with neurologic changes (irritability, tremors, twitching, and/or seizures) and cardiac arrhythmias. Prematurity, perinatal depression, and concomitant hypomagnesemia may worsen the hypocalcemia. Serum calcium levels should be monitored in infants of diabetic mothers daily during the first 72 to 96 hours of age.

A complete blood count and C-reactive protein are not indicated in this infant with low risk factors for perinatal bacterial infection and no other clinical signs of sepsis. Since the infant is feeding well, hyponatremia is less likely to be a cause of her seizures. Imaging of the head in an infant with a nonfocal neurologic examination is not warranted.

(Page 197, Section 5: Newborn)

Answer 5-56. e

The nonvigorous infant in this vignette requires intubation and aspiration of the trachea for aspirated meconium from the amniotic fluid. He demonstrates signs of secondary apnea at birth (apnea, hypotonia, and bradycardia [heart rate 50 beats/min]), putting him at risk for meconium aspiration syndrome. This baby requires endotracheal intubation and suctioning on arrival at the delivery room table. Suctioning of the mouth and nose of a meconium-stained infant would be performed only if the infant was vigorous (ie, demonstrating normal respiratory effort, muscle tone, and heart rate [over 100 beats/min]). Chest compressions and umbilical vein catheterization (for epinephrine administration) are indicated only if the infant remains

bradycardic after tracheal aspiration and ventilation. Nasogastric tube placement would be indicated to decompress the stomach after prolonged bag–mask ventilation.

(Page 166-167, Section 5: Newborn)

Answer 5-57. b

The infant in this vignette has a normal abdominal examination and, in the absence of any other abnormal physical findings, should be discharged home with her parents. The finding of a liver edge 1-2 cm below the costal margin is unremarkable. The umbilical stump in a neonate should be dry; moisture around the umbilical stump may be due to a patent urachus or a mucosal cyst. The lower poles of each kidney may be palpable, with the right kidney higher than the left kidney. The baby has a diastasis recti, a gap in the abdominal rectus muscles that is common in the neonatal period and does not require surgical intervention.

(Page 178-179, Chapter 5: The Newborn)

Answer 5-58. e

Cigarette smoking remains a major cause of prenatal, perinatal, and infant morbidity and mortality, including IUGR. Initiation of a smoking cessation program is an appropriate step to reduce the risk of IUGR in this mother. Prenatal alcohol exposure increases the risk of growth restriction, including microcephaly, and should be avoided in pregnancy. Folic acid supplementation reduces development of congenital spine and brain defects but does not reduce the risk of fetal growth restriction. β-Carotene promotes fetal growth and immune development and should be consumed in appropriate amounts in pregnancy. Consumption of a strict vegan diet may place the fetus at risk for poor growth; appropriate supplementation of the diet with nonmeat-derived protein (ie, legumes, soy) is required in pregnancy.

(Page 162-163, Section 5: Newborn)

Answer 5-59. c

Neonatal and infant mortality rates have steadily declined over the past 10 years (see Figure 41-1), largely due to advances in neonatal care. The advent of surfactant therapy and antenatal corticosteroids to decrease the incidence of respiratory distress syndrome has reduced significantly neonatal mortality. Furthermore, mortality among low-birth-weight infants has decreased in NICU centers providing high levels of care and treating high volumes of these at-risk infants. However, certain factors, including male sex, African American ethnicity, late (after the first trimester of pregnancy) or no prenatal care, multiple gestation, and low birth weight, increase the risk of neonatal and infant mortality.

(Page 160-163, Section 5: Newborn)

Answer 5-60. c

Metabolic acidosis is defined as an increase in serum hydrogen (H⁺) ion or a decrease in serum bicarbonate, resulting in a decrease in serum pH. A normal ion gap metabolic acidosis occurs in the setting of renal or gastrointestinal bicarbonate losses and is characterized by hyperchloremia. Preterm neonates (as in case C) often develop a mild, proximal renal tubular acidosis, with urine bicarbonate wasting and a low serum pH. In contrast, an increased ion gap metabolic acidosis develops due to production of lactate (from sepsis, hypoxia–ischemia, tissue damage, or a congenital heart defect) or another anion (from an inborn error of metabolism [IEM]). The other infants have conditions (aortic coarctation, patent ductus arteriosus, IEM, and bacterial sepsis, respectively) that will produce a serum anion gap and metabolic acidosis.

(Page 220-221, Section 5: Newborn)

Answer 5-61. d

The neonate in this vignette has an abnormal neurologic examination, which may occur secondary to abnormalities in levels of serum electrolytes, glucose, or amino acids. However, of the values listed, the serum calcium level is the abnormal laboratory value most associated with this neonate's presentation. His hypercalcemia has occurred secondary to subcutaneous fat necrosis (in the indurated cheek nodules) associated with perinatal trauma. Granulomata in the necrotic fat cause parathyroid hormone (PTH)–independent overproduction of 1,25-dihydroxyvitamin D. Presentation of the hypercalcemia may range from mild neurologic changes seen here to hypertension, seizures, respiratory distress, and nephrocalcinosis. Management includes hydration, increasing urinary calcium excretion, and restriction of dietary calcium intake.

(Page 217-218, Chapter 5: The Newborn)

Answer 5-62. e

The premature neonate in this vignette has signs of systemic hypotension. The cardiovascular system of the preterm infant has adapted in utero to the low-resistance state of the placenta. With the clamping of the umbilical cord, the premature myocardium is exposed to a high-resistance ex utero state, and is generally unable to readily adapt to the change. Initiation of an inotrope (in this case, dopamine) will provide cardiac stimulation and vasopressor effects that will improve blood pressure and perfusion.

The myocardium of the preterm infant is impacted by positive pressure ventilation; increases in the PIP and PEEP will increase intrathoracic pressure, decreasing cardiac output and perfusion. Sepsis is a common cause of hypotension and hypoperfusion in the neonate, but immune globulin has not been shown to reverse the circulatory collapse associated with early onset or late-onset infections. Maintaining the patency of the ductus arteriosus with a PGE1 infusion will allow left-to-right shunting of blood during the cardiac cycle, lowering systemic blood pressure.

(Page 243-244, Section 5: Newborn)

Answer 5-63. b

The infant in this vignette developed anasarca as a result of an in utero tachyarrhythmia. However, delivery room management of this infant does not differ from the management of other infants with ineffective ventilation. This infant may have respiratory failure due to respiratory distress syndrome and pleural effusions (secondary to arrhythmia-induced congestive heart failure). Thus, intubation and mechanical ventilation are the appropriate steps at this point in the resuscitation. Neither blow-by nor nasal cannula oxygen will sufficiently support the degree of respiratory distress in this neonate. Epinephrine only should be administered after adequate ventilation and chest compressions fail to improve neonatal bradycardia. Infusion of adenosine (to convert SVT into a sinus rhythm) is not indicated in delivery room resuscitation of a neonate, including those with fetal SVT.

(Page 166-169, Section 5: Newborn)

Answer 5-64. a

In general, due to the increased surface area of the newborn relative to a newborn's body weight, heat production in the neonate is greater than heat production in the adult.

Nonshivering thermogenesis is generally accepted as the major source of heat generation in neonates. An important protein involved in nonshivering thermogenesis is UCP1, an ion transport protein that generates heat through entry of protons into mitochondria. Brown fat, the major tissue involved in nonshivering thermogenesis, also is relatively more abundant in the neonate than in the adult. Energy generation in neonates is also augmented by intracellular free fatty acids, which are produced by elevated levels of lipoprotein lipase at birth. Circulating free fatty acids replenish depleted intracellular energy stores but do not serve as an acute source of energy.

The neonate, however, has thermogenic disadvantages relative to adults. Due to an increased surface area relative to body weight, newborns must generate more heat to maintain a normal body temperature. Additionally, the absolute extent to which a neonate can maintain a normal body temperature during cold stress is limited.

(Page 171-172, Chapter 5)

Answer 5-65. b

Although preterm delivery can occur in both singleton and multifetal pregnancies, the preterm birth rates for multifetal gestations are significantly greater. Recent data have indicated that most multifetal gestations are born prematurely, with preterm birth rates for twins and triplets reported as 60.5% and 93.7%, respectively (see Table 46-1). These preterm infants are at risk for developing all of the complications typically associated with prematurity, including poor long-term neurodevelopmental outcomes. Twin–twin transfusion syndrome typically occurs in monozygotic twinning when a vascular connection between twins develops in the shared placenta. Dizygotic twins account for two thirds of all spontaneous twin births. In association with the use of assisted fertilization and advanced maternal age, there has been an overall increase in the incidence of multifetal gestations since the 1980s. Fetuses of multifetal gestations are more likely to have breech or other malpresentations at delivery, contributing to a higher rate of cesarean deliveries.

(Page 190, Section 5: Newborn)

Answer 5-66. d

The infant is this vignette has become apneic secondary to ventilatory insufficiency. Surfactant deficiency and increased chest wall compliance have led to atelectasis and diminished gas exchange, which are hallmarks of respiratory distress syndrome. Positive pressure ventilation is necessary until the infant's own respirations can support gas exchange. Endotracheal intubation will also allow for the administration of surfactant. Exogenous surfactant administration can reduce the surface tension of the alveoli and improve functional residual capacity. CPAP and nasal cannula oxygen would not be appropriate modes of ventilation for an apneic patient as they rely on the patient to spontaneously breathe for gas exchange. Tension pneumothoraces can be a complication of mechanical ventilation and should be suspected when asymmetric breath sounds, asymmetric chest wall contours, hypotension, and hypoxia develop acutely. Inhaled nitric oxide, a vasodilator used to reduce the pulmonary vascular tone in infants with persistent pulmonary hypertension of the newborn, is not indicated during delivery room resuscitation.

(Page 258, Section 5: Newborn)

Answer 5-67. c

The infant in this vignette is a preterm infant with respiratory distress syndrome (RDS) and subsequent CO_2 retention. Additionally, she has developed radiographic changes in her lung fields and prolonged ventilator dependency. Over time, infants with RDS develop areas of inflammation, mucous plugging, and airway narrowing. Such infants may experience worsening of respiratory symptoms following extubation, as removal of the positive pressure can reduce airway patency. Without intervention, the infant may develop worsening atelectasis and severe respiratory distress. CPAP delivered noninvasively (via nasal prongs or mask) at pressures of 4 to 8 cm H_2O can often provide enough support to distend the airways and reduce alveolar atelectasis.

Common indications for use of CPAP in neonates include supporting mild RDS or narrowing of the airways, transitioning from mechanical ventilation, and decreasing the incidence or severity of apnea and bradycardia in some preterm infants. If CPAP did not resolve the infant's symptoms (or if symptoms worsened) over a defined period of time, then endotracheal intubation and mechanical ventilation would be appropriate management. As the infant's lung disease was improving with SIMV mode, ventilation with high frequency

is not indicated. Supplemental oxygen may improve the infant's pulse oxygen saturations but would not provide consistent and adequate positive pressure to achieve airway patency.

(Page 258, Section 5: Newborn)

Answer 5-68. e

The infant in this vignette has lung injury secondary to congenital pneumonia. As his pulmonary infection resolves, his lung compliance changes, leading to variable tidal volumes despite stable ventilator settings. With pressure-limited ventilation, the volume of gas delivered depends on the underlying lung compliance (ie, highly compliant lungs will receive a greater volume of gas at a given pressure). Volume-targeted ventilation attempts to deliver consistent volumes of gas into the lungs despite changing lung compliance. For example, if lung compliance abruptly increases, the ventilator will maintain the same inhaled volume of gas by reducing the pressure used during inspiration. Intermittent mandatory ventilation, high-frequency oscillation, and pressure support all are forms of pressure-limited ventilation that would not be able to respond to changes in lung compliance.

(Page 259, Section 5: Newborn)

Answer 5-69. c

The infant in this vignette developed persistent pulmonary hypertension of the newborn (PPHN) secondary to meconium aspiration syndrome. PPHN is characterized by persistently elevated pulmonary vascular tone causing intrapulmonary or extrapulmonary right-to-left shunting. The overall goals of therapy are to optimize lung inflation and lower pulmonary vascular resistance. High-frequency oscillation is being used in this vignette to improve lung inflation. Techniques to reduce pulmonary vascular tone include avoiding hypercarbia, hypoxia, and acidosis. Another therapy is inhaled nitric oxide, a selective pulmonary vasodilator. It increases the activity of soluble guanylate cyclase, leading to increases in cyclic GMP (cGMP), an important promoter of smooth muscle relaxation. Inhaled nitric oxide has become an important therapy in the management of PPHN. Diuretics that block transporters in the nephron (chlorothiazide to block the Na^+–Cl^- symporter or furosemide to block the Na^+–K^+–$2Cl^-$ cotransporter) have a limited role in PPHN. Opiates, which activate mu opioid receptors, may be used for sedating patients who have difficulty tolerating high-frequency ventilation but are not specifically therapeutic in PPHN. Albuterol, a β_2-adrenergic agonist, is used for patients with airway hyperresponsiveness and has a role in the management of chronic lung disease.

(Page 207, 260, Section 5: Newborn)

Answer 5-70. c

Infants with SIP clinically present with pneumoperitoneum, making the differentiation between SIP and advanced NEC challenging. The infant in this vignette has several features and risk factors to suggest that the intestinal perforation is a consequence of a SIP, including timing of the perforation (7-10 days) after indomethacin and glucocorticoid exposure, poor intrauterine growth, and extremely low birth weight. Conversely, infants who develop NEC typically have received enteral feeds prior to presentation and may demonstrate radiographic features such as portal venous gas or pneumatosis intestinalis.

The mucosal margins of the intestinal perforation appear healthy in a SIP (as opposed to the coagulation necrosis observed in NEC). This histopathologic difference also helps to distinguish the 2 entities. Additionally, infants with SIP have decreased mortality compared with infants with NEC-related intestinal perforation. Volvulus and duodenal atresia in the newborn period require surgical management; however, they typically present with symptoms of intestinal obstruction, including vomiting and bilious aspirates. As with NEC, cow's milk protein allergy can present with hematochezia and feeding intolerance, but this illness does not involve intestinal perforation.

(Page 247, Section 5: Newborn)

Answer 5-71. a

The infant experienced delayed cord clamping during his home delivery, which allowed for the transfusion of excess red blood cell volume. Polycythemia, defined as a central venous hematocrit of greater than 65%, can result in hyperviscosity syndrome, or organ dysfunction due to impaired blood flow. Symptoms include neurologic changes (as described in the vignette), respiratory impairment, feeding difficulty, and thrombocytopenia. A cranial sonogram can be used to diagnose intracranial causes of neonatal irritability and lethargy such as acute hemorrhage and sinus venous thrombosis. Congenital hypothyroidism can present with hypotonia, lethargy, and poor feeding, but the symptoms often present days to weeks after birth. A stool occult blood test can help determine a source of bleeding in an anemic infant but is not a useful test for polycythemia. A chest radiograph would be helpful to rule out alternative causes of the infant's respiratory distress but would not be helpful for the diagnosis of polycythemia.

(Page 227, Section 5: Newborn)

Answer 5-72. e

Given the risk of kernicterus in the newborn period, significant efforts should be made to identify all infants with pathologic serum bilirubin levels. Risk factors for hyperbilirubinemia include a family history of neonatal jaundice, East Asian ethnicity, male gender, blood extravasation (ie, cephalohematoma), prematurity, exclusive breast-feeding, and postnatal weight loss. The infant in this vignette has multiple risk factors for hyperbilirubinemia, making a total serum bilirubin level an appropriate screening test. Screening for

iron deficiency anemia with a hemoglobin level is done at 9 to 12 months of age. Vitamin D supplementation is often needed to reach the recommended amount of vitamin D intake, 400 IU daily; however, screening serum vitamin D levels is not recommended. C-reactive protein can be used as a screening test for sepsis in the neonatal period. Screening for lead toxicity is performed between 1 and 2 years of age for infants with risk of environmental lead exposure.

(Page 231, Section 5: Newborn)

Answer 5-73. b

Factors such as prematurity and being the infant of a diabetic mother contribute to increased bilirubin production in this infant, leading to neonatal jaundice. Based on the AAP practice guidelines for infants with hyperbilirubinemia (see Figure 53-3), phototherapy should be initiated in this infant. Phototherapy converts the bilirubin to lumirubin for excretion. If the bilirubin level rises too quickly (greater than 0.2 mg/dL/h) despite intensive phototherapy, IV Ig or exchange transfusion may be needed to decrease any circulating antibodies that cause hemolysis and/or reduce the serum bilirubin concentration. The infant is well hydrated, voiding, stooling, and does not have excessive weight loss; therefore, IV hydration or discontinuation of breast-feeding is unnecessary at this time.

(Page 232, Section 5: Newborn)

Answer 5-74. c

This infant's fetal anemia, bilious amniotic fluid, and features of hydrops suggest erythroblastosis fetalis, resulting from the hemolysis of fetal red blood cells by maternally derived Rh antigens. Mothers who are Rh-negative may become sensitized to the most significant Rh protein, anti-D antigen, if Rh-positive fetal blood cells enter into the maternal circulation. However, Rh sensitization has been largely decreased in the United States thanks to the use of anti-D immune globulin given to Rh-negative mothers at 28 weeks' gestation and after the birth of an Rh-positive infant.

Viruses such as parvovirus and cytomegalovirus are significant causes of fetal hydrops, but the associated anemia results from decreased erythrocyte production rather than hemolysis. Complex congenital heart disease and supraventricular tachycardia may cause fetal hydrops but do not typically involve hemolytic anemia.

(Page 226, Section 5: Newborn)

Answer 5-75. e

Thrombocytopenia in the neonate can result from either decreased production or increased destruction of platelets. Kasabach-Merritt syndrome, also known as giant hemangioma syndrome, is characterized by the presence of a vascular tumor that sequesters platelets, leading to significant thrombocytopenia. In this case, the trapping of platelets and consumptive coagulaopathy end in platelet destruction. There may also be a microangiopathic hemolytic anemia associated with the presence of the mass. Trisomies 13 and 18, Fanconi syndrome, and TAR syndrome all may present with thrombocytopenia but are not associated with the presence of vascular malformations.

(Page 228, Section 5: Neonatology)

Answer 5-76. b

When labor begins, sodium–potassium exchange occurs at the basolateral membrane of the lung epithelium allowing for active transport of sodium across the apical surface via sodium channels. Subsequently, water is drawn from the air spaces into the lung interstitium, clearing fetal lung fluid in anticipation of air exchange. This process is activated by a surge of catecholamines and other hormones during labor.

The infant in this vignette was born by cesarean section without a period of labor, which increases his risk for transient tachypnea of the newborn (TTN). The mild respiratory alkalosis and radiographic changes noted in this vignette support this diagnosis. Chemical pneumonitis can occur as a result of meconium aspiration syndrome, which did not occur in this case. Ascending infection through the birth canal can cause congenital pneumonia, which is less likely in this neonate due to the rupture of amniotic membranes at delivery. Increased pulmonary vascular tone results in persistent pulmonary hypertension of the newborn, which is less likely in this case given the normal pulse oximetry readings. High alveolar surface tension due to surfactant deficiency can result in respiratory distress syndrome (RDS). However, the absence of a supplemental oxygen requirement and traditional radiographic findings (bilateral granular lung fields) make RDS less likely in this case.

(Page 201, Section 5: Newborn)

Answer 5-77. a

The infant in this vignette has a pneumothorax, one type of air leak syndrome. Pulmonary air leaks can result from any lung disease in newborns, particularly in those who require mechanical ventilation. The size of the pneumothorax at presentation can vary, as does the degree of clinical compromise. Pneumothoraces can cause significant respiratory distress, hypoxemia, hypercarbia, or hypotension, warranting emergent decompression. If the infant's clinical deterioration precludes chest tube placement in a controlled setting, needle decompression of the affected hemithorax should be performed immediately as a temporizing measure. Increasing the mean airway pressure will not resolve the infant's pneumothorax and may contribute to worsening air leak.

Pericardiocentesis is indicated for a pneumopericardium (air collection in the pericardial space) associated with cardiac tamponade, which this infant does not demonstrate based on clinical examination and radiographic data. Stabilization of the airway, drainage of gastric contents, and surgical consultation are initial steps in the management of congenital diaphragmatic hernia, which is demonstrated radiographically by bowel (or other abdominal contents) in the thorax. Intubation of the right main stem bronchus may cause decreased left-sided breath sounds and respiratory insufficiency; however, this infant's endotracheal tube is appropriately placed as visualized on the x-ray.

(Page 206, Section 5: Newborn)

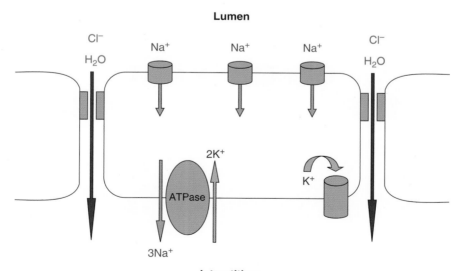

FIGURE 50-1. Model of fetal lung fluid absorption by epithelial cells. Fluid absorption results from vectorial transport of Na+, driven by Na+/K+-ATPase. The resultant electrochemically increased gradient leads to passive Na+ absorption via apical Na+-permeant channels that is extruded by Na+/K+-ATPase out of the cell. Cl and water passively follow the Na+ ions through paracellular or intracellular pathway. (Reproduced, with permission, from Rudolph CD, Rudolph A, Lister G, First L, Gershon A. *Rudolph's Pediatrics*. 22nd ed. New York: McGraw-Hill, 2011.)

Answer 5-78. a

The infant in this vignette has developed idiopathic persistent pulmonary hypertension of the newborn (PPHN). Constriction of the fetal ductus arteriosus by nonsteroidal anti-inflammatory drug exposure is 1 possible cause of idiopathic PPHN. Findings of idiopathic PPHN include cyanosis and respiratory distress within hours of birth, differential cyanosis or pulse oximetry indicating right-to-left shunt, and reduced arterial oxygenation despite relatively normal pco_2 and/or metabolic acidosis. X-rays of the chest may reveal undervascularized lung fields with hyperlucency (depending on the presence or absence of additional lung pathology). Echocardiography with Doppler flow studies can confirm features of PPHN such as intracardiac right-to-left shunts and tricuspid valve regurgitation, which suggest elevated right-sided pressures. Serial blood gas sampling and pulse oximetry are important clues to the diagnosis of PPHN and are useful in ongoing management, but are nonspecific and do not estimate pulmonary vascular resistance. Tracheal aspirates and blood cultures may identify an infectious etiology for an infant with PPHN but do not assess pulmonary vascular pressures.

(Page 207, Section 5: Newborn)

Answer 5-79. d

Pulmonary hemorrhage, a potentially fatal complication, is a chief cause of death in 9% of neonatal autopsies. It most commonly occurs between days 2 and 4 of life. Left ventricular failure is thought to be an inciting factor in pulmonary hemorrhage, as increased pressures are transmitted to the lung capillaries and generate injury. Conditions that precipitate left heart failure such as cocaine exposure, sepsis, asphyxia, and congenital heart disease are associated with pulmonary hemorrhage. However, preterm infants with persistence of a large patent ductus arteriosus (PDA) are at particular risk for pulmonary hemorrhage. In neonates with large PDAs, exposure of the lungs to high pressure and high blood flow results in microvascular injury that leads to hemorrhage.

(Page 203-204, Section 5: Newborn)

Answer 5-80. a

The infant in this vignette has developed a pulmonary hemorrhage following the administration of surfactant, which is a recognized risk factor. As pulmonary hemorrhage is a potentially fatal event, rapid measures should be taken to stabilize the patient and correct any known causes of the hemorrhage. Specific measures to treat pulmonary hemorrhage include maintaining adequate mean airway pressure to support lung volume and gas exchange, restoring circulating blood volume, and ameliorating coagulopathy. Management of predisposing factors also should be considered, such as closure of a large patent ductus arteriosus with indomethacin. However, without a patent airway none of these interventions will sufficiently provide adequate cardiorespiratory support for the patient. Therefore, the first step in the management of this infant is to suction and secure the airway.

(Page 203-204, Section 5: Newborn)

CHAPTER 6 | Principles of Adolescent Care

Lauren B. Hartman and Sara M. Buckelew

6-1. A 17-year-old boy presents to your office for an acute care visit. He has come without his parents' knowledge or consent. He recently started having sexual intercourse and has not always been using a condom. He would really prefer that his parents not know that he has started having sex. He states that he has had some yellow discharge from his penis and is concerned he may have a sexually transmitted infection. Your next step is to:

a. Call his parents and explain the situation without telling him that you are calling.

b. Call his partner and explain the situation without telling him that you are calling.

c. Tell him that you cannot see him without notifying his parents.

d. Explain the rules of confidentiality in the state where you practice, and offer confidential STI testing and treatment as able.

e. Explain to him that under federal law, you cannot treat him for an STI without notifying his parents.

6-2. A 14-year-old African American male presents to your office for an urgent care visit. He presents with sudden onset of severe left-sided hip and thigh pain and is unable to bear weight. Of note, he is obese (BMI 35). You are concerned he might have a slipped capital femoral epiphysis (SCFE). If he does in fact have SCFE, which sexual maturity rating (SMR) would you expect on physical examination?

a. SMR 1

b. SMR 3

c. SMR 4

d. SMR 5

e. SMR 6

6-3. Which hormone is the most influential in affecting breast development during puberty?

a. Progesterone

b. Thyroxine

c. Luteinizing hormone

d. Insulin

e. Estrogen

6-4. At what mean age and mean sexual maturity rating does spermarche occur?

a. 12 years; 2 SMR

b. 13 years; 3 SMR

c. 13.5 years; 2.5 SMR

d. 14.5 years; 3.5 SMR

e. None of the above

6-5. A patient presents for a physical examination for school. Overall he reports that things are going well. On your HEADSSS assessment, he reports that he lives with his parents. While they get along well generally, they have been fighting more because he has been staying out later than they would like. He states he is attracted to females, and just recently began dating for the first time. He reports that he and the girl broke up, and his friends were his main support. He reports he has used alcohol, as all of his friends drink as well. As a result, he is unclear if he really wants to stop drinking at this time. You note that he has never driven in a car with someone who is drinking. When thinking about his biopsychosocial development, what stage would you estimate him to be?

a. Early adolescence (age 10-13)

b. Middle adolescence (age 14-16)

c. Late adolescence (age 17-21)

d. Young adulthood (age 21-24)

e. None of the above

6-6. A 14-year-old girl, new patient, presents for a physical examination. You obtain a medical history and want to do a social history. You decide to complete a HEADSSS assessment. You ask the parent to leave the room so you can ask the patient about these sensitive topics. After mom has left, you begin. Which of the following is true about the HEADSSS assessment model?

a. It is a good model in order to assess the health and well-being of the adolescent in a number of different domains.

b. You must report all the information obtained back to her parent.

c. If you complete a HEADSSS assessment, you do not need to complete a physical examination.

d. You should not ask the patient about suicidal ideations as that might lead them to have thoughts about suicide.

e. HEADSSS is a series of questions used to definitively diagnose specific conditions.

6-7. A 16-year-old male presents for a physical examination. Overall, he seems to be healthy and doing well. His last physical examination was so long ago that he cannot remember the date of the visit. His mother wants to make sure he is caught up in his immunizations but she did not bring his immunization records. What will you advise the patient and his mother about immunizations?

a. If it has been more than 5 years since he received any vaccines, he should receive a TdAP, given recent concern about tetanus outbreaks.

b. If it has been more than 5 years since he received any vaccines, he should receive a TdAP, given recent concern about pertussis outbreaks.

c. Adolescents typically do not require any vaccinations, even though he hasn't had any in at least 5 years.

d. He needs his third measles–mumps–rubella (MMR) immunization at 16 years of age.

e. He needs to repeat all of his vaccines since his mother did not bring his vaccination records.

6-8. You are asked to give a presentation to a local group of high school students. The school has asked that you present information related to adolescent health. One teacher reports that they recently had a student in the school who died, and the students have been quite upset about this. The teachers would like to be sure that you mention the major causes of adolescent mortality. Which of the following should you report to them as the leading cause of death in teens?

a. Suicide

b. Homicide

c. Late effects from the treatment of childhood neoplasms

d. Malignant neoplasms

e. Unintentional injuries, including motor vehicle accidents

6-9. A 13-year-old male presents for a physical examination. You notice on review of his chart that he is overweight, and has been overweight since he was about 3 years old. You want to discuss your concerns about the health consequences of being overweight with him. What will be your next step in managing this patient about his weight?

a. Say nothing, since he is so young that there are no health consequences to his current weight.

b. Document the BMI for now and track over time. Most overweight adolescents do not become overweight or obese adults.

c. Discuss with him some of the health consequences that are associated with overweight and obesity such as diabetes, hypertension, and high cholesterol.

d. Counsel him that he shouldn't worry, given that only 25% of overweight adolescents become overweight or obese adults.

e. Advise him that he will never get a date unless he loses weight.

6-10. What percentage of adolescents uses contraception at their first intercourse?

a. 10%

b. 25%

c. 50%

d. 75%

e. 95%

6-11. A 14-year-old male is brought into the ER by his friends. His friends explain that the patient had been with them at a party earlier that night when he suddenly lost consciousness. They are not exactly sure what he had ingested. After his airway is secured and IV fluids are administered, his labs return and you learn that his blood alcohol level is 250 mg/dL of ethanol. With severe alcohol intoxication, what other laboratory abnormalities can you expect to find?

a. Hyperkalemia

b. Hyperglycemia

c. Elevated osmolar gap

d. Metabolic alkalosis

e. Hyponatremia

6-12. A mother presents to clinic with her 15-year-old daughter. The mother is concerned because her daughter used to be very close with the rest of the family, an excellent student, and captain of the soccer team. However, over the past few months she has been refusing to join the family at dinner, her grades are deteriorating, and she has been missing soccer practice. You meet with the patient alone. On examination, she is tachycardic and appears anxious. Her pupils are dilated and she has injected conjunctiva, and she has poor coordination and balance. What is the patient's diagnosis?

a. Panic disorder

b. Schizophrenia, paranoid type

c. Opiate intoxication

d. Ethanol intoxication

e. Cannabis intoxication

6-13. Which of the following statements correctly describes the American Academy of Pediatrics position on drug testing of adolescents?

a. Adolescents can be tested for drugs of abuse involuntarily with their parent's consent.

b. With few exceptions, involuntary testing of adolescents for drugs of abuse should not be done.

c. Adolescents can be tested for drugs of abuse if their parent, teacher, or doctor suspects that they are using drugs.

d. Involuntary testing of adolescents for drugs of abuse can be done if the results are kept confidential.

e. Involuntary testing of adolescents for drugs of abuse can be done on a case-by-case basis.

6-14. A 16-year-old girl presents complaining of symptoms such as depressed mood and worthlessness. She states, "nothing matters." Her parents report that her performance in school has declined over the course of this year, and she no longer seems interested in her school clubs, which she used to greatly enjoy. Both the patient and parents are interested in starting a treatment that may help her. What is your next step in the management of this patient?

a. You ask them to follow up with you in 3 months.

b. Medications are not recommended for the management of depression in adolescents, so you refer them for therapy.

c. You discuss options for medications, including potential risks and benefits, and reach a decision with the patient and family.

d. You ask her specific questions in order to assess her risk of suicide in order to determine the acuity of her depressive symptoms.

e. You order a hemoglobin level and thyroid-stimulating hormone (TSH) levels to screen for anemia and hypothyroidism.

6-15. A 15-year-old female presents to the emergency department for chest pain. She reports that she was at school and she began to feel dizzy and light-headed and then noticed that her heart felt like it was beating so hard it was going to pop out of her chest. She reports that she felt like she was going to die of a heart attack. She has a family history positive for asthma, but she herself has no other significant medical history and her physical examination is within normal limits. What is your next step in the management of this patient?

a. Order echocardiography and an electrocardiogram in order to rule out a myocardial infarction.

b. Discharge home with an albuterol inhaler.

c. Recommend and prescribe lorazepam for her to use regularly.

d. Refer her for a psychological assessment for cognitive behavioral therapy and psychiatric evaluation for medication.

e. Review the results of your examination with the parents and patient. Reassure them that nothing is wrong. No further treatment is needed.

6-16. The mother of a 17-year-old patient of yours calls you to express her concerns about her son. She is crying when she speaks to you. She reports that he was caught shoplifting and seems to have no understanding of the potential consequences. His mom reports that she feels like he is out of control for the last week, staying up all night playing music. He has started talking about being a rock star. She feels like she can't get a word in when she speaks to him as he speaks so quickly. You are reviewing the chart when you speak with her. You notice last year when you saw him for his annual physical examination, you were concerned that he was depressed. Currently, in speaking with mom, you are most concerned that:

a. He is having a manic episode, which untreated may put his safety at risk.

b. He is abusing alcohol, which untreated may put his safety at risk.

c. He has symptoms of barbiturate abuse, which may put his safety at risk.

d. He has symptoms of posttraumatic stress disorder, which will be difficult to treat.

e. This episode of shoplifting may put his chances of being accepted into a competitive university at risk.

6-17. A 12-year-old girl is brought in by her parents as they are worried about her. About a month ago, the house was burglarized at night while the family was home asleep. Your patient woke up to get a drink of water, and saw the burglars who threatened her and her family if she told anyone what she had seen prior to their fleeing the home. Since then, she has had nightmares and hasn't wanted to sleep in her room by herself. She is jumpy and hypervigilant. Her parents are looking to you for what they should do next for their daughter. You:

a. Prescribe a sleeping pill such as zolpidem.

b. Criticize the parents for involving the police given the threat to their safety.

c. Refer the patient and her family for a psychological assessment for appropriate therapy.

d. Inform the parents that this condition is transient and will improve with time, especially if the police catch the burglars.

e. Inform the parents that this condition is less common among females than among males.

6-18. A 15-year-old female presents for her annual physical examination. You review her growth chart prior to seeing her and notice that both her weight and body mass index (BMI) have dropped significantly since you saw her last year (from the 50th percentile to the 10th percentile). On history, she reports that she is on the cross-country team and running many miles weekly. Additionally, she reports that while onset of menarche was at age 12, she has not had a period in the last 6 months. She denies sexual activity, substance use, and any other physical complaints and is doing very well in school. Her mother reports that she has been worried about her daughter's recent weight loss and social isolation, particularly around meal times. Your next step is to:

a. Obtain vital signs, including a resting heart rate, blood pressure, and body temperature, as you are concerned she may require hospitalization.

b. Order lab tests, including a complete blood count and serum electrolyte levels.

c. Reassure mom that dieting is normal adolescent behavior.

d. Call her coach to see if the coach has any concerns.

e. Hospitalize the patient.

6-19. A 19-year-old female presents to your office for a physical examination. Her weight and BMI are at the 60th percentile. Her heart rate and blood pressure are within normal limits. She reports that overall things are going well at home and at school. She does endorse that she is experimenting with alcohol and marijuana. She also states that she wishes that she were thinner,

and that she has been dieting. You proceed to your physical examination. Which of the following physical examination findings would make you more concerned that the patient is engaging in disordered eating behaviors?

a. Acanthosis nigricans on her neck and axillae

b. Russell sign on her hands

c. Dilated pupils

d. Hyperthermia

e. Kayser-Fleischer rings

6-20. A 16-year-old female presents to your office having recently been hospitalized for medical complications due to anorexia nervosa. She was hospitalized for 2 weeks and was able to gain weight in the hospital. Since hospital discharge, she has been eating better, including 3 meals and 3 snacks, and has limited her physical activity. Her parents would like her to start mental health treatment and would like some next steps in finding appropriate treatment for her. You make the following recommendation, thinking it has the strongest evidence base in the treatment of anorexia nervosa:

a. You refer her to a psychiatrist to begin psychotropic medication, such as an antidepressant.

b. You refer her to a nutritionist, as the studies show she has the best chance to do well if she can reach a higher weight.

c. You refer her to an individual therapist, as research demonstrates she will do better if the parents play a minimal role in treatment.

d. You refer her to a family-based therapist, as this psychotherapeutic modality has the strongest evidence base.

e. None of the above.

6-21. A 14-year-old female presents for her annual physical examination. During the review of systems, she says that she has bilateral breast pain, in the upper outer quadrants of her breasts. On physical examination, you find diffuse cordlike thickening, as well as discrete mobile lesions throughout her breasts. Which additional piece of history or examination finding would aid in confirming the diagnosis?

a. The pain begins in the premenstrual phase of the menstrual cycle.

b. The pain begins in the ovulatory phase of the menstrual cycle.

c. She has a positive family history for *BRCA-1* genes.

d. She is having fevers.

e. She was recently in a car accident and was wearing a seat belt overlying her breasts.

6-22. A 14-year-old male presents to your clinic with the chief complaint of breast development. He and his mother explain that they first noticed the enlargement of his breasts 1 year ago. You obtain a detailed history and physical examination and determine that he has pubertal gynecomastia. Which of the following about pubertal gynecomastia is a true statement?

   a. It is common, and occurs in 90% of boys.

   b. It peaks in incidence during Tanner stage (or SMR) 5.

   c. It is a permanent condition.

   d. Spontaneous resolution occurs in 90% of boys.

   e. Medications such as danazol, tamoxifen, and testolactone are recommended.

6-23. A 14-year-old previously healthy male presents with severe left-sided scrotal pain. In addition, he complains of nausea and fever. On physical examination, the left scrotum is erythematous with moderate swelling. His cremasteric reflex is absent. What is the best treatment for this patient?

   a. Empiric treatment with antibiotics.

   b. Supportive treatment including analgesics, anti-inflammatory agents, and scrotal elevation.

   c. Surgical exploration and detorsion.

   d. Surgical exploration and detorsion, as well as scrotal orchiopexy.

   e. Additional testing is required prior to treating this patient.

6-24. A 16-year-old male presents with fever, abdominal pain, and pain in his right scrotum. In reviewing his history, you learn that he has no other significant past medical history, but that 1 week ago he had parotitis. What is the most common cause of this patient's diagnosis in adolescent males?

   a. *Chlamydia trachomatis*

   b. *Staphylococcus aureus*

   c. Coxsackievirus

   d. Adenovirus

   e. Mumps virus

6-25. An 18-year-old male presents for his annual physical examination. He is otherwise healthy, but does report that over the past few months, his right scrotum has been swollen. He denies any pain. On his testicular examination, you note a firm irregular mass that does not transilluminate. The examination is also significant for gynecomastia. Which of the following is a risk factor for this patient's diagnosis?

   a. Cryptorchidism

   b. An uncircumcised penis

   c. Anabolic steroid use

   d. Obesity

   e. Unprotected intercourse

6-26. Which of the following choices best describes a spermatocele?

   a. It is an inflammatory disease of the epididymis.

   b. It is the result of fluid tracking down into the tunica vaginalis.

   c. It is a dilation of the pampiniform venous plexus within the scrotum.

   d. A cystic accumulation of sperm within the epididymis.

   e. It is a dilation of the pampiniform venous plexus within the epididymis.

6-27. A 16-year-old female presents to your clinic for her annual physical examination. During the history, you learn that despite having a history of regular periods, she has not had a period in 3 months. After you complete the history and physical examination, what test would you order next?

   a. A DEXA scan to evaluate her bone density

   b. A qualitative urine human chorionic gonadotropin test

   c. Follicle-stimulating hormone (FSH) and luteinizing hormone (LH)

   d. A karyotype

   e. A urine drug screen

6-28. A 15-year-old female with cystic fibrosis presents to your clinic with the concern of amenorrhea. You do a pregnancy test, which is negative. You suspect that the patient has amenorrhea from nutritional deficiencies secondary to having a chronic disease. What labs would confirm your suspicion?

   a. High luteinizing hormone (LH), high follicle-stimulating hormone (FSH), and low estrogen

   b. High LH, high FSH, and high estrogen

   c. Low LH, low FSH, and low estrogen

   d. High gonadotropin-releasing hormone (GnRH), high LH, and high FSH

   e. Low GnRH, high LH, and high FSH

6-29. A 15-year-old female presents to your clinic with 6 months of painful menstrual periods. She is otherwise healthy and had menarche at age 13. Unfortunately, the painful periods have led to missing a significant amount of school. You begin to counsel your patient about managing dysmenorrhea. Which of the following would *not* help your patient in managing her symptoms?

a. Avoid dietary omega-3 polyunsaturated fatty acids.

b. Take ibuprofen 1 to 2 days before the onset of menses.

c. Take combination oral contraceptive pills.

d. Avoid smoking.

e. Take mefenamic acid 1 to 2 days before the onset of menses.

6-30. You receive a phone call from your colleague informing you that one of your patients has been admitted to the hospital. You learn that the patient is a 14-year-old female with menorrhagia who requires hospitalization for excessive menstrual bleeding. Your patient is undergoing an evaluation to determine the etiology of the bleeding. What is the most common cause of excessive menstrual bleeding requiring hospitalization?

a. Polycystic ovarian syndrome

b. Spontaneous abortion

c. Hemangioma

d. Bleeding disorder

e. Cervical polyps

6-31. A 15-year-old female presents to your clinic with concern that she may be pregnant. She explains that she had unprotected intercourse with her boyfriend 2 weeks ago. You perform a urine pregnancy test, which confirms that she is pregnant. Which of the following statements about teenage pregnancy is correct?

a. Only 50% of adolescents who maintain a pregnancy to term decide to parent the child themselves.

b. Confidentiality does not apply to adolescents who become pregnant.

c. A pelvic examination is not part of the evaluation of a possible pregnancy for an adolescent.

d. Urine B-HCG testing at 1 week postimplantation is unlikely to be positive.

e. Unusual vaginal bleeding is a sign of a possible pregnancy.

6-32. A 17-year-old female presents to the emergency room with the chief complaint of severe lower abdominal pain. You begin interviewing the patient and learn that she hasn't had a period in 2 months. On physical examination, she has abdominal tenderness, and adnexal tenderness. You send some labs and her B-HCG is positive and you are concerned that your patient may have an ectopic pregnancy. Which of the following is *not* a risk factor for developing an ectopic pregnancy?

a. Urinary tract infection

b. Previous pelvic surgery

c. Early sexual debut

d. Multiple sexual partners

e. Cigarette smoking

6-33. A 16-year-old healthy female presents for routine primary care. While talking alone with the patient, she discloses to you that she is sexually active with her boyfriend. She has been using condoms, but wants to start taking oral contraceptive pills. You discuss her history and side effects of the medication and determine that she is a good candidate for this method. Her last menstrual period was 2 days ago.

When should the patient begin taking the pill?

a. At the time of her next menses

b. After you have discussed the plan with the patient's parents

c. Immediately

d. After she has a negative pregnancy test

e. After she has a normal pelvic examination

6-34. A 15-year-old female presents for follow-up after being treated for a deep venous thrombosis in her left calf. In reviewing her history, you learn that the patient is sexually active with her boyfriend and is taking oral contraceptive pills. What is an appropriate management step for you to take?

a. Discontinue her current oral contraceptive pills and start the patient on a lower-dose pill.

b. Discontinue her current oral contraceptive pill and start the patient on depot medroxyprogesterone acetate (DMPA).

c. Discontinue her current oral contraceptive pill and advise to abstain from having sex.

d. Do not change her medication regimen while the patient is sexually active.

e. Discontinue her current oral contraceptive pill and start the patient on the hormonal patch or vaginal ring.

6-35. A 17-year-old female presents to your clinic. She appears anxious as she explains to you that she had unprotected intercourse 3 days ago with her boyfriend. You perform a urine pregnancy test, which is negative. You explain the results to the patient, and she is relieved. Which of the following management steps would be most indicated at this time?

a. Progestin-only emergency contraception (EC)

b. Reassurance, and offering counseling to the patient

c. Estrogen–progestin EC

d. A pelvic examination

e. Providing condoms and asking the patient to follow up in 1 week

6-36. A 16-year-old female presents for her annual physical examination. While discussing her social history, you learn that she is sexually active with her boyfriend. She is interested in starting contraception. You discuss the different options and together decide that depot medroxyprogesterone acetate (DMPA) would be an appropriate method for the patient. Before starting the method you discuss the side effects. Which of the following is a side effect of DMPA?

a. Nausea

b. Breast tenderness

c. Weight loss

d. Amenorrhea

e. Increased bone mineral density

6-37. Which of the following is the most common reported bacterial STI in the United States?

a. *Chlamydia trachomatis*

b. Human papillomavirus (HPV)

c. *Neisseria gonorrhoeae*

d. *Trichomonas vaginalis*

e. Bacterial vaginosis

6-38. A 17-year-old sexually active female presents with 1 week of abnormal vaginal discharge. She describes the discharge as being thin in consistency and white in color. You sample the discharge, and note a pH of 8 and an amine odor. No additional findings are seen on the wet prep. What is the best treatment for this patient?

a. Azithromycin 1 g orally × 1 dose.

b. Ceftriaxone 250 mg IM × 1 dose and doxycycline 100 mg orally twice daily × 7 days.

c. Metronidazole 500 mg orally b.i.d. for 7 days.

d. Fluconazole 150 mg orally × 1 dose.

e. Additional workup is necessary prior to determining treatment.

6-39. A sexually active 15-year-old male presents with a 3-hour history of left-sided testicular pain. He reports no history of trauma. In addition, he is complaining of dysuria. On examination, the scrotum is painful and red. The patient does report pain relief when you elevate the testis. Which of the following diagnostic tests can help confirm your diagnosis?

a. A Doppler ultrasound

b. Nucleic acid amplification tests for *Chlamydia trachomatis*

c. A complete blood count (CBC)

d. Dark field microscopy

e. Radionuclide imaging

6-40. A 15-year-old male presents to your clinic with the concern that he had acquired a sexually transmitted infection (STI). On examination, he has multiple grouped vesicles with an erythematous base on the shaft of his penis that are very painful along with tender inguinal adenopathy. You suspect that he has genital herpes. Which of the following statements can you tell your patient about genital herpes?

a. Most genital herpes infections are symptomatic.

b. Herpes simplex virus type 1 (HSV-1) is now the most common cause of genital herpes in the United States.

c. Stress and sexual intercourse can precipitate recurrences.

d. Close to 90% of genital herpes infections occur in people younger than 19 years old.

e. Seroepidemiologic studies show that 75% of adults in the United States are seropositive for herpes simplex virus type 2 (HSV-2).

6-41. A 17-year-old female presents to the emergency department with fever and lower abdominal pain. She is sexually active and occasionally uses condoms. On physical examination, you note a temperature of 38.4°C, and lower abdominal and pelvic tenderness. She has vaginal discharge, as well as cervical motion tenderness. You suspect pelvic inflammatory disease (PID). What treatment is recommended for PID?

a. Doxycycline 100 mg PO b.i.d. for 14 days with metronidazole 500 mg PO b.i.d. for 14 days

b. Ceftriaxone, 250 mg IM

c. Cefotetan 2 g IV q 12 h plus metronidazole 500 mg PO b.i.d.

d. Cefotetan 2 g IV q 12 h plus doxycycline 100 mg IV q 12 h

e. Clindamycin 900 mg IV q 8 h

6-42. You answer a call for your clinic and speak with a 16-year-old female who is concerned about a vaginal infection. She explains her symptoms to you over the phone and you suspect that she has vaginal candidiasis. You ask that she come to clinic to be examined prior to initiating any treatment. Which of the following is *not* consistent with vaginal candidiasis?

a. Pruritis

b. Vaginal pH >5.0

c. Pseudohyphae in KOH preparation

d. White lesions on vaginal mucosa

e. Erythematous vaginal mucosa

6-43. A 15-year-old female presents for her annual physical examination. The patient's mother would like to make sure she is screened for scoliosis. The patient denies any concerns including back pain. You complete a HEADSSS psychosocial screening, which demonstrates that she is making a number of healthy choices and avoiding risky health behaviors. On her physical examination, her vital signs are stable and both her weight and height are at the 60th percentile for age. In order to screen her for scoliosis, your next step would be:

a. To order an MRI of the entire spine.

b. To obtain a standing posteroanterior and lateral x-ray views of the spine.

c. To perform an Adam forward bend test during your examination.

d. Given the patient has no back pain, she is unlikely to have scoliosis and does not require screening.

e. None of the above.

6-44. A 19-year-old male presents for an acute care visit for back pain. He states that he just got a new job and is doing a lot of lifting. Previously, he was in fairly good physical shape, and has not previously had any back pain. On further history, which complaint would prompt you to obtain a radiograph?

a. He reports that his pain is the worst at the end of the work day.

b. He reports that his pain radiates to the lower extremities.

c. He reports that his pain improves with rest.

d. He reports that his pain is localized to his lower back.

e. Radiographs are not indicated for back pain.

6-45. A 14-year-old male athlete comes to your office 2 days after a championship soccer game. He explains that during the game, while running he twisted his leg. He immediately felt pain in his left ankle. On examination, he has swelling and pain along the ligament. You suspect a grade I or II ankle sprain. Which of the following does *not* describe appropriate management for a grade I or II sprain?

a. Treat your patient with the RICE protocol.

b. During the initial 72 hours after the injury, begin range of motion exercises.

c. During the initial 72 hours after the injury, begin weight bearing.

d. Slowly return to activity as pain and swelling resolve.

e. Refer your patient to a musculoskeletal specialist for further evaluation.

6-46. A 17-year-old male presents to your office because of concerns about his acne. He has never been treated previously but would like to start. On physical examination, he has mild comedonal acne centralized on his face, particularly his nose and forehead. He has no lesions on his chest or back. He has no cysts and no evidence of scarring. You decide the first line of treatment for this patient would be:

a. Topical benzoyl peroxide

b. Oral minocycline

c. Oral isotretinoin

d. Oral adapalene

e. Referral to a dermatologist

6-47. A 17-year-old female presents with moderate acne over her forehead and cheeks, and with several lesions on her back with no evidence of scarring. For the last 6 months she has been using topical tretinoin and benzoyl peroxide with minimal improvement. As a result, she is very interested in additional treatment. She is still quite embarrassed by her acne and really would like her skin to look better. Which is the next best step in management of her acne?

a. Instruct her to make changes to her diet, such as removing chocolate and pizza.

b. Recommend she continue her topical treatment, as she has not given it enough time to work.

c. Insist at this point that she should start oral isotretinoin as nothing else will help.

d. Discuss adding a combined estrogen/progesterone oral contraceptive pill to her current treatment regimen.

e. Referral to a dermatologist.

6-48. A 15-year-old boy presents to your office concerned about a rash. He said it started with a single large, well-circumscribed lesion on his trunk (back), and about a week later he has developed a number of oval salmon-colored flat patches. He says it has been itchy. On physical examination, you notice a number of lesions on his back that resemble the branches of a Christmas tree. He also has lesions in his axillae. He has no lesions on the palms of his hands. He has no past medical history of any skin conditions and is on no medications. You recommend the following next steps in order to manage his rash:

 a. You prescribe a 5-day course of an oral corticosteroid.

 b. You prescribe topical clotrimazole.

 c. You prescribe oral doxycycline.

 d. You recommend oatmeal baths to help with the itching and reassure him that it should self-resolve.

 e. You administer an intramuscular injection of penicillin in the office.

6-49. A 14-year-old male presents to clinic for his physical examination. You complete a HEADSSS interview, and find that he is making very healthy choices. On his physical examination, his vital signs are stable and both his height and weight are at the 50th percentile. On your physical examination, you notice that he has a rash on his chest. He has noticed it but is unsure how long it has been there. The rash includes sharply demarcated and hypopigmented macules and papules with some scaling. He says that sometimes it might be a little itchy, and he thought it got worse this summer following his job as a lifeguard. Your next step in diagnosing this rash would most likely be:

 a. A potassium hydroxide (KOH) examination of scrapings from the lesions

 b. A bacterial culture of scrapings from the lesions

 c. A rapid plasma regain (RPR)

 d. A scabies preparation of scrapings from the lesions

 e. A skin biopsy

6-50. A 17-year-old female presents for an acute care visit. She is concerned that she has "lumps in her armpits." She is afebrile, her vital signs are stable, and she is overweight. On physical examination, you notice she has several large and tender cysts in both axillae. She reports that she has had these before, but they were milder and resolved on their own. You perform a culture, which is negative for growth. Your next step in managing these lesions is:

 a. Oral isotretinoin

 b. Oral diphenhydramine

 c. Topical clindamycin

 d. Immediate surgical excision

 e. Skin biopsy with potential surgical excision

ANSWERS

Answer 6-1. d

In the 1960s, in order to prevent foregone treatment of adolescent sexually transmitted infections, all state legislatures enacted statutes allowing minors to receive treatment for STIs without parental involvement. These laws vary in specifics state to state and are not mandated by federal law. You should be able to see an adolescent and discuss their concerns confidentially without parental involvement, and thus do not need to call the parent to discuss these issues. Billing for these services however may not be confidential depending on the insurance carrier and state regulations.

(Pages 24-25, Section 1: Fundamentals of Pediatrics, Chapter 9: Law, Ethics, and Clinical Judgment)

Answer 6-2. b

The musculoskeletal system is affected significantly by the biological changes of puberty. The growth spurt typically occurs at SMR 2 to 3 for girls and SMR 4 for boys. SCFE typically occurs during the period of maximal skeletal growth, such as occurs concurrently with puberty at SMR 3. SMR 1 is prepubescent (prior to growth spurt or developmental changes), and SMR 5 is complete adult development (postpubertal). SMR 6 does not exist.

(Pages 265-266, Section 6: Principles of Adolescent Care, Chapter 63: Somatic Growth and Development)

Answer 6-3. e

Estrogen is the most influential hormone affecting breast development during puberty. It binds to the breast tissue resulting in stimulation of the glandular ductal system, whereas progesterone is linked to alveolar growth. Other hormones, such as insulin, prolactin, thyroxine, and cortisol, do play an important role in breast development, particularly in their interactions with estrogen. Luteinizing hormone and follicle-stimulating hormone are released by the ovaries and stimulate ovarian growth, not breast development.

(Page 267, Section 6: Principles of Adolescent Care, Chapter 64: Reproductive Growth and Development in the Female Adolescent)

Answer 6-4. c

"Spermarche," or the onset of spermatogenesis, occurs relatively early in puberty. It typically corresponds with a time of rapid increase in testicular weight, as well as in seminiferous tubular diameter, length, and relative volume. Testosterone initiates and maintains the process of spermatogenesis in humans.

(Pages 269-270, Section 6: Principles of Adolescent Care, Chapter 65: Reproductive Growth and Development in Males)

Answer 6-5. b

In middle adolescence, teenagers are now able to understand complex concepts, and have begun to question the thinking and behavior of adults. They begin to think in more abstract terms, which allows for shifts from same-sex relationships/friendships to romantic dating. Risky health behaviors are of critical importance in middle adolescence, as peer norms include engaging in risky behaviors, as individuals make more independent choices.

Early adolescents typically focus on their developing bodies and on their peer group, and their concerns are often around acceptance and conformity.

During late adolescence, individuals are less egocentric and self-centered, are better at understanding others' points of view, and have greater ability to self-reflect and be insightful. Identity exploration/life roles begin to be defined. At this point, physical maturation is complete, and body image and gender role definition clearer. A description of the different stages of adolescence is listed in Table 66-1.

(Pages 271-272, Section 6: Principles of Adolescent Care, Chapter 66: Psychological Development)

TABLE 66-1. Biopsychosocial Development During Adolescence/Emerging Adulthood

Characteristics	Impact
Early adolescence (age 10-13 years)	
Onset of puberty; becomes concerned with developing body	Major questions concerning normality of physical maturation; often concerned about the stages of sexual development and how the process relates to peers of same gender. Occasional masturbation. Important to normalize differences and explain range of normal development
Begins to expand social relationships beyond family and to concentrate on relationships with peers	Encourage teens to begin to take responsibility for their own health and contact with health professionals, in consultation with parents (eg, part of visit time alone with health provider)
Beginning of transition from concrete to abstract thinking	Shift in health provider's focus from anticipatory guidance to parents to risk reduction and prevention education to adolescent. Concrete thinking requires dealing with most health situations in an explicit manner with simple language
Middle adolescence (age 14-16 years)	
Pubertal development usually complete, and sexual drives emerge	Explores ability to attract others. Sexual experimentation (same and opposite sex) begins. Masturbation increases
Peer group sets behavioral standards, although family values usually persist	Peer group influences engagement in positive and negative health behaviors; peers rather than parents may also offer key support. Important to emphasize role of teen in making good choices and taking responsibility
Conflicts over independence	Increased assumption of independent action, together with continued need for parental support and guidance; able to discuss and negotiate changes in rules. Increased involvement of teen in setting health-related goals and being clear on how to handle health situation (eg, time to take medication). Reinforce adolescents' growing competencies
Emergence of abstract thinking with new cognitive competencies	Increased ability to process information, see other perspectives, and reflect. Often leads to questioning adult behavior. While may consider broader range of possibilities/options, may not yet be able to integrate into real life. Important to be clear that individual understands and knows what he or she needs to do regarding health concerns
Late adolescence/emerging adulthood (age 17-21 years)	
Physical maturation complete; body image and gender role definition clearer	Begins to feel comfortable with relationships and decisions regarding sexuality and preference. Individual relationships become more important than peer group
Individuals less egocentric and self-centered; better at understanding others' points of view; greater ability to self-reflect and be insightful	More open to questioning regarding their behavior. More able to work with clinician on setting goals and changing behavior
Idealistic	Idealism may lead to conflict with family or authority figures
Identity exploration/life roles begin to be defined	People most likely to be exploring options in their lives; often interested in discussion of life goals
Cognitive development nearing completion	Most are capable of understanding a full range of options for health issues. Important to help them become competent in negotiating the health care system

Reproduced, with permission, from Rudolph CD, Rudolph A, Lister G, First L, Gershon A. *Rudolph's Pediatrics*. 22nd ed. New York: McGraw-Hill, 2011.

TABLE 67-1. HEADSSS Assessment for Psychosocial Concerns: Screening History

Assessment Area	Questions
Home	How is the adolescent's home life? How are his or her relationships with family members? Where and with whom does the patient live? Is his or her living situation stable?
Education (or employment)	How is the adolescent's school performance? Is he or she well behaved, or are there discipline problems at school? If adolescent is working, is he or she making a living wage? Is the adolescent financially secure?
Eating (incorporates body image)	Does the patient have a balanced diet? Is there adequate calcium intake? Is the adolescent trying to lose weight, and if so, is it in a healthy manner? How does the patient feel about his or her body? Has there been significant weight gain or loss recently?
Activities	How does the patient spend his or her time? Is he or she engaging in dangerous or risky behavior? Is the adolescent supervised during free time? With whom does the adolescent spend most of his or her time? Do they have a supportive peer group?
Drugs (including alcohol and tobacco)	Does the patient drink caffeinated beverages (including energy drinks)? Does the patient smoke? Does the patient drink? Has the patient used illegal drugs? If there is any substance use, to what degree, and for how long?
Sex	Is the patient sexually active? If so, what form of contraception (if any) is used? How many partners has the patient had? Has the patient ever been pregnant or fathered a child? Does the patient get routine reproductive health checks? Are there any symptoms of a sexually transmitted infection? Does the patient identify as heterosexual, homosexual, or unsure? Does the patient feel safe discussing sexuality issues with parents or other caregivers?
Suicidality (including general mood assessment)	What is the patient's mood from day to day? Has he or she thought about or attempted suicide?
Strengths	Inquire about assets. What does the patient enjoy doing? What are the patient's life goals?

Reproduced, with permission, from Rudolph CD, Rudolph A, Lister G, First L, Gershon A. *Rudolph's Pediatrics.* 22nd ed. New York: McGraw-Hill, 2011. Data from Goldenring JM, Rosen DS. Getting into adolescent heads: an essential update. *Contemp Pediatr.* 2004;21(1):64–90.

Answer 6-6. a

The HEADSSS (Home, Education or Employment, Eating, Activities, Drugs, Sex, Suicidality, Strengths) assessment tool is based on the biopsychosocial model of adolescent development (see Table 67-1). HEADSSS is a screening tool, not a diagnostic tool. It allows clinicians to assess a variety of domains; however, a positive HEADSSS assessment is not diagnostic. More specific questions and investigation are necessary for a specific diagnosis.

Certain topic areas are confidential, and confidentiality and its limits should be explained to both parent and adolescent at the start of the visit. The HEADSSS is part of the history, but does not take the place of a physical examination. There is no evidence to support that asking an adolescent about suicidal thoughts will lead to suicidality.

(Page 273, Section 6: Principles of Adolescent Care, Chapter 67: The Adolescent Visit)

Answer 6-7. b

The adolescent visit is an important time to make certain that teens have received all their necessary vaccines. The current recommendations are that all adolescents should receive a TdAP 5 years after their previous tetanus vaccine. Additionally all adolescents should have documentation of 2 MMR vaccines, and 3 hepatitis B vaccines if not given earlier. Adolescent vaccines now also include vaccines for meningococcal disease, varicella, hepatitis A, human papillomavirus, and influenza. For an adolescent female, it is important to determine possibility of pregnancy prior to giving vaccines as some are contraindicated. In general, adolescents do not need an MMR if they have received 2 MMR immunizations earlier during childhood.

(Page 275, Section 6: Principles of Adolescent Care, Chapter 67: The Adolescent Visit)

Answer 6-8. e

Unintentional injuries account for about 45% of adolescent deaths. The majority of these are motor vehicle accidents. Other etiologies of unintentional injuries include drowning, fires, burns, falls, and poisoning. Alcohol is a cofactor in injuries associated with boating, swimming, bicycles, and skateboards. Additionally male adolescents and young adults have a higher unintentional injury rate than females, and this disparity increases with age. Homicide is the second leading cause of death in adolescents and young adults, and suicide is third. Malignant neoplasms lead to almost 6% of adolescent mortality.

(Page 277, Section 6: Principles of Adolescent Care, Chapter 68: Mortality)

Answer 6-9. c

The percentage of adolescents who are overweight and obese has more than tripled over the past 25 years. With this major increase, associated health consequences of obesity such as diabetes, hypertension, and high cholesterol have begun occurring at much younger ages and at much higher rates. It is important that teens understand the associated health consequences as this knowledge may help to motivate some behavior change. Overweight adolescents have a 70% chance of becoming overweight or obese adults. Young people with obesity may be targeted by bullying due to their weight, and advising him about dating may be damaging to an already potentially low self-esteem.

(Page 278, Section 6: Principles of Adolescent Care, Chapter 69: Morbidity)

Answer 6-10. d

Over the past 15 years, fewer adolescents have initiated sexual intercourse and more adolescents are using effective contraception when they initiate sexual activity. Approximately 75% of adolescents report using some form of contraception at first intercourse. Given rates of younger (middle-school) adolescents' sexual activity are low, with a major increase at the start of high school (ninth grade), this may be an important time to counsel teens about available contraceptive methods so that they are prepared at the time of onset of sexual behavior.

(Page 278, Section 6: Principles of Adolescent Care, Chapter 70: Sexual Behavior)

Answer 6-11. c

The patient in the vignette has moderate-to-severe alcohol intoxication. Laboratory findings that you may find include an elevated osmolar gap, hypoglycemia, hypokalemia, and metabolic (lactic) acidosis. You would not expect to see hyponatremia with alcohol intoxication.

(Page 279, Section 6: Principles of Adolescent Care)

Answer 6-12. e

The patient in the vignette has intoxication effects from cannabis/marijuana. Patients typically experience euphoria, tachycardia, postural hypotension, anxiety, psychosis, time–space distortion, impaired balance and coordination, confusion, panic, and increased appetite. Eye findings include dilated pupils and injected conjunctiva.

Although patients with panic disorder and schizophrenia may become more socially isolated, you would not expect to see dilated pupils, injected conjunctiva, or impaired balance and coordination with these diseases. Patients with opiate intoxication typically have constricted pupils, not dilated. Although patients with ethanol/alcohol intoxication may present with impaired coordination, you would not expect patients to be anxious or with dilated pupils. Instead, patients with ethanol intoxication present with altered cognition,

disinhibition, and euphoria. Typical eye findings with severe ethanol intoxication include nystagmus, but normal pupil size.

(Pages 278-280, Section 6: Principles of Adolescent Care)

Answer 6-13. b

The American Academy of Pediatrics opposes involuntary testing of adolescents for drugs of abuse. "Testing adolescents requires their consent, unless (1) a patient lacks decision-making capacity; or (2) there are strong medical indications or legal requirements to do so" (AAP, 1996). Laboratory testing for drugs under any circumstances is improper unless the patient and clinician can be assured that the test procedure is valid and reliable and that patient confidentiality is ensured.

(Page 281, Section 6: Principles of Adolescent Care)

American Academy of Pediatrics, Committee on Substance Abuse. Testing for drugs of abuse in children and adolescents. *Pediatrics.* 1996;98:305–307 [the statement was reaffirmed by the AAP in 2006].

Answer 6-14. d

Based on the history given here, the patient most likely suffers from symptoms of depression and may have major depressive disorder. In an adolescent suffering from major depressive disorder, it is critical to assess potential risk for suicide, including obtaining a history about suicidal ideation, a potential suicide plan (if they have thought about any mechanism by which they would commit suicide), history of suicide in family or friends, and prior suicide attempts. This approach will assist in determining level of acuity and if the patient is safe to go home or potentially requires an acute psychiatric hospitalization. If it has been determined that the patient is safe to go home, discussing options for treatment including medications and therapy (in particular cognitive behavioral therapy) is appropriate. Close monitoring and follow-up is important with children and adolescents with depression in order to ensure they are receiving appropriate treatment and tolerating medications if prescribed.

(Page 283, Section 6: Principles of Adolescent Care, Chapter 72)

Answer 6-15. d

This patient most likely had a panic disorder. Panic disorder presents with episodes of increasing anxiety typically lasting for about 10 minutes. Patients typically feel a sense of doom and often believe they are about to die. Patients often present to the emergency department due to these symptoms. Panic disorder is best treated with cognitive behavioral therapy to educate patients about how to respond to possible triggers and strategies for self-soothing. Medications also have a role in treatment of panic disorder both as prophylaxes against panic episodes (selective serotonin reuptake inhibitors) and to immediately relieve a panic episode (benzodiazepines). Benzodiazepines should be closely monitored due to their potential for dependency and abuse; therefore, they should not be prescribed for regular use in an emergency department that cannot provide regular follow-up care.

(Page 286, Section 6: Principles of Adolescent Care, Chapter 72)

Answer 6-16. a

Bipolar disorders can begin at any age, but most often between the ages of 15 and 19 years. This teen's sensation-seeking behavior (shoplifting), rapid speech, and prolonged period of excitation (staying up all night) are all potential symptoms of a manic episode. Other symptoms include grandiosity, euphoria, and racing thoughts. Depressive symptoms in adolescent with bipolar disorder include hypersomnia, psychosis, and very low energy. Adolescents with bipolar disorder are more likely than adults to present with rapid cycling (moods shifting rapidly between depression and mania), sometimes presenting with symptoms of both in the same day. Diagnosis of bipolar disorder is based on careful history and mental status examination. The goal of treatment is mood stabilization and typically includes medication, such as lithium. Alcohol is a central nervous system depressant, and abuse would typically not present with the symptoms of rapid speech and grandiosity the mother describes. Posttraumatic stress disorder typically presents with patients being hypervigilant, easily startled, depersonalization, and derealization. Barbiturate use is unlikely in this case, as it is associated with sedation, pinpoint pupils, bradycardia, hypothermia, as well as central nervous system and respiratory depression.

(Pages 283-284, Section 6: Principles of Adolescent Care, Chapter 72)

Answer 6-17. c

The patient has had a significant stressor, and may be experiencing posttraumatic stress disorder (PTSD). PTSD occurs following experiencing or witnessing a terrifying physical or emotional event in which life is lost, injured, or threatened (as in this case). The symptoms of PTSD include frequent and persistent thoughts, memories, nightmares, and flashbacks. People with PTSD are hypervigilant and easily aroused. PTSD is twice as common among women, compared with men. Combat is reported to be the most common source of PTSD among men, versus sexual assault for women.

The diagnosis of PTSD is established by a thorough and careful assessment by a skilled clinical professional, as the interview itself may be traumatic. Therapy, particularly cognitive behavioral therapy and other therapeutic modalities such as exposure therapy, is effective. Certain medications (such as selective serotonin reuptake inhibitors) may have a role with associated symptoms such as anxiety and depression, and other medications may help reduce the hyperarousal symptoms. A sleeping medication, such as zolpidem, has little role on its own in the treatment of PTSD.

(Pages 286-287, Section 6: Principles of Adolescent Care, Chapter 72)

Answer 6-18. a

You are concerned that this patient has anorexia nervosa, given her severe weight loss, amenorrhea, and her mother's concerns. The majority of patients with anorexia nervosa may express denial of the seriousness of being at such a low weight or the degree of weight gain. The first step in your management is to determine if the patient is medically stable, so obtaining vital signs is the next step. In the setting of severe weight loss, you may see bradycardia, orthostatic changes by pulse or blood pressure, hypotension, and hypothermia. Depending on the severity of vital sign changes, the patient may require hospitalization. Assuming the patient is medically stable, you may then consider ordering lab tests, including a complete blood count, serum electrolyte levels, a pregnancy test, thyroid hormones, liver function tests, and an electrocardiogram. Reassuring the patient's mother and calling the coach are not appropriate steps at this time given your concerns.

(Pages 288-292, Section 6: Principles of Adolescent Care, Chapter 73: Disorders of Eating)

Answer 6-19. b

The patient is expressing body dissatisfaction by her desire for thinness and dieting behaviors, despite having a weight and BMI in the healthy range. Given this, it is important to evaluate for signs or symptoms of disordered eating/eating disorder. Russell sign is callusing on the back of the hand due to abrasions from self-induced vomiting. Other symptoms and findings that may be seen with disordered eating include hypothermia (not hyperthermia), bradycardia, hypotension, fatigue, growth stunting, delayed puberty, irregular periods (oligomenorrhea and amenorrhea), lanugo and hair loss, brittle nails and hair, tooth decay and gingivitis, and salivary gland enlargement. Acanthosis nigricans is seen in patients with insulin resistance. Dilated pupils may be seen with certain substance use such as marijuana but are not classically seen in eating disorders. A Kayser-Fleischer ring is a brown-green ring at the edge of the cornea. Kayser-Fleischer rings are associated with disorders of copper accumulation, such as Wilson disease.

(Pages 290-292, Section 6: Principles of Adolescent Care, Chapter 73: Disorders of Eating)

Answer 6-20. d

Family-based treatment/family therapy has the strongest evidence base as a psychotherapeutic modality in the treatment of adolescents with anorexia nervosa. Malnutrition alone can worsen anxiety and depression symptoms, so restoring nutrition is critically important. A nutritionist may assist with this, and it may be important to have a nutritionist as a part of an interdisciplinary treatment team; however, there is no evidence that a nutritionist alone can provide the necessary support needed for an optimal outcome. Antidepressant medication, particularly selective serotonin reuptake inhibitors, may be beneficial in treating coexisting symptoms of depression or anxiety, but have little evidence in treating the anorexia nervosa itself, so are not first-line management without a patient also being in therapy.

(Page 291, Section 6: Principles of Adolescent Care, Chapter 73: Disorders of Eating)

Answer 6-21. a

The patient described in the vignette was fibrocystic breast change (benign proliferative breast change), which is a physiological response of breast tissue to cyclic hormonal activity. The pain begins in the premenstrual phase of the menstrual cycle and subsides thereafter. Supportive care, including nonsteroidal anti-inflammatory agents for pain and a well-fitting supportive bra, is primary treatment modality. In addition, oral contraceptives reduce symptoms in 70% to 90% of cases.

The pain from fibrocystic breast changes begins in the premenstrual phase, not the ovulatory phase of the menstrual cycle. A positive family history of *BRCA-1* and *BRCA-2* genes is associated with the development of breast cancer, not fibrocystic breast change. Fevers would aid in the diagnosis of infection. However, fibrocystic breast changes are not associated with fevers. Obtaining a history of a recent car accident would aid in the diagnosis of fat necrosis.

(Pages 292-293, Section 6: Principles of Adolescent Care)

Answer 6-22. d

Pubertal gynecomastia does spontaneously resolve in 90% of boys within 3 years. This is usually not a permanent condition. Pubertal gynecomastia is a common condition, seen in 40% to 60% of 10- to 16-year-olds. It peaks in incidence at SMR 2 to SMR 4 (age 14 years), not SMR 5. The medications listed in answer choice e are generally not recommended because of their side effect profiles, lack of documented efficacy, and frequent return of breast tissue after the drug is discontinued.

(Page 294, Section 6: Principles of Adolescent Care)

Answer 6-23. d

The patient in the vignette has testicular torsion. Common presentation includes abrupt onset of severe scrotal pain, with associated nausea, vomiting, fever, and abdominal pain. On examination, if the adolescent presents early, the testicle may have a horizontal lie with minimal swelling. Typically, the adolescent presents later, and the scrotum is swollen, tender, erythematous, and difficult to examine. The cremasteric reflex is usually absent. Testicular torsion is a surgical emergency, and time is of the essence with treatment because testicular viability declines to zero after 24 hours. Treatment involves prompt surgical exploration and detorsion. Given the high incidence of retorsion, as well as torsion of the contralateral testis, once detorsed, the affected testis and the contralateral testis are fixed to the scrotum in a procedure called scrotal orchiopexy.

Empiric antibiotics are not necessary for this patient because he does not have epididymitis. Patient with epididymitis often present with scrotal pain and swelling, but not with an absent cremasteric reflex as described in this patient. Supportive treatment including analgesics, anti-inflammatory agents, and scrotal elevation is the appropriate management for torsion of testicular or epididymal appendage, but not for torsion of the testis. Diagnosis of testicular torsion can be made by physical examination alone. A Doppler ultrasound can assist in the diagnosis, but should not delay treatment and is not necessary if there is a high index of suspicion.

(Page 294, Section 6: Principles of Adolescent Care)

Answer 6-24. e

The patient in this vignette has orchitis. The mumps virus is the most common cause of orchitis. Mumps orchitis usually follows parotitis by about 4 to 8 days, but presentation up to 6 weeks later has been reported. The typical presentation includes edema, erythema, and tenderness of testicle. In addition, you may see constitutional symptoms (eg, fever, nausea, and lower abdominal pain). Other viruses (coxsackievirus, echovirus, adenovirus, varicella) or bacteria may cause orchitis, but not as commonly as mumps. Bacterial orchitis is usually associated with an epididymal infection.

(Page 295, Section 6: Principles of Adolescent Care)

Answer 6-25. a

The patient in the vignette has a testicular tumor, the most common solid tumor seen in males aged 15 to 34 years. Patients present with painless scrotal swelling of gradual onset. On physical examination, you see a firm irregular mass that is opaque to transillumination. Gynecomastia can be present because stromal tumors tend to produce androgens and/or estrogen, which can cause feminization in a pubertal male. Cryptorchidism is the absence of 1 or both testes from the scrotum. About 1 in 500 males born with 1 or both testes undescended develops testicular cancer, roughly a 4- to 40-fold increased risk.

An uncircumcised penis does not increase a patient's risk for cancer. Anabolic steroids can cause gynecomastia in males, but do not increase their risk for testicular cancer. Obesity increases the risk of developing many medical conditions, including but not limited to hypertension, diabetes, and hyperlipidemia. It does not, however, increase the risk of developing testicular cancer. Unprotected intercourse puts patient at risk of developing sexually transmitted infections (STIs). Human papillomavirus, and STI, is associated with cancer of the anus and penis, but not with testicular cancer.

(Page 294, Section 6: Principles of Adolescent Care)

Answer 6-26. d

Spermatocele refers to the accumulation of sperm within the head of the epididymis. They are benign cysts that do not require intervention unless symptomatic. On palpation, they are predominantly smooth, soft, well circumscribed, and found on the superior aspect of the testicle.

Epididymitis is an inflammatory disease of the epididymis. A communicating hydrocele is an abnormality that develops when fluid tracks down the inguinal canal into the tunica vaginalis. A varicocele is a dilation of the pampiniform venous plexus within the scrotum, not within the epididymis.

(Page 295, Section 6: Principles of Adolescent Care)

Answer 6-27. b

Pregnancy is the most common cause of secondary amenorrhea. Therefore, the most important test to order next is the urine human chorionic gonadotropin test to check for pregnancy.

Patients with amenorrhea secondary to nutritional deficiencies, such as anorexia nervosa, can develop osteopenia and osteoporosis and be at an increased fracture risk. Obtaining DEXA scans in these patients can be useful to evaluate their bone density. FSH and LH levels are useful in evaluating amenorrhea. Low levels of these hormones indicate inadequate hypothalamic–pituitary stimulation. High levels of these hormones can result from ovarian failure. Although these hormone levels are useful in diagnosing the etiology of amenorrhea, a pregnancy test is still the next best test to order. A karyotype is also a useful test in the workup of amenorrhea, and can help diagnose Turner syndrome (45, XO) or androgen insensitivity (46, XY), but is not more important than a pregnancy test in the workup of amenorrhea. Certain medications and illicit drugs, such as phenothiazine derivatives, methadone, and heroine, can result in amenorrhea. If any of these drugs are suspected, a drug screen can be useful. However, a urine pregnancy test is still the next best test to order in the evaluation for secondary amenorrhea.

(Page 296, Section 6: Principles of Adolescent Care)

Answer 6-28. c

Hypogonadotropic hypogonadism indicates inadequate hypothalamic–pituitary stimulation of the ovary and is characterized by low levels of FSH, LH, and estrogen. Hypothalamic amenorrhea results from partial or complete inhibition of GnRH release. This may be associated with constitutional delay of puberty; nutritional deficiencies secondary to chronic diseases such as regional enteritis, cystic fibrosis, poorly controlled anorexia nervosa, and excessive exercise resulting in malnutrition, stress, and isolated GnRH deficiency; endocrinopathies such as hypothyroidism, congenital adrenal hyperplasia, and Cushing disease; and specific drugs.

Answer choice a correlates with hypergonadotropic hypogonadism, which is characterized by high levels of LH and FSH and low estrogen. Hypergonadotropic hypogonadism would result from ovarian failure, not from a chronic disease. Answer choices b, d, and e, all with high levels of hormones, would not be expected in a patient with amenorrhea from a chronic disease.

(Page 296, Section 6: Principles of Adolescent Care)

Answer 6-29. a

(Page 299, Section 6: Principles of Adolescent Care)

Your patient should be counseled to increase, not decrease, her dietary omega-3 polyunsaturated fatty acids, as it has been found to have a beneficial effect on adolescents with dysmenorrhea. In addition, treating dysmenorrhea focuses on inhibiting the synthesis or action of prostaglandins. Standard therapy includes ibuprofen, naproxen sodium, or mefenamic acid taken 1 to 2 days before the onset of expected menses. Combination oral contraceptive pills also improve symptoms in 90% of young women with dysmenorrhea, but may take 3 cycles to achieve maximum therapeutic benefit. Patients should be told to avoid smoking, as it is one of the risk factors leading to dysmenorrhea.

Answer 6-30. d

The most common cause of excessive menstrual bleeding requiring hospitalization is a bleeding disorder. Abnormal bleeding at the time of menarche might be the initial manifestation of a bleeding disorder. The most common bleeding disorder is von Willebrand disease, which has a prevalence of 1%.

The remainder of the choices, polycystic ovarian syndrome, a spontaneous abortion, a hemangioma, and cervical polyps, are all causes of abnormal vaginal bleeding. However, bleeding disorders are more likely to require hospitalization.

(Page 298, Section 6: Principles of Adolescent Care)

Answer 6-31. e

Unusual vaginal bleeding or amenorrhea should alert the physician to the possibility of pregnancy. In addition to menstrual changes, other symptoms of pregnancy include nausea, vomiting, breast tenderness, unexplained weight gain, urinary frequency, and fatigue.

Close to 800,000 adolescents between 15 and 19 years old in the United States experience a pregnancy each year, with 30% of pregnancies terminated by therapeutic abortion, 14% resulting in spontaneous abortion, and the balance resulting in a live birth. Of those who maintain the pregnancy to term, about 95% of adolescents decide to parent the child. Confidentiality should be offered to the adolescent and maintained at the request of the adolescent, based on state minor consent laws, as appropriate.

During the evaluation for a possible pregnancy, a physical assessment, including a pelvic examination, should be done. In addition, a pregnancy test should be done. Urine testing using monoclonal antibodies to B-HCG provides an accurate, sensitive, easy, and inexpensive screening tool to detect early pregnancy. In fact, testing performed as early as 1 week postimplantation will be positive for 98% of women.

(Pages 299-300, Section 6: Principles of Adolescent Care)

Answer 6-32. a

Ectopic pregnancy is an expanding problem for young, sexually active women. The most common factor that predisposes the young woman to tubal damage and therefore ectopic pregnancy is acute salpingitis, especially chlamydial infection, not a urinary tract infection.

Other predisposing factors include previous pelvic or abdominal surgery, and prior ectopic pregnancies. Other factors linked to ectopic pregnancy include multiple sexual partners and early sexual debut, as well as cigarette smoking, and vaginal douching. Endometriosis is also a risk factor for ectopic pregnancy.

(Page 300, Section 6: Principles of Adolescent Care)

Answer 6-33. c

Effective use of a hormonal method is enhanced if the adolescent can initiate her contraceptive method right away rather than waiting for her next menses. This is termed the "quick start" approach and means starting the patient on their method immediately. Waiting for the patient's next menses is not necessary and delays the patient's use of an effective contraceptive method. With the quick start method, a pregnancy test is only necessary if it has been greater than 5 days since the last menstrual period. Since the patient in the vignette had a period 2 days ago, a pregnancy test is unnecessary.

The primary reason adolescents hesitate or delay obtaining family planning or contraceptive services is concern about confidentiality. Without confidentiality, adolescents may forego necessary health care, especially those teens at greatest risk. As a result, professional health organizations recommend that clinicians provide confidential contraceptive care. Therefore, the provider does not need to discuss the plan for prescribing oral contraceptive pills prior to initiating the method. A pelvic examination is not necessary prior to initiating oral contraceptive pills.

(Page 303, Section 6: Principles of Adolescent Care)

Answer 6-34. b

Absolute contraindications for use of estrogen–progestin combination contraception include abnormal vaginal bleeding of unknown cause, estrogen-dependent tumor, liver disease, thromboembolic disease, and cerebrovascular disorders. The patient's history of having a deep venous thrombosis constitutes thromboembolic disease, and should prompt the clinician to discontinue this medication. An appropriate method is one that does not contain any estrogen.

DMPA is an appropriate progestin-only method that would be safe for this patient. Starting the patient on a lower-dose combination oral contraceptive pill would not be appropriate, as all estrogen-containing methods may increase the patient's risk for another clot. The hormonal patch and vaginal ring also contain estrogen and are therefore inappropriate methods for the patient. Advising the patient to abstain from sex is not an appropriate next step, and instruction that the patient may not be able to follow. Instead, providing a safe contraceptive method will ensure that the patient is protected from pregnancy.

(Pages 301-302, Section 6: Principles of Adolescent Care)

Answer 6-35. a

Progestin-only EC products are more efficacious and easier to dose, and have fewer side effects than combined oral contraceptive pills. They are indicated for use after unprotected or underprotected intercourse. EC is extremely time sensitive with an increased risk of pregnancy as the time from unprotected intercourse to EC use increases. Although you may provide reassurance and offer counseling to the patient if you determine it is indicated, it should not delay the use of EC. FDA approval of EC is to provide it within a 72-hour window, but clinical practice is to use it up to 5 days. Asking the patient to follow up in 1 week is inappropriate as it will delay the use of EC and increase her chances for pregnancy. A pelvic examination is not indicated unless the patient is complaining of vaginal or pelvic symptoms.

(Page 303, Section 6: Principles of Adolescent Care)

Answer 6-36. d

DMPA appeals to adolescents because it is comparably long lasting, easy to use, and invisible to parents and partners. However, there are some significant side effects associated with the method. The 3 main side effects are weight gain, irregular bleeding/amenorrhea, and a reduction in bone mineral density. Nausea and breast tenderness are common side effects with combined hormonal contraceptives.

(Page 302, Section 6: Principles of Adolescent Health)

Answer 6-37. a

C. trachomatis is the most common reported bacterial STI in the United States, and the rates of *Chlamydia* are highest in adolescent women. An estimated 2.8 million infections occur annually in the United States. Underreporting is substantial because most people with *Chlamydia* are not aware of their infections and do not seek testing.

HPV is common in the United States with an annual incidence of 5.5 million. However, HPV is a virus and therefore an incorrect answer to this question. *N. gonorrhoeae* is the second most commonly reported bacterial STI in the United States. *T. vaginalis* is a protozoan infection, not bacterial. Bacterial vaginosis is the most common cause of abnormal vaginal discharge, but the transmission is not clearly from a direct sexual route. It is therefore not the correct answer to this question asking about STIs.

(Page 928, Section 17: Infectious Diseases)

Answer 6-38. c

Bacterial vaginosis (BV) results from replacement of normal vaginal flora with a number of anaerobic bacteria in high concentrations, including *Bacteroides* species, *Mobiluncus* species, and other bacteria such as *G. vaginalis* and *Mycoplasma hominis*. Symptoms include pruritus, irritation, and a thin white vaginal discharge with a "fishy" odor. With BV, vaginal pH is >4.5, and when KOH is added, there is a fishy amine odor noted. Treatment with metronidazole 500 mg orally BID for 7 days yields a 95% cure rate.

Azithromycin and ceftriazone plus doxycycline is the treatment for *Chlamydia trachomatis* and *Neisseria gonorrhoeae*, respectively. Neither of these infections would present with a basic vaginal discharge with a fishy amine odor. Additionally, you would expect to see polymorphonuclear leukocytes on the wet prep with these infections. Fluconazole is appropriate treatment for candidal vaginitis. With candidal vaginitis, vulvar pruritus is the dominant feature. There is often little or no discharge; that which is present is typically white and clumpy, not thin in consistency as described above. The vaginal pH is typically 4 to 4.5, which also distinguishes it from BV. In addition, with candidal vaginitis, you would expect to see pseudohyphae on the wet prep.

(Page 931, Section 17: Infectious Diseases)

Answer 6-39. b

The patient in the vignette has epididymitis. In addition to scrotal pain and edema, patients with epididymitis can present with abdominal or flank pain, urethral discharge, or dysuria. The lessening of pain with scrotal elevation (ie, a positive Prehn sign) may help to distinguish epididymitis from testicular torsion. Epididymitis is a clinical syndrome of inflammation of the epididymitis caused by infection or trauma. *C. trachomatis* and *Neisseria gonorrhoeae* are the most common organisms causing epididymitis in sexually active adolescents. Evidence of urethritis, with a positive test for *C. trachomatis* or *N. gonorrhoeae*, can help confirm the diagnosis.

A Doppler ultrasound would help confirm the diagnosis of testicular torsion by showing decreased testicular perfusion. With testicular torsion, you would not expect the patient to have dysuria. Dysuria is expected with urethritis, as seen with this patient. Although the white blood count may be elevated in a patient with epididymitis, a CBC would not confirm the diagnosis. Dark field microscopy is a helpful test to see treponemes, if a diagnosis of syphilis was suspected. However, the patient in the vignette does not have signs or symptoms of syphilis. Radionuclide imaging can reveal a "hot dot" sign to help diagnose torsion of the appendix testis. This would not help in the diagnosis of epididymitis.

(Section 17: Infectious Diseases)

Answer 6-40. c

Factors implicated in precipitating recurrences include emotional stress, menses (in females), and sexual intercourse. Most genital herpes infections are actually asymptomatic. In fact, only 10% to 25% of people with HSV-2 antibodies have a history of genital herpes. There is an increasing prevalence of HSV-1 and it has become the predominant cause of genital

herpes in some countries. However, in the United States, HSV-2 remains the most common cause of genital herpes. At least 30%, not 90%, of genital herpes infections occur in people 19 years old or younger. Seroepidemiologic studies show that 17% of adults, not 75%, in the United States are seropositive for HSV-2.

(Page 1151, Section 17: Infectious Diseases)

Answer 6-41. d

Based on history and physical examination, this patient most likely has PID. PID can be challenging to diagnose as there is no single historical, physical, or laboratory finding that is definitely diagnostic. Diagnostic criteria for PID are shown in Table 233-3.

There are multiple different antibiotic regimens recommended for the treatment of PID, for both inpatient and outpatient treatment (Table 233-4). All regimens used to treat PID should be effective against *N. gonorrhoeae* and *C. trachomatis* because

TABLE 233-3. Diagnostic Criteria for Pelvic Inflammatory Disease (PID)

Diagnostic criteria

Treat empirically if all are present:

    Lower abdominal tenderness or pelvic tenderness

    No cause can be identified other than PID

    Cervical motion tenderness

        Or uterine tenderness

        Or adnexal tenderness

Additional criteria

The following criteria help in differential diagnosis and increase the specificity of the diagnosis:

    Oral temperature >38.3°C

    Abnormal cervical or vaginal discharge

    Elevated erythrocyte sedimentation rate

    Laboratory-documented *Neisseria gonorrhoeae* or *Chlamydia trachomatis* cervical infection

    Abundant WBC on saline wet prep

Definitive criteria (selected cases)

The following criteria are based on findings consistent with PID delineated during additional testing when appropriate and available:

    Evidence of endometritis on biopsy

    Tubo-ovarian mass on transvaginal ultrasound or other imaging techniques

    Laparoscopic findings of PID

From CDC, Workowski KA, Berman SM. Sexually transmitted diseases treatment guidelines, 2006. *MMWR Recomm Rep.* 2006;55(RR-11):1–94. (Check www.cdc.gov/STD/treatment/ for the most current updates to the treatment guidelines.)

even negative endocervical screening for these organisms does not rule out upper reproductive tract infection. Cefotetan 2 g IV q 12 h plus doxycycline 100 mg IV q 12 h would effectively treat both *N. gonorrhoeae* and *C. trachomatis*.

The other answer choices do not treat both organisms. Doxycycline 100 mg PO b.i.d. for 14 days with metronidazole 500 mg PO b.i.d. for 14 days does not treat *N. gonorrhoeae*. Ceftriaxone, 250 mg IM, does not treat *C. trachomatis*. Cefotetan 2 g IV q 12 h plus metronidazole 500 mg PO b.i.d. does not treat *C. trachomatis*. Clindamycin 900 mg IV q 8 h does not treat *N. gonorrhoeae*.

(Page 932, Section 17: Infectious Diseases)

Answer 6-42. b

Patients with discharge seen with vaginal candidiasis have a pH <4.5. This helps to distinguish it from the basic discharge seen in bacterial vaginosis and trichomonas vaginitis.

The remainder of the answer choices correctly described vaginal candidiasis. It is characterized by pruritus and a white or watery discharge. The vaginal mucosa is erythematous with white lesions like those seen in thrush.

(Page 927, 1117, Section 17: Infectious Diseases)

Answer 6-43. c

Idiopathic scoliosis is the most common type of scoliosis, and is often seen in adolescent girls. Patients do not typically present with pain, but with an observed deformity noticed by family members or school nurses. The Adam's forward bend test is performed by having the patient bend forward at the waist with the arms dangling in front, which allows rotational deformity of the spine to be easily visualized (see Figure 216-5). Significant curves require referral to an orthopedist and x-rays of the spine. An MRI may be required in infantile and juvenile scoliosis when there more likely is concern regarding a potential underlying diagnosis.

(Pages 857-858, Section 16: The Musculoskeletal System, Chapter 216: Disorders of the Neck and Spine)

Answer 6-44. b

Back pain in adolescents is common. Mechanical back pain results from muscle spasm as the paraspinal muscles fatigue during or following activities. Treatment for mechanical back pain includes core strengthening and physical therapy. Common features of mechanical back pain include worsened pain at the end of an active day, localized pain to the lower back without radiation to lower extremities, improvement with rest, and no association with bowel or bladder symptoms. Concerning symptoms for another etiology of back pain that may warrant a radiograph include radiation to the lower extremities, night pain that awakens the patient from sleep, constitutional symptoms such as fever, and pain with palpation of the bone.

(Page 861, Section 16: The Musculoskeletal System, Chapter 216: Disorders of the Neck and Spine)

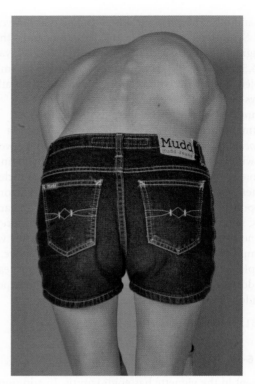

FIGURE 216-5. The Adam's forward bend test is used to visualize the axial plane deformity seen in idiopathic scoliosis. (Reproduced, with permission, from Rudolph CD, Rudolph A, Lister G, First L, Gershon A. *Rudolph's Pediatrics*. 22nd ed. New York: McGraw-Hill, 2011.)

Answer 6-45. e

Sprains are classified into 3 clinical grades. Grade I sprains involve pain along a ligament, but no laxity in comparison to the contralateral joint. Grade II sprains involve some detectable degree of asymmetry in laxity testing. Grade III sprains describe injuries to a ligament that result in greater than 10 mm of laxity in comparison to the contralateral joint. Most sprains are grade I or grade II injuries with minimal fiber injury and are appropriately treated by the RICE protocol. The RICE protocol consists of rest, ice, compression, and elevation and is appropriate for most nonbony injuries.

In addition to the RICE protocol during the initial 72 hours, low-grade sprains benefit from early range of motion and weight bearing as tolerated. Slow return to activity is allowed as pain and swelling resolve over 3 to 4 weeks. However, *only* suspected grade III sprains and lower-grade sprains that fail to improve following the initial 3 weeks should be referred to a musculoskeletal specialist for further evaluation. Therefore, answer e does not describe appropriate management.

(Page 868, Section 16: The Musculoskeletal System)

Answer 6-46. a

Benzoyl peroxide is a suitable first-line choice for the treatment of mild inflammatory acne. It is particularly effective given its bactericidal nature and use inhibits the development of bacterial resistance. Side effects include irritation and erythema, and bleaching of clothing or towels. Other topical options may also be beneficial in this case including topical retinoids (such as tretinoin, adapalene, and tazarotene). Topical antibiotics may also be first-line therapy and may be used together in combination with topical benzoyl peroxide for maximal efficacy. Oral antibiotics, including doxycycline and tetracycline, may be tried if a patient does not respond to topical therapy, presents with moderate to severe acne, or presents with acne on the back that may be more difficult to reach with topical medications. Minocycline may be more efficacious, but is more expensive and has more serious associated side effects. Oral isotretinoin is highly effective but is typically only used for very severe acne with concerns for significant scarring given its side effect profile.

(Section 18: Disorders of Skin)

Answer 6-47. d

Typically patients with acne who begin topical treatment should begin to see some results after 4 to 6 weeks of therapy. Since she has been using the medications consistently by her report for 6 months without improvement; it makes sense to consider another agent. Starting either an oral contraceptive pill or an oral antibiotic would make sense in this case. Oral contraceptives have been shown to be efficacious in adolescent females with moderate to severe or persistent inflammatory acne. Oral antibiotics such as doxycycline and tetracycline may also be of benefit in the management of her acne. Oral isotretinoin is highly effective, but given its significant side effects, including teratogenicity, its use is typically limited to patients with severe scarring acne or who have failed adequate trials of conventional therapy.

(Section 18: Disorders of Skin)

Answer 6-48. d

The patient in the scenario most likely has pityriasis rosea, a common, generalized, and self-limited dermatosis. The etiology of the rash is unclear. Typically, it presents with a single patch, as described in the case, known as a *herald patch*, which may be mistaken for nummular eczema (which may require treatment with topical steroids) or tinea corporis (which you would treat with an antifungal, such as clotrimazole). Days

to weeks following the development of the herald patch, patients with pityriasis rosea develop a progressive eruption of numerous lesions as described above. Pityriasis rosea typically spares the face, hands, and feet, differentiating it from secondary syphilis, which typically affects the palms and soles. Treatment of pityriasis rosea is typically not necessary, as it will self-resolve in 4 to 6 weeks. Treatment of syphilis would include an intramuscular injection or penicillin.

(Page 1262, Section 18: Disorders of the Skin, Chapter 358: Disorders of the Epidermis)

Answer 6-49. a

This patient's most likely diagnosis is *tinea versicolor*, a superficial skin infection caused by the fungus *Malassezia furfur*. This infection typically occurs on the chest, back, and face. It is diagnosed by KOH examination of the scrapings, demonstrating short stubby hyphae that appear like "spaghetti and meatballs." Culture is not useful because *M. furfur* is a normal skin inhabitant. An RPR would be the test for secondary syphilis, which presents differently from the rash above. Scabies is extremely pruritic and typically is located at the wrists, finger web spaces, and waistline. Often scabies burrows appearing like a threadlike trail of scale on the skin are present.

(Section 18: Disorders of the Skin, Chapter 367: Skin Infections)

Answer 6-50. c

Based on the case, this patient likely has *hidradenitis suppurativa*. This condition is a chronic inflammatory disease of the apocrine gland–bearing areas of the body. It can be mild or more severe that can cause formation of sinus tracts and fistulas. Typically, first-line treatment may include topical antibacterials, such as topical clindamycin and/or benzoyl peroxide, incision and drainage, or intralesional steroids. Other treatment options may include systemic steroids or, in severe cases that are recalcitrant to other treatments, surgical excision. The fact that she is afebrile and the culture was negative makes an abscess much less likely. The treatment of choice for an abscess would be incision and drainage. Oral isotretinoin is used for severe scarring acne but has not been described as a treatment for *hidradenitis suppurativa*.

(Section 18: Disorders of the Skin)

CHAPTER 7 | Development and Behavior

Martin T. Stein and Julie Stein O'Brien

7-1. The development of "basic trust" is among the most important psychosocial tasks of the first year of life. It is the process whereby predictable events and people lead to a sense of inner certainty. Basic trust in infants is most closely associated with which aspect of early development?

   a. Separation anxiety

   b. Attachment

   c. Autonomy

   d. Object constancy

   e. Parallel play

7-2. During a well-child visit, you asked, "Why does the sun come up in the morning?" The response was, "So mommy to work." Using Piaget's framework of cognitive development in children, what stage of development would you place this child in?

   a. Concrete operational

   b. Preoperational

   c. Sensorimotor

   d. Formal operations

   e. Informal operations

7-3. There are 4 phases of brain development. Which 2 phases occur in both the prenatal and postnatal periods?

   a. Neural tube construction and neurogenesis

   b. Neurogenesis and cell migration

   c. Myelination and cell migration

   d. Synaptogenesis and myelination

   e. Synaptogenesis and cell migration

7-4. You are supervising a resident who is seeing a newborn in their clinic for the first visit at 2 weeks. The resident observed the absence of a red reflex on the right. There is a family history of congenital cataracts. You confirm the resident's examination. In addition to an urgent referral to ophthalmology, which of the following would be appropriate anticipatory guidance for the parents?

   a. Congenital cataracts do not require intervention as they will recede spontaneously.

   b. Surgery may be required, only if the child has a retinoblastoma.

   c. It is important to correct the pathology to improve visual acuity.

   d. The child's vision will be unaffected by the timing of the intervention.

   e. Visual acuity is determined by prenatal brain development.

7-5. The American Academy of Pediatrics (AAP) recommends using a standardized developmental screening tool to screen for developmental delays at 3 well-child visits before the age of 3. Which of the following visits are recommended?

   a. 4, 9, and 24 months

   b. 6, 12, and 24 months

   c. 9, 18, and 24 months

   d. 9, 18, and 30 months

   e. 9, 18, and 36 months

7-6. You are part of a new group of pediatricians and have been assigned to organize a developmental screening program for well-child visits in the first 3 years of life. The program needs to be accurate, efficient, and cost-effective. Among the choices below, which idea about developmental screening should guide your decisions?

   a. Encourage clinicians to ask about development at each clinical encounter.

   b. Print 5 milestones in the medical chart for each well-child visit.

   c. Make a policy for the office nurse or medical assistant to ask the parent about a child's development when the child is taken to the examination room.

   d. Ask the parent about their concerns in each developmental and behavioral category.

   e. Use the Denver Developmental Screening Test at each well-child visit.

7-7. You are evaluating an almost 4-month-old, full-term infant whose parents are concerned about excessive crying. After a careful history and complete physical examination, you conclude that the baby has infant colic. You note clusters of more than 3 hours of crying usually in the late afternoon and early evening without other symptoms. In addition, the baby is feeding well and growing appropriately. Which of the following points will be included in your discussion about colic with the baby's parents?

   a. The long-term prognosis for infants with typical colic is no different from those without colic.

   b. Formula-fed babies may cry more and have more colic than breastfed babies.

   c. Changing from breast-feeding to a formula may reduce the crying.

   d. Too much parental responsiveness to a baby may encourage the development of colic.

   e. Crying is usually caused by a wet diaper.

7-8. Which of the following statements concerning frequent crying in infants (colic) is correct?

   a. Breastfed babies cry less than formula-fed infants.

   b. Changing from breast-feeding to formula feeding often reduces crying.

   c. An overly responsive parent promotes colic.

   d. A physical cause is usually found with a detailed evaluation.

   e. Growth, development, and general health are not affected by typical 3-month colic.

7-9. Maria is 10 years old and her teacher reports to her parents that Maria is hyperactive in the classroom with a poor attention span. She often blurts out answers to questions before the teacher completes the question. The teacher recommended "an ADHD evaluation." What is the most important part of the evaluation for attention-deficit/hyperactivity disorder (ADHD) in this case?

   a. Formal educational testing by a teacher who has not yet assessed the patient

   b. Documentation of specific ADHD behaviors by both the parents and teacher

   c. A blinded electroencephalogram (EEG) assessment

   d. An evaluation by a pediatric psychiatrist

   e. A trial of ADHD medication for 1 week

7-10. Which characteristic of an evaluation for attention-deficit/hyperactivity disorder (ADHD) is an important part of a comprehensive diagnosis?

   a. Ascertainment of the genetic etiology (eg, comprehensive family history)

   b. Demonstration of the child's hyperactivity in the office setting

   c. Documentation of delayed language skills

   d. Abnormal neurologic examination (eg, repetitive alternating movements, assessment of gait and station)

   e. Screening for coexisting conditions (eg, mental health conditions and learning disabilities)

7-11. You have just diagnosed a school-age patient in your practice with ADHD. You decide to prescribe only an evidence-based treatment for your patient. Which treatment plan best fits your therapeutic goal?

   a. A stimulant medication and behavior modification

   b. Cognitive behavioral therapy

   c. Play therapy

   d. Hypoallergenic diet

   e. Participation in a team sport

7-12. Patrick's parents are concerned that he is not doing well in school. Patrick is a healthy, active 10-year-old boy with no history of developmental delays. He states that he enjoys school and likes to read. His teacher describes him as an active participant in class, engaged, and cooperative. He has difficulty completing his homework assignments, particularly for English class, and his grades have decreased recently. He has always struggled with penmanship. What is the most likely diagnosis?

   a. Dyslexia

   b. Dyscalculia

   c. Dysnomia

   d. Dysgraphia

   e. Pragmatic language disorder

7-13. Beth is going to start school this fall. Her mom wants to know how to determine if she is "ready" to go to school. Beth is an active 5-year-old; she plays independently, and is able to be away from her mother without significant distress. She is learning to tie her shoes independently. She can copy a triangle, and can tell a story with a clear beginning, middle, and end. You are concerned about the possibility of dyslexia based on which of the following additional findings?

   a. Difficulty rhyming words, confusing words that sound alike

   b. Reversal of b and d when writing her name

   c. Difficulty counting past 10

   d. Does not know the days of the week

   e. Cannot tell which words do not belong in a group

7-14. Marsha was recently diagnosed with dyslexia. Her parents have many questions and are concerned about her future ability to perform well in school and go on to college. What is the most appropriate response to Marsha's parents' concerns?

   a. There is no biologic evidence for dyslexia; children with this diagnosis should not be given any additional services or accommodations.

   b. With appropriate intervention, children with dyslexia can do well academically in high school and go on to do well in postgraduate education.

   c. Children with dyslexia have persistently lower reading comprehension scores compared with their peers.

   d. Dyslexia affects higher-order language, processing, and cognition.

   e. Children with dyslexia have the same outcome as children with reading deficiency.

7-15. Which of the following is a known risk factor for language delay?

   a. Female gender

   b. High socioeconomic status

   c. Bilingual household

   d. Term delivery

   e. Family history of reading delay

7-16. Which of the following is a concerning "red flag" for language development?

   a. A 12-month-old who does not understand 2-step commands

   b. A 2-year-old who does not understand the concept of "same" and "different"

   c. A 2.5-year-old who uses 3- to 4-word sentences

   d. A 3-year-old who has less than a 200-word vocabulary

   e. A 6-year-old who struggles to pronounce the "th" sounds in *think*

7-17. Maria is a 15-month-old child who is seen in your clinic for her well-child appointment. Mom is concerned that she only has 5 to 10 words and is not putting words together. She points to body parts by name and follows 1-step commands without gestures. What is the most appropriate next step?

   a. Referral to audiology

   b. Referral to speech-language pathologist

   c. Comprehensive developmental assessment

   d. Reassurance

   e. Group language therapy

7-18. Timmy is an 18-month-old toddler whose mother is concerned about "fainting" episodes occurring about 3 times each month for the past 3 months. When you explore the history further, his mother states that prior to fainting he is always upset and cries for various periods of time. His face turns blue and he falls to the ground and becomes unresponsive. After a brief period, he awakens, his color returns to normal, and he continues to play as usual. Timmy had a normal prenatal and neonatal history, and developmental milestones in motor, language, and social skills are normal. Following a normal complete physical examination, you inform his mother that the episodes are consistent with breath-holding spells (BHS).

As part of the education for Timmy's mom about BHS, which fact should you discuss?

   a. A BHS typically occurs in early infancy.

   b. 25% of children have at least 1 BHS by the time they are 2 years old.

   c. A few children with BHS have tonic–clonic movements before awakening.

   d. If they occur frequently, BHS may cause brain injury and epilepsy.

   e. Apnea can be prolonged and children may require external stimulus to reinstitute respirations and normal behavior.

7-19. Jessie is an 8-year-old boy who has been a challenge to his parents for several years. As a toddler and preschool-age child, he had frequent tantrums often occurring without a clear precipitating event. During the past year, he is often disruptive at school, home, and in restaurants. During his prolonged tantrums, he frequently throws an object or breaks a piece of furniture. His mother says that he does not feel remorse after one of his outbursts. Jessie does not have any close friendships. Which of the following conditions is consistent with Jessie's presentation?

   a. Autistic spectrum disorder associated with anger

   b. Fetal alcohol syndrome

   c. Conduct disorder (CD; undersocialized type)

   d. Attention-deficit/hyperactivity disorder

   e. Depression

7-20. When counseling the parent of a toddler with disruptive behaviors, a useful tool to include when talking to the parent is:

a. Discuss the range of normal developmental expectations at this age with regard to tantrums and oppositional behaviors.

b. Point out that occasional tantrums should never be seen as a reflection of a toddler's quest for autonomy.

c. Physical punishment such as spanking brings an immediate halt to a tantrum and therefore should be used by parents. Point out that it is more effective than behavior management techniques.

d. Behavior management of tantrums is limited to time-outs.

e. Use of the technique of "active listening" (eg, teaching a parent to not say anything when a child has a disruptive behavior) should be reserved only for older school-age children.

7-21. Jason is an 8-year-old boy who comes to a health supervision visit. His mother is concerned that "he worries a lot"—about grades, friends, safety issues at home, and the health of his parents. Jason's early developmental history and, until recently, peer relations and school achievement have been normal. He has always had significant difficulty separating from his mother, especially in new situations. His mother is now concerned that her son's worrying is increasing and beginning to affect relationships with friends and family. What is the most likely diagnosis?

a. Atypical social development complicated by panic disorder

b. Depression complicated by obsessive–compulsive disorder

c. Panic disorder and anhedonia

d. Separation anxiety disorder and a generalized anxiety disorder

e. A typically developing school-age boy

7-22. You are seeing a 6-year-old well-known patient for his well-child visit. He has always been a shy child, but his mother is particularly concerned because he is not doing well in first grade, not answering the teachers' questions and refusing to read aloud in class. Which of the following features is concerning for social anxiety disorder?

a. Child participates in only familiar activities.

b. Child has friends at the school, but struggles to make new friends.

c. Child tends to "warm up" to new situations and become more comfortable over time.

d. Child seems to have excessive concern for embarrassment and negative feedback.

e. Child has recurrent panic attacks and avoids situations that cause concern.

7-23. Paul is brought to your clinic for his 10-year-old well-child visit. He has been healthy and developing normally, but his parents are concerned about unusual movements Paul has been making for the last 3 months. He seems to grimace and blink sporadically. It is not associated with pain or irritation. This movement occurs multiple times a day and seems to happen more often when Paul is tired or distressed. What is the most likely diagnosis?

a. Obsessive–compulsive disorder

b. Tourette syndrome

c. Transient tic disorder

d. Absence seizures

e. Normal development

7-24. Jenny is 3 years old and sucks her thumb at night to go to sleep. Parents are concerned about this continued behavior and have heard that it may signal a more serious psychological problem or insecurity. What is the most appropriate advice for Jenny's parents?

a. Reassure Jenny's parents that thumb sucking is common and usually self-limited.

b. Advise Jenny's parents to punish her when she engages in the behavior.

c. Refer Jenny to a psychiatrist as this behavior at this age is atypical.

d. Recommend aversive treatments such as bitter nail polish to discourage the behavior.

e. Refer Jenny to a dentist as her thumb sucking may have orthodontic consequences.

7-25. A 5-year-old boy is seen in your office because his mother is concerned about excessive interest in genitalia. A developmental history with a focus on gender identification, inappropriate exposure to nude adults (in person or on screen), or child abuse does not raise any concerns. As you think further about this situation, you ask yourself, which of the following behaviors are seen in the majority of 2- to 5-year-old boys?

a. Touching sexual (private) parts when at home

b. Touching sexual (private) parts when in public places

c. Trying to look at people when they are nude or dressing

d. Touching or trying to touch their mother's or other woman's breasts

e. Standing too close to people

7-26. A mother comes to your clinic with her 2-year-old son who was born at 25 weeks' gestation, weighing 1200 g at birth. The child has significant motor, language, and cognitive delays. She is thinking about having another child and wants to know more about what caused her child's intellectual disabilities. Which of the following should be a part of the discussion with this mother?

    a. Postnatal injury is the most likely etiology for her child's delays.

    b. Congenital infections and early meningitis cause a large percentage of developmental delay.

    c. Cocaine exposure is the most common teratogen known to causes intellectual disability.

    d. Low birth weight (<1500 g) is associated with a 3-fold risk of cognitive and developmental delay.

    e. Cognitive delays are unaffected by psychosocial or environmental factors.

7-27. John's first-grade teacher is concerned about his performance in school. He is struggling to keep up with his classmates in reading and writing. The teacher feels he is not qualified to move on to second grade. Physical examination is unremarkable; he is not dysmorphic, has a normal head circumference, and a normal neurologic examination. Screening for visual acuity and hearing is normal. If you are now considering an intellectual disability, which of the following tests may be indicated?

    a. Brain MRI

    b. Urine organic acids and serum amino acids

    c. High-resolution karyotype and testing for fragile X syndrome

    d. Serum copper and ceruloplasmin

    e. Bone marrow biopsy

7-28. You are seeing a 4-year-old in your clinic for a well-child visit. He recently moved to your area and has not seen a primary care doctor since he was an infant. Mom says that he has about 50 to 100 words and uses 2-word sentences. You are only able to understand 50% of what he says. After discussing your concerns about his language development and referring him to audiology, his mother asks if there are any services he could get at school. This child would likely need which of the following?

    a. An individualized family service plan (IFSP)

    b. An individualized education plan (IEP)

    c. Disability insurance

    d. Special education classes

    e. A specialized aid for Language Arts and English classes

7-29. You are seeing a 2-year-old girl in your office for a well-child visit. Her mother is concerned that she is not talking much. She only says 5 words, but she knows her body parts and follows simple directions. According to the mother, she doesn't seem interested in playing with other children. You are aware that a language delay and atypical social development may be early signs of autism. Among the following, which question, if answered negatively by the mother, would be the most revealing about a possible diagnosis of an autistic spectrum disorder (ASD)?

    a. If you point to a toy in a room, does your child look at it and then look at you?

    b. Does your child enjoy playing peek-a-boo?

    c. Does your child understand what people say to her?

    d. Does your child have sensitivities to particular foods or fabrics?

    e. Does your child often seem to worry when in new situations?

7-30. The etiology and pathogenesis of most cases of autistic spectrum disorders are unknown. Which of the following statements is correct?

    a. Autism can be caused by some immunizations.

    b. Autism is due to an immune dysregulation caused by cow's milk protein or gluten ingestion.

    c. Between birth and 14 months of age, the majority of children with autism experience brain overgrowth (head circumference in the upper quartile).

    d. Autism is a result of inadequate mothering skills in the first year of life often seen in women with postpartum depression.

    e. Known genetic conditions are not associated with autism.

7-31. Mark is a 4-year-old boy who is brought to your office because of parental concerns about his development. His mother describes a typical birth history with no significant medical problems. She says that Mark always seems "a little behind" other kids his age. His language development has always been delayed; he had no words until he was 30 months old and continues in speech therapy. She states that Mark has trouble making eye contact and has no friends at preschool. She finds him playing by himself, always doing the same activity even when there are new toys or games. What is the most likely diagnosis?

    a. Autistic disorder

    b. Asperger disorder

    c. Pervasive developmental disorder-NOS

    d. Rett syndrome

    e. Childhood disintegrative disorder

7-32. Theo is a 7-year-old boy with autism. He has been followed in your clinic for the last 2 years. He has been receiving educational and behavioral interventions; however, mom feels like his behavior has not improved. He is having increasing difficulty falling asleep and staying asleep, which seems to make him more prone to act out during the day. He is increasingly aggressive and irritable, often injuring himself. The school is concerned he may injure another student. Theo's mom is interested in pharmacologic therapy. Which of following would you recommend?

a. Propanolol

b. Risperidone

c. Lamotrigine

d. Phenobarbital

e. Midazolam

7-33. The diagnosis of dysthymia in children and adolescents differs from the diagnosis in adults by which of the following criteria?

a. Mood may be described as irritable; duration of symptoms must be at least 1 year.

b. Mood must be described as depressed; duration of symptoms must be at least 1 year.

c. Mood may be described as irritable; duration of symptoms must be at least 2 years.

d. Mood must be described as depressed; duration of symptoms must be at least 2 years.

e. Children and adolescents can have a major depressive episode within the 2-year period.

7-34. Mary is 7 years old and has juvenile idiopathic arthritis (JIA) for which she is treated with systemic corticosteroids. After presenting with sleep disturbances, change in mood, weight gain, and a deterioration in school performance over the last 4 weeks, she was recently diagnosed with major depressive disorder. Her mother has a history of depression. Which of the following is the greatest risk factor for this patient's diagnosis of major depressive disorder?

a. Female sex

b. Glucocorticoids

c. Systemic illness

d. Prepubertal age

e. Parental history

7-35. Josie is a 16-year-old girl who has been diagnosed with major depressive disorder. She has recently begun treatment with fluoxetine. She has a history of 3 failed suicide attempts in the last year. Which of the following is most effective in preventing suicide in this patient?

a. Discontinuing fluoxetine

b. Creating a "no-suicide" contract

c. Removing firearms from the home

d. Avoiding questions about suicidality

e. Promising confidentiality

7-36. A 2-year-old child is admitted to the hospital for a diagnostic workup for recurrent vomiting. The child meets all developmental milestones, but she is falling off her growth curve, failing to gain weight in the last 6 to 9 months. Her mother describes daily vomiting—often several times a day. However, when the child is admitted, the health care providers do not witness any episodes of vomiting when her mother is not present. Her mother is very anxious and wants "some sort of scope." Of the following, which is most suspicious for factious disorder by proxy (FDP)?

a. Vomiting leading to failure to thrive.

b. First-time hospitalization for ongoing problem.

c. Signs and symptoms of the child's illness do not occur when parent is absent.

d. Normal developmental milestones in the setting of a chronic illness.

e. Mother's lack of medical terminology.

7-37. Which of the following statements is consistent with childhood schizophrenia?

a. The onset is usually prior to 5 years of age.

b. Hallucinations and delusions are rare.

c. Auditory hallucinations are more common than visual hallucinations.

d. Having a parent with schizophrenia does not put a child at risk for schizophrenia.

e. Medications are not prescribed for children with schizophrenia.

7-38. Which of the following is the most accurate description of modern family life?

a. Issues of family structure are irrelevant to the care of children or their health.

b. There is a proven family structure that results in the best outcomes for children.

c. Most children live in families with a single income.

d. Most single-parent homes are headed by men.

e. Less than half of families in the United States consist of a mother and a father living with their biologic children.

7-39. Jake is being seen for his 6-month well-child visit. He is growing well and meeting all his developmental milestones. While in your office, Jake's mom becomes teary-eyed as she states that she is returning to work and looking to put Jake in day care. She has read that early development is critical and is worried that Jake's development will suffer in a day care setting. Which of following is true of nonparental childcare?

a. The benefits of mother–child play and maternal sensitivity cannot be matched by nonparental caregivers.

b. Quality childcare has been linked to improved cognitive and social skills regardless of family background.

c. There are no good research studies investigating the impact of childcare on children's development.

d. There are no national standards or accreditation bodies for day care facilities.

e. Child–staff ratios are not a valid measure by which to assess the quality of the day care environment.

7-40. Emily is 2-year-old girl who you have seen in your clinic since she was born. She has a past medical history significant for prematurity, born at 30 weeks' gestation, and also had a patent ductus arteriosus (PDA) that required surgical closure. Since her hospital discharge she has been in good health without any significant complication. However, Emily's mother frequently brings her in with multiple concerns about her health. You attempt to provide reassurance that Emily is now a very healthy 2-year-old. Which of the following features would be consistent with diagnosis of vulnerable child syndrome?

a. Multiple upper respiratory tract infections in 1 year with prolonged cough lasting 1 to 2 weeks

b. Normal development with child–parent interactions and separation

c. Separation difficulty and overindulgent/ overprotective parental behaviors

d. Fabrication of symptoms and intentionally misleading providers regarding the severity of illness

e. Multiple missed follow-up appointments

7-41. You are seeing a child with cystic fibrosis in your clinic. She was recently hospitalized for a severe pulmonary infection. When you ask her about her hospitalization, she states that she "got a bad infection from some bug," but does not relate it to her cystic fibrosis. Based on her developmental response to illness, how old is this child?

a. 3 to 4 years old

b. 5 to 7 years old

c. 9 to 10 years old

d. 12 to 15 years old

e. 16 to 19 years old

7-42. Megan is an otherwise healthy 7-year-old with evidence of obstructive sleep apnea on polysomnography. She is going to be admitted to the hospital for a T&A. Her mom is wondering if there is anything she can do to help make the hospitalization less stressful. Which of following is most helpful?

a. Avoid all conversation about the hospitalization.

b. Facilitate a prehospitalization tour, coloring books, or videos.

c. Avoid homework, chores, and big family activities prior to the hospitalization.

d. Avoid all conversation of the disease process.

e. While inpatient, do not have child participate in school programs or other activities.

7-43. You have just started a practice in a community clinic in a major urban center. Most of your patients are below the Federal Poverty Line and receiving food stamps and state financial assistance. They are primarily Latino with working parents. Which of the following characteristics describes the majority of children living in poverty in the United States?

a. Working parents

b. Urban environment

c. Latino descent

d. African American descent

e. English as a second language

7-44. Bobby is 6 years old and comes to your clinic to establish care. He recently moved to the city with his mother. His mother is currently not working and they are receiving federal and state assistance. They are staying with a friend temporarily while his mom is looking for more permanent housing. The friend has a 1-bedroom apartment in a good neighborhood. Bobby is enrolled in the first grade. His mother has a high school education. This social history is missing which of the following key components?

a. Income

b. Housing

c. Education

d. Literacy

e. Safety

7-45. Your new patient is an 8-year-old girl who is now living with her aunt and uncle. Until recently, she lived with her parents who verbally and physically fought with each other for many years under the influence of alcohol. Your patient has never been abused and has not had any educational problems in school. Further history does not reveal other risk factors. You decide to talk about resiliency in children as a way to support her aunt and uncle. Research evidence about resiliency in children supports which of the following statements?

a. Most children at psychological risk do poorly as adolescents and young adults.

b. Even in the presence of poverty, family conflict, perinatal stress, and abuse, one third of children develop well personally, socially, and educationally.

c. Resiliency in children is not associated with secure early attachment, a calm temperament, and higher intelligence.

d. Studies do not support optimism and the development of a sense of purpose as protective against adverse childhood events.

e. The concept of resilient children is no longer applicable in our understanding of child development.

7-46. You are seeing Mary for her 9-month well-child visit. Her mother is worried that Mary is not developing appropriately. Which of the following would raise concern for developmental delay?

a. Mary is able to pull herself to stand, but does not take independent steps.

b. Mary turns to sounds and follows a point, but does not point at objects to express interest.

c. Mary bangs 2 objects together, but does not throw the objects.

d. Mary laughs and coos, but does not babble with consonants, and does not say Mama or Dada.

e. Mary turns to her name, but does not follow 1-step commands.

7-47. You are seeing a new patient in your clinic. When you walk into the room, his mom is talking on the phone and unable to introduce herself or her son. You begin to observe the child playing; he is opening and closing the examination room door by turning the knob without difficulty. To distract him, you offer him a ball and he throws it overhand back to you. When you toss it back to him, he then kicks it down the hall. You show him how to walk on his toes, but he cannot imitate you. He refers to himself as "Andy" and is able to point to pictures of various animals. When you ask him where is the picture of the dog *under* the bridge or *on* the table, he is not able to find the right picture. How old is this child?

a. 22 months

b. 24 months

c. 28 months

d. 33 months

e. 36 months

7-48. A child prefers to use his right hand to pick up objects, runs and is beginning to climb steps, says about 15 words, and can feed himself with a spoon. The developmental age of this child is most consistent with:

a. 10 months

b. 15 months

c. 18 months

d. 24 months

e. 30 months

7-49. Your patient is a 5-year-old boy who is about to enter kindergarten. Screening for developmental competency should include which of the following:

a. Phonetic awareness

b. Ability to add with 1 number

c. Repeating 4 random numbers in order

d. Copying a diamond

e. Drawing a person with more than 12 body parts

7-50. Juanita is able to play games with explicit rules, reads simple sentences with fluency and understanding, copies a diamond, and has an ability to know right from wrong most of the time. Her developmental age is consistent with:

a. 4 years

b. 6 years

c. 8 years

d. 10 years

e. 12 years

ANSWERS

Answer 7-1. b

Attachment refers to the process by which a young child experiences a sense of security and positive self-worth in response to a caregiver's predictable responses to an infant's feelings. Secure attachment with a small number of caregivers is the foundation for basic trust in individuals and events that provides for healthy cognitive, social, and emotional development. Separation anxiety is a normal response of an infant from about 9 to 15 months of age when he or she appears upset when a new person enters the environment. Autonomy refers to the psychological independence that develops gradually between 1 and 3 years. Object constancy is a developmental marker of early cognitive maturity when, beginning at about 9 months, an infant is able to detect a hidden object ("out of site is no longer out of mind"). Parallel play refers to playing with another child in close proximity but not interactively.

(Page 307, Section 7: Developmental and Behavioral Pediatrics, Part 1: General Concepts, Chapter 80)

Answer 7-2. b

Children are programmed from early infancy to learn about the world from their own actions and the construction of mental representations from their experiences. Piaget's theory of cognitive development includes 4 discrete stages (sensorimotor, preoperational, concrete operational, formal operations). The child who was asked, "Why does the sun come up in the morning?" responded in a typical way of the child in the *preoperational stage* of development (18 months to 7 years of age). This stage is characterized by representational, egocentric, and magical thinking. At this stage, the inanimate world is perceived as responding to the child's own needs or perceptions. In the first stage (sensorimotor: birth to 18 months), knowledge is gained through the infant's motor activities and sensory experiences. In the third stage (concrete operational: 7-11 years), logical mental manipulations are possible including the ability to understand several dimensions of an issue at the same time (eg, learning math and rules of games that lead to cooperative competitive play). The final stage (formal operations: typically begins in early adolescence) is characterized by abstract thinking leading to the ability to manipulate ideas and no longer be confined to concrete thinking (eg, discussing morality, values, and philosophic principles).

(Page 308, Section 7: Developmental and Behavioral Pediatrics, Part 1: General Concepts, Chapter 80)

Answer 7-3. d

Early development of the neural tube consists of the forebrain, midbrain, hindbrain, and spinal cord; the neural tube completes its closure by the end of the third prenatal week.

Neuron and supporting tissue (glia) development comprises neurogenesis and is mostly completed by the end of the third trimester; the only exception is postnatal development in the olfactory bulb and the hippocampus. Cell migration that forms the 6 layers of the cerebral cortex is complete by the end of the second trimester. Synaptogenesis is the process by which axons reach out to neighboring cells to form synaptic connections that allow communication between cells. Importantly, synaptogenesis in the visual and auditory cortexes is not complete until 3 to 4 months postnatally. Myelination refers to the production of myelin that insulates cells and increases conduction velocity. Myelination reaches its peak at 20 years of age. Both synaptogenesis and myelination occur prenatally and postnatally when they are influenced by the environment including diet (myelination) and the behavioral milieu (synaptogenesis).

(Pages 311-312, Section 7: Developmental and Behavioral Pediatrics, Part 1: General Concepts, Chapter 81)

Answer 7-4. c

Although the initial development of the visual cortex occurs prenatally and is independent of experience, the full elaboration and differentiation of the development of vision is dependent on experience. Infants who have congenital cataracts removed within the first few months of life have significantly better outcomes in visual acuity compared with infants whose lenses are replaced later in infancy. Prompt intervention is necessary to improve vision. Congenital cataracts do not resolve spontaneously.

(Page 312, Section 7: Developmental and Behavioral Pediatrics, Part 1: General Concepts, Chapter 81)

Answer 7-5. d

The AAP recommends screening at 9, 18, and 30 months. These ages were chosen because they are times when development achievements in particular domains can be assessed. At 9 months, gross and fine motor skills, stranger anxiety, and object permanence can be assessed. At 18 months, language and social reciprocity can be evaluated, which is also an important screening mechanism for autistic spectrum disorders. At 30 months, expressive and receptive language skills are more established and therefore better assessed. Importantly, using a standardized screening tool provides validity and reproducibility.

(Page 313, Section 7: Developmental and Behavioral Pediatrics, Part 1: General Concepts, Chapter 82)

Answer 7-6. d

The most effective way to begin screening for developmental and behavioral problems is to ask a parent if he or she has any *concerns* about his or her child. This general question can be followed by asking about concerns in each developmental category (language, motor, and social skills), concerns about behavior, and concerns about early learning skills. The specific word "concern" has been shown in several studies and in different languages to correlate with areas of development that may need further evaluation. This novel screening procedure has been standardized in the Parents' Evaluation of Development Status (PEDS) test. Methods of early developmental screening that are not accurate and reproducible include casually asking about development ("How's the baby developing" or "Tell me about her development—talking and motor skills") and inquiring about a few age-specific milestones printed on the medical chart. Although the Denver II Developmental Screening Test was used by pediatricians for many years, psychometric qualities are poor. In addition to consistently asking about concerns, other standardized screening tests that rely on questions answered by parents have an acceptable sensitivity and specificity (eg, Ages and Stages Questionnaires [ASQ] and the Cognitive Adaptive Test/Clinical Linguistic Auditory Milestone Scale [CAT/CLAM]).

(Pages 313-318, Section 7: Developmental and Behavioral Pediatrics, Part 1: General Concepts, Chapter 82)

Answer 7-7. a

When a diagnosis of typical colic is secure, the literature supports the idea that there are no long-term, adverse physical or behavioral outcomes related to colic. Clinicians can be assisted in the diagnosis by using Wessel "rule of 3s": crying more than 3 hours a day for more than 3 days per week for more than 3 weeks. There is no evidence that formula-fed babies may cry more and have more colic than breastfed babies or that changing from breast-feeding to a formula may reduce the crying. Similarly, parental responsiveness to a baby is not associated with colic. Crying associated with wet diapers is not a cause of colic.

Importantly, children whose crying is persistent and increasing past the age of 4 months have been associated with negative outcomes, including sleep disturbances, eating disorders, parent–infant relationships, hyperactivity, and cognitive difficulties.

(Pages 318-320, Section 7: Developmental and Behavioral Pediatrics, Part 2: Developmental Variation to Disorder, Chapter 83)

Answer 7-8. e

Colic is defined as crying more than 3 hours per day for more than 3 days per week for more than 3 weeks. It typically begins during the second week of life, peaks at 6 weeks, and resolves by the end of the third month. Colic infants experience normal growth, development, and general health. Colic occurs equally in breastfed and bottle-fed babies. Changing from breast to a formula rarely changes the crying pattern. Parents who respond to a crying baby do not promote colic. Frequent paroxysms of crying before 4 months of age that are not acute and/or

associated with fever are rarely due to an organic disease. Some uncommon causes include cow's milk protein intolerance, maternal fluoxetine hydrochloride (Prozac) via breast milk, infantile migraine, and anomalous left coronary artery.

(Pages 320-321, Section 7: Developmental and Behavioral Pediatrics, Part 2: Developmental Variation to Disorder, Chapter 83)

Answer 7-9. b

ADHD is a neurobehavioral condition that requires the presence of specific behaviors consistent with hyperactivity/impulsivity and/or inattention in both the school and the home; behaviors must occur frequently and impairment in school achievement and/or social function must be documented. A standardized behavioral questionnaire, teacher narrative, and an interview with the parents are the acceptable methods of acquiring this information. Formal educational testing is done when a problem with cognition is considered (ie, a learning disorder or intellectual disability); a psychiatric evaluation may be considered when there is concern about coexisting severe anxiety, depression, conduct disorder, or autistic spectrum disorder. An EEG is not a part of an ADHD evaluation unless there is a suspicion in history of a seizure disorder. Medication is not used "as a trial" prior to establishing the diagnosis.

(Page 321, Section 7: Developmental and Behavioral Pediatrics, Part 2: Developmental Variation to Disorder, Chapter 84)

Answer 7-10. e

The diagnosis of ADHD requires the presence of specific behaviors described as hyperactive/impulsive and/or inattentive occurring both at school and at home, occurring for at least 6 months, and documentation of impairment in either school work or social relationships. In a less distractible and less demanding environment like a medical office, these behaviors may not be seen. Although there is a 2- to 8-fold increase in the risk for ADHD in parents and siblings, it is not part of the diagnostic criteria. Most children with ADHD do not have a history of delayed language skills. The neurologic examination is normal in most children with ADHD. Screening for mental health conditions (oppositional defiant disorder, anxiety, depression, and conduct disorder) and learning disabilities is an important part of an ADHD evaluation because they co-occur at a high frequency.

(Pages 312-323, Section 7: Developmental and Behavioral Pediatrics, Part 2: Developmental Variation to Disorder, Chapter 84)

Answer 7-11. a

Evidence-based therapy refers to a treatment that has been consistently effective following several, independent, well-designed randomized controlled trials (RTC). The more RTCs published usually suggest a stronger evidence base.

Other criteria include a dose–response relationship, biologic plausibility, consideration of alternative explanations, and consistency with other knowledge (Bradford-Hill, 1965). Over 200 scientific studies support stimulant medications (methylphenidate and amphetamine) as effective in reducing core symptoms of ADHD in children and adolescents. Nonstimulant medicines may improve core symptoms, but the evidence base (number of RCTs and effect size) is not as strong as stimulants. Nonstimulants include atomoxetine, tricyclic antidepressants, clonidine, and guanfacine. Behavior management for ADHD refers to parent training to achieve consistent and positive interactions with their child, learn about developmentally normal behaviors, limit negative interactions such as arguing, provide appropriate consequences, and become more empathic. Behavior management has been demonstrated to be effective in RCTs in children with ADHD. It is most effective when used in combination with medication.

Cognitive behavioral therapy, play therapy, and hypoallergenic diets have not been shown to significantly reduce core ADHD behaviors. Encouraging participation in a team sport is often recommended as a way to enhance social relations; it has not been studied rigorously as a treatment for children with ADHD.

(Pages 325-327, Section 7: Developmental and Behavioral Pediatrics, Part 2: Developmental Variation to Disorder, Chapter 84)

Bradford-Hill A. The environment and disease: association or causation? *Proc R Soc Med.* 1965;58:295–300.

Answer 7-12. d

Dysgraphia is defined as difficulty expressing thoughts on paper. This condition is often associated with unreadable penmanship, or problems gripping or manipulating a pencil. A history of difficulty drawing (eg, distorted shapes, missing details) is not uncommon. Fine motor skills may be delayed or performed awkwardly. In contrast, dyslexia is difficult in word recognition and word decoding (the ability to translate letters and letter patterns into sound with precision and speed). Patients with dyscalculia have problems with perception of shapes and confusions of arithmetic symbols, often manifesting as difficulty with simple mathematical functions. Dysnomia is the inability to recall names or words for common objects. Pragmatic language disorder is used to describe individuals with difficulty with the use of language in social contexts, such as nonverbal aspects of speech—including tone and rate—that may lead to impulsive social interactions.

(Pages 328-329, Section 7: Developmental and Behavioral Pediatrics, Part 2: Developmental Variation to Disorder, Chapter 85)

Answer 7-13. a

Risk factors for dyslexia in preschool children include a history of language delay, trouble rhyming, confusing words that sound alike, difficulty learning to recognize letters, and a family history of dyslexia. A child with dyslexia may not know the letters of alphabet by kindergarten and may not read until the first grade. They lack the ability to focus on phonemes, the speech sounds in spoken syllables and words. Phonemic awareness manifests as the ability to rhyme or figure out which word begins or ends with same sound. Early intervention, using evidence-based, phonologic-processing techniques, can remediate or even prevent reading difficulties. The reversal of b or d can be normal up to age 7. Counting past 10, knowing the days of the week, and identifying words belonging to a group are all developmental milestones appropriate for a 6-year-old.

(Pages 329-331, Section 7: Developmental and Behavioral Pediatrics, Part 2: Developmental Variation to Disorder, Chapter 85)

Answer 7-14. b

Dyslexia is a persistent weakness in phonologic processing, the ability to analyze and synthesize phonemes. Importantly, early intervention in developing phonologic processing and decoding is essential to providing children with the best chance of achieving academic success and preventing loss of self-esteem. With appropriate intervention using evidence-based, phonologic-processing techniques, reading difficulty can be prevented in primary school students and remediated in older children. Dyslexia does not have any impact on high-order processing or cognition. It is persistent and should be distinguished from a developmental lag in acquiring reading skills.

Neurobiologic research has identified 3 neural systems involved in reading: (1) Broca's area, which is involved in articulation and word analysis; (2) the parietotemporal area that is responsible for word analysis; and (3) the occipitotemporal area that helps in the rapid, automatic, fluent identification of words. Dyslexia has been shown to be a disruption in the left hemisphere posterior brain systems. Functional imaging studies have shown brain changes normalizing in children with dyslexia after intensive phonologic training.

(Pages 329-331, Section 7: Developmental and Behavioral Pediatrics, Part 2: Developmental Variation to Disorder, Chapter 85)

Answer 7-15. e

The cause of language delay is multifactorial. It can be due to biologic factors, such as hearing loss or cognitive difficulties, autism, or environmental causes. Children whose first-degree relatives have a history of language, speech, or reading delays are at greater risk for language disorders. Other known risk factors include premature birth, male gender, and low socioeconomic status. There is no evidence to support a relationship between speech delays and birth order, history of otitis media, or multilingual environments.

(Page 332, Section 7: Developmental and Behavioral Pediatrics, Part 2: Developmental Variation to Disorder, Chapter 86)

Answer 7-16. d

A 3-year-old should have a vocabulary of greater than 200 words. Other red flags at this age include more than 75% of speech unintelligible to strangers, not following 2-step commands, or responding to questions with echolalia.

At 12 months, a child would not be expected to follow 2-step commands, but would likely follow simple requests. A 2-year-old typically follows 2-step commands, has 3- to 4-word sentences, and asks "what" questions. The concepts of "same" and "different" are mastered until ~4 years old. At 6 years old, most children will pronounce most sounds correctly but may still have difficulty with *sh* and *th* sounds as well as *l* and *r*. See Table 86-1 for language milestones and red flags.

(Page 333, Developmental and Behavioral Pediatrics, Part 2: Developmental Variation to Disorder, Chapter 86)

TABLE 86-1. Language Milestones and Red Flags

Age	Receptive Skills	Expressive Skills	Red Flags
Birth	Turns to source of sound Shows preference for voices Shows interest in faces	Cries	Lack of response to sound Lack of interest in interaction with people
2-4 months		Coos Takes turns cooing	Lack of any drive to communicate
6 months	Responds to name	Vocalizations (screeching, babbling) Differential cries	Loss of the early ability to coo or babble Lack of responsiveness
9 months	Understands verbal routines (wave bye-bye)	Points Says *ma-ma, da-da*	No verbal routines
12 months	Follows a verbal command Understands names of family members and familiar objects Understands simple requests ("give me the _____")	Uses jargon Says first words Uses gestures (pointing, head shaking)	No verbal routines Failure to use *ma-ma* or *da-da* Loss of previous language or social milestones
15 months	Points to body parts by name Understands instructions without gestural cues ("go get your _____")	Learns words slowly	No single words Not using 3 words Does not follow simple directions ("get your shoes")
18-24 months	Understands sentences	Learns words quickly Uses 15-20 words Uses phrases of 2-3 words	Less than 50 words Less than 50% of speech intelligible to strangers No 2-word phrases
24-36 months	Answers questions Follows 2-step commands ("put the _____ on the chair, and the _____ under the table")	Phrases 50% intelligible Uses phrases of 3-4 words Asks "what" questions	Does not verbally respond or nod/shake head to questions
36-48 months	Understands much of what is said commensurate with cognitive level Follows 2- or 3-step commands	Phrases 75% intelligible Asks "why" questions Masters the early acquired speech sounds: *m, b, y, n, w, d, p,* and *h* May experience developmental dysfluency ("Mommy, I was, I was, um, um, I was . . .")	Vocabulary less than 200 words More than 75% of speech unintelligible to strangers Does not follow 2-step directions Echolalia to questions

(continued)

TABLE 86-1. Language Milestones and Red Flags (*Continued*)

Age	Receptive Skills	Expressive Skills	Red Flags
48-60 months	Understands concept of "same" and "different"	100% intelligible Creates well-formed sentences Tells stories	Stuttering of initial sounds or parts of words Inability to participate in conversation or tell a simple story
6 years		Pronounces most speech sounds correctly; may have difficulty with *sh* and *th* as in "think," *s*, *z*, and *th* as in "the," *l*, *r*, and the *s* as in "treasure"	Immature or inaccurate speech sound production
7 years		Pronounces speech sounds correctly, including consonant blends such as *sp*, *tr*, and *bl*	Immature or inaccurate speech sound production

Reproduced, with permission, from Rudolph CD, Rudolph A, Lister G, First L, Gershon A. *Rudolph's Pediatrics.* 22nd ed. New York: McGraw-Hill, 2011.

Answer 7-17. d

The child described in the vignette has receptive and expressive skills appropriate for her age. At 15 months the child should be learning words slowly, typically having 15 to 20 words by the time they are 18 months old. Children this age are able to point to body parts when named and understand simple commands.

Children with language delays should receive a full age-appropriate audiology assessment. Children with normal hearing, but with evidence of cognitive impairment should receive a comprehensive development assessment, often including evaluation by a psychologist and a neurologist or development and behavioral pediatrician. Children who are otherwise developing normally should be referred to a speech-language pathologist for further evaluation and treatment. Group therapy, especially involving interaction with typically developing children, is helpful for children with language delays.

(Pages 333-334, Section 7: Developmental and Behavioral Pediatrics, Part 2: Developmental Variation to Disorder, Chapter 86)

Answer 7-18. c

BHS usually occur at the initiation of a temper tantrum. Fear, anger, or frustration triggered by some environmental event is usually the cause. BHS are common; they occur in 5% of children most often in the second year of life; occasionally they may be seen as early as 6 months of age. There is often a positive family history for BHS. A cyanotic and a pallid type of BHS refers to the facial color during the breath-holding episode, the latter associated with vasovagal syncope.

Rigid, arching posture or tonic–clonic movements may occur with BHS, but they do not alter the prognosis. BHS are not associated with hypoxic brain injury of seizures. These children have a normal developmental and behavioral trajectory.

(Pages 335-338, Section 7: Developmental and Behavioral Pediatrics, Part 2: Developmental Variation to Disorder, Chapter 87)

Answer 7-19. c

Children with a CD have disruptive behaviors that are repetitive, persistent (at least 6 months), and violate the rights of others or their property. They typically do not respond with guilt or remorse when confronted with their misconduct. Stealing and lying are often seen in children with CD.

Two types of CD have been described: *undersocialized* CD where there is impairment in interpersonal relationships, lack of close friendships, and social isolation; *socialized* CD characterized by participation in antisocial behaviors (eg, criminal acts, school truancy) in the context of peer groups. Attachments with peers are strong and binding compared with confrontation with adult authority.

A child with an autistic spectrum disorder, fetal alcohol syndrome, ADHD, or depression may have a coexisting CD. However, the available information about Jessie does not point to these conditions. Autism is associated with language impairment, atypical social patterns, and an inflexible, repetitive behavior pattern. Many children with fetal alcohol syndrome have a CD, but we are not informed about prenatal exposure to alcohol or physical signs associated with prenatal alcohol exposure (eg, microcephaly, hypoplastic philtrum, or narrow upper lip). Children with ADHD exhibit hyperactivity, impulsivity, and inattention that impair learning and/or social development. Depression in a school-age child is associated with mood irregularity (sadness and/or irritability) and anhedonia (unable to experience joy in activities that were previously joyful).

(Page 336, Section 7: Developmental and Behavioral Pediatrics, Part 2: Developmental Variation to Disorder, Chapter 87)

Answer 7-20. a

The education of parents about disruptive behaviors should start with a discussion about normal developmental expectations. Using terms that will be understood by the parent, it is often useful to point out that toddler tantrums frequently reflect the child's developmental stage of autonomy—seeking independence during play and exploration of his or her environment. Within family and cultural context, toddlers should be encouraged to be more independent. Although spanking often terminates a tantrum, there is no evidence that it is more effective than correctly applied behavior management techniques that have more lasting value.

Behavior management consists of anticipating disruptive behaviors, learning parent–child communication skills, distracting the child, and time-out and behavioral reinforcement ("catching them when they're good" with a rewarding smile and positive words). In addition, active listening is another tool that a parent can utilize. To use this technique, a parent is taught to reflect with words on a child's emotional state (eg, "You seem real upset now") followed by a moment of silence that allows the child to reflect on what was said by his or her parent.

(Pages 337-338, Section 7: Developmental and Behavioral Pediatrics, Part 2: Developmental Variation to Disorder, Chapter 87)

Answer 7-21. d

Separation anxiety that persists beyond toddler years may impair autonomy and social development. When it persists into the school-age period, it is frequently associated with calamitous thoughts about what will happen to a parent or the child. This is one form of an anxiety disorder. Generalized anxiety disorder occurs with multiple worries that are difficult to control. Atypical social development refers to absence of social reciprocity and significantly ineffective relations with peers and family. Depression often coexists with anxiety disorders, but the child in this vignette does not have evidence of mood symptoms (eg, sadness) or anhedonia (absence of joy in things he likes doing). Typically developing school-age children have some worries and fears, but the extent and emerging impairment of this child's worries are not a part of normal development. Panic attacks are recurrent episodes of panic followed by worry or change in behavior because of the attacks.

(Pages 338-339, Section 7: Developmental and Behavioral Pediatrics, Part 2: Developmental Variation to Disorder, Chapter 88)

Answer 7-22. d

Social anxiety disorder is marked by excessive concern about embarrassment in front of others. This often manifests as avoiding speaking in class, lack of friends, refusal to participate in activities, loneliness, and low self-esteem. Importantly this is distinguished from shyness, which is common in childhood.

Shy children may participate only in familiar activities, struggle to make new friends, and take time to "warm up" to new social situations. Shyness does not cause impairment in social functioning. Panic disorder is characterized by recurrent panic attacks followed by changes in behavior in an effort to avoid future episodes. See Table 88-1 for the hallmark features of childhood anxiety disorders.

(Pages 338-339, Section 7: Developmental and Behavioral Pediatrics, Part 2: Developmental Variation to Disorder, Chapter 88)

Answer 7-23. c

The behavior described in the vignette is most consistent with a transient tic disorder, which is characterized by a single or multiple motor and/or vocal tics, lasting at least 4 weeks and up to 12 months. A tic is a brief, rapid, coordinated movement or vocalization that can be easily mimicked. Motor tics are typically brief clonic movements of eyes, face, neck, or shoulder—such as eye blinking, facial grimacing, or head jerking. Vocal tics include repetitive throat clearing or grunting. Complex tics are more elaborate involving multiple movements or vocalizations. Transient tic disorders typically involve simple tics.

In contrast, Tourette syndrome is characterized by multiple motor and vocal tics lasting a period of at least 1 year, with no more than 3 consecutive tic-free months. Children with complex and distressing tics are more likely to develop Tourette syndrome. Obsessive–compulsive disorder is defined by obsessional anxiety and compulsive behaviors; common compulsive behaviors include counting, matching, and hand washing. In absence seizures, consciousness is altered and typically the child is staring and unresponsive during the time of seizure (usually <30 seconds). Automatisms (eg, rubbing the face or licking the lips), jerky movements of the hands, and head nods may also occur with staring during an absence seizure. Although simple tics are very common in childhood (5%-13% of children experience a transient tic disorder), this is not considered normal development.

(Pages 343-344, Section 7: Developmental and Behavioral Pediatrics, Part 2: Developmental Variation to Disorder, Chapter 89)

Answer 7-24. a

Habits are very common in normal healthy children. Common habits include nail biting, head banging, hair twirling, teeth grinding, and thumb sucking. Most habits serve a self-soothing function. Thumb sucking occurs in approximately 15% to 30% of children under the age of 4; its incidence tends to peak between 18 and 21 months. Persistent thumb sucking into adolescence occurs more often in girls and may indicate more underlying insecurities or psychological problems. At the age of 3, reassurance and explanation that Jenny's behavior is benign and self-limited is the most appropriate advice. Attempts to punish or dissuade the behavior often cause more

TABLE 88-1. Hallmark Features of Child Anxiety Disorders

Child Anxiety Disorder	Hallmark Feature	Duration (for Diagnosis)
Separation anxiety disorder	Extreme fears on separation from primary attachment figures and calamitous thoughts about what will happen to parent or child when separated	1 month
Social anxiety disorder (social phobia)	Extreme fears of embarrassment in social situations and negative evaluation; includes performance and social interactions	6 months
Selective mutism	Fails to speak in at least 1 situation (eg, school) despite ability to speak in other situations (eg, at home). Often very similar to social anxiety disorder	1 month (not limited to first month of school)
Generalized anxiety disorder	Worries excessively about many things, including school, grades, friends, health, current events, family matters, etc. Difficult to control worries	6 months
Specific phobia (simple phobia)	Excessive and irrational fear of a specific object or situation	6 months
Obsessive–compulsive disorder	Obsessive thoughts (usually somewhat bizarre and nonsensical) and repetitive behaviors beyond child's control. Compulsions often performed to neutralize obsessions	Not specified
Panic disorder with or without agoraphobia	Recurrent and unexpected panic attacks followed by worry or changes in behavior because of panic attacks. Significant avoidance behavior noted by agoraphobia diagnosis	1 month
Posttraumatic stress disorder	Traumatic event leading to flashbacks (also nightmares, persistent memories), avoidance of trauma-related triggers, and hyperarousal (irritability, sleep difficulties, poor concentration)	1 month

Note: For all anxiety problems, clinically significant impairment at home, school, with friends, or with family or subjective distress must be confirmed. Reproduced, with permission, from Rudolph CD, Rudolph A, Lister G, First L, Gershon A. *Rudolph's Pediatrics*. 22nd ed. New York: McGraw-Hill, 2011.

anxiety and can reinforce the behavior. Aversive treatments can be helpful but only if they are not punitive. It is recommended that parents praise the child when not engaging in the behavior. Although thumb sucking can be associated with orthodontic and speech problems, these complications are rare before the age of 4.

(Pages 343-345, Section 7: Developmental and Behavioral Pediatrics, Part 2: Developmental Variation to Disorder, Chapter 89)

Answer 7-25. a

Between 4 and 6 years old, boys and girls show an increasing interest in their body, especially focusing on their genitals. This is a period of emerging gender identification when differences in the appearance of genitalia in boys and girls become more prominent. Curiosity about these differences manifests in various ways. Touching their own genitalia when at home as a form of body exploration occurs in over 60% of preschool-age boys compared with a frequency of about 25% in public places. Looking at people when they are nude or dressing and standing too close to people occurs in about one quarter of boys at this age. As many as 40% of 2- to 5-year-old boys attempt to touch the breasts of their mother or other woman.

(Page 346, Section 7: Developmental and Behavioral Pediatrics, Part 2: Developmental Variation to Disorder, Chapter 90)

Answer 7-26. d

A variety of both prenatal and postnatal events affect cognition and both biologic and psychosocial factors affect cognition. The brain requires appropriate stimulation for development. In this vignette, the most likely etiology for the child's development delay is his gestational age and low birth weight. Low-birth-weight infants (<1500 g) have a 3-fold risk for intellectual disability. There is no history of postnatal injury; moreover, congenital infections and postnatal infections, such as encephalitis or meningitis, cause only a small percentage of cases. Genetic abnormalities are the most commonly identified biologic cause of intellectual disability. Alcohol is the most common teratogen known to cause intellectual disability. Children living in poverty who are more likely to receive poorer schooling and have increased psychosocial stressors are at increased risk for cognitive delays.

(Page 349, Section 7: Developmental and Behavioral Pediatrics, Part 2: Developmental Variation to Disorder, Chapter 91)

Answer 7-27. c

Only 20% to 30% of children with developmental delays will have findings on history or physical examination that suggest a specific diagnosis. When a comprehensive history and physical examination do not suggest an etiology, additional tests should be considered. Consensus guidelines recommend that

TABLE 91-2. Indications for Metabolic Testing

Prenatal

Parental consanguinity

Family history of unexplained deaths in infancy

Acute fatty liver of pregnancy (fatty acid oxidation disorders)

HELLP syndrome (fatty acid oxidation disorders)

Postnatal

Newborn screening not done or done in state with limited screening

Regression in skills

History of hypoglycemia or unexplained acute encephalopathy

Extreme reaction to seemingly mild illnesses such as gastroenteritis

Protein aversion (urea cycle defects)

Developmental delay with hearing or vision loss

Seizures in newborn period (nonketotic hyperglycinemia, peroxisomal disorders, sulfite oxidase/molybdenum cofactor deficiency)

Hepatosplenomegaly (storage diseases)

Unusual odors (organic acid disorders)

Reproduced, with permission, from Rudolph CD, Rudolph A, Lister G, First L, Gershon A. *Rudolph's Pediatrics.* 22nd ed. New York: McGraw-Hill, 2011.

the genetic evaluation of children with intellectual disability should include a high-resolution karyotype and testing for fragile X syndrome. The yield on these tests is between 3% and 10%. Structural brain abnormalities can be detected using MRI; however, imaging should be reserved for those patients with significant microcephaly, macrocephaly, seizures, loss of skills, or focal neurologic deficits. Testing for inborn errors of metabolism (with urine organic acids, serum amino acids) or metabolic diseases such as Wilson disease (answer choice d) or storage diseases (answer choice e) is not indicated unless there are concerning features on history or physical examination (see Table 91-2, page 350). As mentioned in the clinical vignette, hearing and vision should be evaluated in all children with concerns for cognitive delays. Sensory deficits can result in cognitive delay and importantly children with intellectual disabilities are at a 10-fold higher risk of having a hearing or vision deficit compared with the general population.

(Page 350, Section 7: Developmental and Behavioral Pediatrics, Part 2: Developmental Variation to Disorder, Chapter 91)

Answer 7-28. b

The *Individuals with Disabilities Education Improvement Act (IDEA) of 2004* requires that for children aged 3 to 21, a multidisciplinary team, including school professionals and the child's parents, develop an IEP. This plan describes measurable annual goals for the child with details of what services or accommodations the child needs. The plan could include

special education classes or aids, but the most appropriate next step for this child would be to develop an IEP. For children aged 0 to 3, an *IFSP* is developed.

(Page 350, Section 7: Developmental and Behavioral Pediatrics, Part 2: Developmental Variation to Disorder, Chapter 91)

Answer 7-29. a

Children with ASD have a deficit in 3 core areas of development: a delay in communication (delayed language milestones or awkward use of language in social situations), atypical social skills, and interests characterized as rigid and inflexible (often with repetitive or stereotypic movements). One of the most revealing developmental milestones that is absent in toddlers with ASD is joint attention—when an infant shares his or her gaze between an object or event and another person by looking back and forth between the 2. Joint attention can be seen just after the first birthday; it should be established by 18 months. Limited joy when playing peek-a-boo, delayed receptive language, and sensory hypersensitivities are seen in many children with ASD, but they are not consistently present. Excessive worry in a toddler is usually an expression of a shy, slow-to-warm-up temperament; it may or may not be an early clue to anxiety.

(Pages 352-355, Section 7: Developmental and Behavioral Pediatrics, Part 3: Major Psychopathologic Disorders, Chapter 92)

Answer 7-30. c

Although a genetic etiology has not been found for most cases of autism, there are as many as 10% of cases with a genetic condition. Examples include fragile X syndrome, Angelman syndrome, 15q duplication, 22q11 deletion, and Rett syndrome. The role of cow's milk protein and gluten has not been proven as a cause or autism; eliminating these proteins has not been proven to alter the symptoms of autism. There is no evidence base for a link between immunizations and the development of autism. The "refrigerator mother" (distant, overintellectual, and unable to express appropriate affect with an infant) has been disproven as an etiology of autism. Serial MRI imaging studies and head circumference measurements have documented postnatal overgrowth of the brain in infants with autism. It may be used by clinicians as an early clue to an autistic spectrum disorder.

(Pages 352-355, Section 7: Developmental and Behavioral Pediatrics, Part 3: Major Psychopathologic Disorders, Chapter 92)

Answer 7-31. a

The child described in this vignette most likely has autistic disorder as he has symptoms of disability in socialization, communication, and fixed repetitive interests and routines. Table 92-1 details the DSM IV criteria for autistic disorder as well as Asperger. The key distinguishing factor is that children with Asperger disorder do not have any significant language delay or cognitive disability. Pervasive development disorder-NOS is characterized by impairment in the same 3 areas of social interaction, communication, and stereotyped behaviors; however, children with PDD-NOS do not meet all the criteria for autism. More specifically, children with PDD-NOS often have less impairment in social skills and intellectual deficits less common. Rett syndrome is more common in girls and is characterized by normal development until 6 to 18 months and then regression. Notably, there is a decrease in head growth and loss of language and motor skills. The diagnosis can be confirmed in about 80% of cases with DNA testing for methyl-CpG-binding protein 2 (MECP2). Childhood disintegrative disorder also presents with loss of developmental milestones in at least 2 of the following areas: language, social skills or adaptive behavior, bowel or bladder control, play, and motor skills.

(Pages 353-355, Section 7: Developmental and Behavioral Pediatrics, Part 3: Major Psychopathologic Disorders, Chapter 92)

Answer 7-32. b

There are many adjunctive pharmacologic therapies used in the treatment of autistic spectrum disorders (see Table 92-2). Importantly, risperidone, an atypical antipsychotic, has been improved by the FDA to treat irritability, aggressive behavior, self-injury, and temper tantrums in children and adolescents with autism. Additionally, risperidone can be used as a sleep aid. Many children with autism have sleep disturbances that can impact their daytime functioning as well.

Propanolol and other β-blockers can be used to treat aggression and irritability but not typically first line and do not have the additional sleep benefits. Lamotrigine and phenobarbital are antiepileptics. These specific antiepileptic medications are not often used to treat autism; in contrast, valproate has been shown to be effective in the treatment of repetitive and compulsive behavior. Midazolam is an anxiolytic. It is sedating and has not been shown to be effective in the management of autism.

(Page 355, Section 7: Developmental and Behavioral Pediatrics, Part 3: Major Psychopathologic Disorders, Chapter 92)

Answer 7-33. a

Dysthymia is defined as depressed mood for most of the day for at least 2 years in adults. In children and adolescents, mood can be described as irritable and duration must be at least 1 year. In order to meet the DSM-IV criteria for dysthymia, 2 or more the following symptoms must be present: poor appetite or overeating, insomnia or hypersomnia, low energy or fatigue, low self-esteem, poor concentration, and feelings of hopelessness. During the 1- to 2-year period of time, the patient is not without symptoms for more than 2 months at time, there are no major depressive episodes during this time, there are no manic or hypomanic episodes, and the symptoms cannot be attributed to a psychotic disorder, substance, or medical condition. Finally, these symptoms must cause significant distress or impairment.

Of note, major depressive disorder is distinguished from dysthymia by the presence of 5 or more of the following symptoms within 2-week period of time: (1) depressed mood (may be described as irritable in children/adolescents); (2) diminished interest in activities; (3) weight change; (4) insomnia or hypersomnia; (5) psychomotor agitation or retardation; (6) feelings of worthlessness or guilt; (7) impaired concentration; (8) recurrent thoughts of death.

(Page 357, Table 93-1, Section 7: Developmental and Behavioral Pediatrics, Part 3: Major Psychopathologic Disorders, Chapter 93)

Answer 7-34. e

The single most important risk factor associated with developing an early depressive illness is having a depressed parent. This risk is quadrupled with 2 depressed parents. Parental depression contributes to the illness of the child through both genetic and environmental sources. Child and adolescent depression has been associated with medications (such as glucocorticoids, immunosuppressives, antivirals), in addition to chronic illness; however, this effect is not as significant as parent history. Depression is less common in prepubertal children, 1.5% to 2.5% compared with 3% to 8% in adolescence. There are no gender differences in depression in prepubertal children; however, there is significant increase in major depression in females in adolescence (female:male ratio is 3:1).

(Page 356, Section 7: Developmental and Behavioral Pediatrics, Part 3: Major Psychopathologic Disorders, Chapter 93)

Answer 7-35. c

According to the Youth Risk Behavior Surveillance System, a survey of high school students across the United States in 2005, 16.9% of adolescents had considered suicide and 8.4% had attempted it within the past year. Suicide remains the third leading cause of death among adolescents aged 10 to 24 years. Approximately 50% of completed suicides occur following previous suicidal threats or attempts. Therefore, the patient described in this clinical vignette is at high risk. Any child or adolescent who is thought to be at risk for suicidal thoughts should be questioned directly.

Pediatricians should avoid promises of confidentiality that they are likely to break to protect and treat the patient. "No-suicide" contracts, in which the patient agrees not to harm himself or herself, are not helpful in preventing suicide in children or adolescents. A child who is actively suicidal is rarely in a position to understand or abide by the contract's ramifications. In 2006, an FDA meta-analysis concluded that children and adolescents taking SSRIs for depressive symptoms had a 2-fold risk for suicidal tendencies when compared with those taking a placebo. A subsequent meta-analysis found a 14:1 ratio between those children who benefited from SSRI treatment and those who became suicidal during treatment. It remains prudent to follow these patients closely; however, discontinuation of the medication

TABLE 93-2. Risk Factors for Suicidal Behavior in Adolescents

Psychiatric difficulties, including depression, conduct problems, psychosis, or past suicidal threats or attempts

Poor social adjustment, including school failure, legal problems, and social isolation with severe interpersonal conflicts

Severe family or environmental discord

Family history of psychiatric disorder or suicide

Significant interpersonal loss, abuse, or neglect

The availability of firearms in the home

Reproduced, with permission, from Rudolph CD, Rudolph A, Lister G, First L, Gershon A. *Rudolph's Pediatrics.* 22nd ed. New York: McGraw-Hill, 2011.

is not indicated. Among risk factors for suicidal behaviors in adolescents (see Table 93-2), the availability of firearms in the home is readily modifiable.

(Pages 359-360, Section 7: Developmental and Behavioral Pediatrics, Part 3: Major Psychopathologic Disorders, Chapter 93)

Answer 7-36. c

FDP, also known as Munchausen by proxy, is a diagnostic description for abuse through fabrication—this includes exaggeration, falsification, or induced medical problems. FDP occurs when a caretaker abuses a child for personal psychological motivations. Approximately 140 new cases of the most serious forms of FDP are diagnosed each year, often presenting as suffocation or poisonings. Other common presentations include failure to thrive, vomiting, ALTEs, or dermatologic conditions. Typical clinical profiles that are suspicious for FDP include a child who presents with medical problems that do not respond to treatment, signs and symptoms that fail to occur in the parent's absence, a parent who is unusually medically knowledgeable, a parent who appears unusually calm in the face of serious illness, and discrepancies in the medical history (see Table 94-1). Diagnosis of FDP is often challenging. A careful review of all the medical records is important as well as identifying the motivation for falsification.

(Pages 360-361, Section 7: Developmental and Behavioral Pediatrics, Part 3: Major Psychopathologic Disorders, Chapter 94)

Answer 7-37. c

Childhood schizophrenia is rare (2 in 10,000). The clinical profile includes hallucinations (mostly auditory and persecutory in content; less frequently visual), delusions,

and problems with thought process (loose associations; illogical thinking). The onset is usually after 5 years of age. Genetic aspects of schizophrenia are supported by higher rates among children whose parents have the disorder. Multimodal treatment includes medication, psychotherapy, educational intervention, and family support.

(Pages 361-362, Section 7: Developmental and Behavioral Pediatrics, Part 3: Major Psychopathologic Disorders, Chapter 95)

Answer 7-38. e

The "traditional nuclear family," consisting of a mother and a father living with their biologic children, is becoming more rare; according to the US Bureau of the Census only 25% of households fit this description. There are many single-parent families, mostly headed by women. There are blended families from remarriage. In fact, although only 25% of families consist of both parents with their biologic children, approximately 70% of children live with married parents. In over 66% of households both parents work. The majority of children who are reared in any particular family type (eg, single parent, grandparent as primary caretaker, divorced, blended, and gay families) will thrive in a loving, supportive environment. Family structure plays an important role in a child's development, and the clinician who has trusting relationship with a child and family can play a key role in helping a family overcome the challenges of raising children.

(Pages 363-364, Section 7: Developmental and Behavioral Pediatrics, Part 4: Psychosocial Context of Development and Behavior, Chapter 96)

Answer 7-39. b

There are multiple types of nonparental childcare, most commonly center-based (childcare centers, preschools), home-based, or school-age care (before or after school programs). Research in early brain and child development has shown that although maternal sensitivity and mother–child play is associated with positive peer competence in later years, children who spend time in nonparental childcare may have improved cognitive and social skills. These effects were sustained for most children through kindergarten. These effects are more closely associated with higher-quality classroom practices (including appropriate child–staff ratios and staff trained in early childhood development). There have been several large research studies detailing these findings, including the National Institute of Child Health and Human Development (NICHD) Study of Early Child Care. Moreover, there are national standards for child-to-staff ratios based on the age of the children.

Many parents experience guilt, frustration, or sadness when considering childcare options. Families can be encouraged to observe several childcare facilities before making a decision and clinicians can recommend several guidelines for observation and specific questions to ask (see Table 97-1).

(Pages 364-366, Section 7: Developmental and Behavioral Pediatrics, Part 4: Psychosocial Context of Development and Behavior, Chapter 97)

Answer 7-40. c

Vulnerable child syndrome is the extreme manifestation of persistent and unfounded parental perception of medical vulnerability after a real or perceived health threat to a child. This parental perception can lead to increased use of acute medical care, increased attention to behavioral and developmental problems, and parental distress. As in this vignette, vulnerable child syndrome often develops after an event near birth. The early the event, the less severe the event needs to be. However, in this case the patient's prematurity and heart disease were the likely triggers. The clinical centerpiece of vulnerable child syndrome is the distorted parental perception of the child's health that leads to an alteration in the child–parent relationship. Many parents are overly protective or overly indulgent due to their own anxiety about the child's health. Children may sense their parent's worries and fears and may respond by staying inappropriately attached to their parents, by becoming more defiant or detached, or by developing functional somatic symptoms (eg, headaches, stomachaches).

Multiple upper respiratory tract infections are not atypical in this age. Fabrication of symptoms is more consistent with factious syndrome. Multiple missed follow-up appointments are not consistent with the high parental perception of child vulnerability that is the hallmark of this process.

(Pages 366-367, Section 7: Developmental and Behavioral Pediatrics, Part 4: Psychosocial Context of Development and Behavior, Chapter 98)

Answer 7-41. c

It is important to appreciate how children of various ages interpret illness differently depending on their developmental stage. By age 9 to 10, children can typically understand the concepts of contagion and germs as a source of infection; however, they are rarely able to articulate the mechanisms of disease or understand complex relationships. Very young children often rely on magical thinking to explain illness. Children aged 5 to 7 are beginning to understand the concept of contagion, but tend to extend this to not infectious illnesses. Older children, aged 12 to 13, begin to appreciate complicated causes of illness and recovery from illness. It is not until adolescence that children are able to associate seemingly unrelated symptoms or different stages of illness.

(Page 368, Section 7: Developmental and Behavioral Pediatrics, Part 4: Psychosocial Context of Development and Behavior, Chapter 99)

Answer 7-42. b

Hospitalization is often a stressful event for children and their families. There is anxiety around the separation of the child from her family, disruption of normal routines, unfamiliarity with the surroundings and people, and fear around the illness and any pain that may result from treatment. Prior to the hospital stay, tours, videos, and other educational materials can help prepare the child. Avoiding conversations about the hospitalization or the disease process is usually counterproductive, and providing age-appropriate information about the illness and hospitalization can be helpful. Maintaining normal routines and normal expectations is also important to minimizing the stress and impact of a hospital stay. This is particularly important for children hospitalized for prolonged stays (see Table 99-3).

(Pages 369-370, Section 7: Developmental and Behavioral Pediatrics, Part 4: Psychosocial Context of Development and Behavior, Chapter 99)

Answer 7-43. a

In 2009, it is estimated that 15 million children live below the Federal Poverty Line; unfortunately this number continues to grow. Contrary to many assumptions, almost two thirds of poor children have working parents. The majority of poor children live in suburbs or rural areas. Importantly, there are racial disparities in poverty with greater proportion of African American and Latino children living in poverty, but there are a larger number of poor Caucasian children.

(Pages 370-371, Section 7: Developmental and Behavioral Pediatrics, Part 4: Psychosocial Context of Development and Behavior, Chapter 100)

Answer 7-44. d

Table 100-2 and the mnemonic "I HELLP" can be used as an outline for obtaining a social history, with particular focus on the basic needs that affect health. These include income, housing, education, legal status, literacy, and personal safety. Importantly, literacy refers to not only the child's but also the parents' literacy level. This assessment can help guide future interaction between the provider and the parent and improve communication.

(Page 372, Section 7: Developmental and Behavioral Pediatrics, Part 4: Psychosocial Context of Development and Behavior, Chapter 100)

Answer 7-45. b

Resiliency is the ability to rebound from real, experienced adversity. It refers to an individual's inner strengths (biologic endowment) and external resources (environmental influences) to overcome adverse or traumatic circumstances and to continue a healthy developmental trajectory. Resiliency in children is seen more frequently in kids with a tranquil, calm temperament and higher intelligence. A secure early attachment with a parent or other caretaker is an additional protective factor. Studies on resiliency show that even with significant psychological risk (including child abuse and

TABLE 100-2. Examples of Potential Social History Questions: "I HELLP" to Address Basic Needs

Domain	Areas	Examples of Questions
Income	General	Do you ever have trouble making ends meet?
	Food income	Ever a time when you don't have enough food?
		Do you have WIC? Food stamps?
Housing	Housing	Is your housing ever a problem for you?
	Utilities	Do you ever have trouble paying your electric/heat/phone bill?
Education	Appropriate school placement	How is your child doing in school?
		Is he/she getting the help to learn what he/she needs?
	Early childhood program	Is your child in Head Start or preschool or other early childhood enrichment?
Legal status	Immigration	Do you have questions about your immigration status?
		Do you need help accessing benefits or services for your family?
Literacy	Child literacy	Do you read to your child every night?
	Parent literacy	How happy are you with how you read?
Personal safety	Domestic violence	Have you ever taken out a restraining order?
		Do you feel safe in your relationship?
	General safety	Do you feel safe in your home? Neighborhood?

Reproduced, with permission, from Kenyon C, Sandel M, Silverstein M, Shakir A, Zuckerman B. Revisiting social history for children. *Pediatrics.* 2007;120(3):e734–e738.

severe family conflicts), poverty, and perinatal stress, one third of children will have normal social and educational outcomes. Children who are raised in an environment that supports optimism and a sense of purpose may be protected against adverse childhood events. For school-age children and adolescents, a "mentor" (eg, teacher, coach, religious leader, relative) who provides consistent guidance over several years may also be a reliable protective factor.

(Pages 372-374, Section 7: Developmental and Behavioral Pediatrics, Part 4: Psychosocial Context of Development and Behavior, Chapter 101)

Answer 7-46. d

At 9 months, a child who is not babbling with consonants likely has an expressive language delay. Typically children will begin to babble at 5 months with vowels and add consonants by 6 to 7 months. By 8 months, children use "Dada" nonspecifically for both of their parents, and by 9 months, also begin to use "Mama" nonspecifically.

Mary's gross motor and fine skills seem developmentally appropriate; children pull to stand or "bear walk" by crawling with their limbs straight at 9 months. Typically, children will be able to take independent steps at 12 months. She is banging blocks together, but would not be expected to throw objects until 10 to 11 months. Socially, Mary is able to follow gestures at this age, but the ability to point to express interest is more typical at 12 months old. Her receptive language is normal as

she orients to her name, but does not follow commands, which again would be more typical for 12-month-olds.

(Section 7: Developmental and Behavioral Pediatrics)

Answer 7-47. b

This child is most like 24 months old. He is able to throw overhand, kick without demonstration, and open a door using the knob. He refers to himself by name and points correctly to pictures. At 22 months, the child would likely need to be shown how to kick the ball before he would initiate that activity. At 28 months, the child would likely be able to walk on his toes after the demonstration. At 33 months, children are beginning to understand prepositions. By 36 months, children are able to balance on 1 foot and name parts of pictures (eg, the door of the car).

(Section 7: Developmental and Behavioral Pediatrics)

Answer 7-48. c

Infants are ambidextrous until about 18 months when handedness becomes apparent. Running occurs between 15 and 20 months. Expressive language is highly variable in the first 2 years of a child's life. At 18 months, a child can say 5 to 30 words. Self-feeding is a sign of emerging independence. A spoon is usually used effectively between 15 and 20 months.

(Section 7: Developmental and Behavioral Pediatrics)

Answer 7-49. c

Phonetic awareness refers to the ability to produce a sound for letter and then combine the sounds that are created by 2 or more letters. It is the foundation for reading and occurs in most children between 5.5 and 7 years of age. Adding numbers at kindergarten entry is dependent on preschool and home educational experience. As a test of working memory, a 5-year-old child should be able to repeat 4 random numbers, copy a square (a diamond at 7 years), and draw a person with at least 8 body parts.

(Section 7: Developmental and Behavioral Pediatrics)

Answer 7-50. c

The ability to make use of rules in interactive games is a reasoning skill that emerges between 7 and 9 years of age. It is a reflection of cognitive development and an example of "concrete operations." An awareness of "right from wrong" can be demonstrated by 8 years old. Reading sentences with fluency and good comprehension occurs between 7 and 8 years of age. A child should be able to copy a diamond by 7 years of age.

(Section 7: Developmental and Behavioral Pediatrics)

CHAPTER 8 | The Acutely Ill Infant and Child

Christine S. Cho, Jerusha Pearson-Lev, and Cornelia Latronica

8-1. Which of the following statements is true about the regulation of respiration in healthy children?

   a. Changes in PCO_2 are interpreted by chemoreceptor cells in the carotid bodies that can cause downstream changes in work and the pace of breathing.

   b. Adaptations (such as nasal flaring, increased diaphragmatic contraction, and intercostal and subcostal retractions) are all voluntary changes.

   c. Changes in PCO_2 have more influence than changes in PO_2 in causing compensatory changes during respiratory distress.

   d. Central chemoreceptors sense changes in PO_2, while peripheral chemoreceptors sense changes in PCO_2.

   e. Tachypnea and retractions are not common physiologic adaptations to respiratory distress in children.

8-2. A 7-year-old girl with a history of poorly controlled moderate-persistent asthma presents to the Emergency Department. Her mother says she has had a cold for 2 days, which has worsened over the past 24 hours. She has run out of her beta-agonist and lost her controller medicine months ago. She is audibly wheezing and unable to speak in complete sentences. When her shirt is removed, abdominal breathing and subcostal retractions are observed. Her initial vitals are: RR 42, HR 135, O_2 saturation 89% on room air (RA). On exam she is wheezing throughout and is moving air poorly bilaterally. Her expiratory phase is prolonged. A chest radiograph is obtained and shows hyperinflation with a flat diaphragm and hilar peribronchial thickening, suggestive of gas trapping. Why does intrathoracic obstructive lung disease cause the phenomenon of gas trapping?

   a. Tachypnea allows for increased air movement and subsequent hyperinflation of the lungs.

   b. Alveoli do not empty fully at the end of expiration and their volume therefore increases.

   c. Increased deadspace due to slower expiratory times increases lung volume.

   d. A decrease in transmural pressure on the airways causes collapse and traps air.

   e. Turbulent airflow in the airways resulting from the obstruction causes more gas to remain in the lungs.

8-3. Which of the following statements is true regarding ventilation–perfusion inequality ($V–Q$ mismatch)?

   a. $V–Q$ mismatch is the least common mechanism of hypoxemia and hypercapnea, both in children and in adults with respiratory disease.

   b. Gravity does not contribute to $V–Q$ mismatch in normal lungs even though it acts to direct a larger share of blood flow to more dependent areas.

   c. $V–Q$ mismatch arises from several different pathways, including true anatomic shunts, diffusion defects, and incomplete oxygenation of blood flowing through parts of the lung with a low ventilation-to-perfusion ratio (virtual shunts).

   d. Hypercapnea, instead of hypoxemia, is a prominent feature of respiratory failure. This phenomenon occurs because alveolar-capillary units with *low V–Q* ratios have increased PCO_2 and therefore cannot remove CO_2 from the blood effectively.

   e. Alveolar-capillary units that have a *high* ventilation–perfusion ratio are the main cause for hypoxemia in $V–Q$ mismatch because the end-capillary blood is not fully saturated with oxygen.

8-4. A 1-month-old girl born at term by C-section is brought in by her parents to the Emergency Department for concerns about breathing. The baby has been growing and developing well until 2 days prior to presentation when she started to have increased congestion. An older sibling has a URI at home. The infant now has significant clear rhinorrhea and a cough with posttussive emesis. As per the mother, she is unable to finish her bottles and seems more tired than usual. She has been afebrile at home. On exam she is breathing 80 times per minute with significant subcostal and intercostal retractions. Her oxygen saturation is 85% on RA. Which statement below is true regarding mechanical dysfunction of respiratory muscles and respiratory effort in young infants?

a. Limited ossification of the rib cage and short axial dimension of the thorax make the small infant's chest wall prone to distortion, which can decrease respiratory muscle efficiency.

b. Inward distortion of the infant rib cage decreases the energy used by the diaphragm, thereby decreasing the work of the diaphragmatic muscle.

c. The area of apposition of the diaphragm and the rib cage is larger proportionally in an infant, and results in wasted work of the diaphragm on abdominal organs.

d. Inward distortion of the rib cage in an infant allows for more effective respiratory effort and increases lung volume on inspiration.

e. Respiratory muscle efficiency is higher in infants than in adults, allowing them to compensate better during times of increased demand.

8-5. A 7-month-old female presents to the Emergency Department with vomiting and diarrhea for the past 36 hours. Vital signs reveal a temperature of 37.9°C, heart rate of 179, respiratory rate of 40, blood pressure 90/42, O_2 saturation of 99% on RA. The patient appears tired and pale, is tachypneic with clear lung fields, tachycardic without a gallop, there is no hepatosplenomegaly, her skin is cool and there is delayed capillary refill. Which of the following statements is TRUE?

a. Mean blood pressure is a sensitive measure of circulatory dysfunction. This patient has a normal blood pressure and is therefore not in shock.

b. This patient appears to be in compensated hypovolemic shock, and requires immediate intravenous fluid resuscitation.

c. Children frequently suffer from hypovolemic shock because they lack mechanisms to sense intravascular volume.

d. Patient's immediate adaptation to hypovolemic shock is activation of the Renin–Angiotensin–Aldosterone-System (RAAS).

e. Children are less susceptible to the development of hypovolemic shock.

8-6. A 1-month-old infant is brought to the Emergency Department. The triage nurse brings the patient back immediately stating that the patient is ill appearing, tachycardic to 188, and hypotensive with a BP 50/35. The patient's skin is mottled and the capillary refill is 6 seconds with weakly palpable pulses in all 4 extremities. The patient's abdomen is distended and the liver edge is palpable well below the costal margin. You obtain blood and urine studies, a chest radiograph, and begin a 20 mL/kg intravenous fluid bolus. Reassessment following the bolus reveals that the patient has developed rales and is now arousable only to stimulus. The next step in the management of this patient would be:

a. Repeat fluid bolus 20 mL/kg.

b. Administer ampicillin and cefotaxime.

c. Begin dopamine IV infusion.

d. Give 1 mEq/kg sodium bicarbonate IV.

e. Administer calcium chloride 10–20 mg/kg.

8-7. A 3-week-old male presents for poor feeding. The mother notes that the patient has not fed well for the last day and has decreased urine output. He has not been exposed to any sick contacts or exhibited any signs of upper respiratory tract infection. He has not had any vomiting, diarrhea, or fever. Vital signs reveal a temperature of 38.7°C, heart rate of 166, respiratory rate of 55, mean arterial pressure of 45 mm Hg, O_2 saturation of 99% on RA. The patient is sleeping and latches when placed to the breast but quickly falls asleep, fontanel is soft and flat, skin is warm. You perform a complete work-up to rule out sepsis. Labs are remarkable for a WBC of 4000, hemoglobin of 8.0, platelets of 149,000. Sodium is 149, CO_2 is 16, BUN is 48, creatinine is 1.1, and glucose is 40. A chest X-ray is unremarkable , though incidentally reveals diffuse gaseous distention of the bowel throughout the abdomen without air fluid levels.

Which of the following statements is TRUE?

a. The patient is in hypovolemic shock and has decreased urine output and an elevated BUN/Cr.

b. The patient is in septic shock with evidence of multisystem organ dysfunction.

c. The patient is exhibiting symptoms of shock from cardiac tamponade.

d. The patient should not be given excessive intravenous fluids, due to increased vascular permeability seen in sepsis,

e. The patient should not be given antibiotics until all appropriate cultures are drawn.

8-8. Which of the following statements is TRUE regarding alterations in the level of consciousness?

  a. Normal consciousness is maintained exclusively by the reticular activating system within the brain.

  b. Patients presenting with altered mental status may be classified as altered or normal.

  c. Only primary processes originating from the central nervous system should be considered in the differential of patients with altered mental status.

  d. Careful history may help guide the choice of diagnostic testing in patients presenting with altered mental status.

  e. Alterations in mental status are often secondary to a benign condition and rarely indicate a serious medical problem.

8-9. A 14-year-old female is found in the locker room after gym class to be unresponsive. You have been informed that several students have been caught for alcohol consumption earlier that day. Which of the following statements is TRUE regarding the next step in her management?

  a. The priority in her management is to administer glucose, as it is likely that she is hypoglycemic since her gym glass immediately precedes lunch and she has had nothing to eat for the past 4 hours.

  b. This patient should be taken immediately to the CT scanner before further assessment to rule out intracranial bleed from a trauma sustained during the gym class.

  c. This patient should be immediately defibrillated as history reveals she has a known history of SVT for which she has probably experienced a reoccurrence due to exertion during gym class.

  d. This patient has probably been drinking alcohol. Workup should start with a serum alcohol level, as well as a serum blood glucose level.

  e. The priority in her management is to assess her airway, breathing, and circulation followed by a careful neurologic assessment and secondary survey.

8-10. A 3-month-old term infant presents to the Emergency Department with a 1-day history of fever, irritability, poor feeding, and lethargy. You suspect meningitis. Which of the following statements is TRUE?

  a. CNS infections present only with generalized findings. A focal finding is suggestive of a different distinct diagnosis.

  b. As the patient is older than 2 months, you may be able to defer lumbar puncture if there are no signs of nuchal rigidity.

  c. Lumbar puncture is contraindicated in cases of parameningeal infection due to risk of herniation.

  d. Normal CSF studies can exclude all infectious etiologies of altered mental status and obviate the need for empiric antibiotic therapy.

  e. Antibiotics should always be delayed until lumbar puncture is performed as it is not possible to diagnose the causative organism following empiric therapy.

8-11. Brain death occurs when all cerebral functions are irreversibly absent. Criteria for the diagnosis of brain death include:

  a. Two detailed examinations by an experienced clinician followed by formal documentation of apnea. EEGs or a cerebral perfusion scan may alternatively be used in children under 1-year-old.

  b. Spinal motor reflexes must be absent. Decorticate or decerebrate posturing may be present and are not a sign of central motor function.

  c. Vestibular and oculomotor functions are tested with the instillation of cold water into the ear canal. Failure to elicit a response is sufficient to document lack of brain stem function.

  d. Confounding factors such as hypotension, hypothermia, and sedating medications are not relevant to the brain death exam.

  e. Established practice guidelines must be rigidly followed.

8-12. A 35-day-old term infant presents to the Emergency Department with a history of 1 day of fussiness, slightly decreased eating, and congestion. Rectal temperature is 38.4°C. The baby was born by routine vaginal delivery and all maternal laboratory tests, including Group B streptococcus screening were negative. The infant up until this point has been growing well. There is a 3-year-old sibling at home with viral upper respiratory symptoms. The baby is sleepy and has mild upper airway congestion on exam but is otherwise well-appearing. Additional vitals are: RR 55, HR 153, O_2 saturation 98% on RA. The following statement represents the best management according to the most reliable clinical prediction tools:

a. Obtain a CBC with differential, a blood culture, and a CRP and give the infant IV antibiotics and admit for observation.

b. Obtain viral cultures and a chest x-ray. If CXR is negative, send home with strict return precautions.

c. Obtain CBC with differential, blood culture, urinalysis with microscopy, urine culture, CSF gram stain, and culture. Start antibiotics and admit.

d. Obtain CBC with differential, blood culture, urinalysis with microscopy, urine culture, CSF gram stain, and culture. If WBC <15 K/mm, urinalysis is normal and CSF gram stain is negative and WBC <8/mm³, send home without antibiotics with a 24-hour return visit.

e. Obtain a CBC with differential, a urine analysis with microscopy, and blood and urine cultures as well as a CXR. If WBC <15 K/mm, urine has <10 WBC/hpf, and CXR is negative, send home without antibiotics with a 24-hour return visit.

8-13. A 2 ½-month-old infant presents to the Emergency Department with a rectal temperature of 39°C. He was born at term by normal spontaneous vaginal delivery and has been growing well. He has been fussy for the past 24 hours but eating well and otherwise acting normally. His fever has responded to antipyretics at home. He is febrile, but well-appearing, with a flat fontanel, normal tympanic membranes, and clear lungs. Which of the following statements is true regarding his risk for having a serious bacterial infection?

a. An elevated CRP would indicate bacterial infection.

b. He likely has a viral illness and there is no concern for bacterial infection.

c. Occult bacteremia is less likely now given routine immunization for *Haemophilus influenza* type B and *Streptococcus pneumoniae*.

d. He likely has a viral infection, however the most likely bacterial co-infection would be a urinary tract infection so a urine sample should be obtained via a bag.

e. If his CBC and urinalysis look normal, it would be reasonable to defer empiric antibiotics while cultures are pending.

8-14. A 2-year-old fully vaccinated female presents to the Emergency Department. She is febrile to 40°C and is sleepy. Her parents report that the fever started the previous day and it did not respond to 1 dose of acetaminophen at home. She has had no cough, no rhinorrhea, no diarrhea, but she has vomited 3 times. She responds to your exam by fussiness and is consoled by her mother. She is flushed and tachycardic but has clear lung sounds. Her tympanic membranes are red but not bulging. Her neck is supple with no meningismus. Which of the following statements is true?

a. Her fever did not respond to antipyretics so she must have a bacterial infection.

b. She needs blood and urine studies to rule out a bacterial infection.

c. She likely has a viral infection and can be sent home with close follow-up.

d. She needs a CXR and a lumbar puncture and should be admitted for observation.

e. Occult bacteremia can be identified by clinical exam and she should be treated with antibiotics.

8-15. Arterial pulse oximetry estimates the relative fraction of oxygenated hemoglobin through differential absorption of 2 different wavelengths of light through a digit. Pulse oximetry has become the most common method of monitoring arterial blood oxygenation. Which of the following is an advantage of pulse oximetry?

a. It is accurate even when there is motion or poor perfusion in the extremity.

b. It is the only method of estimating oxygen content during carbon monoxide poisoning.

c. It is most accurate in the setting of methemoglobinemia.

d. It gives accurate readings regardless of the quality and quantity of external light.

e. It is a noninvasive, nonpainful method of estimating hemoglobin oxygen saturation.

8-16. A 12-year-old girl arrives at the Emergency Department with a complaint that her "heart feels funny." She walks into the patient room with her mother. The nurse places her on an electrocardiogram (ECG) monitor to continuously monitor her rhythm and rate. The heart rate on the monitor reads 210. Which of the following is TRUE?

a. The monitor detects heart rate from the frequency of the atrial contraction (the "p" signal).

b. When the voltage of a signal is large, both the P and QRS waves may be detected as beats and the rate may be falsely read as twice normal.

c. It is common for monitors to fail to detect a signal when there is artifact such as a moving patient.

d. Obtaining a complete ECG is unnecessary as monitors are accurate, and it is more important to begin resuscitation.

e. The diagnosis is likely supraventricular tachycardia. Intravenous access should be obtained and adenosine should be administered as a first priority.

8-17. A 4-year-old boy presents with a fever of 40°C, HR 160, and RR 40. He is lethargic, with poor respiratory effort and mottled extremities. You suspect sepsis, and initiate bag-valve-mask ventilation and aggressive fluid and antimicrobial therapy after obtaining cultures. Blood pressure measurements are difficult to obtain through the automated machine, so you are asked to take a manual blood pressure. Of the following, which is TRUE?

a. The most sensitive indicator of shock is decrease in systolic blood pressure.

b. The blood pressure cuff of a sphygmomanometer should be 2/3 the length of the limb segment it is encircling.

c. When measuring blood pressure with a blood pressure cuff, a stethoscope should be used to auscultate Korotkoff sounds. Palpating the pulse is not an appropriate way to measure blood pressure.

d. Arterial blood pressure can be continuously monitored by a central venous catheter.

e. Upper and lower extremity blood pressures have the same normal values.

8-18. A 14-month-old boy with 3 days of abdominal pain, vomiting, and diarrhea arrives at the Emergency Department via ambulance. He appears lethargic with a temperature of 38.5°C, pulse 150, respiratory rate 30, blood pressure 100/60, and oxygen saturation 98% on RA. He has sunken eyes and dry mucous membranes. Breath sounds are equal and normal, and he has no evidence of flaring or retractions. His abdomen is tender and capillary refill time is 4 seconds. After administering supplemental oxygen, your next priority in management is:

a. Obtaining blood cultures and administering antibiotics for likely bacterial sepsis.

b. Endotracheal intubation and mechanical ventilation for impending respiratory failure.

c. Getting a detailed history from the parents regarding potential toxic ingestions.

d. Intravenous access and initiation of fluids for compensated hypovolemic shock.

e. Immediate consultation with general surgery for management of his abdominal pain.

8-19. An infant is brought into the Emergency Department apneic and asystolic. Bag-valve mask ventilation and chest compressions are being performed. You decide that intraosseous (IO) access is indicated and palpate the insertion site at the surface of the tibia about 1 cm below and medial to the tibial tuberosity. You manually insert the IO needle with a twisting motion. One sign that suggests that you have achieved successful IO cannulation is when:

a. The needle remains upright at the skin surface without any support.

b. You administer IO fluids and see successful expansion of the subcutaneous space.

c. You feel resistance as you enter the bony cortex.

d. None of the IO needle is visible above the surface of the skin.

e. You can no longer aspirate the bone marrow from the IO catheter with a syringe.

8-20. A 6-year-old girl with congestive heart failure and cardiogenic shock from viral myocarditis is transported to the critical care unit. She has 1 peripheral 20 gauge IV in a left antecubital vein, but is in need of additional intravenous access. One advantage of central venous cannulation over a peripheral IV is:

a. Administering medications via a peripheral IV is more caustic to the vasculature because the catheter is shorter than a central venous catheter.

b. Sterile technique is not needed to insert a central venous catheter.

c. Air embolism is a common complication of peripheral IVs.

d. Hemodynamic monitoring can be performed with a central venous catheter.

e. A central venous catheter can usually be inserted more easily and quickly than a peripheral IV.

8-21. A 2-year-old child requires a blood draw in the Emergency Department. She is very fearful and cries every time anyone other than the mother or father is in the room. Of the following, which is the best course of action?

   a. Child life resources should be called upon: Music, distraction, toys, and other tools to minimize stress can be helpful.

   b. Defer the blood draw despite the clinical necessity.

   c. Call the operating room to arrange for anesthesia to sedate the child for the blood draw.

   d. Topical anesthetic creams have no use in alleviating pain.

   e. The child should be strapped down while the parents wait in the waiting room, and the blood draw done quickly before she can object any longer.

8-22. Which of the following is true about pediatric cardiopulmonary arrest?

   a. Respiratory arrest results most commonly in arrhythmias such as VT and fibrillation.

   b. Sudden cardiac events are the most common causes of arrest in infants and children

   c. Of the prehospital arrests, more victims are found to be in asystole and pulseless electrical activity than VT or fibrillation.

   d. The 2005 American Heart Association recommends using pediatric resuscitation guidelines up to 8 years of age.

   e. The most common cause of cardiopulmonary arrest in infants below the age of 6 months is trauma.

8-23. Which of the following is NOT a reversible cause of pulseless electrical activity (PEA) in children?

   a. Tension pneumothorax

   b. Commotio cordis

   c. Hypovolemia

   d. Cardiac tamponade

   e. Pulmonary embolus

8-24. A 10-month-old baby with an unknown genetic syndrome is brought in by ambulance in cardiorespiratory arrest. He has a tracheostomy and is receiving positive pressure ventilation. No pulse is palpable so CPR is initiated. Monitor electrodes are placed on the chest and the monitor displays a VT. Which of the following is TRUE?

   a. Children presenting to the hospital with VT have lower survival than those who present with asystole.

   b. This patient has stable VT and attempts should be made to administer antiarrhythmic medications

   c. Untreated pulseless VT will rapidly progress to asystole then VF.

   d. CPR should be discontinued in this patient, as there is a very low chance of survival.

   e. When VT develops, the arterial oxygen content of the blood is initially normal; oxygen delivery to the brain is limited by blood flow more than by oxygen content.

8-25. The AHA Pediatric Advanced Life Support (PALS) guidelines were updated to enhance the treatment approach to the pre-arrest, CPR, and post-arrest intervals of pediatric cardiopulmonary arrest. Which of the following statements is correct about the delivery of high-quality CPR, which optimizes blood flow and oxygen delivery?

   a. Advanced life-support interventions, such as drug delivery and intubation, are organized around 3-minute intervals.

   b. Compression-to-ventilation ratios should be 15:2, regardless of the number of rescuers, to optimize oxygen delivery, as the vast majority of pediatric arrest is due to asphyxia, rather than arrhythmias.

   c. Bradycardia (HR <60 beats/minute with poor perfusion despite adequate oxygenation and ventilation) should be recognized early and treated with chest compressions.

   d. AEDs should be used in children aged 1–8 years, ideally with pediatric AED pads, at an initial dose of 2 J/kg.

   e. Epinephrine should be administered in a standard dose every 3–5 minutes in cardiac arrest with the optimal routes being intravenous, intraosseus, or endotracheal.

8-26. A 17-month-old boy has 5 days of worsening cough and fever and presents to the hospital with severe respiratory distress. He has a temperature of 39°C, heart rate of 175, respiratory rate of 50, blood pressure of 95/35 mm Hg, and oxygen saturation of 88% on RA. Supplemental oxygen is provided via a non-rebreather mask and portable chest x-ray shows a large left lower lobe opacity with pleural effusion. Intravenous fluids and antibiotics are initiated; however, the patient becomes more tachypneic, tired, and less responsive. Of the following which is TRUE?

   a. This patient should be admitted to the critical care unit given that the clinical trajectory is headed towards circulatory failure and need for cardiac transplant.

   b. ECMO (extracorporeal membrane oxygenation) is the most widely used and versatile technique that allows thousands of patients to recover from respiratory failure every year.

   c. Intensive care unit outcomes from respiratory failure have dramatically improved in the last decade due to the innovation of implantable ventricular assisting devices.

   d. Supplemental oxygen is potentially toxic to the lung and should be removed from this patient.

   e. Although positive pressure ventilation will not perfectly simulate healthy lung mechanics, it is the primary option for treating respiratory failure.

8-27. In patients with ventilation/perfusion inequality, the most rapid and predictable way to increase arterial PO_2 in a patient is to:

   a. Endotracheally intubate the patient.

   b. Increase inspired FiO_2.

   c. Start bag-valve mask ventilation.

   d. Increase respiratory rate.

   e. Increase tidal volume.

8-28. A 2-year-old boy contracts influenza and presents with a 5-day history of cough that has worsened over the past 2 days. His fever has been as high as 40°C, with a heart rate of 180 beats per minute, respiratory rate of 44, and blood pressure of 100/60 mm Hg. His chest x-ray is consistent with a multilobar pneumonia that you suspect is a bacterial superinfection. After being admitted to the critical care unit, he progresses to respiratory failure requiring the initiation of mechanical ventilation. Of the following which is TRUE?

   a. High-frequency ventilation can be initiated in this patient, however this requires higher airway pressures than traditional modes of mechanical ventilation and puts the patient at risk for trauma to the lungs

   b. In young children, sedation and neuromuscular blockade are not necessary given that pain receptors are not yet developed and patients can be easily restrained with soft restraints tied to their arms.

   c. Noninvasive methods of support (such as continuous positive airway pressure, CPAP) should not be used as the first-line support in pediatrics as it has not been studied and has not been shown to be useful.

   d. Settings of mechanical ventilation should be aimed at minimizing pressure and volume trauma that occurs with excessive stress and stretching of the lung.

   e. Permissive hypercapnea should not be allowed during mechanical ventilation as it leads to carbon dioxide toxicity.

8-29. Which of the following statements regarding mechanical ventilation is TRUE?

   a. Synchronized intermittent mandatory ventilation (SIMV) and pressure support ventilation are rarely used when weaning a patient off a ventilator.

   b. Tidal volume can be controlled by setting the volume or the pressure generated when the airway is opened.

   c. Airway leaks around the endotracheal tube do not play a role in ultimate tidal volume delivered to the lung.

   d. Positive end-expiratory pressure (PEEP) increases the workload of the respiratory muscles by exerting an additional pressure on alveoli and by closing them and decreasing the functional residual capacity.

   e. During assist-control ventilation, patient-initiated breaths are not completed by the ventilator.

8-30. Which of the following statement is TRUE regarding the stabilization and transport of children?

   a. Complex, high-acuity services for children are distributed evenly throughout the United States in order to simplify transport systems.

   b. Only critically ill children require transport by a professional team as all others may be transported by a private vehicle.

   c. Consideration of the insurance status is important in the determination of where an acutely ill child should be sent.

   d. Telemedicine has been fully incorporated into consultation with large referral centers and is the standard of care.

   e. Communication is paramount providing optimal care for acutely ill children and is often a source of misunderstanding.

8-31. A mother brings her 3-day-old newborn male into a community hospital Emergency Department for respiratory distress. The child is brought back immediately and you observe a cyanotic and lethargic infant. While staff call the nearest pediatric referral center, you place the patient on oxygen and continue your assessment. The patient's color improves on oxygenation, and when monitoring is established, you observe the patient to have an O_2 saturation of 90% on 100% O_2 by facemask. The patient has periods of apnea requiring bag-mask ventilation. The patient has palpable brachial pulses; however; you are unable to obtain a measurable blood pressure. You consider possible etiologies to be sepsis, a ductal dependent cardiac lesion, a primary respiratory illness such as bronchiolitis or congenital adrenal hyperplasia and discuss your assessment over the phone with the accepting physician. You are informed that a skilled pediatric critical care transport team is 5 minutes away, and that they will be transporting the patient 30 miles by ground to the referral center. Your best next step in preparation for transport of this child is:

a. Obtain venous access and intubate the newborn.

b. Request antibiotics, prostaglandin E1, and hydrocortisone from the pharmacy for transport.

c. No further intervention, additional procedures will only delay transport. The patient ventilates easily with BVM, and has palpable pulses. Antibiotics may be given intramuscularly.

d. Call back to the accepting physician and request that the patient be flown to the referring facility.

e. Explain to the mother the critical nature of the patient and obtain permission for transport.

8-32. Which of the following statements about cerebral edema is FALSE?

a. Cerebral edema is classified as either vasogenic, cytotoxic, or interstitial, depending on the etiology, and in most clinical situations, cerebral edema results from a combination of more than 1 of these mechanisms.

b. The blood–brain barrier protects the brain from exposure to potentially toxic circulating molecules and from excessive accumulation of water.

c. Interstitial cerebral edema results exclusively from increased capillary permeability and disruption of the blood–brain barrier following injury.

d. Cerebral edema results in increased intracranial pressure (ICP) that can reduce cerebral perfusion pressure below the autoregulation range of the cerebral blood vessels, resulting in ischemia.

e. Cerebrospinal fluid (CSF) production remains constant and declines only slightly with ICP, while the rate of absorption of CSF increases linearly with increased ICP.

8-33. A 7-year-old male presents to the Emergency Department by ambulance after being hit by a car while riding his bicycle. He was not wearing a helmet and was found unconscious on the ground immediately after the crash. He was intubated in the field for apnea and has been unresponsive en route. His pupils are 3 mm and appear to be minimally reactive. He withdraws to painful stimulus. A CT scan in the emergency department shows a skull fracture and an epidural bleed with diffuse swelling of his brain. Based on consensus statement for managing pediatric intracranial hypertension, which of the following is <u>NOT</u> a recommended treatment for severe traumatic brain injury?

a. Hyperventilation

b. Barbiturates

c. Hyperosmolar therapy

d. Corticosteroids

e. Hypothermia

8-34. A 3-week-old boy has a 2-week history of projectile, nonbloody, nonbilious emesis after every feed. His current medications include ranitidine. He has failed to gain weight, and appears dehydrated on exam. He sucks vigorously and has a normal neurologic, cardiac, and respiratory exam. On abdominal exam, you palpate an olive-shaped mass. His electrolytes are notable for a hypochloremic, hypokalemic, metabolic alkalosis. After fluid resuscitation and electrolyte correction, a pyloromyotomy is planned to correct his pyloric stenosis. Which of the following is TRUE?

a. The current medication that the infant is taking has no effect on the selection of anesthetic agent for the surgery.

b. If this infant was born at 39 weeks gestation, then he is at low-risk of postoperative complications from anesthesia, and does not need to be admitted for hospitalization for monitoring after his surgery.

c. In all procedures (including those where minimal blood loss is expected), a routine preoperative blood count should be performed on all patients prior to surgery.

d. Prior to surgery, it is important that the infant has nothing to eat or drink for 6 hours.

e. The ASA (American Society of Anesthesiology) anesthetic risk assessment class is determined by the general state of health of the patient and the complexity of the surgery.

8-35. A 1-year-old boy is scheduled for elective bilateral inguinal hernia repair. Although routine laboratory screening tests are not recommended for otherwise healthy children scheduled for minor surgery, which of the following situations should prompt you to obtain preoperative hemoglobin?

- **a.** Family history of iron deficiency anemia
- **b.** History of sickle cell disease
- **c.** Breast-fed infant
- **d.** Formula-fed infant
- **e.** Full-term infant

8-36. A 6-year-old boy is scheduled for umbilical hernia repair. On the day before his surgery, he develops nasal congestion. Which of the following would prompt most anesthesiologists to reschedule this elective procedure?

- **a.** Wheezing on physical exam
- **b.** Clear nasal discharge
- **c.** History of being born at 36 weeks gestation, as there is risk for apnea.
- **d.** Drinking apple juice 5 hours ago
- **e.** History of nasal congestion alone.

8-37. A 3-year-old girl is brought to the postanesthesia care unit after successful endoscopic removal of a quarter she swallowed yesterday. Prior to surgery she had no airway compromise. She is sleeping with normal vital signs. When would the child be considered stable for discharge?

- **a.** She can be discharged while still sleeping as long as her vital signs are within normal limits.
- **b.** This child should be admitted as she is at high risk for postoperative apnea.
- **c.** She can be discharged after 1 additional dose of intravenous narcotics for her pain.
- **d.** She can be discharged based on the results of established scoring systems, which take into account activity, respirations, circulation, consciousness, color, and movement.
- **e.** Nausea and vomiting are infrequent concerns in the postoperative course and are not considered in the assessment for discharge.

8-38. A 6-day-old term infant presents to the Emergency Department with erythema and swelling of his right leg. The patient's mother states that baby has been extremely fussy and inconsolable. The patient is afebrile and vitals are within normal limits, except for a heart rate of 180 while crying. As you enter the room you note the infant to be crying. There is decreased movement of his right leg, mild swelling and warmth, and tenderness to palpation of the entire right leg. The following statement is TRUE regarding pain in neonates:

- **a.** Treatment of pain in children is often inadequate despite numerous reports of under-treatment.
- **b.** Neonates do not show signs of distress and have a reduced ability to experience pain.
- **c.** There are no reliable measures of pain in preverbal children.
- **d.** Pain is a necessary experience for normal child development and maturation.
- **e.** The pathophysiology of pain is a simple and well-defined process.

8-39. A 20-month-old female presents to your office with a burn to the dorsum of her left hand and forearm after pulling a pot of hot water off of the stove. On physical examination, she is crying inconsolably in her mother's arms. She has blistering and open superficial partial thickness burns over the back of her left hand and forearm. How would you best manage this child's pain?

- **a.** Ask that child's mother to try and comfort her.
- **b.** Give the child a dose of ibuprofen.
- **c.** Give the child a dose of acetaminophen with codeine.
- **d.** Give the child a dose of acetaminophen with oxycodone.
- **e.** Apply topical lidocaine cream and send the patient to the ED for additional management.

8-40. A 3-year-old male presents to an urgent care 30 minutes after sustaining a laceration to his right temporal area. The preschool teacher told the mother that the patient fell from a stool, hitting his head on the corner of the table. The patient did not lose consciousness, has not vomited, and is behaving normally. On physical examination there is a 2-cm oblique laceration adjacent to the right eye. The wound is slightly gaping and is continuing to ooze. You determine that sedation should be administered for repair of his laceration and plan to give the patient 5 mg oral midazolam followed by local infiltration with buffered 1% lidocaine with epinephrine. Which of the following statements is TRUE regarding procedural sedation?

   a. If you are certified to provide sedation and have a protocol in place to access emergency services as needed, you do not need to have all of the drugs and equipment necessary to rescue the patient immediately.

   b. Procedural sedation is appropriate in this scenario, as you feel you will not be able to safely perform the repair without sedation.

   c. Apnea, aspiration, and hypotension are almost never seen with the use of benzodiazepines at moderate doses; therefore, these side effects should not be discussed with the patient's mother when obtaining consent for this procedure.

   d. In assessing whether a patient is an appropriate candidate for sedation, the patient's last oral intake is not relevant, as you are not planning on performing endotracheal intubation.

   e. The administration of 2 mg of morphine intramuscularly would be an acceptable alternative to oral midazolam for procedural sedation in this scenario.

8-41. Which of the following facts should prompt you to suspect an underlying inborn error of metabolism in a critically ill child?

   a. No past medical history, need for medications, or hospitalizations.

   b. A history of multiple sick contacts with similar symptoms currently in the family.

   c. Normal laboratory values including glucose, urinalysis, and pH.

   d. A patient whose symptoms present after their first prolonged fast.

   e. A patient who has fever and signs of septic shock.

8-42. A 2-week-old baby girl presents to the Emergency Department with decreased feeding for 2 days and a decreased level of alertness for 1 day. She has had a problem with vomiting after feeds since birth and has already gone through 2 formula changes. Her pediatrician sent her to the ED with concern for lethargy and dehydration. On arrival, the baby is minimally responsive to painful stimuli and is immediately taken to the resuscitation room. Oxygen is administered and intravenous access is attempted. A fingerstick blood glucose is found to be low at 25. Which of the following would be a useful additional step in the diagnosis and management of this infant?

   a. Check her urine for the presence of ketones.

   b. Immediately feed the child formula to support her hypoglycemia.

   c. Stop attempts at intravenous access as it places undue stress on the body and could worsen her hypoglycemia.

   d. Wait for a confirmatory blood glucose result from the laboratory before giving intravenous dextrose.

   e. She likely has gastroesophageal reflux (GERD), and hypoglycemia is commonly found in cases of GERD.

8-43. A 6-month-old girl with 2 days of fever and nasal congestion presents to the Emergency Department with a hypoglycemic seizure that responds to glucose infusion. She was previously in good health, until 2 days ago when she seemed to have contracted a viral illness that her older sister brought home from school. The night prior to having a seizure she slept through the night for the first time without feeding. You are concerned about an inborn error of metabolism given the hypoglycemic seizure after a prolonged fast, which seems unusual for a 6-month-old who presents with fever and upper respiratory infection. Which of the following statements regarding diagnosis of inborn errors of metabolism is TRUE?

   a. Additional laboratory testing is not useful in the diagnosis of inborn errors of metabolism as it is a diagnosis based on history and physical exam.

   b. A normal newborn screen rules out any possibility of inborn errors of metabolism.

   c. Inborn errors of metabolism are a group of varying diseases that have different physical exam and laboratory result profiles.

   d. There is no urgency in making the diagnosis since inborn errors of metabolism are a chronic disease and treatment is unnecessary in the acute presentation.

   e. Radiologic studies are the primary method of diagnosis.

8-44. A 12-year-old boy presents to the Emergency Department because of ataxia. Review of systems reveals he has had vomiting for the past 2 days. His symptoms began after eating a large hamburger at a fast food restaurant. His past medical history is remarkable for headaches that his pediatrician has diagnosed as migraines. There are no sick contacts and no family history of significant illness. On physical exam, he has decreased responsiveness to verbal stimulation, tachycardia, tachypnea, and normal blood pressure. His cranial nerves are intact, but he has truncal ataxia as well as inability to perform rapid alternating movements. His laboratory evaluation is notable for a mild respiratory alkalosis and elevated ammonia level. Which of the following is TRUE?

a. This patient's presentation is consistent with a diagnosis of an inborn error of metabolism, which if left untreated, could lead to seizures, cerebral edema, and coma.

b. The likely diagnosis is food poisoning and ataxia due to dehydration from vomiting.

c. His past history of migraine headaches makes the diagnosis of an inborn error of metabolism unlikely.

d. A normal family history makes the diagnosis of an inborn error of metabolism unlikely.

e. Ataxia is a common complaint in children that rarely indicates a concerning diagnosis.

8-45. A 10-year-old male presents to his primary care physician with the complaint of an enlarging red, painful, hard bump on his left buttock. The lesion began as a small pimple and has gotten worse over the past 2 days. Some purulent material has drained from the lesion. The boy cannot sit down secondary to the pain and had a tactile low-grade fever the night before presenting. The exam is normal with normal vitals with the exception of the left buttock which has a 2 cm by 3 cm indurated, red, tender nodule with a central pustule from which a small amount of purulent material can be expressed with light palpation. There is surrounding warmth and erythema. The process by which this inflammation occurs is best described by which of the following statements?

a. This infection was recognized initially by multiple cell types that reside in the tissues prior to the onset of infection, primarily neutrophils, and lymphocytes.

b. This represents an endogenous microbial inducer of inflammation, releasing damage-associated molecular patterns (DAMPs) and thereby triggering inflammation.

c. Macrophages engulf the bacteria in this infection based on detection via pattern recognition and the release of pro-inflammatory cytokines leads to the recruitment of inflammatory cells to the site of infection and elimination of the microbe.

d. The release of proinflammatory mediators at the site of the infection cause changes in the endothelial cells of nearby blood vessels, making them less permeable to neutrophils and plasma proteins.

e. The activation of Toll-like receptors (TLRs) by the pathogen-associated molecular patterns carried by the bacteria in this infection must be suppressed in order that commensal microorganisms that normally reside in the patient's body do not become a source of additional inflammation.

8-46. A 4-year-old female is brought into the Emergency Department by paramedics following a rollover motor vehicle crash on the highway. The patient was appropriately restrained in the backseat and was removed from the vehicle by medics. There is no report of loss of consciousness. As the patient is brought into the trauma bay you observe an agitated girl in cervical spine immobilization. Your primary survey reveals a patent airway, midline trachea and symmetric breath sounds; palpable femoral pulses bilaterally; GCS 15, and moving all extremities. Heart rate is 130 beats per minutes, blood pressure 92/48, respiratory rate 21, and O_2 saturation of 100% on RA. As you begin your secondary survey the patient becomes quiet and arousable only to painful stimulus. Repeat vitals are heart rate of 149, blood pressure of 63/29. Your next step in management is to:

a. Place an 18 French chest tube on the right side, 6th intercostal space, midaxillary line, for suspected hemothorax.

b. Accompany the patient to radiology to obtain computed tomography of the head and obtain an emergent neurosurgical consultation for her decline in mental status.

c. Ensure intravenous access, begin fluid resuscitation, and prepare the patient for probable emergent exploratory laparotomy.

d. Send a type and screen to the blood bank and send a complete blood count to determine the need for transfusion.

e. Perform a diagnostic peritoneal lavage to determine whether the patient needs to be taken to the operating room.

8-47. Which of the following is TRUE regarding trauma management?

    a. Airway, breathing, and circulation are the only three elements of the primary survey.

    b. Cervical spine injury is rarely seen and therefore stabilization is selectively applied as determined by prehospital personnel based on mechanism of injury.

    c. Bag-valve mask ventilation is often sufficient to maintain oxygenation and ventilation and is preferred to endotracheal tube placement when a difficult airway is anticipated or providers have little experience with intubation.

    d. Needle decompression through the 2nd intercostal space, midclavicular line, is the first-line treatment for hemothorax.

    e. In the setting of suspected intra-abdominal injury, a minimum of 2 intravenous lines placed in the patient's lower extremities, or a single subclavian line are necessary for fluid resuscitation.

8-48. An 18-month-old female, rescued from a house fire, arrives in the Emergency Department. As you begin your assessment you note that she is alert and crying due to pain. Her head, neck, and face are not burned, there is no carbonaceous sputum, no stridor, normal work of breathing, and clear breath sounds. Her pajamas are burned and she has superficial and deep partial thickness burns over the majority of her posterior trunk, buttocks, and left thigh. You suspect a full thickness burn approximately the size of the patient's palm in the middle of the left buttock. You estimate the extent of burn surface area to be 28%. Which of the following statements is TRUE regarding the patient in this scenario?

    a. The patient will not require intubation during her illness because she lacks burns to her head or neck, increased work of breathing, or circumferential burns on her chest.

    b. After airway assessment, immediate management should include removal of all clothes, placement of the patient into an ice bath to prevent ongoing thermal injury, treatment of pain, IVF resuscitation, and confirmation of tetanus immunization.

    c. Transfer to a burn center for admission is not indicated as she does not have a circumferential burn, chemical or electric burn, or burns involving the hands, feet, face, or genitalia.

    d. Regarding wound management, this patient should initially be dressed with dry gauze; further management may include debridement, topical antibiotics, nonadherent dressings, silver impregnated dressings, and potentially skin grafting to achieve wound coverage.

    e. The pattern of burn described in this scenario is highly suspicious for child abuse and Child Protective Services must be notified.

8-49. Which is TRUE regarding burns in children?

    a. Chemical burns, from common household cleaners, are the most common type of burns in children.

    b. The modified Lund–Browder surface area chart should be used to approximate the burned surface area.

    c. Children are more likely to be burned because of a larger body surface area to body mass ratio.

    d. It is very easy to distinguish partial thickness from full-thickness burns.

    e. Because patients with severe burns are hospitalized and relatively immobile they have decreased caloric requirements.

8-50. A 7-year-old boy presents to your office after being bitten by his pet cat. He has puncture wounds to the dorsal and volar aspects of his hand. There are no signs of infection. Which of the following is TRUE?

    a. Cat bites are the most common type of animal bite.

    b. Your next step in management is to irrigate and suture the patient's wounds.

    c. You should obtain x-rays to rule out fracture.

    d. This patient will require rabies immunization.

    e. Amoxicillin/clavulanate should be prescribed to prevent infection.

8-51. Which of the following is TRUE regarding the epidemiology of submersion injury?

    a. Unintentional injuries such as submersion are second only to childhood cancers as the most common cause of childhood mortality.

    b. The peak of pediatric submersion injury occurs in the 10–14 year-old age range.

    c. Toddlers most commonly suffer from submersion injury in oceans where the strength of the tides overpowers their strength.

    d. Submersion injury is more common in males than females.

    e. Alcohol is rarely involved in submersion injury.

8-52. A mother checks on her 12-year-old daughter in the bathroom and finds her submerged in the bathtub. The girl had been in her usual healthy state before going to the bathroom to take a bath. Her mother calls 911 and begins CPR. When EMS arrives, they find the girl limp with shallow respirations and a weak pulse. Bag-valve mask ventilation is begun as she is brought to the ED. Which of the following is TRUE?

   a. It is common to have serum electrolyte shifts due to the significant hypotonic fluid aspiration.

   b. Patients with epilepsy, prolonged QT syndrome, or a history of cardiac arrhythmias are counseled not to take baths alone.

   c. A Glasgow Coma Score of less than 15 on arrival to the ED predicts a poor neurologic outcome.

   d. It is rare for water to be aspirated into the lungs as laryngospasm prevents movement of water in that direction.

   e. By current definitions, this is a case of near drowning.

8-53. A 15-year-old boy was with friends on a camping trip. The youths were drinking heavily and the boy slipped from a tree branch into a river. By the time the friends were able to pull him from the water, he suffered a prolonged submersion. Rescue workers were called, and the boy was ultimately transported to a local emergency department. Which of the following is TRUE about the effects of submersion on the body?

   a. Most severe submersion victims have intact neurologic status after recovery. Initially they present with decreased consciousness but the condition usually resolves in the first hour after the event.

   b. Cardiac dysrhythmias, cardiac dysfunction, and hypotension are caused primarily by direct myocardial hypoxia or ischemia.

   c. Victims rarely swallow water during submersion.

   d. Freshwater drowning results in water absorption into the vascular space from the lungs through osmosis and resultant hypervolemia and hemolysis.

   e. Laryngospasm prevents the water from being aspirated into the lungs and most drownings are considered dry drownings.

8-54. A 14-month-old toddler is found floating face down in the family pool. Which of the following regarding prevention of submersion injury is TRUE?

   a. Only a minority of submersion injury deaths are preventable.

   b. Parental supervision of toddlers near bodies of water has little effect on prevention of submersion.

   c. Four-sided fencing which isolates the pool has higher risk of submersion injury because children cannot easily get away from the pool.

   d. Soft and rigid covers are both effective at preventing pool submersion injury.

   e. Pool alarms are an effective method of preventing submersion injury.

8-55. According to the National Safety Council, choking is a prominent cause of unintentional injury-related death in infants and young children. Which age group is the most likely to aspirate a foreign body (FB)?

   a. Age 0–1 year

   b. Age 1–2 years

   c. Age 2–3 years

   d. Age 3–10 years

   e. Older than 10 years

8-56. A 2-year-old female is brought in by ambulance for a choking episode. She was playing on the floor with her older brother. Her mother found her coughing and gagging and seemingly unable to breathe. The mother performed rescue breaths and CPR and EMS was called. By the time the paramedics arrived, the girl was persistently coughing but had a normal oxygen saturation. She was transported via ambulance on 100% O_2 by mask and the cough has subsided. Her respiratory rate was elevated at 30 breaths per minute and her O_2 saturation was 92% on RA. Which of the statements below is true regarding the pathogenesis of a FB aspiration such as this?

   a. When a FB is first aspirated, the discomfort and irritation cause the child to cough and cry and the child exhales, causing impaction within the airway.

   b. The FB creates a valve-like effect in the airway, increasing resistance to inspiration but not expiration.

   c. A cough reflex results from the stimulation of surface motor receptors of the respiratory mucosa.

   d. Mucosal receptors in the airway can become adapted to pressure caused by a lodged FB over time and the initial cough will subside.

   e. With time after FB aspiration, the airway mucosal receptors will not be restimulated, resulting in a latent period free of cough.

8-57. A 4-year-old female presents to the Emergency Department with a complaint of 1 month of cough and wheeze. She has been seen 3 other times in the past month and has received a single-view chest x-ray and a trial of a bronchodilator with minimal change in her symptoms. On the day of this ED visit she coughed up a small amount of blood and her parents are very worried. She has otherwise been in her normal state of health, able to eat and attend school, although her cough is exacerbated with activity and seems to bother her throughout the day and evening. She has had no fever, no rhinorrhea or other viral upper respiratory symptoms, and has no history of reactive airways disease. On exam she is well-appearing with normal pulse oximetry and a normal respiratory rate. She has occasional right-sided wheeze but her lungs are otherwise clear and she has no signs of increased work of breathing. The physician suspects an impacted FB and orders films. Which of the following statements is true about the diagnosis and management of impacted foreign bodies?

a. Inspiratory and expiratory films are easy to obtain and frequently lead to the diagnosis of impacted FB.

b. The majority of all FB aspiration cases are diagnosed more than 1 month after the event.

c. Radiographic findings associated with impacted bronchial foreign bodies most commonly show obstructive asymmetric hyperinflation.

d. Lateral decubitus films are the gold standard for diagnosis of impacted FB and they have a high diagnostic predictive value.

e. Diagnostic endoscopy should only be undertaken if radiographic evidence of foreign-body aspiration is unequivocal.

8-58. An 11-month-old male is found by his mother at home unconscious and not breathing. He had been eating a cut up hotdog for lunch just prior to the event and she stepped out of the room to answer a phone call. She came back to find him slumped in his high chair with blue-tinged lips and face. She activates the emergency medical system and while she waits for them to arrive, which of the following describes the best course of action?

a. Back blows face down

b. Blind finger sweep of his mouth

c. Heimlich maneuver

d. CPR

e. Subdiaphragmatic thrusts with head down

8-59. Which of the symptoms below is NOT included in the 1986 National Institutes of Health (NIH) consensus definition of an apparent life-threatening event (ALTE)?

a. Eyes rolling back

b. Cyanosis

c. Limpness

d. Apnea

e. Gagging

8-60. A 10-day-old infant male is brought in by EMS to the Emergency Department for an episode of not breathing and choking for which the parents initiated CPR. As per the mother, the infant was sleeping in his car seat when she looked over he appeared not to be breathing and had blue lips for 2 minutes. After picking him up, he made high-pitched choking sounds that resolved once the infant received rescue breaths from his mother. Upon EMS arrival at the home, the infant was saturating and breathing normally and did not require interventions en route to the hospital. The infant is the product of a full-term first pregnancy to a 19-year-old mother and has been growing and developing well up until this point. When the ED physician has the mother sit quietly for 1 minute, she rethinks that perhaps the period of apnea was closer to 20–30 seconds, although it felt as if it might be longer at the time.

Which of the statements below is true regarding the process of establishing whether or not symptoms are consistent with an ALTE?

a. The ability of caretakers to provide an accurate history for an ALTE is improved by the fact that they may have been frightened and panicking.

b. Reports of a baby turning blue are not consistent with a genuine ALTE.

c. A previous history of life-threatening events in the infant or a sibling is diagnostic and indicates that the event was real or that child abuse might be playing a role.

d. Episodes involving choking and color change are often related to seizure or cardiac pathology.

e. Because of the absence of persistent symptoms or sequelae it is sometimes difficult to establish that an ALTE actually occurred; a careful and thorough history must be taken.

8-61. A 20-day-old infant born at 36 weeks by Cesarean section presents to the Emergency Department for concerns about an event during which he stopped breathing, his eyes rolled back and he had a color change. He has been taking 4 ounces of formula every 3 hours and is gaining weight well. His mother is a 29-year-old G2P2 with a 3-year-old at home. She states that the baby often vomits after feeds but this event was not associated with a feed. The baby was sleeping and seemed to choke and stopped breathing for what she thinks was 60 seconds. She slapped the baby on the back and blew in his face and eventually he began to breathe. He has had several days of upper airway congestion and trouble with feeds secondary to mucus. His older sibling has a cold. The infant is well-nourished with normal color and tone at the time of exam and is congested with slight retractions, a respiratory rate of 75, and an oxygen saturation of 94% on RA; the rest of his vitals are normal.

Which of the following does not fit in the differential diagnosis for the cause of this patient's ALTE based on history and physical exam?

a. Respiratory infection

b. Seizure

c. Gastroesophageal reflux

d. Child abuse

e. Periodic breathing

8-62. An infant is brought into the Emergency Department with the parental concern for an ALTE. Once the history and physical is completed, which of the following represents a reasonable management strategy for a possible ALTE?

a. If the episode can be attributed to misinterpreted normal behavior or minor coughing/gagging, the patient should be admitted overnight for observation and the parents should be trained in CPR.

b. If the episode is convincing, the patient should be admitted and a work-up should be directed at the plausible problems based on history and physical.

c. If the episode is convincing and appears to be idiopathic after a workup in the ED, the family should be reassured and sent home, as it is unlikely the episode was a true ALTE.

d. If the episode is convincing and there were persistent symptoms, the infant should be admitted and have cardiorespiratory monitoring in the hospital until symptom free for 2 days.

e. If the episode is convincing and an identifiable cause is determined in the ED, the family should be sent home with reassurance and advice related to strategies for avoiding future episodes.

8-63. The mother of a 2-year-old (12 kg) male calls your office distraught after discovering her son with an open, 4 oz bottle of liquid Tylenol (160 mg/5 mL). She thinks that the bottle was almost entirely full and notes that there is only about an ounce remaining. She wonders if he has ingested a dangerous amount and what she should do now? Which of the following statements is TRUE regarding acetaminophen overdose in children?

a. N-acetyl-p-benzoquinoneimine (NAPQI), the toxic metabolite of acetaminophen responsible for hepatic injury, is produced ONLY in cases of overdose.

b. Acute ingestion of more than 150 mg/kg in children is potentially hepatotoxic. The patient described is at risk for hepatoxicity.

c. An immediate serum acetaminophen level should be obtained and plotted on the Rumack–Matthew nomogram to guide your treatment decision.

d. In toxic overdoses, hepatic injury is evident by serum testing of markers of liver function immediately after ingestion.

e. Antidotal therapy with N-acetylcystine (NAC) is such an effective antidote that it may be beneficial even if started up to 72 hours after ingestion.

8-64. A one-and-half-year-old female presents to the Emergency Department lethargic, diaphoretic, and tremulous. Her heart rate is 156, respiratory rate 24, BP 98/56, O_2 saturation 99%, and temperature 37.9°C. There is no history of recent illness or fever, no history of trauma; her mother went to arouse her from a nap and discovered her this way. On further questioning she had been cared for by her grandmother that morning; she has multiple medical conditions and is on a number of different medications. This patient's presentation is most consistent with which of the following ingestions and what would you do next?

a. Oral hypoglycemic agent: obtain a finger-stick glucose, prepare to give dextrose and possibly octreotide.

b. Tricyclic antidepressant: intubate, administer charcoal via nasogastric tube, obtain an EKG to evaluate for QRS widening.

c. Opioid overdose: perform a pupillary assessment, administer naloxone, and reassess the patient for improvement in mental status.

d. Beta-blocker: obtain an EKG, begin IV fluid resuscitation and whole bowel irrigation, and consider a glucagon infusion.

e. Carbon monoxide poisoning: start intravenous fluids and oxygen by nasal cannula, send a carboxyhemoglobin (COHb) level using co-oximetry, and consider hyperbaric oxygen therapy.

8-65. A 1-year-old female is brought into the Emergency Department after being found with an open bottle of furniture polish. Her mother states that the child vomited once en route and on exam smells of lemon cleaning solution. You do not note any lesions within the oropharynx or any respiratory distress by observation and auscultation. Which of the following statements is TRUE?

a. Hydrocarbon exposures are rare in children and therefore the cleaner ingested is unlikely to cause symptoms.

b. CNS depression is commonly seen in cases of true hydrocarbon ingestion due to efficient absorption from the gastrointestinal tract.

c. A stat ECG is indicated as cardiovascular toxicity is common after accidental hydrocarbon ingestion or aspiration and is your primary concern.

d. Children with presumed hydrocarbon ingestion should be observed for 6 hours from the time of ingestion for the development of respiratory symptoms.

e. Activated charcoal should be administered to all patients who have ingested hydrocarbons.

8-66. A 4-year-old is brought in to the Emergency Department after drinking antifreeze that was stored in a large soda bottle on the floor of the back seat of the family's car. Which of the following statements is TRUE regarding ethylene glycol poisoning?

a. Toxicity is diminished as ethylene glycol is metabolized.

b. On laboratory evaluation, an initial increased anion gap metabolic acidosis gives way to a significant osmolar gap.

c. There is no antidote, only supportive care and hemodialysis can be used for treatment.

d. The lethal dose of ethylene glycol is very high.

e. Symptoms of toxicity may include ataxia, seizures, altered mental status, coma, myocardial depression, hypotension, hypocalcemia, vomiting, and renal failure.

8-67. Which of the following is TRUE about heat-related illness?

a. Heat syncope is usually due to peripheral vasoconstriction and dehydration.

b. Heat stroke is the second most common cause of death in athletes.

c. Heat cramps are due to dehydration and overuse of muscles.

d. Rhabdomyolysis is a common side effect of heat cramps.

e. Systemic inflammatory response and multisystem organ failure will occur with heat exhaustion.

8-68. A 14-year-old soccer player is practicing outside with her team on a hot, sunny day. The outside temperature is 100°F. Of the following, which is the principal method of physiologic heat elimination?

a. Conduction

b. Convection

c. Radiation

d. Evaporation

e. Sublimation

8-69. A 3-week-old baby is found in a car on a hot summer day. An ambulance brings the infant into the Emergency Department. Her temperature is 41°C, HR 170, and RR 8. She is minimally responsive and has hot dry skin. Which of the following statements is TRUE?

a. The infant is suffering from heat exhaustion.

b. Acetaminophen and/or ibuprofen should be administered immediately to start reducing the temperature.

c. Ice water immersion may not be the ideal form of cooling because shivering and peripheral vasoconstriction may increase heat production.

d. Evaporative cooling by spraying the body with lukewarm atomized water and fanning is much less effective than cold water immersion.

e. First-line measures should be invasive cooling with cardiopulmonary bypass and gastric, peritoneal, or pleural lavage should be implemented immediately.

8-70. A 17-year-old varsity football player arrives in the Emergency Department on a hot summer day for symptoms of heat exhaustion. He is treated with rest and intravenous fluids. His father asks what are some steps they can take to prevent heat exhaustion and heat stroke in the future. Which of the following would be a useful message to impart?

a. Outdoor football practice in the summer should be discontinued.

b. Speaking with the coach about instituting preventive measures will not be helpful.

c. When signs of heat exhaustion develop, there is nothing that can be done to prevent it from developing into heat stroke

d. Ready access to water and regular rest in between exertion should be scheduled during training.

e. Reassure them that heat exhaustion and stroke are uncommon conditions and therefore no further counseling is necessary.

8-71. A 6-year-old male presents to your office with facial swelling, rash and abdominal pain after being stung by a bee at school during recess. The patient's mother notes that he has been stung before but not previously developed the symptoms presently seen. Which of the following statements is true regarding the management of hymenoptera (bee, hornet, yellow jacket, wasp, and ant) stings?

a. This patient's symptoms are not life threatening and no immediate treatment is indicated. An allergy referral should be made.

b. This patient's symptoms are consistent with a local reaction and may be treated with a cold compress and comfort measures.

c. This patient's symptoms will resolve once the stinger and venom sac are carefully removed with tweezers.

d. This patient is almost certain to develop worsening symptoms and therefore requires immediate intubation to protect his airway.

e. This patient's symptoms are consistent with anaphylaxis and should be treated with intramuscular epinephrine, corticosteroids, H1/H2 blockers and intravenous fluids as needed.

8-72. A 5-year-old boy is bit on his right hand by a rattlesnake while playing in his backyard. The patient is brought to the Emergency Department. Triage vitals are within normal limits and on exam the patient is alert but uncomfortable and diaphoretic and has begun vomiting. On the dorsum of his right hand you see 2 puncture marks separated by approximately 1 cm, there is swelling, erythema, and ecchymosis extending to the patients distal forearm. Before the medics leave they inform you that the rattlesnake was successfully captured, killed, and identified. Which statement regarding rattlesnake bites is TRUE?

a. Members of the Crotalidae (pit viper) family are distinguished by the heat-sensitive organs, pits on the sides of their triangularly shaped heads, their vertical elliptical pupils, and curved fangs.

b. An arterial tourniquet should be applied in all cases of venomous snakebites; incision and suction should be used in the prehospital setting to remove as much venom as possible.

c. Rattlesnake venom, designed to digest prey, contain enzymes that cause only local tissue injury, and therefore mortality from envenomations is low.

d. This patient's symptoms are likely at their peak and would be classified as mild on the envenomation grading system.

e. Equine IgG antivenin is more efficacious and less antigenic than Crotalidae polyvalent immune Fab (CroFab®), and is the preferred treatment for moderate to severe bites requiring antivenin.

ANSWERS

Answer 8-1. c

Children, especially, infants are at increased risk for issues associated with respiratory distress and respiratory failure due to immaturity of neural control of breathing, small airway caliber, and limited respiratory reserve. In healthy individuals, respiratory and circulatory functions are linked to tissue metabolic activity by a regulatory system that translates neural and biochemical signals in order to make adjustments to cardiac output, vascular tone, and minute ventilation. These adjustments ensure that the body receives sufficient O_2 without accumulating excessive CO_2. The system works by way of central and peripheral circulatory reflexes that are sensitive to alterations in PO_2, PCO_2, and pH. Answers a and d are not correct, as the carotid bodies are peripheral chemoreceptors that have cells that sense PO_2, while the reticular nuclei of the medulla oblongata are the central chemoreceptors that sense PCO_2 and pH. Answer b is not correct, as increases in PCO_2 (and only if sufficiently large, decreases in PO_2) are sensed by the chemoreceptors and can result in the recruitment of respiratory muscles. Nasal flaring, increased vocal cord abduction, and dilation of the pharyngeal passages during inspiration are all adaptations that occur but may be less noticeable to the observer. Finally, Answer e is not correct as alterations in breathing frequency and retractions, however, are prominent in almost every child with acute respiratory distress.

(Reference: Section 8: The Acutely Ill Infant and Child; Part 1: Assessment of the Acutely Ill Infant and Child, Chapter 102, p 375–376)

Answer 8-2. b

Obstructive lung disease is characterized by impairments in expiration, inspiration, or both. The physical findings of intrathoracic obstruction are more prominent during expiration. The expiratory phase is prolonged while the decrease in pleural pressure during inspiration helps to relieve the obstruction. The preferential impairment of expiratory gas flow may not be compensated entirely by the prolonged expiratory phase. If so, the alveolar spaces

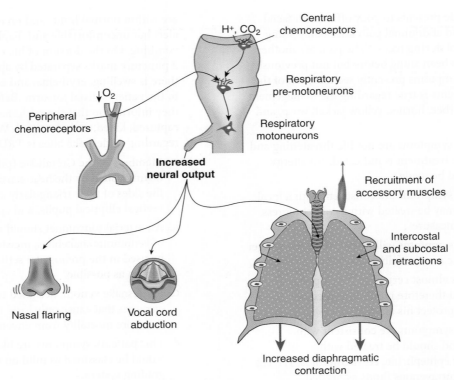

FIGURE 102-1. Genesis of the signs of respiratory distress. Changes in blood–gas tensions are sensed by chemoreceptor cells in the carotid bodies (O_2) and in the reticular formation of the medulla oblongata (CO_2). The nerve signals originating in the chemoreceptors are integrated and processed by a complex medullary neuronal network that also receives inputs from mechanoreceptors in the lungs and chest wall and from other areas of the brain. Increases in arterial PCO_2 and, if sufficiently large, decreases in arterial PO_2 sensed by the chemoreceptors activate neural programs that result in the progressive recruitment of a variety of respiratory muscles, as shown in the bottom of the figure. Nasal flaring (from contraction of the dilators of the alae nasae), increased vocal cord abduction, and dilation of the pharyngeal passages during inspiration may not be apparent to the observer. However, alterations in the breathing frequency (usually tachypnea) or intercostal and subcostal retractions (from the subatmospheric pleural pressures generated by the forceful contractions of the diaphragm) are prominent in almost every child with acute respiratory disease. (Reproduced, with permission, from Rudolph CD, Rudolph AM, Lister GE, First LR, Gershon AA. *Rudolph's Pediatrics.* 22nd ed. New York: McGraw-Hill, 2011.)

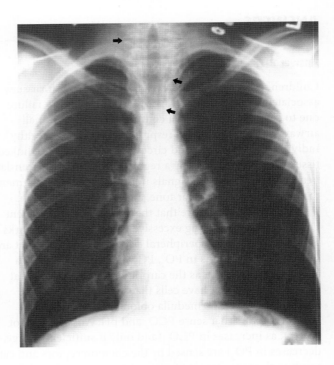

Example of a chest x-ray of a child with an acute asthma exacerbation which shows hyperinflation (abnormally lucent lungs). In addition, the diaphragm is flattened and relatively small and air is present within the mediastinum. (Reproduced, with permission, from Strange GR, Ahrens WR, Schafermeyer RW, Wiebe RA. *Pediatric Emergency Medicine.* 3rd ed. New York: McGraw-Hill, 2009.)

subtended by the obstructed airways do not empty entirely before the next inspiration starts, and the volume of the affected alveoli at end-expiration increases—leading to gas trapping, as suggested by hyperinflation and a flat diaphragm on chest radiograph. However, the alveolar volume increase is limited by the effects of distention on lung recoil, which dictate an equilibrium whereby the increased recoil limits tidal volume and accelerates exhalation enough to compensate for the low expiratory flow. The development of lung distention in patients with intrathoracic airway obstruction adds a restrictive component to the manifestations of their lung disease. This effect may be one of the reasons why children with asthma or other forms of bronchial obstruction have tachypnea as a prominent sign.

(Reference: Section 8: The Acutely Ill Infant and Child; Part 1: Assessment of the Acutely Ill Infant and Child, Chapter 102, p 379)

Answer 8-3. c

Arterial blood gas concentrations result from a mixture of 2 sources: systemic venous blood that bypasses the alveoli and does not participate in gas exchange and blood that undergoes perfect exchange with alveolar gas. The blood that bypasses the alveoli, that which is shunted, arises from several different, discrete pathways. True anatomic shunts represent anatomic communications between the arterial and venous sides of circulation and can be found in normal individuals and those with cardiac or lung disease. Diffusion defects are either due to problems with the alveolar capillary membrane or by blood being forced through the capillaries too quickly to equilibrate with the alveolar gas. Incomplete oxygenation of blood circulating through areas of the lung with a low ventilation–perfusion ratio creates virtual shunts.

Answer a is not correct, as the ventilation–perfusion inequality is the most common mechanism of hypoxemia and hypercapnea in both adults and children with respiratory failure. Answer b is not correct. The parallel organization of the bronchial and arterial networks of the lungs allows for numerous $V–Q$ ratios to exist in the same lung and gravity contributes a certain degree of $V–Q$ inequality by directing a larger share of blood flow to more dependent areas. Answer e is not correct. The cause of hypoxemia in $V–Q$ inequality lies primarily with the alveolar-capillary units that have a low $V–Q$ ratio because renewal of the alveolar gas cannot keep up with O_2 uptake by the blood resulting in end-capillary blood that is not fully loaded with O_2; this creates substantial venous admixtures.

Answer d is not correct. Alveolar-capillary units with low $V–Q$ ratios cannot decrease their alveolar PCO_2 and their ability to remove CO_2 from the blood is therefore impaired. However, this is offset by lung units with a high $V–Q$ ratio and allows for compensation that makes hypercapnea a less

prominent feature than hypoxemia in the infant or child that has sufficient reserve to support an increase in ventilation.

(Reference: Section 8: The Acutely Ill Infant and Child; Part 1: Assessment of the Acutely Ill Infant and Child, Chapter 102, p 380–381)

Answer 8-4. a

Efficiency of the respiratory system is the proportion of energy consumed by the respiratory muscles in pressure–volume work and is estimated to be 15% in adults but only 5% in infants. Respiratory efficiency is affected by respiratory pattern, the conditioning of the respiratory muscles, and configuration of the chest wall. The diaphragm can increase its work with small increases in O_2 consumption and blood-flow needs, while other accessory respiratory muscles have higher energy demands. In newborns and small infants, limited ossification of the rib cage and a short axial dimension of the thorax make their chest wall prone to distortion, which decreases respiratory muscle efficiency. (See Figure 102-6.)

The area of contact between the lateral surface of the diaphragm and the internal surface of the rib cage (the area of apposition) facilitates lung inflation by converting the increase

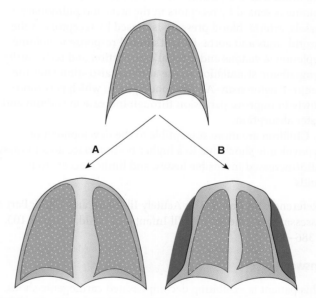

FIGURE 102-6. Effect of rib cage distortion on lung volume change and diaphragmatic displacement. Inward distortion during inspiration is common in the newborn and small infant, particularly when pleural pressure is decreased to overcome lung disease. The upper panel shows the chest in expiration, with the diaphragm displaced upward. The diagram shows how the same inspiratory displacement of the diaphragm is applied entirely to inflate the lungs in the absence of distortion (**A**) and divided between the inward volume change of the rib cage (shaded area) and lung inflation when chest wall distortion exists (**B**). (Reproduced, with permission, from Rudolph CD, Rudolph AM, Lister GE, First LR, Gershon AA. *Rudolph's Pediatrics.* 22nd ed. New York: McGraw-Hill, 2011.)

in intraabdominal pressure into outward directed force on the rib cage. The area of apposition in infants is small because of their relatively wide lower chest that spreads out the costal insertions of the diaphragm, resulting in wasted work by the diaphragm. Inward distortion of the infant rib cage increases the shortening of phrenic fibers as they generate volume change in the lungs, causing the volume displaced by the diaphragm to be divided between the volume increase of the lungs and the volume created by the inward movement of the ribcage. The energy used in the process of distorting the rib cage is wasted by the diaphragm, therefore making the muscle more prone to fatigue.

(Reference: Section 8: The Acutely Ill Infant and Child; Part 1: Assessment of the Acutely Ill Infant and Child, Chapter 102, p 381–382)

Answer 8-5. b

This patient is in compensated hypovolemic shock. Mean blood pressure is an insensitive measure of circulatory function in children because they do not have to be hypotensive to be in shock. As shock progresses from compensated to decompensated, patients may develop lassitude, hypotension, delayed capillary refill, and pallor. Blood is redistributed away from the skin and gut, but is preserved to the heart and brain where O_2 extraction is maximized. Intravascular volume is sensed by receptors in the atria and pulmonary vessels, arterial blood pressure is sensed by receptors in the carotid sinus and aorta. Patient's initial response to volume depletion is venous and arterial constriction and tachycardia. Sympathetic stimulation of the adrenals also stimulates the Renin–Angiotensin–Aldosterone-System, which acts more slowly to improve perfusion through increase in sodium and water absorption.

Children are more susceptible to the development of hypovolemic shock due to a higher body surface area to mass ratio/increased insensible losses, and limited access to free fluids.

(Reference: Section 8: The Acutely Ill Infant and Child; Part 1: Assessment of the Acutely Ill Infant and Child, Chapter 103, p 386–389)

Answer 8-6. c

This patient is exhibiting decompensated cardiogenic shock. Shock is a state in which tissue perfusion is impaired and systemic blood flow is inadequate to sustain vital functions. It is an unstable condition and if left untreated causes progressive multi-organ system failure, lactic acidosis, and death. When considering the treatment of this patient, fluid bolus worsened this patient's clinical status. The next step in management is to improve systemic perfusion through improved cardiac output. Cardiac output is improved by improving the heart rate and contractility or stroke volume. This may be achieved with dopamine infusion. In the differential for this patient is

septic shock and therefore the patient will also likely receive antibiotics, however this would not be the appropriate next step. Sodium bicarbonate may be used in cases of profound acidosis to restore cellular function and calcium chloride may be used in patients not responding to inotropes and vasoactive medications, however, these would also not be the next immediate steps in management.

(Reference: Section 8: The Acutely Ill Infant and Child; Part 1: Assessment of the Acutely Ill Infant and Child, Chapter 103, p 386–390)

Answer 8-7. b

The above scenario portrays an infant in septic or distributive shock. This patient may have adequate cardiac function and blood volume; however, abnormal vascular tone can lead to decreased preload and inadequate cardiac output. The elevation in BUN and creatinine, along with the decrease in urine output, is an indication of inadequate perfusion of the kidneys. Although these signs may also be present in hypovolemia, the patient's exam—including an elevated temperature, flat fontanel, and warm skin—are also consistent with distributive shock.

Symptoms of cardiac tamponade include: jugular venous distention, muffled heart sounds, and pulsus paradoxus and are not exhibited by this patient. The priority in a patient's initial resuscitation is to give fluids liberally to maintain tissue perfusion and if this is not achieved with fluids, vasopressor infusion should be initiated. Given that there are multiple etiologies of septic shock, including bacterial, viral, or toxin-mediated shock, it is helpful but not necessary to draw cultures before empiric antibiotics are initiated. This patient is in decompensated septic shock and therefore antibiotics should be administered as soon as possible.

(Reference: Section 8: The Acutely Ill Infant and Child; Part 1: Assessment of the Acutely Ill Infant and Child, Chapter 103, p 386–389)

Answer 8-8. d

A complex network of interactions within the brain mediates arousal. This includes, but is not limited to, the reticular activating system, cerebral cortex, thalamus, hypothalamus, and all major sensory systems. Alteration of the mental status is a continuum from lethargy, to obtundation, to stupor, to coma.

Because terminology is inconsistently used among observers, the Glasgow Coma Scale (GCS) may be used to score patients in 3 categories: eye opening, verbal response, motor response. GCS is useful in documenting changes in mental status over time. Both primary processes originating within the central nervous system as well as secondary processes should be considered in the differential of patients presenting with altered mental status as respiratory failure, cardiac rhythm disturbances, sepsis/shock, and metabolic

TABLE 11–5. Glasgow Coma Scale[a]

Eye opening response

Spontaneous	4
To speech	3
To pain	2
None	1

Verbal response: Child (Infant modification)[b]

Oriented (*Coos, babbles*)	5
Confused conversation (*Irritable cry, consolable*)	4
Inappropriate words (*Cries to pain*)	3
Incomprehensible sounds (*Moans to pain*)	2
None	1

Best upper limb motor response: Child (Infant modification)[b]

Obeys commands (*Normal movements*)	6
Localizes pain (*Withdraws to touch*)	5
Withdraws to pain	4
Flexion to pain	3
Extension to pain	2
None	1

[a]The appropriate number from each section is added to THE total between 3 and 15. A score less than 8 usually indicates CNS depression requiring positive-pressure ventilation.

[b]If no modification is listed, the same response applies for both infants and children.

disorders may all be potential etiologies. Given the broad differential, a careful history and physical exam may help guide the practitioner's choice of testing. Alterations in mental status should always be assumed to indicate a serious medical problem and should receive prompt and comprehensive evaluation.

(Reference: Section 8: The Acutely Ill Infant and Child; Part 1: Assessment of the Acutely Ill Infant and Child, Chapter 104, p 391–392)

Answer 8-9. e

While hypoglycemia, acute intracranial bleed, cardiac rhythm disturbance, or toxic ingestion are all possible etiologies in the presentation of altered mental status, a systematic and comprehensive evaluation must be performed before determining the etiology. This evaluation should focus on ensuring that the patient is able to maintain and protect her airway, is breathing sufficiently to maintain both oxygenation and ventilation, and establish that she has adequate perfusion

by means central pulse palpation, assessment of heart rate and blood pressure and perfusion. If any of these vital functions are compromised on initial assessment, they must be addressed before moving forward with the secondary survey or treatment of a presumed etiology. All cases of altered mental status should be assumed to indicate a serious problem and comprehensive evaluation is warranted even in cases of suspected alcohol abuse.

(Reference: Section 8: The Acutely Ill Infant and Child; Part 1: Assessment of the Acutely Ill Infant and Child, Chapter 104, p 391–392)

Answer 8-10. c

CNS infections typically present with generalized findings. Diagnosis requires a lumbar puncture.

However, in cases of parameningeal infection, lumbar puncture should be deferred in favor of surgical drainage due to the risk of herniation. Parameningeal foci of infection typically present with focal neurological findings.

In children younger than 18–24 months, signs of meningeal irritation such as nuchal rigidity or the Kernig or Brudzinski signs may be absent. While bacterial meningitis will likely present with a CSF pleocytosis, other causes of CNS infection such as herpes encephalitis may present with normal CSF findings. Antibiotics should not be delayed in cases of suspected meningitis. In cases in which there has been pretreatment of the CSF, latex agglutination may identify a bacterial organism.

(Reference: Section 8: The Acutely Ill Infant and Child; Part 1: Assessment of the Acutely Ill Infant and Child, Chapter 104, p 393–394)

Answer 8-11. a

The diagnosis of brain death may be made by 2 careful examinations conducted by an experienced physician. The exam consists of documenting lack of central motor response to stimuli including decorticate and decerebrate posturing, though spinal motor reflexes may persist. Documentation of lack of brain stem function should be done by individually testing all cranial nerves and finally by performing an apnea test. All efforts to eliminate confounders such as hypotension, hypothermia, and sedating medications must be made. As an alternative to the documentation of 2 exams, 2 EEGs or a cerebral perfusion scan may be used in children under 1-year-old. Guidelines have been put in place to provide a process and uniformity but are nonbinding and should take into consideration individual factors such as mechanism, patient age, and the presence of other organ systems dysfunction.

(Reference: Section 8: The Acutely Ill Infant and Child; Part 1: Assessment of the Acutely Ill Infant and Child, Chapter 104, p 396)

Answer 8-12. d

It has been the practice of the majority of clinicians in the United States to aggressively work up any infant who presents with fever before 2–3 months of age, including a broad laboratory investigation for bacterial disease, hospitalization, and empirical parenteral administration of antibiotics. This approach has been tempered by a series of large clinical studies that established new screening tools to identify febrile infants at low risk of having a serious bacterial infection. Of the 3 screening tools developed, the Rochester Criteria, the Philadelphia Criteria, and the Boston Criteria, the model created at the Children's Hospital of Philadelphia was the most conservative and demonstrates the highest negative predictive value. The Philadelphia rules are for infants between the ages of 29 and 60 days with a temperature greater than 38.2°C who are well-appearing on exam and have no evidence of ear/bone/skin infection. Infants are considered low-risk if their peripheral WBC was <15 K/mm, their UA was <10 WBC/hpf, their CSF had <8 WBC/mm^3, and gram stain was negative and their CXR was negative. Low-risk infants could be sent home with no antibiotics and mandatory follow-up and these rules have a negative predictive value of 99.7%. A CXR is not a component of the standard work-up.

(Reference: Section 8: The Acutely Ill Infant and Child; Part 1: Assessment of the Acutely Ill Infant and Child, Chapter 105, p 397–398)

Answer 8-13. e

The minimum diagnostic testing for evaluating fever in young infants consists of a complete blood count with differential, blood culture, urinalysis with microscopy, urine culture, and usually spinal fluid analysis and culture. A lumbar puncture is indicated in febrile infants less than 1 month of age and in any ill-appearing older infants. The necessity of a lumbar puncture in well-appearing febrile infants who are 1–2 months of age is controversial. Some studies suggest that lumbar puncture can be delayed or omitted provided that the infant meets all low-risk clinical and laboratory criteria and that the parents are reliable observers and have appropriate follow-up skills. However, recent data has shown that infants who had bacterial meningitis often had total WBC counts in the normal range and that screening tools to predict infants at low risk for meningitis failed most consistently in infants younger than 2 months old.

Acute phase reactants such as C-reactive protein (CRP) and procalcitonin (PCT), produced by the liver in response to cytokines like tumor necrosis factor alpha and interleukin-6, are often used as predictors of bacterial infection. Their values increase and peak within hours after the onset of fever. While valuable as a screening tool, none of these acute phase reactants is reliable as a sole predictor of bacterial infection.

Young infants can test positive for two infecting agents at the same time so identification of a viral agent does not rule out the possibility of bacterial infection. Studies of febrile infants and preschool-age children have consistently demonstrated that 6–7% will test positive for the simultaneous presence of viral and bacterial pathogens. In infants who have documented viral disease, the most common location for simultaneous bacterial infection is the urinary tract. A urine bag sample is not the gold standard for diagnosis. Importantly, bacteremia occurs in approximately 1% of infants who test positive for the presence of common viral infections.

(Reference: Section 8: The Acutely Ill Infant and Child; Part 1: Assessment of the Acutely Ill Infant and Child, Chapter 105, p 397–398)

Answer 8-14. b

The rates of bacterial infection in toddlers are lower than those of younger infants but higher than those in school-age children, and the urinary tract is the most likely locus of infection when it is bacterial. Given that the child in the vignette does not have a focal source of fever and has some signs of ill appearance, blood and urine studies are indicated. It is important to note that in this era of pneumococcal vaccination, the practice of routine blood cultures in well-appearing febrile children to evaluate for occult bacteremia is unlikely to continue as a recommended practice.

Contrary to a belief among many parents, responsiveness of a fever to antipyretics is not correlated with incidence of bacterial disease. Although viral sources of fever are the most common, given the ill appearance of the child, reassurance alone is not sufficient. Clinical exam, as in the case with younger infants, is not reliable for identifying all instances of bacterial infection and while clinical prediction tools are good, they are not perfect. The white blood cell count has been used to predict the probability of bacterial infection, but the sensitivity of that test alone is only 21%. In any toxic-appearing toddler or infant, a thorough work-up for bacterial infection, including lumbar puncture, should be performed and parenteral antibiotics should be started; the patient should be admitted.

(Reference: Section 8: The Acutely Ill Infant and Child; Part 1: Assessment of the Acutely Ill Infant and Child, Chapter 105, p 398–399)

Answer 8-15. e

Arterial pulse oximetry is a noninvasive, nonpainful method of estimating hemoglobin oxygen saturation and is more common than directly measuring arterial blood PO_2. Some disadvantages of pulse oximetry are that it can be less reliable when there is movement or poor perfusion in the extremity, interference from external light, and an inaccurate portrayal of oxygen content in carbon monoxide poisoning or methemoglobinemia.

(Reference: Section 8: The Acutely Ill Infant and Child; Part 2: Stabilization and Management of the Acutely Ill Infant and Child, Chapter 106, p 402–403)

Answer 8-16. c

Electrocardiographic electrodes placed on the chest can monitor the ECG continuously, and a cardiotachometer determines the heart rate from the frequency of the "QRS" signal. Although an invaluable tool for monitoring and for observing responses to therapy, there are important sources of error. When the signal is large, the T wave and QRS may both be detected, and the cardiotachometer may show a value that is twice normal. Failure to detect a signal can occur when the QRS amplitude changes—for example, with respiration, repositioning of the leads, or changes in posture. Finally, it is essential to recognize that the ECG recording used in patient monitoring is filtered to help reduce the amount of artifact and does not provide a complete view of cardiac forces. It is quite easy to misinterpret rhythm disturbances or even fail to detect them by observing the monitor or by reading a single "rhythm strip."

Whenever an arrhythmia is suspected or the rate of the peripheral pulse does not concur with the monitor, a complete ECG should immediately be obtained unless instability of the patient's clinical status must be addressed first. In this case, the patient's heart rate may possibly be due to supraVT, but it also may be a false reading. If the diagnosis is SVT and the patient is stable, vagal maneuvers may be attempted. Obtaining intravenous access is recommended, but attention to airway, breathing, circulation, and stabilization should be prioritized first.

(Reference: Section 8: The Acutely Ill Infant and Child; Part 2: Stabilization and Management of the Acutely Ill Infant and Child, Chapter 106, p 403)

Answer 8-17. b

Arterial blood pressure can be measured by a sphygmomanometer—a blood pressure cuff should be 2/3 the length of the segment of the limb it is encircling. After inflating the cuff beyond the pressure that occludes the arterial pulse, Korotkoff sounds can be auscultated as the cuff is deflated. Alternatively the arterial pulse can be palpated or detected using a pulse oximeter or Doppler ultrasound. There is a range of normal values that differs in children versus adults. It is normal for upper extremity systolic blood pressure (brachial and radial arteries) to be lower than the legs, and diastolic blood pressures to be higher. An indwelling arterial catheter, not a central venous catheter, can measure continuous arterial blood pressure invasively. Shock is the impaired perfusion of end organ tissues and is a clinical state that does not rely solely on the measurement of the blood pressure. Importantly, blood pressure can be near normal until very late stages of shock.

(Reference: Section 8: The Acutely Ill Infant and Child; Part 2: Stabilization and Management of the Acutely Ill Infant and Child, Chapter 106, p 403–404)

Answer 8-18. d

The child described in the vignette is in compensated shock from hypovolemia due to vomiting, diarrhea, and likely poor oral intake. Airway, breathing, and circulation are the management priorities in any emergency situation. This patient's airway and respiratory status are, for the time being, stable. Supplemental oxygen is being administered. Timely vascular access and initiation of fluids is the priority. Endotracheal intubation is not necessary at this time given minimal evidence of respiratory distress. Although obtaining blood cultures, getting a detailed history, and potentially getting a surgical consultation may be necessary in the management of this patient, they are not the next priority in a patient who is in need of resuscitation with intravascular fluids.

(Reference: Section 8: The Acutely Ill Infant and Child; Part 2: Stabilization and Management of the Acutely Ill Infant and Child, Chapter 107, p 404)

Answer 8-19. a

IO infusions can be preformed rapidly and reliably (see Figure 107-1 below).

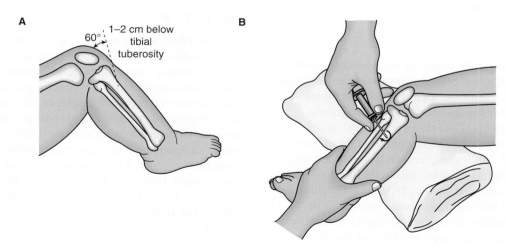

FIGURE 107-1. (A) Preferred site for intraosseous cannulation in infants. (B) Technique for insertion of the trocar. Note that the trocar is advanced with a twisting movement and in a caudal direction to avoid injuring the tibial growth plate. (Reproduced, with permission, from Rudolph CD, Rudolph AM, Lister GE, First LR, Gershon AA. *Rudolph's Pediatrics.* 22nd ed. New York: McGraw-Hill, 2011.)

When manually inserting an IO needle, the ability of the needle to remain upright without support is 1 sign of successful IO cannulation. Fluid will expand the subcutaneous space when the IO catheter is not in the correct space causing extravasation into the tissue. Feeling resistance is common while inserting an IO needle, but once the needle enters the marrow it will "give" because of lack of resistance of the marrow; this "give" indicates successful placement of an IO. The amount of needle visible above the skin is not a reliable method to measure IO cannulation. Aspirating bone marrow is a sign of successful IO needle placement; however, the IO catheter may be in place even if the marrow is not aspirated.

(Reference: Section 8: The Acutely Ill Infant and Child; Part 2: Stabilization and Management of the Acutely Ill Infant and Child, Chapter 107, p 405–406)

Answer 8-20. d

One advantage of a central venous catheter is that you may be able to use it for hemodynamic monitoring such as measuring central venous pressure, cardiac output, mixed venous saturation, and pulmonary artery pressures. Vasoactive medications are more safely administered through central venous catheterization because the increased flow of blood in the larger vessels dilutes and protects the endothelial vasculature. The length of the catheter does not affect the tolerance to medications. Central venous catheters should be inserted using sterile technique. Sterile techniques in addition to the use of systematic checklists have reduced the incidence of catheter-related infections. Air embolism is a life-threatening risk during insertion of a central venous catheter as well as when it is removed, but not a complication of peripheral IV's. Compared to peripheral IVs, central venous catheter insertion takes more skill and time.

(Reference: Section 8: The Acutely Ill Infant and Child; Part 2: Stabilization and Management of the Acutely Ill Infant and Child, Chapter 107, p 406–408)

Answer 8-21. a

An important yet frequently neglected issue for any invasive procedure on a child is that of pain management and sedation. In the nonemergency situation, topical or local anesthetics should be used as they can minimize pain. Management of anxiety is also important and the psychological milieu during the procedure should also be optimized. Music, toys, and interaction with family members can be important tools for improving comfort, thereby increasing the likelihood of cooperation and technical success. Separating the child from the family and holding them down would likely be traumatizing. Minimizing discomfort during the procedure generally encourages better cooperation during the next potentially painful procedure for that child. Child life services should be employed when available. For this type of minor procedure, sedation by an anesthesiologist is unnecessary

with the potential risks of sedation outweighing the benefit of comfort. If the blood draw is clinically necessary it should not be postponed.

(Reference: Section 8: The Acutely Ill Infant and Child; Part 2: Stabilization and Management of the Acutely Ill Infant and Child, Chapter 107, p 408)

Answer 8-22. c

Initial pediatric advanced life support guidelines were introduced in 1986 and since then research and registry data have provided information about epidemiology, presentation, and outcome of pediatric cardiopulmonary arrest. In a 1987 study of prehospital arrest, paramedics found the pediatric victim's rhythms on arrival were predominantly asystole (80%) and PEA (10%) rather than VF or VT (9%) and this distribution is most characteristic of pediatric cardiac arrest.

Asphyxic arrest is the most common type of arrest in infants and children, which ultimately leads to bradycardia and pulseless electrical activity. Sudden cardiac arrest results from an arrhythmia; ventricular tachycardia (VT) and ventricular fibrillation (VF) are the most common rhythms associated with sudden cardiac arrest. Sudden cardiac arrest is more common in adults. Respiratory arrest occurs with apnea in the presence of spontaneous circulation; treatment of respiratory arrest can prevent progression to cardiopulmonary arrest. Between the ages of 0 and 6 months, sudden infant death syndrome (SIDS) is the leading cause of cardiopulmonary arrest (CPA) and death, while trauma is the leading cause of CPA and death in children older than 6 months. The 2005 American Heart Association guidelines recommend using pediatric basic life support guidelines for children up to the age of 12 and emphasize priorities based on the circumstances of the arrest.

(Reference: Section 8: The Acutely Ill Infant and Child; Part 2: Stabilization and Management of the Acutely Ill Infant and Child, Chapter 108, p 408–409.)

Answer 8-23. b

PEA describes cardiac electrical activity that fails to provide sufficient function to generate a central pulse. It is a term usually reserved for those patients with narrow QRS complexes that do not produce a palpable pulse. There are several reversible causes of PEA in children, which if promptly treated can prevent progression to asystole. These are: tension pneumothorax, hypovolemia, cardiac tamponade, and occasionally, pulmonary embolus. Commotio cordis is a blow to the chest that results in sudden cardiac arrest from a ventricular arrhythmia that can then progress to VT and fibrillation. It is occasionally seen in athletes and requires a shock in order to revert to a normal rhythm.

(Reference: Section 8: The Acutely Ill Infant and Child; Part 2: Stabilization and Management of the Acutely Ill Infant and Child, Chapter 108, p 409–410)

Answer 8-24. e

Children who present with VT or VF in the prehospital or in-hospital settings typically have higher survival rates than those presenting with PEA or asystole. CPR was correctly initiated in this patient and should be continued until return of a normal sinus rhythm, return of palpable pulses, or termination of the code. Untreated pulseless VT will rapidly progress to VF, and untreated VF will deteriorate to asystole. Given this patient had no pulse, this patient is not considered stable. Defibrillation should be performed without delay. Medical conversion for VT should be tried only when a patient with VT has a pulse, and is stable (has unlabored spontaneous respirations, normal mental status, normal blood pressure). When VF or pulseless VT develops suddenly, the alveolar oxygen tension and arterial oxygen content should initially be normal. During the first minutes of sudden VT or VF arrest, oxygen delivery to the heart, brain, and other organs is limited more by blood flow than by oxygen content.

(Reference: Section 8: The Acutely Ill Infant and Child; Part 2: Stabilization and Management of the Acutely Ill Infant and Child, Chapter 108, p 410)

Answer 8-25. d

The AHA CPR guidelines emphasize effective chest compressions for all victims and the PALS guidelines recommend that advanced life support interventions be performed at 2-minute intervals of uninterrupted CPR. The AHA recommends a 30:2 compression-to-ventilation ratio for single rescuers and a 15:2 ratio for 2 or more rescuers, based on expert consensus and the prevalence of asphyxial arrest in children. These ratios were established to optimize myocardial and systemic blood flow by minimizing interruptions in chest compressions while maintaining adequate arterial oxygen content. If treated early before it progresses to arrest, bradycardia has a high survival rate with chest compressions. Compressions should be initiated for a HR of <60 BPM with poor perfusion despite adequate oxygenation and ventilation. If a shock is indicated it should be delivered within 10 seconds or less of the last chest compression and an AED is recommended for children aged 1–8 years suffering from cardiac arrest. Pediatric pads are ideal, although the adult pads may be used if necessary. The current recommendation is an initial 2 J/kg shock, although this dose may be inadequate in arrests of longer duration and larger doses can be used.

Although no drug increases survival from pediatric cardiac arrest, vasoconstrictors do increase blood pressure and therefore coronary and cerebral blood flow and return to spontaneous circulation in animal models. The AHA recommends a standard dose of IV epinephrine every 3–5 minutes for cardiac arrest. High-dose epinephrine is no longer recommended for routine resuscitation as it was found to be associated with decreased survival and neurological outcomes in an RCT. Intravenous and intraosseus routes of drug administration are preferred to endotracheal routes, as drug absorption by the ETT is poor and unpredictable and optimal drug doses are not known.

(Reference: Section 8: The Acutely Ill Infant and Child; Part 2: Stabilization and Management of the Acutely Ill Infant and Child, Chapter 108, p 411–412)

Answer 8-26. e

Mechanical ventilation is the most widely used and versatile technique that allows thousands of patients to recover from respiratory failure every year; ECMO is becoming more popular and widespread in its adoption and efficacy as its protocols are refined and disseminated. This patient is suffering from respiratory failure and CO_2 retention. Positive pressure ventilation is the best next step in treating his tiring respiratory status. Although excessive oxygen can be toxic to the lungs, this patient should receive supplemental oxygen for hypoxemia.

The critical care unit is where this patient should be admitted, however, the clinical indication is for the impending respiratory failure that will likely require positive pressure ventilation via endotracheal intubation. This patient may have a degree of cardiac compromise, but they do not meet criteria for cardiac transplantation or a ventricular assistance device. Ventricular assistance devices are utilized in uni- or biventricular heart failure with patients with no intrinsic abnormalities in lung function. In recent years, increasingly smaller ventricular assistance devices have been developed. These devices can be used to support the function of one or both ventricles and have considerably improved the autonomy and quality of life of many pediatric heart transplantation candidates. Ventricular assistance devices have no role in treating respiratory failure.

(Reference: Section 8: The Acutely Ill Infant and Child; Part 2: Stabilization and Management of the Acutely Ill Infant and Child, Chapter 109, p 412)

Answer 8-27. b

The fastest and most reliable way to increase arterial PO_2 is to increase the inspired concentration of oxygen. Increasing the respiratory rate, tidal volume, or initiating positive pressure ventilation or endotracheal intubation would allow for better access of the airway and improved ventilation and therefore may also increase the arterial PO_2, but higher concentration of inspired oxygen is the most rapid and predictable way to increase PaO_2.

(Reference: Section 8: The Acutely Ill Infant and Child; Part 2: Stabilization and Management of the Acutely Ill Infant and Child, Chapter 109, p 413)

Answer 8-28. d

Mechanical ventilation for respiratory failure can be a lifesaving mode of ventilatory support in children. However, both mechanical ventilation and positive pressure ventilation can have negative effects due to the stress and strain caused by excessive pressure and volume on the lungs. Ventilation settings should be adjusted to minimize pressure and volume during mechanical ventilation. Permissive hypercapnea is 1 strategy to minimize strain on the lungs and does not lead to deleterious effects. High-frequency ventilation is an alternate method of mechanical ventilation that decreases pressure trauma to the lungs, although may only be appropriate in certain clinical scenarios. Noninvasive methods of support (CPAP, BiPAP, etc.) are useful adjuncts that should be tried in children who exhibited signs of respiratory fatigue. Just as in adults, children should be sedated and given pharmacologic neuromuscular blockade during mechanical ventilation to both address their pain and to minimize complications associated with spontaneous movements, such as endotracheal tube dislodgement.

(Reference: Section 8: The Acutely Ill Infant and Child; Part 2: Stabilization and Management of the Acutely Ill Infant and Child, Chapter 109, p 413–416)

Answer 8-29. b

Tidal volume can be controlled during mechanical ventilation either by setting the volume or setting the pressure generated during the airway opening. In a volume-controlled setting, the tidal volume generated by the ventilator is always greater than the tidal volume delivered to the lungs. This is due to airway leaks around the endotracheal tube; and therefore this leak must be considered in calculating tidal volumes. PEEP acts to increase functional residual capacity, and does so by exerting pressure at the end of expiration preventing the alveoli from collapsing and helping to recruit collapsed alveoli. SIMV and pressure support ventilation are common modes of ventilation used when weaning a patient off the ventilator. In SIMV, ventilator breaths are delivered at a preestablished rate, but with a variable interval—allowing the patient an opportunity to initiate some breaths independently. In the pressure support mode, the ventilator complements the early phase of the patient's own inspiratory effort with a set inspiratory pressure. In assist-control ventilation, all breaths (whether initiated by the ventilator or the patient) are completed by the ventilator.

(Reference: Section 8: The Acutely Ill Infant and Child; Part 2: Stabilization and Management of the Acutely Ill Infant and Child, Chapter 109, p 413–415)

Answer 8-30. e

Specialized care is expensive and there are a limited number of personnel qualified to provide specialized care, which are concentrated at referral centers. Not all transports are of critically ill children; however, it is still preferred to entrust transport to a professional team than impose upon families to assume the risk. Level of care required, cost, distance, and availability of an appropriate transport team help guide the decision. The decision of where to send a patient should be based on perceived acuity and not extraneous considerations such as insurance. In addition, personal reasons for transport

must be carefully balanced against risk to the child and team of the transport. Telemedicine is increasingly being used in the consultation of physicians specializing in the care of critically ill children but has not yet become the standard of care. Explicit understanding by both referring and receiving parties of the patient's status, plan of care, and individual responsibilities is necessary. Patient's status may change and frequent communication is necessary by the referral facility and transport team so that the receiving facility may be prepared.

(Reference: Section 8: The Acutely Ill Infant and Child; Part 2: Stabilization and Management of the Acutely Ill Infant and Child, Chapter 110, p 417–418)

Answer 8-31. a

This scenario portrays an ideal situation in which the severity of the child is recognized early, communication with a referral center and activation of a transport team is almost immediate, and an initial diagnostic evaluation is made. In this case, the next step in preparation for transport is stabilization of the child from a respiratory, circulatory, and neurologic standpoint. Patients may be categorized as stable, stable/critical or unstable (see Table 110-1). Stable patients are those who require transport, but do not require initial resuscitation. Patients who are critical but stable are those who have required initial resuscitation but have little risk of deterioration during transport.

In this case, the patient is an unstable child who meets multiple criteria for intubation. Indications for intubation prior to transport include progressive respiratory distress, apnea, unstable circulatory system, altered mental status, and/or a progressive neuromyopathy. Venous access should be established, through IV or IO placement; a central line is not necessary as this may be time-consuming and delay transport. The referral center must attempt to anticipate and prepare the transport team to respond to deterioration en route, however, stabilization of the patient should be the next step in management. While the receiving facility often arranges for transportation, it is the choice and responsibility of the referring center to determine the type of the transport team. Reasons to transport this unstable child by ground may include distance <60 mi, unfavorable weather conditions, or increased space needs. Alternatives for transport include helicopter or fixed wing transport, but these pose other risks to the patient and transporting team that must be balanced against the stability of the patient. The parents or guardians should be informed; however, consent for transport should not take priority over stabilization.

(Reference: Section 8: The Acutely Ill Infant and Child; Part 2: Stabilization and Management of the Acutely Ill Infant and Child, Chapter 110, p 418–419)

Answer 8-32. c

Cerebral edema can be either vasogenic, cytotoxic, or interstitial, and usually results from a combination of these mechanisms. Vasogenic edema is caused by increased capillary leak after injury. Cytotoxic edema is caused by alterations in membrane function of neurons, glia, and endothelial cells after injury. Interstitial edema is caused by an alteration or disruption in the flow of transependymal fluid in the ventricular system, when CSF absorption is blocked or production is increased.

Cerebral edema, along with hemorrhage, acute hydrocephalus, and rapidly growing tumors, causes in intracranial hypertension. The most immediate and dangerous result of ICP is a reduction in cerebral blood flow, and ultimately, cerebral ischemia. Blood flow in the brain is autoregulated and is designed to maintain blood flow over a wide range of perfusion pressures, but intracranial hypertension can reduce cerebral perfusion pressure below the autoregulation range of the cerebral blood vessels. Cerebrospinal fluid production is also dynamic, with a fairly constant rate of formation despite increase in ICP, but the rate of absorption of CSF increases as the pressure increases in a linear fashion. A specialized system regulates water and solutes in and out of the brain, and specialized endothelial cells without fenestrations that have an extensive network of tight-junctions form the blood–brain barrier. This barrier is designed to selectively transfer nutrients and metabolic products while keeping out potentially toxic circulating molecules and preventing excessive accumulation of water. The capillary basement membrane is made of pericytes and aquaporin-4-expressing astrocytic foot processes to form a sheath around each blood vessel in order to accomplish this barrier.

(Reference: Section 8: The Acutely Ill Infant and Child; Part 2: Stabilization and Management of the Acutely Ill Infant and Child, Chapter 111, p 420–421)

Answer 8-33. d

Treatment of intracranial hypertension (ICH) is aimed at preventing further brain injury from focal or global ischemia. There are limited therapies and even less data to support improved outcomes in children. In 2003, a consensus statement was published regarding the management of pediatric traumatic brain injury. Hyperosmolar therapy with either mannitol or hypertonic saline has been used in treatment of ICH for decades, and both have some evidence of being effective. Hyperventilation has also been used for years in the treatment of ICH and is now thought to be most effective in cases of life-threatening neurological deterioration, such as herniation or in refractory ICH. Barbiturates can be effective in lowering intracranial pressure in patients with ICH, probably by lowering cerebral oxygen consumption. Hypothermia lowers cerebral metabolism thereby reducing the cerebral oxygen demand and has been shown to be effective in neonates with hypoxic-ischemic injury and in adults after cardiac arrest. Corticosteroids have been used to treat ICH because of their anti-inflammatory properties but multiple adult studies have not documented any beneficial effect on the

outcome. A large, randomized, controlled trial on steroid use after significant head injury (CRASH trial) was stopped early because of increased mortality in the steroid-treatment group. Finally, an emerging treatment of TBI in adults and children is decompressive craniectomy, but there are still insufficient data to establish guidelines for using this technique.

(Reference: Section 8: The Acutely Ill Infant and Child; Part 2: Stabilization and Management of the Acutely Ill Infant and Child, Chapter 111, p 421–422)

Answer 8-34. e

The ASA classification is determined by 2 factors: the general health of the patient and the complexity of the surgery. See Table 112-3 for details about the various ASA physical status classifications. Premature infants born at less than 37 weeks who are less than 56 post-conceptual age at the time of surgery are at the greatest risk of postanesthesia complications. Full-term infants are at highest risk when they are less than 44 weeks postconceptual age, which is true for the infant in this clinical scenario. Postanesthesia complications include: apnea, periodic breathing, and bradycardia. Infants at higher risk should be admitted post-surgery for monitoring. In children, a routine preoperative complete blood count should be obtained for surgeries with the potential for large blood loss, or higher-risk patients (premature infants or those with chronic disease). In routine, minor, elective surgeries a preoperative blood count is not required. Fasting guidelines for procedures are listed in Table 112-2; for elective procedures the ASA recommends no solid food or nonhuman milk for 6 hours prior to the procedure. Clear liquids are allowed up to 2 hours prior to the procedure. All medications that the patient is taking must be considered when selecting anesthetic agents, given the potential for interactions.

(Reference: Section 8: The Acutely Ill Infant and Child; Part 2: Stabilization and Management of the Acutely Ill Infant and Child, Chapter 112, p 422–425)

Answer 8-35. b

Because of low predictive value and cost-effectiveness, many centers no longer perform routine laboratory screening tests in otherwise healthy children scheduled for minor elective surgery. However, important baseline values (eg, hemoglobin level determination) in anticipation of major blood loss are still performed. At present, there are no universal guidelines concerning preoperative laboratory testing; many anesthesiologists follow institutional protocols or their own personal preferences. Mild anemia (Hb ≥ 9.5 g/dL) has been reported in up to 2% of pediatric patients undergoing elective surgery. No studies to date have shown justification to modify the perioperative management in otherwise healthy children who have a borderline low hemoglobin concentration, and therefore routine hemoglobin determinations are usually not necessary. However, it is reasonable to obtain preoperative hemoglobin values in (1) former preterm infants due to the risk of postoperative apnea, (2) patients with chronic illness, (3) children with sickle cell disease (including sickle cell anemia, sickle Hb C disease, and the sickle thalassemias), and (4) those instances where having a baseline hemoglobin value may be useful (along with blood typing and cross-matching) in anticipation of significant surgical loss.

(Reference: Section 8: The Acutely Ill Infant and Child; Part 2: Stabilization and Management of the Acutely Ill Infant and Child, Chapter 112, p 423–425)

Answer 8-36. a

Anesthesiologists and surgeons often face decisions regarding children who are experiencing respiratory symptoms at the time of a scheduled surgery. Upper respiratory infections (URI) are very common in children, averaging 5–10 episodes per year. Some studies indicate significant risk for laryngospasm, bronchospasm, arterial O_2 desaturation, and postextubation stridor in children who are suffering from a URI, whereas other studies did not show major increased risk. There is still controversy among pediatric anesthesiologists on whether to proceed with surgery in the presence of a current or recent URI. The decision often depends on the experience of the anesthesiologist and the type and urgency of the surgery. Most anesthesiologists postpone elective surgery if the patient exhibits 1 or more of the following: fever, ill appearance, purulent rhinorrhea, tachypnea, or involvement of the lower respiratory tract. If this child had wheezing, this would indicate lower respiratory tract involvement and most anesthesiologists would postpone the case.

Infants born prior to 37 weeks gestational age who are less than 56 weeks postconceptional age at the time of surgery are at greater risk of anesthetic complications than full-term infants. This child is now 6 years old, so the fact that he was a premature infant is no longer relevant for apnea risk. Clear liquids are allowed in children up to 2–4 hours prior to surgery.

(Reference: Section 8: The Acutely Ill Infant and Child; Part 2: Stabilization and Management of the Acutely Ill Infant and Child, Chapter 112, p 425)

Answer 8-37. d

The main goal of postoperative care is to ensure smooth recovery from anesthesia and surgery to the patient's baseline state. The initial recovery period is critical; up to 13% of all reported adverse events occur at this time. Staff should maintain constant surveillance of airway patency, ventilation, and circulatory function. A patient is usually deemed stable enough for discharge when consciousness is fully recovered, postoperative nausea and vomiting are controlled, and pain is relieved. There are several scoring systems for determining discharge readiness in the post-anesthesia care unit (PACU), including the Aldrete recovery score (see Tables 112.2 and 112.3). Established scoring systems take into account activity, respirations, circulation, consciousness, color, and movement in determining readiness for discharge. This patient should not be

discharged while sleeping unless she has demonstrated readiness in all areas. She is unlikely to have postoperative apnea given her healthy status and does not need to be admitted for that reason.

(Reference: Section 8: The Acutely Ill Infant and Child; Part 2: Stabilization and Management of the Acutely Ill Infant and Child, Chapter 112, p 426)

Answer 8-38. a

The first reports of undertreatment of pain in children were published approximately 30 years ago; despite numerous subsequent studies, inadequate treatment of pain in children remains a problem. While it was initially believed that neonates had the reduced ability to experience pain, animal studies suggest that they may actually be more sensitive to noxious stimuli than older children. Effective pain management requires accurate initial assessment and ongoing reassessment. Older children may be able to self-report pain using the Faces Pain Scale, Oucher or Visual Analogue Scales. Children under 3 years of age require assessment with observational scales, such as the FLACC and CHEOPS scales, both of which have well-established reliability for use in acute pain (see Table 113-1).

Pain is not a necessary experience for normal child development. Due to the plastic nature of young children's central nervous systems, repeated painful stimulus may lead to abnormal reorganization and sensitization. Pain recognition is a complex process involving local tissue damage leading to release of inflammatory mediators that lead to peripheral sensitization of nociceptors, transduction, transmission, modulation, and recognition. Overall pain experience is affected by maturity, attitude, emotion, environment, and culture. Left untreated, pain can lead to social withdrawal, anxiety, developmental delay, growth failure, immunosuppression, and increased morbidity.

(Reference: Section 8: The Acutely Ill Infant and Child; Part 2: Stabilization and Management of the Acutely Ill Infant and Child, Chapter 113, p 426–428)

Answer 8-39. d

Oxycodone can be administered to patients for moderate pain, such as the child described in this clinical scenario. Acetaminophen has central and peripheral effects and may potentiate opioids when used in combination.

Nonpharmacological interventions such as rocking, stroking, patting, and cuddling may be quite effective but should not replace pain medications. Ibuprofen may be administered but will likely not adequately control the patient's pain. Codeine is a weak analgesic and is not recommended as between 4% and 12% of patients lack the enzyme required to convert it to its active form, morphine. Local anesthetics, such as lidocaine, block sodium channels preventing depolarization and propagation of the nerve signal. Topical lidocaine should not be used over large areas or in areas of severely burned or abraded skin, as there may be increased systemic absorption.

Signs of lidocaine toxicity may include CNS depression, seizure, and cardiac arrhythmia.

(Reference: Section 8: The Acutely Ill Infant and Child; Part 2: Stabilization and Management of the Acutely Ill Infant and Child, Chapter 113, p 428–431)

Answer 8-40. b

Procedural sedation is indicated in this scenario if you feel you will not be able to safely perform the repair without sedation, have determined the patient is an appropriate candidate through your presedation assessment, and have obtained informed consent. A presedation assessment should include adherence to NPO guidelines for nonemergent procedures such as laceration repair, review of the patient's past medical history to ensure that any chronic conditions are well controlled, and a focused evaluation of the airway. The risk of apnea, aspiration, hypotension, and paradoxical excitement should all be discussed when obtaining informed consent for procedural sedation. To provide sedation you must not only be certified to do so and have a protocol in place to access emergency service, but be capable of rescuing the patient from sedation 1 level deeper than the anticipated level and have the drugs and equipment necessary to do so. Sedation should not be confused with analgesia; thus, large doses of analgesic medication (such as opiates), which have the side effect of causing drowsiness, should not be used as a substitute for sedation or anxiolysis.

(Reference: Section 8: The Acutely Ill Infant and Child; Part 2: Stabilization and Management of the Acutely Ill Infant and Child, Chapter 113, p 431–432)

Answer 8-41. d

Signs and symptoms of an inborn error of metabolism can be nonspecific and vague. In particular, clues to suspecting an inborn error of metabolism can include: children who have a clinical status worse than expected given the history of present illness; children who do not respond to conventional therapies like most children with a similar presentation; unexpected metabolic abnormalities on laboratory investigation (eg, hyperammonemia, metabolic acidosis, hypoglycemia); multiple episodes of similar presentations in the past, family history of unexplained death, evidence of chronic disease (eg, failure to thrive, liver or renal failure, hearing loss, developmental delay); or symptoms that present after an inciting event including change in diet or prolonged fast.

(Reference: Section 8: The Acutely Ill Infant and Child; Part 2: Stabilization and Management of the Acutely Ill Infant and Child, Chapter 114, p 432–433)

Answer 8-42. a

A lethargic patient who presents with hypoglycemia should be given intravenous dextrose as soon as possible. Confirmatory lab testing is useful in the diagnosis and management, but should not delay treatment. Although intravenous access can be difficult to obtain and places stress on the patient, it is vital to the patient's survival to gain access for fluids and medication as prolonged hypoglycemia can result in the loss of neurons. The patient should be given a dextrose bolus dose of 0.5–1 g/kg, followed by frequent serum glucose monitoring and a follow-up infusion of continuous dextrose if indicated. If intravenous access cannot be obtained, IO access is a viable alternative. Given the child's lethargy and minimal responsiveness, oral feeds are contraindicated. Airway and gag reflexes may be impaired, gut perfusion may be compromised, and the stomach should be kept as empty as possible in anticipation for emergency procedures such as endotracheal intubation.

Testing for urine (or serum) ketones would be useful in the diagnosis of this patient to assess specifically for disorders of fatty acid oxidation. In this inborn error of metabolism, the inability to utilize fatty acids leads to the notable absence of ketone production. In normal individuals, significant hypoglycemia leads to breakdown of fatty acids as a fuel source and increased ketone production.

(Reference: Section 8: The Acutely Ill Infant and Child; Part 2: Stabilization and Management of the Acutely Ill Infant and Child, Chapter 114, p 432)

Answer 8-43. c

Inborn errors of metabolism comprise a group of varying diseases that have different laboratory profiles (see Table 114-3). Although history and physical exam can be useful in screening for inborn errors of metabolism, it is through laboratory testing that a definitive diagnosis can be made. Newborn screens may be useful in identifying some inborn errors of metabolism; however, they do not screen for all the different types of diseases. Radiologic studies have limited utility in diagnosing inborn errors of metabolism. It is of utmost importance to suspect inborn errors and diagnose them in a rapid fashion as supportive care, removal of offending agents, and potential detoxification is crucial early in the management. Unfortunately, many children with inborn errors of metabolism do not survive their first episode of metabolic decompensation.

(Reference: Section 8: The Acutely Ill Infant and Child; Part 2: Stabilization and Management of the Acutely Ill Infant and Child, Chapter 114, p 432–434)

Answer 8-44. a

This patient has signs and symptoms consistent with the diagnosis of late-onset urea cycle disorders. Patients with urea cycle defects can exhibit symptoms during episodes of metabolic stress (eg, illness, fasting) or during periods of inappropriately high protein intake. In urea cycle disorders, the inability to metabolize protein leads to a buildup of toxic ammonia. Without removal of the ammonia, neurologic sequelae can develop. Headache and vomiting are mild symptoms, but more serious neurologic problems including ataxia, seizures, cerebral edema, and coma are possible. Various urea cycle defects can be inherited through an X-linked recessive or autosomal recessive fashion, but a normal family history does not rule out urea cycle disorders. This patient has likely had headaches because of his mild urea cycle defect, and in this case presented with worsening symptoms after eating a high-protein load. Ataxia in a child should be taken seriously and worked up for a variety of potential concerning diseases.

(Reference: Section 8: The Acutely Ill Infant and Child; Part 2: Stabilization and Management of the Acutely Ill Infant and Child, Chapter 114, p 434)

Answer 8-45. c

The initial recognition of infection is mediated by multiple cell types that reside in the tissues before the onset of infection, most importantly, tissue-resident macrophages and mast cells. These cells are the primary gatekeepers of the innate immunity system. Macrophages and mast cells recognize inducers of inflammation, which can be exogenous or endogenous. The infection described in this vignette releases exogenous inducers. Once the tissue macrophages and mast cells have recognized the source of the infection, they engulf the microorganism and produce a variety of inflammatory mediators that lead to recruitment of inflammatory cells to the site of infection. The local release of these proinflammatory mediators can cause changes in endothelial cells of nearby blood vessels, selectively increasing the extravasation of neutrophils and plasma proteins, converting infected tissues from a normal to an inflamed state.

Exogenous microbial inducers include pathogen-associated molecular patterns (PAMPs) and virulence factors. Non-infectious inflammatory triggers, such as necrosis, release endogenous adjuvants called damage-associated molecular patterns (DAMPs) that trigger an inflammatory response, similar to the PAMPs seen with infectious inflammation. PAMPs have conserved molecular patterns carried by all microorganisms, both pathogenic and commensal microbes can potentially induce inflammation. The body actively suppresses the activation of TLRs by the commensal bacteria that resides in the gut. However, as described in the vignette, the TLRs would not be suppressed in the setting on an active infection with a pathogenic microbe.

(Reference: Section 8: The Acutely Ill Infant and Child; Part 3: Injuries and Untoward Events, Chapter 115, p 436–437)

Answer 8-46. c

The patient has deterioration in her mental status in conjunction with a drop in blood pressure and increase in heart rate suggestive of poor cerebral perfusion. While you would likely send a CBC and other diagnostic studies, this patient should be given normal saline or O-negative blood until additional units can be cross-matched by the blood bank. In this case, the patient is unstable with evidence of decompensated hypovolemic shock. By the time children present with decompensated shock they have lost at least 20% of their circulating blood volume. At least 2 points of IV access should be obtained, with 1 in the upper extremity if possible, rapid volume resuscitation should be started and the patient will likely need to be taken directly to the operating room for exploratory laparotomy.

In children 1 month to 18 years old, trauma accounts for 50% of all deaths, more than deaths from cancer, heart disease, and infections combined. The vast majority of injuries result from blunt trauma. Due to the elastic nature of children's skeletons, visceral injury without fractures is more commonly seen in children compared to adults. Although inadequate oxygenation and ventilation are common causes of arrest after trauma, in this scenario, the patient has no evidence of pneumothorax or hemothorax. The patient's elevated heart rate and low blood pressure are more consistent with hypovolemia rather than primary head injury. Diagnostic peritoneal lavage is rarely performed, as the presence of free blood is not an automatic indication for surgery.

(Reference: Section 8: The Acutely Ill Infant and Child; Part 3: Injuries and Untoward Events, Chapter 116, p 440–442)

Answer 8-47. c

Inadequate oxygenation and ventilation are the most common causes of arrest after trauma in children. Therefore, primary attention should be focused on assessing the child's airway and efficiency of breathing. The presence of respiratory distress or insufficient respiratory effort is usually an indication to take over the patient's airway. Bag-valve mask is an invaluable skill and may provide adequate ventilation under many difficult circumstances. It is preferred to repeated or unsuccessful attempts at intubation, particularly if laryngeal or tracheal injuries are suspected.

The primary survey includes airway, breathing, and circulation, but also disability and exposure and should be performed in the first several minutes. Cervical spine injury is assumed and thus stabilization should be universally applied until injury is excluded. Needle decompression may be performed in the case of tension pneumothorax, however a large bore chest tube placement is more appropriate when hemothorax is suspected. In the setting of intraabdominal injury, 2 IVs, with at least 1 in the upper extremity is ideal. For suspected abdominal injuries, in which the IVC may be involved, fluid administered via lower extremity IV access will not reach the heart or improve perfusion to critical organs including the heart, lungs, and brain. Subclavian lines carry the risk of iatrogenic hemothorax and pneumothorax, and are time-consuming to place. If IV access is not rapidly obtained during the time it takes to complete the primary survey, an IO should be placed.

(Reference: Section 8: The Acutely Ill Infant and Child; Part 3: Injuries and Untoward Events, Chapter 116, p 440–442)

Answer 8-48. d

Burn injuries are the third most common cause of death due to trauma in children, the majority of which occur in children under 2 years of age. Immediate burn treatment involves removing any ongoing source of injury, and wrapping the burn in a clean dry cloth, cool water may be applied; however, cold water or ice baths may diminish perfusion and worsen the injury. Wound care for burns can ultimately involve debridement, topical antibiotics, nonadherent dressings, silver impregnated dressings, and potentially skin grafting.

Burn patients with signs of respiratory distress including stridor, dyspnea, and hypoxemia should be given supplemental oxygen and endotracheal intubation should be considered early in their management. Supraglottic injuries are usually thermal in nature whereas subglottic injuries are due to chemical damage. In addition, patients with more than 25–30% BSA affected are at significant risk for the development of pulmonary edema secondary to a systemic inflammatory response. Therefore, even though the patient described in this vignette does not show immediate signs of respiratory compromise, she may require ventilatory support during the course of her treatment. Further management includes, intravenous fluid resuscitation initially at 4 ml/kg/BSA burned, with a goal urine output of 1 mL/kg/hr. Patients with myoglobinuria require larger urine outputs and urine alkalinization should be considered. Criteria for hospital admission in the pediatric patient include partial thickness burns >5–10%, full-thickness burns >1%, inhalation injury, chemical injury, electrical burn, circumferential burns, and burns involving the hands, feet, face, genitalia, or major joints (see Table 116-1). This patient should be hospitalized at a burn center due to her extensive partial-thickness burns, which will require careful wound care to prevent infection and sepsis. Prevention of burns through safety education is essential.

(Reference: Section 8: The Acutely Ill Infant and Child; Part 3: Injuries and Untoward Events, Chapter 116: p 442–445)

Answer 8-49. b

Integral to burn assessment is the estimation of burned surface area using a Modified Lund–Browder chart (Figure 116-1). This replaces the "rule of nines" used in adults—where each upper extremity and the anterior and posterior surfaces of the chest, abdomen, and lower extremity each represent 9% of the total body surface area. In children, particularly children under 1 year of age, the head and neck account for much more of the total surface area. The Modified Lund–Browder chart provides the most accurate estimate based on age. Alternatively the palm of a child's hand represents a body surface area of approximately 1%.

Burn injuries may be the result of thermal, electric, chemical, or radiation mechanisms. Hot liquids, resulting in a type of thermal injury, are the most common cause of burns in children under 3. Fire is a common cause of burns in older children and adolescents. The severity of tissue damage is related to temperature, duration of exposure, area of the body burned, and the age of the patient. While it is true that children have a larger body surface area to body mass ratio as compared to adults making them more vulnerable to fluid and heat losses, it does not make them more likely to be burned. Compared to adults, children's skin is less thick so the same duration of contact with comparable heat sources may result in a deeper burn in children. Burns are classified as either partial (superficial, deep) or full thickness, replacing the previous nomenclature of first second-, third-, and fourth-degree burns. It may be very difficult to distinguish deep partial-thickness and full-thickness burns from one another. In some cases, classification is determined based on whether they heal or require grafting. Burn patient's caloric requirements may be increased by as much as 50%. When possible, nutrition

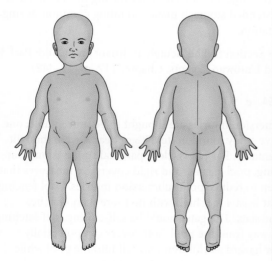

Area	Age–Years					% 2°	% 3°	% Total
	0–1	1–4	5–9	10–15	Adult			
Head	19	17	13	10	7			
Neck	2	2	2	2	2			
Ant. trunk	13	13	13	13	13			
Post. trunk	13	13	13	13	13			
R. buttock	2–1/2	2–1/2	2–1/2	2–1/2	2–1/2			
L. buttock	2–1/2	2–1/2	2–1/2	2–1/2	2–1/2			
Genitalia	1	1	1	1	1			
R. U. arm	4	4	4	4	4			
L. U. arm	4	4	4	4	4			
R. L. arm	3	3	3	3	3			
L. L. arm	3	3	3	3	3			
R. hand	2–1/2	2–1/2	2–1/2	2–1/2	2–1/2			
L. hand	2–1/2	2–1/2	2–1/2	2–1/2	2–1/2			
R. thigh	5–1/2	6–1/2	8–1/2	8–1/2	9–1/2			
L. thigh	5–1/2	6–1/2	8–1/2	8–1/2	9–1/2			
R. leg	5	5	5–1/2	6	7			
L. leg	5	5	5–1/2	6	7			
R. foot	3–1/2	3–1/2	3–1/2	3–1/2	3–1/2			
L. foot	3–1/2	3–1/2	3–1/2	3–1/2	3–1/2			
					Total BSA Burn			

Modified from Lund and Browder

• Hand method for nonuniform burns—palm of child's hand approximates 1 percent of child's total BSA burn.

FIGURE 116-1. Lund–Browder body surface area chart. (Reproduced, with permission, from Rudolph CD, Rudolph AM, Lister GE, First LR, Gershon AA. *Rudolph's Pediatrics.* 22nd ed. New York: McGraw-Hill, 2011.)

should be given enterally to avoid infections associated with intravenous nutrition.

(Reference: Section 8: The Acutely Ill Infant and Child; Part 3: Injuries and Untoward Events, Chapter 116, p 442–444)

Answer 8-50. e

Infection occurs in approximately 30% of hand wounds, with cat bites carrying the highest risk of infection. Cat bite wounds are often deep puncture wounds and common infecting organisms are *Pasteurella multocida* and *Staphylococcus aureus; Bartonella hensaelae*, which causes cat scratch fever is less common. Amoxicillin/clavulanate prophylaxis is therefore recommended in most cases of hand wounds due to bites.

Approximately 80–90% of animal bites are inflicted by dogs, with only 5–15% being inflicted by cats. In the case of dog bites, 75% of bites are inflicted by the family pet or a neighbor's dog. Wounds are typically left open due to the risk of abscess formation. Contamination, length of time since the injury, signs of infections, and location of the wound all contribute to management. Dog bites in contrast to cat bites, tend to be more crushing, and may be associated with tissue loss or even underlying fracture. Rabies is uncommon in domesticated pets within the United States and rabies postexposure prophylaxis will likely not be necessary.

(Reference: Section 8: The Acutely Ill Infant and Child; Part 3: Injuries and Untoward Events, Chapter 116, p 446)

Answer 8-51. d

Unintentional injury is the leading cause of mortality in children aged 1–19 years, and is more common in males. After motor vehicle crashes, submersion injuries are the 2nd most common cause of unintentional injury. There is a bimodal age distribution of submersion injury with 2 peaks in toddlers (1–4 years) and teens (15–19 years). Toddler submersion is most common in unsupervised pool settings. Teens are more likely to drown in natural freshwater bodies—where they may be participating in risky recreational activities and possibly under the influence of drugs or alcohol. Alcohol has been shown to be associated with 25–50% of submersion injuries in teens and adults.

(Reference: Section 8: The Acutely Ill Infant and Child; Part 3: Injuries and Untoward Events, Chapter 117, p 446–447)

Answer 8-52. b

Older children with epilepsy are counseled to take showers instead of baths to reduce the risk of submersion injury. This is also true for children with prolonged QT syndrome or other cardiac disease with the potential for loss of consciousness in a bath that might lead to submersion injury. Near drowning is one of the several terms that have fallen out of common use since the consensus conference developed unified definitions. The term *drowned* refers to one who has died from drowning. *Submersion* is defined as the entire body, including the airway,

being under water. *Immersion* is defined as any part of the body being covered in water. For drowning to occur, the face and airway need to be immersed.

Most of the time submersion leads to aspiration of water into the lungs; however, it is rare to get electrolyte abnormalities. Patients with a GCS of less than 5 have poor neurologic outcome.

(Reference: Section 8: The Acutely Ill Infant and Child; Part 3: Injuries and Untoward Events, Chapter 117, p 447)

Answer 8-53. b

Submersion initiates a complex sequence of behavioral and reflex responses and has respiratory, neurologic, and cardiovascular manifestations. Cardiac dysrhythmias, cardiac dysfunction, and hypotension are caused primarily by hypoxemic or ischemic hypoxia of the myocardium.

The neurologic manifestations of submersions are secondary to hypoxia. Decreased consciousness is very common in all patients who have suffered a severe insult and rarely resolve in the first hour following a submersion event. Coma, decreased respiratory drive, decorticate and decerebrate responses, and seizures can also be found. These effects can been seen for days or weeks. It was traditionally thought that the respiratory effects of submersion occur as seawater draws water from the intravascular spaces into the lungs by osmosis, resulting in fluid-filled alveoli and hypovolemia, and freshwater results in water absorption into the vascular space and hypervolemia and hemolysis. This hypothesis was based on physiologic reasoning; however, it was rarely found to be true in clinical cases. Most survivors do not aspirate sufficient volumes of liquid to justify these changes. However, aspiration of fluid into the lungs is common and is not prevented by laryngospasm. In addition, the term dry drowning has fallen out of favor. Victims may often swallow large amounts of water during the submersion event. A distended stomach makes vomiting common during the resuscitation.

(Reference: Section 8: The Acutely Ill Infant and Child; Part 3: Injuries and Untoward Events, Chapter 117, p 447–448)

Answer 8-54. e

Many submersion injuries are thought to be preventable; one retrospective study found up to 85% of deaths were thought to be preventable. For pools, close parental supervision, four-sided fencing, pool alarms, and rigid covers are measures that can be taken to reduce pool submersion injuries. Pool fencing should be at least 4 feet high with no more than 4 inches between the slats. The gate should be self-closing, self-latching, and open away from the pool. Soft covers can potentially be a greater hazard as children may fall into the pool while attempting to walk across them. In addition, a child can be trapped in the pool under the cover, and not be visible to bystanders.

(Reference: Section 8: The Acutely Ill Infant and Child; Part 3: Injuries and Untoward Events, Chapter 117, p 449)

Answer 8-55. b

Choking was the fourth leading cause of unintentional injury-related death in the United States in the year 2000 and the leading cause of death for children under 12 months. Although all children are at risk for choking/aspirating, most of the documented aspirations of foreign bodies involve preschoolers. The approximate distribution by ages is <1 year 10–15%; 1–2 years 40–50%; 2–3 years 15–25%; >3 years 15–20%. Boys aspirate objects twice as much as do girls and most choking episodes are actually nonfatal. Sixty percent of the nonfatal choking episodes were associated with nonfood items, with coins being involved in almost 20% of all choking-related ED visits for children aged 1–4 years.

(Reference: Section 8: The Acutely Ill Infant and Child; Part 3: Injuries and Untoward Events, Chapter 118, p 449)

Answer 8-56. d

When a FB enters the posterior pharynx the child coughs or cries secondary to the discomfort and the child will deeply inspire, causing the FB to become impacted within the airway, anywhere from the level of the oropharynx to the hypopharynx. The lodged FB will increase resistance to both inspiration and expiration and creates a valve-like effect if in the intrathoracic airway, producing gas trapping. The surface sensory receptors of the respiratory mucosa are stimulated, producing a strong reflex cough that can last for several minutes up to half an hour. If the FB does not move in the airway secondary to this initial cough, the mucosal receptors adapt to the pressure and the cough will subside until other sensory receptors are stimulated by movement of the FB or by mucus production. This latent period free of cough can last from hours to months and can be a diagnostic quandary for clinicians if patients present with a cough remote from the time of the actual FB aspiration event.

(Reference: Section 8: The Acutely Ill Infant and Child; Part 3: Injuries and Untoward Events, Chapter 118, p 449–450)

Answer 8-57. c

The diagnosis of FB aspiration is frequently delayed and as many as 15–20% of cases are diagnosed more than 1 month after the event. Many children who have a late diagnosis of FB aspiration will present without clinical symptoms or radiographic signs. This delay may be attributed to a lack of a suspicious history, minimal symptoms, incorrect diagnosis (such as asthma), or limited access to care. Many aspirated FBs are radiolucent, but radiographs, including PA and lateral chest as well as AP and lateral soft tissue neck films, are useful in the initial diagnosis. For bronchial FBs, the most common radiographic abnormality on chest radiograph is obstructive asymmetric hyperinflation, present in up to 65% of cases. A radiopaque FB is found in only 5–10% of chest radiographs. Inspiratory and expiratory and decubitus films are recommended in the workup for suspected impacted FB, but their diagnostic utility is modest and they are often difficult to obtain in the age groups that most commonly present with aspirated FBs. Ten to 25% of children diagnosed with foreign bodies have no abnormality on plain chest radiography. Other diagnostic techniques can be employed if a FB is suspected but not visualized, including fluoroscopy, spiral and 3-D computed tomography and virtual bronchoscopy. If the history or physical examination strongly suggests FB aspiration, the diagnostic standard is bronchoscopy, even if the radiographic evidence is negative or equivocal.

(Reference: Section 8: The Acutely Ill Infant and Child; Part 3: Injuries and Untoward Events, Chapter 118, p 450)

Answer 8-58. a

The management of FB aspiration depends on the presentation and age of the patient, but if the patient has complete obstruction of the airway as indicated by being unconscious and cyanotic, a rescuer should intervene prior to seeking care in a hospital for removal of the FB. An experienced rescuer can attempt a tongue-jaw lift or a jaw thrust in order to relieve the obstruction. For infants under the age of 1 year, the recommendation of the American Heart Association is to hold the infant face down along the rescuer's arm and deliver sharp back blows between the scapulae. Children over the age of 1 year should receive the Heimlich maneuver as the first method of intervention. Blind finger sweeps are now no longer recommended in infants and young children as they can cause the FB to be pushed further back in the airway and can cause further obstruction. If these methods fail to dislodge the FB and reestablish ventilation, a surgical airway such as a tracheotomy or cricothyroidotomy distal to the suspected site of obstruction should be considered.

(Reference: Section 8: The Acutely Ill Infant and Child; Part 3: Injuries and Untoward Events, Chapter 118, p 450–451)

Answer 8-59. a

In 1986, the NIH Consensus Development Conference on Infantile Apnea and Home Monitoring came up with a definition for an ALTE as "an episode that is frightening to the observer and that is characterized by some combination of apnea (central or occasionally obstructive), color change (usually cyanotic or pallid but occasionally erythematous or plethoric), marked change in muscle tone (usually limpness), choking, or gagging." Although more than 20 years have passed since this original definition of an ALTE, the epidemiology, clinical course, and prognosis of ALTEs remain limited and there is no single mechanism that has been identified to explain ALTEs. ALTEs are difficult to study and characterize because there is heterogeneity in their clinical presentation, patients often present to care after the symptoms have resolved, caretakers are unable to accurately describe the signs or symptoms due to anxiety, and there is always a possibility that the signs or symptoms could be fabricated or inflicted.

(Reference: Section 8: The Acutely Ill Infant and Child; Part 3: Injuries and Untoward Events, Chapter 119, p 451)

Answer 8-60. e

Usually infants with an ALTE are no longer experiencing respiratory or circulatory dysfunction by the time they are first seen by medical professionals. The clinician, therefore, must identify the events that actually transpired with a careful history; the accuracy of the caretaker's history might be diminished by the fact that they were frightened to the point of panic. Establishing characteristics of the event include determining if the baby was making breathing efforts or whether there was an irregular breathing pattern—this helps to determine if there was an episode of airway obstruction or if the infant was demonstrating normal periodic breathing. Establishing whether or not there were changes in the infant's color is also helpful. Reports of the baby turning blue are consistent with a genuine life-threatening event, but it is important to distinguish between perioral cyanosis and general cyanosis. Abnormal body movements, especially a loss of tone, are frequently associated with ALTEs, although sleeping infants can appear hypotonic. Establishing whether the event was associated with feeding, choking, or emesis may help to suggest gastroesophageal reflux, issues with feeding technique, swallowing discoordination, or possible airway obstruction. Symptoms that resolved within 30–60 seconds, especially if no or minimal intervention was required, should generally not be considered life-threatening. In addition to the health status of the infant, a previous history of life-threatening events or a history of life-threatening events, sudden infant death syndrome, or inborn errors of metabolism in other family members should be considered, but are not diagnostic. In the end, the clinician must make a judgment regarding whether or not the episode was an ALTE and in the absence of persistent symptoms or sequelae, it is difficult to be confident that a life-threatening event actually occurred.

(Reference: Section 8: The Acutely Ill Infant and Child; Part 3: Injuries and Untoward Events, Chapter 119, p 452)

Answer 8-61. e

In cases when an infant has truly experienced a life-threatening event, the clinician must do a careful investigation to identify a cause. Some of the most common potential causes of an ALTE relate to alterations in respiratory control or mechanical function of the respiratory system, including: infection (ie, respiratory syncytial virus); seizures; central nervous system tumors; gastroesophageal reflux; drug-induced respiratory depression; poisoning; post-anesthetic depression; upper-airway obstruction; arrhythmias; inborn errors of metabolism; child abuse. Periodic breathing, where the infant has up to a 20-second pause in breathing, is a normal finding in young infants.

(Reference: Section 8: The Acutely Ill Infant and Child; Part 3: Injuries and Untoward Events, Chapter 119, p 452–453)

Answer 8-62. b

There is considerable variation in the management of infants admitted for ALTEs across US hospitals, but a general strategy for managing these infants has been determined based on the fact that in the majority of cases, a careful history and physical examination will suggest whether an event is misinterpreted normal behavior or minor choking. In these cases, the families can be discharged home after reassurance and advice regarding childcare practices that will decrease the likelihood of recurrence. The majority of infants who present with a possible ALTE appear well within minutes and will have no subsequent problems. If, however, findings are suggestive of a truly life-threatening event, further evaluation in the hospital is warranted and will determine further management. If a specific cause for the ALTE is identified, then the treatment plan is directed to that specific entity. If a cause is not identified and the ALTE is deemed idiopathic, there are 2 management strategies depending on whether or not there are persistent symptoms or sequelae, concerns about the social situation, or if the infant was born premature. If none of these conditions are met, it is reasonable to reassure the family and provide advice related to strategies for assessing and avoiding future episodes. If any of the above conditions are met in the case of an idiopathic ALTE, it is reasonable, based on the 1986 NIH Consensus Statement on ALTEs, to recommend home cardiorespiratory monitoring for 2 months. This can be discontinued if there are no further ALTE recurrences and must continue with an ongoing search for an underlying cause should the ALTEs persist (see Figure 119-1).

(Reference: Section 8: The Acutely Ill Infant and Child; Part 3: Injuries and Untoward Events, Chapter 119, p 453–454)

Answer 8-63. b

Analgesics, including acetaminophen, are the most common pharmaceutical exposure in young children and account for 10% of calls to poison control. *N*-acetyl-*p*-benzoquinoneimine (NAPQI) is a toxic metabolite that is normally produced in the metabolism of acetaminophen. It is eliminated by conjugation to glutathione but in the case of overdose, NAPQI exceeds the detoxification mechanism. An initial serum acetaminophen level may be obtained but levels drawn at or after 4 hours are used in guiding treatment decisions. This level can be plotted on the Rumack–Matthews nomogram (see Figure 120-2)

Often treatment decisions may be made on history alone. Ingestions greater than 150 mg/kg are at risk of hepatotoxicity. This patient has ingested up to 240 mg/kg. The antidote for acetaminophen overdose is *N*-acetylcystine (NAC) which functions both as a glutathione precursor to replenish depleted glutathione stores and as a glutathione substitute that directly binds to NAPQI. NAC should be started within 8 hours of drug ingestion because its efficacy for preventing fulminant hepatic failure diminishes thereafter.

There are 4 phases typically described in the course of acetaminophen toxicity. *Phase I* occurs during the first few hours after ingestion, and is characterized by gastrointestinal symptoms of nausea, vomiting, and abdominal pain, some patients are asymptomatic. *Phase II* occurs within 24 hours and is manifested by upper-right quadrant abdominal tenderness

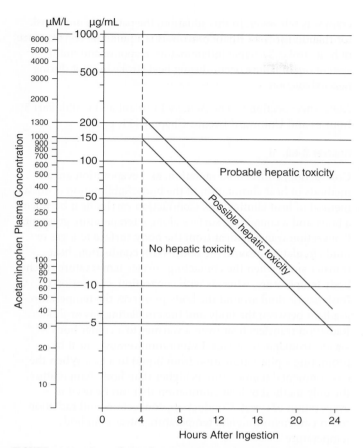

FIGURE 120-2. Rumack–Matthews nomogram showing the risk of hepato-toxicity based on the relationship between plasma acetaminophen concentration and time after ingestion. The range between the red lines represents a 25% chance of clinically significant disease. (Reproduced, with permission, from Rudolph CD, Rudolph AM, Lister GE, First LR, Gershon AA. *Rudolph's Pediatrics.* 22nd ed. New York: McGraw-Hill, 2011.)

and elevation of laboratory markers of liver injury. *Phase III* is the period of maximal hepatotoxicity, usually occurring within 72–96 hours. *Phase IV* is the period of hepatic recovery, which may occur over a week or longer.

(Reference: Section 8: The Acutely Ill Infant and Child; Part 3: Injuries and Untoward Events, Chapter 120, p 458)

Answer 8-64. a

This patient's presentation is most consistent with hypoglycemia from oral hypoglycemic overdose. Sulfonylureas bind to receptors on pancreatic β-cells, stimulating release of insulin. They also enhance peripheral insulin sensitivity and reduce gluconeogenesis. The signs and symptoms of hypoglycemia include confusion, lethargy, and seizures and are caused by neuroglycopenia. Additional signs such as anxiety, tremors, diaphoresis, tachycardia, and vomiting are caused by the accompanying catecholamine release. Hypoglycemia may be severe and prolonged. Treatment with intravenous dextrose is usually adequate; however in severe

cases octreotide is used to inhibit release of insulin from the pancreas.

Tricyclic antidepressant overdose is characterized by the combination of anticholinergic signs, coma, seizures, hypotension, and a widened QRS interval. Treatment consists of gastric decontaminant and supportive care for presenting symptoms, which may include airway protection and respiratory support, IVF, blood pressure support, and serum alkalinization. This patient has diaphoresis and does not have signs of anticholinergic toxicity. Opioid overdose typically presents with coma, respiratory depression, and miosis. While we do not know the papillary exam on this patient, there is no evidence of respiratory depression. Beta-blocker poisoning manifests with bradycardia, impaired cardiac contractility, hypotension, and profound shock. Altered mental status is usually caused by cerebral hypoperfusion, but in the case of beta-blockers may also be caused by hypoglycemia. This patient has neither hypotension nor bradycardia. The symptoms of carbon monoxide poisoning are nonspecific and caused by tissue hypoxia. In mild exposures, patients present with malaise, nausea, vomiting, dyspnea, headache, dizziness, and confusion. Severe poisoning is characterized by syncope, seizures, coma, cardiorespiratory depression, and death. This patient's presentation is not consistent with carbon monoxide poisoning.

(Reference: Section 8: The Acutely Ill Infant and Child; Part 3: Injuries and Untoward Events, Chapter 120, p 460–465)

Answer 8-65. d

Hydrocarbon exposures are a frequent cause of pediatric morbidity and mortality. Hydrocarbons are found in many common household and automotive cleaning products. The most important concern with hydrocarbon exposure is aspiration and chemical pneumonitis, due to their low viscosity and volatile nature. Hydrocarbon aspiration may result in bronchospasm, bronchial inflammation, lipid solubilization, and disruption of the surfactant layer, and may result in edema, exudates, hemorrhage, decreased lung compliance, alveolar collapse, and/or necrosis. Most patients with hydrocarbon aspiration will have immediate symptoms of coughing and gagging, but other patients have more gradual development of respiratory distress. Therefore, it is important to monitor patients for 6 hours, after which they are unlikely to have pulmonary aspiration and may be safely discharged.

Most hydrocarbons are poorly absorbed from the gastrointestinal tract after ingestion and lack systemic toxicity. Systemic effects, such as central nervous system depression may occasionally be seen due to absorption across the alveolar-capillary membrane. Cardiovascular toxicity is an unusual complication of hydrocarbon ingestion or aspiration but may be seen in cases of intentional inhalational abuse of aromatic hydrocarbons. Gastric decontamination with activated charcoal is not indicated as it has poor adsorptive capacity for most hydrocarbons.

(Reference: Section 8: The Acutely Ill Infant and Child; Part 3: Injuries and Untoward Events, Chapter 120, p 466–467)

Answer 8-66. e

Both ethylene glycol and methanol toxicity result from toxic metabolites formed during metabolism by alcohol and aldehyde dehydrogenases (see eFigure 120-3). The principal toxic metabolites of ethylene glycol are glycolic and oxalic acid. Oxalic acid causes precipitation of calcium oxalate leading to renal failure, hypocalcemic seizures, altered mental status and coma, prolonged QT interval, and ventricular dysrhythmias.

Suspected ethylene glycol ingestions must be taken very seriously as the lethal dose is very low. An initial osmolar gap gives way to an anion gap metabolic acidosis. The antidotes—ethanol or fomepizole—are competitive inhibition of alcohol and aldehyde dehydrogenase reducing the formation of the toxic metabolites of ethylene glycol, oxalic, and glycolic acid. Hemodialysis may still be indicated.

(Reference: Section 8: The Acutely Ill Infant and Child; Part 3: Injuries and Untoward Events, Chapter 120, p 467–468)

Answer 8-67. b

Heat stroke is the most severe form of heat-related illness. It is the second cause of death in athletes after closed head injury. Heat syncope usually occurs because of dehydration coupled with peripheral vasodilation due to high ambient temperatures. Heat cramps are muscle cramps that occur often in the legs after vigorous exercise and sweating. They are due to hyponatremia resulting from large volume salt loss in sweat with concurrent fluid replenishment in the form of water. The treatment for heat

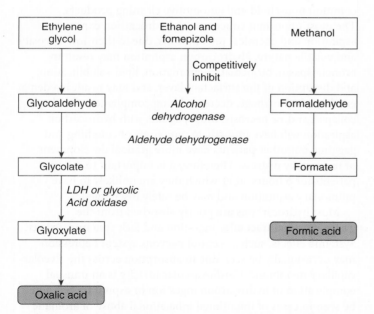

eFIGURE 120-3. Mechanism of action of fomepizole and ethanol in ethylene glycol and methanol poisoning. Both antidotes compete for the alcohol dehydrogenase, limiting the metabolism of both alcohols to more toxic products. (Reproduced, with permission, from Rudolph CD, Rudolph AM, Lister GE, First LR, Gershon AA. *Rudolph's Pediatrics.* 22nd ed. New York: McGraw-Hill, 2011.)

cramps is salt water. In this situation, the patient is not at risk for rhabdomyolysis. Rhabdomyolysis is a potential consequence of heat stroke. Systemic inflammatory response and multi-system organ failure occur during heat stroke but not during heat exhaustion.

(Reference: Section 8: The Acutely Ill Infant and Child; Part 3: Injuries and Untoward Events, Chapter 121, p. 470)

Answer 8-68. d

Conduction, convection, radiation, and evaporation are all methods of heat elimination in the body. Sublimation is not a method of heat elimination. Conduction carries heat between a body and a contacting surface along a temperature gradient. Convection transfers heat from the body surface to a gas or fluid circulating around the body. With conduction, heat transfer stops when the contacting surface temperature reaches body temperature, whereas with convection, circulation of fresh gas or fluid around the body preserves the temperature gradient between the body and the circulating gas or fluid. Radiation transfers heat from a warmer to a colder body via electromagnetic waves. Evaporation removes heat by promoting a phase transition from liquid to a gas. When the environmental temperature is higher than body temperature, the only method of heat elimination that can be used is evaporation of sweat. Conduction, convection, and radiation rely on an environmental temperature lower than body temperature.

(Reference: Section 8: The Acutely Ill Infant and Child; Part 3: Injuries and Untoward Events, Chapter 121, p 470)

Answer 8-69. c

The infant in this scenario is suffering from heat stroke. This is the most severe form of heat-related illness and carries a high morbidity and mortality unless cooling measures are instituted quickly. Water immersion is a quick and effective method of reducing body temperature, however, ice water immersion may be counterproductive because shivering and peripheral vasoconstriction may work towards increasing heat production. Evaporative cooling with atomized lukewarm water and fanning is another effective way of cooling a patient. These and other noninvasive cooling measures should be instituted immediately and are first-line therapies. Antipyretic medications should not be given in heat stroke. These medications may potentiate organ damage and are not effective in heat stroke.

(Reference: Section 8: The Acutely Ill Infant and Child; Part 3: Injuries and Untoward Events, Chapter 121, p 471)

Answer 8-70. d

Heatstroke is a preventable disease caused by circumstances largely under human control. Prevention requires an awareness of risk factors as well as appropriate behavioral responses to heat stress. Anticipatory guidance should focus on education of parents, young athletes, and coaches about the need for both rest in between exertion and appropriate hydration when exercising in warm environments. Athletic events should be planned with environmental conditions and the need for ready access to water in mind. Finally, parents, coaches, and childcare supervisors need to be aware of the signs of heat-related illness to allow detection prior to the full manifestation of heatstroke. Heat-related illnesses are common, especially in teens who are involved in rigorous team sport training in hot weather.

(Reference: Section 8: The Acutely Ill Infant and Child; Part 3: Injuries and Untoward Events, Chapter 121, p 472)

Answer 8-71. e

The patient described above is experiencing a systemic allergic reaction. Patients with systemic reactions may experience cutaneous, mucocutaneous, respiratory, cardiovascular, and gastrointestinal symptoms. Patients who experience symptoms in 2 or more or of the above categories after receiving a sting meet criteria for anaphylaxis that may be severe and in some cases fatal. Anaphylaxis should be treated with epinephrine, H1 and H2 blockers, steroids, and observation. Immediate intubation is not indicated in all cases of anaphylaxis. Patients who have been observed for anaphylaxis should be sent home with epinephrine to be administered in the event of a subsequent sting and should receive referral to an allergist. Prompt removal of barbed honeybee stinger and venom sac may decrease the dose of venom received but alone is insufficient to resolve this patient's systemic symptoms.

(Reference: Section 8: The Acutely Ill Infant and Child; Part 3: Injuries and Untoward Events, Chapter 122, p 475–476)

Answer 8-72. a

Crotalidae and Elapidae families are indigenous to the United States. They are correctly identified as described above by the shape of their head, fangs, and eyes. Their venom is a mixture of enzymes designed to immobilize and digest prey and as such their effects include not only local tissue damage but also systemic neurotoxic, cardiotoxic, nephrotoxic, and hemotoxic effects. The natural progression of injury following envenomation is the onset of pain within 5–10 minutes, followed by progressive swelling and edema that may continue for up to 24 hours. Bites on limbs must be monitored closely for the development of compartment syndrome. Patients may experience systemic symptoms including perioral numbness and paresthesias, nausea, vomiting, chills, sweating, progressive weakness, hypotension, and shock, depending on the nature of the bite and host characteristics.

Venous tourniquets may be used in select cases when transport to the receiving medical facility will take over 30–60 minutes. There has not been any benefit demonstrated by the study of suction devices, and therefore incision and suction are not recommended. This patient has systemic symptoms and therefore at minimum has moderate grade of envenomation (see Table 122-1). This patient should be admitted for pain control and monitoring for compartment syndrome and/or systemic effects. The antivenin CroFab® is preferred to the older equine antivenin as it is less antigenic, equally effective, and safe in children as well as adults. Bites occur primarily in the southeast and southwest between the months of April and October, when treated early and properly the mortality is low.

(Reference: Section 8: The Acutely Ill Infant and Child; Part 3: Injuries and Untoward Events, Chapter 122, p 476–478)

TABLE 122-1. Crotalidae (Pit Viper) Envenomation Grading System (AAPCC)

Grade of Envenomation	Local Findings	Systemic Findings	Laboratory Abnormalities
None	Little or no pain; no swelling after 4 hours	None	None
Mild	Pain, tenderness, and swelling within 10 cm of the bite; possible slight bluish discoloration around the bite	None	None
Moderate	Same as in mild envenomation, with progressive swelling; may have bluish discoloration of entire limb	Nausea, vomiting, weakness, perioral and scalp paresthesias, and fasciculation	Thrombocytopenia, hypofibrinogenemia, and hemoconcentration
Severe	Rapidly progressing pain and swelling; development of vesicles/bullae and ecchymoses	Same as in moderate envenomation, with hypotension, shock, bleeding diathesis, and respiratory distress	Thrombocytopenia, hypofibrinogenemia, anemia, and metabolic acidosis

Note: AAPCC, American Association of Poison Control Centers.

CHAPTER 9 | The Chronically Ill Infant and Child

John I. Takayama and Sunitha V. Kaiser

9-1. In 1987, the former US Office of Technology Assistance defined the medically fragile, technology-dependent child as one who needs:

  a. A medical device to compensate for the loss of a vital body function

  b. A chronic care facility for continuous care

  c. Substantial ongoing nursing care to avert death and further disability

  d. Both a medical device to compensate for the loss of a vital body function and substantial ongoing nursing care to avert death or further disability

  e. Care for a chronic illness that is associated with increased health-care cost

9-2. Common features of medically complex and fragile children with special health-care needs (CSHCN) include needs for multiple medical and nonmedical services, technological supports, and effective care coordination. The level of and time involved in care coordination depend both on their medical complexity and fragility. Among the following examples, which children would require the highest level of care coordination?

  a. A 7-year-old child with congenital hypothyroidism and intellectual disability who is able to walk to school under adult supervision and has not required more than several visits to the pediatrician every year.

  b. A 5-year-old girl with trisomy 21, hypothyroidism, glaucoma, intellectual disability, and partially corrected congenital heart disease who requires oxygen at night for mild pulmonary hyptertension. She is monitored every 4 months by a pediatric pulmonologist and every year by a pediatric cardiologist. Her pediatrician sees her for both routine care and acute illnesses.

  c. A 12-year-old girl with a perinatal diagnosis of hypoxic ischemic encephalopathy who has cerebral palsy, severe developmental delay, seizure disorder, cortical blindness, loss of hearing, scoliosis, and severe contractures of her extremities. She is dependent upon gastrostomy-tube feeding for nutrition; her parents transport her in a wheel chair. In the last year, she has been hospitalized once for pneumonia. She is followed by 8 subspecialists.

  d. A 16-year-old adolescent with uncontrolled diabetes who does not have a primary care pediatrician and presents to the emergency room over 6 times per year for diabetic ketoacidosis.

  e. A 3-month-old infant who was born 12 weeks preterm and who has just been discharged from the Intensive Care Nursery; the family lives 20 miles from the nearest tertiary care center and must rely on others for transportation. Although he required oxygen and mechanical ventilation initially, he is currently gaining weight and is on high calorie formula. He will be followed on a regular basis by the hospital-based Intensive Care Nursery follow-up clinic and has already been referred to an early developmental intervention center.

9-3. Common features of medically complex and fragile CSHCN include needs for multiple medical and nonmedical services, technological supports, and effective care coordination. While the level of and time involved in care coordination depend on both their medical complexity and fragility, a variety of nonmedical factors may further impact access to needed services. Which of the following nonmedical factors will increase the level of care coordination intensity.

  a. Consistent and reliable health-care seeking behaviors

  b. Availability of adequate home care assistance

  c. Limited fluency in English

  d. Close proximity to a tertiary care center

  e. Adequate insurance coverage

9-4. Families, providers, and organizations seeking to improve health care have identified poor care coordination as a major problem in the care of medically complex and fragile CSHCN. Which of the following is an example of a model of care developed to address this problem?

   a. Fragmented community and hospital-based services

   b. Tertiary center-based subspecialty clinics

   c. The "medical home"

   d. Hospitalist-based inpatient units

   e. Separated inpatient and outpatient services

9-5. A 5-year-old girl with cerebral palsy from perinatal hypoxic ischemic encephalopathy, chronic restrictive lung disease and spasticity of her lower extremities presents to your clinic. Which one of the following will facilitate independent function in the domain of mobility?

   a. Orthoses

   b. Peripherally inserted central catheter

   c. Suctioning and cough assist devices

   d. Pulse oximetry

   e. Home apnea monitor

9-6. A 3-year-old child with muscular dystrophy, recurrent aspiration pneumonia, and poor weight gain is being considered for gastrostomy tube placement. Which of the following is the MOST important reason for considering assistive technology, such as a gastrostomy tube, in the care coordination needs assessment.

   a. Availability of a particular technology

   b. Particular technology is consistent with parents' goals for their child

   c. Technology will not alter the course of a child's ability to meet a goal

   d. Several subspecialists offer strong advice on the merits of the technology

   e. Therapists, vendors, and insurers ensure that the technology is appropriate

9-7. You are the primary medical care provider for a 6-year-old girl with cerebral palsy, spastic hemiparesis, and vision impairment. Which of the following addresses problems with neuromuscular dysfunction, sensory perception, psychosocial competence, and fine motor delay as they influence the child's ability to participate in self-care, play, and school activities.

   a. Physical therapy

   b. Occupational therapy

   c. Speech and language pathology

   d. Orthopedics

   e. Orthotics

9-8. An infant with chronic lung disease is being discharged from the hospital because his oxygen requirement has now decreased to 35% FiO_2 to maintain oxygen saturations at an appropriate level. At home, 100% oxygen is delivered and the required FiO_2 is achieved by varying the flow rate by nasal cannula. As a general rule, the FiO_2 likely reaches or exceeds 35% when oxygen flow through a nasal cannula exceeds how many liters per minute in infants?

   a. 1 L per minute

   b. 1.5 L per minute

   c. 2 L per minute

   d. 2.5 L per minute

   e. 3 L per minute

9-9. You are counseling a parent regarding suctioning through a tracheostomy tube that was recently placed in a 10-year-old boy with muscular dystrophy. Which of the following is CORRECT regarding suctioning in children with tracheostomies?

   a. Children with tracheostomies generally require suctioning once or twice a day

   b. The size of the suction catheter is fixed and independent of the size of the tracheostomy tube

   c. During suctioning, the catheter tip should be inserted deep enough to meet resistance from the carina to assure complete clearance

   d. Applying suction pressure both on insertion and withdrawal of the suction catheter should be avoided because this may injure the lining of the airway

   e. Following suctioning, many children with tracheostomy tubes may benefit from a few manual ventilation breaths to re-recruit the lung

9-10. You are the primary medical care provider for a 16-year-old with cystic fibrosis whose parents express concern about decline in school performance and antisocial behaviors. Which of the following are functional domain factors that can contribute to poor psychosocial adjustment:

   a. Positive self-image

   b. Dependence in functioning for basic self-help needs

   c. Peer acceptance

   d. Participation in activities of childhood

   e. Diagnosis

9-11. You are caring for a 4-year-old girl who suffers from a severe neurological impairment following near-drowning. Which of the following is an important risk factor for parental adjustment difficulties when they must care for children with special health-care needs?

 a. Child's disability status

 b. Burden associated with medical treatment management

 c. Loss of parent career opportunities

 d. Child's intellectual functioning

 e. Child's age

9-12. A 14-year-old boy with type-I diabetes is being hospitalized for DKA for the second time in the past 6 months. Which of the following is associated with poor diabetes self-care behaviors and metabolic control?

 a. Family support

 b. Family conflict

 c. Family size

 d. Family immigration status

 e. Family professional status

9-13. Which of the following is TRUE related to paternal involvement in improving the adjustment of patient or family adjustment to chronic illness?

 a. Increased paternal involvement has not been shown to be associated with improvement in maternal psychological functioning

 b. Increased paternal involvement in disease management relates to more favorable outcomes in marital satisfaction but not family functioning

 c. Increased paternal involvement in disease management relates to more favorable outcomes in family functioning but not marital satisfaction

 d. Decreased paternal involvement in the care of an adolescent with chronic illness has demonstrated positive influence on treatment adherence

 e. Increased paternal involvement in the care of an adolescent with chronic illness has demonstrated positive influence on treatment adherence

9-14. You are the primary medical care provider for a 2-year-old boy with recurrent infections who was recently diagnosed with severe combined immunodeficiency (SCID). Which of the following is the BEST example of a potential way that pediatricians can assess the needs of the family and mobilize resources:

 a. Emphasize the importance of extended family involvement in the medical management of the child and in the daily activities of the child

 b. Assist in the education of the school staff regarding the child's condition, medical device management, and troubleshooting as well as anticipated treatment needs

 c. Make statements, such as "I know what you may be feeling or enduring," which are often considered to be empathetic and may improve communication with parents

 d. Schedule standard timeslots for visits with these patients, allowing time only for focusing on acute needs and illnesses.

 e. Refer to a family support group

9-15. You are caring for a 10-year-old healthy boy whose parents inform you that their second child, a 4-year-old girl, was recently diagnosed with leukemia. Which of the following is TRUE related to the impact of children with chronic conditions on their siblings?

 a. Although families may need to carry out demanding care plans for their children with chronic illness, they are usually able to attend equally to the needs of well siblings

 b. Siblings may function as a care provider for children with chronic illness

 c. Siblings of children with chronic illness are less likely than their peers to experience problems with psychosocial adjustment

 d. Siblings may seek attention through externalizing behavior (oppositional or defiant) much more so than internalizing symptoms of anxiety and depression

 e. The severity of the child's illness is associated with the risk for negative psychological effects on siblings.

9-16. You are the primary medical care provider for a 15-year-old healthy boy whose parents inform you that their second child has been diagnosed with Down Syndrome. Pediatricians can play an important role in helping siblings of children with chronic conditions. Which of the following is the BEST example of a suggestion to families to address the potential needs of the 15-year-old child?

a. Older siblings, particularly adolescents, should be trained to fill the parenting role. Given the hardships that parents often face when caring for children with chronic illness, it is natural for older siblings to take on more responsibility, even if it means sacrificing their own needs.

b. Younger siblings should be prepared for environmental restrictions to accommodate the needs of the child with chronic illness; while these restrictions can impact play and family vacations, children are resilient and can easily overcome such restrictions.

c. Families may benefit from maintaining an open communication about feelings, worries, and concerns since these communications can help address emotional stressors and resolve potential conflict.

d. Although inequities in care and attention are often present, age-appropriate responses of anger, jealousy, and resentment are rare. Exhibition of such emotion by the sibling should be discouraged as these will lead to anxiety in the child with chronic illness.

e. Sibling discussion groups have not been found to be helpful since group participants often are not able to express themselves in such settings.

9-17. You are part of a group practice in a rural area with few community resources. You are the primary medical care provider for a 5-year-old boy with muscular dystrophy. Families have suggested which of the following to improve services for children with chronic conditions:

a. Variety of types of support groups

b. Child and family counseling

c. Respite care

d. Availability of recreational and community-based activities

e. All of the above

9-18. Which of the following chronic diseases of childhood accounts for the GREATEST number of deaths during childhood?

a. Chronic lung and respiratory diseases

b. Diseases of the heart

c. Cerebrovascular diseases

d. Malignant neoplasms

e. Congenital malformations and chromosomal anomalies

9-19. You are treating a 12-year-old boy with muscular dystrophy who has developed cardiac failure. You decide the best course of action is to discuss comfort care with the family. Which of the following BEST describes the goals of comfort care?

a. To prolong life with evidence-based medical therapies

b. To cure the underlying illness with experimental therapies

c. To discover alternate curative treatment options through additional diagnostic testing

d. To support the parents and family with psychological counseling

e. To maximize physical comfort and quality of life, but not cure the underlying illness

9-20. You are caring for an 8-year-old boy with severe cystic fibrosis who wants to discuss death. Which of the following BEST describes the understanding of death to expect in a child this age?

a. All interactions with the world are sensory and motor and there is no concept of death.

b. Orientation is self-centered and reality is not limited by logic. The concept of all things dying is not yet developed and imagination and magic play a large influence, such that many beings may be considered immortal.

c. Reasoning is based on direct observation and concepts of death are present. Concerns of death are of separation and less about afterlife.

d. Full intellectual capacities have developed including adult concepts of death.

e. Thoughts of death mainly center around questions of the afterlife.

9-21. You are taking care of a 4-year-old girl with an infiltrative CNS neoplasm that has now been deemed terminal due to lack of response to therapy. Which of the following strategies for discussing death is MOST developmentally appropriate for a child this age?

a. Discuss detailed plans of care and reassure the child that they will not suffer or be in pain

b. Avoid any discussion of death due to the child's lack of the capacity to understand

c. Address misperceptions about death and allay fears of separation or abandonment by facilitating consistent caretaker presence

d. Empathize with the child's concerns about changes in appearance and physical limitations as compared to their healthy peers

e. Limit parental involvement in discussions around death so as to preserve the child's autonomy

9-22. You are caring for an 11-year-old boy with acute lymphoblastic leukemia that has failed multiple treatment attempts. He and his family have opted for comfort care at home. Which of the following scenarios describes the best environment for end-of-life care at home?

   a. A multifamily home in which the child will be sleeping in a common living area

   b. A single-family home in a rural area that is a 3-hour drive from the nearest medical facility

   c. A single-family home in which there is another child with chronic illness and a single parent as the caretaker

   d. A multi-family home in which the child will be sleeping in a common area, but multiple adult caretakers are available

   e. A single-family home in which there is a private, comfortable space for the child as well as multiple caretakers

9-23. In order to develop a palliative care plan, providers often categorize a child's disease trajectory. Which of the following best describes an example where curative therapy is available but may fail?

   a. A 16-year-old boy with end-stage renal disease awaiting renal transplant

   b. A 12-year-old girl with severe cystic fibrosis requiring frequent hospitalizations

   c. An 8-year-old boy with muscular dystrophy who is wheelchair-bound

   d. A 1-year-old girl with infantile spasms and developmental regression

   e. An 11-year-old with Crohn disease and chronic malnutrition

9-24. You are a member of a multidisciplinary palliative care team engaged in the treatment of a 10-year-old child with metastatic rhabdomyosarcoma. Which of the following best describes the role of social workers as members of a palliative care team?

   a. To provide psychosocial assessment and supportive counseling for the child and family adjusting to changes along with identifying community services.

   b. To provide skills in facilitating communication with children through activities that assist with emotional distress and can provide important understanding of the child's fears and wishes.

   c. To support faith traditions and spiritual values that promote healing and hope and support families as they face change, loss, or grief.

   d. To bring expertise in symptom management and serve as mediators between the medical teams and families.

   e. All of the above

9-25. The family of a 5-year-old boy with refractory acute lymphoblastic leukemia speaks to you about participating in a Phase I clinical trial. They wish to know what percent of patients derive significant clinical benefit from participating in such trials. Which is the MOST appropriate answer?

   a. Between 5 and 10% of patients

   b. Between 20 and 30% of patients

   c. Between 30 and 50% of patients

   d. Between 50 and 70% of patients

   e. Over 80% of patients

9-26. You are discussing different treatment options with the parents of a 10-year-old boy with severe cerebral palsy from hypoxic brain injury at birth. Which of the following interventions has the BEST evidence-base at this time to suggest potential benefit?

   a. Gastrostomy tube

   b. Nissen fundoplication

   c. Anti-reflux medications

   d. Tracheostomy

   e. Salivary gland ligation

9-27. You are taking care of a boy with terminal cancer who is complaining of bony pain. You would like to use a 0–10 numerical (as opposed to a pictorial) pain rating scale to have him quantify his pain level to assist in pain management. At what age are children reliably able to use a numerical pain scale?

   a. 5–6 years old

   b. 7–8 years old

   c. 9–10 years old

   d. 11–12 years old

   e. 12 years old

9-28. A 15-year-old boy with osteosarcoma complains of sharp stabbing pain at the site of his tumor. This type of pain is best characterized as:

   a. Somatic nociceptive pain

   b. Neuropathic pain

   c. Psychogenic pain

   d. Visceral nociceptive pain

   e. Radicular pain

9-29. You are trying to manage an acute pain crisis in a 13-year-old with a newly diagnosed Ewing sarcoma of his left distal humerus. He rates his pain as severe, so you would like to treat with an opioid. Which of the following choices should be avoided in children?

   a. Morphine

   b. Fentanyl

   c. Hydromorphone

   d. Codeine

   e. Oxycodone

9-30. You are caring for an 8-year-old boy with end-stage renal disease awaiting transplant. He complains of severe pain, and you choose to use an opiate given the severity of his pain. Which of the following opiates should be avoided in children with renal impairment?

a. Fentanyl

b. Hydromorphone

c. Oxycodone

d. Morphine

e. Tramadol

9-31. A 14-year-old girl with cystic fibrosis has developed depression and her symptoms are worsening despite having regular counseling sessions with a psychologist for several months. You decide to start treating her depression with an SSRI (selective-serotonin reuptake inhibitor). Which if the following statements regarding counseling the patient and family about this drug is CORRECT?

a. They can expect to see positive effects from the drug in 7–10 days

b. Side effects include hypersalivation, diarrhea, and urinary frequency

c. They should monitor for suicidal thoughts; worsening symptoms such as agitation and irritability can be precursor signs

d. There are no potential drug interactions

e. The family can abruptly stop the drug anytime

9-32. A 12-year-old girl with terminal CNS tumor is in your care. You discuss with her parents that it is necessary to stop giving her enteral nutrition due to risks of vomiting. What is the BEST estimate you can give the family of the time it takes for death to occur after the discontinuation of artificial nutrition and hydration?

a. 1–2 days

b. 3–5 days

c. 5–7 days

d. 7–10 days

e. 10–14 days

9-33. You are caring for a 3-year-old boy who suffered from a stroke that has left significant brain damage and he is sustained by artificial ventilatory support. You deem further interventions to be medically futile, however, his family insists you provide additional treatments. What is the BEST first step in management?

a. Do not provide any additional treatments and inform the family of your decision

b. Obtain a court order to remove the child from ventilator support

c. Discuss with the family their goals of care

d. Call Child Protective Services to discuss placing the child in alternate custody

e. Ask the parents to sign a Do Not Resuscitate order

9-34. Which of the following statements CORRECTLY describes the rights of adolescents regarding medical treatment decisions?

a. All states allow minors to refuse participation in research, without possibility of parental override.

b. All states allow a minor to sign durable power of attorney or a living will.

c. All states have consent statutes stating that at a specific age (14–16 years) a minor can consent to any medical treatment, including abortion.

d. All states allow minors to refuse life-saving care.

e. All states permit adolescents to confidentially seek care for sexually transmitted infections without parental knowledge.

9-35. A 13-year-old boy with refractory acute myelogenous leukemia (AML) and chronic pain is started on around-the-clock morphine. Which of the following side effects of opiate medications can be expected to improve over time without dose adjustment or additional intervention?

a. Respiratory depression

b. Constipation

c. Nausea

d. Hypotension

e. Allergic reaction

9-36. You are caring for a 12-year-old boy with terminal AML who has become anorexic and cachectic. Which of the following treatments to stimulate appetite should be used with greatest caution?

a. Corticosteroids

b. Dronabinol

c. Megestrol

d. Hypnosis

e. Behavioral counseling

9-37. Which of the following medications has a slow elimination phase that may lead to drug toxicity?

a. Morphine

b. Hydromorphone

c. Fentanyl

d. Oxycodone

e. Methadone

ANSWERS

Answer 9-1. d

A small but increasing subpopulation of children with special health care needs (CSHCN) can be described as "medically complex and fragile" with chronic conditions requiring technologic assistance. A medically fragile, technology-dependent child is defined as a child "who needs both a medical device to compensate for the loss of a vital body function and substantial ongoing nursing care to avert death or further disability." With advances in medical knowledge and technology, there are great numbers of technology-dependent children living longer and living at home with technological assistance. Given the lack of home nursing care and increased expertise of parents in providing health care, the dual requirement of technology and nursing has now become an inadequate definition of medical fragility.

(Section 9: The Chronically Ill Infant and Child. Chapter 124: The Technology-Dependent Child, p 484)

Answer 9-2. c

The level of care coordination intensity can be categorized as low, moderate, or high based upon the following combination of medical complexity and medical fragility.

	Low	Moderate	High
Medical Complexity			
Organ systems	<3	3–5	>5
Specialists	<5	5–7	>7
Diagnosis and disease trajectory	Known	Unknown	Disputed
PCP involvement	Provides routine and acute care	Provides routine care	Uninvolved
Coordination	Comprehensive tertiary center coordination	Disease/condition specific coordination	No tertiary center coordination
Fragility			
ER visits/yr	<4	5–10	>10
Clinic visits/yr	<5	5–10	>10
Hospital visits/yr	1	2–3	>3
Hospital days/yr	<5	5–10	>10
Technology Dependence	Function enhancing technology, ie, wheelchair	For nutrition, ie, gastrostomy tube	For sustaining life, ie, oxygen

Based on criteria used by the Special Needs Program of the Children's Hospital of Wisconsin.

For the child in choice a, the level of care coordination intensity can be considered low since this 7-year-old has a condition that affects fewer than 3 organ systems, is followed only by his pediatrician, and does not require frequent ER or hospital services. For the child in choice b, the level of care coordination intensity can be considered moderate to high since this 5-year-old girl has a condition that affects 5 organ systems (moderate) and is followed by several subspecialists (moderate). Her pediatrician provides both routine and acute care (low). She is dependent on oxygen at night (high). For the child in choice c, the level of care coordination intensity can be considered high since this 12-year-old has conditions that affect more than 5 organ systems (high) and is followed by more than 7 subspecialists (high). For the child in choice d, the level of care coordination intensity can be considered mild to moderate since this 16-year-old has only a condition with limited organ involvement at this time (low); however, given the frequency of ER visits (moderate), the care coordination required falls into the mild to moderate intensity. For the child in choice e, the level of care coordination intensity can be considered mild since this 3-month-old infant does not have a condition with 3 or more organs involved at this time. The level of care coordination intensity must be re-assessed on a regular basis, at least once per year and especially with changes in medical complexity or fragility.

(Section 9: The Chronically Ill Infant and Child. Chapter 124: The Technology-Dependent Child, p 485)

Answer 9-3. c

The level of and time involved in care coordination depend on both the medical complexity and fragility of the child with special health-care needs as well as a variety of nonmedical factors that impact access to needed services. The level of care coordination intensity can be categorized as low, moderate, or high based upon the combination of medical complexity, medical fragility and nonmedical factors such as family structure and capacity, location of residence, and insurance.

(Section 9: The Chronically Ill Infant and Child. Chapter 124: The Technology-Dependent Child, p 485)

Answer 9-4. c

Caregivers of CSHCN often face the daunting task of identifying and negotiating the maze of community and hospital-based services; the children require multiple medical services and frequent hospitalizations, but care is often partitioned with limited communication among providers, contributing to duplicated or unnecessary investigations and therapies, the potential for costly medical errors, and frustration for families.

Stakeholders have identified poor care coordination as a major problem in the care of medically complex and fragile CSHCN. The American Academy of Pediatrics and others advocate the Medical Home, a concept of accessible, continuous, comprehensive, family-centered, coordinated, compassionate, and culturally effective primary care delivered by a primary care clinician. Many tertiary care centers have developed disease- or condition-specific programs that provide care coordination for medically complex and fragile CSHCN (eg, diabetes programs, tracheostomy/ventilator programs). Some centers provide predominantly ambulatory or hospitalist-based inpatient "complex care services." Finally, a few programs offer integrated inpatient and outpatient services, some in collaboration with local primary care pediatricians.

(Section 9: The Chronically Ill Infant and Child. Chapter 124: The Technology-Dependent Child, p 485)

Answer 9-5. a

Chronic illness and significant injury in childhood can result in impairment, defined by the World Health Organization (WHO) as any loss or abnormality of psychological, physical or anatomic structure, or function. Disability is the limitation in activity caused by impairment. Handicap exists when an impairment or disability limits or prevents participation in a role that is normal for age and gender, within the social and cultural milieu.

Orthoses, transfer aids and lifts, wheelchair and wheelchair ramps are all devices that can be used to improve mobility. Orthoses can be applied to or around a body segment to prevent involuntary movement or movement from abnormal tone, maintain joint alignment to facilitate body mechanics, and stabilize a joint. Wheelchairs can be used to facilitate developmentally appropriate independence and functional activity. Poor positioning and restriction of movement can result in pressure areas and musculoskeletal deformity; therefore, mobility devices are often combined with customized positioning or seating systems. Many medically fragile and complex CSHCN will attain close to adult size and weight. Some are able to bear weight but need assistance to move from one surface to another. Transfer aids should be considered for any child who weighs more than 25 kg and cannot be safely transferred by 1 caregiver alone. Aids should also be considered for children with inconsistent ability to assist in transfers. Home adaptations can also improve the child's ability to participate in social and avocational activities within the community. A wheelchair ramp is an example of home remodeling that can improve access between the outside and inside. Peripherally inserted central catheter (PICC) can provide central venous access for nutrition and medication; however, it does not directly facilitate independent function in the domain of mobility.

(Section 9: The Chronically Ill Infant and Child. Chapter 124: The Technology-Dependent Child, p 490)

Answer 9-6. b

When a care coordination needs assessment is conducted, assistive technology may be raised as a consideration. Families must be involved in the decision to adopt a particular technology because they can appropriately assess its consistency with their overall goals for their child. Just because a particular technology exists does not mean that it should be acquired, especially if adoption will not alter the course of a child's ability to meet a goal.

If assistive technology is desired, the choice of support or device requires input from the family and members of the coordination team. Parents may rely on the expertise of the primary care physician and subspecialists to understand both the benefits and limitations of a specific technology. Additional input from specialists, therapists, teachers, vendors, durable medical equipment companies, and insurers may also be helpful to assure that the technology is appropriate.

(Section 9: The Chronically Ill Infant and Child. Chapter 124: The Technology-Dependent Child, p 486)

Answer 9-7. b

Given their role in coordinating care, physicians must understand the roles and functions of physical and occupational therapists and speech language pathologists. Physical therapy addresses problems associated with neuromuscular dysfunction and gross motor delay as they impact on the child's ability to be mobile within an environment. Occupational therapy addresses problems with neuromuscular dysfunction, sensory perception, psychosocial competence, and fine motor delay as they influence the child's ability to participate in self-care, play, and school activities. Speech and language pathology address problems of communication as well as neurologic, respiratory, and digestive disorders that affect speech and swallowing. Orthopedics addresses abnormalities of the bone or joint that may limit mobility. Orthoses are custom-fitted devices applied to or around a body segment that are designed to meet specific musculoskeletal goals such as stabilization of a joint.

(Section 9: The Chronically Ill Infant and Child. Chapter 124: The Technology-Dependent Child, p 487)

Answer 9-8. c

The amount of air entrained within each breath determines the actual FiO_2 received by the infant. As a general rule, the FiO_2 likely exceeds 35% when oxygen flow through a nasal cannula exceeds 2 L per minute in infants or 3–4 L per minute in older children; when Venturi-type valves calibrated for greater than 30% O_2 are used; when nonbreather masks are used; and when flow exceeds 4 L per minute on a home ventilator. It may be helpful to measure the relationship between flow and FiO_2 prior to discharging the child from hospital.

(Section 9: The Chronically Ill Infant and Child. Chapter 124: The Technology-Dependent Child, p 488)

Answer 9-9. e

Children with tracheostomies usually require suctioning at least three to four times per day and more frequently when they acquire respiratory illnesses. Rattling mucus sounds, tachypnea, secretions pooling at the opening of the tracheostomy tube or signs of respiratory distress are all indications for initiating suctioning. Instilling normal saline drops immediately before suctioning may help to loosen thick secretions or elicit a cough. The size of the suction catheter depends on the size of the tracheostomy tube. While a size 8 French suction catheter is appropriate for a 3.5–4.5 mm diameter Shiley pediatric tracheostomy tube, a smaller size 5 or 6 French catheter is necessary for a 3.0-mm diameter tube. Shallow suctioning removes secretions at the opening of the tracheostomy; suctioning just past the tip of the tracheostomy tube allows complete clearance. Suctioning until the catheter meets resistance from the carina should generally be avoided as this may injure the lining of the airway. Applying suction pressure both on insertion and withdrawal of the suction catheter facilitates removal of secretions. Following suctioning, many children with tracheostomy tubes may benefit from a few manual ventilation breaths to re-recruit the lung.

(Section 9: The Chronically Ill Infant and Child. Chapter 124: The Technology-Dependent Child, p 489)

Answer 9-10. b

Children are resilient and can adjust to difficult conditions appropriately; yet children with chronic illness have been found to be at least twice as likely as the general population to develop a behavioral or psychiatric disorder. Poor adjustment, the most common type of psychological or behavioral difficulty seen in children with chronic conditions, can lead to problem interactions with peers, low self-esteem, and externalization (such as oppositional behavior) as well as internalization of symptoms (such as anxiety). Adjustment to illness can affect adherence to treatment and influence perception of quality of life for both the child and the family.

When caring for children with chronic conditions, pediatricians should be sensitive to factors that influence child adjustment, such as functioning or participation in activities of childhood (play, school performance, communication, and interpersonal skills); self-image; independence in functioning for basic self-help needs; peer acceptance; perception of high self-efficacy in an area important to the child and peers; presence of pain or other disruptive symptoms (diarrhea, cough, tics, seizures, etc.); and ability to choose or navigate through remaining choices (in medical treatment plan, school, or daily tasks) with a sense of control. By asking questions related to these functional domains, pediatricians can more likely identify and understand adjustment problems than by analyzing or sorting only by diagnosis or severity of condition.

(Section 9: The Chronically Ill Infant and Child. Chapter 123: Psychological and Behavioral Responses, p 479)

Answer 9-11. c

Parental adjustment to their children with special health-care needs may vary greatly within domains of adjustment, such as coping with loss, processing stress, changing the focus of control, and managing financial and care-related responsibilities. Studies have suggested greater need for mental health services in parents of CSHCN. Neither disease parameters, such as a child's disability status or intellectual functioning, nor the burden associated with medical treatment management has been found useful in predicting adjustment of caregivers. On the other hand, a range of events, such as hospitalization and loss of career opportunity related to the child's illness, has been found to cause psychosocial distress in caregivers. Role restriction is defined as the extent to which a caregiver of a child with a chronic condition feels unable to pursue his/her own personal or career interests. The perception of role restriction contributing to adjustment difficulties was associated with low social support, suggesting that caregivers with poor adjustment and loss of career opportunities may benefit from greater social support.

(Section 9: The Chronically Ill Infant and Child. Chapter 123: Psychological and Behavioral Responses, p 480)

Answer 9-12. b

High levels of family conflict are related to poorer self-care behaviors in children with diabetes. The disruptive effect of family conflict is one of the most consistent findings across studies; positive family attributes, such as support, warmth and cohesion, are related to better behaviors and outcomes. For illnesses in which compliance with medical regimens is critical to optimal outcomes, presence of family conflict should be determined.

(Section 9: The Chronically Ill Infant and Child. Chapter 123: Psychological and Behavioral Responses, p 481)

Answer 9-13. e

Paternal involvement has been reported to be associated with improved maternal psychological functioning, parental stress, marital satisfaction, and family coping with disease management. Paternal involvement in the care of a child or adolescent with chronic illness has demonstrated a positive influence on treatment adherence in the adolescent with chronic illness. Increased involvement of fathers in disease management relates to more favorable outcomes in marital satisfaction and family functioning. Pediatricians should emphasize the importance of paternal involvement in the medical management of the child and in the daily activities of the child. Suggestions for alternative activities that do not revolve around sports or other physical interactions may be helpful if the child is unable to participate in these activities. Reframing expectations for paternal involvement in medical management and in interactions with the child is helpful to both the child and the family.

(Section 9: The Chronically Ill Infant and Child. Chapter 123: Psychological and Behavioral Responses, p 481)

Answer 9-14. b

Social support and coordination of care at school are identified as interventions that contribute to the support of families with chronically ill children. Direct involvement in the development of the Individualized Educational Plan and plans for medical management during the school day is ideally provided by the pediatrician. The pediatrician can assist in the education of the school staff regarding the child's condition, medical device management, and troubleshooting as well as anticipated treatment needs. When school staff is informed and comfortable with the child's medical management, the burden of some of the child's medical care can be distributed to the school, relieving the parents from providing such care during the school day. Parents who are able to pursue other activities during the school day, including exploring roles other than those of the primary caregiver, can become better adjusted through the support that such activities yield. Inquiry about parental engagement in meaningful activities or supportive interactions should be pursued during pediatric visits.

Involvement of the father in the care of the child or adolescent with chronic illness can have a series of positive outcomes including improved treatment adherence in the adolescent with chronic illness, better maternal psychological functioning, decreased parental stress, and more effective family coping with disease management. Pediatricians, therefore, should emphasize the importance of paternal but not necessarily extended family involvement in the medical management of the child and in the daily activities of the child.

Regardless of the nature of the chronic condition, if any of these areas are problematic, support should be sought to lessen the burden. Perceived needs or inequities are to be taken as objective measures of parental experience; individual parents will experience identical conditions in very different ways. Although there may be trends within certain groups of patients, careful listening to identify needs is critical. Physician statements, intended to be empathetic, such as "I know what you may be feeling or enduring," may be heard as dismissive or may lead to loss of physician credibility from the parent or caregiver's perspective—even if that physician has substantial experience with the same condition in similar family settings. Hence, it may be better to allow enough time during visits to ask well-focused questions about events, functioning, and adjustment and then to listen carefully to gain the understanding required to address needs.

(Section 9: The Chronically Ill Infant and Child. Chapter 123: Psychological and Behavioral Responses, p 483)

Answer 9-15. b

Siblings may be forgotten by families in the process of carrying out demanding care plans; they may function as a care provider; or they may be overlooked if their needs are overshadowed by the urgent-care needs of the child. Parental resources, such as financial, temporal, and emotional, may be unduly shifted to the "sick" child; the "well" sibling may seek needed attention more often through internalizing symptoms of anxiety and depression and less through externalizing behavior (oppositional or defiant) if his or her needs are not met. Other environmental restrictions are often imposed to accommodate the needs of the sick child; these restrictions

can impact play, family vacations, and other activities related to mobility such as changing jobs or changing school districts. Aside from sibling–parent time limitations, there may also be a relative unavailability of the mother to attend to the emotional needs of all family members.

Siblings of children with chronic illnesses are 2–3 times more likely than their peers to experience problems with psychological adjustment, as reported in siblings of cancer patients before and after diagnosis. Additional stressors for siblings include limited access to information about their ill sibling's condition, negative peer reactions, and disruptions in social activities. The risk for negative psychological effects in siblings appears to be related to the functional status of the chronic illness and the attentional needs from the parent. The risk for negative psychological effects is not related to the severity of disease.

(Section 9: The Chronically Ill Infant and Child. Chapter 123: Psychological and Behavioral Responses, p 483)

Answer 9-16. c

Assessment of sibling psychosocial behavioral functioning should be undertaken to determine the presence of the following features in siblings: anxiety; presence of oppositional defiant disorder or other externalizing behaviors; difficulty in peer relationships; parental attention and focus on the well-sibling; inappropriate sibling responsibility and participation in the care of the chronically ill sibling; and need for information or assistance with understanding of the condition of the chronically ill sibling.

Often, well children have an unstated resentment, fear, or guilt about thoughts of their chronically ill sibling. Inequities in care and attention are often present and age-appropriate responses of anger, jealousy, and resentment, which are often not discussed, can lead to regret and conflict. Siblings often report worrying about suffering or death in the chronically ill child. These siblings assume a more adult or mature role than other age-matched siblings in families without illness.

Families who have open communication about feelings, worries, and concerns often resolve emotional stressors and overall experience less conflict. Direct inquiry by the pediatrician about the sibling's perceptions of their role, attentional needs, and family condition may lead to understanding important aspects of the family functioning necessary to direct care or referral. Facilitated sibling discussion groups are reported to be highly valuable and can help encourage open expression of emotions and contribute to adjustment.

(Section 9: The Chronically Ill Infant and Child. Chapter 123: Psychological and Behavioral Responses, p 483)

Answer 9-17. e

Chronic illness in a child presents a variety of challenges, some of which may result in an imbalance between demands and resources to cope with those demands. Recommendations suggested by families to improve services for children with chronic conditions include developing a variety of types of support groups, providing child and family counseling if needed, increasing availability of recreational and community-based activities, providing more parent-to-parent support in a variety of settings, providing opportunities for family-to-family support, making support groups and activities more accessible, ensuring quality of support provided in support groups, and providing opportunities for youth to meet adults with chronic conditions. Interventions to assist in adjustment or preventative measures to reduce maladjustment are needed to support optimal outcomes for children and adolescents with chronic conditions and their families. While evidence indicates that the majority of children and their families adjust satisfactorily, it is likely that even those who have accommodated could benefit from bolstering interventions due to the dynamic and development of the child and disease process.

(Section 9: The Chronically Ill Infant and Child. Chapter 123: Psychological and Behavioral Responses, p 484)

Answer 9-18. d

In 2005, 5 of the 10 leading causes of death in children in the United States were chronic diseases. In order of their frequency, these diseases included: malignant neoplasms, congenital malformations and chromosomal abnormalities, diseases of the heart, cerebrovascular diseases, and chronic lung and respiratory diseases. Cancer is the chronic disease of childhood that accounts for the greatest number of deaths during childhood. Despite remarkable improvements in survival since the advent of intensive and combination chemotherapy about 1200 children die from cancer each year in the United States. Childhood cancers are generally more rapidly growing and aggressive than adult carcinomas. Once the disease becomes resistant to therapy, the course to death is also shorter and more fulminant than that observed in adults.

(Section 9: The Chronically Ill Infant and Child, Chapter 125: Caring for Children Dying from Chronic Disease, p 494)

Answer 9-19. e

When curing illness is no longer a possible outcome of treatment, a discussion should be had with the patient and caregivers that treatments are still available. Options include palliative treatment with a goal to prolong life as long as acceptable quality of life is possible, palliative treatment with the goal to achieve maximum comfort but not to prolong life, or in some cases participation in clinical trials whose purposes are to advance knowledge about possible future drugs or procedures. These are some of the most difficult discussions to have with patients and families. When comfort care is pursued, the patient, family, and physician must be convinced that comfort treatment *is* in reality the optimal treatment and that it should not be considered giving up or lessening treatment.

(Section 9: The Chronically Ill Infant and Child, Chapter 125: Caring for Children Dying from Chronic Disease, Page 495)

Answer 9-20. c

Children acquire an understanding of death over time, influenced by many factors in the cultural and family environment as well as their own psychological and cognitive makeup. Choice a here describes children under 2 years of age; Choice b describes children between ages 2 and 7 years; and Choice d describes children 12 years and older, with whom discussions around death should be honest and direct. Choice c best describes children 7–11 years of age, so would best fit the child in this vignette.

(Section 9: The Chronically Ill Infant and Child, Chapter 125: Caring for Children Dying from Chronic Disease, p 496)

Answer 9-21. c

When discussing impending death with children, their cognitive understanding of death should be considered. Under age 2, no discussion of death will be understood and, therefore, the focus should be physical comfort measures including holding and hugging. For children aged 2–7, death is seen as temporary, reversible, and possibly magical. Children of this age may attempt to correct misperceptions about the cause of their illness, and may experience feelings of guilt and self-blame. Beginning around age 7, children begin to perceive reality and causation. They need to know the details of how their pain and symptoms will be treated. With adolescents, it is important to address concerns about physical changes as well as give them the opportunity to express their anger.

(Section 9: The Chronically Ill Infant and Child, Chapter 125: Caring for Children Dying from Chronic Disease, p 496)

Answer 9-22. e

Providing end-of-life care at home is an enormous responsibility for any family. They must have some basic resource available including a telephone, transportation, and a space for the sick child that offers quiet and privacy. The physician for the child and home health-care services should be readily accessible. Respite facilities can be essential to providing families needed breaks.

Children are more comfortable in their own home environment; families can also carry on some aspects of their normal activities at home. When family members have the opportunity to participate in the care of the child, it allows families a greater sense of control. There is an opportunity for strengthening of relationships prior to the child's death.

(Section 9: The Chronically Ill Infant and Child, Chapter 125: Caring for Children Dying from Chronic Disease, p 498)

Answer 9-23. a

Patients for whom palliative care should be considered are (1) those where treatment is possible but may fail, (2) those requiring intensive long-term treatment aimed at maintaining the quality of life, and (3) those with a severe disability resulting in vulnerability to health complications and progressive decline in health and function. Answers b–e above describe conditions for which there is currently no curative therapy available.

(Section 9: The Chronically Ill Infant and Child, Chapter 126: Hospice and Palliative Care, p 501)

Answer 9-24. a

Palliative care teams can assist the health-care team in managing the distress that can come with caring for a child with a serious illness. Interdisciplinary teams can assure that the physical, emotional, spiritual, and practical needs of children and families are identified and met and that a supportive environment is provided for health-care team members. Choice a above describes the role of social workers; Choice b, the role of child life specialists; Choice c, the role of Chaplains; and Choice d, the role of physicians and advanced practice nurses.

(Section 9: The Chronically Ill Infant and Child, Chapter 126: Hospice and Palliative Care, p 502)

Answer 9-25. a

Parents of children with terminal illness may inquire about pursuing experimental options such as phase I clinical trials. Generally, the likelihood of significant benefit from phase I trials is limited, typically under 8%. Misconceptions about the purpose of phase I trials are common, including the belief that the purpose of such a trial is to benefit them personally, rather than to benefit future patients. Clarity about the purpose of a clinical trial is important to allow parents and children to make informed decisions about whether such therapy will help to meet their goals.

(Section 9: The Chronically Ill Infant and Child, Chapter 125: Caring for Children Dying from Chronic Disease, p 495)

Answer 9-26. d

Some of the more common interventions for children with severe developmental disability include gastrostomy feeding tube, anti-reflux surgery, and tracheostomy. However, there is limited evidence available for these interventions. The benefit of a tracheostomy is unclear. A review of tracheostomy identified 27% mortality in neurologically impaired patients compared with 11% or less mortality for conditions of airway obstruction. This likely reflects greater benefit for those with airway obstruction than with chronic pulmonary aspiration.

Although the improvement in life expectancy for the most medically fragile children with cerebral palsy is felt to be a result of gastrostomy feeding tubes, there are no studies to guide which children benefit. Anti-reflux surgery does not routinely alter respiratory symptoms or frequency of pneumonia, although it is still offered for this purpose. Salivary duct ligation decreases drooling but does not alter the frequency of pneumonia or respiratory symptoms in children with chronic pulmonary aspiration.

(Section 9: The Chronically Ill Infant and Child, Chapter 126: Hospice and Palliative Care, p 503 (only in e-version))

Answer 9-27. e

Pain assessment involving rating of pain must be appropriate to the child's cognitive level. This involves discussions with parents and caregivers to determine a child's developmental age, then using a validated pain rating system appropriate for that stage of development. Pain rating tools appropriate for children aged 5–6 years include poker chips and Oucher scale. Children from ages 7 to 10 can begin using tools to quantify pain, such as the Wong–Baker FACES® Pain Rating Scale. Adolescents can use a numerical 1–10 pain rating scale.

(Section 9: The Chronically Ill Infant and Child, Chapter 126: Hospice and Palliative Care, p 503)

Answer 9-28. a

Somatic nociceptive pain is caused by stimulation of nociceptors as a result of tissue injury. Nociceptive somatic pain is well localized and described as sharp, aching, squeezing, stabbing, or throbbing. Neuropathic pain is caused by abnormal functioning of damaged sensory nerves. Neuropathic pain is usually described as burning, shooting, or tingling. Visceral nociceptive pain is caused by stimulation of nociceptors and stretch receptors in the viscera; it is usually poorly localized and often described as dull, crampy, or achy. Radicular pain usually occurs in a dermatomal distribution. Since this boy has a known etiology for his pain, there is no reason to suspect psychogenic pain.

(Section 9: The Chronically Ill Infant and Child, Chapter 126: Hospice and Palliative Care, p 505)

Answer 9-29. d

The World Health Organization (WHO) analgesic ladder provides general guidelines for choosing the drug based on the degree of pain. Nonopioids such as acetaminophen and NSAIDs can be used for mild pain, tramadol for moderate pain, and opioids for severe pain. Nonopioids used for mild pain should always be considered as adjuvant therapy when using opioids for moderate to severe pain. Morphine, fentanyl, hydromorphone, and oxycodone are all acceptable choices for opiates to be used in the management of severe pain. However, codeine should be avoided because it is ineffective in approximately one third of individuals due to a genetic variation in its metabolism to morphine.

(Section 9: The Chronically Ill Infant and Child, Chapter 126: Hospice and Palliative Care, p 505)

Answer 9-30. d

The World Health Organization (WHO) analgesic ladder provides general guidelines for choosing the drug based on the degree of pain. Nonopioids such as acetaminophen and

NSAIDs can be used for mild pain, tramadol for moderate pain, and opioids for severe pain.

Children with renal impairment merit special consideration due to their impaired abilities to metabolize and excrete opiates. Fentanyl and methadone are considered the safest opiates, oxycodone and hydromorphone should be used with caution, and morphine sulfate should be avoided.

(Section 9: The Chronically Ill Infant and Child, Chapter 126: Hospice and Palliative Care, p 506)

Answer 9-31. c

Psychopharmacologic treatment should be considered in patients whose symptoms of depression and anxiety persist despite nonpharmacologic interventions, in patients that meet diagnostic criteria, or have disorders of greater severity. When using pharmacologic treatment, it is important to continue to offer supportive counseling and psychosocial interventions to assist the child in reducing symptoms.

Important points to keep in mind when using SSRIs include:

1. Anticipation of 2–4 weeks to see benefit.
2. Patients may experience side effects that can include dry mouth, constipation, urinary retention, sedation, anxiety, agitation, insomnia, irritability, impulsivity, akathisia, and hypomania.
3. Providers must monitor for suicidal thoughts.
4. Discontinuation syndrome occurs when SSRIs are stopped abruptly with symptoms including anxiety, irritability, dizziness, nausea, fatigue, myalgias, and chills.
5. There is a risk of serotonin syndrome, usually with drug–drug interaction.

(Section 9: The Chronically Ill Infant and Child, Chapter 126: Hospice and Palliative Care, p 508)

Answer 9-32. e

It is permissible to discontinue artificial nutrition and hydration when it is contributing to suffering. Its discontinuation can lessen discomfort due to decreased oral and airway secretions, leading to less choking and dyspnea. Ketosis also produces a sense of well-being, analgesia, and mild euphoria. When artificial nutrition and hydration are discontinued, it is helpful for families to estimate the length of time that may pass until death occurs, usually 10–14 days. This time period can be shorter when there is organ malfunction and longer when fluids are used for flushes after medication administration.

(Section 9: The Chronically Ill Infant and Child, Chapter 126: Hospice and Palliative Care, p 510)

Answer 9-33. c

While certain treatments may seem futile to providers because they will not improve the outcome of the fatal illness, these treatments may seem vital to families for whom they allow prolonged time with their child. In such cases, taking the time to find out what the parents think, correcting misconceptions, and building trust may lead to agreement on a treatment plan, and thus should always be the first step in approaching the situation. While it may ultimately be necessary to involve the courts or establish a DNR order, it would be inappropriate to do so without attempting discussion with the family in advance around goals of care. Avoiding discussions around the topic or involving CPS are inappropriate choices.

(Section 9: The Chronically Ill Infant and Child, Chapter 127: Law, Ethics, and Caring Near End of Life, p 510)

Answer 9-34. e

Currently all states in the United State allow minors to confidentially obtain treatment for sexually transmitted infections, and alcohol and drug problems without parental knowledge. This consideration is based on ample evidence that teenagers would not seek treatment for these conditions if parental involvement were required.

Minors have the right to refuse to participate in research, but if there is a prospect of direct benefit to the child and no alternative therapy is likely to be as effective, a parent may override the child's refusal. Minors are currently unable to sign a durable power of attorney or a living will. About half the states in the United States allow minors at a specified age (14–16) to consent to any medical care without parental involvement, but many state legislatures exempted abortions from their minor consent statutes. Courts in only a few states have held that if a minor clearly understands the consequences of refusing treatment, he or she may do so even if that consequence is death.

(Section 9: The Chronically Ill Infant and Child, Chapter 127: Law, Ethics, and Caring Near End of Life, Page 511)

Answer 9-35. c

Acute adverse effects of opiates such as respiratory depression and hypotension must be addressed immediately and subsequent dosing of the drugs should be titrated to avoid these side-effects. For other side effects of opiates, such as sedation and nausea, symptom improvement may occur after several days even without dose adjustment. Laxative regimens should be started whenever opioids are prescribed to prevent constipation.

(Section 9: The Chronically Ill Infant and Child, Chapter 126: Hospice and Palliative Care, p 506)

Answer 9-36. c

Anorexia and cachexia are common in children with advanced cancers. Contributors include poor nutritional intake, increased metabolic demands, impaired taste, and depression. When possible, treatment should be directed at identifiable causes. Choices for pharmacologic interventions to increase appetite include corticosteroids and cannabinoids such as dronabinol and megestrol acetate. Megestrol acetate should be used with caution because it is associated with severe adrenal suppression in children with cancer. Some practitioners even recommend routine steroid replacement therapy for children who have been prescribed megestrol acetate.

(Section 9: The Chronically Ill Infant and Child, Chapter 126: Hospice and Palliative Care, p 507)

Answer 9-37. e

Unless pain is infrequent, an opioid should be given on an around-the-clock schedule based on the duration of analgesic effect of the specific opioid. Once the opioid requirement is determined, it can be converted to a sustained release given 2 or 3 times daily and a fast-acting medication can be used as needed for breakthrough pain.

Methadone is an important long-acting option and is available as a liquid. However, titration of methadone can be complicated by its slow elimination phase (half-life 4.2–130 hours). This long duration can result in drug accumulation and toxicity 2–5 days after starting or increasing methadone. Morphine, hydromorphone, fentanyl, and oxycodone do not have an extended elimination phase.

(Section 9: The Chronically Ill Infant and Child, Chapter 126: Hospice and Palliative Care, p 506)

CHAPTER 10 | Transplantation

Marie H. Tanzer and David B. Kershaw

10-1. You are seeing a 26-month-old boy with ESRD secondary to dysplastic kidneys, currently managed on peritoneal dialysis. He is in the clinic with his parents for kidney transplant evaluation. His parents are asking about complications of transplant and would like to know his risk factors for development of post-transplant lymphoproliferative disorder (PTLD). Which of the following is an associated risk factor for development of PTLD?

a. EBV seronegative status pretransplant

b. Female gender

c. Age >5 years old

d. CMV seropositive status pretransplant

e. Asian race

10-2. A 13-year-old girl presents to your clinic with low-grade fever and URI symptoms for 3 days. She has a history of end-stage kidney disease secondary to reflux nephropathy, s/p transplant 6 years ago. Her kidney function has been stable over the past few years with a baseline creatinine of 0.8. Her medications include prednisone, tacrolimus mycophenolate mofetil (eg, CellCept, myfortic) and ferrous sulfate. She does not require any medicine for blood pressure.

For her acute illness, you decide to start her on treatment with azithromycin. Four days later, her Mom calls to report that her fever and respiratory symptoms have improved, but now she is feeling shaky and her blood pressures have increased from her baseline of 110s/70s to 140s/90s. Her diet has not changed and she continues to drink her usual 2.5 L of fluid daily. Her Mom is concerned about her kidney function so you order labs with the following results: Sodium 138, potassium 6, Chloride 102, CO_2 22, BUN 27, creatinine 1.2, glucose 70, calcium 9, phosphorus 4.2.

What is your next step in evaluation of this patient?

a. Obtain a history of caffeine consumption

b. Order a renal ultrasound with dopplers

c. Check a tacrolimus level

d. Check fractionated serum metanephrines

e. Check serum and urine electrolytes for a FeNa

10-3. You are seeing a 4-year-old boy in your primary care clinic for routine well child care. He has a history of hypoplastic left heart and he received a heart transplant at 18 months of age. His transplant is functioning well and his cardiologist is happy with his progress. His current medications include prednisone and tacrolimus. Mom is asking whether he needs any vaccines today. You review his chart and note that he is due for a number of vaccines.

Which of the following vaccines is contraindicated for this patient?

a. DTaP

b. MMR

c. PPSV

d. IPV

e. MCV4

10-4. All of the following medications may contribute to the development of renal dysfunction in patients with solid organ (heart, liver, kidney, intestine) or hematopoietic cell transplant EXCEPT…

a. Tacrolimus

b. Ganciclovir

c. Sirolimus

d. Vancomycin

e. Mycophenolate mofetil

10-5. The mother of an 8-year-old boy with a history of biliary atresia, s/p liver transplant at 7 months of age, calls your clinic. Her son was at a sleepover party 2 nights ago with a friend who was diagnosed with chicken pox the next day. His current immunosuppression includes tacrolimus and prednisone. The mom reports her son is well, without any signs of illness. What is the appropriate management of this patient?

   a. Monitor for chicken pox lesions and give varicella immune globulin if he develops any

   b. Measure serum IgM and IgG levels to varicella and prescribe immune globulin if IgM positive

   c. Prescribe antibiotics to prevent superinfection of any developing varicella lesions

   d. Administer varicella immune globulin and continue to monitor for signs of illness

   e. Monitor for signs of chicken pox and treat symptoms of illness

10-6. A 7-year-old girl presents to the emergency department (ED) with severe diarrhea for the past 4 days. She received a kidney transplant 5 years ago for dysplastic kidneys.

His mother reports she has been maintaining her usual daily fluid goal of 2 L and drinking above that to keep up with the diarrhea. Her urine output has not changed. Her mother reports that she has also been more hypertensive over the past 24 hours, with blood pressures ranging in the 130s mm Hg systolic, though she is usually stable in the 100–110s mm Hg systolic. She has continued to take all her usual immunosuppression medications including prednisone, tacrolimus, and cellcept.

You obtain the following labs in the ED:

Sodium 134, potassium 6, chloride 94, HCO_3 16, BUN 48, creatinine 0.8 (baseline 0.5), glucose 82, calcium 11, phos 5.8. Stool studies are pending.

Which of the following pieces of information will help you diagnose the most likely cause of this child's acute kidney injury?

   a. Serum tacrolimus level

   b. Kidney biopsy

   c. Transtubular potassium gradient

   d. Stool studies

   e. Urine culture

10-7. You are seeing a 15-year-old boy for routine well-child care. He has a history of liver transplant 10 years ago for Alagille syndrome. He is maintained on prednisone and tacrolimus for immunosuppression.

For this patient on chronic immunosuppression, which of the following examinations/evaluations is NOT required on a routine basis?

   a. Eye exam

   b. Skin exam

   c. Blood pressure measurement

   d. Lipid panel

   e. Hearing evaluation

10-8. A 13-year-old boy s/p liver transplant 9 years ago comes to your office with complaint of daily right hip pain for the past few weeks.

His liver function was stable when checked 1 month ago. He had a runny nose and fever a week ago, but this has resolved. His current immunosuppression consists of daily prednisone and tacrolimus. He is on a regular daily multivitamin. His mother is concerned that "he is short" compared to all his friends. Physical exam is remarkable for height and weight <3rd percentile for his age and mild pain with internal and external rotation of his right hip, otherwise it is normal.

Of the following, you are most concerned that this boy's symptoms are being caused by the following conditions?

   a. Septic arthritis due to immunosuppression

   b. Chronic steroid use

   c. Chronic malnutrition

   d. Medication nonadherence and graft failure

   e. Growth hormone deficiency

10-9. An 11-month-old boy underwent liver transplant for cholestatic liver disease 6 days ago. He received a deceased-donor split liver. Initially his LFTs were trending down, but in the past day they have started to trend up and his total bilirubin level is also rising. This morning he developed a fever and abdominal distension, thus he was made NPO. An abdominal ultrasound is ordered, which demonstrates abdominal free fluid and minimal arterial signal on doppler evaluation over the hepatic artery.

What is the PRIMARY process leading to these complications?

   a. Acute cellular rejection

   b. Acute bacterial cholangitis

   c. Hepatic artery thrombosis

   d. Primary graft nonfunction

   e. Post-transplant coagulopathy

10-10. A 15-week-old boy presents to the emergency room for evaluation of poor appetite, weight loss, abdominal distension, and decreased energy. Labs reveal elevated AST, ALT, and total bilirubin. Stool patterns have changed and are now described as "pale" in color.

What is the most common reason for liver failure and need for liver transplantation in patients this age?

a. Wilson disease

b. Autoimmune hepatitis

c. Viral hepatitis

d. Biliary atresia

e. Tylenol-induced hepatic necrosis

10-11. You are seeing a 16-year-old boy for follow-up in a transplant clinic. The patient had a history of end-stage renal disease of unknown etiology, and had been anuric, managed on hemodialysis for 6 months.

Two weeks ago he received a living unrelated kidney transplant. The surgery was uncomplicated and his creatinine came down from a pretransplant level of 4.5 mg/dL to 0.7 mg/dL at the time of discharge. He was discharged 1 week ago and presents today for his first follow-up visit. He reports he is drinking 2.5 L of fluid daily, voiding every few hours, and taking all his medications as directed. He reports that he is feeling well without any fevers or dysuria, but he has had lower extremity edema for the past 2 days.

His labs demonstrate the following:

Serum: Na 136, K 4, Cl 101, CO_2 23, BUN 27, Cr 1.0, Alb 2.4, glu 91, Ca 8, phos 3.2, C3 115 (normal)

Urine: S.G. 1.015, (+) LE, 500 protein, 25 blood.

Statistically, which of the following was the most likely cause of this patient's *initial* kidney failure?

a. Membranoproliferative glomerulonephritis

b. Hemolytic uremic syndrome

c. IgA nephropathy

d. Focal segmental glomerulosclerosis

e. Anti-GBM nephritis

10-12. You are seeing a 17-year-old girl in your primary care clinic for evaluation for depression. She has a history of end-stage kidney disease secondary to renal dysplasia and received a deceased donor kidney transplant at age 2.

Over the past few months, she has been having increasing fatigue and depression. She agrees school has been particularly stressful lately as she has been working on college applications, preparing for college entrance examinations, and participating on the swim team. As a result, she had not followed up with her nephrologist in the last 6 months.

When she went back last week, her nephrologist told her that she would have to "go on dialysis soon." She reports that she has been adherent with her transplant medications and meets her daily total fluid goal of 2.5 L. She has been eating, voiding, and stooling normally. She is upset and does not understand why her kidney is failing.

Statistically, which of the following is the most likely cause for graft loss?

a. Chronic allograft nephropathy

b. Acute rejection

c. Medication nonadherence

d. Vascular thrombosis

e. BK nephropathy

10-13. A 5-year-old boy comes in with intestinal failure and evaluation for intestinal transplant. In discussing outcomes with the family you explain that 1 year outcomes for intestinal transplant recipients are excellent at around 90% but the 5-year survival is only about 60%.

You also explain that the leading cause of death in intestinal transplant patients is:

a. Rejection of intestinal allograft

b. Post-transplant lymphoproliferative disease

c. Infection

d. Surgical complications

e. Cardiac arrest due to electrolyte complications

10-14. A 15-year-old girl with a history of T-cell lymphoma received a hematopoietic stem cell transplant after a myeloablative conditioning regimen 100 days ago. Her early course was unremarkable except for mild CMV infection. She presents to the office with a cough, low grade fever, and dyspnea. She has tachypnea and her chest radiograph is normal. She reports she has been missing one of her medications for the past 2 months.

This medication is most likely:

a. Acyclovir

b. Ferrous sulfate

c. Prednisone

d. Tacrolimus

e. Trimethoprim-sulfamethoxazole

10-15. A 17-year-old boy develops dyspnea and exercise intolerance 5 years after receiving a cardiac transplant for a dilated cardiomyopathy. He and his family have been adherent with his immunosuppressive regimen and he has had an uneventful course except for an early CMV infection. His EKG shows ischemic changes and his ECHO shows decreased function with focal wall abnormalities. He undergoes a cardiac catheterization and biopsy.

Which of the following processes is most likely to be present?

a. Acute cellular rejection

b. Carnitine deficiency

c. CMV cardiomyopathy

d. Graft vasculopathy

e. Recurrent disease

10-16. A 5-year-old boy with a history of ALL who failed to attain remission received an allogeneic stem cell transplant from his non-HLA identical sibling 2 years ago. He had an early complicated course with moderate sinusoidal obstruction and acute GVHD. At this time, he demonstrates weight loss, rash, restrictive lung disease, and elevated liver enzymes. Bowel biopsy shows chronic GVHD. He does not respond to methylprednisone and is placed on mycophenolate mofetil.

In talking with the family, you can tell the family that they can expect that 1 year from now:

a. His disease may progress despite treatment

b. He has over a 80% chance of being alive

c. He will be off antibiotics

d. He will be off immunosuppression

e. Other organs will not become involved

10-17. A 4-year-old with a history of acute lymphoblastic leukemia who has relapsed is being evaluated for hematopoetic cell transplant. His parents, along with a twin sibling and 2 other older siblings, are potential donors. Which source of stem cells will present the highest risk of graft versus host disease:

a. Bone-marrow transplant from an unrelated donor with a HLA genetic match

b. Bone-marrow transplant from an identical twin

c. Cord blood transplant from an unrelated donor with a HLA antigen match

d. Peripheral blood stem cell transplant from a sibling with a HLA antigen match

e. Peripheral blood stem cell transplant using pooled donations from parents

10-18. A 15-year-old girl who had a stem cell transplant at 20 months of age comes in for well child care. She was transplanted for a nonmalignant condition without prior chemotherapy. She had problems with chronic GVHD that required prolonged steroid therapy.

In reviewing the potential late effects of her transplant, the least likely complication would be:

a. Alopecia

b. Cataracts

c. Deceased bone mineral density

d. Pulmonary disease

e. Thyroid disorder

10-19. The wait-list mortality in pediatric solid organ transplant varies by organ and age.

Overall, which organs represent the highest and lowest waitlist mortality, respectively?

a. Heart highest, liver lowest

b. Heart highest, kidney lowest

c. Intestine highest, kidney lowest

d. Intestine highest, liver lowest

e. Liver highest, intestine lowest

10-20. A 16-month-old girl with a history of liver failure due to biliary atresia, status post liver transplant 2 months ago, presents for routine follow-up. Her post-transplant course has been fairly unremarkable. Her routine labs are all within normal limits apart from a hemoglobin of 8.8 and WBC 2.7. She has no evidence of active bleeding and stool hemoccult is negative and no evidence of active infection. You suspect that one of her medications is causing the anemia.

Which of the following medications prescribed to this patient is least likely to be responsible for this anemia?

a. Trimethoprim and sulfamethoxazole (Bactrim)

b. Fluconazole

c. Tacrolimus

d. Mycophenolate mofetil

e. Valganciclovir (Valcyte)

ANSWERS

Answer 10-1. a

The majority of PTLD cases are associated with primary EBV infection post transplant, either from an EBV (+) graft or from community acquired infection. By adulthood, most people have been exposed to EBV and have developed immunity to it. This immunity is protective as immunosuppression post transplant leads to significant T-cell suppression, making it difficult to mount an immune response to a new EBV infection. On the other hand, children are more likely to be EBV negative, putting them at risk of developing EBV viremia with exposure to an EBV positive organ or EBV infection from the community.

Option b is incorrect as PTLD is associated with male gender. Option d is incorrect as primary CMV infection is associated with greater risk for PTLD development. Options c and E are incorrect as children < age 5 and of Caucasian race are associated with higher risk for development of PTLD in kidney transplant recipients.

(Chapter 128, p 516 "Post Transplant Lymphoproliferative Disorder" and p 520 "Management Issues in the Renal Transplant Patient")

Answer 10-2. c

The patient in this vignette has all the signs and symptoms consistent with tacrolimus toxicity: hyperkalemia, acute kidney injury, hypertension, and tremors. Tacrolimus and cyclosporine (calcineurin inhibitors) are metabolized by the cytochrome p450 enzyme system. In a patient on a stable immunosuppression regimen, many medications that interact with this system can lead to increased or decreased metabolism of tacrolimus.

Common medications that decrease tacrolimus metabolism and lead to increased serum levels include fluconazole, ketoconazole, and macrolide antibiotics. Metoclopromide and cimetidine can also increase tacrolimus levels. Ideally, one should try to avoid these medications in patients taking a calcineurin inhibitor. However, if the medication is absolutely necessary, care must be taken to adjust the dose of the tacrolimus and cyclosporine at the start of therapy with the interfering agent, as well as follow drug levels until the interfering medication is completed.

Options a, b, and d are all appropriate evaluations to perform in someone with new onset hypertension and option e is an appropriate evaluation to perform in someone with acute kidney injury. However, this patient has been stable for some time and she is demonstrating a classic presentation for tacrolimus toxicity. Consequently, before performing a more involved evaluation of hypertension and acute kidney injury, it is appropriate to start with evaluation of the tacrolimus level. If the level is normal, proceeding to these other tests would be appropriate.

(Chapter 128, p 518 "Drug Interactions")

Answer 10-3. b

MMR is a live-virus vaccine which is contraindicated in patients receiving immunosuppressive therapy. These vaccines may be administered up to 1 month prior to transplantation, but should not be given post transplant. It is for this reason that it is critical to make sure any child undergoing evaluation for transplant receives all appropriate vaccines, particularly live-virus vaccines.

All of the remaining vaccines are inactivated vaccines and are safe for administration post transplant. It is recommended that children with transplants continue to receive all the usual recommended vaccines for children of their age (apart from live-virus vaccines). It is notable that in patients on chronic immunosuppression, vaccines will be less immunogenic. For this reason, it is recommended that vaccines not be given in the first 6 months post transplant when immunosuppression is at its highest. Otherwise all routine vaccines should be administered as any immunity conferred by vaccines is better than no immunity in an otherwise immunosuppressed patient.

PPSV and MCV4 are not absolutely indicated for well-children, but for this child who is chronically immunosuppressed, it would be indicated to administer these vaccines if he has not yet received them.

In immunosuppressed transplant patients, influenza vaccination with the inactivated form is indicated annually.

(Chapter 128, p 518 "Vaccinations")

Answer 10-4. e

Tacrolimus and other calcineurin inhibitors (immunosuppressive agents) are the most common cause of nephrotoxicity in transplant patients. These medicines lead to an acute reduction in renal blood flow and long-term chronic changes such as tubular atrophy and interstitial fibrosis. Ganciclovir (used to treat CMV infection) is associated with interstitial changes and reduction in GFR. Sirolimus (an immunosuppressive agent) can lead to proteinuria. Vancomycin (for acute bacterial infections) is associated with tubular toxicity. Mycophenolate mofetil is not generally associated with any renal toxicity.

(Chapter 128, p 517 "Renal Complications")

Answer 10-5. d

It is notable that the boy in this vignette received his transplant prior to his first birthday, thus it is unlikely that he ever received live-virus vaccines such as MMR and varicella. Consequently, it is imperative to administer the immune globulin as quickly as possible. Given the severity of infection that can occur in these patients, it is not appropriate to delay treatment by monitoring for symptoms or checking labs (Answers a, b, and d). An immunocompromised patient is at higher risk of bacterial superinfection of varicella lesions;

however, until evidence of this occurs, it is not appropriate to prescribe antibiotics (Answer c).

(Chapter 128, p 518 "Vaccinations")

Answer 10-6. a

Diarrheal illnesses can have a significant impact on immunosuppression absorption, particularly for calcineurin inhibitors. Diarrhea can lead to poor absorption of cyclosporine, but increased absorption of tacrolimus. The girl in this vignette has had significant diarrhea for several days and is maintained on tacrolimus. As a result, she is at risk for developing supratherapeutic levels of tacrolimus, leading to the acute kidney injury, hypertension, and hyperkalemia. In this case, it is imperative to measure a tacrolimus level.

A kidney biopsy may be indicated if the creatinine does not improve with hydration and adjustment of the tacrolimus. Fractional excretion of sodium will help you determine whether this child has significant intravascular volume depletion, though the mother reports she is drinking well and she has been hypertensive, so this is less likely. Stool studies may help identify the cause of the diarrhea, but will not immediately address the acute kidney injury. Urine culture is also indicated in transplant patients with acute kidney injury to evaluate for infection, but there is nothing in the history to support this as the most likely etiology of her acute kidney injury.

(Chapter 128, p 518 "Intercurrent Illness Management")

Answer 10-7. e

Chronic immunosuppression may lead to a variety of complications, requiring routine surveillance monitoring; however, hearing changes are not generally associated with chronic immunosuppression therapy.

Steroids lead to glaucoma and cataracts, requiring annual ophthalmologic evaluations. They also lead to hypertension and hyperlipidemia requiring regular lipid screening and blood pressure monitoring. Patients on chronic immunosuppression such as tacrolimus are at risk for developing skin malignancies, thus routine monitoring for new or changing skin lesions is critical.

(Chapter 128, pp 516–518 "Long-Term Management of Solid Organ Recipient")

Answer 10-8. b

The child in this vignette is demonstrating evidence of poor bone growth and bone demineralization secondary to chronic steroid use. He has been on steroids for most of his life and he has poor growth secondary to the chronic steroid use. Specifically, one should have a high suspicion for avascular necrosis, which can occur in up to 1% of transplant patients secondary to chronic steroid use.

Septic arthritis would have a more toxic presentation. Chronic malnutrition and growth hormone deficiencies are

considerations for the poor growth, but would not explain the hip pain. Nothing in this vignette indicates the patient is nonadherent and there are no symptoms of graft failure.

(Chapter 128, p 517 "Bone and Growth Complications")

Answer 10-9. c

The patient in this vignette has signs of bile leak and peritonitis secondary to hepatic artery thrombosis. His liver ultrasound demonstrates minimal arterial signal, consistent with a primary diagnosis of hepatic artery thrombosis (HAT), seen in up to 10% of pediatric liver recipients. Children <1 year of age are at highest risk of developing HAT. Other risk factors include poor arterial influx, graft edema, and hypercoagulable conditions. Sequelae of HAT include biliary necrosis leading to biliary leak or stricture, as seen in the patient in this vignette.

Acute cellular rejection is incorrect as one would not expect diminished arterial flow on doppler evaluation, though one may see a bump in LFTs and bilirubin in acute cellular rejection. This child may develop bacterial cholangitis as sequelae, but it is not the primary process in this case. Primary graft nonfunction would be seen in the immediate post-transplant period; this child has been recovering well for several days prior to this presentation. Post-transplant coagulopathy is not an entity.

(Chapter 130, p 524 "Complications of Liver Transplantation")

Answer 10-10. d

The majority of children are referred for liver transplantation due to cholestatic liver disease. Of these, biliary atresia accounts for approximately 45% of children undergoing liver transplant. Wilson disease, autoimmune hepatitis, viral hepatitis, and Tylenol-induced hepatic necrosis are also causes of transplant, but less commonly than cholestatic disease.

(Chapter 130, p 522, "Indications for Liver Transplantation")

Answer 10-11. d

While all of the listed glomerular diseases may recur in a renal transplant, the one with the highest rate of symptomatic recurrence is FSGS. Rates of recurrence of FSGS in pediatric kidney transplants can be as high as 50% and can be seen days to weeks following transplant. In the clinic, this patient demonstrates a low serum albumin, proteinuria, edema, and an increase in creatinine, all consistent with recurrence of FSGS. This diagnosis can be confirmed by kidney biopsy.

(Chapter 129, p 520 "Recurrence of Original Disease in Allograft")

Answer 10-12. a

Chronic allograft nephropathy is the leading cause of graft failure (41%). As per North American Pediatric Rental Trials and Cooperative Studies (NAPTRCS) data, the 5-year graft survival for deceased donor transplants is 68% in children.

This patient with a deceased donor graft has had it for 15 years, placing her at high risk for having chronic allograft nephropathy.

Untreated acute rejection, medication nonadherence, and BK nephropathy are causes of graft failure, but are less likely from an epidemiologic standpoint. Vascular thrombosis tends to occur in the immediate post-transplant period.

(Chapter 129, p 519 "Graft Survival")

Answer 10-13. c

The main cause of readmissions and death for intestinal transplant recipients is infection. In the early post-transplant period, bacterial and fungal infections are common. After the initial postoperative period, infectious enteritis is common and can be due to viral or bacterial pathogens. Infections seen in other organ transplant recipients are also prevalent. Prophylaxis and/or surveillance for *Pneumocystis jiroveci*, Epstein–Barr, and Cytomegalovirus is recommended.

Recipients of intestinal transplantation face a number of other specific risks due to a narrow effective therapeutic window for immunosuppression, inherent bacterial colonization of graft, perioperative nutritional issues, and technical surgical considerations. Complications such as obstruction or perforation can be a manifestation of a surgical complication, graft dysfunction, or post-transplant lymphoproliferative disease. Many of these processes, or their treatment, may be complicated by infection.

(Chapter 131, p 527 "Infections")

Answer 10-14. e

Pulmonary complications are a leading cause of death in hematopoietic cell transplant recipients occurring in 40–60% of patients. In the first month post-transplant, noninfectious causes such as pulmonary edema, pulmonary hemorrhage, and idiopathic pneumonia syndrome may occur and antimicrobial prophylaxis is used to prevent infection. At this time, the patient has persistently decreased cellular immunity and is at risk for bacterial and nonbacterial infections.

Her presentation with fever, cough, dyspnea, and tachypnea is concerning for a number of processes including viral infections, bacterial infections, and bronchiolitis obliterans. Her lack of infiltrates on her CXR at this time makes these less likely. Definitive diagnosis may require specimen obtained by bronchoalveolar lavage. At this time point she is at high risk for *Pneumocystis jiroveci*, especially if her prophylaxis (commonly Trimethoprim-sulfamethoxazole or pentamidine) was not taken. The early course of *Pneumocystis jiroveci* infection in a non-HIV infected immunocompromised host can be indolent and include minimal clinical signs and symptoms (dry cough and tachypnea with a normal chest radiograph). Definitive diagnosis is made by showing the organism in sputum or bronchoalveolar lavage specimens by immunofluorescence or staining.

(Chapter 133, p 534 "Infections following Hemopoietic Cell Transplantation")

Answer 10-15. d

Heart transplant has complications similar to other transplants (eg, technical problems, infections, and medication side effects) but also the added complication of accelerated atherosclerotic heart disease and graft vasculopathy. This patient's early CMV infection puts him at higher risk of graft vasculopathy. His symptoms of decreased cardiac function could be due to a late rejection but the ischemic changes on EKG and focal wall motion changes on ECHO would make graft vasculopathy more likely. The other possibilities listed (Carnitine deficiency, CMV cardiomyopathy, and recurrent disease) are much less likely than graft vasculopathy (17% prevalence at 5 years) and would usually cause a uniform decrease in function.

(Chapter 132, p 530 "Graft Vasculopathy")

Answer 10-16. a

This patient has chronic GVHD which has failed to respond to glucocorticoids. Chronic refractory GVHD requires prolonged immunosuppressive therapy and antibiotic prophylaxis to prevent morbidity and mortality from infection. Unfortunately, patients with refractory chronic GVHD requiring secondary agents may have progressive organ complications and 35% mortality at 2 years.

(Chapter 133, p 536 "Treatment of GVHD")

Answer 10-17. e

Stem cell sources are ranked from lowest to highest risk for development of graft versus host disease as follows: (1) A syngeneic (identical twin) donor or HLA identical sibling. (2) Unrelated donors with HLA antigen match. (3) Umbilical cord blood can allow less stringent HLA matching between donor and recipient (ie, some mismatch). (4) Peripheral blood stem cells from a parent can be used with difficulty (by definition haploidentical) but using pooled donations from both parents would be not be done due to presence of multiple mismatch HLA antigens.

(Chapter 133, p 531 "Stem Cell Source" and "Donor Type")

Answer 10-18. a

The late complications of hematopoietic cell transplantation can involve many organs and may be related to myeloablative chemotherapy, radiation, chronic steroid or immunosuppressive use, infections, or GVHD. This patient is at risk for complications of her prolonged steroid therapy (cataracts, and decreased bone mineral density). Pulmonary disease develops in 15–25% and thyroid abnormalities are observed in 10–40% of patients after hematopoietic cell transplantation. Patients who undergo hematopoietic cell transplantation for nonmalignant disease without prior chemotherapy are unlikely to have permanent alopecia.

(Chapter 133, p 537 "Late Effects after Hematopoietic Cell Transplantation")

Answer 10-19. c

The limited supply of size-matched deceased donors for pediatric intestinal transplant candidates leads to the highest waitlist mortality of any group waiting for a solid organ transplant. Mortality on the pediatric transplant liver waitlist is approximately a third of that of the pediatric intestinal waitlist, but is strongly influenced by high mortality in the <1-year-old waitlist candidates. The waitlist mortality for pediatric heart recipients is between 10% and 31%. The kidney transplant waitlist mortality is low due to the availability of effective organ replacement therapy (dialysis).

(Chapter 131, p 525 "Epidemiology")

Answer 10-20. b

Trimethoprim and sulfamethoxazole (Bactrim) can be associated with anemia due to hemolysis or aplastic anemia as well as leukopenia. Tacrolimus can cause calcineurin-associated hemolytic uremic syndrome with anemia. Mycophenolate mofetil is associated with overall marrow suppression, though particularly neutropenia. Valganciclovir (Valcyte) is associated with pancytopenia. Fluconazole is the only agent not associated with any marrow suppression.

(Chapter 128, p 514 "Immunosuppression" and pp 516–517 "Long-Term Management of the Solid Organ Recipient")

CHAPTER 11 | Disorders of Metabolism

Ayesha Ahmad

11-1. Most inborn errors of metabolism (IEM) are inherited by an autosomal recessive mode of inheritance. An example of an inborn error of metabolism with X-linked recessive inheritance and significant variability in clinical phenotype is:

   a. Ornithine transcarbamylase (OTC) deficiency

   b. Propionic acidemia

   c. Methylmalonic acidemia

   d. Biotinidase deficiency

   e. Citrullinemia

11-2. The next 2 questions relate to the following clinical vignette:

A 3-day-old male neonate presents to the emergency department (ED) with a 1-day history of poor feeding. He was born to a 21-year-old primigravida after a normal pregnancy and delivery. In the ED you note that he is lethargic. Vitals reveal normal temperature and normal blood pressure for age. During your evaluation, he is noted to become increasingly lethargic. Arterial blood gas reveals a respiratory alkalosis, normal glucose, and normal lactic acid level.

Of the following, which is the most important next diagnostic test?

   a. Urine organic acids

   b. Plasma amino acids

   c. Urine reducing substances

   d. Plasma ammonia level

   e. Plasma acylcarnitine profile

11-3. In the above case, you have just completed a normal saline bolus of 20 mL/kg. Repeat vital signs are age-appropriate and normal.

What type of fluids do you now order?

   a. Normal saline at maintenance rate

   b. Ringers lactate at maintenance rate

   c. 5% Dextrose at maintenance rate

   d. 10% Dextrose at maintenance rate

   e. 10% Dextrose at 150% (1.5 times) maintenance

11-4. Which of the following scenarios should prompt you to evaluate further for a possible underlying metabolic disorder:

   a. A previously healthy 2-year-old with increasing fever for 5 days, poor oral intake for 2 days, and metabolic acidosis

   b. A neurocognitively normal, healthy 3-year-old, in the care of his grandmother, with sudden onset of lethargy and increased anion gap metabolic acidosis

   c. A 3-week-old with feeding intolerance, increased anion gap metabolic acidosis, and significant ketosis (urinary ketones 4+)

   d. A 5-year-old with lethargy, increased anion gap metabolic acidosis, and blood glucose of 354 mg/dL

   e. A 7-month-old with a 3-day history of persistent diarrhea and hyperchloremic, normal anion gap, metabolic acidosis

11-5. You are meeting with a pregnant couple for a prenatal visit. They request information on current newborn screening (NBS). Which statement are you *most* likely to include in your discussion?

   a. A positive newborn screen is almost always diagnostic for a specific condition and confirmatory testing is often not needed

   b. The advent of newer technology now allows for the detection of over 40 different metabolic disorders by NBS

   c. Only disorders that are fatal, if left untreated, are included in NBS

   d. Blood spot cards for NBS have to be collected immediately after birth, within the first 6 hours

   e. Only disorders that have an incidence of greater than 1 in 10,000 births are included in NBS

11-6. You have just been informed by your state NBS laboratory of a positive newborn screen for phenylketonuria (PKU) on one of your patients. This is a healthy, term, 5-day-old male child. You have scheduled an appointment to see the patient and meet with the parents who are of Caucasian descent.

Which of the following statements about PKU do you include in your discussion with the parents?

a. PKU is an extremely rare genetic disorder and is especially rare in Caucasians

b. After you evaluate the newborn, if he has a normal physical examination and is feeding well, he is unlikely to have PKU

c. PKU can be exclusively treated by dietary manipulation and its effects entirely prevented by NBS and timely intervention

d. This is most likely a false-positive NBS results and no further action is needed at this time

e. About 50% of individuals with untreated PKU develop severe mental disability

11-7. A 35-year-old woman gives birth to a female infant who is growth restricted, microcephalic, and has a congenital heart defect. She has had 1 prior miscarriage and reports that she has a 3-year-old son with mental impairment. She also recalls being on a special diet as a child which she subsequently discontinued. Which of the following maternal conditions is most consistent with this history?

a. Fragile X syndrome

b. Alkaptonuria

c. Myotonic dystrophy

d. Type 1 diabetes mellitus

e. PKU

11-8. A 2-year-old new patient presents to your clinic for initial evaluation. Her mother reports 2 prior episodes of unsteady gait associated with viral illness with resolution of symptoms when well. She also reports an intermittent "sweet caramel-type" odor to her skin. Past medical history is otherwise normal. Neurodevelopmental parameters are age-appropriate. Current growth parameters and physical examination are normal. What is your current recommendation?

a. Further evaluation for a biotin responsive disorder

b. Further evaluation for a branched chain amino acid disorder

c. Limiting the amount of fruit juices in her diet as that may be causing the sweet odor

d. Referral and an evaluation by an infectious disease specialist

e. MRI of the brain to ensure no intracranial abnormalities

11-9. A 5-day-old term neonate presents to the ED. Her parents report a 2- to 3-day history of poor feeding and a 1-day history of increasing lethargy. She has increased anion gap metabolic acidosis and a glucose level of 24 mg/dL. Urinalysis reveals the presence of large urinary ketones. Which of the following laboratory evaluations, is MOST likely to lead to an underlying diagnosis?

a. Urine organic acids

b. Free and total carnitine levels

c. Very long chain fatty acids

d. Urine reducing substances

e. Urine amino acids

11-10. IEM can be associated with a characteristic odor/smell. Select the correct association.

a. MSUD and a sour smell

b. Propionic acidemia and a mousy odor

c. Isovaleric acidemia and a smell of sweaty feet

d. Methylmalonic acidemia and a sweet smell

e. 3-methlglutaconic aciduria and a fishy odor

11-11. An 18-year-old with a history of cognitive impairment is referred for evaluation from an ophthalmologists' office with a diagnosis of subluxation of the ocular lens.

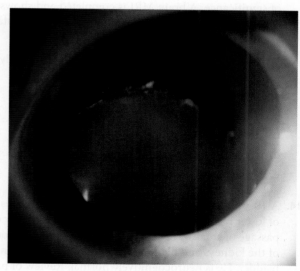

(Reproduced, with permission, from Lueder GT. *Pediatric Practice Ophthalmology.* New York: McGraw-Hill, 2011.)

Which of the following tests is most likely to be abnormal and lead to an underlying diagnosis?

a. Chromosomal analysis

b. Free and total carnitine levels

c. Urine organic acids

d. Total homocysteine level

e. Acylcarnitine profile

11-12. A term neonate is admitted to the neonatal intensive care unit, transferred from the well-baby nursery secondary to onset of seizures noted at 16 hours of age.

He was born after a normal pregnancy and no complications during delivery were noted. He appeared normal at birth; however, at 16 hours of age he developed myoclonic seizures and recurrent hiccoughs. A sepsis evaluation was completed and IV antibiotics were initiated. All cultures were negative at 24 hours. Over the next day he develops apnea. He is unresponsive and has continued seizure activity. You suspect a possible inborn error of metabolism.

Which of the following disorders MOST typically presents with early neonatal seizures?

a. Homocystinuria

b. Glutathione synthase deficiency.

c. Hyperprolinemia type 1

d. Hyperlysinemia

e. Nonketotic hyperglycinemia

11-13. A 5-month-old, previously healthy infant followed in your clinic has sudden onset of hypotonia and dystonia after an intercurrent illness. She was born with macrocephaly. You have followed her in your clinic since birth without other medical problems of significance. A brain MRI is completed and shows degeneration of the caudate and putamen with frontal atrophy.

Which of the following diagnostic tests is most likely to reveal the underlying diagnosis?

a. Galactose-1 phosphate level

b. Urine organic acids

c. Ceruloplasmin level

d. Copper level

e. Urine mucopolysaccharides

11-14. A 10-year-old male presents with recurrent episodes of lower back and abdominal pain. He has a history of passage of stones. He is on a regular diet. An ultrasound of the kidneys and bladder reveals stones in the urinary bladder. He is neurocognitively normal. Review of past medical history reveals no other medical problems. What is the most likely diagnosis.

a. Cystinuria

b. Cystinois

c. Lysinuric protein intolerance

d. Hartnup disease

e. Creatine metabolism defect

11-15. Trichorrhexis nodosa (a node-like appearance of fragile hair that breaks easily), is pathognomonic for which urea cycle disorder?

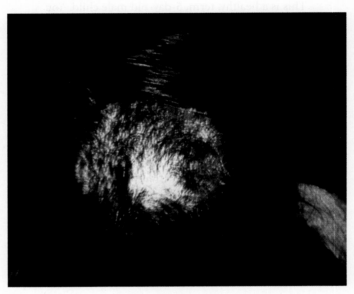

(Reproduced, with permission, from Weinberg S, Prose NS, Kristal L. *Color Atlas of Pediatric Dermatology.* 4th ed. New York: McGraw-Hill, 2008.)

a. OTC deficiency

b. Carbamyl phophate synthetase deficiency

c. Citrullinemia type 1

d. Argininosuccinic aciduria

e. Argininemia

11-16. A 3-day-old comatose male neonate is noted to have an ammonia level of 550 µmol/L. What is the next most critical treatment option that should be initiated emergently to provide the best neurocognitive outcome?

a. Administer a bolus of IV arginine

b. Make immediate arrangements to initiate hemodialysis

c. Administer lactulose for gut sterilization

d. Start a 20 mg/kg bolus of normal saline

e. Administer IV sodium benzoate

11-17. A 4-month-old male with OTC deficiency is followed in your clinic. He was diagnosed at the age of 2 days with severe hyperammonemic coma requiring hemodialysis for management and a hospital stay of 10 days. Since discharge, parents have been very compliant with management recommendations made by your biochemical genetics colleagues. Nevertheless, he had been admitted 3 additional times with ammonia levels ranging between 150 and 200 µmol/L, managed with IV arginine and IV sodium benzoate and IV sodium phenylacetate (Ammonul) as alternate pathways for nitrogen excretion. He has mild head lag at present age but you have no additional concerns on current physical or developmental evaluation. What is the most appropriate consideration at this stage?

a. Referral for liver transplantation

b. Increase the dose of oral nitrogen excretion drugs like sodium phenylbutyrate

c. Reduce protein intake to well below RDA level

d. Initiate gut sterilization with daily lactulose

e. Discussion with the parents regarding poor prognosis based on poor response to standard therapy

11-18. Several IEM respond dramatically to treatment with vitamins which act as co-enzymes. An example of an inborn error of metabolism responsive to treatment with vitamin therapy is:

a. D-2-hydroxyglutaric acidemia

b. GABA transaminase deficiency

c. Cobalamin c disease

d. Glycine encephalopathy (GCE)

e. Sulfite oxidase deficiency

11-19. A 6-month-old male is hospitalized for evaluation of increased anion gap metabolic acidosis and seizures. He is noted to have alopecia and a periorificial skin rash. These features should prompt you to evaluate for which disorder.

a. Homocystinuria

b. Galactosemia

c. Fatty acid oxidation disorder

d. Glycogen storage disease

e. Biotinidase deficiency

11-20. A 7-month-old previously healthy female infant is brought to the ED. Her mother reports a 2-day history of poor oral intake associated with diarrhea and vomiting. Her mother found the 7-month-old in the crib this morning limp and lethargic and immediately came to the ED. A glucose level is collected and is noted to be 25 mg/dL. A dextrose bolus is initiated. No hepatomegaly is noted on physical examination. Electrolytes reveal a bicarbonate level of 18 mg/dL and glucose level of 25 mg/dL, without other significant abnormalities. A stat ammonia level is noted to be normal. Urinalysis reveals specific gravity 1030, negative glucose, negative protein, and negative ketones. What is the most likely underlying diagnosis?

a. Organic acidemia

b. Fatty acid oxidation disorder

c. Hypoglycemia related to viral gastroenteritis

d. Glycogen storage disease

e. Urea cycle disorder

11-21. A 5-month-old presents with a history of 2–3 previous episodes of fasting hypoglycemia. Laboratory evaluations collected during these episodes at a local ED are available for your review and indicate hypoketotic hypoglycemia with mild acidosis, mild hyperammonemia, and elevated liver transaminases during episodes of hypoglycemia.

What is the optimal diagnostic modality to establish an underlying diagnosis?

a. Urine organic acids

b. Plasma amino acids

c. Free and total carnitine levels

d. Plasma acylcarnitine profile

e. VLCFAs

11-22. A 2-year-old patient relocates to your practice from another state. She has a diagnosis of medium chain acyl Co-A dehydrogenase (MCAD) deficiency made by NBS.

Which of the following statements regarding MCAD deficiency is correct?

a. NBS for MCAD deficiency is advocated based on the responsiveness to treatment and the frequency of death following the initial episode

b. The use of medium-chain triglycerides is often beneficial in the management of patients with MCAD deficiency

c. MCAD deficiency is a fatty acid oxidation defect that is inherited in an X-linked recessive fashion

d. Many patients with MCAD deficiency have significant cognitive impairment as adults

e. Analysis of plasma acylcarnitines by tandem mass spectrometry reveals elevation of long-chain acylcarnitines in patients with MCAD deficiency

11-23. You are evaluating a 4-month-old infant, currently hospitalized for evaluation of a history of hypoglycemia. Parents report that he typically feeds every 3 hours. On physical examination you note hepatomegaly with a liver edge palpable about 5–6 cm below the costal margin. Spleen tip is also palpable. You order laboratory evaluation, which reveals an elevated lactic acid level, elevation of uric acid, and elevated triglycerides.

What is the most likely diagnosis?

a. Glycogen storage disease

b. Pompe disease

c. Gaucher disease

d. Tay Sachs disease

e. Krabbe disease

11-24. You are evaluating a 5-month-old male child in your clinic in a follow-up to a recent hospitalization. During his hospitalization, he was diagnosed with glycogen storage disease type 1a. In your discussion with the parents, what is the most appropriate mechanism to prevent night-time hypoglycemia in this infant?

a. Administration of a dose of glucagon

b. Adding corn starch to all his feeds

c. Providing continuous night-time nasogastric feeds

d. The parents should feed this child *ad lib*

e. The parents should feed him every 6–7 hours overnight

11-25. A 17-year-old patient of Caucasian descent complains of muscle cramps and muscle pain with exercise. He reports 1 incident of tea-colored urine after a 400-m sprint. He denies any other medical problems. He reports, if he rests at the first sign of pain, he can resume exercise at a slower pace. You check a CPK level which is mildly elevated; electrolyte levels, renal function, and AST/ALT levels are normal. You suspect a diagnosis of McArdle disease.

Which of the following diagnostic modalities would you recommend to establish the diagnosis?

a. Plasma acycarnitine profile

b. Liver biopsy for enzymatic analysis

c. An ischemia exercise test

d. Urine organic acid analysis

e. Mutation analysis

11-26. A 3-month-old male infant is noted to have severe cardiomegaly on chest X-ray. He has a history of hypotonia and poor weight gain. Physical examination reveals macroglossia and hepatomegaly. Cardiology consultation is pursued, EKG reveals high-voltage QRS complexes and shortened PR interval. Echocardiogram reveals hypertrophic cardiomyopathy. Laboratory evaluation reveals elevated CPK, elevated AST and ALT levels.

What is the most likely underlying diagnosis?

a. McArdle disease (muscle phosphorylase deficiency)

b. Pompe disease (acid glucosidase deficiency)

c. X-linked phosphorylase kinase deficiency

d. Glycogen synthase deficiency

e. Muscle phosphofructokinase deficiency

11-27. A 2-week-old neonate is admitted with sepsis. Blood cultures reveal sepsis due to *Escherichia coli* (*E. coli*). On physical examination she is lethargic, skin appears icteric, and she has hepatomegaly. Testing on urine reveals the presence of nonglucose reducing substances.

What is the most likely underlying diagnosis?

a. Glycogen storage disease

b. MSUD

c. Organic acidemia

d. Galactosemia

e. Urea cycle defect

11-28. A 6-month-old female develops new-onset seizures. Physical examination reveals hypotonia without other abnormalities. Interictal EEG is normal. MRI brain reveals no structural abnormalities. Cerebrospinal fluid analysis reveals a low CSF glucose level of 35 mg/dL. CSF analysis is otherwise normal and not indicative of infection.

Which of the following conditions would you include in your differential diagnosis?

a. Congenital glucose galactose malabsorption

b. Renal glucosuria

c. Glucose transporter-1 deficiency

d. Fanconi–Bickel syndrome

e. Arterial tortuosity syndrome

11-29. The respiratory chain is the terminal pathway of mitochondrial metabolism, where most energy is produced as adenosine triphosphate (ATP). Which statement best describes mitochondrial genetics?

a. The rules of mitochondrial genetics are the same as the rules of Mendelian genetics

b. Each cell contains 2–10 copies of mitochondrial DNA which distribute randomly among daughter cells at cell division

c. At cell division the proportion of mutant mitochondrial DNA in daughter cells always remains constant

d. A male carrying a mitochondrial point mutation will transmit it to all his progeny

e. At fertilization, all mitochondrial DNA is derived from the oocyte

11-30. A 15-year-old female presents with a 4- to 6-month history of recurrent vomiting and migraine-like headaches, and 2 stroke-like episodes associated with hemiparesis. Early developmental milestones are normal. MRI brain reveals "infarcts" not corresponding to the distribution of major vessels. Molecular analysis reveals a mitochondrial mutation in the tRNA gene.

Which of the following statements is correct?

a. This patient is likely to have an elevated lactic acid level

b. Opthalmoplegia is a characteristic finding in this disorder

c. This condition is an autosomal recessive disorder

d. This patient will most likely develop cataracts in the next 2–3 years

e. Treatment for this condition with mitochondrial co-factors is well established

11-31. A 1.5-year-old patient with Hurler syndrome is followed in your practice. Which of the following statements is important to review with her parents?

a. Anesthesia is particularly difficult in patients with Hurler syndrome and surgery should only be performed in centers with access to anesthesiologists used to dealing with difficult pediatric airways

b. Most patients with Hurler syndrome do not survive beyond the age of 3–5 years and parents should consider involvement of hospice services

c. This is an autosomal dominant disorder. Recurrence risks with future pregnancies for the parents of this child may be as high as 50%

d. Patients with Hurler syndrome are at very high risk for intercurrent illness due to impaired immune function

e. This is a progressive, lysosomal storage disorder, without any effective treatment options

11-32. The mucopolysaccharidosis (MPSs) are a group of inherited disorders caused by defects in the catabolism of glycosaminoglycans. Which of the following MPS disorders is inherited in an X-linked manner?

a. Hurler syndrome (MPS1)

b. Hunter syndrome (MPS II)

c. Sanfillipo syndrome (MPS III)

d. Morquio syndrome (MPS IV)

e. Maroteaux-Lamy syndrome (MPS VI)

11-33. A 9-year-old female presents with a history of recurrent bruising. She also reports chronic bone pain, especially in her legs, worse at night. No developmental or neurocognitive concerns are identified. Examination reveals painless hepatosplenomegaly. Neurologic examination is normal. Complete blood counts (CBC) reveal a low platelet level and mild anemia. You recommend a referral to hematology/oncology. Extensive evaluation by this service, including a bone marrow examination, does not reveal a malignancy or primary hematologic disorder.

Which of the following conditions should be on your differential diagnosis?

a. Sandhoff disease

b. Multiple sulfatase deficiency

c. Metachromatic leukodystrophy

d. Gaucher disease

e. GM-1 gangliosidosis

11-34. What therapy would you recommend for the most effective treatment of the hematologic complications for Gaucher disease?

a. There is no effective therapy for this disorder

b. Surgical referral for splenectomy

c. Bone marrow transplantation

d. Liver transplantation

e. Enzyme replacement therapy (ERT)

11-35. A couple of Ashkenazi Jewish descent asks you for advice regarding carrier testing before pursuing a pregnancy. Which of the following disorders is included in Ashkenazi Jewish carrier testing panels?

a. Ornithine transcarbomylase deficiency

b. Fabry disease

c. Tay Sachs disease

d. Hurler syndrome

e. Sanfillipo syndrome

11-36. Peroxisomes are single-membrane bound organelles present in cells that contain enzymes which participate in a variety of metabolic processes. Prominent among these are enzymes that catalyze β-oxidation. β-oxidation also occurs within the mitochondria.

Which of the following statements is true about the difference in β-oxidation systems between the peroxisomes and the mitochondria?

a. There is no difference between the β-oxidation systems within the peroxisomes and mitochondria

b. Only the peroxisomal system oxidizes VLCFAs with carbon chain lengths of 20–26 (C20–C26)

c. The first step in the mitochondrial oxidation system, and not in the peroxisomal system, leads to the formation of hydrogen peroxide (H_2O_2)

d. The mitochondrial matrix enzymes, unlike peroxisomal enzymes, are also involved in synthesis of cholesterol, bile acids, and ether lipids such as plasmalogen

e. Medium-chain fatty acid oxidation (C6–C12) occurs exclusively in the peroxisome

11-37. A 1-month-old female is hospitalized for evaluation of conjugated hyperbilirubinemia and failure to thrive. She is noted to have a large and high forehead, large anterior fontanelle, epicanthal folds, a small nose, broad nasal bridge, and micrognathia. She is profoundly hypotonic. Previous ophthalmology evaluation revealed cataracts and a pigmentary retinopathy.

Which of the following evaluations is most likely to be abnormal and provide a diagnosis?

a. Plasma very long chain fatty acids (VLCFAs)

b. Serum free and total carnitine levels

c. Plasma amino acids

d. Biotinidase enzyme assay

e. Urine organic acids

11-38. Glycosylation is an important post-translational protein modification. A growing family of genetic disorders, called congenital disorders of glycosylation (CDG), is due to defects in protein glycosylation.

Which of the following statements best describes the phenotype associated with CDG's?

a. Most CDG are benign disorders with normal neurocognitive development

b. The majority of CDG can be easily treated with ERT

c. Most CDG are severe multisystem disorders with neurological involvement

d. Most CDG show an X-linked mode of inheritance

e. Important tools in the diagnostic evaluation of suspected CDG include VLCFA analysis

11-39. A 25-year-old primigravida delivers a term male infant with severe intrauterine growth retardation. Prenatal maternal screening revealed low estriol levels. On physical examination the newborn is microcephalic, growth restricted, has a cleft palate, and 2–3 toe syndactyly. A heart murmur is auscultated. Genital examination reveals cryptorchidism.

What is the most likely underlying diagnosis?

a. Desmosterolosis

b. Mevalonic aciduria

c. Chondrodysplasia punctate

d. Smith Lemli Opitz syndrome

e. CHILD syndrome

11-40. Disorders of lipid and lipoprotein metabolism are characterized by dyslipidemia (elevated or low levels of one or more of the major lipoprotein classes). Which of the following statement best describes dyslipidemias?

a. The most frequent cause of dyslipidemias is the result of expression of a mutation in a single gene that plays a paramount role in lipoprotein metabolism

b. Environmental influences (like excessive intake of fat and calories, limited physical activity, obesity) can contribute significantly to dyslipidemias

c. The major clinical complication of dyslipidemias is their association with impairment in neurocognitive development and varying degrees of developmental delay

d. A number of clinical, epidemiologic, metabolic, genetic and randomized clinical trials support the tenet that the risk factors associated with dyslipidemia most often begin in early adulthood

e. Children with inherited disorders of lipid and lipoprotein metabolism may manifest profound hypertriglyceridemia, which can lead to episodes of severe and acute abdominal pain as a result of pseudo-obstruction

11-41. You have arranged a meeting with other pediatricians in your practice to review policy for screening for dyslipidemia for children followed in your practice. Which of the following best reflects current recommendations for screening?

   a. Based on the increased incidence of obesity in children and youth, recommendations should include general screening for all children and adolescents

   b. Recommend a lipoprotein profile in youth whose parents and/or grandparents required coronary artery bypass surgery or balloon angioplasty prior to age 65 years

   c. Recommend a lipoprotein profile in youth with a family history of myocardial infarction, angina pectoris, peripheral or cerebral vascular disease, or sudden death prior to the age of 65 years

   d. A total cholesterol in those whose parents have high total cholesterol levels of greater than 240 mg/dL

   e. A lipoprotein profile should be collected in all youth whose biological parental or grandparental family history is unknown

11-42. You identify a 6-year-old patient with primary dyslipidemia with elevated total cholesterol level. What is the first form of therapy you recommend?

   a. A diet containing decreased amounts of fat, cholesterol, and simple sugars but increased amount of complex carbohydrates with no decrease in total protein

   b. A diet containing decreased amounts of fat, cholesterol, and total protein but increased amounts of simple sugars to maintain adequate caloric intake

   c. Increase amount of physical activity with no dietary modification at present age with consideration of dietary modification by age 10 years if total cholesterol remains elevated

   d. Initiation of pharmacologic therapy with use of inhibitors of HMG CoA reductase (the statins)

   e. Initiation of pharmacologic therapy with use of bile acid sequestrants (BAS)

11-43. Disorders affecting LDL receptor (LDLR) activity lead to elevations in LDL-cholesterol. Which of the following statements best describes familial hypercholesterolemia (FH), a disorder that results from mutations in the LDL receptor?

   a. FH is an X-linked disorder that presents in adolescence

   b. Heterozygosity for FH affects about 1 in 50,000 people

   c. 25–50% of untreated adults with heterozygous FH will develop cardiovascular disease (CVD) by age 50

   d. Patients who are homozygotes for FH have milder manifestations than heterozygous FH

   e. About 1 in 5000 individuals are homozygous for FH

11-44. You follow a 9-year-old girl with a diagnosis of lipoprotein lipase deficiency. She has significantly elevated triglyceride levels that exceed 1000 mg/dL. What is the most important acute medical concern for this patient?

   a. Sudden cardiac death

   b. Early stroke

   c. Potential for myocardial infarction in the first decade of life

   d. Severe hypertension

   e. Recurrent episodes of pancreatitis

11-45. Which of the following statements best describes the porphyrias (disorders of heme biosynthesis)?

   a. The enzyme deficiencies leading to the porphyrias are all inherited as autosomal recessive disorders

   b. These disorders are primarily classified as hepatic or erythropoietic, depending on the primary site of overproduction or accumulation of the porphyrin

   c. Manifestations of the erythropoietic porphyrias characteristically include abdominal pain, neuropathy and mental disturbance

   d. Manifestations of the hepatic porphyrias characteristically include cutaneous photosensitivity

   e. There are currently *no* known environmental factors involved in the pathophysiology of these disorders

11-46. A 15-year-old, otherwise healthy boy, presents with a 1-year history of fatigue and muscle weakness. He reports myalgia and muscle cramps with exercise and 1 prior episode of red urine following exercise raising your concern for myoglubinuria. A forearm ischemic exercise test is performed. After 2 minutes of ischemic forearm exercise, venous ammonia level is normal.

What is the most likely diagnosis?

a. Purine nucleoside phosphorylase deficiency

b. Phosphoribosylpyrophosphate synthase superactivity

c. Myoadenylate deaminase deficiency

d. Adenylosuccinase deficiency

e. Xanthine oxidase deficiency

11-47. A 1-year-old boy presents with a history of irritability and generalized muscle weakness. His mother reports a history of "brownish-red sand" in his diapers. She reports normal development in the first 4 months of life with concern for developmental delay and low muscle tone noted around 6 months of age. Your review of prior laboratory tests reveals an elevated uric acid level.

What is the most likely diagnosis?

a. Purine nucleoside phosphorylase deficiency

b. Phosphoribosylpyrophosphate synthase superactivity

c. Adenosine deaminase deficiency

d. Hypoxanthine–Guanine phosphoribosyltransferase deficiency (Lesch–Nyhan disease)

e. Deoxyguanosine kinase deficiency

11-48. Dihydropyrimidine dehydrogenase deficiency is an inherited disorder of pyrimidine catabolism with very variable clinical symptoms. In older individuals, partial deficiency of this enzyme, causes severe hypersensitivity to which drug?

a. 5-fluorouracil

b. Nonsteroidal anti-inflammatory drugs (NSAID's)

c. Valproic acid

d. L-arginine

e. L-carnitine

11-49. Metals are indispensable elements of cell biology. They function as cofactors in many specific proteins and are involved in all major metabolic pathways. Clinical presentations of disorders of metal metabolism are diverse and involve all major organs and systems. A 3-month-old presents with persistent diarrhea and severe periorificial dermatitis.

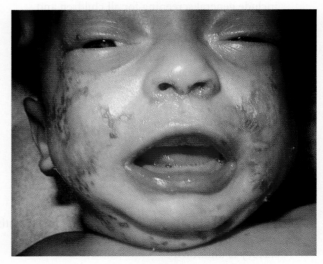

(Reproduced, with permission, from Weinberg S, Prose NS, Kristal L. *Color Atlas of Pediatric Dermatology.* 4th ed. New York: McGraw-Hill, 2008.)

What is the most likely metal deficiency associated with these symptoms?

a. Copper

b. Iron

c. Zinc

d. Magnesium

e. Manganese

11-50. A 3-month-old male infant presents with loss of developmental milestones, hypotonia, seizures, and failure to thrive. He has short, sparse, and twisted hair. What is the most likely metal metabolism defect associated with these symptoms?

a. Copper

b. Iron

c. Zinc

d. Magnesium

e. Manganese

ANSWERS

Answer 11-1. a

Most IEM are inherited as autosomal recessive conditions. A significant minority are inherited as X-linked recessive and a few as dominant disorders. However, in developed countries, where consanguinity is rare and the size of sibships small, many cases appear to be sporadic with a negative family history. It is important to remember OTC deficiency, the most common urea cycle defect, is an X-linked disorder with a very variable phenotype in females that can lead to fatal hyperammonemia in both affected males and females.

(P 542 "Genetics" and Table 134-1 p 544)

Answer 11-2. d

The neonate has a limited repertoire of responses to severe illness and IEM may present with nonspecific symptoms. Consider IEM in parallel with other more common conditions like sepsis. Rapid clinical deterioration is concerning for IEM. Isolated hyperammonemia can occur and an elevated ammonia level alone can induce respiratory alkalosis. Respiratory alkalosis is rare in septic neonates who usually present with metabolic acidosis. A finding of respiratory alkalosis in a neonate that appears "septic" should prompt rapid evaluation for hyperammonemia.

(P 542: "Acute Encephalopathy and Metabolic Crash" and p 544: "Initial Approach to Investigation", Figure 134-2, p 545)

Answer 11-3. e

First ensure adequate cardiorespiratory function (ABCs). Adequate hydration is essential to maintain good urine output because many of the offending metabolites in IEMs are freely filtered at the glomerulus. Fluid therapy should be judicious as cerebral edema can occur. During resuscitation of patients with suspected metabolic disease, it is also critical to reverse the catabolic state. 10% dextrose run intravenously at 150% maintenance will provide about 9–10 mg/kg/min of glucose to neonates and infants. The other fluids listed above do not provide an adequate glucose infusion rate (GIR) to reverse catabolism.

(P 545: "Approach to Therapy")

Answer 11-4. c

Metabolic acidosis can result from a large variety of acquired conditions, including infections (patient described in "A"), severe catabolic state, severe dehydration and intoxication (patient described in "C"). Evaluation of patients with metabolic acidosis includes calculating the anion gap. In patients with metabolic acidosis caused by loss of bicarbonate (GI or renal loss), the plasma chloride is elevated and the anion gap normal (patient described in "E"). The patient described in "D" most likely has diabetic ketoacidosis.

Metabolic acidosis in IEMs often develops as a result of accumulation of a fixed anion, like lactate, ketone bodies, organic acid, or a combination of these, leading to increased anion gap metabolic acidosis. Ketonuria should always be considered abnormal in a neonate and when associated with metabolic acidosis should prompt evaluation for metabolic disease.

(P 554: "Metabolic Acidosis and Ketosis")

Answer 11-5. b

The application of tandem mass spectrometry to NBS has greatly changed both NBS and the diagnosis of many IEMs. This technology allows for detection of many disorders at one time. A positive newborn screen is considered a screening test and must be confirmed, false-positive results can occur. It is recommended the sample for NBS be collected after 24 hours of age to allow for oral intake of formula or breast milk which may be necessary to show characteristic elevations of metabolites. Current NBS panels include several conditions with a much lower frequency than 1 in 10,000 and many of the disorders screened for are NOT fatal.

(P 559: "Newborn Screening Program")

Answer 11-6. c

PKU has a very distinct role in the field of metabolic disorders. It is the first genetic disease that could be treated exclusively by dietary manipulation and entirely prevented by universal NBS and presymptomatic dietary intervention.

It is one of the most common inherited metabolic diseases and has a higher incidence in Caucasians than people of African descent, Hispanics, or Asians. Children with severe hyperphenylalaninemia do not show any symptoms at birth. If untreated, symptoms usually appear after 6 months of age. NBS for PKU is fairly specific, false-positives are more often seen in premature or sick babies. All positive newborn screens must be promptly followed by confirmatory testing. For patients with PKU, initiation of treatment before the age of 2 weeks is recommended. Approximately 90% of individuals with untreated PKU have severe mental disability. The damage to the brain is believed to occur from direct toxicity of phenylalanine and depletion of tyrosine, tryptophan, and other large neutral amino acids that compete with phenylalanine for uptake into the brain.

(Pp 561–563: "Hyperphenylalaninemias")

Answer 11-7. e

Intrauterine exposure of an unborn child to elevated phenylalanine concentrations due to maternal PKU can disrupt embryo-fetal development. Effects include facial dysmorphism resembling fetal alcohol syndrome, microcephaly, mental impairment, and malformations especially of the heart. None of the other maternal conditions listed above would lead to the clinical features described in this vignette. Maternal diabetes leads to macrosomia not growth restriction.

(Pp 561–563: "Hyperphenylalaninemia")

Answer 11-8. b

The 3 essential branched-chain amino acids (BCAA); leucine, isoleucine, and valine; encompass about 25% of human protein. The most frequent inborn errors affecting the BCAA catabolic pathway are maple syrup urine disease (MSUD), isovaleric, propionic, and methylmalonic acidemias. In the typical patient with MSUD, symptoms appear at 3–5 days of age and can progress rapidly to death. Early manifestations include poor feeding, irregular respirations, lethargy, muscle rigidity, and ophistotonus. The characteristic maple syrup odor can be detected in the urine, skin, hair, or ear wax. Milder intermittent forms of the disease can occur and present with episodic ataxia or episodes of lethargy, which can progress to coma without mental retardation. These episodes are often precipitated by intercurrent illness. Early diagnosis is essential as treatment with special diets with closely controlled intake of the BCAA leads to normal neurocognitive outcome. Intake of fruit juices does not cause a maple-syrup type smell. A referral to a geneticist is appropriate to evaluate for MSUD, not an ID referral. An MRI brain will most likely be normal and will not add towards establishing the underlying diagnosis.

A biotinidase deficiency usually presents in infancy with periorificial dermatitis resembling acrodermatitis enteropathica patchy alopecia, neurologic abnormalities, and metabolic acidosis related to impaired activity of the carboxylases, which use biotin as a cofactor.

(P 565, Chapter 137: Disorders of Branched Chain Amino Acids: Maple Syrup Urine Disease")

Answer 11-9. a

Most organic acidemias present in the newborn period with lethargy or encephalopathy, metabolic acidosis (with an increased anion gap), hypoglycemia, and ketosis. Characteristic, diagnostic metabolites are noted on urine organic acids, especially if collected during an acute event. Free and total carnitine levels will indicate a carnitine deficiency and possible need for carnitine supplementation but are not diagnostic. Alternatively, an acylcarnitine profile (which is a different test from free and total carnitine levels and is not one of the choices above), uses tandem mass spectrometry to quantitate specific acylcarnitines, and is an extremely useful adjunct diagnostic test for organic acidemias.

Very long chain fatty acids (VLCFAs) are used in the diagnosis of peroxisomal disorders, not organic acidemias. Urine reducing substances would not lead to a diagnosis and

amino acids are best sampled in plasma not urine as they are effectively cleared by the kidneys.

(Pp 566–568. Disorders of Organic Acid Metabolism: Isovaleric, Propionic, Methylmalonic and Other Rare Organic Acidemias)

Answer 11-10. c

Isovaleric acidemia was the first condition recognized as an organic acidemia when the odor of sweaty feet in an infant with episodic encephalopathy was shown to be caused by isovaleric acid. MSUD, as the name suggests causes a maple-syrup odor to emanate from the urine and skin. Propionic, methylmalonic and 3-methylglutaconic aciduria are not noted to have characteristic odors. Carnitine supplementation used in the management of many organic acidemias can cause a fishy odor.

(Pp 565–568: "Disorders of Branched Chain Amino and Organic Acid Metabolism")

Answer 11-11. d

Classical homocystinuria (CBS deficiency). Classical homocystinuria presents as a multisystem disease with dysplasia of connective tissue, a predisposition to thromboembolism, and mental retardation. The most characteristic feature of this disorder is subluxation of the ocular lens, which occurs in almost all untreated individuals until adulthood. Severe hyperhomocysteinemia is identified with homocysteine levels in the range of 80–300 µmol/L. Plasma amino acids can be collected once hyperhomocystenemia has been detected, and generally reveal high methionine and low cysteine levels.

Subluxation of the ocular lens can also be seen in Marfan syndrome, but patients with Marfan syndrome do not have cognitive impairment. Chromosome analysis would be normal in both Marfan syndrome and homocystinuria. The other tests listed above would also be nondiagnostic. Presence of cognitive impairment in patients with marfanoid skeletal features and/or lens subluxation should prompt evaluation for homocystinuria.

(P 569: "Disorders of Sulfur-Containing Amino Acid Metabolism")

Answer 11-12. e

Glycine encephalopathy (GCE) is an inherited metabolic disorder in which large amounts of glycine are found in body fluids, without further metabolic derangement. GCE typically presents with severe neonatal epileptic encephalopathy, like the clinical picture described above, recurrent hiccoughing is common. EEG shows a typical burst suppression pattern. It is caused by defects in the mitochondrial glycine cleavage system.

Diagnosis is made by documentation of elevated CSF glycine levels and a characteristic CSF/plasma glycine ratio (by collecting CSF and plasma amino acids). There is no effective treatment and prognosis is generally poor. The other disorders listed above do not present with neonatal seizures. Patients with hyperprolinemia type 1 and hyperlysinemia are typically asymptomatic. Glutathione synthase deficiency presents with hemolytic anemia.

(Chapter 139, p 572: "Glycine Encephalopathy (nonketotic hyperglycinemia)")

Answer 11-13. b

Glutaric acidemia type 1 is caused by defects in glutaryl-CoA dehydrogenase. Many patients are born with macrocephaly and develop normally until they suddenly develop hypotonia and dystonia after an intercurrent illness. MRI scans show frontal and cortical atrophy and after the onset of dystonia, degeneration of the caudate nucleus and putamen. Urine organic acids are often diagnostic and show increased excretion of glutaric acid and 3-hydroxyglutaric acid. Diagnosis can also be made by collecting a plasma acylcarnitine profile that shows elevation of glutarylcarnitine. Most patients are now diagnosed by NBS. Effective treatment is possible with early diagnosis.

Galactose-1-phosphate levels are used in diagnosis and follow-up of patients with galactosemia. Copper and ceruloplasmin levels are used in the diagnosis of Wilson disease. Assessment of urine mucopolysaccharides are used in the diagnosis of the mucopolysacaccharidosis.

(Chapter 140, p 574: "Glutaric acidemia type 1")

Answer 11-14. a

Inherited defects in amino acid transport at cell membranes (Figure 143-1) are expressed as selective renal aminoaciduria and impaired intestinal absorption. Their symptoms result from excess of certain amino acids in the urine or lack of them in the tissues. Examples of disorders in this category include cystinuria (not cystinosis), lysinuric protein intolerance, and Hartnup disease.

Cystinuria leads to formation of cystine stones secondary to high urinary concentration of poorly soluble cystine and can be detected by checking urine amino acids. Nephropathic cystinosis is characterized by renal tubular Fanconi syndrome, poor growth, hypophosphatemic rickets,

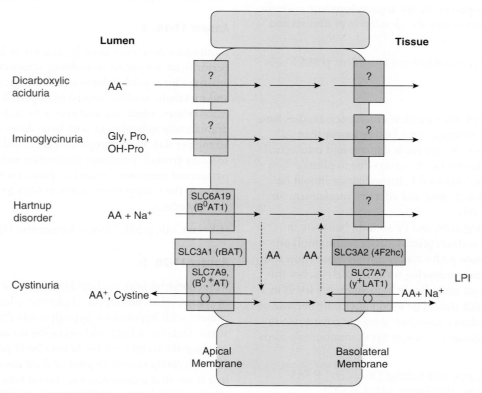

FIGURE 143-1. Simplified schematic representation of amino acid transport in proximal tubular epithelial cell. Transport systems for negatively charged dicarboxylic amino acids (AA⁻), imino acids (glycine, proline, and hydroxyproline); neutral amino acids (AA); and cystine and positively charged dibasic amino acids (AA⁺) are shown. The special transporters, some of which are formed of light and heavy subunits, act on the luminal and basolateral membranes of the epithelial cell. In man, the transporters for neutral amino acids (B⁰AT1/SLC6A19), for cationic dibasic amino acids and cystine at the luminal surface (formed by subunits b⁰,⁺AT/SLC7A9 and rBAT/SLC3A1), and for dibasic amino acids at the basolateral surface (formed by subunits ⁺LAT1/SLC7A7 and 4F2hc/SLC3A2) have been characterized at the genetic and molecular level. The subunits that carry mutations that cause Hartnup disorder, cystinuria, and lysinuric protein intolerance are shown in red. (Reproduced from Rudolph CD, Rudolph AM, Lister GE, First LR, Gershon AA. *Rudolph's Pediatrics.* 22nd ed. New York: McGraw-Hill, 2011.)

impaired glomerular function, and accumulation of cystine crystals in almost all cells, leading to tissue destruction. The typical untreated child has short stature, growth failure noted between 6 and 9 months, rickets, and photophobia. Prior to the use of renal transplantation and cystine-depleting therapy, the lifespan in nephropathic cystinosis was no longer than 10 years.

In lysinuric protein intolerance, the transport of dibasic amino acids is impaired, leading to lack of the urea cycle intermediates arginine and ornithine, with resultant hyperammonemia and protein intolerance. Deficiency of tryptophan, the precursor to niacin, leads to a pellagra-type dermatitis and ataxia in Hartnup disease. The main clinical symptoms seen in creatine metabolism defects include mental retardation, pronounced speech delay, autistic behavior, and seizures.

(Chapter 143: "Disorders of Amino Acid Transport Across Cell Membranes")

Answer 11-15. d

In addition to hyperammonemia symptoms, several hyperammonemic disorders have other more specific clinical abnormalities. Trichorrhexis nodosa, a node-like appearance of fragile hair, is pathognomonic for argininosuccinic aciduria. Patients with this disorder can also develop liver fibrosis and cirrhosis.

(Chapter 145, Urea Cycle and Related Disorders, p 584.)

Answer 11-16. b

Hyperammonemia presents a medical emergency. Studies have shown that hyperammonemic coma lasting longer than 72 hours invariably leads to severe brain damage and intellectual disability. When newborns are in a coma due to plasma ammonia levels above 200 μmol/L, hemodialysis should be initiated. This is the most rapid and effective mechanism for reducing ammonia levels.

Intravenous (IV) arginine, and IV sodium benzoate in combination with IV sodium phenylacetate (Ammonul) are used to provide alternate pathways for nitrogen excretion and should be initiated while preparing for hemodialysis, but this therapy does not reduce exceedingly high ammonia levels in a timely fashion. IV fluids should be used judiciously because of the risk for cerebral edema. Lactulose does not have a role in the emergency management of severe hyperammonemic coma in neonates.

(Chapter 145: "Urea Cycle and Related Disorders". P 585: "Treatment Approaches", also Figure 145-4, p 587)

Answer 11-17. a

For the most severe cases, which are not amenable to standard therapy, liver transplantation currently offers the only curative therapy. With the reduced mortality and morbidity from this procedure, it is now considered the treatment of choice

for neonatal onset CPS and OTC deficiencies and is usually performed between 3 and 6 months of age.

(Chapter 145: "Urea Cycle and Related Disorders". Pp 586–587: "Long-term Therapy")

Answer 11-18. c

Vitamins are organic molecules that are present in trace amounts in the diet and act as co-enzymes, or co-enzyme precursors. Several inborn errors respond dramatically to treatment with vitamins. Because treatment of these conditions with vitamins may be life-saving it is important that they be thought of and recognized early in patient evaluation. Cobalamin c disease (p 589 and Table 147-1) results in combined methylmalonic aciduria and homocystinuria because cobalamin serves as the cofactor for both methylmalonyl Co-A mutase (deficiency of which leads to methylmalonic acidemia) and methionine synthase (which catalyzes the methylation of homocysteine to methionine and deficiency of which leads to hyperhomocysteinemia). This disorder is treated with large doses of cobalamin administered intramuscularly. There is no effective therapy for the other disorders listed above.

(Chapter 146, p 588: "Inborn Errors of Water Soluble Vitamins")

Answer 11-19. e

Biotinidase deficiency usually presents in infancy with periorificial dermatitis resembling acrodermatitis enteropathica, patchy alopecia, neurologic abnormalities and metabolic acidosis related to impaired activity of the carboxylases, which use biotin as a co-factor. Patients respond dramatically to treatment with large doses of biotin, usually at 10 mg per day. Early recognition is critical because it can be so easily treated. Untreated biotinidase deficiency can lead to permanent neurologic sequelae. Based on these factors, most states in the United States perform NBS by enzymatic assay for this disorder.

(Chapter 148, p 591: "Biotin Responsive Disorders")

Answer 11-20. b

Mitochondrial fatty acid oxidation provides the main source of energy when the supply of glucose is limited. Patients present with hypoketotic hypoglycemia during fasting or stress. Defects in fatty acid oxidation do not allow generation of adequate acetyl CoA for ketone body production. Hypoglycemia related to poor oral intake and increased loss from viral gastroenteritis, should lead to an appropriate physiological ketone body response in patients with a normal fatty acid oxidation pathway (note negative urinary ketones in the urinalysis).

Organic acidemias would also lead to significant ketonuria. GSDs are most often associated with hepatomegaly. Ammonia level would be elevated in urea cycle defects.

(Chapter 150. P 594. Disorders of Fatty Acid Oxidation)

Answer 11-21. d

This vignette describes the typical; hepatic presentation of fatty acid oxidation disorders (FAODs), characterized by fasting-related hypoketotic hypoglycemia. Diagnosis may be difficult even when the presentation is characteristic. Probably the most important single diagnostic test is analyzing acycarnitine esters in plasma or serum by tandem mass spectrometry (plasma acylcarnitine profile). Urine organic acids and free and total carnitine levels are useful but not diagnostic. Plasma amino acids are usually normal in patients with FAODs. "Very long chain fatty acids" is a test for peroxisomal disorders as the VLCFAs are metabolized in peroxisomes, unlike fatty acid oxidation which occurs in mitochondria.

(Chapter 150, p 594: "Disorders of Fatty Acid Oxidation")

Answer 11-22. a

In patients with a clinical diagnosis of MCAD deficiency, initial episode is fatal in about 25% of patients. Combined with the simplicity of treatment of this condition (avoidance of fasting and use of IV glucose during intercurrent illnesses which impair appetite), most states now advocate and complete NBS for this disorder.

Use of medium-chain triglycerides is contraindicated in MCAD deficiency as the block in this condition is at the level of medium-chain fatty acids. Medium-chain triglycerides are beneficial in the management of long-chain fatty acid oxidation disorders. MCAD deficiency and the other disorders of fatty acid oxidation are inherited in an autosomal recessive fashion. Most patients with MCAD deficiency, especially if the diagnosis is known and made presymptomatically by NBS, have normal neurocognitive development. The best diagnostic modality for fatty acid oxidation disorders is plasma acylcarnitines by tandem mass spectrometry, which reveals elevation of medium-chain acylcarnitines in patients with MCAD deficiency. Long-chain acylcarnitine elevations are seen in the long-chain fatty acid oxidation defects, like VLCAD.

(P 596: "Defects of B-oxidation and MCAD deficiency")

Answer 11-23. a

Type 1 GSD is due to a defect in glucose-6-phosphatase in the liver, kidney, and intestine. Patients with GSD type 1 typically present with hypoglycemia and hepatomegaly at 3–4 months of age. The biochemical hallmarks of the disease are hypoglycemia, lactic acidosis, hyperuricemia, and hyperlipidemia. The other disorders listed above are lysosomal storage disorders which do not lead to the classic biochemical abnormalities described above including hypoglycemia, hyperuricemia, lactic acidosis, and hyperlipidemia.

(GSD Type 1, p 601)

Answer 11-24. c

Treatment of GSD type 1 is designed to maintain normal blood glucose levels and is achieved by continuous nasogastric infusion of glucose or oral administration of uncooked cornstarch. Nasogastric feeds, especially at night, are used in infancy and may consist of an elemental formula or a glucose polymer to maintain normoglycemia during the night. Frequent meals with a high carbohydrate content are given during the day. Uncooked cornstarch acts as a sustained release form of glucose but can only be used after the age of 9 months when pancreatic amylase activity is mature. Administration of glucagon causes little or no rise in glucose but increases lactate levels significantly. Adlib feeding or feeds spaced out more than about every 4 hours would most likely lead to hypoglycemia in this disorder.

(P 599: "Carbohydrate Metabolism. Disorders of Glycogen Metabolism". GSD Type 1 p 601)

Answer 11-25. e

Symptoms of GSD V are characterized by exercise intolerance and muscle cramps. Brief periods of intense activity or less intense but sustained activity lead to symptoms. Most patients report a "second wind" phenomenon, like described by the patient in the above vignette. About half of patients report burgundy-colored urine after exercise, the consequence of myoglobinuria secondary to rhabdomyolysis. Intense myoglobinuria after vigorous exercise can cause renal failure. Serum creatine kinase is usually elevated at rest and increases more after exercise. This is an autosomal recessive disorder. One common mutation (R49X) accounts for 90% of North American patients with this disorder. Lack of an elevated blood lactate level and exaggerated ammonia elevations are noted after ischemia exercise test.

The abnormal exercise test, however, is NOT limited to type V GSD and can be seen in other defects of glycogenolysis or glycolysis. Definitive diagnosis is made by enzymatic assay in muscle tissue (not liver) or by mutation analysis of the myophosphorylase gene. Mutation analysis offers the least invasive test to establish a diagnosis. Plasma acylcarnitine profile and urine organic acids are normal in patients with GSD. These tests are used in the diagnosis of fatty acid oxidation disorders, some of which can also present with exercise intolerance.

(P 605: "Muscle Glycogenoses. Type V GSD, McArdle disease")

Answer 11-26. b

The above vignette describes the typical infantile presentation of Pompe disease. This disease is also a lysosomal storage disease and is characterized by accumulation of glycogen in lysosomes as opposed to its accumulation in the cytoplasm in other GSD's. The disorder encompasses a range of phenotypes with severe infantile form as described above (which includes skeletal, cardiac, and smooth muscle involvement) and a late onset form characterized by skeletal muscle manifestations. It is important to establish the correct diagnosis, as enzyme replacement therapy (ERT) is currently available for Pompe disease and leads to improved cardiac and skeletal muscle function, although response to ERT is variable.

The other GSD's listed above have a primary liver (hepatomegaly) or skeletal presentation (exercise intolerance), without cardiomegaly.

(P 606: "GSD Type 2, Pompe disease")

Answer 11-27. d

Classic galactosemia is due to deficiency of galactose-1-phosphate uridyltransferase. Incidence is approximately 1 in 60,000. Symptoms typically appear by the first to second week of life for newborns receiving breast milk or regular formulas (with lactose). Manifestations include jaundice, hepatomegaly, feeding intolerance. Patients are at increased risk for *E. coli* sepsis. A preliminary diagnosis of galactosemia is made by demonstrating reducing substances in urine (both glucose and galactose are reducing substances, it is easy to exclude glucosuria as contributing to the presence of reducing substances by completing a urinalysis to check for glucose in urine).

Only patients with galactosemia receiving lactose will have positive reducing substances. Enzymatic testing for galactose-1-phosphate uridyltransferase in erythrocytes or molecular analysis confirms the diagnosis. Treatment includes elimination of galactose from the diet with use of galactose free formulas (lactose free/soy-based formulas). Most patients with galactosemia are now diagnosed by NBS.

(P 607: Disorders of Galactose Metabolism. Galactosemia)

Answer 11-28. c

Glucose and other monosaccharides are hydrophilic substances that cannot easily cross the lipophilic bilayer of the cell membrane. Since carbohydrates are most important for supplying energy to essentially all cell types, specific transport mechanisms have evolved. To date, 5 congenital defects of monosaccharide transport are known (listed above: A–E). Their clinical presentation is a consequence of tissue-specific expression of the transporter and its substrate specificity. Glucose transporter (GLUT) 1 exclusively facilitates glucose transport across the blood brain barrier. GLUT 1 deficiency results in low glucose levels in CSF.

The above vignette describes a typical clinical presentation for this disorder. GLUT 1 deficiency should be suspected in any patient with a low CSF glucose level (less than 45 mg/dL) with a normal blood glucose level. Diagnosis can be confirmed by molecular analysis. Treatment includes high-fat, low-carbohydrate diet. Ketone bodies derived from fat metabolism restore brain energy metabolism since ketone transport into the brain is not dependent on GLUT1. The other glucose transport disorders listed above are reviewed in pages 610–613.

(Pp 610–613: "Disorders of Glucose Transporters")

Answer 11-29. e

The rules of mitochondrial genetics differ from those of Mendelian genetics in the following ways. Each cell contains hundreds of thousands (not 2–10) of copies of mitochondrial DNA which distribute randomly among daughter cells at cell division. In normal tissues, all mtDNA molecules are identical (homoplasmy). Most deleterious mtDNA mutations affect some, not all mtDNA within a cell, tissue, or individual (heteroplasmy). The clinical expression is determined by the relative proportion of normal and mutant mtDNA. A minimum critical number of mtDNA is required to cause mitochondrial dysfunction (threshold affect).

At cell division the proportion of mutant mitochondrial DNA in daughter cells may shift and change the phenotype (mitotic segregation). At fertilization, all mitochondrial DNA derives from the oocyte. A mother carrying a mitochondrial point mutation will transmit it to all her children, male and female. But only her daughters will transmit it to their progeny.

(Respiratory Chain Disorders, p 614)

Answer 11-30. a

Clinical Features in Mitochondrial Disease due to Mitochondrial DNA mutations. This vignette describes a patient with MELAS (mitochondrial encephalomyopathy, lactic acidosis and stroke like episodes). Opthalmoplegia is not seen in MELAS, it is a feature of the Kearnes Sayre syndrome. Inheritance is maternal as discussed in question 11-29. Cataracts are NOT typically seen in patients with MELAS. Therapy for mitochondrial disorders including MELAS is still inadequate.

(Pp 615–620, Table 158-1)

Answer 11-31. a

All MPS disorders are multisystem diseases and effective management depends on a multidisciplinary approach. The pediatrician has a major role in orchestrating the various members of the therapeutic team. Anesthesia is particularly difficult in patients with the Hurler syndrome and surgery should only be performed in centers with access to anesthesiologists used to dealing with difficult pediatric airways. Many patients survive through adolescence, into adulthood and careful planning of transition from pediatric to adult services is necessary.

MPS1 (Hurler syndrome) is an autosomal recessive disorder with a recurrence risk of 25% for parents of an effected child. Hurler syndrome is not associated with increased risk for infections or immune dysfunction. There are several effective treatment options including bone marrow or stem cell transplantation for patients that are less than 2 years of age. ERT is also available and leads to improvement in endurance, respiratory status, hepatosplenomegaly and cardiac status. ERT does not cross the blood–brain barrier and the only option for a good neurologic outcome is stem cell/bone marrow transplantation often in combination with ERT.

(Chapter 160, pp 622–629)

Answer 11-32. b

Hunter syndrome is inherited as an X-linked condition. All the other MPSs are autosomal recessive (like most IEM). Males with Hunter syndrome present fairly similar to patients with Hurler syndrome. Hunter syndrome is not associated with corneal clouding, which is part of Hurler. It is important to check for carrier status in mothers of affected males with Hunter syndrome to establish appropriate recurrence risks.

(Table 160-1: The Mucopolysaccharidosis, p 623)

Answer 11-33. d

Gaucher disease is an example of how sphingolipid storage diseases may present at any age. Gaucher disease can present in the neonatal or early infantile period with severe CNS impairment and hepatosplenomegaly. However, the most common presentation is in late childhood or adulthood (Type 1 Gaucher disease) without CNS impairment. A typical presentation is described above. All the other disorders listed above are examples of shingolipidoses; however, the presentation for these disorders includes CNS impairment.

(Table 161-1. pp 634–637: "Clinical features of shingolipidoses")

Answer 11-34. e

ERT has emerged as one of the most important advances in the treatment of shingolipidoses. ERT with biweekly infusions of recombinant human glucocerebrosidase is invariably effective in reversing the hematologic and early skeletal complications of Gaucher disease. None of the other options listed above are valid treatment options for Gaucher disease.

(P 637: "Clinical features of shingolipidoses")

Answer 11-35. c

Clinical features of shingolipidoses. Large-scale carrier detection for Tay Sachs disease is used among high-risk populations like the Ashkenazi Jewish population (page 637). The incidence of this disorder is much higher in Ashkenazi Jews compared to the general population. None of the other disorders listed above have a higher incidence among Ashkenazi Jews.

(Table 161-1. Pp 634–637)

Answer 11-36. b

Peroxisomes are single membrane bound organelles present in all cells except erythrocytes, which contain enzymes which participate in a variety of metabolic processes. β-oxidation systems within the peroxisomes and mitochondria have distinct substrate specificities. VLCFA oxidation, C20–C26, occurs only in peroxisomes. The mitochondrial system oxidizes fatty acids with carbon chain lengths from C18 to C4. Choices c, d, and e are false in that the first step in only the peroxisomal oxidation system leads to the formation of hydrogen peroxide (H_2O_2);

peroxisomal enzymes, not mitochondrial, are also involved in synthesis of cholesterol, bile acids, and ether lipids such as plasmalogen; and medium-chain fatty acid oxidation (C6–C12) occurs in the mitochondria not peroxisome (a defect in this pathway leads to MCAD deficiency: medium-chain acyl Co-A dehydrogenase deficiency).

(Pp 637–638. Chapter 162: "Peroxisomal Disorders")

Answer 11-37. a

The Zellweger syndrome spectrum accounts for about 80% of peroxisomal biogenesis disorders (PBD) patients. Listed from most to least severe this spectrum includes Zellweger syndrome (which presents with the phenotype described in the above vignette), neonatal adrenoleukodystrophy, and infantile Refsum disease. The most frequently utilized diagnostic laboratory test for PBD includes VLCFAs. VLCFAs are abnormally increased in patients with Zellweger syndrome. None of the other tests listed above would show any significant abnormalities or be diagnostic in PBD patients.

(Pp 638–640: "Peroxisomal Biogenesis Disorders (PBD), Clinical Phenotypes and Laboratory Diagnosis")

Answer 11-38. c

Glycosylation is an important posttranslational protein modification that occurs in cytoplasm, the endoplasmic reticulum, and Golgi. A rapidly growing group of genetic disorders, collectively called CDG, is due to defects in N or O glycosylation. Most CDG are severe multisystem disorders with neurological involvement.

There is no effective treatment for the majority of patients with CDG; ERT is not available for this group of disorders. CDG 1b (which is much rarer than CDG1a) is the only known CDG that is efficiently treatable with oral mannose. Many CDGs show autosomal recessive inheritance, not X-linked. The most important initial diagnostic tool is transferrin isoelectric focusing not VLCFA analysis (which is used in the diagnostic evaluation of patients with peroxisomal disorders).

(Chapter 163: "Congenital Disorders of Glycosylation." Pp 642–644.)

Answer 11-39. d

All the disorders listed above are disorders of cholesterol synthesis; however, the phenotype described above is most consistent with Smith Lemli Opitz syndrome. Cholesterol is an important constituent of cell membranes and has important interactions with signaling proteins involved in embryogenesis and development. Disorders of this pathway lead to dysmorphic features and malformations of internal organs.

The signs and symptoms of Smith Lemli Opitz syndrome vary in severity. Typical features include intrauterine growth restriction with low maternal estriol levels. At birth, dysmorphic features include microcephaly, ptosis, anteverted nares, cleft palate, other midline defects such as congenital heart disease, genital abnormalities, and 2–3 toe syndactyly. Hypotonia, feeding problems and failure to thrive are common. Patients with IUGR, microcephaly, and 2–3 toe syndactyly warrant further evaluation for this disorder. This is an autosomal recessive disorder. Diagnosis requires analysis of plasma sterols and shows elevated concentration of 7-dehydrocholesterol.

(Pp 645–647. Chapter 164: "Disorders of Cholesterol Synthesis")

Answer 11-40. b

Disorders of lipid and lipoprotein metabolism are characterized by dyslipidemia, which is defined as either elevated or low levels of one or more of the major lipoprotein classes: chylomicrons, very-low-density lipoproteins (VLDL), low-density lipoproteins (LDL), and high-density lipoproteins (HDL). Dyslipidemias can result from the expression of a mutation in a single gene that plays a paramount role in lipoprotein metabolism.

More often, dyslipidemias reflect the influence of multiple genes with a significant contribution of environmental influences (as listed in Choice b). The major clinical complication of dyslipidemias is their predilection to atherosclerosis starting early in life and leading to cardiovascular disease (CVD) in adulthood. Dyslipidemias are not usually associated with developmental delay. A number of clinical, epidemiologic, metabolic, genetic, and randomized clinical trials support the tenet that the origins of atherosclerosis and CVD risk factors begin in early childhood and treatment should begin early in life. Children with inherited disorders of lipid and lipoprotein metabolism may manifest profound hypertriglyceridemia, which can lead to episodes of severe and acute abdominal pain as a result of pancreatitis not pseudo-obstruction.

(P 651. Chapter 166: "Disorders of Lipid and Lipoprotein Metabolism")

Answer 11-41. d

In 1992, the National Cholesterol Education Program (NCEP) Expert Panel on Blood Cholesterol Levels in Children and Adolescents recommended that selective, not general screening be performed. Universal lipid screening for all children is controversial. Current NCEP guidelines recommend a lipoprotein profile in youth whose parents and/or grandparents required coronary artery bypass surgery or balloon angioplasty prior to age 55 years (not 65 years).

Other NCEP guidelines for screening include: a lipoprotein profile in youth with a family history of myocardial infarction, angina pectoris, peripheral or cerebral vascular disease, or sudden death prior to the age of 55 years (not 65 years); a total cholesterol in those whose parents have high total cholesterol levels of greater than 240 mg/dL ; a lipoprotein profile if the biological parental or grandparental family history is unknown *and* the patient has 2 or more other risk factors for CAD.

(P 653: "Screening for Dyslipidemia in Youth")

Answer 11-42. a

The first form of therapy for children with dyslipidemia is a diet containing decreased amounts of fat, cholesterol, and simple sugars but increased amount of complex carbohydrates. No decrease in total protein is recommended.

Recent data from randomized trials indicate that a diet low in total fat, cholesterol and saturated fat may be instituted safely under medical supervision at 6 months of age. The statins and BAS are the 2 main classes of pharmacologic agents currently used in children over 10 years of age who have sufficiently elevated LDL-C; however, they are not generally used as first line of therapy.

(P 655–656: "Guidelines for Treating Dyslipidemia in Children and Adolescents")

Answer 11-43. c

Heterozygous FH is an autosomal dominant disorder that presents at birth and early in life with 2–3 fold elevations in LDL-C. Heterozygosity for FH affects about 1 in 500 people and is due to more than 900 different mutations in LDLR. 50% of male adults with untreated heterozygous FH and 25% of female adults with untreated heterozygous FH, will develop CVD by age 50.

Patients who are homozygotes for FH have significantly more severe manifestations than heterozygous FH and can die from CVD in the second decade. About 1 in a million individuals are homozygous for FH.

("Familial hypercholesterolemia (FH). Pp 657–658)

Answer 11-44. e

Most disorders of hypertriglyceridemia in children are due to VLDL overproduction. A few rare disorders like of lipoprotein lipase deficiency are expressed as marked hypertriglyceridemia with TG levels exceeding 1000 mg/dL. Pancreatitis is the major medical concern with significantly elevated TG levels.

(P 660: "Disorders of Marked Hypertriglyceridemia")

Answer 11-45. b

The porphyrias are a group of inherited and acquired metabolic disorders, each resulting from the deficient activity of a specific enzyme in the heme biosynthetic pathway. These disorders are inherited as autosomal dominant, autosomal recessive, and sporadic (porphyria cutanea tarda) conditions. They are primarily classified as hepatic or erythropoietic, depending on the primary site of overproduction or accumulation of the porphyrin precursor or porphyrin.

Manifestations of the *hepatic* porphyrias characteristically include abdominal pain, neuropathy, and mental disturbance. Manifestations of the *erythropoietic* porphyrias characteristically include cutaneous photosensitivity.

The porphyrias are ecogenic disorders in which environmental, physiologic, and genetic factors interact to cause disease. Steroid hormones, drugs, and nutrition influence the production of porphyrin precursors and porphyrins, thereby precipitating or increasing the severity of some porphyrias.

(P 662. Chapter 167: "Disorders of Heme Biosynthesis: The Porphyrias" and Table 167-1, p 663)

Answer 11-46. c

All the disorders listed above are defects in purine metabolism. Main presenting clinical signs and laboratory data in inborn errors of purine and pyrimidine metabolism are summarized in Table 168-1. Myoadenylate deaminase deficiency has been found in 1–2% of the Caucasian population; however, many deficient patients may remain asymptomatic. It can manifest with muscle weakness and cramps following exercise. Patients should be advised to exercise with caution.

Adenylosuccinase deficiency can also present with myopathy but is also associated with seizures, mild to profound neurocognitive impairment and autistic features. In normal individuals, 2 minutes of ischemic forearm exercise leads to a several fold elevation of venous ammonia level, this is absent in myoadenylate deaminase deficiency.

(Pp 668–671 and Table168-1, pp 669–670. Purine Metabolism)

Answer 11-47. d

Lesch–Nyhan disease is an incapacitating neurological disorder that is typically limited to males based on X-linked inheritance. It is characterized by choreoathetosis, spasticity, compulsive self-mutilation, and 3- to 4-fold elevations in plasma and urine uric acid levels.

The first indication of the disease may be brownish to red "sand" (crystals of uric acid tinged with blood) in diapers especially with dehydration. Infants show normal development in the first 4–6 months, followed by irritability (possible related to renal colic) and hypotonia. These events are followed in the 2nd year of life by choreiform movements, development of spasticity, and subsequently by onset of self-mutilatory behavior. Severely affected children are never able to walk. The excessive production of uric acid in HPRT deficiency is explained by an enhanced purine synthesis rate. Milder and intermediate variants have been described.

(P 671: "Disorders of Purine Salvage. Hypoxanthine–Guanine phosphoribosyltransferase deficiency (HPRT deficiency/ Lesch–Nyhan disease)"

Answer 11-48. a

Dihydropyrimidine dehydrogenase deficiency has been found in subjects with very variable clinical symptoms including children with seizures, autistic features, and neurocognitive impairment; and asymptomatic relatives or subjects presenting with toxic reactions to the anticancer drug, 5-flourouracil (5-FU). The deficiency leads to accumulation of uracil and thymine and blocks the catabolism of 5-FU. Discontinuation of 5-FU results in a slow resolution of its toxicity.

(Pp 671–672: "Pyrimidine Metabolism: Disorders of Pyrimidine Catabolism: Dihydropyrimidine dehydrogenase deficiency")

Answer 11-49. c

Zinc is the cofactor for over 100 enzymes and as such is involved in all major metabolic pathways. Patients with mutations in the intestinal zinc specific transporter, SLC30A2 develop acrodermatitis enteropathica characterized by diarrhea and severe periorificial dermatitis. Diagnostic tests include a low zinc level followed by DNA testing. Treatment includes high doses of zinc sulfate.

(Pp 673–675 and Table 169-1, p 674. Disorders of Metal Metabolism. Zinc)

Answer 11-50. a

The above vignette describes the characteristic presentation of classic Menkes disease, which is due to mutations in the ATP7A gene that encodes a copper-transport protein required for the efflux of copper from cells.

Diagnostic tests include low levels of copper and ceruloplasmin in serum, followed by DNA-based testing. Subcutaneous injections of copper histidine or copper chloride before age 10 days normalizes developmental outcome in some children and improves the neurologic outcome in others.

(Pp 673–675 and Table 169-1, p 674. Disorders of Metal Metabolism. Copper)

CHAPTER 12 | Clinical Genetics and Dysmorphology

Angela Scheuerle

12-1. You are seeing a 47-year-old woman for a prenatal visit. She is expecting her first child and she is concerned whether her future infant will be at risk for any genetic conditions. Which common aneuploidy is NOT associated with increasing maternal age?

   a. Down syndrome

   b. Edwards syndrome

   c. Patau syndrome

   d. Turner syndrome

   e. All of the above

12-2. A 5-year-old boy presents for his first well-child visit to your practice. In terms of past medical history, you learn from his mother that he was diagnosed with autism spectrum disorder. He was conceived by artificial reproductive technologies because his mother has premature ovarian failure. A quick family history reveals that his maternal grandfather was diagnosed with Parkinson disease at the age of 55.

   Mutation of which gene is most likely responsible for this family's presentations?

   a. *AR*

   b. *FMR1*

   c. *HD*

   d. *PARK2*

   e. *UBE3A*

12-3. A 2-month-old female is diagnosed with phenylketonuria (PKU), which is caused by a deficiency in phenylalanine hydroxylase (PAH). She has a 10-year-old brother who is clinically normal. Assuming that the brother is not affected with PKU, his risk of carrying a mutation affecting PAH activity is:

   a. 1/4

   b. 1/3

   c. 1/2

   d. 2/3

   e. 3/4

12-4. You are attending in the nursery and suspect that the child pictured below has Down syndrome. Which of the following statements is correct?

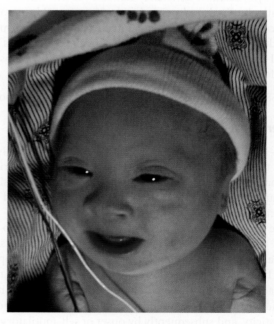

(Reproduced, with permission, from Rudolph CD, Rudolph AM, Lister GE, First LR, Gershon AA. *Rudolph's Pediatrics.* 22nd ed. New York: McGraw-Hill, 2011.)

   a. Down syndrome is relatively rare and occurs in 1 in 8000 infants

   b. All individuals with Down syndrome have three copies of the entire chromosome 21

   c. The presence of a single transverse crease is pathognomic for Down syndrome

   d. Physical examination is likely to reveal hypertonia and exaggerated primitive reflexes

   e. Referral for echocardiogram is not necessary for routine health supervision for children with Down syndrome

12-5. A newborn female weighs 4.6 kg. She has a large tongue and an umbilical hernia. She is noted to have facial hemangiomata, pits on the backs of her ear helices, and double creases in her earlobes. Abdominal ultrasound reveals enlarged, lobulated kidneys. Her likelihood of having cognitive impairments is most related to the presence of:

a. Hemihyperplasia

b. Hypoglycemia

c. Jaundice

d. Obstructive apnea

e. Wilms tumor

12-6. A newborn has a round, flattened face, accessory fontanelle, small ears and mouth, upslanted palpebral fissures, a short rib cage, short fingers, bilateral transverse palmar creases, widely spaced 1st and 2nd toes, and generalized hypotonia. Echocardiogram reveals an ostium primum atrial septal defect. Radiographic examination of the chest and abdomen reveals a "double bubble" sign. In order to provide the parents with complete diagnostic and recurrence risk counseling, the most appropriate genetic test is a:

a. Chromosome breakage study

b. Cytogenomic microarray analysis

c. Flourescence *in situ* hybridization

d. Routine karyotype

e. Whole exome sequencing

12-7. A newborn is noted to have a large anterior fontanelle, low set ears, bifid left thumb, imperforate anus, and undescended testes. In investigating possible causes, which 2 defects have the highest likelihood of generating a useful list of differential diagnoses when used together in a search?

a. Bifid left thumb and imperforate anus

b. Large anterior fontanelle and low-set ears

c. Low-set ears and undescended testes

d. Imperforate anus and large anterior fontanelle

e. Undescended testes and bifid thumb

12-8. You are seeing a 2-year-old who has an open neural tube defect. The mother has heard that taking folic acid can decrease the chance of having another child with this condition. She asks your advice about folic acid supplementation. The recommendation is:

a. 0.4 mg (400 mcg) of folic acid daily beginning preconceptionally

b. 0.4 mg (400 mcg) of folic acid daily from the diagnosis of pregnancy

c. 4.0 mg (4000 mcg) of folic acid daily beginning preconceptionally

d. 4.0 mg (4000 mcg) of folic acid daily from the diagnosis of pregnancy

e. Any dosage of folic acid as long as it is started before the end of the first trimester

12-9. Animal studies of drug X have shown no apparent increased risk of birth defects in rabbits and non-human primates, but a slight increased risk of cleft lip in rats. How would you interpret this information for a pregnant woman who has been on drug X and is at the 12th week of gestation?

a. The data are reassuring because the risk in non-human primates was not elevated

b. There are too many variables to extrapolate to humans from animal models

c. She has a high risk of having a fetus with a cleft lip

d. Clefting of the lip in rats has a different embryogenesis than clefting in humans.

e. The fetus is at no risk as long as the medication is discontinued immediately

12-10. The embryonic stage that determines laterality and creates 3 tissue layers is

a. Gastrulation

b. Implantation

c. Induction

d. Neurulation

e. Pattern Formation

12-11. In embryonic limb development, the structure that drives proximal/distal growth is the

a. Apical ectodermal ridge

b. Neural crest cell

c. Pharyngeal pouch

d. Progress zone

e. Zone of polarizing activity

12-12. Abnormality of chromosome number (i.e., aneuploidy) is the leading known cause of:

a. Cognitive impairment

b. Growth aberration

c. Heritable disorders

d. Major malformations

e. Spontaneous abortion

12-13. Hereditary conditions are those that…

    a. are present from the time of conception

    b. can be transmitted during reproduction from the parent to the offspring

    c. manifest equally in all affected persons

    d. originate by mutation of the nuclear but not mitochondrial genome

    e. present in more than 1 member of the family

12-14. With regard to the inheritance of genetic conditions, the concept of *penetrance* refers to the

    a. clinical diagnosis assigned when more than one condition is caused by mutations in the relevant gene (ie, allelic conditions)

    b. degree of variation or severity among people who express the phenotype

    c. incidence of familial cases as compared to cases caused by de novo genetic mutation

    d. percentage of affected individuals within a given generation of a family

    e. proportion of individuals with the genotype who manifest any part of the phenotype

12-15. With regard to inheritance of genetic conditions, the concept of *expressivity* refers to the

    a. clinical diagnosis assigned when more than one condition is caused by mutations in the relevant gene (i.e., allelic conditions)

    b. degree of variation or severity among people who express the phenotype

    c. incidence of familial cases as compared to cases caused by de novo genetic mutation

    d. percentage of affected individuals within a given generation of a family

    e. proportion of individuals with the genotype who manifest any part of the phenotype

12-16. A genetic condition is caused by a repeated triplet base pair sequence (CAG). With each generation in a family, the repeated segment enlarges, leading to earlier symptom onset. This phenomenon is known as:

    a. Anticipation

    b. Increased penetrance

    c. Mutagenesis

    d. Pleiotropy

    e. Variable expressivity

12-17. Collagen protein is comprised of 3 intertwining strands. Most commonly there are two identical strands ("A" strands) and 1 nonidentical strand ("B" strand). A and B strands are coded by separate genes. A mutation in the gene for the B strand will interfere with structure of that polypeptide so that the final collagen protein will be abnormal. This is an example of which mechanism of mutation?

    a. Dominant negative

    b. Gain of function

    c. Haploinsufficiency

    d. Imprinting

    e. Pleiotropy

12-18. A 3-year-old girl with a history of autism presents for a second opinion. She has delayed language development. You note paroxysmal laughter and tongue thrusting. On examination, you note prognathism, and an abnormal gait. Examination is negative for any rash. What is the most likely diagnosis?

    a. Angelman syndrome

    b. Prader–Willi syndrome

    c. Rett syndrome

    d. Tuberous sclerosis

    e. Fragile X syndrome

12-19. A 3-year-old child is diagnosed with Angelman syndrome. When taking the family history, you learn that his first cousin – his mother's sister's child – also has been diagnosed with Angelman syndrome. Both mothers are normal and there is no other history of the condition in the family.

The most likely explanation for this familial occurrence of Angelman is:

    a. Coincidence

    b. Deletion of the Prader–Willi/Angelman region on the maternal chromosome 15

    c. Maternally inherited *UBE3A* mutation

    d. Nonpaternity

    e. Uniparental disomy of chromosome 15

12-20. For each mother, what is the risk that her next child will have Angelman syndrome?

    a. Less than 1%

    b. 25%

    c. 50%

    d. 66%

    e. Depends upon the sex of the child

12-21. A 3-year-old boy presents to your clinic for the first time. He is a former full-term infant, who was originally noted to have hypotonia and had a poor swallow. He has since recovered; however, he is now noted to have a BMI approaching the 90th percentile. He learned how to walk at 15 months of age. His language development is delayed. On examination he has almond-shaped eyes, as well as small hands and feet. The remainder of the examination is unremarkable.

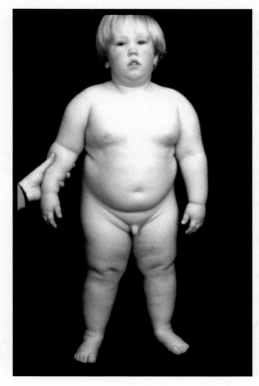

(Reproduced, with permission, from Kappy MS, Allen DB, Geffner ME. *Pediatric Practice: Endocrinology.* New York: McGraw-Hill, 2010.)

What is the most likely diagnosis?
a. Angelman syndrome
b. Prader–Willi syndrome
c. Rett syndrome
d. Tuberous sclerosis
e. Fragile X syndrome

12-22. Heteroplasmy is the state of having 2 or more different populations of mitochondrial DNA. Heteroplasmy arises by
a. absence of heterozygosity in the mitochondrial genome
b. functional differentiation of mitochondria by tissue type

c. inheritance of different mitochondria from the parents
d. mutations in the mitochondrial genome
e. post-zygotic mitochondrial fusion

12-23. Tay Sachs disease is an autosomal recessive degenerative neurologic disease. It is relatively common in the Cajun population of Louisiana. Cajuns descend from a group of French-speaking immigrants (Acadians) from eastern Canada in the 18th century. It is postulated that one of them was a man who was a carrier for the Tay Sachs mutation. His descendants carry the mutation and intermarriage has led to appearance of the disease. This phenomenon of a mutation originating with a single individual is known as:
a. Consanguinity
b. Endogamy
c. Decreased fitness
d. Founder effect
e. Genetic drift

12-24. The recurrence of a multifactorial condition or birth defect in the family varies based on a variety of factors. How does male or female sex influence the recurrence risk?
a. Risk is higher if an affected parent is of the opposite sex
b. Risk is higher if the proband is the first sibling of that sex.
c. Risk is higher if the proband is of the less commonly affected sex
d. Risk is lower if the proband has more than 1 unaffected sibling of the same sex
e. Risk is lower if the only other affected family member is in the paternal lineage

12-25. For autosomal dominant disorders, recurrence risk decreases by one-half for each successive degree of a relationship. Comparably, recurrence risk for multifactorial disorders:
a. Falls off more rapidly as genetic distance increases
b. Increases with descendent generations
c. Is inherited only through the maternal line
d. Is not affected by degree of relationship
e. Remains above background for all relatives of the more commonly affected sex

12-26. By studying twins, monzygotic versus dizygotic, it is possible to estimate the relative contribution of genetics to a given trait or birth defect. The best type of study design to indicate the difference between environmental and genetic influences involve:

a. Children born to mothers who are themselves monozygotic twins

b. Dizygotic twins discordant for structural birth defects.

c. Dizygotic twins of the same sex

d. Monozygotic twins who are raised apart

e. Triplets comprised 1 set of monozygotic twins and an independent triplet

12-27. Diagnosis and management of a genetic condition, particularly one that is rare, includes recognition of signs/symptoms, adequate history taking, detailed physical exam, triage of testing to look first for treatable conditions, coordination of medical surveillance and management, and appropriate counseling and support of the family. In this way, genetic medicine differs from all other branches of medicine in what aspect?

a. History taking

b. Recognition of signs

c. Directed testing

d. Care coordination and counseling

e. None of the above

Questions 12-28 to 30.

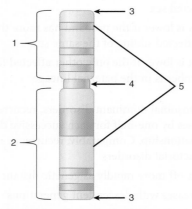

FIGURE 1. (Questions 12-28 to 30)

12-28. For the chromosome labeled in Figure 1, what is represented by the numeral 2?

a. Bands

b. Centromere

c. p arm

d. q arm

e. Telomere

12-29. For the chromosome labeled in Figure 1, what is represented by the numeral 3?

a. Bands

b. Centromere

c. p arm

d. q arm

e. Telomere

12-30. For the chromosome labeled in Figure 1, what is represented by the numeral 5?

a. Bands

b. Centromere

c. p arm

d. q arm

e. Telomere

12-31. What karyotype would represent the following description: A male with unbalanced translocation between chromosomes 1 and 3 with breakpoints at 1p22 and 3q13.1 resulting in partial monosomy 1p and partial trisomy 3q.

a. 46,XY,der(1;3)(p22;q13.1)

b. 46,XY,t(1;3)(p22;q13.1)

c. 46,XY,t(1p22;3q13.1)

d. 46,XY,der(1)t(1;3)(p22;q13.1)

e. 46,XY,der(1;3)(p22-;q13.1+)

12-32. A newborn has routine nondisjunction trisomy 21 causing Down syndrome. The mother is 28 years of age. Her risk of having another child with Down syndrome in the next 5 years is:

a. 1/800

b. 1/100

c. 1/6

d. Age-dependent

e. Dependent upon parental carrier state

12-33. A 3-year-old comes to the office as a new patient. She has right-sided microtia and facial asymmetry with the right side of her mandible being small relative to the left. She has no history of chronic or recurrent health problems. Hearing has been tested within the previous 6 months and is normal in the left ear. She is developmental appropriate for her age. Renal ultrasound was normal in the newborn period. What additional testing should be considered?

a. Adaptive behavior evaluation

b. Cytogenomic microarray

c. Electroencephalogram

d. Spine radiographs

e. Visual evoked potentials

12-34. A child is born with bilateral microtia, colobomata of the lower eyelids, absent zygomata, micrognatia, and a high but intact palate. What is the most likely diagnosis?

    a. Pierre Robin sequence

    b. Smith–Lemli–Opitz syndrome

    c. Goldenhar syndrome

    d. Treacher Collins syndrome

    e. CHARGE syndrome

12-35. A child is born with bilateral microtia, colobomata of the lower eyelids, absent zygomata, micrognatia, and a high but intact palate. A diagnosis of Treacher Collins syndrome is made. The most important intervention that should be done to maximize speech development is:

    a. Hearing aid placement

    b. Mandibular distraction

    c. Pharyngeal flap surgery

    d. Sign language training

    e. Speech therapy

12-36. Osteogenesis imperfecta is caused by mutations in the genes for type I collagen (*COL1A1* and *COL1A2*). Mutations that decrease polypeptide synthesis typically result in less severe disease than point mutations that change a single amino acid. Why?

    a. Amino acid changes almost always involve *COL1A2*

    b. Epigenetic factors are more important in the context of missense mutations

    c. Mutations deleting a gene are less likely to be inherited

    d. Null mutations are more likely to result in spontaneous abortion

    e. Point mutations interfere with tertiary protein structure

12-37. Thanatophoric dysplasia, achondroplasia, and hypocondroplasia are caused by different mutations in the Fibroblast Growth Factor Receptor 3 gene (*FGFR3*). This phenomenon is an example of:

    a. Allelic heterogenity

    b. Co-dominance

    c. Locus heterogenity

    d. Reduced penetrance

    e. Variable expressivity

12-38. A child is born with micrognathia, glossoptosis, and a U-shaped cleft palate. This combination of findings is most appropriately classified as a:

    a. Association

    b. Disruption

    c. Field defect

    d. Sequence

    e. Syndrome

12-39. A 12-year-old presents as a new patient to your clinic. She has a diagnosis of intellectual disability with autism spectrum disorder. Her general physical health is good. Her mother requests referral to dermatology because the patient has facial acne that has been resistant to therapy (Figure 360-4), including dermabrasion, a bumpy rash over the left scapula, and "fungus" of the toenails.

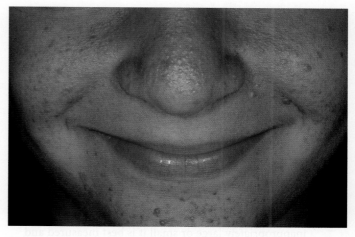

FIGURE 360-4. (Reproduced, with permission, from Rudolph CD, Rudolph AM, Lister GE, First LR, Gershon AA. *Rudolph's pedistrics.* 22nd Ed. New York: McGraw-Hill, 2011.)

On physical exam you also note 3 areas of hypopigmentation on the abdomen. The most appropriate next step in patient management is:

    a. Biopsy of the facial lesions

    b. Brain magnetic resonance imaging

    c. Prescription of isotretinoin

    d. Referral to dermatology

    e. Technicium nuclear medicine evaluation

12-40. A child is brought to the clinic by her father. She is clinically well. The father reports that he was recently diagnosed with von Hippel–Lindau syndrome. He wants to know whether his daughter is also affected. What do you need to know to best answer his question?

    a. If there was more than one tumor present at diagnosis.

    b. How old he was when he was diagnosed

    c. Location of his presenting tumor

    d. Results of his mutation analysis

    e. Whether there are other affected members of the family

12-41. There are 5 clinical types of von Hippel–Lindau syndrome differentiated by their mutation and tumor types. It has been recognized that patients with missense mutations are more likely to have pheochromocytoma than patients with complete gene deletion. This phenomenon, in which the clinical presentation of a specific condition varies with the underlying mutation type is

a. Allelic heterogenity

b. Genotype:phenotype correlation

c. Pleiotropy

d. Reduced penetrance

e. Variable expressivity

12-42. Hutchinson–Gilford syndrome (short stature, sparse hair, osteopenia), Hallerman–Streif syndrome (short stature, sparse hair, premature cataracts), and cutis laxa (loose, unelastic skin) are all what type of condition?

a. Collagenopathies

b. Disorders of accelerated aging

c. Ectodermal dysplasias

d. Laminopathies

e. Nucleotide excision repair disorders

12-43. In order to determine whether a child's head size is inappropriately large or small it is best measured and compared against what other growth parameter?

a. Arm length

b. Chest circumference

c. Height or length

d. Inner canthal distance

e. Weight

12-44. A woman with PKU has been under moderate control since she was diagnosed in infancy. Her unaffected husband is not a carrier of the condition. She became unexpectedly pregnant: her pregnancy was identified at 8 weeks post conception. At that time, she began restricting her diet to what she had been on as a child. What are the risks to the baby?

a. Microcephaly with a 25% risk of PKU

b. Microcephaly with a 50% risk of PKU

c. Microcephaly with a >99% risk of PKU

d. Microcephaly alone

e. PKU alone

12-45. A male patient appears with a family history of the following conditions: his mother has breast cancer, his maternal aunt had a foot amputation in a machinery mishap, his father sneezes when going out into the sun, his paternal uncle has asbestosis, his sister has had multiple miscarriages. Of these conditions, which is not of genetic concern?

a. Amputation

b. Asbestosis

c. Breast cancer

d. Recurrent miscarriage

e. Sneezing

12-46. A healthy 2-week-old baby presents for routine newborn pediatric evaluation. Her mother reports that the baby has been diagnosed with a balanced chromosomal translocation involving chromosomes 2 and 13. The mother also has this translocation having been diagnosed after her third miscarriage. The birth weight was 3450 g with Apgar scores of 7 and 9. She went home with her mother in 36 hours and has had no subsequent hospitalizations. She is breast feeding without problems and has good weight gain. There is a normal red reflex and the child is not dysmorphic. There is no heart murmur or abdominal mass. The genitalia and extremities are normal. The most likely reason that the newborn was found to have the balanced translocation is:

a. Amniocentesis because of the maternal diagnosis

b. Evaluation because of intrauterine growth restriction

c. Placental testing after complicated delivery

d. Prenatal diagnosis of a structural heart defect.

e. Umbilical cord blood testing for stem cell banking

12-47. Congenital contractures are caused by:

a. Any factor that diminishes movement

b. Autosomal dominant Mendelian mutations

c. Constricting maternal anatomy

d. Environment such as maternal nutritional state

e. Epigenetic factors

12-48. There are estimated to be 20,000–25,000 genes in the human genome. It is observed that some genes have variable splicing and that a single stretch of DNA may produce more than one gene depending upon the direction of transcription. Additionally, there are polymorphisms that lead to hundreds of normal variant base pair differences between even closely related people. The ultimate source of person-to-person variation in the genome is:

  a. Epigenetic factors

  b. Fertilization

  c. Recombination

  d. Meiotic crossover

  e. Mutation

12-49. The number of descendants produced by a person possessing a given genotype or phenotype is a description of that person's:

  a. Fertility

  b. Fitness

  c. Genetic drift

  d. Reproducibility

  e. Zygosity

12-50.

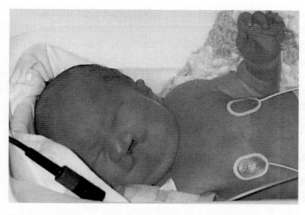

Figure for questions 12-50 and 12-51. (Reproduced, with permission, from Jorde LB, Carey JC, Bamshad MJ, White RL. *Medical Genetics*. 2nd ed. St Louis: CV Mosby; 2000.)

The baby in the picture was diagnosed prenatally with intrauterine growth restriction, facial malformations, and structural abnormalities of the brain and heart. Based upon the child's facial features, what is the most likely brain malformation affecting the child?

  a. Dandy–Walker malformation

  b. Holoprosencephaly

  c. Hydrocephalus

  d. Polymicrogyria

  e. Schizencephaly

12-51. What genetic test is appropriate to confirm the baby's diagnosis?

  a. 7-dehydrocholesterol level

  b. Cytogenomic microarray analysis

  c. Routine karyotype

  d. Sequencing of the *SHH* gene

  e. Whole exome sequencing

12-52. A patient presents for a routine 3-year-old follow-up. He has been a patient in your clinic since birth. You last saw him at 2½ years when you noted that his height measurement was lower than expected and his head circumference had "crossed a curve" upward. His general health has been average. His mother is concerned that the child is not using language as much as previously. On exam at this visit, his height again shows no gain and his head is now frankly macrocephalic. His liver is mildly enlarged and he is hypertonic.

You are concerned about a storage disease. As part of the evaluation, you recommend an ophthalmologic exam. What finding would you specifically wish the ophthalmologist to look for?

  a. Cataracts

  b. Cherry red spot

  c. Iridodonesis

  d. Retinal detachment

  e. Retinitis pigmentosa

12-53. A 2-year-old female presents for routine pediatric evaluation. Her general health has been good. At her last visit she was developmentally normal. She walked at 11 months and had 5 words by her first birthday. Her mother is now concerned that the child has autism because of decreased use of language and social interaction. The child now says only "mama" and "ba," meaning "bottle". There are also some self-stimulation/ stereotypic behaviors such as midline hand grasping and wringing and blowing "raspberries." The mother has also noticed breath-holding spells. On exam, it is noted that her head circumference is static compared to the 18 month visit. She is unsteady in her gait and hyperreflexic. The most likely diagnosis is:

  a. Angelman syndrome

  b. Autism spectrum disorder

  c. Mowatt–Wilson syndrome

  d. PKU

  e. Rett syndrome

12-54. You see a patient in an urgent care center and notice the presence of microbrachycephaly and micrognathia. The patient has a low hairline, synophrys, arched eyebrows, long eyelashes, a thin upper lip and low-set ears. In examining the patient's extremities, you note spade like hands, 2–3 syndactyly of toes. What is the most likely syndrome?

a. Moebius sequence

b. Sturge–Weber syndrome

c. Cornilia de Lange syndrome

d. Beckwith–Wiedemann syndrome

e. Cleidocranial dysplasia

12-55. Which of the following syndromes is not associated with craniosynostoses?

a. Crouzon syndrome

b. Apert syndrome

c. Carpenter syndrome

d. Cleidocranial dysplasia

e. Pfeiffer syndrome

12-56. A newborn male is diagnosed with achondroplasia. He was born to unaffected parents and it is presumed that his case represents a de novo mutation in *FGFR3*. The mother was 37 at the time of conception and smoked 1 pack per day of cigarettes. She worked in a manufacturing plant during the pregnancy. The father was 41 at the time of conception, had congenital hip dysplasia at birth, and worked as a contract engineer during the first Gulf War. The mother is 5 feet, 4 inches tall. The father is 5 feet, 10 inches tall. It is reported that the paternal grandmother was under 5 feet tall. Of these factors, which is most associated with the manifestation of achondroplasia in the infant?

a. Environmental exposure in a war zone

b. Grandparental height

c. Hip dysplasia

d. Paternal age

e. Smoking

ANSWERS

Answer 12-1. d

Turner syndrome is most commonly related to abnormalities of the sperm – failure of the sperm to have a sex chromosome. This fact is important for genetic counseling. Down (Trisomy 21), Patau (Trisomy 13), and Edwards (Trisomy 18) are all associated with advanced maternal age.

(Chapter 173: "Mechanism of Formation of Abnormal Chromosomes and Clinical Consequence")

Answer 12-2. b

FMR1 mutations are associated with many phenotypes, including Fragile X syndrome, autism spectrum disorder, premature ovarian failure, and Fragile X Associated Tremor/Ataxia Syndrome (FXTAS).

Fragile X syndrome is caused by the triplet repeat expansion mutation of *FMR1*. Full triplet repeat expansion mutations (>200 repeats) in *FMR1* cause mental retardation. In addition, *FMR1* mutations are a common cause of autism in males, with approximately 20% of autism in males estimated to be caused by *FMR1* mutations (Boyle, 2010). Women who are carriers of an *FMR1* pre-mutation (50–200 repeats) are at high risk of premature ovarian failure. Males who are hemizygous for a permutation-sized allele are at risk for Fragile X associated tremor/ataxia syndrome (FXTAS), which is often mis-diagnosed as Parkinson disease.

The androgen receptor (*AR*) expansion repeat causes Kennedy spinal and bulbar muscular atrophy. Point mutations cause androgen insensitivity. *HD* expansion mutations cause Huntington disease. *PARK2* mutations cause juvenile Parkinson disease. *UBE3A* mutations cause Angelman syndrome when inherited from the mother.

(Boyle L, Kaufman WE. The behavioral phenotype of FMR1 mutations. *Am J Med Genet C Semin Med Genet.* 2010;154C: 469–476.)

(Chapter 170: "Mechanisms of Mutation")

Answer 12-3. d

All forms of PKU affecting PAH activity are inherited in an autosomal recessive manner.

If "R" represents a normal allele and "r" represents a recessively mutated allele, the parents are R r and R r. Offsprings of these parents can be RR (normal), Rr (carriers), or rr (affected). The ratio is 1 RR : 2 Rr : 1 rr risk for each pregnancy.

	R	r
R	RR	Rr
r	Rr	rr

The affected child is rr. The normal brother cannot be rr (because if he were, he would have the disease). So that possibility drops out so there are three remaining possible combinations for him:

	R	r
R	RR	Rr
r	Rr	rr

Of these three, the likelihood that he is a carrier (Rr) is 2/3 [Chapter 170: Monogenic Conditions: Single-Gene Disorders]

(Chapter 170: "Key Principles in Human Genetics: Monogenic Conditions". Chapter 135: "Hyperphenylal-Aninemias")

Answer 12-4. c

Although the overall phenotypic pattern of Down syndrome is characteristic and identifiable, specific physical examination findings can be found in patients without Down syndrome. For example, the presence of a single transverse crease is a non-sensitive and nonspecific physical examination finding for Down syndrome.

Down syndrome is the most common autosomal chromosomal abnormality, with a frequency of 1 in 800 infants. Physical examination is likely to reveal hypotonia in approximately 90% of infants with Down syndrome. Congenital cardiac issues occur in 40% of infants with Down syndrome. As a result, an echocardiogram is commonly a part of routine health supervision for Down syndrome.

Over 90% of infants with Down syndrome have three separate copies of chromosome 21; however, approximately 10% have trisomy due to a translocation of only a part of the long arm of chromosome 21.

(Chapter 174: Chromosome disorders)

Answer 12-5. a

The child has Beckwith–Wiedemann syndrome. These patients generally do quite well cognitively unless there are problems with untreated hypoglycemia in infancy. The other features on the list are possible complications of Beckwith–Wiedemann, but have not been associated with the development of cognitive impairment.

(Chapter 176: "Syndromes of Multiple Congenital Anomalies/ Dysplasias: Introduction" and Chapter 177: "Craniofacial Disorders: Introduction")

Answer 12-6. d

The baby has Down syndrome, caused by trisomy of chromosome 21. It is a clinical diagnosis. Genetic testing is necessary to evaluate for a translocation trisomy as this has implications for higher recurrence and indicates a need to test the parents. Flourescence *in situ* hybridization (FISH) studies do not differentiate free from translocation trisomy and are not indicated in this situation. The other testing is inappropriate for the question being asked.

(Chapter 174: "Common Trisomy Syndromes")

Answer 12-7. a

Large anterior fontanelle, low-set ears, and undescended testes are common, nonspecific findings that are considered minor malformations. Using any of them to search for an underlying diagnosis will lead to an extended list of diagnostic possibilities that will be overwhelming.

The imperforate anus is a major malformation with a more limited scope. Bifid left thumb is also a major malformation and is much more rare. The combination of bifid thumb (major and rare) and imperforate anus (major and uncommon) has the best chance of generating a short differential diagnosis list.

(Chapter 178: "Clinical Practice")

Answer 12-8. c

This folic acid regimen is the CDC recommendation. For women with no history of an NTD-affected pregnancy, the recommended daily folic acid dosage is 0.4 mg (400 mcg): the amount found in a standard multivitamin. After the birth of a child with an NTD, the mother should take 4.0 mg (4000 mcg) of folic acid daily prior to conception. Since 50% of all pregnancies are unplanned, it is recommended that all women, regardless of the recommended dosage, be on folic acid as long as they are of childbearing potential.

(Chapter 183: "Counseling Patients about Teratogens")

Answer 12-9. b

Known variables include differences in pharmacokinetic profiles and placental biology. Unknown variables are probably many. It is noted that some animal models in thalidomide trials showed no increased risk of birth defects. On the other hand, a minority of fetuses exposed to any drug are likely to develop malformations, so she is not at a "high risk" of anything. Embryology is the same even if pathogenesis is different. It is rarely appropriate to recommend an abrupt discontinuation of any maternal medication without the input of the physician who prescribed the medication. Stopping the medication may affect the fetus and the maternal condition being treated may confer a risk greater than that of the medication.

(Chapter 183: "Factors used to Determine Teratogenic Risk")

Answer 12-10. a

Implantation is the placement of the zygote/blastula against the uterine wall. Induction is the chemical signaling between cells. Neurulation is the formation of the hollow neural tube. Pattern formation is the process by which ordered spatial arrangements of differentiated cells create tissues and organs.

(Chapter 175: "Pattern Determination")

Answer 12-11. a

Neural crest cells derive from the area of closure of the neural tube and go on to form the head, face, some heart components, melanocytes, and ganglion cells. They are not involved in limb formation. Pharyngeal pouches are structures involved in head and neck development. The progress zone is a population of mesodermal cells underneath the apical ectodermal ridge, which respond to signals from it. The zone of polarizing activity is responsible for medial/lateral and anterior/posterior positioning along the limb bud.

(Chapter 175: "Formation of Organs and Appendages")

Answer 12-12. e

Chromosomal aneuploidy is thought to account for the majority of early-pregnancy loss. While important in all of the other signs and symptoms, most genetic disease is not chromosomally based and so chromosomal aneuploidy as a whole is not the single leading cause of any of the other conditions.

(Chapter 170: "Classification of Genetic Disorders")

Answer 12-13. b

This is the definition of hereditary. It is differentiated from genetic conditions that are present at the time of conception (A). The manifestation (phenotype) of different individuals is separate from the hereditary nature of a condition (C) and can be widely variable. Genetic conditions can arise from mutations in either the nuclear or mitochondrial genome (D). Both genetic and nongenetic conditions can be present in more than 1 member of the family (E).

(Chapter 170: "Key Principles in Human Genetics")

Answer 12-14. e

This is the definition of penetrance. Answer b is the definition of expressivity. The other statements are not standard definitions of common terms.

(Chapter 170: "Key Principles in Human Genetics")

Answer 12-15. b

This is the definition of expressivity. Answer e is the definition of penetrance. The other statements are not standard definitions of common terms.

(Chapter 170: "Key Principles in Human Genetics")

Answer 12-16. a

This statement is the definition of molecular and clinical anticipation. Molecular anticipation refers to the expansion of triplet repeats in a subset of neuromuscular disease including myotonic dystrophy, Huntington disease, Fragile X syndrome, and others. Clinical anticipation is the concept that a condition is easier to diagnose in subsequent generations of a family. All conditions with molecular anticipation have clinical anticipation, but the reverse is not true.

(Chapter 170: "Key Principles in Human Genetics")

Answer 12-17. a

This situation describes a dominant negative mutation, which is, itself, a type of loss-of-function mutation. Haploinsufficiency results when 50% of the gene product is insufficient for normal development and/or function. The other 2 are not mechanisms of mutation.

(Chapter 170: "Mechanisms of Mutation")

Answer 12-18. a

Although Angelman syndrome, Rett syndrome, tuberous sclerosis, and Fragile X syndrome can be associated with autism, the phenotype of prognathism, paroxysmal laughter, and tongue thrusting make Angelman syndrome more likely. Angelman syndrome occurs when a mutated *UBE3A* is inherited through the mother. Prader–Willi syndrome results if the gene is inherited from their father. Methylation testing for UPD15 can help confirm the diagnosis.

(Chapter 170: "Nontraditional Mechanisms of Disease")

Answer 12-19. c

Both mothers/sisters inherited a mutated *UBE3A* from their father. Since it is inactive when inherited from the father, the mutation is silent and the women are healthy. But, when they conceived their own children, the mutated gene became active again. Inheritance by their children of the mutated gene will result in Angelman syndrome. The children will have no active/normal copy of the gene because the allele inherited from the father will be inactive. Coincidence and uniparental disomy of 15 are possible, but much less likely. Deletion of the entire region would either have to have occurred separately in each pregnancy – highly unlikely – or be carried by both women as inherited from a parent.

If the women had inherited the deletion, they would have one of the conditions. Specifically, they would have Angelman syndrome if inherited from their mother and Prader–Willi syndrome if inherited from their father (see Figure 170-4).

Nonpaternity is irrelevant to this condition as the paternal gene is inactive.

(Chapter 170: "Nontraditional Mechanisms of Disease")

Answer 12-20. c

Since the *UBE3A* gene will be active from the mother, regardless of which allele is passed on, it can be considered as a typical dominant condition. There is a 50% likelihood of passing on the mutated allele to each child, thus a 50% risk of Angelman syndrome in each pregnancy for each of the women. The sex of the child is irrelevant to the inheritance risk.

(Chapter 170: "Nontraditional Mechanisms of Disease")

Answer 12-21. b

Prader–Willi syndrome is caused by a deletion of 2–4 Mb of chromosome 15. When the deletion is inherited from the father, the child will have Prader–Willi syndrome. The phenotype includes severe neonatal hypotonia, obesity, small hands and feet, and mental retardation. Although infants may be described as having a "failure to thrive" during infancy due to the initial hypotonia, the syndrome is also associated with polyphagia and subsequent obesity.

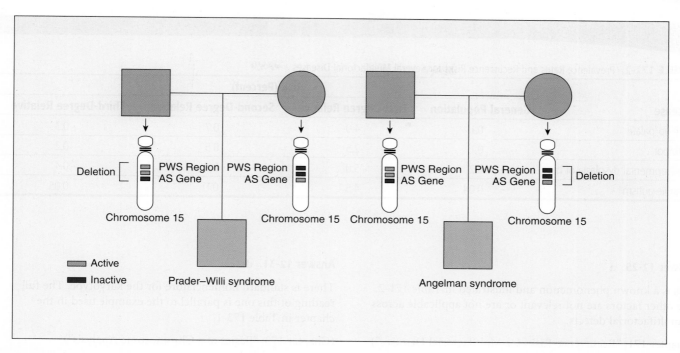

FIGURE 170-4. Pedigrees illustrate the inheritance pattern of the chromosome 15 deletion and the activation status of genes in the critical region. Inheritance of the deletion from the father produces Prader–Willi syndrome (PWS), and inheritance of the deletion from the mother produces Angelman syndrome (AS). (Reproduced, with permission, from Jorde LB, Carey JC, Bamshad MJ, White RL. *Medical Genetics*. 3rd ed. St Louis: CV Mosby; 2006.)

Angelman syndrome is also caused by a microdeletion on chromosome 15. When this microdeletion is inherited via the mother, Angelman syndrome results, which has a different phenotype.

Answer 12-22. d

This is the definition as provided by the chapter. It is important to know that all mitochondria are inherited from the mother. The other answers are invented distractors: There is no heterozygosity in the mitochondrial genome. It is haploid and, therefore, cannot demonstrate heterozygosity. There is no evidence of functional differentiation of mitochondrial by tissue type and there is no such thing as post-zygotic mitochondrial fusion.

(Chapter 170: "Nontraditional Mechanisms of Disease")

Answer 12-23. d

This scenario is considered a standard example of the Founder effect; however, other factors must come into play for the Founder effect to manifest. Endogamy (marriage within the group) and consanguinity (mating between related individuals) are part of the process perpetuating the mutation. Also a population "bottleneck" occurred. Tay Sachs does confer decreased fitness, but that is not what is driving the increased prevalence. Genetic drift is random fluctuation in gene frequencies and is essentially the opposite of this situation.

Answer 12-24. c

This is a known phenomenon that holds true for those conditions in which there is a baseline difference is birth prevalence by sex such as cleft lip, cleft palate, pyloric stenosis, and autism. The other factors are not relevant or are not applicable across all multifactorial defects.

For example, pyloric stenosis is thought to be multifactorial and affects approximately 1 in 1000 females and approximately 1 in 200 males. Those females affected may have more "liability factors" than affected males. As a result, affected females who have pyloric stenosis are more likely to produce affected offspring that affected fathers (See Table 171-1).

(Chapter 171: "Recurrence Risks for Multifactorial Diseases")

TABLE 171-1. Recurrence Risks for Offspring of Individuals Affected with Pyloric Stenosis

Affected Parent	Male	Female
Affected sons	5.5%	19.4%
Affected daughters	2.4	7.3

Data from Kidd KK, Spence MA. Genetic analyses of pyloric stenosis suggesting a specific maternal effect. *J Med Genet*. 1976;13:290–294.

TABLE 171-2. Prevalence Rates and Recurrence Risks for Several Multifactorial Diseases

Disease	Risk (Percent)			
	General Population	**First-Degree Relative**	**Second-Degree Relative**	**Third-Degree Relative**
Cleft lip/palate	0.1	4.0	0.7	0.3
Clubfoot	0.1	2.5	0.5	0.2
Developmental dysplasia of hip	0.2	5.0	0.6	0.4
Infantile autism	0.04	4.5	0.1	0.05

Answer 12-25. a

This is a known phenomenon and illustrated in Table 171-2. The other factors are not relevant or are not applicable across all multifactorial defects.

(Chapter 171: "Recurrence Risks for Multifactorial Diseases")

Answer 12-26. d

These are the best twin studies because the children are presumed to be genetically identical (or near-identical) but they have been exposed to different postnatal environments. This works for behavioral and psychological studies, but not, obviously, for studies of birth defects. For that, the studies compare MZ and DZ twins, but that is not one of the choices. The other choices are not relevant to this question.

(Chapter 171: "Twin Studies: Gauging the Relative Influence of Genetics and Environment")

Answer 12-27. e

Genetic medicine is no different in form from any other branch of medicine, but it is a separate specialty with its own language. Pediatricians should be as familiar with aspects of genetics as they are with aspects of other specialties such as surgery and ophthalmology.

Answer 12-28. d

It is always a small letter "q". The key for this and the two following questions is:
    1 = p arm
    2 = q arm
    3 = telomere(s)
    4 = centromere
    5 = bands

(Chapter 173: "Basics of a Chromosome Analysis")

Answer 12-29. e

Answer 12-30. a

Answer 12-31. d

There is standard nomenclature for the karyotype. The full reading of this one is parallel to the example used in the chapter in Table 173-1.

(Chapter 173: "Basics of a Chromosome Analysis")

Answer 12-32. b

This estimate is the recognized risk. The baseline risk for anyone in the population is about 1/800 or 0.125%, so the recurrence risk after 1 affected child represents an 8–16 fold increase in risk. Nondisjunction trisomy is a sporadic event and no testing of the parents is indicated.

(Chapter 174: "Common Trisomy Syndromes")

Answer 12-33. d

It is estimated that 25–30% of children with hemifacial microsomia (CFM) have vertebral abnormalities. Cytogenomic microarray is interesting academically but is not medically indicated. There is no clinical evidence that would suggest the need for behavioral evaluation, EEG, or VEP testing.

(Chapter 177: "Brachial Arch Derivative Anomalies")

Answer 12-34. d

The description is most consistent with Treacher Collins syndrome. Persons with Treacher Collins syndrome are typically cognitively normal, but they often have conductive hearing loss (see Figure 177-2).

Goldenhar syndrome, or Oculoauriculovertebral (OAV) syndrome, is also associated with anomalies involving the head and neck. The phenotype includes hemifacial microsomia and anomalies of the pinna with associated deafness. Other findings include ear tags, vertebral anomalies, and Arnold–Chiari type I malformations (herniation of the cerebellum into the cervical spinal canal).

Pierre Robin sequence is characterized by a triad of cleft palate, micrognathia and glossoptosis.

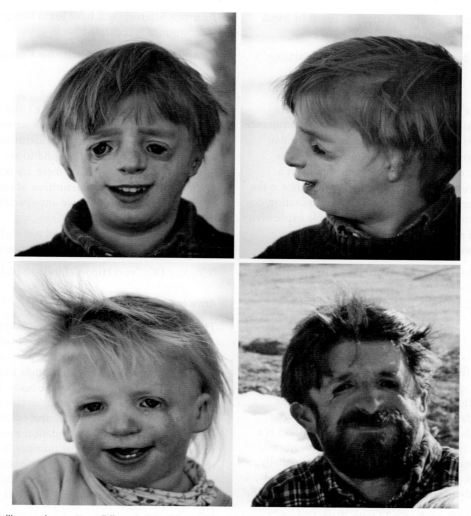

FIGURE 177-2. Treacher Collins syndrome. Two siblings (top and lower left) with variable manifestations of autosomal dominant Treacher Collins syndrome. Their father (lower right panel) was the first individual in his family known to have Treacher Collins syndrome. Both children were born with cleft palate, but their father has an intact palate. (Reproduced, with permission, from Rudolph CD, Rudolph AM, Lister GE, First LR, Gershon AA. *Rudolph's Pediatrics.* 22nd ed. New York: McGraw-Hill, 2011.)

Smith Lemli Optiz syndrome is associated with cleft palate, micrognathia, short nose, ptosis, high square forehead, microcephaly, hypospadias, cryptorchidism, VSD, TOF, hypotonia, mental retardation, postaxial polydactyly, 2–3 toe syndactyly, and defect in cholesterol biosynthesis.

CHARGE syndrome consists of **C**oloboma of the eye, **h**eart malformations, **a**tresia (choanal), **r**etardation, **g**enital anomalies, **e**ar abnormalities and/or deafness, facial palsy, cleft palate, dysphagia.

(Chapter 177: "Brachial Arch Derivative Anomalies")

Answer 12-35. a

People with Treacher Collins are typically cognitively normal, but they often have conductive hearing loss. The single most important intervention is placement of bone conduction hearing aids as young as possible. Other hearing assisting

devices can be explored over time. Palate surgery is not indicated at this time in this child. The mandible may need to be distracted and the child may need speech therapy, but those are not of urgent importance. Sign language training may be useful depending upon the situation, but it may slow rather than assist spoken language development.

(Chapter 177: "Brachial Arch Derivative Anomalies")

Answer 12-36. e

The collagen I protein is a triple helix consisting of 2 A1 polypeptides and 1 A2 poly peptide. As with twisted fibers of a rope, abnormality of 1 polypeptide—A1 or A2—will interfere with the structure of the final protein. Deletions or other mutations that lead to decreased polypeptide synthesis result in decreased but otherwise normal protein. Epigenetic factors are not relevant to this question. Gene deletions are more likely to be inherited, because they are less likely to result in lethal disease or spontaneous abortion.

(Chapter 179: "Disorders of Structural Proteins of Cartilage")

Answer 12-37. a

These are examples of a situation in which mutations in a single gene cause clinically distinct phenotypes. Co-dominance results when all alleles manifest, even if they are dissimilar, (eg, the ABO blood groupings). Locus heterogenity is the presence of a specific clinical phenotype resulting from a change in any of more than 1 gene. Reduced penetrance is the concept that some persons who have a dominant mutation do not manifest any features of the condition. Variable expressivity is the dissimilarity in manifestation of a given disease phenotype from person to person.

(Chapter 179: "Skeletal Dysplasias Caused by Mutations in Transmembrane Receptors"; Chapter 184: "Disorders of Accelerated Aging: Introduction (definition of allelic heterogeneity)")

Answer 12-38. d

The combination of findings describes the Pierre Robin Sequence. It is not a syndrome because it does not have a single consistent etiology. It is a sequence of embryologic events starting with failure of the jaw to grow. The tongue then prevents the palatal folds from fusing. A disruption is a chemical or physical interference of a structure with normal primary embryogenesis. A field defect results from spatially related abnormalities. An association is a set of defects that occur more frequently together than expected by chance alone

(Chapter 178: "Approach to the Child with Birth Defects")

Answer 12-39. b

This child presents with autism spectrum disorder and skin findings. Her clinical presentation is consistent with a diagnosis of tuberous sclerosis. The child has adenoma sebaceum , which is composed of numerous angiofibromas (skin-colored to red papules) over the central face. They continue to increase in size and number with age.

The 1–4 cm hypopigmented macules can be shaped like "ash leaves" (eg, "ash leaf spots") but they can also be round, oval, irregular, or confetti-like in their appearance. The presence of 3 or more hypomelanotic macules at birth should raise suspicion for tuberous sclerosis and warrants further evaluation.

Connective-tissue nevi, which includes a fibrous forehead plaque and shagreen patches (collagenomas, a type of connective-tissue nevus), may also aid in early diagnosis, especially when the fibrous forehead plaque is present at birth. Other cutaneous findings of tuberous sclerosis include periungal fibromas and gingival fibromas.

While dermatology referral may useful, there is no directed treatment that will cure the skin and nail findings. Brain MRI or CT is indicated because 75% or more of patients with

Tuberous Sclerosis will have brain hamartomata. None of the other options is indicated.

(Chapter 182: "Tuberous Sclerosis Complex")

Answer 12-40. d

In order to determine whether the child inherited the condition from the father, it is first necessary to know whether the father's mutation is identifiable. If it is, then it is straightforward to test the child to see if she inherited the mutation. Knowing whether there are other affected members of the family will help in definition of whether this is sporadic or inherited, but will not give any specific information about the child's risk.

The father's tumor status and age at diagnosis are relevant to his health and management, but do not impact heritability.

(Chapter 182: "von Hippel–Lindau Syndrome")

Answer 12-41. b

This is the definition of genotype: phenotype correlation. Allelic heterogeneity results when mutations in one gene cause 2 or more clinically distinct conditions. Pleiotropy is the phenomenon in which a single mutant allele may influence more than 1 part of the body. For example, a single mutation in the fibrillin gene in Marfan syndrome can have effects on the skeletal, cardiac, and ophthalmologic systems. Reduced penetrance is a population measure of the disease manifestations relative to the number of people who have the mutation. Variable expressivity is variation from person to person of mutations in a particular gene, but without specific indication that the variation is based on the type of mutation.

(Chapter 182: "von Hippel–Lindau Syndrome")

Answer 12-42. b

These are all disorders of accelerated aging: the point being that they all have features which are generally associated with normal advanced age: loss of hair, loose skin, osteopenia, cataracts, etc. None of these is a disorder of collagen or a nucleotide excision repair disorder, though some of the diseases of accelerated aging fall in that group. They are not ectodermal dysplasias. Cutis laxa is not a laminopathy and the causative gene for Hallerman–Streif has not been identified.

(Chapter 184: "Disorders of Accelerated Aging: Introduction")

Answer 12-43. c

Height or length is the best comparator. Weight is too variable with environmental factors. The other parameters are not useful in a 2-year-old. Age is not a growth parameter, though comparison of the child's head circumference against growth standards can be useful to determine whether the problem is an overall growth deficiency or just microcephaly.

(Chapter 185: "Microcephaly")

Answer 12-44. d

PKU is an autosomal recessive condition. PKU is a strong teratogenic condition causing microcephaly and severe intellectual disability. While some restriction is better than none, metabolites concentrate in the fetus so it is necessary for women with PKU to be on a severely restricted diet at least 3 months prior to conception. Restriction to standard pediatric levels is insufficient. As her spouse is unaffected and is not a carrier, all of her children will be carriers, but none will be affected with PKU.

(Chapter 170: "Monogenic Conditions: Single-Gene Disorders"; Chapter 185: "Microcephaly")

Answer 12-45. a

Conditions exist on a spectrum from fully genetic to fully acquired. Of this list, only the amputation is a fully acquired condition. Sneezing when going into the sun (eg, a photic sneeze reflex, photoptarmosis, or the "Achoo syndrome'") is a dominant condition. Breast cancer and asbestosis are both conditions with a combination of genetic and environmental influences. Recurrent miscarriage is highly likely to have an underlying genetic cause. The fact that he is a male does not eliminate his genetic risk related to breast cancer or infertility.

(Chapter 172: "Principles of Care: Introduction")

Answer 12-46. a

Balanced translocations are those in which there is no net gain or loss of genetic material. It is not unusual for otherwise healthy fetuses/newborns to be diagnosed by amniocentesis because of maternal issues such as advanced maternal age. In these instances, the finding is coincidental. Umbilical cord blood testing because of stem cell banking is a possible way to find the translocation, but is much less likely than the amniocentesis diagnosis. The other items are not indicated as the child did not have any of those findings.

(Chapter 173: "Mechanism of Formation of Abnormal Chromosomes and Clinical Consequence")

Answer 12-47. a

Any factor that decreases joint mobility—intrinsic genetic neuromuscular abnormality, teratogen, or mechanical construction—will lead to joint contractures.

(Chapter 180: "Congenital Contractures: Introduction")

Answer 12-48. e

It is true that no 2 people have exactly the same genome—identical twins coming the closest. However, for the vast majority of genes there is a standard sequence, which varies little if at all from person to person. This level of variation is nonpathogenic. The way that this base-pair variation

happens is through the various mechanisms of mutation. The mutation stays in the population through failure of DNA repair mechanisms AND the fact that the variation does not negatively impact the reproductive fitness of the individual. All of the other possible answers do create person-to-person variation, but do not cause change in the primary base pair sequence of the genome.

(Chapter 170: "Population Variation, Consanguinity, and Inbreeding")

Answer 12-49. b

This is the definition of fitness. Fertility is the ability to become or father a pregnancy during a particular menstrual cycle. Genetic drift refers to population-level random fluctuations in gene frequencies from generation to generation. Reproducibility is the ability to recreate a particular outcome or set of outcomes in an experiment. Zygosity is the way that multiple gestations are defined.

(Chapter 170: "Key Principles in Human Genetics")

Answer 12-50. b

The child has a midline cleft lip: cleft with absence of the prolabium represents a primary mildline craniofacial defect and is on the holoprosencephaly spectrum. When midline cleft lip is present, the child should be assumed to have holoprosencephaly until it is ruled out. While any of the other brain malformations can occur with facial abnormalities, holoprosencephaly is the most likely.

(Chapter 174: "Common Trisomy Syndromes")

Answer 12-51. c

The baby has Trisomy 13. The infant has a midline cleft and postaxial polydactyly as noted in the photo. In addition, there is IUGR and structural abnormalities of the heart and brain. The appropriate test to confirm Trisomy 13 is a routine karyotype.

(Chapter 174: "Common Trisomy Syndromes")

Answer 12-52. b

In a subset of lysosomal storage diseases that have CNS involvement, there is storage of lipid in the retina except at the fovea. This causes paleness of the retina with the bright red foveal "cherry red" spot. Cataracts are a feature of some of these conditions, but are more of a delayed finding. Iridodonesis is a "shaking" of the iris which is visible by routine physical exam and is seen in Marfan syndrome. Retinal detachment and retinitis pigmentosa are not features of storage diseases.

(Chapter 574: "Lysosomal Storage Disease affecting the Central Nervous System")

Answer 12-53. e

The period of normalcy with deterioration is consistent with Rett syndrome. The hand wringing and abnormal breathing are stereotypical for Rett syndrome as is the acquired microcephaly. This is caused by a mutation in the *MECP2* gene. The other conditions are in the differential diagnosis, but would have shown abnormalities since birth and have other physical abnormalities. Autism spectrum is a symptom complex that can be seen in a variety of conditions and does not constitute a single diagnosis.

(Chapter 575: "Rett Syndrome (*MECP2*-Related Disorders): Introduction")

Answer 12-54. c

This patient most likely has Cornelia de Lange syndrome.

Moebius sequence is associated with congenital facial palsy, cranial nerve VI and VII palsy, distal limb deficiencies, occasional arthrogryposis, and/or mental retardation

Sturge–Weber syndrome is associated with hemangiomata in the distribution of the trigeminal nerve, glaucoma, and seizures

Beckwith–Wiedemann syndrome is associated with coarse facial features, macroglossia (often with secondary maxillary and mandibular deformity), ear lobe creases, posterior auricular pits, mid face hypoplasia, omphalocele, generalized overgrowth or hemihypertrophy, visceromegaly, Wilms tumor (and other malignancies), cryptorchidism, and cardiomyopathy.

Cleidocranial dysplasia is associated with brachycephaly, frontal and parietal bossing, wormian bones, persistent open anterior fontanelle, maxillary hypoplasia, delayed eruption of deciduous and permanent teeth, supernumerary and fused teeth, hypoplastic to absent clavicles, brachydactyly, and joint laxity.

(Chapter 177: "Craniofacial Disorders")

Answer 12-55. d

Cleidocranial dysplasia is associated with brachycephaly, frontal and parietal bossing, wormian bones, persistent open anterior fontanelle, maxillary hypoplasia, delayed eruption of deciduous and permanent teeth, supernumerary and fused teeth, hypoplastic to absent clavicles, brachydactyly, and joint laxity

(Chapter 177: "Craniofacial Disorders")

Answer 12-56. d

"Advanced paternal age" is associated with de novo mutation in dominant conditions: conditions in which a single base pair change leads to the disease phenotype. This was first noted with achondroplasia and has subsequently been shown with other dominant conditions. Empirically, a father is considered to have "advanced paternal age" at 37 1/2 years of age.

(Chapter 170: "Key Principles in Human Genetics")

CHAPTER 13 | Immunologic Disorders

Hilary M. Haftel

13-1. A 3-year-old boy returns to your office with his sixth upper respiratory infection this year. Which of the following factors would increase your index of suspicion for an underlying immunodeficiency?

　a. The child is in daycare 4 days per week.

　b. The child's tonsils are grossly enlarged

　c. He was hospitalized 3 times last year for infections

　d. His thymic shadow is visualized on chest radiograph

　e. He is maintaining steady growth at the tenth percentile for height and weight.

13-2. Of the following options, the best initial test for a workup for immunodeficiency is:

　a. Serum levels of IgG, IgM, IgA, IgE

　b. A complete blood count with differential

　c. Peripheral T-cell phenotyping

　d. Erythrocyte sedimentation rate

　e. Postimmunization immunoglobulin levels

13-3. A 5-month-old child is brought to your office for evaluation of failure to thrive. His mother reports that he has been suffering from constant diarrhea and failure to gain weight. On exam you note that the child is in the 50% percentile for a 1-month-old. Physical exam reveals diffuse erythroderma, a distended, tympanitic abdomen, and a palpable liver and spleen. In addition to lymphopenia, what other abnormality would you expect to find on assessment of a complete blood count?

　a. Macrocytosis

　b. Small platelets

　c. Neutrophilia

　d. Basophilic stippling

　e. Eosinophilia

13-4. A 7-month-old child is brought to your office for evaluation for an immune deficiency. Her mother reports that she has had several bouts of diarrhea in the last few months and has had difficulty gaining weight. She was recently hospitalized for pneumonia. Physical exam demonstrates absence of tonsillar tissue and a thymic shadow is absent on chest radiograph. Her mom also reports that several family members died in infancy from infection and she had been told they had "some enzyme deficiency."

Which of the following physical findings would provide further evidence that this child has adenosine deaminase deficiency?

　a. Cupping and flaring of the costochondral junctions

　b. Shortening of the forearms

　c. Bowing of the legs

　d. Midface hypoplasia

　e. Epicanthal folds

13-5. An 8-month-old male is diagnosed with Severe Combined Immunodeficiency after presenting with failure to thrive and chronic infections. Genotyping reveals a mutation in the gene coding for Janus-type protein tyrosine kinase (JAK3).

Your advice to his parents would include which of the following?

　a. Only the patient's female offspring can be carriers

　b. Given time, the patient's T- and B-cell function should return to normal

　c. The disorder is due to failure of mature T cells to properly recognize the antigen

　d. The patient may not have normal B-cell function even after bone marrow transplantation

　e. The patient's splenic function will be impaired

13-6. ZAP70 is a protein tyrosine kinase expressed in T lymphocytes and is critical in the pathway for activation of T cells. In addition to impaired responses to antigenic stimulation, the following can also be found on cell analysis:

a. Lack of circulating CD8+ T cells

b. Lack of circulating CD4+ T cells

c. Lack of CD4+CD8+ thymocytes

d. Lack of circulating CD3+ B cells

e. Lack of B-cell precursors

13-7. A male infant is noted at birth to have a broad and depressed nose and broad nasal filtrum and a cleft palate. At 12 hours of life, he becomes jittery and is noted to have a serum calcium level of 6.8 mg/dL. Chest radiograph demonstrates absence of a thymic shadow and a complete blood count demonstrates lymphopenia. Subsequent flow cytometry demonstrates normal numbers of B cells with moderately low T-cell numbers.

Over time, which of the following would be expected of this patient's immunodeficiency?

a. T-cell numbers will continue to fall unless the patient undergoes thymic transplantation

b. The patient will develop a sustained neutrophilia

c. The patient's T cell numbers will rise and T-cell function will improve

d. Despite normal B cell numbers, the patient will remain dependent on intravenous immunoglobulin therapy

e. The degree of T-cell dysregulation is dependent on the degree of cardiac involvement.

13-8. An 8-year-old girl presents to your office for follow-up of a recent bout of pneumonia. This episode of pneumonia is the sixth respiratory infection the patient has had this year. You note that the time between illnesses has been decreasing, as has her baseline respiratory function. Her mother also mentions to you at this visit that she has noticed that the child has been more clumsy lately and that her gait has always been different from her peers. Physical exam reveals a thin, cooperative child. Respiratory exam demonstrates coarse rhonchi and decreased bibasilar breath sounds. Neurologic exam reveals a mildly staggering gait and she is unable to perform cerebellar maneuvers with her legs. Skin exam reveals dilation of small blood vessels around her neck, ears, and antecubital fossae.

Which of the following tests would provide the most sensitive indicator of the underlying disease?

a. A complete blood count

b. Measurement of serum amyloid A

c. Biopsy of the rash

d. Measurement of serum alpha-fetoprotein

e. Measurement of serum IgG, IgM, and IgA

13-9. Given the underlying defect in Ataxia Telangiectasia (AT), which of the following tests should be avoided in a patient with the disorder?

a. Chest radiography

b. Bone marrow biopsy

c. In vitro lymphocyte proliferation assays

d. Flow cytometry for T-cell subsets

e. MR imaging of the brain

13-10. A 6-month-old boy is brought to your office for evaluation of failure to thrive and persistent eczema. The child has had several upper respiratory infections and has been hospitalized for pneumonia twice in the last 2 months. He has not gained weight since the age of 2 months despite adequate intake, although his mother has made him switch from cow's milk based- to soy-based formula in the hope of improving his severe eczema. Physical exam reveals an irritable child with an extensive eczematous rash on his trunk and legs. He has moderate hepatosplenomegaly and a few petechiae on his legs.

The most likely finding that might be seen on a complete blood count and smear would be which of the following?

a. Low numbers of neutrophils

b. Thrombophilia

c. Microcytosis

d. Low platelet volumes

e. Lymphoblasts

13-11. Patients with hyper IgE syndrome, or Job syndrome, can have infections resulting in severe tissue damage without features of fever, localized erythema, or warmth. The immune defect thought to be responsible for this abnormality is which of the following?

a. Elevated IgE levels

b. Defective neutrophil chemotaxis

c. Impaired intracellular killing of organisms

d. Eosinophilia

e. Abnormal antibody cross-linking

13-12. Patients with disorders of B-cell development are susceptible to infections from encapsulated organisms and enteroviral infections. These patients typically become symptomatic at what age?

a. In the second decade of life

b. Between the ages of 5 and 10

c. In the first three months of life

d. Between the first 6 and 12 months of life

e. In the immediate postpartum period

13-13. A 7-month-old male presents to your office with chronic enteroviral infection and failure to thrive. The mother is very concerned as multiple family members have died of infection in infancy in the past. A complete blood count demonstrates a normal total white blood cell count, but further investigation with flow cytometry detects normal numbers of T cells and the absence of any circulating B cells.

The patient's diagnosis is most likely to be which of the following?

a. Severe combined immunodeficiency

b. 22q11 syndrome

c. X-linked agammaglobulinemia

d. Adenosine deaminase deficiency

e. Vertically transmitted HIV infection

13-14. You are evaluating a 1-year-old male in your office in post-hospitalization follow-up. He was admitted with *Pneumocystis jiroveci* pneumonia 2 weeks ago. You also note that he has had several respiratory infections with *H. influenza* and pneumococcus despite being immunized. Laboratory evaluation notes a normal CBC. Flow cytometry demonstrates normal numbers of T and B lymphocytes, but quantitative immunoglobulins show significantly decreased IgG and IgA levels, although IgM levels are elevated.

This immunodeficiency in most likely caused by which of the following?

a. Maturation arrest of B cell precursors

b. Abnormal function of CD4+ T helper cells

c. Abnormal NK cell function

d. Elevated levels of IgE

e. Impaired class-switch recombination of immunoglobulins

13-15. A 12-year-old girl presents to your office for initial evaluation. She has had a long history of chronic pulmonary infections with bronchiectasis, failure to thrive, and chronic diarrhea. The patient had been noted to have lesions in her liver on abdominal CT scan and a liver biopsy demonstrated non-caseating granulomata. Further evaluation reveals normal numbers of circulating T and B cells but profoundly low levels of IgG, IgM, and IgA.

Which of the following would be appropriate advice to provide the child and family?

a. Over time, immunoglobulin levels should rise and the patient will no longer be susceptible to infection

b. The patient is at risk to develop autoimmune diseases such as rheumatoid arthritis

c. The patient's gastrointestinal symptoms are due to Celiac disease

d. The patient will need a bone marrow transplant

e. The patient has cystic fibrosis

13-16. A 14-year-old male with X-linked lymphoproliferative disease is admitted to the hospital with fulminant Epstein–Barr viral infection, hepatitis, and respiratory failure. He is currently intubated, on ventilator and pressor support in the Pediatric Intensive Care Unit. He has received 2 g/kg of intravenous immunoglobulin.

Should he survive this current illness, you would expect which of the following?

a. He is at great risk for extranodal lymphoid malignancy

b. He will have a reactive, sustained polyclonal hypergammopathy

c. He will develop chronic, active hepatitis

d. His female offspring will be at great risk for fulminant EBV infection

e. He will suffer significant neurologic impairment

13-17. A 7-month-old infant is brought to your office because his mother believes that he has been "sick for months." The child appears to have bilateral otitis media as well as coarse rhonchi in his lungs, but he is active and appears to be gaining weight. A complete blood count reveals normal numbers of T and B cells, but quantitative immunoglobulins demonstrate profoundly low levels of IgG, IgM, and IgA.

Your next step would be which of the following?

a. Refer the patient for bone marrow transplant

b. Start scheduled intravenous immunoglobulin administration

c. Initiate prophylactic antibiotic therapy

d. Reassure the mother that the child should recover from immune function

e. Anticipate that the child will develop chronic lung disease

13-18. Patients with IgA deficiency should be given which of the following with caution?

a. Packed RBCs

b. Intravenous Immunoglobulin

c. GM-CSF

d. Pneumococcal immunization

e. Folic acid supplementation

13-19. A 6-year-old male with juvenile idiopathic arthritis is brought to your office by his mother because she is worried that his arthritis medicine "keeps making him sick." He is currently taking naproxen, calcium, and vitamin D. On review of his medical records, you note that he has had multiple respiratory infections in the past several years, as well as a history of chronic otitis media requiring tympanostomy tube placement which pre-dates his arthritis diagnosis. You suspect that he might have an underlying immunodeficiency.

Your advice to the mother would be which of the following?

a. The arthritis medication is worsening his immunodeficiency and will need to be stopped

b. The arthritis and the immunodeficiency are unlikely to be related

c. More aggressive treatment of his arthritis may increase the patient's risk of infection

d. Treatment of the arthritis will result in an improvement in his immunodeficiency

e. The patient will require IgA supplementation

13-20. The immune dysregulation associated with hereditary polyendocrinopathies is due to which of the following?

a. B-cell maturation arrest in the bone marrow

b. Failure of T regulatory cells to suppress immune responsiveness

c. Lack of appropriate T-cell responses to regulate endocrine gland function

d. Failure of CD8+ T cells leaving the thymus

e. Failure of immunoglobulin class switching

13-21. A 12-year-old boy is seen in your office for complaints of recurrent facial swelling. His father reports that the boy has had several episodes of spontaneous lip swelling, as well as 1 recent episode of tongue swelling and difficulty swallowing. The father reports that the mother died several years ago after a respiratory arrest after having similar symptoms. Physical exam demonstrates edema of the lower lips and right cheek without erythema or tenderness. Based on the history, family history, and exam, you initiate a workup for hereditary angioedema.

You would expect to find which of the following abnormalities?

a. Increased levels of C4 (complement component 4)

b. An elevated CH50

c. Decreased levels of bradykinin

d. Elevated levels of IgE

e. Decreased levels of C1(complement component 1)-inhibitor

13-22. Recurrent infection with *Neisseria* is related to which of the following complement deficiencies?

a. C5 deficiency

b. C1-inhibitor deficiency

c. C2 deficiency

d. C3 deficiency

e. C1q deficiency

ANSWERS

Answer 13-1. c

The severity of recurrent infection can be a clue for an underlying immunodeficiency. While children in daycare are frequently ill with viral upper respiratory tract infections, over 3 hospitalizations for severe bacterial infection should raise concern for a larger immune-mediated dysfunction. Absence of tonsillar tissue, adenoidal tissue, or thymic tissue, either by direct visualization or on radiograph may be a clue to an underlying B-cell or T-cell dysfunction. Hypertrophy of these tissues, in contrast, is not uncommon in immunocompetent children. Failure to thrive can also be a sign of an underlying immune dysregulation, but this child was growing and maintaining his height and weight, not crossing percentiles, as would be seen in a failure to thrive.

(Chapter 187: "Undue Susceptibility to Infection", pp 755–756)

Answer 13-2. b

The initial step in the workup of a child with a suspected immunodeficiency should always include a complete blood count and differential, as this test will reveal disorders involving lymphopenia (particularly T-cell lymphopenias) and neutropenia. Other hints can be found by the CBC, including small platelets associated with the Wiskott–Aldrich syndrome, anemias, and evidence of eosinophilia.

An erythrocyte sedimentation rate is a nonspecific marker of inflammation and would not point to a specific immunodeficiency. While quantitative immunoglobulins, peripheral T-cell phenotyping, and lack of antibody response to standard immunizations would all be part of an immunodeficiency investigation, these would not be considered first steps in the evaluation.

(Chapter 187: Undue Susceptibility to Infection, pp 755–756)

Answer 13-3. e

This patient has Omenn syndrome, caused by abnormalities in the RAG1/2 lymphoid-specific recombination activating genes. This condition leads to failure of both T-cell and B-cell development and subsequent severe combined immunodeficiency. The presence of erythoderma and eosinophilia are clues to this diagnosis, which is not associated with neutrophilia. Macrocytosis, while seen in disorders of folic acid metabolism, is not seen in this disorder. Basophilic stippling is characteristic of sideroblastic anemia or lead toxicity. Small platelets are found in the Wiskott–Aldrich syndrome, but not in the Omenn syndrome.

(Chapter 188: "Primary Immunodeficiencies," pp 758–759)

Answer 13-4. a

Abnormalities of the purine salvage pathway account for up to 20% of severe combined immunodeficiency cases.

The most common is adenosine diaminase deficiency in which deoxyadenosine and the metabolite deoxyadenosine triphosphate accumulate and are toxic to thymocytes. Skeletal abnormalities such as cupping and flaring of the costochondral junctions are seen in ADA deficiency.

Shortening of the forearms can be seen in TAR syndrome (thrombocytopenia with absent radii) and bowing of the legs seen in disorders causing osteomalacia, such as rickets. Midface hypoplasia is seen in midline disorders such as DiGeorge syndrome, which also affects thymic development. Epicanthal folds are seen in numerous disorders, but are not specific to ADA deficiency.

(Chapter 188: "Primary Immunodeficiencies," p 759)

Answer 13-5. d

Severe combined immunodeficiency due to mutation in JAK3 results in failure of T cells and NK cell to develop, resulting in low numbers of circulating T and NK cells while B-cell numbers can be normal or elevated. These abnormalities are permanent and do not recover over time. While T-/B+ SCID can be X-linked, the inheritance pattern associated with JAK3-related SCID is autosomal recessive, resulting in a carrier state or disease state for all offspring. The treatment of choice for JAK3 deficiency is bone marrow transplantation, which will restore normal T-cell function, but frequently fails to restore B-cell function, resulting in the need for lifelong intravenous immunoglobulin therapy.

(Chapter 188: "Primary Immunodeficiencies," p 759)

Answer 13-6. a

ZAP70 is an autosomal recessive disorder resulting in chronic recurrent infection and impaired cellular and humoral responses. The thymus contains CD4+CD8+ thymocytes, but no CD8+ thymocytes and no CD8+ T cells are present in the peripheral circulation. While there are CD4+ thymocytes and circulating T cells, these cells function poorly, resulting in the global immune dysfunction. B-cell dysfunction is a result of the impaired T-cell responses, rather than a specific abnormality in B-cell development.

(Chapter 188: "Primary Immunodeficiencies," p 760)

Answer 13-7. c

This patient has mid-face hypoplasia and a low calcium, indicative of hypoparathyroidism. The absence of a thymus on chest radiograph and low numbers of lymphocytes suggest that he has a form of 22q11 deletion syndrome, known in the past as DiGeorge syndrome.

Given the fact that he has some circulating lymphocytes, it can be presumed that his thymus is not completely absent, or he has had extrathymic maturation of T cells. This condition tends to improve over time, leading to resolution of the immune defect in both T cells and B cells. As a result, patients with partial forms of the disorder rarely need lifelong immunoglobulin supplementation. As immune function improves over time, patients will not require thymic transplantation, although this therapy can be successful in patients with the complete form of the disease. While many patients with 22q11 syndrome have cardiac defects, the extent of cardiac disease does not directly correlate with the extent of immune dysfunction.

(Chapter 188: Primary Immunodeficiencies, pp 760–761)

Answer 13-8. d

This patient's clinical features of chronic respiratory infections, ataxia, and telangiectasias are consistent with Ataxia telangiectasia (AT). AT is an autosomal recessive disease that leads to progressive neurologic dysfunction, chronic infection, and a high risk of malignancy, caused by a genetic mutation leading to defective DNA repair. Usually the ataxia appears (around 1 year of age) well before the telangiectasias become apparent (around 5 years of age). It is important to consider the diagnosis of AT early and not wait for the presence of telangiectasias before measuring serum alpha-fetoprotein levels.

The immune defects in AT occur in both T and B lymphocytes. The thymus is small and T-cell numbers reduced. B-cell numbers are normal, but immunoglobulin class switching is altered with low levels and IgA and IgE, loss of IgG subclasses, and elevated levels of IgM. While abnormalities can be found on the complete blood count and quantitative immunoglobulin analysis, these are not necessarily specific for AT. Serum levels of onco-feto-proteins are elevated in this disorder, and elevated levels of alpha-fetoprotein in a patient with the appropriate clinical picture provides the most sensitive test. Serum amyloid A can be elevated in many inflammatory conditions and is not specific to AT and a biopsy of a telangiectasia would not ascertain the diagnosis.

(Chapter 188: "Primary Immunodeficiencies," p 761)

Answer 13-9. a

The genetic defect in AT, the ATM gene, leads to impairment of DNA repair. Patients with AT are thus highly sensitive to ionizing radiation, and are at significantly increased risk for developing malignancies, particularly of lymphoid origin. Exposure of patients to ionizing radiation or radiomimetic agents should be strictly limited, including standard radiography.

(Chapter 188: "Primary Immunodeficiencies," p 761)

Answer 13-10. d

This patient's history of chronic and recurrent infection and failure to thrive raises suspicion for an underlying immunodeficiency. The accompanying features of severe eczema, hepatosplenomegaly, and petechiae point towards a diagnosis of Wiskott–Aldrich syndrome. Wiskott–Aldrich syndrome is an X-linked disorder characterized by eczema, increased risk of infection, and small platelets with thrombocytopenia.

There is no particular effect on either numbers of neutrophils or red cell volumes. The underlying cause of WAS is a mutation in the WASP (Wiskott–Aldrich syndrome protein) gene, leading to abnormalities in intracellular signal transduction. Patients with WAS are at high risk for hematologic malignancy, but the presence of lymphoblasts on peripheral smear would not be the most common finding seen in the disorder.

(Chapter 188: Primary Immunodeficiencies, pp 761–762)

Answer 13-11. b

Hyper-IgE syndrome has both an autosomal dominant and autosomal recessive form. The autosomal dominant form includes eczema, skeletal and vascular abnormalities, while both forms display the immunologic defects, including elevated levels of IgE, increased risk of viral infections and autoimmunity. Impairment of neutrophil chemotaxis leads to failure to migrate to the site of infection and therefore lack of a local inflammatory response, such as erythema, warmth, or release of cytokines leading to production of a fever.

Impaired intracellular killing of organisms leading to granuloma formation is not a feature of Job syndrome, nor is eosinophilia or antibody cross-linking abnormalities.

(Chapter 188: "Primary Immunodeficiences", p 762)

Answer 13-12. d

Disorders of B-cell development result in maturation arrest of B cells and lack of mature B cells in the peripheral circulation. This condition results in agammaglobulinemia. The affected child depends on maternal immunoglobulin for humoral immune system protection; however, once maternal immunoglobulin decays (typically by 6 months of age), the child has no protection against infections with encapsulated bacteria or viruses, such as enterovirus, leading to chronic recurrent infection.

(Chapter 188: Primary Immunodeficiences, pp 762–763)

Answer 13-13. c

Normal T-cell numbers but absent B cells indicate a primary disorder of the humoral immune system leading to B-cell maturation arrest. The most common of these is X-linked agammaglobulinemia, which accounts for over 80% of these disorders. The significant family history of early death from infection is a clue that this patient's disorder may be genetic in origin. XLA is caused by an abnormality in Bruton's tyrosine kinase resulting in a block preventing maturation past the CD19+ pro-B cell stage. The lack of B cells in the periphery leads to susceptibility with typical organisms dependent on humoral immune system function. The other listed disorders all result in T-cell abnormalities, which ultimately cause abnormalities in B-cell function, but cause disorders in both cellular and humoral immune system function.

(Chapter 188: Primary Immunodeficiencies, pp 762–763)

Answer 13-14. e

The elevated levels of IgM and profoundly low levels of IgG and IgA indicate a failure in immunoglobulin class-switching, making the patient susceptible to encapsulated organisms. The most common of these disorders is X-linked hyper-IgM syndrome which causes an abnormality in the gene encoding the CD40 ligand on T cells leading to failure of CD40 on B cells leading to blockade of the class-switch process. CD40 is also present on macrophages and dendritic cells, leading to susceptibility to opportunistic organisms such as *P. jiroveci*.

(Chapter 188: "Primary Immunodeficiencies", p 763)

Answer 13-15. b

The patient's clinical picture is consistent with an immunodeficiency, but presentation in the second decade, and in a female, indicates a less profound immune dysregulation than in seen in X-linked agammaglobulinemia. The presence of granulomata and low levels of immunoglobulin point toward Common Variable Immunodeficiency as the most likely diagnosis. These patients are affected by the same organisms seen in other disorders of humoral immunity but survive long enough to develop granulomata and other disorders of immunoregulation, such as autoimmune diseases and hematologic disorders. The chronic diarrhea seen in these patients is commonly due to bacterial overgrowth and villous atrophy, rather than gluten intolerance. While patients can present similarly to cystic fibrosis, patients with CF do not have the same degree of hypogammaglobulinemia. Treatment of common variable immunodeficiency centers on replacement of immunoglobulin and vigilance for autoimmune disease and hematologic malignancy. Bone marrow transplantation does not have a role in treatment of this disorder.

(Chapter 188: "Primary Immunodeficiencies," pp 763–764)

Answer 13-16. a

X-linked lymphoproliferastive disease is due to a mutation in *SH2D1A*, which encodes the protein SAP (signaling lymphocyte activation molecule-associated protein), which regulates T cell response to EBV infection. Patients can develop overwhelming EBV infection, which is fatal in over 50% of patients infected. Survivors have sustained hypo- or agammaglobulinemia and can often develop extranodal lymphoid malignancies, particularly of the Burkitt type. Other than as residua of severe infection, there are no specifically

associated neurocognitive abnormalities and patients do not develop chronic hepatitis.

(Chapter 188: "Primary Immunodeficiencies," p 764)

Answer 13-17. d

This patient has hypogammaglobulinemia, leading to chronic infection now that the placentally-acquired immunoglobulin from his mother has decayed. As contrasted with X-linked agammaglobulinemia, however, this patient has normal circulating numbers of B cells and the low levels of immunoglobulin are due to a delay in onset of Ig production. This disorder is called transient hypogammaglobulinemia of infancy. As depicted by the title, this disorder is not permanent; spontaneous recovery is expected by 2 to 4 years of age. Prophylactic antibiotics are not indicated, nor is prophylactic intravenous immunoglobulin administration unless the patient continues to have serious recurrent infection.

(Chapter 188: "Primary Immunodeficiencies," p 764)

Answer 13-18. b

IgA deficiency is the most common primary immunodeficiency, occurring in approximately 1 in 600 people. While most people with selective IgA deficiency are asymptomatic, some develop recurrent infections at mucosal barriers, such as the respiratory and gastrointestinal tracts. Some patients with IgA deficiency develop anti-IgA antibodies and are at risk for anaphylaxis when they receive any blood product containing IgA, the most common of which is pooled intravenous immunoglobulin.

(Chapter 188: "Primary Immunodeficiencies," pp 764–765)

Answer 13-19. c

Given the chronic recurrent respiratory tract infections in an otherwise healthy child with arthritis, this patient is likely to have IgA deficiency. The relationship of autoimmune disease and IgA deficiency has been well described, particularly with juvenile idiopathic arthritis and celiac disease. There is no treatment for IgA deficiency and treatment of the arthritis will not improve IgA production. Given the destructive nature of untreated JIA, the medication cannot be stopped. More aggressive treatment for arthritis, such as with methotrexate, steroids, or biologic agents will lead to further immunosuppression and the patient will need to be monitored for infection and treated aggressively when present.

(Chapter 188: "Primary Immunodeficiencies", pp 764–765)

Answer 13-20. b

The hereditary polyendocrinopathies are associated with immune dysregulation and autoimmunity due to abnormalities in T regulatory cell differentiation. T_{reg} cells leave the thymus as CD4+ cells and are responsible for controlling exuberant T-cell responses as well as identifying and helping clear autoreactive T cells in the peripheral blood. Failure of T_{reg} cell differentiation leads to T-cell over-responsiveness and persistence of autoreactive cells, which can lead to autoimmune disease. While B-cell function is affected by T-cell function, these disorders are not due to B-cell lineage dysfunction. T-cell responsiveness is critical in controlling infection and in immune surveillance, but are not directly responsible for the endocrine gland function.

(Chapter 188: "Primary Immunodeficiencies," p 765)

Answer 13-21. e

Hereditary angioedema is an autosomal dominant disorder that results from an absolute or functional deficiency in C1-inhibitor. Uncontrolled C1 activity leads to production of bradykinin, which drives the clinical features. Patients with this disorder have low C4 levels, which is a reasonable screening test for the disorder. Patients have abnormalities of the classical complement pathway, leading to a low or normal CH50, but alternative pathway (AH50) function and late complement components (C5–C9) are normal.

(Chapter 189: "Complement Disorders," p 767)

Answer 13-22. a

Disorders of the alternative complement pathway and terminal complement deficiencies have all been associated with increased risk of pyogenic infections, particularly *Neisseria*. Terminal complement component deficiencies, such as C5 deficiency lead to infection by affecting the ability to make a membrane attack complex and thereby lyse the bacteria. Disorders of the classical pathway can lead to infection, but are more commonly associated with autoimmune disease, particularly systemic lupus erythematosus.

(Chapter 189: "Complement Disorders," p 767)

CHAPTER 14 | Allergic Disorders

Alan P. Baptist and Aimee Leyton Speck

14-1. A 6-year-old girl presents with a history of a rash 6 hours earlier in the day. The rash was raised, erythematous, and pruritic. The rash was primarily on the trunk, arms, and exposed parts of the legs. On examination, the child is comfortable and in no respiratory distress. She is afebrile. According to the mother, the rash seems to be fading.

The diagnosis of urticaria is typically based on which of the following?

a. Careful physical examination

b. History and description of the rash

c. Dietary history

d. Skin biopsy

e. IgE level

14-2. Which of the following is an example of an IgE-mediated hypersensitivity reaction?

a. A 13-month-old child with recurrent, fever, nasal congestion, and wheeze

b. An infant with emesis and bloody stools after bottle feeding

c. A 6-year-old with recurrent rash at the umbilicus in the area of his belt buckle

d. A 13-year-old with facial flushing and pruritis after consuming sesame dressing

e. A 15-year-old with indigestion and abdominal pain after consuming ice cream

14-3. An 8-year-old child presents to the clinic with chief complaints of sneezing, nasal congestion, and nasal discharge. Symptoms are present on most days and seem worse after playing in his bedroom. He is doing well in school and sleeping well at night. On physical exam, he has mild clear rhinorrhea and pale nasal turbinates. Skin-prick testing reveals a large reaction to dust mite.

What is the best initial therapeutic intervention for this patient?

a. Avoidance measures: mite-proof coverings, removal of carpet from bedroom

b. Oral anti-histamine

c. Oral phenylephrine

d. Leukotriene receptor antagonist (LTRA)

e. Immunotherapy with allergenic extracts

14-4. Which of the following oral antihistamine medications would most likely cause sedation in a preschool age child?

a. Loratidine

b. Cetirizine

c. Fexofenadine

d. Hydroxyzine

e. Levocetirizine

14-5. A 15-year-old girl with symptoms of perennial AR undergoes skin-prick testing. She has positive results to dust mite and mold. She has a negative reaction to cat. Which of the following is the most accurate statement regarding her symptoms?

a. Her symptoms are most likely due to dust mite exposure

b. Her symptoms are most likely due to mold exposure

c. Her symptoms are most likely due to dust mite and mold exposure

d. Her symptoms are most likely due to cat dander exposure

e. Her symptoms are unlikely to be due to cat dander exposure

14-6. Which of the following physical exam findings on nasal exam is most consistent with allergic rhinoconjunctivitis (ARC) in a 5-year-old child?

a. Pale, enlarged nasal turbinates and clear rhinorrhea

b. Erythematous nasal mucosa with crusty secretions

c. Nasal polyps and clear rhinorrhea

d. Unilateral, bloody nasal discharge

e. Erythematous nasal mucosa and purulent nasal discharge

14-7. A 14-year-old boy is referred to your clinic due to recurrent sneezing, nasal congestion, and ocular pruritus. His symptoms occur every spring and fall. On exam, he is overall well-appearing. He has pale, enlarged nasal turbinates, clear rhinorrhea, and erythema of the conjunctiva bilaterally.

Which medication will provide the best long-term monotherapy for the patient's symptoms?

  a. Intranasal corticosteroid spray (eg, fluticasone nasal spray)

  b. Oral antihistamine (eg, loratidine)

  c. Oral LTRA (eg, montelukast)

  d. Saline nasal washes

  e. Topical oxymetazoline

14-8. A 7-year-old girl presents to the emergency department with sudden onset of wheezing, generalized hives, facial flushing, and abdominal pain after eating cookies at a friend's birthday party. Which of the following laboratory tests would confirm the suspected diagnosis?

  a. White blood cell count with differential 1 hour after the anaphylactic event

  b. Platelet count 1 hour after the anaphylactic event

  c. Tryptase level 1 hour after the anaphylactic event

  d. Erythrocyte sedimentation level (ESR) 1 hour after the anaphylactic event

  e. Histamine level 1 hour after the anaphylactic event

14-9. A 10-year-old girl was stung by a hornet 20 minutes prior to arrival at the emergency department, and now presents with wheezing, generalized urticaria, tongue angioedema, and repeated episodes of vomiting.

What is the most important initial medical therapy to administer in this setting?

  a. IV diphenhydramine

  b. IV fluids

  c. IV methylprednisolone

  d. IV/IM epinephrine

  e. Inhaled albuterol

14-10. A 12-year-old girl presents to the Emergency Department with acute onset of facial flushing, abdominal pain, diffuse pruritis, diaphoresis, and shortness of breath. The symptoms started minutes after eating almonds at a friend's house. She has never had similar symptoms. She is stabilized and observed for 12 hours in the Emergency Department without any recurrence of symptoms.

Which of the following discharge instructions is most appropriate?

  a. Instruct her to start daily diphenhydramine to prevent another episode

  b. Instruct her to start daily loratidine to prevent another episode

  c. Instruct her to use inhaled fluticasone if another such episode occurs

  d. Instruct her to use injectable epinephrine if another such episode occurs

  e. Instruct her to use inhaled albuterol if another such episode occurs

14-11. Which of the following is an example of a kinin-mediated condition?

  a. A patient with hereditary angioedema

  b. A patient with acute urticaria

  c. A patient with pruritus and angioedema immediately after eating shrimp

  d. A patient with acute anaphylaxis

  e. A patient with ARC

14-12. A 17-year-old girl presents to your clinic, and states that she has been having random episodes of angioedema of the lip, face, and hands. When you inquire about her family history, she notes that her father and paternal grandmother have had similar episodes, also starting in their teenage years.

You suspect the condition that she has is due to a mutation in which of the following?

  a. C1-inhibitor (*C1INH*) gene

  b. *CFTR* gene

  c. Dystrophin gene

  d. *FBN1* gene

  e. *HFE* gene

14-13. For a patient with urticaria, how long must the patient display near daily symptoms for the condition to be considered chronic?

  a. 4 weeks

  b. 6 weeks

  c. 8 weeks

  d. 12 weeks

  e. 16 weeks

14-14. An 8-year-old girl with no significant history presents to your clinic for acute urticaria over the past 3 days. When discussing her history, you determine that she had a viral infection approximately 1 week prior to the onset of the urticarial lesions. Which of the following is the most appropriate initial medication for the treatment of acute urticaria lasting for more than 3 days?

a. Prednisone

b. Montelukast

c. Diphenhydramine

d. Cetirizine

e. Ranitidine

14-15. A 13-year-old boy comes to you for evaluation of a food allergy to soy. His first reaction consisted of urticaria and angioedema when he ingested soy. The subsequent reaction was similar to the first, though his mother thinks the hives were somewhat more severe. His mother asks you how severe her son's reaction will be if he consumes soy-containing foods. Which of the following statements is appropriate?

a. The patient will experience only urticaria if he consumes soy

b. The patient will experience urticaria and angioedema if he consumes soy

c. The patient will experience, urticaria, angioedema, and shortness of breath if he consumes soy

d. The patient will experience, urticaria, angioedema, shortness of breath, and abdominal cramping if he consumes soy

e. There is currently no way to reliably predict the severity of a food allergic reaction

14-16. A 3-year-old girl is girl is seen in clinic after a new diagnosis of a peanut allergy. Her mother asks you if her other children (the patient's siblings) are likely to develop a peanut allergy. Which of the following is an appropriate response?

a. Her other children will definitely also develop a peanut allergy

b. Her other children are 2 times more likely than the general population to develop a peanut allergy

c. Her other children are 6 times more likely than the general population to develop a peanut allergy

d. Her other children are 10 times more likely than the general population to develop a peanut allergy

e. Her other children have no increased risk for developing a peanut allergy compared to the general population

14-17. An exclusively breastfed infant is brought to clinic due to the passage of frequent mucousy stools, which sometimes contain blood. The infant is well-appearing with appropriate weight gain since the last visit 1 week prior. He has never experienced urticaria, angioedema, nausea, vomiting, or shortness of breath while breast feeding.

Which of the following is the most appropriate initial step in management?

a. Perform patch testing on the infant to cow's milk and soy

b. Perform prick testing on the infant to cow's milk and soy

c. Instruct the mother to eliminate cow's milk and soy from her own diet and continue breastfeeding

d. Discontinue breastfeeding and switch the infant to a soy-based formula

e. Discontinue breast feeding and switch the infant to an amino-acid based formula

14-18. A 15-year-old boy develops mouth and throat pruritus after eating cantaloupe at a family picnic. He has not had these symptoms previously with cantaloupe, but on further questioning does note similar symptoms with watermelon over the past 3 years. He had consumed both of these foods as a young child without any such symptoms, but has not eaten them in many years. He has a history of seasonal allergies, but no other significant medical problems. What is the most likely cause of his current symptoms?

a. An IgE-mediated food allergy to cantaloupe

b. An IgE-mediated food allergy to watermelon

c. A condition of the small bowel and colon leading to diffuse inflammation of the gastrointestinal tract, mild villous atrophy, and crypt abscesses

d. A prior pollen sensitization to ragweed

e. An increased number of eosinophils in the esophageal tissue

14-19. A 17-year-old girl has recurrent choking, coughing, and difficulty swallowing with both liquid and solid intake. She states that she often feels like her food is "getting stuck" after she swallows and complains of an uncomfortable feeling in her chest. At times, she has had to force herself to vomit in order to clear her esophagus. She has kept a food diary, but symptoms do not seem to correlate with any particular foods. She has a history of seasonal AR, but no other significant past medical history. Which of the following is the most appropriate initial diagnostic/therapeutic intervention?

   a. A 1-month trial of an antacid

   b. Use of an albuterol inhaler PRN

   c. An upper endoscopy with biopsy

   d. A dairy elimination diet

   e. Flexible laryngoscopy

14-20. Which of the following tests is the gold standard for diagnosing a suspected IgE-mediated food allergy?

   a. Skin prick testing

   b. Intradermal skin testing

   c. Measurement of serum food-specific IgE antibodies

   d. Oral food challenge

   e. Patch testing

14-21. A 5-year-old boy ate peanut butter, and within 5 minutes developed shortness of breath, tongue swelling, generalized urticaria, and vomiting. He underwent IgE-specific food testing, which came back very elevated for peanut. The parents are very concerned, and want to do everything possible to prevent a future reaction.

   Which of the following should be recommended for the patient's treatment?

   a. Careful elimination of peanut from the child's diet, but no other daily treatment

   b. Daily oral antihistamine use

   c. Daily injectable epinephrine use

   d. Oral glucocorticoids in the event of an acute food allergic reaction

   e. Oral immunotherapy for desensitization

14-22. Which of the following Hymenoptera is least likely to sting if unprovoked?

   a. Yellow Jackets (*Vespula dolichovespula*)

   b. Hornets (*Vespa* spp)

   c. Wasps (*Polistes*)

   d. Honeybees (*Apis mellifera*)

   e. Africanized honeybees (*Apis mellifera* scutellata)

14-23. A 14-year-old boy presents to the emergency department 2 days after sustaining a wasp sting to his right ankle. On exam, he has erythema, swelling, and tenderness of his entire right leg. He is able to converse with you easily. He complains of tenderness to palpation of the right leg. He denies any hives, angioedema, or shortness of breath with this reaction. He is afebrile and heart rate, respiratory rate, and blood pressure are within normal limits. A complete blood count with differential is normal. What is the most appropriate initial treatment?

   a. Injectable epinephrine

   b. IV fluids

   c. Oral corticosteroids

   d. IV clindamycin

   e. Ice and oral pain relief

14-24. For which of the following patients should hymenoptera venom immunotherapy be indicated?

   a. A 12-year-old with swelling, erythema, and pain at the site of a honeybee sting

   b. An 8-year-old with swelling, erythema, and tenderness involving the entire right low extremity after a wasp sting on the right ankle

   c. A 4-year-old with generalized urticaria after being stung by a yellow jacket

   d. A 10-year-old with rhabdomyolysis after being stung by 50 Africanized honey bees

   e. A 6-year-old with angioedema and vomiting after being stung by a hornet

14-25. One of your patients will be undergoing a surgical procedure in the near future. For which of the following patients would you recommend evaluation for latex sensitization prior to the surgical procedure?

   a. A newborn with hypoplastic left heart syndrome underdoing a Norwood procedure

   b. A 16-year-old with a history of shellfish allergy who will be undergoing wisdom teeth removal

   c. A 12-year-old with a history of anaphylaxis to honey bee sting undergoing open reduction internal fixation due to femur fracture

   d. A 2-year-old with a history of spina bifida undergoing a vetriculoperitoneal shunt revision

   e. A 5-year-old with a history of anaphylaxis to peanut undergoing tympanostomy tube placement

14-26. A dental assistant presents to your clinic with a chief complaint of a rash and irritation on her hands bilaterally, in the distribution in which she wears her gloves. She states that she notices her symptoms the day after she works. She denies any other symptoms.

Which of the following is the most appropriate test to confirm the diagnosis?

a. Latex-specific IgE skin prick testing

b. Latex-specific IgE intradermal skin testing

c. Serum radioallergosorbent latex-specific IgE testing

d. Atopy patch testing

e. Latex contact exposure challenge

14-27. An 11-year-old girl has generalized urticaria, angioedema, laryngeal edema, and bronchospasm after blowing up a balloon. You send off a latex-specific IgE level, which comes back elevated.

In addition to recommending a medical alert bracelet and prescribing self-injectable epinephrine, which of the following instructions is most appropriate to tell her?

a. She should take diphenhydramine if she experiences similar symptoms in the future

b. She should not undergo routine medical and dental checkups to minimize potential latex exposure

c. She should avoid kiwi, banana, papaya, avocado, potato, tomato, and chestnut

d. She should begin latex immunotherapy

e. She should carry her own supply of nonlatex gloves for use for medical or dental care

14-28. Which of the following most likely represents an immunologically-mediated drug reaction?

a. A 14-year-old with infectious mononucleosis who develops a rash after receiving amoxicillin

b. A 16-year-old girl with acute renal failure while receiving vancomycin

c. A 12-year-old boy with nausea and vomiting while receiving penicillin

d. A premature infant boy with ototoxicity after receiving gentamicin

e. A 15-year-old girl with rash and fever while receiving minocycline

14-29. A G1P0 woman, currently at 38 weeks gestational age, tests positive for Group B streptococcus bacteria. She has a history of nausea and vomiting when receiving penicillin, but no rash or shortness of breath.

Which of the following antibiotics would be the most appropriate treatment during her labor for intrapartum antibiotic GBS prophylaxis?

a. IV clindamycin

b. IV vancomycin

c. IV ampicillin

d. IV erythromycin

e. IV gentamicin

14-30. A 17-year-old girl has a history of adverse reactions to multiple antibiotics, and claims previous reactions to clindamycin, doxycyline, cephalexin, penicillin, and erythromycin. She is referred to your clinic to assess which antibiotics are associated with a type I hypersensitivity reaction.

For which of the following antibiotics can skin testing be used to determine IgE sensitivity?

a. Clindamycin

b. Doxycycline

c. Cephalexin

d. Erythromycin

e. Penicillin

14-31. A woman currently at 28 weeks gestational age is diagnosed with syphilis (*Treponema pallidum*) via treponemal antibody test (FTA-ABS). She has a history of hives when she received penicillin 2 years ago. Which of the following is an appropriate strategy?

a. Doxycyline

b. Tetracycline

c. Azithromycin

d. Penicillin at a full strength dose

e. Penicillin after a desensitization protocol

14-32. A 15-year-old boy has a history of an IgE-mediated hypersensitivity to penicillin. Which of the following medications is LEAST likely to cause a hypersensitivity reaction?

a. Imipenem

b. Aztreonam

c. Ceftazadime

d. Cefazolin

e. Ampicillin

14-33. A 6-year-old boy with a history of hydrocephalus is started on a new medication. He subsequently develops skin erythema, fever, lymphadenopathy, eosinophilia, and elevated liver enzymes. His symptoms are most likely secondary to which of the following medications?

a. Clonezapam

b. Phenytoin

c. Valproic acid

d. Ampicillin

e. Bactrim

14-34. A 13-year-old girl has a history of sneezing, nasal congestion, rhinorrhea, and ocular pruritus. Her symptoms occur year round. Oral antihistamines are somewhat effective, but she still has symptoms on most days during the year.

Which of the following is most likely the cause of this girl's symptoms?

a. Recurrent upper respiratory tract infections

b. Seasonal AR

c. Perennial AR

d. Chronic sinusitis

e. Adenoid hypertrophy

14-35. A 13-month-old child is seen by her pediatrician for a health maintenance examination. She has a history of an egg allergy, with anaphylaxis symptoms after ingestion. She is due for immunizations. On physical exam, the girl is well-appearing. Which of the following is the appropriate course of action in clinic today?

a. Give her the measles, mumps, and rubella (MMR), and influenza vaccinations

b. Wait until she is 15 months to give her the MMR and influenza vaccines

c. Give her the MMR vaccine only

d. Give her the influenza vaccine only

e. Do not vaccinate her

14-36. A 6-year-old girl was dining with her family at an all-you-can-eat seafood buffet when she developed acute onset of wheezing, hives, and tongue swelling. She is transported to your Emergency Department 20 minutes later.

A delay in the administration of which of the following medications has been strongly associated with mortality from this condition?

a. Epinephrine

b. IV fluids

c. Diphenhydramine

d. Methylprednisolone

e. Inhaled albuterol

14-37. Allergic responses are caused by antigen uptake and a skewing of the immune response to the TH2 lineage. Which immunoglobulin class is activated in allergic responses?

a. IgA

b. IgG

c. IgM

d. IgD

e. IgE

14-38. A 6-year-old girl presents to your office for upper airway complaints. She has symptoms of sneezing, congestion, and itchy, watery eyes. Her mother wants to know if the symptoms are due to AR or frequent viral infections. The most common finding on physical examination of the nose in AR is:

a. Pale, enlarged turbinates with clear rhinorrhea

b. Nasal polyposis

c. Erythematous mucosa with crusting

d. Erythematous mucosa with purulent discharge

e. Small, retracted turbinates

14-39. A 15-year-old boy with moderate to severe allergic asthma and ARC presents to your office. They have tried multiple medications, but inevitably end up requiring oral steroids for treatment. The family is interested if there are any approved novel therapies currently available for use. You let them know that:

a. There is an FDA-approved therapy against IL-4

b. There is an FDA-approved therapy against the soluble IL-4 receptor

c. There is an FDA-approved therapy against IL-13

d. There is an FDA-approved therapy against IgE

e. There are no FDA-approved biological therapies currently available

14-40. A parent comes to your clinic and is interested in starting her child on montelukast for seasonal AR. She asks how the medication works. You tell her that montelukast:

a. Blocks the H1 histamine receptors

b. Redirects the immune response toward a tolerant state

c. Blocks the leukotriene receptor

d. Inhibits the synthesis of leukotrienes

e. Stabilizes mast cells to prevent their degranulation

ANSWERS

Answer 14-1. b

Urticarial lesions are also called "hives" or "nettle rash." They are classically transient and "migratory" as individual lesions last from minutes to hours.

Due to its evanescent quality, urticaria may not be present at the time of a clinical visit. As a result, diagnosis is usually established by a careful history. Although a dietary history may be helpful in some cases, many nondietary exposures can trigger urticaria. Lab testing (eg, IgE level or skin biopsy) is not required.

(P 778: Section 14: Allergic Disorders)

Answer 14-2. d

The immediate type hypersensitivity reaction is IgE-induced. It is reversible and usually subsides within 2 hours of initiation. The immediate type hypersensitivity reaction in an atopic individual is characterized by vasodilation, edema, and smooth muscle contraction. In skin, this reaction manifests with the "wheal and flare" urticarial skin reaction when the skin is scratched with an allergic substance. In the airways, allergen inhalation induces mucosal edema, mucous production, and smooth muscle contraction leading to reduced air flow and wheezing. If the antigen encounter occurs in the gut, the result is abdominal cramping and diarrhea due to the contraction of smooth muscles. An IgE-mediated food allergic reaction is characterized by flushing, pruritis, angioedema, and urticaria with or without GI manifestations.

In a young toddler, nasal congestion and wheezing are often due to respiratory infections and less likely manifestations of allergy. Recurrent emesis or bloody stools in a bottle-fed infant is suggestive of a cow's milk protein allergy. Recurrent rash with exposure to belt buckles is likely allergic contact dermatitis due to nickel. Contact dermatitis is a Type IV hypersensitivity reaction and is not antibody mediated, but instead a cell-mediated response. A teenager with abdominal pain and indigestion after consuming a milk-containing product is suggestive of lactose intolerance secondary to deficiency of the enzyme lactase. The lack of cutaneous symptoms makes an IgE-mediated food reaction less likely.

(Pp 773, 774: Section 14: Allergic Disorders)

Answer 14-3. a

The child in the vignette above has perennial allergic rhinitis (AR) secondary to dust-mite allergy. Management of the allergic child requires a multifaceted approach that includes minimizing exposure to the allergic trigger as well as using medications that can control an established allergic reaction (antihistamines, epinephrine) or limit the development of an allergic reaction (corticosteroids, leukotriene inhibitors).

The first line of treatment for this patient should be education and allergen avoidance measures such as allergen-proof bed and pillow covers, washing bedding weekly, washing stuffed animals, regular vacuuming, and carpet removal.

Histamine is a primary amine produced by mast cells and basophils that orchestrates many aspects of the allergic response by binding to specific receptors present on the surface of its target cells. The 4 types of histamine receptors are H1, H2, H3, and H4. Signals induced via the H1 receptor (and to a lesser extent the H2 receptor) mediate many of the acute symptoms and signs of allergic disease. Histamine receptor antagonists are widely used for the treatment of allergic disorders and many antihistamines are acceptable for use in children.

Oral phenylephrine is a decongestant. Decongestants work by constricting the blood vessels lining the nose. Their long-term use is discouraged due to the risk of rebound nasal congestion. Oral decongestants are also not recommended in children due to their cardiovascular (high blood pressure) and CNS (nervousness, excitability, difficulty sleeping) side effects.

Cysteinyl leukotrienes induce the migration and activation of white blood cells involved in allergic inflammation as well as smooth muscle and asthma. The effectiveness of LTRAs is comparable to that of oral antihistamines. The safety profile makes them a suitable alternative for patients who cannot receive steroids or who are wary of their side effects.

Allergen specific subcutaneous immunotherapy (SCIT) is an effective therapy for AR. It is currently the only treatment that modifies the course of AR by redirecting the immune system toward a tolerant state. Its clinical benefits may be sustained for years after discontinuation of treatment. SCIT is a time-consuming therapy that requires long-term commitment (minimum of 2 years). The subcutaneous administration is an added drawback for children who are fearful of injections.

While medications may become necessary, avoidance measures should be the first line of treatment given the patient's mild symptoms.

(Pp 771, 774, 775, 777: Section 14: Allergic Disorders)

Answer 14-4. d

H1 receptor antagonists are widely prescribed for the treatment of allergic disorders. Pretreatment with oral H1 antihistamines reduces early response to allergen and administering the medication during the course of an allergic response curbs the symptoms triggered by acute allergic inflammation. First-generation H1 blockers (diphenhydramine, brompheniramine, cyproheptadine, chlorpheniramine, hydroxyzine, promethazine) are lipophilic and readily penetrate the CNS causing sedation, and in some patients a paradoxical excitation.

Second-generation H1 antihistamines (loratadine, cetirizine, fexofenadine, and levocetirizine) penetrate the CNS poorly and therefore are less likely to cause sedation.

(P 775: Section 14: Allergic Disorders)

Answer 14-5. e

Skin-prick tests are in-office tests routinely performed and results can be obtained within minutes. Sensitization however, does not always correlate with clinical allergy and therefore these tests should be considered confirmatory only in the context of a documented or highly probable reaction following exposure.

The positive predictive value for these tests has been estimated to be approximately 40% and the negative predictive value of it is approximately 90% or greater. Skin-prick tests are therefore very useful for ruling out a particular allergen as the trigger for an allergic reaction than ruling it in.

Although this patient's symptoms could be secondary to dust mite, mold exposure or both, her lack of a reaction to cat dander makes it unlikely that her symptoms are secondary to cat dander exposure.

(P 774: Section 14: Allergic Disorders)

Answer 14-6. a

AR is a chronic inflammatory disease of the upper airway caused by IgE sensitization to airborne allergens. The clinical presentation is usually associated with frequent sneezing, nasal congestion, and nasal discharge. The majority of patients with AR complain of or display ocular symptoms (itchy/watery eyes) and thus it is termed ARC.

Pale, enlarged nasal turbinates and clear rhinorrhea are usually a sign of ARC. Erythematous mucosa with either crusty or purulent secretions is suggestive of acute infection, either viral or bacterial. Nasal polyps in a young child should prompt one to search for a cystic fibrosis or aspirin sensitivity in an older child. Unilateral, bloody nasal discharge is suggestive of a nasal foreign body or digital trauma.

(Pp 775, 776: Section 14: Allergic Disorders)

Answer 14-7. a

The symptoms described for the boy in the vignette are consistent with seasonal ARC.

Fluticasone nasal spray is an intranasal corticosteroid (INC). As monotherapy, INCs are more efficacious than antihistamines, LTRAs, or their combination in the management of symptoms or ARC. Local side effects are usually mild. When used at the recommended doses, INCs are not usually associated with clinically-significant effects on the hypothalamic–pituitary–adrenal axis, ocular pressure or cataract formation, or bone density.

Loratidine is a second-generation oral H1 antihistamine. Second-generation H1 antihistamines are preferred over first-generation antihistamines because of their reduced risk to cause sedation and/or anticholinergic effects. These medications are particularly effective for the ocular symptoms of ARC. As monotherapy, however, they are not as effective as INCs.

Montelukast is a LTRA. The effectiveness of LTRAs in the treatment of ARC is comparable to that of oral antihistamines.

As monotherapy, they are less effective than INCs for the treatment of ARC, but should be considered in patients with concomitant asthma or in those whom corticosteroids are contraindicated or unwelcome.

Nasal saline washes are of benefit in reducing symptoms in patients with ARC or rhinosinusitis. They can be used as either single or adjuvant agents. As monotherapy, however, they are not as effective as INCs for the treatment of ARC.

Oxymetazoline is a topical decongestant, which works by constricting the blood vessels lining the nose. Topical decongestants may provide temporary relief, but long-term use is discouraged due to the risk of rebound nasal congestion that sets in within 5–7 days of repeated use.

(P 777: Section 14: Allergic Disorders)

Answer 14-8. c

The patient in the above vignette has symptoms consistent with acute anaphylaxis. Her symptoms are likely secondary to a component of the cookies she ate at the party. Anaphylaxis is most commonly the result of IgE-mediated mast cell activation resulting in the release of histamine, leukotrienes, and other mast cell activators. Anaphylaxis is a clinical diagnosis. Symptoms of anaphylaxis usually appear within minutes of antigen exposure, but occasionally symptom onset may be delayed for several hours after oral ingestions.

Although anaphylaxis is a clinical diagnosis, confirmatory testing is sometimes useful to confirm systemic mast cell activation. Tryptase, a protease specific to mast cells, reaches a serum peak level 30–120 minutes after the anaphylactic event and remains elevated for 6 hours making it helpful to confirm systemic mast cell activation.

A serum histamine level would be helpful for confirming systemic mast cell activation, however, histamine is detectable in plasma for only 15–30 minutes after the anaphylactic event making appropriate collection difficult.

A white blood cell count with a differential would be helpful for assessing a viral or bacterial infection in a patient, but would not confirm systemic mast cell activation.

Platelets are an acute phase reactant. Reactive thrombocytosis is thrombocytosis in the absence of a chronic myeloproliferative or myelodyspastic disorder, in patients who have a medical or surgical condition likely to be associated with an elevated platelet count. Reactive thrombocytosis most frequently occurs secondary to infection, post-surgical status, malignancy, post-splenectomy, acute blood loss or iron-deficiency anemia. An elevated platelet count is not a specific marker for confirming mast cell activation.

ESR defined as the rate (mm/hour) at which erythrocytes suspended in plasma settle when placed in a vertical tube, reflects a variety of factors. ESR is a non-specific marker for chronic inflammation and is slow to change as a patient's condition worsens or improves. It is not used to confirm mast cell activation.

(P 778: Section 14: Allergic Disorders)

Answer 14-9. d

This patient meets the clinical diagnostic criteria for anaphylaxis. The approach to treating anaphylaxis should focus on maintaining the airway, breathing, and circulation. Mortality from anaphylaxis results from asphyxiation due to upper airway angioedema, respiratory failure from bronchial obstruction, or cardiovascular collapse.

Epinephrine is a sympathomimetic catecholamine that acts on both alpha- and beta-adrenergic receptors. It is the most potent alpha receptor activator and causes vasoconstriction through its effect on alpha-adrenergic receptors to counter vasodilation and increases in vascular permeability. It also induces relaxation of the bronchial smooth muscle by acting on beta-adrenergic receptors to alleviate wheezing and shortness of breath. Epinephrine is the most important initial medical therapy in treating acute anaphylaxis. It is most effective when administered within 30 minutes of onset of symptoms. Mortality from anaphylaxis is strongly associated with delays in epinephrine therapy.

H1 and H2 histamine receptor antagonists (eg, diphenhydramine, ranitidine) are adjunctive medications that should be given to reduce pruritis and urticaria. Antihistamines without epinephrine are insufficient to adequately treat anaphylaxis. Corticosteroids, such as methylprednisolone, are frequently given to attenuate the potential late-phase inflammatory reaction and prevent recurrence of symptoms 8–12 hours after the initial onset. Corticosteroids are not effective in treating the initial acute phase of anaphylaxis. Large volume fluid resuscitation may be required if hypotension is present, but unlikely to be effective if epinepherine is not simultaneously administered. If respiratory compromise or bronchospasm is present, inhaled bronchodilators (albuterol) should be administered. Bronchodilators are not, however, the most important initial therapy in treating anaphylaxis.

(P 778: Section 14: Allergic Disorders)

Answer 14-10. d

The patient in the above vignette most likely presented with an acute anaphylactic reaction after consuming almonds at a friend's house. The approach to treating anaphylaxis should focus on maintaining the airway, breathing, and circulation. Mortality from anaphylaxis results from asphyxiation due to upper airway angioedema, respiratory failure from bronchial obstruction, or cardiovascular collapse.

Epinephrine is a sympathomimetic catecholamine that acts on both alpha- and beta-adrenergic receptors. It is the most potent alpha receptor activator and causes vasoconstriction through its effect on alpha-adrenergic receptors to counter vasodilation and increases in vascular permeability. It also induces relaxation of the bronchial smooth muscle by acting on beta-adrenergic receptors to alleviate wheezing and shortness of breath. Epinephrine is the most important initial medical therapy in the treatment of acute anaphylaxis and thus the patient should be discharged with injectable epinephrine for home use and receive appropriate instructions on how to administer the medication. Epinephrine is most effective when administered within 30 minutes of onset of symptoms. Mortality from anaphylaxis is strongly associated with delays in epinephrine therapy.

While oral H1 antihistamines and inhaled bronchodilators can be used adjunctive medications in an acute anaphylactic reaction, they are not sufficient to adequately treat an acute anaphylactic reaction as monotherapy. Daily use of oral H1 antihistamines is not indicated after an anaphylactic reaction. Corticosteroids are frequently given to attenuate the potential late-phase anaphylactic inflammatory response, however, inhaled corticosteroids are not indicated in acute anaphylaxis.

(P 778: Section 14: Allergic Disorders)

Answer 14-11. a

Anaphylaxis, urticaria, and angioedema most commonly result from IgE-mediated mast cell activation resulting in the release of histamine, leukotrienes, and other mast cell mediators into the superficial dermis (urticarial) and deep dermis (angioedema). Urticaria and angioedema are isolated to mucocutaneous symptoms whereas anaphylaxis is an acute systemic reaction. The majority of urticaria and angioedema are mast cell-mediated conditions.

Angioedema in the absence of urticaria and/or pruritis, however, may be caused by mediators other than histamine. In particular, hereditary angioedema is classified as a kinin-related angioedema, with bradykinin recognized as the most important mediator in this condition.

AR is a chronic inflammatory disease of the upper airway caused by IgE sensitization to airborne allergens in genetically susceptible individuals. AR is not a kinin-mediated condition.

(Pp 775, 777, 778, 779: Section 14: Allergic Disorders)

Answer 14-12. a

Hereditary angioedema is caused by mutations in the C1-inhibitor (C1INH) gene leading to low C1INH levels and/or activity. The inheritance pattern is autosomal dominant. C1INH is a primary inhibitory protein for steps leading to bradykinin production. Therefore, C1INH deficiency leads to increased tissue bradykinin which results in vasodilation, increased vascular permeability, and angioedema.

A mutation in the CFTR (cystic fibrosis transmembrane conductance regulator) gene is the most common gene mutation responsible for cystic fibrosis; an autosomal recessive disease. The CFTR gene is required normal transport of chloride and sodium across epithelium. The mutation leads to thick, viscous secretions affecting the lungs, gastrointestinal tract, and pancreas.

A mutation in the dystrophin gene leads to Duchenne muscular dystrophy (DMD); an X-linked recessive form of muscular dystrophy. The dystrophin gene codes for the protein dystrophin, which is an important structural component within muscle tissue. DMD results in muscle degeneration, difficulty in walking, and breathing.

FBN1 is the gene responsible for Marfan Syndrome; a genetic disorder of connective tissue. The *FBN1* gene encodes fibrillin-1, a connective protein. Clinical features associated with the syndrome usually involve the skeleton, skin, and joints, although there may be considerable clinical variability in features. Marfan syndrome is inherited as an autosomal dominant trait.

The *HFE* gene is the gene responsible for hereditary hemochromatosis; an autosomal recessive disease characterized by an accelerated rate of intestinal iron absorption and progressive iron deposition in various tissues.

(P 779: Section 14: Allergic Disorders)

Answer 14-13. b

Over two thirds of urticaria/angioedema cases are self-limited with symptoms resolving in less than 6 weeks. Approximately one third of patients will have daily or near daily symptoms lasting for more than 6 weeks. Urticaria/angioedema lasting for more than 6 weeks is deemed chronic, and a more thorough diagnostic evaluation may be indicated including evaluation for thyroid autoantibodies, autoimmune conditions, and chronic viral infections may be considered.

(Pp 778, 779: Chapter 14: Allergic Disorders)

Answer 14-14. d

The majority of urticaria and angioedema are mast cell-mediated conditions resulting in the release of histamine, leukotrienes, and other mast cell mediators into the superficial dermis (urticaria) and deep dermis (angioedema). In children, common viral or bacterial infections account for 80% of acute urticaria. Treatment of acute urticaria and angioedema should focus on identifying and discontinuing any underlying triggering process and symptom suppression until resolution of the acute episode.

Symptom suppression can often be achieved with administration of H1 antihistamine receptor antagonists. It is most efficient to maximize the H1-receptor antagonist therapy prior to adding additional medications. The use of first-generation H1-receptor antagonists, such as diphenhydramine, is limited by their sedating and anticholinergic side effects. Cetirizine, a second-generation H1-receptor antagonist, is preferable for controlling urticarial symptoms that persist for more than a few days.

H2-receptor antagonists (ranitidine) and leukotriene inhibitors (montelukast) are useful adjunctive medications. Short courses of oral steroids (prednisone) can be used to control severe urticaria that is refractory to high dose antihistamines, but should not be prior to a trial of antihistamine therapy.

(P 779: Section 14: Allergic Disorders)

Answer 14-15. e

Food allergies, defined as adverse immune responses to food proteins, are becoming more common in the pediatric age group. Food allergy is a spectrum of clinicopathological disorders and its manifestations differ significantly depending on the immune mechanism involved and the affected target organ. Manifestations can range from acute urticaria/angioedema to chronic conditions including eczema and failure to thrive.

Currently, there are no tests that can reliably predict the severity of a food allergic reaction, which may vary with similar exposures. Teenagers are particularly vulnerable because they are more likely to take food-consumption risks and may ignore warming signs of an impending severe reaction.

(P 780: Section 14: Allergic Disorders)

Answer 14-16. c

Food allergies have a strong genetic component. Siblings of a peanut allergic child are 6 times more likely to develop a peanut allergy. 64% of monozygotic twins share a peanut allergy compared to 3% of dizygotic twins.

(P 780: Section 14: Allergic Disorders)

Answer 14-17. c

In non-IgE-mediated food hypersensitivity reactions, T-cell mediated mechanisms provide the predominant pathogenic stimulations that drive clinical symptoms. Symptoms of type I hypersensitivity reactions (urticaria, angioedema, flushing,) are usually not present.

This infant is well-appearing and thriving as evidenced by appropriate interval weight gain. The infant is exclusively breastfed and presenting with mucousy, bloody stools. The infant's symptoms are most likely secondary to dietary protein proctocolitis, which is a T-cell mediated food hypersensitivity disorder. Cow's milk and soy products are the most commonly implicated allergens associated with allergic proctocolitis. Some breastfed infants with allergic proctocolitis become sensitized as a result of maternally ingested protein excreted in the breast milk. Elimination of cow's milk and soy from the maternal diet usually results in the resolution of symptoms.

Since cow's milk and soy are the most common causes of allergic proctocolitis in infants, switching to cow's milk formula or soy formula may not be helpful. In addition, due to the positive immunologic effects of breastfeeding as well as maternal–infant bonding, a trial of food elimination from the mother's diet is appropriate before switching the infant to an amino acid based-formula.

Patch testing is a method for eliciting cellular mediated hypersensitivity reactions in sensitized subjects. Patient skin is exposed to the allergen usually for 48 hours and reactions are usually interpreted at 72 hours. Patch testing is used for the assessment of contact allergen sensitization, but is only recently being evaluated for cellular-mediated food hypersensitivity disorders. While patch testing has shown promise for the diagnosis of non-IgE mediated food allergy, there are currently no standardized reagents, application methods, or guidelines for interpretation. Prick testing is useful to evaluate for

IgE-mediated food reactions, such as urticaria, angioedema, nausea, vomiting, or shortness of breath.

(Pp 781, 782: Section 14: Allergic Disorders)

Answer 14-18. d

The patient in the above vignette is experiencing an oral-allergy syndrome. Oral-allergy syndrome develops exclusively in older children or teenagers with prior pollen sensitization. It is due to heat-labile cross-reactive antigens present in plant and food antigens. Usually, these foods are well-tolerated when cooked. Given the patient's history of seasonal allergies, his symptoms are most likely secondary to pollen sensitization to ragweed as cantaloupe and watermelon both have cross reactivity with ragweed.

In IgE-mediated food allergies, patients exhibit the characteristic pattern of type I hypersensitivity reactions, which are the result of release of mast cell granules. Manifestations typically include flushing, urticaria, and/or angioedema, but some patients may present with only respiratory or gastrointestinal symptoms. Patients may progress to anaphylaxis or cardiovascular collapse. The patient's history of seasonal allergies and previous tolerance of both cantaloupe and watermelon makes an oral-allergy syndrome a more likely diagnosis than a primary IgE-mediated food allergy.

Food protein-induced enterocolitis (FPIES) affects both the small bowel and colon, with diffuse inflammation of the gastrointestinal tract, mild villous atrophy, and crypt abscesses. It is typically triggered by ingestion of cow's milk, but can be triggered by soy and solid food proteins. Patients usually present with profuse vomiting and diarrhea, which develop within a few hours of ingestion of the allergic food. FPIES is an example of a delayed onset food hypersensitivity reaction.

Eosinophillic esophagitis (EE) typically affects older children or adolescents. Patients often experience recurrent vomiting and abdominal pain. Coughing and choking are found in the early stages progressing to overt dysphagia and, in severe cases, food impaction. In patient's suspected of having EE, the initial test is typically an upper endoscopy with esophageal biopsies. The majority of patients have at least 15 eosinophils per high power field in at least one biopsy specimen. EE is also an example of a delayed onset food hypersensitivity reaction.

(P 781: Section 14: Allergic Disorders)

Answer 14-19. c

The patient in the above vignette has symptoms consistent with EE). EE is typically a disease of children and adolescents, but symptoms may develop as early as the second or third year of life. Patients often complain of recurrent vomiting and abdominal pain. Coughing and choking are found in the initial stages. Symptoms progress to overt dysphagia, and in severe cases, food impaction. Many patients with EE have concomitant symptoms of environmental allergies.

In patients suspected of having EE, the initial diagnostic test is usually an upper endoscopy with esophageal biopsies following 1–2 months of treatment with a proton pump

inhibitor. Esophageal biopsies from patients with EE show an increased number of eosinophils.

Albuterol is an inhaled bronchodilator used to treat asthma symptoms. While the patient is experiencing frequent coughing and chest discomfort, her symptoms are associated with food intake, and do not seem to be primarily respiratory in nature.

Patients who have lactose intolerance, secondary to deficiency of the enzyme lactase, often experience abdominal pain and indigestion after consuming a milk-containing product. Patients with lactose intolerance, however, would not complain of dysphagia or food impaction.

Flexible laryngoscopy would be the appropriate test to evaluate for paradoxical vocal cord motion. Paradoxical vocal cord motion refers to inappropriate movement of the vocal cords resulting in functional airway obstruction and stridorous breathing. Patients may present with significant respiratory distress and inspiratory stridor. In addition to dyspnea, patients may complain of throat tightness, a choking sensation, dysphonia, and cough. Onset of symptoms may be spontaneous or induced by exercise or irritant exposure. The presence of dysphagia and food impaction in the above vignette, are more suggestive, however, of EE.

(P 781: Section 14: Allergic Disorders)

Answer 14-20. d

Food allergies can be grouped into 2 general categories: IgE-mediated and non-IgE-mediated. IgE-mediated reactions are typically of rapid onset with clinical symptoms usually developing within minutes to a few hours of ingestion of the offending food. These reactions are due to release of mast cell granules and present with the typical characteristics of type I hypersensitivity reactions (flushing, urticaria, and/or angioedema).

The diagnostic workup for a suspected IgE-medicated food allergy includes a skin prick test and/or measurement of serum food-specific IgE antibodies. Both of these tests have sensitivity estimated to be >85%. Specificity, however, is <40%, since both tests measure allergic sensitization and may not correlate with clinical allergy. Clinical allergy can only be assessed by an oral food challenge. For some common food allergens, studies have suggested cut-off values for serum food-specific IgE antibodies that can predict the likelihood of developing systemic allergic reactions in a particular patient.

Intradermal skin testing requires a small amount of the allergen solution is injected into the skin. An intradermal skin test may be done when a substance does not cause a reaction in the skin prick test, but is still a suspected allergen for a given patient. The intradermal test is more sensitive than the skin prick test, but also has more false-positive results. It is not used for the diagnosis of IgE-mediated food allergy, but rather for the evaluation of seasonal and perennial AR.

The atopy patch test is used to elicit cellular mediated hypersensitivity reactions in sensitized subjects. Patient skin is exposed to the allergen usually for 48 hours and reactions are usually interpreted at 72 hours. Patch testing is used for the assessment of contact allergen sensitization, but is only recently being evaluated for cellular-mediated food hypersensitivity disorders. While patch testing has shown promise for the diagnosis of non-IgE mediated food allergy, there are currently no standardized reagents, application methods, or guidelines for interpretation.

(Pp 781, 782: Section 14: Food Allergies)

Answer 14-21. a

Current management of food allergies relies on the careful elimination of the offending food from the diet, including instruction on reading of labels and often requires education of the parents by a dietician. Institution of therapeutic measures to stall the development of severe reactions in the case of an accidental food exposure is also necessary. All patients with a history of a systemic reaction to food should be prescribed injectable epinephrine and instructed on its use. The drug should be employed quickly in the case of an impending anaphylactic reaction. Daily use, however, is not indicated.

Milder food allergic reactions, those involving the skin or the gastrointestinal system exclusively, can be treated with oral antihistamines. Oral antihistamines should be used for symptoms only and daily use is not indicated.

The indication of glucocorticoids for the treatment of acute food allergic reactions is controversial. There is no consistent evidence that glucocorticoids prevent the development of late-phase reactions and are not routinely indicated.

The use of oral immunotherapy for desensitization to food allergens is currently an area of investigation. The safety and efficacy of this approach has not been established in infants and children.

(Pp 781, 782: Section 14: Allergic Disorders)

Answer 14-22. d

Up to 3% of the general population has bee sting allergy. The different families of hymenoptera have different behaviors and degrees of aggressiveness. Honeybees are minimally aggressive and only sting if attacked. Alternatively, yellow jackets and hornets are more aggressive and will sting with less provocation. Wasps tend to build their nests near buildings and under attics, making them more likely to encounter people and therefore contribute to a larger number of stings than yellow jackets an hornets. Africanized honeybees, which are indistinguishable from ordinary honeybees, are much more aggressive about defending their territory than ordinary honeybees, making toxic envenomations much more likely.

(P 782: Section 14: Allergic Disorders)

Answer 14-23. e

The patient in the above vignette is experiencing a reaction to a hymenopterid sting. Four types of reactions to hymenopterid stings occur. A normal reaction results in swelling, redness, and pain at the site of the sting with rapid onset and resolution within hours.

More significantly, some patients may develop a second type of reaction called a large, local reaction. A large local reaction

extends beyond the site of the sting to involve the entire limb. In these reactions, swelling, erythema, and tenderness develop slowly over approximately 48 hours and resolve over days. While it often looks alarming, it is generally no more serious than a normal reaction. Treatment for localized reactions may be managed with ice, pain relief, and antihistamines.

Direct toxic reactions to hymenoptera venom are a third type of reaction, which occur with large doses hymenoptera venom. These reactions have been reported to occur in as few as 50 stings. Anyone who sustains more than 50 stings should be monitored for the complications of hymenoptera venom overdose, which include rhabdomyolysis and myocardial infarction.

The final type of reaction is a systemic, IgE-mediated reaction, leading to anaphylaxis. Systemic reactions typically develop rapidly, within 30 minutes of the sting and may consist of urticaria, angioedema, wheezing, laryngeal edema, hypotension, tachycardia, and diarrhea or vomiting. Systemic reactions can be distinguished from large, local reactions by the involvement of organs distant from the site of the sting and by the rapidity at which a systemic reaction develops.

Systemic reactions to hymenoptera stings should be managed by securing a stable airway, early use of epinephrine, a short course of corticosteroids, and antihistamines. Late-phase reactions are less common in insect stings, but do still occur. Patients should therefore be monitored for at least 4 hours after the sting. All patients should also be given an epinephrine autoinjector with instructions on proper use and referral to an allergist for evaluation for immunotherapy.

Given the slow onset of his symptoms and lack of involvement in sites and organs distant from the sting, the patient in the above vignette is presenting with signs and symptoms consistent with a large, local reaction. Treatment with ice, pain relief, and antihistamines is appropriate. IV clindamycin would be appropriate treatment for cellulitis. While the patient in the above vignette has diffuse erythema of his leg, he is afebrile and given the history of a wasp sting, a large local reaction to the sting is more likely.

(Pp 782, 783: Section 14: Allergic Disorders)

Answer 14-24. e

Systemic reactions to hymenoptera stings should be managed the same as other anaphylactic reactions, by securing a stable airway, early use of epinephrine, short course of corticosteroids and antihistamines. All patients with a systemic reaction to an insect sting should be given epinephrine autoinjectors with instructions on proper use and a referral to an allergist for evaluation and possible immunotherapy.

Venom immunotherapy is one of the most effective therapies available for managing allergic disease and greatly improves the outcome of subsequent stings. While all adults with systemic reactions should be offered venom immunotherapy, children with only cutaneous manifestations do not require desensitization (choice c). Children with only cutaneous reactions appear to be unlikely to go on to have more significant reactions. Children with reactions that are not limited to the skin, however, greatly benefit from immunotherapy.

Venom immunotherapy is only effective for IgE-mediated disease and therefore, venom immunotherapy is not recommended for large local reactions (choice b) or for those that do not have evidence of IgE-mediated reactions.

The patient in choice a is experiencing a normal reaction to an insect sting. This reaction is not IgE-mediated and venom immunotherapy would not be indicated. The patient in choice d is experiencing a direct toxic reaction due to a large dose of hymenoptera venom. The direct toxic reaction is not IgE-mediated. Rhabdomyolysis and myocardial infarction are complications of hymenoptera venom overdose. The patient's rhabomyolysis should be treated supportively, but venom immunotherapy is not indicated.

(Pp 782, 733: Chapter 14: Allergic Disorders)

Answer 14-25. d

Natural rubber is a highly processed plant product of the commercial rubber tree. Most true allergic reactions to natural rubber latex occur with exposure to "dipped" products, such as gloves or balloons. These products are made from liquid latex rubber and have a large number of soluble proteins capable of binding IgE.

Life-threating allergic reactions may be the presenting sign of latex allergic in up to 30% of latex-sensitive children. The majority of latex-allergic individuals are highly atopic with histories of AR or asthma.

Studies have shown a higher prevalence of latex sensitization in certain high-risk groups with frequent exposure to latex including health care workers and children with spina bifida. Children with spina bifida undergo repeated urologic and neurologic surgical procedures. Children with spina bifida have the highest prevalence of latex sensitization, ranging from 18% to 73%. Risk factors in this population include more than 5 surgeries and a history of atopy. The 2-year-old in answer choice d is undergoing a shunt revision and has likely already undergone multiple other surgical procedures.

The high rate of latex sensitization and the potential severity of reactions suggest that all patients with spina bifida be evaluated for their individual risk of latex allergy prior to surgical procedures to minimize complications.

While latex allergy has been associated with several fruits and vegetables, including avocado, kiwi, banana, potato, tomato, chestnut, and papaya, it has not been associated with shellfish or peanut. Latex allergy has also not been associated with bee sting allergy.

While the infant with congenital heart disease will likely undergo multiple procedures in the future, patients with spina bifida have the highest prevalence of latex sensitization.

(P 783: Section 14: Allergic Disorders)

Answer 14-26. d

A detailed history of adverse reactions to latex product exposure is the most important first step in properly assessing for a latex allergy. IgE-mediated latex allergy may cause various symptoms consistent with mast cell-mediated reactions including, urticaria, angioedema, acute rhinitis, bronchospasm, and anaphylaxis. Symptoms generally appear within 15 minutes of exposure.

When IgE-mediated latex allergy is suspected, diagnostic testing for latex-specific IgE should be pursued. Specific-IgE testing for latex can be accomplished by allergy skin resting or radioallergosorbent testing. Presently in the United States, there is no commercially available standardized reagent for skin testing making latex allergy skin testing challenging. Some allergists perform skin testing using solutions extracted from rubber latex gloves. This approach is complicated by variability in the concentration of specific latex allergens and the sensitivity and specificity of this type of testing has not been established. Serum testing for latex-specific IgE is commercially available with immunoassays licensed by the US FDA.

IgE-mediated latex allergy must be differentiated from dermatitis that occurs with rubber glove exposure. Latex rubber products can induce both irritant and allergic contact dermatitis. Allergic contact dermatitis is a delayed-type inflammatory cutaneous reaction caused by specific T-cell activation. The cell-mediated reaction (type IV reaction) may be caused by a variety of chemical accelerators to antioxidants added to the rubber mixture during glove production. This delayed dermatitis is generally not due to IgE sensitization to latex.

The atopy patch test is used to elicit cellular mediated hypersensitivity reactions in sensitized subjects. Patient skin is exposed to the allergen usually for 48 hours and reactions are usually interpreted at 72 hours. Patch testing may be helpful to diagnose sensitization to low-molecular-weight chemicals in rubber products. Given the timing of her symptoms and lack of typical symptoms associated with a mast cell-mediated reaction (urticaria, angioedema, bronchospasm, anaphylaxis), the patient in the above vignette most likely has allergic contact dermatitis from a component in the rubber glove mixture and allergy patch testing may be diagnostic.

Intradermal skin testing requires a small amount of the allergen solution to be injected into the skin. An intradermal skin test may be done when a substance does not cause a reaction in the skin prick test, but is still a suspected allergen for a given patient. The intradermal test is more sensitive than the skin prick test, but also has more false-positive results. Since the patient in the above vignette most likely has a cell-mediated reaction, intradermal testing is not indicated.

If an IgE-mediated latex allergy is suspected, specific IgE testing for latex can be accomplished by allergy skin testing or serum radioallergosobent testing (as stated above). A contact latex exposure challenge poses unnecessary risks for the patient including risk of anaphylaxis and is not indicated to diagnose a latex allergy.

(P 784: Chapter 14: Allergic Disorders)

Answer 14-27. e

Acute allergic reactions to latex are managed in the same manner as other IgE-mediated reactions based on specific symptoms. The patient should be removed from the source of latex exposure to prevent further exacerbations of the allergic reaction. Anaphylaxis is treated primarily with epinephrine, although IV fluids and corticosteroids may be required. Mild urticaria and angioedema can be treated with oral antihistamines, but are not the primary treatment for anaphylaxis.

Once a diagnosis of latex allergy has been established, the long-term management of such patients requires latex avoidance and education of the patient. Minimization of exposure to dipped rubber products. Patients should consider medical alert bracelets. Although the health care system is often equipped with appropriate rubber-free products, it is advisable for patients to have a personal supply of nonlatex gloves for use when they require medical or dental care. Patients should also carry self-injectable epinephrine.

Patients diagnosed with latex allergy should also be educated about allergic signs or symptoms when consuming the foods included in the latex-fruit syndrome (those listed in answer choice c). If patients tolerate these foods without symptoms, there is no reason to avoid them. Latex-allergic patients, however, should be cautious when eating these foods for the first time.

A variety of immunotherapies for latex allergy are under investigation. None of these, however, are yet adequate for routine use.

(P 784: Chapter 14: Allergic Disorders)

Answer 14-28. e

Drug reactions can be classified into immunologic and nonimmunologic etiologies. The majority (75–80%) of adverse drug reactions are predictable, nonimmunologic effects, including: reactions due to overdose, toxicity, pharmacologic side effects, indirect side effects, and drug-drug interactions. The remaining 20–25% of adverse drug events are due to unpredictable effects, which may or may not be immune-mediated. Immune-mediated reactions constituting true drug hypersensitivity account for 5–10% of all drug reactions.

Drug hypersensitivity reactions commonly manifest with dermatologic symptoms. Typically an erythematous, maculopapular rash develops within 2 weeks of drug initiation, originating on the trunk with eventual spread to the limbs. Pruritis and low-grade fever may accompany the drug eruption.

Nephrotoxicity and ototoxicity are known dose-dependent side of effects of vancomycin and gentamicin respectively. Nausea and vomiting is a common adverse drug reaction to certain antibiotics, but nausea and vomiting do not represent an immunologic drug reaction.

Infectious mononucleosis is most commonly secondary to infection with the Epstein–Barr virus. A rash is a relatively common adverse effect of amoxicillin treatment in patients with acute Epstein–Barr virus. It is a nonimmunologically mediated reaction. Amoxicillin is not indicated for the treatment of viral infections including the Epstein–Barr virus.

(Pp 784–785: Section 14: Allergic Disorders)

Answer 14-29. c

Group B streptococcus (GBS) are a gram positive bacteria that cause illness most commonly in newborns and pregnant women. GBS is the leading cause of sepsis, meningitis, and pneumonia in newborns in the United States with attendant substantial short- and long-term morbidity and mortality. Since, intrapartum prophylactic antibiotics significantly reduce mother-to-child GBS transmission, in 1996, the CDC, American College of Obstetricians and Gynecologists, and the American Academy of Pediatrics recommended that hospitals adopt a formal GBS prevention policy.

The efficacy of both penicillin and ampicillin as intravenously administered intrapartum agents for the prevention of early-onset neonatal GBS disease was demonstrated in clinical trials. The dosages of penicillin and ampicillin used for intrapartum GBS prophylaxis are aimed at achieving adequate levels in the fetal circulation and amniotic fluid rapidly while avoiding potentially neurotoxic serum levels in the mother or fetus. In contrast, data on the ability of clindamycin, erythromycin and vancomycin to reach bactericidal levels in the fetal circulation and amniotic fluid are very limited; available data suggest that erythromycin and clindamycin provided to pregnant women do not reach fetal tissues reliably.

Since the patient in the above vignette has a nonimmunologic mediated reaction to penicillin, it is most appropriate to use ampicillin as intrapartum antibiotic prophylaxis as data on erythromycin, clindamycin, and vancomycin is very limited and these antibiotics may not provide effective prophylaxis against GBS disease. Gentamicin is an aminoglycoside antibiotic. Gentamicin provides effective treatment for many gram negative organisms, but does not provide appropriate coverage for Group B streptococcus.

(P 785: Section 14: Allergic Disorders (and the CDC website))

Answer 14-30. e

Drug hypersensitivity reactions commonly manifest with dermatologic symptoms, frequently as morbilliform rashes or exanthems. Type I hypersensitivity reactions require the presence of antigen-specific IgE. Skin testing is a particularly useful diagnostic procedure. Skin testing is standardized for penicillin, but not for other antibiotics. While positive skin testing confirms the presence of antigen-specific IgE and is supportive of a type I hypersensitivity reaction, negative skin testing is only helpful for penicillin skin testing because the test specificity has been adequately established. With other drug agents, a negative skin test does not effectively rule out the presence of IgE.

Due to the frequent lack of drug-specific testing, the diagnosis of drug hypersensitivity is often based on clinical judgment. It is important to distinguish between immune-medicated hypersensitivity reactions and other predictable adverse drug reactions.

(P 785: Section 14: Allergic Disorders)

Answer 14-31. e

Intrauterine infection with *Treponema pallidum* can result in stillbirth, hydrops fetalis, or preterm birth or may be asymptomatic at birth. Infected infants can have hepatosplenomegaly, snuffles, lymphadenopathy, mucocutaneous lesions, pneumonia, osteochondritis and pseudoparalysis, edema, rash, hemolytic anemia, or thrombocytopenia at birth or within the first 4–8 weeks of age.

All women should be screened serologically for syphilis early in pregnancy with a nontreponemal test (eg, RPR or VDRL) and preferably again at delivery. The result of a positive nontreponemal antibody test should be confirmed with a treponemal antibody test (eg, FTA-ABS or TP-PA).

Parenteral penicillin G remains the preferred drug for treatment of syphilis at any stage. Parenteral penicillin G is the only documented effective therapy for patients who have neurosyphilis, congenital syphilis, or syphilis during pregnancy and is recommended for HIV-infected patients. According to the American Academy of Pediatrics Red Book Committee, such patients always should be treated with penicillin, even if desensitization for penicillin allergy is necessary.

Data to support the use of alternatives to penicillin in the treatment of early syphilis are limited. However, several therapies might be effective in nonpregnant, penicillin-allergic patients who have primary or secondary syphilis. Doxycycline 100 mg orally twice daily for 14 days and tetracycline (500 mg four times daily for 14 days) are regimens that have been used for many years. Compliance is likely to be better with doxycycline than tetracycline, because tetracycline can cause gastrointestinal side effects. Although limited clinical studies, along with biologic and pharmacologic evidence, suggest that ceftriaxone (1 g daily either IM or IV for 10–14 days) is effective for treating early syphilis, the optimal dose and duration of ceftriaxone therapy have not been defined. Azithromycin as a single 2-g oral dose is effective for treating early syphilis. However, *T. pallidum* chromosomal mutations associated with azithromycin resistance and treatment failures have been documented in several geographical areas in the United States. As such, the use of azithromycin should be used with caution only when treatment with penicillin or doxycycline is not feasible (www.CDC.gov).

In cases where there is no suitable alternative drug that has previously caused an IgE-mediated hypersensitivity reaction, a drug desensitization procedure may be required. Pregnant patients who are allergic to penicillin should be desensitized and treated with penicillin.

(Pp 785, 786: Section 14: Allergic disorders (and the Redbook online and www.cdc.gov))

Answer 14-32. b

Penicillin is the most commonly reported medication allergy. True allergic reactions to penicillin can be severe and penicillin remains a leading cause of fatal drug reactions. Patients who have a history of an IgE-mediated allergic reaction to penicillin should undergo penicillin allergy skin testing prior to drug administration.

Varying degrees of cross-reactivity have been documented between penicillins and structurally related compounds containing a B-lactam ring. Ampicillin is a penicillin-derived beta-lactam antibiotic and administration to patients with confirmed penicillin allergies should be avoided. Imipenem use should generally be avoided in penicillin-allergic patients due to data suggesting a high-rate of cross-reactivity with penicillin.

The rate of cross-reaction between penicillin and second or third-generation cephalosporins has been found to be 5% or less, but significant cross-reactivity occurs with ceftazadime (a third-generation cephalosporin). The rate of cross-reaction between penicillin and first-generation cephalosporins (eg, cefazolin) is greater than that for second and third-generation cephalosporins.

Aztreonam cross-reactivity is extremely rare in penicillin-allergic patients.

(P 786: Chapter 14: Allergic Disorders)

Answer 14-33. b

Anticonvulsant hypersensitivity syndrome, also known as drug rash with eosinophilia and systemic symptoms (DRESS) and drug-induced hypersensitivity syndrome (DIHS) are rare, multisystem disorders that are most often associated with administration of aromatic antiseizure medications. The most commonly involved medications include carbamazepine, phenytoin, lamotrigine, and phenobarbital. Symptoms of erythroderma, fever, and lymphadenopathy are observed in more than half of affected patients. Leukocytosis, eosinophilia, and elevated liver enzymes are characteristic findings.

Initial management of patients begins with early recognition, cessation of the drug, and supportive therapy including intravenous fluids if required and ocular care. Systemic corticosteroids are usually required.

Cross-reactivity to other aromatic anticonvulsant drugs is reported in over half of affected patients such that they should avoid further use of aromatic anticonvulsant drugs. Family members of patients with anticonvulsant hypersensitivity syndrome are at higher risk for the disorder if they require anticonvulsant treatment. Safe anticonvulsant drugs for these patients include valproic acid and benzodiazepines.

(P 786: Section 14: Allergic Disorders)

Answer 14-34. c

AR is a chronic inflammatory disorder of the upper airway caused by IgE sensitization to airborne allergens in genetically susceptible individuals. The clinical presentation is associated with frequent sneezing, nasal congestion, and nasal discharge. The majority of patients with AR also display or complain of ocular symptoms (itchy or watery eyes). Thus, it is termed ARC.

AR has been subdivided into seasonal and perennial types based on the time and duration of symptom occurrence. Seasonal symptoms occur in the fall and spring whereas perennial AR is caused by an allergic response to allergens that are present throughout the year, such as dust mites and pet dander.

Chronic sinusitis often has other clinical features including headache, facial pain, and purulent or green rhinorrhea. Viral upper respiratory infections can cause sneezing, nasal congestion, and rhinorrhea, but they are not usually associated with ocular pruritus. The duration of a viral upper respiratory infection is also brief and would not be expected to be present consistently year round. Adenoid hypertrophy can produce nasal airway obstruction and can lead to significant pediatric morbidity including chronic sinusitis, recurrent otitis media with effusion, and chronic serous otitis media. Ocular pruritus would not be expected with adenoid hypertrophy. In addition, a history of otitis media was not mentioned for the patient in the above vignette.

(Pp 775, 776: Section 14: Allergic Disorders)

Administering influenza vaccine to egg allergic recipients: a focused practice parameter update. *Ann Allergy Asthma Immunol.* 2011;106:11–16.

Answer 14-35. c

In the pediatric population, anaphylactic reactions to vaccines are a concern. True IgE-mediated anaphylaxis to immunizations is rare and more commonly involved IgE to vaccine components rather than the immunizing antigen itself. Gelatin, added to vaccine as a stabilizing agent, has been implicated in anaphylactic reactions to MMR, varicella, influenza, and Japanese encephalitis vaccines.

Children with a history of egg allergy should be seen by a specialist in allergy before receiving influenza and yellow fever vaccines, as egg protein used in these vaccines has been implicated in anaphylactic reactions to these immunizations.

Since the patient in the above vignette has an egg allergy, she should be referred to an allergist prior to receiving the influenza vaccine. She has no contraindication to the MMR vaccine and therefore, the MMR vaccine should be given.

(P 777: Section 14: Allergic Disorders)

Answer 14-36. a

This patient meets the clinical diagnostic criteria for anaphylaxis. The approach to treating anaphylaxis should focus on maintaining the airway, breathing, and circulation. Mortality from anaphylaxis results from asphyxiation due to upper airway angioedema, respiratory failure from bronchial obstruction, or cardiovascular collapse.

Epinephrine is a sympathomimetic catecholamine that acts on both alpha- and beta-adrenergic receptors. It is the most potent alpha receptor activator and causes vasoconstriction

through its effect on alpha-adrenergic receptors to counter vasodilation and increases in vascular permeability. It also induces relaxation of the bronchial smooth muscle by acting on beta-adrenergic receptors to alleviate wheezing and shortness of breath. Epinephrine is the most important initial medical therapy in treating acute anaphylaxis. It is most effective when administered within 30 minutes of onset of symptoms. Mortality from anaphylaxis is strongly associated with delays in epinephrine therapy.

H1 and H2 histamine receptor antagonists (diphenhydramine, ranitidine) are adjunctive medications that should be given to reduce pruritis and urticaria. Antihistamines without epinephrine are insufficient to adequately treat anaphylaxis.

Corticosteroids, such as methylprednisolone, are frequently given to attenuate the potential late-phase inflammatory reaction and prevent recurrence of symptoms 8–12 hours after the initial onset. Corticosteroids are not effective in treating the initial acute phase of anaphylaxis. Large volume fluid resuscitation may be required if hypotension is present, but unlikely to be effective if epinepherine is not simultaneously administered.

If respiratory compromise or bronchospasm is present, inhaled bronchodilators (albuterol) should be administered. Bronchodilators are not, however, the most important initial therapy in treating anaphylaxis.

(Pp 777, 778: Section 14: Allergic Disorders)

Answer 14-37. e

Allergic reactions occur when antigen presenting cells take up, process, and present antigens to naïve T-cells, which then polarize to the TH2 lineage. These TH2 cells then release cytokines including IL-4 and IL-13, which cause B-cells to class switch into IgE-producing plasma cells. Subsequent exposure to the allergen will cause binding of the allergen by the IgE antibodies. This antibody–antigen complex can then interact with receptors on mast cells, causing mast cell degranulation and triggering an allergic reaction.

(P 770: Section 14: Allergic Disorders)

Answer 14-38. a

The physical examination of children with AR can be very beneficial to determine the cause of upper airway complaints. Classical signs include allergic shiners, allergic salute, and allergic crease. The examination of the nasal cavity in AR often reveals pale, enlarged turbinates with clear rhinorrhea.

While nasal polyps can be seen in AR, they are not typically found, and their presence should prompt the search for a different diagnosis, such as cystic fibrosis or aspirin sensitivity.

Erythematous mucosa is often the sign of a viral or bacterial infection, rather than an atopic condition. Finally, small retracted turbinates are seen more commonly in adenoidal hypertrophy.

(P 776: Section 14: Allergic Disorders)

Answer 14-39. d

Novel therapies are being introduced aimed at interrupting key pathways in atopic responses. Anti-IgE monoclonal antibodies block binding of IgE to the FcεRI receptor without inducing immediate hypersensitivity reactions or anaphylaxis. These monoclonal antibodies reduce IgE levels in humans by binding to IgE and removing by immune complex formation. These antibodies attenuate both the early and late-phase responses to inhaled allergens and reduce the associated increase in eosinophils in sputum. Anti-IgE monoclonal antibody therapy (omaluzimab) is currently available and FDA approved for moderate to severe allergic asthma.

Therapies against IL-4, soluble IL-4 receptor, and IL-13 are currently being investigated in allergic diseases such as asthma. While they do show promise, none are currently FDA-approved nor available for clinical use.

(P 771: Section 14: Allergic Disorders)

Answer 14-40. c

Montelukast is approved for the treatment of asthma and for relief of symptoms of perennial allergic rhinitis. Its mechanism of action is as a LTRA. As a single agent, it is less effective than nasal corticosteroids, yet the safety profile of LTRAs make them a suitable alternative for patients who cannot receive steroids or who are wary of their side effects. There are now medications such as zileuton that are able to partially block the synthesis of leukotrienes, and can be used in allergic conditions such as asthma.

Antihistamines block the H1 histamine receptor, and mast cell stabilizers such as cromolyn are also used occasionally in the treatment of allergic diseases. Allergen-specific immunotherapy is the only treatment that can potentially modify the course of ARC by redirecting the immune response toward a tolerant state, and its clinical benefits may be sustained years after discontinuation of treatment.

(Pp 774–775: Section 14: Allergic Disorders)

CHAPTER 15 | Rheumatologic Disorders

Hilary M. Haftel

15-1. Joint stiffness after rest (gelling) associated with arthritis is due to which of the following mechanisms?

a. Increased effusion in the joint during periods of rest

b. Increased inflammation in the synovial lining during rest

c. Lower temperature in the joint during rest

d. Decreased penetration of medications into the joint at rest

e. Increased tone in the surrounding musculature during rest

15-2. Pain in which of these situations should raise suspicion for a disorder other than inflammatory arthritis?

a. A 3-year old girl with joint pain upon awakening in the morning

b. A 5-year-old boy who awakens with pain during the night

c. A 12-year-old girl with pain in cold, damp weather

d. A 4-year-old girl who has joint pain after a long car ride

e. A 10-year-old boy who complains of joint pain during an viral illness

15-3. Which of the following features is more indicative of a chronic arthritis, rather than an acute arthritis?

a. Swelling of the left elbow joint

b. Tenderness to palpation of a swollen right ankle

c. A leg length discrepancy in a child with a swollen left knee

d. Limitation of range of motion of a swollen wrist

e. Warmth on palpation of a swollen right knee

15-4. A 3-year-old child is brought to the emergency room with fever to 39°C and refusal to bear weight for the last several hours. She is ill-appearing and on exam has a swollen, tender right knee with surrounding erythema. Radiographs of the right knee demonstrate an effusion.

Which of the following tests would most likely to ensure a definitive diagnosis?

a. Blood culture

b. Bone culture

c. MRI of the knee

d. Synovial fluid culture

e. Ultrasound of the knee

15-5. Which of the following clinical situations would lead to an artificially low erythrocyte sedimentation rate (ESR)?

a. A 17-year-old girl with her first pregnancy

b. An 18-year-old girl with chronic lung disease and polycythemia

c. A 9-year-old boy with nephrotic syndrome

d. A 13-year-old girl with SLE and hypergammaglobulinemia

e. A 5-year-old boy with iron deficiency anemia

15-6. A 3-year-old boy is brought in by his mother after falling and hurting his knee. She states that he was running on the lawn and tripped. She picked him up and noticed that his right knee was swollen.

Physical exam reveals a semicooperative male. Vitals signs are normal and patient is afebrile. General exam is unremarkable except for the presence of a warm, swollen right knee with a palpable effusion and widening of the medial aspect of the tibia. He is holding his knee slightly flexed, but is willing to run down the hallway. You tell the mother that the patient has chronic arthritis and that the process has been going on for several weeks to months.

Which physical feature is most consistent with your impression of a chronic arthritis?

a. The palpable effusion

b. Warmth of the knee

c. Widening of the tibia

d. The knee being held in flexion

e. Ability to run down the hall

15-7. A 5-year-old girl is brought to your office with a swollen left wrist. There is warmth, erythema, and decreased range of motion of the wrist, all consistent with a diagnosis of oligoarticular juvenile idiopathic arthritis (JIA).

In addition to starting a regular anti-inflammatory medication, the next step should be which of the following?

a. Refer for a daytime splint for the wrist

b. Refer to ophthalmology

c. Refer to orthopedics for a synovial biopsy

d. Refer to social work for school modifications

e. Refer to gastroenterology

15-8. You are reviewing the results of laboratory testing with the family of a child with newly diagnosed polyarticular JIA. The child is already feeling better on regular anti-inflammatory therapy. You share with the family that the child has a negative ANA, a rheumatoid factor that is positive at 150, and antibodies to cyclic citrullinated peptide (anti-CCP) are also positive.

Your advice to the family would include which of the following?

a. Given the negative ANA, the child has no increased risk for uveitis

b. Given her response to the NSAID, she will likely require no additional medications

c. Given her diagnosis of polyarticular JIA, they should prepare her for the reality that she will have progressive disability

d. Given her positive RF and anti-CCP antibodies, her course will be more similar to those with adult-onset rheumatoid arthritis

e. Levels of her RF and anti-CCP do not correspond to severity of disease

15-9. A 10-year-old previously well male is admitted to the hospital with fever for the last 10 days. The fevers are occurring twice daily and the patient feels well between the episodes of fever. During the fevers, however, he feels poorly and the team notes onset of a salmon-colored serpiginous rash on his trunk becomes much more obvious. He has also been noted to have hepatosplenomegaly, but no evidence of arthritis. All cultures to date have been negative. Today, he became dizzy and short of breath. Chest X-ray demonstrated an enlarged heart silhouette and increased interstitial markings. A STAT echocardiogram has been ordered.

This test is most likely to show which of the following?

a. Mitral regurgitation

b. A large VSD

c. Dilated coronary arteries

d. Pulmonary hypertension

e. A large pericardial effusion

15-10. The most common bony finding on a skeletal radiograph in JIA is which of the following?

a. A normal radiograph

b. Periarticular osteopenia

c. Joint space narrowing

d. Erosions

e. Periosteal new bone formation

15-11. A 9-year-old girl with a recent diagnosis of polyarticular JIA returns for follow-up. Six months ago, she was diagnosed and started on an NSAID. Four months ago, she was started on subcutaneous methotrexate (1 mg/kg/week) and folic acid.

In the office today, she reports that she is improved, but still admits to 60–120 minutes of morning stiffness daily and swelling in the small joints of her hands and wrists that is interfering with her schoolwork. Exam confirms the presence of active synovitis in her MCPs and PIPs bilaterally, as well as both wrists.

Your next best step would be which of the following?

a. Continue current therapy for 3 more months and evaluate

b. Change her current NSAID to different NSAID

c. Add an anti-TNF agent

d. Inject all of the affected joints with intra-articular corticosteroids

e. Increase her methotrexate

15-12. A 16-year-old male presents to the office with complaints of heel pain, morning back pain and stiffness, and left knee swelling that have been becoming progressively worse over the last several months. Exam demonstrates loss of lumbar lordosis and decreased forward flexion of the back. His left knee is swollen with warmth and a palpable effusion. Examination of this reveals tenderness and erythema at the insertion of the Achilles' tendon on the calcaneus bilaterally.

Which of the following tests is most likely to provide the definitive diagnosis?

a. A positive HLA-B27

b. Sacroiliitis on dedicated radiographs of the SI joints

c. A positive ANA

d. An elevated ESR

e. Evidence of effusion on radiograph of the knee

15-13. An established patient with inflammatory bowel disease-related arthritis presents to your office with complaints on knee pain. Her disease has been stable and well controlled for months, but on exam you note swelling, warmth, and erythema of both knees.

Your next step would be which of the following?

a. Escalate her disease-modifying medications to control her arthritis.

b. Give her a burst of corticosteroids

c. Refer her back to her gastroenterologist urgently

d. Place her at bed rest

e. Send her for physical therapy.

15-14. A 13-year-old girl is seen in your office with finger and foot pain that has been progressing for the last several months. She reports that 2 of her fingers on her right hand are swollen and painful and she is not able to make a complete fist on that side. She also states that her left foot and ankle have been stiff and sore, particularly when she awakens in the morning.

On exam you note that she has swelling, synovial thickening, and tenderness in the PIP joints of the 3rd and 4th fingers of the right hand, as well as swelling, erythema, and tenderness in the left ankle and the dorsum of the left foot. The rest of her physical exam is unremarkable, except that you note several nail pits on the thumbs bilaterally.

To make a diagnosis, further information that you would want to collect from this patient would be which of the following?

a. Previous history of fungal infections

b. Family history of skin diseases

c. Previous history of strep pharyngitis

d. History of IgA deficiency

e. Family history of cardiovascular disease

15-15. A 6-year-old boy presents to the emergency room with complaints of ankle pain and rash. He is noted on exam to have bilateral ankle swelling, which is periarticular and nonpitting in nature. He has a purpuric rash on his bilateral lower extremities, scrotum; and buttocks; it is nonblanching and nonmigratory (Figure 203-1).

His platelet count and hemoglobin are normal and his WBC count is elevated to 15,000/mm³. PT and aPTT are normal. Urinalysis is negative. You make the diagnosis of Henoch–Schonlein Purpura.

What anticipatory guidance do you provide the family?

a. His ankle swelling should be treated with NSAIDs and will become chronic

b. The risk of nephritis will be present for the next several years and he should be screened regularly during that time

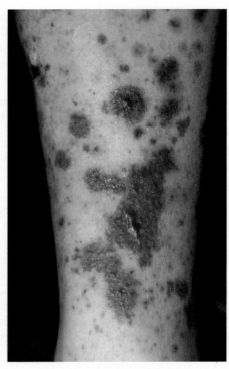

FIGURE 203-1. Classical palpable purpura on the lower legs of a patient with Henoch-Schonlein purpura. (Reproduced, with permission, from Wolff K, Johnson RA. *Fitzpatrick's Color Atlas and Synopsis of Clinical Dermatology.* 6th ed. New York: McGraw-Hill, 2009.)

c. The onset of abdominal pain is most likely from his NSAID and should be treated symptomatically

d. The rash may come and go for weeks to months following the initial presentation

e. The diagnosis of HSP at this time increases his risk for systemic vasculitis as an adult

15-16. A 14-month-old boy is admitted to the hospital following 6 days of unexplained fever and increasing fussiness. The parents states that he had a very red tongue and mouth for the last few days and this morning his eyes appeared "bloodshot." On exam, the child is very irritable. He has a temperature of 40.3°C, bilateral conjunctival injection, dry chapped lips, and a very red tongue. He has palpable anterior and posterior cervical lymphadenopathy, but no palpable hepatosplenomegaly. His hands and feet appear puffy without evidence of frank arthritis. He has a red mildly desquamating rash in his diaper area.

Which of the following would you expect to see on laboratory testing?

a. An elevated platelet count

b. A CSF pleocytosis

c. Red cell casts in the urine

d. A positive blood culture

e. Spherocytes on peripheral smear

15-17. A child hospitalized 2 weeks ago and suffering from Kawasaki disease presents to your office for follow-up. His father reports that the child defervesced within 24 hours of receiving intravenous immunoglobulin and the fever has not recurred. He is now back to his normal activity and disposition, with the exception of swelling of the knees bilaterally that was first noticed while he was in the hospital and is still present.

Your next step would be which of the following?

a. Readmit the patient for another dose of IVIg

b. Change the patient's low dose (5–6 mg/kg/day) aspirin to high dose (80–100 mg/kg/day)

c. Reassure the family that the joint swelling will resolve over time

d. Perform arthrocentesis and corticosteroid injections on both knees

e. Start chronic NSAID therapy

15-18. A 14-year-old girl is admitted to the intensive care unit following a seizure and loss of consciousness. Her parents report that she has been feeling poorly over the last several days, with fever up to 39°C, malaise, and anorexia. Earlier today, she developed a severe headache and subsequently experienced a generalized tonic–clonic seizure and has not regained full consciousness. Exam demonstrates an obtunded female with a blood pressure of 166/96 and a pulse of 108. General physical exam is unremarkable with the exception of livedo reticularis (see the figure below).

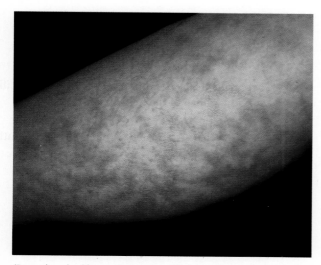

(Reproduced, with permission, from Weinberg S, Prose NS, Kristal L. *Color Atlas of Pediatric Dermatology.* 4th ed. New York: McGraw-Hill, 2007.)

WBC count is 15000 cell per mm³, Hemoglobin is 9 g/dL, and platelet count is 560,000. ESR is 110 and CRP is 9.6 mg/dL. Urinalysis is negative for blood, protein, and casts. All cultures are negative. MRI/MRA of the brain demonstrates changes consistent with hypertensive encephalopathy.

Which of the following tests is most likely to reveal the diagnosis?

a. Lumbar puncture

b. Brain biopsy

c. Skin biopsy

d. Fundoscopic exam

e. Renal angiogram

15-19. A 17-year-old male is admitted with progressive shortness of breath, fever, and malaise that has occurred over the last 2 weeks. Physical exam reveals tachypnea, diffuse rales and rhonchi, and mild stridor. CXR demonstrates diffuse nodular infiltrates in all lung fields. Laboratory studies show elevated inflammatory parameters with an elevated WBC count and a CRP of 16.2 mg/dL. Urinalysis is abnormal with 2+ protein, multiple red blood cells, and red cell casts.

Which of the following antibody tests is likely to be positive in this patient?

a. Anti-neutrophil cytoplasmic antibody

b. Anti-double-stranded DNA antibody

c. Anti Jo-1 antibody

d. Anti-centromere antibody

e. Anti-RNP antibody

15-20. A 17-year-old girl is seen in follow-up for persistent fever and malaise. She has had symptoms of low-grade fevers, headaches, night sweats, and malaise for the last several months. Between today and her last visit 3 weeks ago, she has lost 5 pounds. On exam today, the patient looks mildly ill and tired. You are unable to obtain a blood pressure or a pulse in the right arm, but blood pressure in the left arm is 185/95. Cardiac exam reveals normal S1 and S2, with a III/VI systolic murmur heard in the upper right sternal border.

Your next best step would be which of the following?

a. Start prednisone 2 mg/kg/day

b. Initiate thrombolytic therapy

c. Obtain imaging of the great vessels

d. Start anti-hypertensive therapy

e. Obtain a head MRI

15-21. A 15-year-old girl presents to your office with complaints of painful recurrent mouth sores that have occurred 6 times in the last year. She has also had 1 episode of genital ulceration 2 months ago. She underwent culturing of both the oral and genital lesions, which was negative. You note on exam that the patient has evidence of synovitis in her ankles bilaterally, as well as a pustular rash on her arms.

Which of the following tests is likely to be helpful in ascertaining the diagnosis?

a. A skin biopsy

b. A pathergy test

c. MRI/MRA of the brain

d. C-reactive protein

e. Rheumatoid factor

15-22. A 15-year-old girl with a history of systemic lupus erythematosus and lupus nephritis presents for follow-up. Her disease, which originally manifested with malar rash, arthritis, thrombocytopenia, and constitutional symptoms, has been quite stable over the past 2 years. On evaluation today, however, she reports that she has been having difficulty concentrating at school and that her grades have slipped from A's and B's to C's and D's. Substance abuse and depression screens are negative.

Which of the following statements would be correct?

a. This is unlikely to be due to CNS SLE because the patient has had her disease for over 2 years and has never had prior CNS involvement

b. The negative depression screen makes this unlikely to be secondary to depression as a manifestation of CNS SLE

c. A lumbar puncture may be necessary to eliminate infection as a cause of her cognitive decline

d. If levels of anti-double-stranded DNA antibodies are normal, then she is unlikely to be experiencing CNS SLE

e. Her poor performance in school indicates that she is most likely not taking her medications

15-23. A 10-year-old girl presents to the emergency department with a rash on her lower extremities that has been present for the last several days. Her mother notes that the patient has had a red rash on her face for several weeks that has not responded to topical therapy. Physical exam reveals a cooperative girl with a blood pressure of 95/58, pulse 88, and temp 36.8°C. Skin exam revealed mild diffuse alopecia and a red, raised rash on her cheeks and forehead. She had a petechieal rash on her legs bilaterally. There is a large superficial ulcer and a few petechiae on her soft palate. The rest of the physical exam is unremarkable. Laboratory testing reveals a platelet count of 30,000/mm³, a WBC count of 2.8 and a hemoglobin of 10.9 g/dL. Comprehensive electrolyte panel and urinalysis are unremarkable.

Given your clinical suspicion, which of the following laboratory tests would you expect to be positive?

a. Anti-myeloperoxidase antibody

b. Anti-thyroglobulin antibody

c. Anti-SCL70 antibody

d. Anti-Smith antibody

e. Anti-endomysial antibody

15-24. Of the following medications used in the treatment of systemic lupus erythematosus, which would be considered a long-term maintenance medication?

a. Hydroxychloroquine

b. Prednisone

c. Cyclophosphamide

d. Aspirin

e. Azathioprine

15-25. Patients with mixed connective tissue disease have overlapping features of several rheumatic diseases, including systemic lupus erythematosus, dermatomyositis, scleroderma, and JIA.

These patients, by definition, all possess one specific antibody. Which of the following is the specific antibody?

a. Anti-cyclic citrullinated peptide (anti-CCP) antibody

b. SSA (Ro) antibody

c. Anti- U1RNP antibody

d. Anti-double stranded DNA antibody

e. Anti-histone antibody

15-26. A 5-year-old boy with a recent diagnosis of juvenile dermatomyositis (JDM) presents for follow-up. His mother reports that he is taking his prednisone (2 mg/kg/day) and subcutaneous methotrexate (1 mg/kg/week) and notes that his arm and leg weakness have not progressed. She reports, however, that his voice has started to sound different and wonders if he may be "developing a cold." On exam, the child has a heliotrope rash, Gottrons papules (Figure 205-2), and an erythematous rash on his face.

He has weakness in both his hip and shoulder girdles and is unable to rise from the floor without help. His voice is somewhat nasal and hoarse.

Your next step in his treatment would be which of the following?

a. Provide treatment for thrush

b. Arrange for an outpatient swallowing study

c. Admit the patient to the hospital

d. Lower the patient's steroid dose to 1 mg/kg/day

e. Refer to ENT for direct laryngoscopy

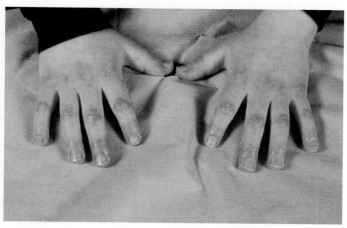

FIGURE 205-2. Gottron papules. Raised erythematous plaques over joint extensor surfaces, here over the finger joints, which are generally symmetric and characteristic of dermatomyositis. (Reproduced, with permission, from Rudolph CD, Rudolph AM, Lister GE, First LR, Gershon AA. *Rudolph's Pediatrics.* 22nd ed. New York: McGraw-Hill, 2011.)

15-27. A 6-year-old boy presents to your office with several months of progressive weakness of the arms and legs. He is now having difficulty climbing stairs, getting out of the bath and lifting his arms over his head. He is on no medications. Physical exam reveals 3+/5 strength in his hip and shoulder girdles and he has a Gowers sign when getting off the floor. The rest of his exam is unremarkable, including the skin exam. Laboratory testing is significant for a CPK of 15,500. You consider that he may have juvenile polymyositis.

Which of the following diagnoses should also be considered?

a. Viral myositis

b. JDM

c. Benign acute myositis

d. Muscular dystrophy

e. Cancer-associated myositis

15-28. The presentation of JDM can be very subtle and it is not until the child has significant muscle weakness that some patients may be identified and treated.

Which of the following is a late complication of JDM that is correlated with a delay in diagnosis?

a. Raynaud phenomenon

b. Dystrophic calcification

c. Vitamin D deficiency

d. Persistent heliotrope discoloration

e. Gottron papules

15-29. Children with juvenile systemic sclerosis are most likely to present with which of the following physical findings?

a. Sclerodactyly

b. Tightening of the skin on the face

c. Pulmonary hypertension

d. Esophageal dysmotility

e. Raynaud phenomenon

15-30. A 16-year-old boy presents to your office with complaints of a rash on his right leg (Figure 206-2; below).

His mother states that the rash started on his upper thigh and has now progressed downwards along the outside of his leg and across his foot. The patient states that it is "a little itchy" and he admits that he is having difficulty fully straightening his right knee. On exam, you note a slightly erythematous, shiny rash that forms a strip from his lateral thigh, across the lateral aspect of his right knee, down his calf, and across the dorsal surface of his left foot. There is no active synovitis in the knee, but the patient has a left knee flexion contracture of about 10 degrees and loss of full flexion. Biopsy results show increased collagen deposition and perivascular infiltration of lymphocytes.

When counseling the family, you tell them which of the following statements?

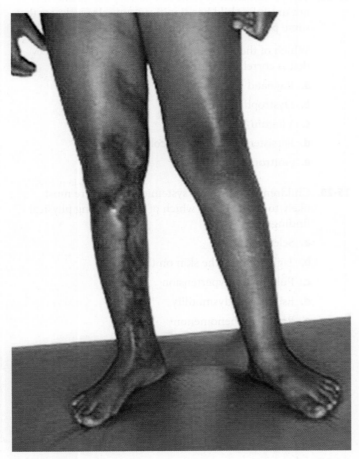

FIGURE 206-2. (Reproduced, with permission, from Rudolph CD, Rudolph AM, Lister GE, First LR, Gershon AA. *Rudolph's Pediatrics.* 22nd ed. New York: McGraw-Hill, 2011.)

a. Outcomes in the disease are determined by the extent of internal organ involvement

b. Since the rash is only affecting one limb, there is no treatment required

c. This form of the disease is much more common in adults than children

d. The left leg may not grow normally due to the rash

e. The rash will become progressively more pigmented over time

15-31. A mother brings her 5-year-old girl to your office with a complaint of leg pain. She states that the child has been complaining of bilateral leg pain almost every night before bed for the last three months. On several occasions, the child has awoken from sleep complaining of pain and has only returned to sleep after her legs were massaged. The child points to both calves as the area of discomfort, but you are not able to elicit any tenderness, nor do you note any joint or muscle swelling, erythema, or limitation of range of motion. The child is growing along the 50th percentile for height and weight, her vital signs are normal and the rest of her physical exam is unremarkable. A CBC and radiographs are unremarkable.

Which of the following is true?

a. The child is likely to develop JIA in the near future

b. The condition will require regular medication into adulthood

c. The condition occurs during the night because of the timing of bone growth

d. The condition will have no long-term sequelae

e. Regular massages during the night will improve the quality of life for the family

15-32. An 8-year-old girl is brought to your office by her mother because the school reported that she has been complaining of leg pain during gym class. There is no significant past medical history except that the patient frequently complains of leg pain after walking distances or standing for long periods of time. Physical exam is unremarkable except for flexible pes planus bilaterally and mild ankle pronation.

Your next step would be which of the following?

a. Prescribe arch supports for both feet

b. Perform radiographs of the feet

c. Refer for physical therapy

d. Exempt the child from gym class for the rest of the school year

e. Provide ankle foot orthotics (AFOs) for both legs

15-33. Parents bring their 9-year-old child in for evaluation after witnessing her "jump through" her interlocked arms at a party. The child has had no complaints of pain or joint swelling, and no history of excessive bruising. She has never dislocated a joint and the rest of her past medical history is unremarkable. Her height has been tracking at the 25–50 percentile. On exam, she has greater than 10 degrees of hyperextension of both elbows and 25 degrees of hyperextension of both knees. She is able to put her palms flat on the floor without bending her knees. Her skin turgor is normal and she has no scars or bruising.

The treatment of this condition would include which of the following?

a. Routine echocardiograms

b. Reassurance and observation

c. Regular analgesics

d. A figure-8 splint to hold her shoulders in place

e. Radiographs of the hips

15-34. A 13-year-old male is brought to your office by his father for complaints of severe pain in his left leg. The patient reports that he sustained an injury to the leg during a soccer game several weeks ago. He applied RICE measures at the time, but has subsequently developed severe pain in the leg, from the site of the injury down to the foot. He is unable to bear any weight on the leg or move the ankle. On exam, you note that he is holding the ankle rigidly in a neutral position and will not move it voluntarily. It is exquisitely painful to even the lightest touch. You also note that the entire area is mildly erythematous and slightly sweaty. Upon questioning, the patient thinks that the toenails are growing faster on the left foot compared to the right.

The most important part of this patient's treatment will be which of the following?

a. Psychological counseling to cope with the pain and disability

b. Mobilization of the leg and ankle joint

c. Analgesic medication

d. Serial casting of the foot and ankle

e. Use of topical medications for hyperhidrosis

15-35. A 14-year-old girl is seen with complaints of fatigue and pain. She reports that she has been "sore all over" for the last 5–6 months to the degree that she has stopped all of her physical activities and after-school activities. She is awakened from sleep at night due to the pain and is tired every morning. She has missed more the 50% of school days this year due to her pain and fatigue. She is taking naps every afternoon for several hours and then having difficulty falling asleep at bedtime. She reports that she is having gassiness and bloating and admits that her mood is poor. Physical exam reveals a cooperative girl with a blunted affect. Her general exam is unremarkable except for multiple tender points along the costochondral junctions, shoulders, upper back, trochanteric bursae, and knees. Laboratory workup including a complete blood count, chemistries, and thyroid function tests is normal.

Which of the following treatment modalities has been found to be efficacious in this disorder?

a. NSAID use

b. Graduated aerobic exercise

c. Thyroid supplementation

d. Vitamin B12 supplementation

e. Scheduled daytime napping

15-36. Which of the following statements regarding chronic fatigue syndrome (CFS) is true?

a. The outcomes in children are worse than those for adults with CFS

b. Cognitive-behavioral therapy has not been found to be helpful in the treatment of CFS

c. Some patients with CFS also have autonomic dysfunction including tachycardia and orthostasis

d. Once the underlying trigger is identified, the treatment of CFS is straightforward

e. Recurrent, tender lymph nodes are a very specific manifestation of CFS

15-37. A 5-year-old boy is brought in by his parents. For the past several months, he has been having episodes of severe abdominal pain and fever. These episodes last 1–3 days and are often accompanied by a rash on his legs and swelling of his knees. The parents state that 2 of his uncles on the father's side, who live in the Middle East, have had similar illnesses. You perform a workup, including genetic testing, which demonstrates a mutation in the *MEFV* gene.

Your next step would be which of the following?

a. Start colchicine 1–2 mg/day

b. Start aspirin 80–100 mg/kg/day

c. Tell the parents that there is no treatment for this disorder

d. Perform abdominal fat pad aspiration for amyloid

e. Start prednisone 2 mg/kg/day

15-38. A mother brings her 11-month-old girl to the office reporting that every time she takes her out in the cold weather, the child gets sick. The mother says that 2–3 hours after any cold exposure, the child develops hives on her extremities and then her trunk, sweating, extreme thirst, and irritability. These symptoms seem to last the rest of the day and resolve within 24 hours.

The mother also reports that there are several paternal family members, including the child's father, paternal uncle, and paternal grandmother who had similar, but worse, symptoms. Both the paternal uncle and paternal grandmother also had hearing loss that developed in adulthood.

The treatment of choice for this condition would be which of the following?

   a. Topical corticosteroids

   b. NSAIDs

   c. Anti-histamines

   d. IL-1 blockers

   e. Methotrexate

15-39. A mother brings in her 4-year-old daughter with complaints of recurrent fever and canker sores. She reports that for the past year, the child has been having episodes of fever every 4 weeks that lasts for 5 days and then resolve. The family can plot, almost to the day, when the next fever will occur. Each time, the child has been worked up for infection, but this has been negative. WBC counts, including neutrophils, have been normal or elevated, but never low.

The child feels poorly during the episodes, but once resolved, the child is back to her baseline activity and is completely well in between episodes. Her growth and development have been completely normal and she has achieved all normal milestones. On exam, the patient is febrile to 39° C. Her lips and buccal mucosa display multiple aphthous ulcers which are painful to touch.

She has mild pharyngeal erythema and tender cervical lymphadenopathy.

Which of the following statements describes the natural history of this illness?

   a. The child will develop decreased saliva and swollen parotids, similar to that seen in Sjogren Syndrome

   b. If left untreated, the child may develop amyloidosis

   c. The periods between febrile episodes becomes longer until the illness resolves

   d. The child will eventually develop polyarticular inflammatory arthritis

   e. The child will develop recurrent genital ulceration and possibly arthritis and rash

15-40. A 10-year-old is admitted to the hospital for complaints of left lower leg pain and fever. MRI is consistent with osteomyelitis in the distal left tibia, as well as in the distal femur. After 5 days of intravenous antibiotics, the patient is still having fever and leg pain and undergoes bone biopsy. The pathologic findings are consistent with osteomyelitis, but there are no organisms identified and the specimen is culture negative. He is treated with a full course of empiric antibiotics for partially-treated osteomyelitis and his pain gradually resolves. Two month later, he is readmitted and MRI at this time shows osteomyelitis in the right distal femur and third left metatarsal. He again undergoes biopsy, which is culture negative.

This presentation is most consistent with which of the following diagnoses?

   a. Subacute bacterial endocarditis

   b. Multiple myeloma

   c. PAPA syndrome

   d. Chronic recurrent multifocal osteomyelitis (CRMO)

   e. Multiple osteochondromas

ANSWERS

Answer 15-1. c

Gelling is a classic finding in children with chronic arthritis. This symptom is typically reported as morning stiffness, but can occur after any period of rest, such as a nap or long car ride. The inflammation of the joint leads to decreased amounts of hyaluronic acid, which in turn leads to decreased lubrication of the joint at normal temperatures.

Once the patient is up and moving around, or has taken or warm bath, the temperature in the joint rises sufficiently to allow the synovial fluid to liquefy and lubricate the joint. There are no specific changes to the amount of effusion or medication

penetration of the synovium while at rest and in some cases, inflammation could be lower while the joint is at rest. In addition, muscles surrounding an inflamed joint tend to relax at rest and during sleep as the joint is not in movement.

(Chapter 199: History and Physical Examination in Rheumatology (pp 792–793))

Answer 15-2. b

Children with inflammatory arthritis have discomfort following periods of rest or in the cold due to decreased lubrication of their joints. Movement of the joints is beneficial to improve lubrication, and therefore children with arthritis have improvement of their symptoms with activity. Children with arthritis may also have increased symptoms in their affected joints during intercurrent illness, most likely due to increased sensitivity of the nerve fibers in the area.

Pain during sleep, however, is not typical of arthritis pain, and should raise warning signs that another process may be present. Considerations would include neuropathic pain, bony pain from malignancy or infection, or functional pain.

(Chapter 199: History and Physical Examination in Rheumatology (pp 792–793))

Answer 15-3. c

The hallmarks of joint inflammation are swelling and tenderness, as well as erythema and warmth due to increased blood supply to the site of inflammation. These can occur in either an acute or chronic arthritis. Limitation of the range of motion can be due to pain and irritability or due to a flexion contracture occurring from chronic lack of full movement of the joint.

A leg length discrepancy is found on exam when the joint has been inflamed for sufficient time to stimulate the growth centers of the surrounding bone, leading to accelerated growth on the affected side. The child then keeps the knee bent to improve stability and over time, the muscles tighten, leading to the flexion contraction. This is a sign of chronicity.

(Chapter 199: History and Physical Examination in Rheumatology (p 794))

Answer 15-4. d

Any child with fever and an inflamed, swollen joint should be considered to have septic arthritis until proven otherwise. It is imperative to obtain synovial fluid for gram stain and culture. In general, for this situation, a synovial fluid culture is most likely to achieve the highest rate of identification of the organism, although this rate is still not 100%. Obtaining blood cultures may increase the yield of identifying the organism, but in the absence of osteomyelitis, bone culture will not be useful. While MRI or ultrasound can document effusion and inflammation and help to determine if there is concomitant osteomyelitis, neither test will yield identification of the actual organism.

(Chapter 199: History and Physical Examination in Rheumatology (pp 794–795))

Answer 15-5. b

The erythrocyte sedimentation rate measures how fast RBCs precipitate in plasma. It is an indirect measure of acute phase response, as the more proteins are present in the serum, the easier it is to bridge the negatively charged RBC and allow rouleux formation.

Patients with polycythemia have more RBCs and the hydrostatic forces associated with those cells lower the ESR.

Conversely, patients with anemia can have an artificially high ESR. Any disorder the increased the amount of serum proteins present in the serum that may moderate the negative charge of the RBCs will prolong the ESR. Such disorders would include nephrotic syndrome, chronic inflammation with immunoglobulin production, such as in SLE, and pregnancy, when circulating serum proteins are also elevated.

(Chapter 200. Diagnostic Testing in Rheumatology (pp 795–796))

Answer 15-6. c

Patients with chronic arthritis rarely complain of pain and do not refuse to bear weight, so it is not unusual that the child in this case was not identified early in his course. He had an intercurrent event, the fall in the yard, at which time the parent noticed the swollen leg. The presence of an effusion, warmth, and the flexed position can be consistent with either an acute or a chronic arthritis. His ability to run down the hall is also not specific to an acute or chronic process.

The widening of the tibia is due to localized growth disturbance at the tibial growth plate leading to accelerated bone formation. This growth could also be contributing to the patient's leg length discrepancy. It takes several weeks to months to be able to appreciate bony changes due to arthritis on exam, thereby indicating that this could be an acute process or due to his recent injury.

(Chapter 201. Juvenile Idiopathic Arthritis (p 803))

Answer 15-7. b

Once the diagnosis of JIA is made, it is imperative that the child be referred to ophthalmology for a slit-lamp exam, due to the risk of asymptomatic uveitis. Uveitis can occur in 20% of children with oligoarticular JIA and is more common in patients with a positive anti-nuclear antibody. Screening is required because although the uveitis can lead to visual disability and blindness, it is initially asymptomatic. Identified early, uveitis can be well treated and visual loss avoided.

The diagnosis of oligoarticular JIA is a clinical diagnosis and synovial biopsy is unnecessary. Referral to gastroenterology is also not required at this time, as the child has no features suspicious for inflammatory bowel disease, which can also be associated with an inflammatory arthritis. Because arthritic joints lose range of motion when immobilized, splinting is not appropriate at this time. It is rarely necessary to make school accommodations for children with oligoarticular JIA.

(Chapter 201. Juvenile Idiopathic Arthritis (p 803))

Answer 15-8. d

Autoantibody testing is helpful in polyarticular JIA and can help predict disease severity and prognosis. The presence of RF or CCP antibodies, particularly in high titer connotes a course similar to those seen in adult Rheumatoid Arthritis, including the possible development of rheumatoid nodules and other sequelae. All patients with inflammatory arthritis are at higher risk for uveitis than the normal population and therefore require screening.

The presence of a positive ANA identified children at even higher risk. These children are screened more often than those JIA patients with a negative ANA. Most patients with polyarticular JIA require a combination of disease-modifying agents to control their disease, so the early response to an NSAID, while gratifying, is not sufficient to predict that she will not require additional therapy. Combination therapy, however, is quite effective and children with polyarticular JIA should expect to live productive, healthy lives.

(Chapter 201. Juvenile Idiopathic Arthritis (p 803))

Answer 15-9. e

This patient has the typical features of systemic onset JIA, with diurnal fevers, an evanescent rash, and hepatosplenomegaly. Patients with SO JIA can develop pericardial effusions which, when large enough, can lead to cardiac tamponade. Bacterial endocarditis, which could cause mitral regurgitation, can present similarly to SO JIA with spiking fevers, rash, and elevated inflammatory parameters. The negative cultures make this less likely.

Given the fact that the patient was well prior to onset of this illness, he is unlikely to have a large VSD. Dilated coronary arteries are seen in Kawasaki disease, which can cause hectic fevers in children under the age of 6. Given the age of the patient and lack of other manifestations of KD, this finding would be unusual. Pulmonary hypertension is seen in patients with chronic lung disease and interstitial lung disease, and would not be expected in this patient.

(Chapter 201. Juvenile Idiopathic Arthritis (pp 803–804))

Answer 15-10. a

Despite the amount of inflammation ongoing in the joint, plain radiography is relatively insensitive in picking up bony changes until late in the disease course. The most common finding on radiograph is normal bone and joint, followed by periarticular osteopenia. Noting osteopenia on radiograph, however, implies that over 50% of the bone mineral content has been lost due to the inflammation. Other findings, such as joint space narrowing, periosteal new bone formation, and most ominous, erosions, are late findings in JIA.

(Chapter 201. Juvenile Idiopathic Arthritis (p 804))

Answer 15-11. c

This patient has significant polyarticular JIA which has not responded to the combination of NSAIDs and methotrexate. The methotrexate is already at the maximum recommended dose and has been given for a sufficient period of time (at least 2 months) to know if it will be sufficient to treat the patient's disease. There are too many joints involved to have the patient under therapeutic arthrocentesis and corticosteroid injection. While low-dose systemic corticosteroids might help as bridging

therapy, given their long-term side effects, cannot be a long-term solution.

It has been well-demonstrated that the addition of an anti-TNF agent to the patient's regimen will decrease joint pain, swelling, and increase the ability to achieve complete remission, thus limiting potential disability.

(Chapter 201. Juvenile Idiopathic Arthritis (pp 800–806))

Answer 15-12. b

This patient has evidence of inflammatory arthritis of the knee, as well as suspicion for inflammatory back arthritis based on the history of morning back pain. He has Achilles' tendon enthesitis bilaterally. This presentation is consistent with enthesis-related arthritis (See Figure 202-1). A significant number of these patients progress to juvenile ankylosing spondylitis, the diagnosis of which would be made by evidence of sacroileitis on radiography.

While greater than 90% of patients with JAS are HLA-B27 positive, this information is only supportive, as a significant number of the normal population also carry B27. There is a high incidence of positive ANA's in the normal population, so its presence or absence does not provide a definitive diagnosis. Likewise, an elevated ESR and effusion on knee films only state that there is joint inflammation, but does not help determine what type.

(Chapter 202. Spondyloarthropathies (pp 807–809))

Answer 15-13. c

This patient with IBD-related arthritis is presenting with a flare of her peripheral arthritis. As opposed to the axial arthritis which can progress or remit unrelated to bowel disease activity, peripheral arthritis tends to flare during periods of bowel disease activity, so this patient is likely having a flare of her IBD. Until her bowel disease is controlled, she may not likely respond to altered treatment for her peripheral arthritis, such as by giving her more disease-modifying medications or a corticosteroid. Patients with inflammatory arthritis should not

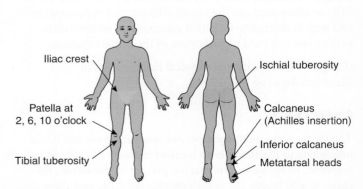

FIGURE 202-1. Common sites of enthesitis in children with enthesis-related arthritis. (Reproduced, with permission, from Rudolph CD, Rudolph AM, Lister GE, First LR, Gershon AA. *Rudolph's Pediatrics.* 22nd ed. New York: McGraw-Hill, 2011.)

be placed at bedrest, as they will get stiffer over time. Sending her for physical therapy before her arthritis is under better condition will not be as helpful compared to a referral when she is feeling better.

(Chapter 202. Spondyloarthropathies (p 809))

Answer 15-14. b

Juvenile psoriatic arthritis is a constellation of different arthritides that are associated with psoriasis. The psoriasis can occur before, at the same time, or following the onset of the arthritis. Clues for considering juvenile psoriatic arthritis would be asymmetric small joint disease, patients with both small and large joint arthritis (both seen in this patient), or the presence of cutaneous findings of psoriasis, such as psoriatic rash, nail pitting, or onycholysis.

A first-degree relative with psoriasis is also frequently found to have psoriatic arthritis and is considered a minor criteria for its diagnosis. Onycholysis can look similar to fungal toe nail disease, but this is unrelated to psoriatic arthritis, as is a family history of cardiovascular disease. While there is an increased incidence of JIA in patients with IgA deficiency, the same relationship is not seen in juvenile psoriatic arthritis. In the past, there has been postulated a relationship with pediatric arthritis with strep, but this has not been borne out in multiple studies.

(Chapter 202. Spondyloarthropathies (pp 807, 810))

Answer 15-15. d

HSP is the most common vasculitis of childhood. It is typically a self-limited condition unrelated to systemic vasculitis seen in adults. The arthritis tends to involve the joints of the lower extremities and is a periarthritis, which does not actually involve the joint space and does not cause chronic deformity. The joint symptoms can be treated acutely with NSAIDs. While the disease is "uniphasic," the rash of HSP can come and go for several weeks to months, but is not indicative of full systemic flare.

One of the late complications of the disease is intussusception, as the previously inflamed bowel may not have normal peristalsis. Any abdominal pain should be considered indicative of intussusception and should be investigated. Most renal involvement will be present within the first month. In the absence of acute nephritis, urine should be screened weekly for the first month and then monthly for the next several months, after which time the risk is significantly reduced.

(Chapter 203. Vasculitides (pp 810–811))

Answer 15-16. b

This child presents with classical Kawasaki disease. During the acute phase, the children are very irritable, thought to be due to aseptic meningitis, as patients who undergo lumbar puncture typically have a CSF pleocytosis. During the acute phase, the platelet count is abnormally low, and then rebounds into a thrombocytosis during the subacute phase. Patients may have a sterile pyuria, but RBC casts would not be present. Likewise, there should be no evidence of other ongoing infection, such as a bacteremia. Spherocytosis is not associated with Kawasaki Disease.

(Chapter 203. Vasculitides (p 812))

Answer 15-17. c

Patients with Kawasaki disease can develop arthritis as part of their disease. The arthritis, which affects approximately 1/3 of patients with KD, usually occurs in the acute phase of the illness and resolves within 3 weeks to 3 months.

The presence of arthritis is not considered a treatment failure and therefore repeat dosing of IVIg is not required. Intermittent NSAID therapy may help joint pain, but chronic treatment is not necessary, with either NSAIDs or aspirin. Intra-articular corticosteroid injections can be helpful in patients with chronic arthritis, but are not indicated in this context.

(Chapter 203. Vasculitides (p 812))

Answer 15-18. e

This patient had onset of fever and constitutional symptoms, followed by severe hypertension and significantly elevated inflammatory parameters. In the absence of infection, systemic vasculitis should be suspected. The diagnosis of vasculitis is definitely made either by tissue biopsy demonstrating vasculitis in an affected organ or by angiography demonstrating vasculitis or nodosa (aneurysm). Given this patient's severe hypertension without evidence of glomerulonephritis, the possibility of renal artery aneurysms due to polyarteritis nodosa warrants a renal angiogram. In the absence of MRI/MRA findings consistent with vasculitis, findings on lumbar puncture or brain biopsy are less likely to reveal a definitive diagnosis. Livedo reticularis, commonly seen in vasculitis, is a nonspecific finding and less likely to be helpful.

(Chapter 203. Vasculitides (p 812))

Answer 15-19. a

This patient presents with a pulmonary–renal syndrome, most likely either Wegener granulomatosus or Goodpasture disease. The nodularity seen on CXR is more common in WG, although both can cause the abnormalities seen in the renal sediment. Patients with WG can have a positive ANCA, typically with cytoplasmic staining (c-ANCA) directed against proteinase 3, which can also be measured directly.

Patients with Goodpasture disease make antibodies directly against the glomerular basement membrane (anti-GBM antibody) that can be measured in the serum and found upon staining of renal biopsy tissue. Anti-double stranded DNA antibodies are found in patients with systemic lupus erythematosus, which could present with glomerulonephritis, but rarely has this degree of pulmonary involvement.

Conversely, patients with mixed connective tissue disease, who have a positive anti-RNP antibody, develop lung involvement, but renal disease is unusual. Jo-1 is a myositis-specific anti-synthetase autoantibody found in patients with dermatomyositis and interstitial lung disease, but is not consistent with this presentation. Anti-centromere antibodies are found in patients with diffuse limited systemic sclerosis (CREST syndrome).

(Chapter 203. Vasculitides (pp 813, 820))

Answer 15-20. c

This patient has had fever, night sweats, weight loss, malaise, and headaches for several months followed by elevated blood pressures and pulselessness in the right arm. The history is suspicious for chronic inflammation and with the pulselessness and hypertension, one should be suspicious for Takayasu Arteritis, a granulomatous vasculitis of the large vessels. Imaging of the great vessels, either through MR angiography, conventional angiography, CT, or ultrasound would be the next step in the workup.

While thrombolytic therapy would be necessary if the patient had an arterial clot, treatment without a diagnosis would be premature.

Once the Takayasu arteritis diagnosis is made, high-dose prednisone would be the treatment of choice. A head MRI might be helpful in the workup of this patient's headache, but it is highly likely due to the elevated blood pressure. This will need to be treated, but given the chronic nature of the symptom, can wait until the workup has been initiated. Lowering of the blood pressure in the face of poor outflow may worsen any ischemic symptoms the patient may have.

(Chapter 203. Vasculitides (pp 813–814))

Answer 15-21. b

This patient has a history of recurrent oral ulceration and at least 1 episode of genital ulceration. She has a rash and arthritis on exam. All of these findings are consistent with a diagnosis of Behcet Disease (BD). The diagnosis requires recurrent oral ulceration (see Figure 203-2) and at least 2 of the following: recurrent genital ulceration, eye disease, skin lesions, and a positive pathergy test. This patient does not fulfill criteria, as she has had only one episode of genital ulceration. A positive pathergy test would provide sufficient evidence to make a diagnosis of BD.

The pustular rash is nonspecific and biopsy would not be definitive. Patients with BD can have CNS involvement, including encephalitis or aseptic meningitis, but the MRI/MRA findings would be nonspecific. A C-reactive protein can be elevated in any systemic inflammation and is not helpful for making a specific diagnosis. This patient, although she has arthritis, is unlikely to have rheumatoid arthritis given her presentation. A positive RF would not be helpful in this case, given the low pretest probability for RA.

(Chapter 203. Vasculitides (p 814))

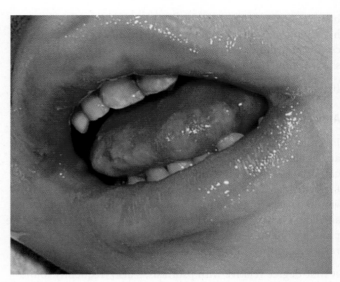

FIGURE 203-2. Behçet disease. Extensive aphthae involving the lips and tongue. (Reproduced, with permission, from Wolff K, Goldsmith LA, Katz SI, et al. *Dermatology in General Medicine.* 7th Ed. New York: McGraw-Hill, 2007.)

Answer 15-22. c

While most manifestation of SLE occur in the first year of disease, the onset of CNS SLE can occur at any time. Features can be overt, such as seizures, severe headache or psychosis, or subtle, with mild cognitive changes that would lead to decreased school performance. Patients with SLE and a suspicion of CNS involvement should be put under neuroradiologic testing followed by lumbar puncture to look for evidence of hemorrhage, vasculitis, or infection. Spinal fluid can be analyzed to look for in situ immunoglobulin production that would be suspicious for CNS SLE.

Depression is not uncommon in patients with SLE and can be the presenting manifestation of CNS involvement or secondary to chronic illness. A negative depression screen in the office cannot absolutely rule out depression nor CNS SLE. While elevated levers of anti-DNA antibodies correlate with nephritis, this is not true of CNS SLE, where these antibodies may remain normal despite active diseases. While non-adherence can be a problem in any chronic illness, there are many factors that could be contributing to this patient's poor school performance.

(Chapter 204. Systemic Lupus Erythematosus, Overlap Connective Tissue Disease, and Mixed Connective Tissue Disease (pp 814–817))

Answer 15-23. d

The malar rash (Figure 105-1), mucosal ulceration, alopecia, thrombocytopenia, and leukopenia all raise suspicion that this child has systemic lupus erythematosus.

Of all the options listed, only the anti-Smith antibody is found in patients with SLE. Although anti-Smith antibodies are only seen in 30% of patients with SLE, they are highly specific

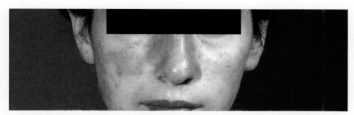

FIGURE 105-1. The characteristic malar rash of systemic lupus erythematosus. Note the extension across the cheeks and the nasal bridge with sparing of the nasolabial folds. (Reproduced, with permission, from Strange GR, Ahrens WR, Schafermeyer RW, Wiebe RA. *Pediatric Emergency Medicine.* 3rd ed. New York: McGraw-Hill, 2009.)

to the disorder and if present, constitute 1 of the 11 criteria for the diagnosis.

Anti-myeloperioxidase antibodies are found in patients with microscopic polyangiitis and account for the perinuclear staining of an anti-neutrophil cytoplasmic antibody (p-ANCA). Anti-thyroglobulin antibodies are seen in patients with Hashimoto thyroiditis. Antibodies directed against SCL70 (topoisomerase I) are seen in patients with systemic sclerosis and anti-endomysial antibodies can be positive in patients with celiac disease.

(Chapter 204. Systemic Lupus Erythematosus, Overlap Connective Tissue Disease, and Mixed Connective Tissue Disease (pp 815–817))

Answer 15-24. a

Treatment of SLE is a balance of benefits of medications against the known toxicities of the drugs used. While prednisone is the mainstay of treatment for significant organ involvement, the side effects of prolonged use, including risk of avascular necrosis, osteoporosis, and growth delay, are significant. Use of prednisone should be minimized, particularly in patients with mild disease, and weaned as fast as is safe for the patient. Steroid-sparing medications, such as cyclophosphamide and azathioprine, have their own toxicities, including bone marrow suppression and risk of malignancy, and are reserved for serious organ involvement. Low-dose aspirin has been used in patients with anti-phospholipid antibodies to decrease clotting risk, but its actual benefit is uncertain.

Hydroxychloroquine, on the other hand, has been shown to decrease the number of lupus flares and increase the time between flares. It also lowers serum lipid levels, a benefit in patients with renal disease and in chronic corticosteroid use.

(Chapter 204. Systemic Lupus Erythematosus, Overlap Connective Tissue Disease, and Mixed Connective Tissue Disease (pp 814–817))

Answer 15-25. c

Patients with undifferentiated connective tissue disease are patients that do not neatly fit into one set of diagnostic criteria.

Rather, these patients have overlapping features of several illnesses. One specific overlap disease, mixed connective tissue disease, is defined as overlapping features of at least 2 diseases and the presence of antibodies against U1RNP.

Anti-CCP antibodies are found in the patients with rheumatoid arthritis and in sero-positive polyarticular JIA patients. SSA (Ro) antibodies are found in several illnesses, including SLE and Sjogren syndrome. Anti-double stranded DNA antibodies are found in patients with SLE and vary based on disease activity. Anti-histone antibodies can be found in patients with SLE, but are also high correlated with drug-induced lupus.

(Chapter 204. Systemic Lupus Erythematosus, Overlap Connective Tissue Disease, and Mixed Connective Tissue Disease (pp 817–818))

Answer 15-26. c

The onset of dysphonia and hoarseness in a patient with JDM is a result of palatal involvement and should be considered a sign of serious disease, necessitating hospitalization for observation and intravenous methylprednisolone.

While the patient could have thrush given his immune suppression, this potential diagnosis would be investigated only after ensuring the patient's safety and the security of his airway. Likewise, any investigation of his upper airway or muscles of swallowing can be accomplished in the hospital if necessary. Given that the dysphonia is a sign of disease progression, it would be inappropriate to lower the patient's steroid dose at this time.

(Chapter 205. Juvenile Dermatomyositis (pp 818–823))

Answer 15-27. d

While juvenile dermatomyositis (JDM) is well described in the pediatric population, Juvenile Polymyositis is quite rare and specific attention must be paid to ensure the diagnosis. JDM presents with progressive proximal muscle weakness, but is accompanied by classical skin features such as heliotrope rash and Gottron papules. When the skin features of JDM are not present and consideration is being given to juvenile polymyositis, then other myopathies must be considered as well. Diseases such as muscular dystrophies, metabolic myopathies, and mitochondrial myopathies can all present similarly, and therefore workup including EMG and muscle biopsy must be performed prior to arriving at the diagnosis of JPM.

Given the history of several months of progressive weakness, this patient is unlikely to have either viral myositis or benign acute myositis, as these are acute onset illnesses that are self-limited. The most common viruses associated with myositis are enterovirus, coxsackievirus, influenza, and parvovirus. Benign acute myositis occurs following an infectious illness and is also self-resolving. While myositis, particularly dermatomyositis, can present as a paraneoplastic syndrome, this is found almost exclusively in adults.

(Chapter 205. Juvenile Dermatomyositis (pp 818–823))

Answer 15-28. b

Patients with JDM can vary greatly in the degree of skin involvement or muscle involvement. Patients with long-term active muscle disease can develop dystrophic calcification in the skin, subcutaneous tissues, or muscle, typically starting several years after diagnosis. The calcinosis can take the form of small deposits, or become quite extensive, leading to joint contractures and skin breakdown.

Raynaud phenomenon is not a typical feature of JDM. While both heliotrope rash and Gottron papules are found in JDM, their presence does not correlate with chronic active disease. Since exposure to the sun can lead to JDM flare, all patients are cautioned to limit their sun exposure, thus potentially leading to vitamin D deficiency. Regardless of length of disease, children with JDM should receive calcium and Vitamin D supplementation.

(Chapter 205. Juvenile Dermatomyositis (pp 818–821))

Answer 15-29. e

Systemic sclerosis is very rare in children, with less than 5% of patients developing their disease before the age of 16 years. In children, the most common presenting feature is Raynaud phenomenon, followed by proximal skin induration that develops later. The figure below shows classic Raynaud phenomenon in a 4-year-old girl. Note the ischemic changes (blanching phase) of the second and fourth fingers and the cyanosis (bluish phase) of the fifth finger.

Internal organ involvement can be significant, but is not typically an early finding. Dysfunction of the esophagus

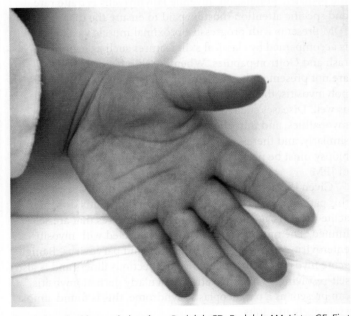

(Reproduced, with permission, from Rudolph CD, Rudolph AM, Lister GE, First LR, Gershon AA. *Rudolph's Pediatrics.* 22nd ed. New York: McGraw-Hill, 2011.)

is the most common gastrointestinal manifestation, seen symptomatically as dysphagia and reflux. Pulmonary involvement can include interstitial fibrosis, pleuritis, or pulmonary hypertension, which can lead to right-sided heart failure.

(Chapter 206. Scleroderma (pp 823–825))

Answer 15-30. d

The description of the rash in the case and the biopsy results are consistent with linear scleroderma, a form of localized scleroderma seen almost exclusively in children. Morphea, or localized scleroderma, are a group of sclerodermatous conditions where the manifestations are localized only to the skin, without any systemic or internal organ involvement. Outcomes in linear scleroderma are determined by the extent to which the sclerodermatous skin binds down the bones and soft tissues under the lesion, thereby preventing normal growth and limiting range of motion.

Over time, lesions will soften, but there may be either hyper- or hypo-pigmentation of the skin. While small lesions may not require intervention other than topical treatment with corticosteroids, more extensive lesions, particularly those that might interfere with joints or limb growth, require treatment. Current therapies include the use of oral or intravenous corticosteroids, as well as a steroid sparing agent, such as methotrexate.

(Chapter 206. Scleroderma (pp 825–826))

Answer 15-31. d

This is a classical presentation of a child with growing pains. Growing pains occur in elementary-school aged children and typically present as nocturnal pain without any physical findings. Growing pains are not correlated with growth, nor do they presage any other illness. Growing pains can be differentiated from disorders like inflammatory arthritis by the lack of morning symptoms of pain and stiffness and the absence of synovitis on physical exam. The treatment of growing pains includes regular stretching, heat, and mild analgesics and will gradually resolve.

While massage may be helpful, the disruption of sleep can affect the quality of life and could lead to behavioral issues later. A regular nighttime routine and set bedtime is the best strategy for minimizing potential problems with the family's interpersonal relationships.

(Chapter 207. Musculoskeletal Pain Syndromes (p 826))

Answer 15-32. a

Pes planus, or flat feet, are very common. While most patients with pes planus are asymptomatic, some patients will develop musculoskeletal pain in the legs or lower back. Most of the time, these symptoms are improved or completely resolved with the addition of arch supports or foot orthotics inserted in their shoes. Physical therapy is rarely required.

If the midfoot of a patient with pes planus is flexible, no other workup is required. If the foot is more rigid, radiographs to investigate for tarsal coalition may be appropriate. Regular exercise and gym participation is important, so the symptoms should be treated with inserts and analgesics if needed to ensure that the child can get regular exercise. Ankle-foot orthotics (AFOs) can be helpful in children with significant isolated ankle pronation and ankle laxity, but this child's pronation should improve with the treatment of her pes planus and AFOs would not be required.

(Chapter 207. Musculoskeletal Pain Syndromes (pp 827–828))

Answer 15-33. b

This child has a Beighton score of 5/9 (2 points for elbows, 2 points for knees, 1 point for palms on the floor) and fulfills criteria for benign hyper mobility (see Figure 207-1). Patients are scored on a 9-point scale, with one point awarded for each hypermobile site as noted in the figure below. A Beighton score of 4 or more points fulfills criteria for hypermobility; however, she does not meet full criteria for benign joint hypermobility Syndrome, which also requires at least 3 months of arthralgia in 4 or more joints.

Most patients do not require any further intervention other than reassurance, although analgesics and/or physical therapy may help symptomatic patients.

This patient does not have Marfanoid habits or physical findings suspicious for Ehlers–Danlos syndrome, so serial Echocardiograms are unnecessary. In the absence of actual joint dislocation, there is no need to splint her shoulders and X-rays of the hips are not indicated. In general, patients with benign hypermobility will improve over time.

(Chapter 207. Musculoskeletal Pain Syndromes (pp 827–828))

Answer 15-34. b

The constellation of hyperesthesia, increased warmth, hyperhidrosis, and immobility is consistent with complex regional pain syndrome, also known as reflex sympathetic dystrophy. The disorder can be precipitated by injury, although in children, an inciting event is not always identified. The affected area becomes very sensitive and painful, to the point where the patient cannot even tolerate light touch. The patient protects the area and the immobilization leads to an increase in symptoms with autonomic dysfunction contributing to the other associated symptoms. The most important aspect of the treatment of CRPS is to mobilize the limb and joints affected. Range of motion exercises, progressive desensitization techniques, and massage are a few of the modalities used to reduce the immobilization that has occurred as part of the illness.

Psychological counseling can be an important part of the treatment regimen, but is secondary to the goal of mobilization. Analgesics may help the patient tolerate range of motion activities. Topical medications that include aluminum may be helpful in cases of extreme hyperhidrosis,

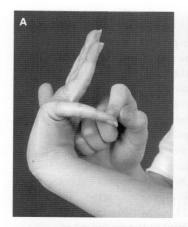
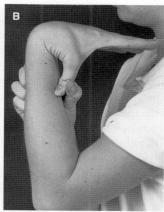
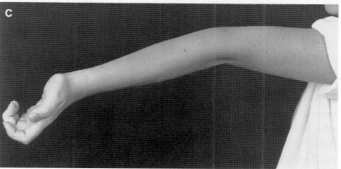
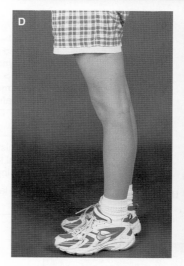
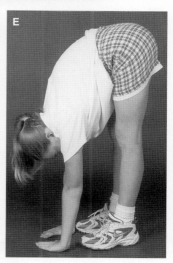

FIGURE 207-1. Demonstrations of Beighton score components. (**A**) Extension of the wrist and metacarpophalangeal joints so that the fingers are parallel to the dorsum of the forearm. (**B**) Passive apposition of the thumb to the flexor aspect of the forearm. (**C**) Hyperextension of the elbows 10 degrees or more. (**D**) Hyperextension of the knees 10 degrees or more. (**E**) Flexion of the trunk with the knees fully extended so the palms rest on the floor. (Reproduced, with permission, from Rudolph CD, Rudolph AM, Lister GE, First LR, Gershon AA. *Rudolph's Pediatrics.* 22nd ed. New York: McGraw-Hill, 2011.)

but treatment of the CRPS should improve the overall autonomic dysfunction. Casting of the limb is clearly contraindicated.

(Chapter 207. Musculoskeletal Pain Syndromes (pp 827–828))

Answer 15-35. b

This patient has multiple tender points and over 3 months of widespread pain, fulfilling the criteria for the diagnosis of fibromyalgia syndrome. Of all the treatment modalities that have been used in juvenile fibromyalgia, cognitive-behavioral therapy and aerobic exercise have been studied and found to be effective. A combination of stretching and graduated aerobic exercise will help not only the pain symptoms, but also the sleep disturbance that commonly accompanies fibromyalgia.

Sleep hygiene is very important, so daytime napping should be actively discouraged. NSAIDs can be helpful in providing some analgesia as the patient becomes more active. There is no evidence that either Vitamin B12 or thyroid supplementation (in the euthyroid patient) is helpful in the treatment of fibromyalgia.

(Chapter 207. Musculoskeletal Pain Syndromes (pp 828–830))

Answer 15-36. c

Chronic fatigue syndrome is characterized by prolonged or relapsing fatigue and constitutional symptoms, the cause of which is unidentified after appropriate investigation. It is thought that the illness is triggered by an intercurrent infection or illness, but by the time symptoms are investigated, it is too late to identify the original trigger. The manifestations of CFS, such as sore throat, tender lymphadenopathy, and joint pain can occur in many other conditions, making the diagnosis of CFS challenging. An association with postural orthostatic tachycardia syndrome (POTS) has been described.

Once other underlying illnesses are excluded, attention should be made to treating the symptoms of CFS (see Figure 208-1). Mental health problems such as depression and anxiety can be co-morbid with CFS and cognitive-behavioral therapy has been found to be helpful in improving affect and function. Outcomes in children with CFS are better than those afflicted as adults with a much higher percent achieving improvement and complete long-term remission.

(Chapter 208. Chronic Fatigue Syndrome (pp 830–832))

Answer 15-37. a

This patient has familial mediterranean fever (FMF), a genetic disorder caused by mutations in the MEFV gene leading to an auto-inflammatory disorder characterized by recurrent fever and serositis, as well as rash and arthritis. The serositis is typically manifest as severe abdominal pain, but pleuritis and pericarditis can occur as well. Amyloidosis due to chronic inflammation has been the primary cause of poor outcomes in FMF. Colchicine is the treatment of choice in FMF, as

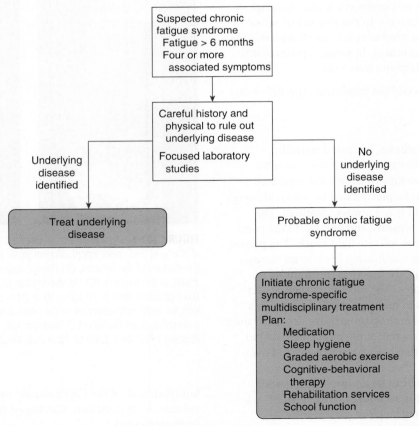

FIGURE 208-1. Algorithm for the evaluation and treatment of suspected chronic fatigue syndrome. (Reproduced, with permission, from Rudolph CD, Rudolph AM, Lister GE, First LR, Gershon AA. *Rudolph's Pediatrics.* 22nd ed. New York: McGraw-Hill, 2011.)

it significantly reduces the number and severity of attacks in FMF, as well as the occurrence of amyloidosis in this population of patients.

Amyloidosis, caused by the accumulation of amyloid in organs, can be diagnosed by renal or GI biopsy, or by abdominal fat pad aspiration. Amyloidosis is a late finding in FMF and would not be expected to be present at this time in the child's course.

(pp 833–834)

Answer 15-38. d

This patient has a serious reaction to the cold. Given the high number of relatives with similar symptoms, one must presume that this is genetic in nature. The cryopyrin-associated periodic syndromes (CAPS) are genetic disorders caused by mutations in the CIAS1/NALP3 gene located on the long arm of chromosome 1, which encodes the protein cryopryin. The spectrum of disease is wide, ranging from familial cold autoinflammatory syndrome (FCAS), described in this child, to Muckle–Wells syndrome, which is associated with hearing loss, to the most severe variant, neonatal-onset multisystem inflammatory disease (NOMID).

In FCAS, the rash is not a true urticaria and NSAIDs and anti-histamines are not effective. Higher doses of oral corticosteroids may help, but topical versions do not, nor does methotrexate play any role. All of the cryopryin-associated periodic syndromes dramatically respond to inhibition of IL-1 and have led to significant improvements in quality of life for these patients.

(Chapter 209. Autoinflammatory Disorders (p 836))

Answer 15-39. c

This patient has periodic fever, aphthous stomatitis, pharyngitis, adenitis (PFAPA) syndrome. This syndrome is characterized by a periodic fever that affects young children. There is no known genetic association, but the illness can run in families. As opposed to other auto-inflammatory syndromes, children with PFAPA are completely well between episodes and grow and thrive normally.

The differential diagnosis includes infection, other inflammatory diseases, and cyclic neutropenia. Initially, the episodes are very stereotypic and occur at regular intervals, 3-4 weeks apart, and then lengthen until the illnesses remit. There is no association with amyloidosis as a late finding. This illness can be differentiated from systemic onset JIA by the lack of daily fever and PFAPA patients do not develop arthritis as a late manifestation of the illnesses. Behcet syndrome, which is characterized by recurrent oral and genetic ulcers, is found in older adolescents and is not periodic in nature.

(Chapter 209. Autoinflammatory Disorders (p 837))

Answer 15-40. d

A patient has pathology consistent with osteomyelitis, but is culture negative and occurs at multiple sites over a period of time most likely has CRMO. This is an auto-inflammatory bone disorder for which antibiotics are ineffective. Treatment is done with anti-inflammatory agents, such as NSAIDs, or if there is no response, more potent immunosuppressing therapy.

Distant infection to bone can occur in endocarditis, but one would expect the patient to be more ill and to respond to antibiotic therapy. Multiple myeloma, which causes lytic bone lesions, would have a typical appearance on radiography as well as characteristic laboratory testing and is quite rare in children. PAPA syndrome (pyogenic sterile arthritis, pyoderma gangrenosum, acne syndrome) is a genetic condition typically presenting in younger children and would include other manifestations. While multiple ostechondromas can cause focal pain at several sites, typically these would be palpable on exam and have a classic appearance on radiographs. One would not expect them to resolve spontaneously.

(Chapter 209. Autoinflammatory Disorders (pp 836–837))

CHAPTER 16 | Musculoskeletal Disorders

Hilary M. Haftel

16-1. A 5-year-old male presents to the emergency department with 24 hours of progressive limp and low-grade fever. His mother reports that he was running on the grass in the front yard 2 days ago and fell, subsequently complaining of shin pain on the left side. Examination reveals a tender, swollen left knee. The patient is holding the knee in flexion and refuses to move it.

Of the following, which is the most sensitive finding that would indicate joint space infection?

a. An elevated C-reactive protein

b. The history of trauma

c. An abnormal radiograph

d. An elevated erythrocyte sedimentation rate (ESR)

e. An elevated WBC count

16-2. A 12-hour-old infant undergoes a physical examination in the newborn nursery. It is noted that there is inward torsion of the forefoot bilaterally that is easily reduced with passive movement of the foot. You diagnose metatarsus adductus.

Given the diagnosis of metatarsus adductus, what other diagnosis should the patient be evaluated for?

a. Clubfoot

b. Myelomeningocele

c. Developmental dysplasia of the hip (DDH)

d. Clavicular fracture

e. Pes planus

16-3. A 6-year-old is brought to the office because her parents are concerned over her clumsiness. They state that she tends to trip over her feet when she walks. On your physical examination, you note an intoeing gait bilaterally. On closer inspection, it appears that her patellae are inwardly deviating as she walks. Her neurologic examination, including muscle strength, is completely normal. The most common cause of this intoeing gait would be:

a. Internal tibial torsion

b. Femoral anteversion

c. Slipped capital femoral epiphysis

d. Metatarsus adduction

e. Bilateral Salter I fractures of the tibia

16-4. In the normal child, genu varum (bowlegs) is maximal at which age?

a. Adolescence

b. Age 10 to 12

c. Newborn period

d. Age 3 to 5

e. Age 6 to 9

16-5. The initial test of choice in an adolescent patient with persistent low back pain despite a regular core stretching program is:

a. EMG of the lower extremities

b. Plain radiographs of the lumbar and sacral spine

c. Urinalysis

d. PA and lateral chest radiographs

e. Stool for occult blood

16-6. A mother brings her 6-year-old daughter to your office for evaluation of her "knock-knees." Your examination demonstrates symmetric valgus deformity of the knees bilaterally, normal range of motion of the hips, knees, and ankles, and no leg length discrepancy. The best next step would be:

a. Radiographs of the legs to exclude fracture

b. Reassurance of the parent

c. Evaluations of serum calcium and phosphate

d. Prescription of orthotics

e. Referral to physical therapy for strength building exercises

16-7. A mother is noted to have oligohydramnios during pregnancy. The infant is born and is noted to have significant hyperdorsiflexion of the right foot, with the dorsal surface of the foot lying against the anterior surface of the tibia (Figure 213-2). There are no other abnormalities noted. The foot is partially moveable at the ankle. You suspect that the patient has a calcaneovalgus deformity.

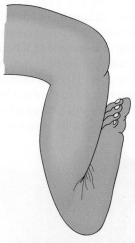

FIGURE 213-2. (Reproduced, with permission, from Rudolph CD, Rudolph AM, Lister GE, First LR, Gershon AA. *Rudolph's Pediatrics.* 22nd ed. New York: McGraw-Hill, 2011.)

In order to confirm this diagnosis, which of the following must be excluded?

a. Pes planovalgus

b. Congenital vertical talus

c. Genu varum

d. Developmental dysplasia of the hip

e. Thrombocytopenia with absent radii (TAR) syndrome

16-8. A 14-year-old female presents to your office with complaints of bilateral leg pain while running that has been present since the track season started this year. Physical examination demonstrates absence of a normal longitudinal arch on the left with decreased movement of the midfoot.

Which of the following features would be more concerning for tarsal coalition than for a diagnosis of pes planovalgus (flat feet)?

a. The presence of pain

b. The gender of the patient

c. The occurrence with exercise

d. The decreased movement of the midfoot

e. The absence of a longitudinal arch

16-9. On delivery, you note that a newborn male has an abnormal right foot, which is severely inverted and does not respond to attempts at passive range of motion. The gastrocnemius muscle is atrophic.

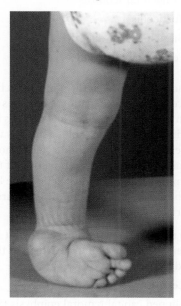

(Reproduced, with permission, from Herring JA, ed. *Tachdjian's Pediatric Orthopaedics.* 4th ed. Philadelphia: Saunders, 2007.)

Which of the following would *not* be a possible treatment of this disorder?

a. Observation

b. Serial casting

c. Physical therapy

d. Soft tissue release

e. Nighttime splinting

16-10. A 16-year-old girl is complaining of pain in her knees for the last several months. She states that it is worst with activity and particularly bad after sitting in class for a prolonged period of time. It is aggravated by climbing up or down steps. There is no morning stiffness, joint swelling, or erythema. She has been using ibuprofen with some relief. Physical examination reveals slight patellar laxity but is otherwise unremarkable.

The most reasonable treatment option is which of the following?

a. Intra-articular corticosteroid injection

b. Targeted physical therapy

c. Patellar tendon shortening

d. Regular NSAID use until growth plate fusion

e. Transcutaneous electrical nerve stimulation (TENS) unit applied to knees and thighs

16-11. Which of the following conditions is associated with developmental dysplasia of the hip?

  a. Tibial torsion

  b. Congenital scoliosis

  c. Torticollis

  d. Branchial cleft disorders

  e. Femoral anteversion

16-12. A mother brings her 13-month-old child into your office for initial evaluation. She states that the child has been walking for the last few months but appears to be clumsier than her 2 older siblings were at this stage. On examination, the child's gait demonstrates listing to the left side and circumduction of the left leg. When examined in the supine position, the left hip is limited in abduction and the left knee appears to be lower than the right when placed at 90°.

The most likely condition to account for this child's physical findings would be which of the following conditions?

  a. Legg-Calve-Perthes disease

  b. Slipped capital femoral epiphysis (SCFE)

  c. Muscular dystrophy

  d. Juvenile dermatomyositis

  e. Developmental dysplasia of the hip

16-13. A 10-year-old boy presents to your office with complaints of right hip pain that has become progressively more severe over the past several months. He is now unable to play sports and the pain is awakening him at night. He is having difficulty sitting in class for more than 10 to 15 minutes without discomfort. Physical examination demonstrates irritability on range of motion of the right hip in all directions and spasm of the surrounding musculature. Plain radiographs of the hips demonstrate flattening and fragmentation of the left femoral head. The right hip is normal in appearance.

Your advice to the family and patient should include which of the following?

  a. The child will not be able to play sports again in the future.

  b. They should expect that he will require surgical correction in the next 2 to 3 years.

  c. It is likely that the contralateral side will be affected as well.

  d. The outcome will be best determined by the shape of the femoral head on resolution of the condition.

  e. He will need to obtain an MRI of the hip in order to confirm the diagnosis.

16-14. A 16-year-old male presents to your office with several weeks of waxing and waning left groin pain, radiating to the knee. Although not particularly an active child, he has further limited his activity and is now only ambulating at home and at school. The patient is lying on your examination table with his left hip held in external rotation. Physical examination demonstrates limited internal rotation of the left hip and abduction on hip flexion. Plain radiographs demonstrate posterior displacement of the left femoral cap (Figure 221-1).

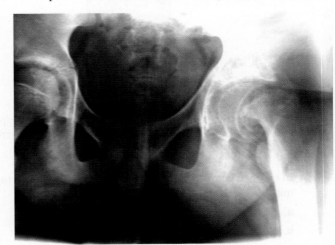

FIGURE 221-1. (Reproduced, with permission, from Rudolph CD, Rudolph AM, Lister GE, First LR, Gershon AA. *Rudolph's Pediatrics.* 22nd ed. New York: McGraw-Hill, 2011.)

Your next step is which of the following?

  a. Have the family take the patient to the hospital to be admitted.

  b. Have the patient return in 1 week to see if symptoms have resolved.

  c. Transport the patient via stretcher to the hospital.

  d. Reassure the patient and family that the symptoms will resolve in the next 12 to 18 months.

  e. Refer the patient for physical therapy.

16-15. A 17-year-old male is brought to the emergency department on a stretcher with severe right hip pain. He reports that he stumbled on the sidewalk and caught himself before he fell, but felt immediately excruciating pain in his right hip. He then fell to the ground in pain and was unable to get back up, necessitating an EMS call. He denies any significant past medical history. Physical examination reveals a male with a reported weight of 135 kg, blood pressure of 148/88, pulse 112, and temperature 37°C. He is sweating profusely, and holding his right hip in abduction. The remainder of his physical examination is unremarkable.

The most likely diagnosis for this patient would be which of the following?

a. Acute slipped capital femoral epiphysis

b. Acute stress fracture of the femoral neck

c. Septic arthritis of the right hip

d. Acute monosodium urate arthropathy (gout)

e. Acute testicular torsion

16-16. A 5-year-old girl is brought to the emergency department by her parents because for the past 24 hours, she has been complaining of progressive right hip pain. This has become severe enough to cause her to limp and she is now refusing to bear weight on the leg. Physical examination demonstrates a cooperative girl with a temperature of 38.6°C and pulse 88. Her general examination is unremarkable except for limitation of range of motion of the right hip due to pain.

The diagnostic test most likely to reveal the diagnosis would be which of the following?

a. Hip ultrasound

b. Blood culture

c. Analysis of synovial fluid

d. C-reactive protein

e. Hip radiograph

16-17. Which of the following is more likely to be true when considering the difference between the presentation of transient synovitis of the hip and septic arthritis?

a. There is more likely to be an antecedent viral infection in septic arthritis.

b. There is more likely to be an elevated temperature in transient synovitis.

c. Inflammatory parameters are more likely to be normal in transient synovitis.

d. There is more likely to be an effusion on hip ultrasound in septic arthritis.

e. Joint aspiration is more likely to be required in septic arthritis.

16-18. A newborn baby is noted to have torticollis, with his head tilted to the left and chin rotated to the right.

Which of the following features would be most consistent with congenital muscular torticollis?

a. A tight sternocleidomastoid muscle on the left

b. A tight sternocleidomastoid muscle on the right

c. Inability to move to chin to midline

d. Cesarean section delivery

e. History of polyhydramnios

16-19. You are seeing a new patient for initial evaluation. She is a 12-year-old female with no significant past medical history. All growth parameters are at 75% for age. You note on examination that she has a relatively low posterior neckline and a short, webbed neck. She is unable to extend her neck and you note on back examination a mild scoliosis and elevation of the right scapula. You order a lateral radiograph, which shows congenital fusion of the cervical spine (Figure 216-2).

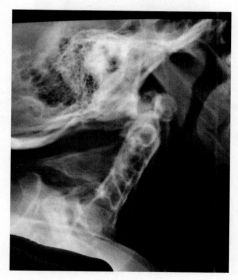

FIGURE 216-2. (Reproduced, with permission, from Rudolph CD, Rudolph AM, Lister GE, First LR, Gershon AA. *Rudolph's Pediatrics.* 22nd ed. New York: McGraw-Hill, 2011.)

Which of the following additional tests should be ordered?

a. Karyotype

b. Renal ultrasound

c. Upper GI series

d. Fundoscopic examination

e. Brain MRI

16-20. You are examining a 14-year-old girl and notice scoliosis with waist, scapula, and shoulder asymmetry (Figure 216-4). The curve is accentuated when she bends forward. There is mild tenderness on palpation of the lower spine.

Which of the following physical findings in an adolescent girl should raise concern for an underlying condition other than adolescent idiopathic scoliosis?

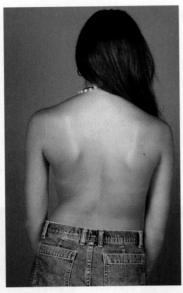

FIGURE 216-4. (Reproduced, with permission, from Rudolph CD, Rudolph AM, Lister GE, First LR, Gershon AA. *Rudolph's Pediatrics.* 22nd ed. New York: McGraw-Hill, 2011.)

a. Waist asymmetry

b. Pain on palpation

c. Increased curve when bending forward

d. Shoulder asymmetry

e. Prominence of the back

16-21. You are following a 13-year-old girl with adolescent idiopathic scoliosis. At her last 2 visits, 6 months apart, she underwent radiography, demonstrating a curve of 18° 12 months ago and 23° 6 months ago. At today's visit, her curve measures 30°.

Your next step would be which of the following?

a. Observe and schedule for repeat radiography in 3 months.

b. Refer for surgical correction.

c. Prescribe a brace to be worn both day and night.

d. Refer for physical therapy.

e. Prescribe a shoe lift for the shorter leg.

16-22. Which of the following clinical scenarios is most likely to require surgery as a final outcome?

a. A 16-year-old female who is 2 years post menarchal and has a scoliosis of 25°

b. A 6-year-old male with a curve of 12°

c. A 13-year-old prepubertal female with a scoliosis of 25°

d. A 9-year-old male with Duchenne muscular dystrophy and a curve of 25°

e. An 18-year-old female with a curve that has been stable at 35° with 2 years of bracing

16-23. A mother brings in her 16-year-old son to your office with complaints that he is "always slouching." Physical examination reveals a tall male adolescent sitting on your examination table in a slouching position. On examination, he has a significant kyphosis of greater than 60° with an exaggerated lumbar lordosis. When requested, he is unable to hyperextend his upper back.

Radiography of the spine is most likely to reveal which of the following?

a. A transitional lumbar vertebra

b. Thoracic compression fractures

c. Anterior wedging of thoracic vertebrae

d. A lytic lesion in a thoracic vertebra

e. A normal spine

16-24. A 12-year-old boy is admitted to the hospital after pinning of a displaced fracture of his radius. During the night, he begins to complain of severe pain in the lower arm, which is worse when he makes a fist.

Evaluation for which of the following would be most appropriate?

a. A compartment syndrome

b. Nonunion of the displaced fracture

c. Posttraumatic anxiety

d. Surgical site infection

e. Missed secondary fracture

16-25. An 8-year-old girl is brought to your office for evaluation of a mass on the dorsal surface of her left wrist. There is full range of motion of the wrist. The mass is nontender to palpation and appears to be cystic when transilluminated. The cystic nature of the mass is confirmed by ultrasound.

The most appropriate treatment for this problem is which of the following?

a. Surgical excision of the lesion

b. Firm compression of the lesion until it is reduced in size

c. Observation without intervention

d. Treatment with regular anti-inflammatory therapy

e. Fine needle aspiration

16-26. A 5-year-old boy is brought to the emergency room after a fall from the monkey bars during recess. The patient is holding his arm in flexion but allows you to examine it. You note tenderness on palpation of the left elbow and radiographs demonstrate no obvious fracture. The radiographs show elevation of the anterior and posterior fat pads.

Which of the following would be the next most appropriate step?

a. Reassurance and observation

b. Immobilization with a cast

c. Aspiration and drainage of the elbow effusion

d. Use of a sling until pain free

e. Surgical fixation

16-27. A 3-year-old boy is brought to your office because he has become irritable and his mother has noticed him to be limping. You note mild swelling and point tenderness in the midtibia on the left and you observe that the child is avoiding bearing weight on this extremity. Radiographs of the tibia and fibula are negative.

The most likely diagnosis is which of the following?

a. Nonaccidental trauma

b. Rickets

c. Osteomyelitis

d. Toddler's fracture

e. Growing pains

16-28. Sprains are ligamentous injuries and are classified into 3 categories based on:

a. Degree of pain

b. Degree of laxity

c. Number of recurrences

d. Degree of bony involvement

e. Age of patient

16-29. A 12-year-old boy is brought to the emergency department with complaints of right elbow pain. His father reports that the pain has been present and worsening for the past several weeks to the point where he is now unable to participate in baseball, where he is the pitcher for his little league team. Physical examination reveals swelling and point tenderness on the medial aspect of the right elbow with full range of motion of the elbow joint.

The most likely diagnosis is which of the following?

a. Distal humeral stress fracture

b. Olecranon bursitis

c. Medial epicondylitis

d. Elbow arthritis

e. Mononeuritis multiplex

16-30. A 15-year-old runner presents to the office complaining of right lower leg pain. She states that the pain started at the beginning of her track season and initially occurred only with activity but is now occurring at night as well. You suspect a tibial stress fracture. A radiograph of the knee is negative.

Your next step would be which of the following?

a. Reassure the patient that there is no fracture and she can continue her athletic activities without restriction.

b. Tell the patient that she should be treated for a stress fracture despite the negative radiograph.

c. Tell the patient to stop running track, as the pain will persist if she continues the sport.

d. Tell the patient to expect that a similar process will occur on the contralateral side.

e. Tell the patient that this warrants further workup for a possible bony malignancy.

16-31. A 15-year-old male presents to your office with the complaint of a mass in his right upper arm that has been growing in size over the past several months. Initially, the mass did not bother him, but lately has been causing discomfort on abduction of his arm and when he bumps it. Physical examination reveals a rough, hard mass palpable in the lateral aspect of the upper right arm and is slightly tender to palpation. Abduction of the right arm is limited. Radiographs demonstrate a calcified irregular mass in the proximal humerus that blends with the cortex of the humerus itself.

Definitive treatment of this problem would include which of the following?

a. Surgical excision of the mass

b. Radioablation

c. Observation with spontaneous regression

d. Combination chemotherapy

e. Wide excision with limb salvage

16-32. The disruption of bony cortex that leads to a nonossifying fibroma typically occurs as a result of which of the following?

a. Following trauma

b. Following radiation exposure

c. Disruption of in utero bone development

d. During rapid bone growth phase of adolescence

e. Chronic hypocalcemia

16-33. Which of the following is true regarding the differences between unicameral bone cysts and aneurysmal bone cysts?

   a. Unicameral bone cysts are symmetric in their expansion and aneurysmal bone cysts are eccentrically expanding.

   b. Only unicameral bone cysts require surgical intervention.

   c. Only aneurysmal bone cysts can grow to the physis (growth plate).

   d. Aneurysmal bone cysts are more likely to recur following treatment.

   e. Unicameral bone cysts are more likely than aneurysmal bone cysts to occur in the second decade.

16-34. A 14-year-old girl is brought to your office with a complaint of persistent left midshin pain. She describes the pain as dull and aching and tends to be worse at night. It is unrelated to position or activity. The pain is not reproducible on examination, but radiographs of the leg reveal a 0.8-cm intracortical lesion in the midtibia, surrounded by dense sclerotic bone.

Initial treatment of this problem would include which of the following?

   a. Directed radiation-beam therapy

   b. Anti-inflammatory (NSAID) therapy

   c. Surgical excision

   d. Antibiotic therapy

   e. Aspirin therapy

16-35. In addition to providing ankle–foot orthoses, early treatment of toe walking in a patient with cerebral palsy could include which of the following?

   a. Gastrocnemius fascial lengthening

   b. NSAID therapy

   c. Serial casting

   d. Botulinum toxin injection

   e. Achilles tendon lengthening

16-36. A family schedules an appointment to see you for a second opinion of a "bent knee." Their previously well 3-year-old child sustained a fracture of the right proximal tibia, which was casted for 4 weeks. The cast was removed a few months ago and they have noted that the child now has significant valgus deformity that was not present prior to the cast being placed. They state that the orthopedic surgeon told them "not to worry, it will correct itself over time." They bring copies of the radiographs (Figure 221-2).

What information is most appropriate to tell this family?

   a. The cast was not placed for long enough and the child should be recasted for at least 4 more weeks.

   b. The valgus deformity was probably there before and they did not notice it until now.

   c. Despite the cast, the fracture has healed improperly and the valgus deformity is a permanent consequence of this.

   d. The valgus deformity is normal and not associated with the fracture and will occur on the other side as well in the near future.

   e. The orthopedic surgeon is correct; the valgus deformity will most likely resolve over time.

16-37. You are seeing a child newly adopted from a foreign country. Her past medical history is unknown. During the visit, you note that the child has very high foot arches bilaterally. The forefeet are plantar flexed with a high arch and there is hindfoot varus deformity. She appears to be walking gingerly and has calluses on the lateral aspect of both feet.

The next step in her evaluation should include which of the following?

   a. Reassurance to the family that the foot deformity is a normal variant

   b. A detailed neurologic examination

   c. Radiographs of the cervical, thoracic, lumbar, and sacral spine

   d. Referral for surgical correction

   e. Karyotyping

16-38. One of your adolescent patients presents at your office with "concerns about my feet." She has noted progressive lateral deviation of the great toes of both feet and now her great toe overlaps with the second toe bilaterally. She states that she cannot find appropriate shoes and is wearing flip-flops instead, regardless of season. Physical examination reveals bilateral hallux valgus deformity with prominent first metatarsal joints.

Correction of what other associated problem could help this patient's hallux valgus without having to refer for surgery?

   a. Tarsal coalition

   b. Pes cavus deformity

   c. Tibial torsion

   d. Pes planovalgus

   e. Metatarsal stress fracture

16-39. A 5-year-old child with a prior history of nursemaid's elbow is sitting in one of your examination rooms holding a toy in his right hand. He is holding his left arm against his chest, flexed at the elbow. He resists attempts to move the elbow in any direction. The rest of the examination is unremarkable. His mother reports that he was playing on the jungle gym outside his school and fell from a height of approximately 5 ft, but there are no abrasions and his clothing is not dirty. When you ask the child how the injury happened, he shrugs and tells you that he "doesn't remember."

In addition to your suspicion that the patient has a nursemaid's elbow, you also consider which of the following diagnoses?

a. Untreated seizure disorder

b. Ehlers-Danlos syndrome

c. Child abuse

d. Benign hypermobility

e. Heart arrhythmia

ANSWERS

Answer 16-1. a

Of the choices, an elevated C-reactive protein is the most sensitive indicator of infection. Previous trauma is reported in up to 35% of patients with infection, but is not specific for septic arthritis. Radiographs in acute joint infection may show soft tissue swelling or a joint effusion, but are not sensitive. The most sensitive radiologic procedure would be an MRI of the affected area. An MRI could also help localize the extent of the infection and whether or not there is adjacent osteomyelitis.

(Page 841, Chapter 211: The Limping Child)

Answer 16-2. c

Metatarsus adductus is one of the most common causes of an intoeing gait and is typically diagnosed in infancy. It is fairly easily distinguished from clubfoot due to flexibility of the foot, as opposed to clubfoot, which cause a rigid deviation of the foot. DDH is found in 10% of patients with metatarsus adductus and diligence must be paid to evaluating for this abnormality. While clavicular fracture can be found in infancy and has an association with DDH, there is no known association with metatarsus adductus. Pes planus, or flat foot, is ubiquitous in infants, as arch development has not yet occurred. Myelomeningocele, while much rarer in the era of folic acid use prior to pregnancy, is still diagnosed peripartum, but is not related to the presence of metatarsus adductus.

(Page 842, 845, Chapter 212: Torsional and Angular Deformities)

Answer 16-3. b

Femoral anteversion is the most common cause of an intoeing gait in children over the age of 4. It is due to excessive internal rotation at the level of the hip, causing the entire leg to be inwardly deviated. In internal tibial torsion, the internal deviation is at the level of the tibia and therefore the patella are noted to be straight on examination, as opposed to femoral anteversion, where they are internally rotated. Metatarsus adductus is a disorder of infants, causing inward deviation of the forefoot. Slipped capital femoral epiphysis is a cause of an out-toeing gait due to medial displacement of the cap of the femur. While fractures can cause a limp, they do not specifically lead to an intoeing gait.

(Pages 842-844, Chapter 212: Torsional and Angular Deformities)

Answer 16-4. c

Babies are born with the maximum amount of varus deformity of the knees. This angular deformity of the knee should improve over time and typically resolves by age 2. Patients whose genu varum persists after this age should be evaluated for other, less typical, cause of varus deformity, including rickets, skeletal dysplasias, or other metabolic bone diseases.

(Pages 843-845, Chapter 212: Torsional and Angular Deformities)

Answer 16-5. b

Low back pain in adolescents is due to muscular tightness that should respond to a regular stretching program. If this does not relieve the discomfort, then further evaluation may be necessary to ascertain the underlying problem. This evaluation should start with radiographs of the lower back. Spinal problems such as spondylolysis, or microfracture of the spine or spondylolisthesis, anterior slipping of a vertebra, should be apparent on lateral films of the spine. Transitional vertebrae, compression fractures, and other bony deformities will also be captured on plain film. While intra-abdominal processes, such as nephrolithiasis or inflammatory bowel disease, can cause referred pain, these should not be reproducible on examination of the back. This finding is also true for upper spine or chest pathology that would be captured on a chest radiograph, unless the back pain also includes the upper spine.

While some of the disorders that lead to chronic low back pain may also affect lower extremity neurologic function, an EMG would not be an initial diagnostic test in the absence of abnormalities on physical examination.

(Page 861, Chapter 216: Disorders of the Neck and Spine)

Answer 16-6. b

Genu valgus is normal between the ages of 3 and 8 and maximal between the ages of 4 and 6. As long as this patient's valgus improves over time, there is no further intervention required and the parent can be reassured.

If the patient has persistent valgus deformity into adolescence, then a workup for previous fracture or metabolic bone disease may be indicated. Neither orthotics nor physical therapy has been shown to be effective in expediting the resolution of genu valgus.

(Pages 844-845, Chapter 212: Torsional and Angular Deformities)

Answer 16-7. b

Calcaneovalgus deformity is due to malpositioning of the foot in utero and can be quite severe. It is generally treated with gentle stretching and usually improves over time. It is important, however, to exclude more serious causes of foot deformities, the most common of which is congenital vertical talus. In this condition, the heel does not descend due to dorsal dislocation of the talonavicular joint and remains in a fixed equinus position leading to the classic "rocket bottom" foot. In calcaneovalgus, the heel should move upwards as the foot is plantar flexed. With congenital vertical talus, the heel has not descended and will not move appropriately with the rest of the foot. This condition will require orthopedic intervention. Congenital vertical talus is teratologic in nature and can be associated with other syndromes, such as trisomy syndromes, arthrogryposis, and myelomeningocele.

Pes planovalgus, or flat feet, is common in infancy, as the arch has not yet developed and is unrelated to calcaneovalgus deformity. TAR syndrome is also unrelated.

It is important to look for developmental dysplasia of the hip in a patient with calcaneovalgus deformity, as the same underlying abnormality (malpositioning in utero) leads to both conditions, but the presence or absence of DDH is not necessary to make the diagnosis of calcaneovalgus deformity.

(Pages 845-846, 849, Chapter 213: Disorders of the Foot)

Answer 16-8. d

The decreased movement of the midfoot significantly raises the likelihood of tarsal coalition, as patients with tarsal coalition develop their symptoms due to rigidity of the midfoot. This condition is typically caused by failure to develop joints between the tarsal bones, which over time calcify and become rigid and painful. Physical examination would demonstrate a decreased longitudinal arch in both conditions.

Both tarsal coalition and pes planovalgus can be causes of leg or foot pain, but pes planovalgus is caused by hyperflexibility. Both conditions can cause pain, which can be worse with activity, although pain from tarsal coalition does not typically occur before the second decade of life. There is no specific gender predilection to either disorder. The

treatment of pes planovalgus is orthotics, but only if the patient is symptomatic. The treatment of tarsal coalition requires a surgical intervention to resect the coalition if conservative measures fail to relieve the pain.

(Page 846, 849, Chapter 213: Disorders of the Foot)

Answer 16-9. a

This case describes a child born with clubfoot, or talipes equinovarus. This is a serious congenital disorder causing dysplasia of the lower leg with dysmorphic bones and subsequent maldevelopment of the surrounding musculature.

Unlike talipes calcaneovalgus, this disorder does not improve with time and requires rapid intervention if corrections are to be made in time for the patient to walk. Initially, nonsurgical techniques are employed, such as serial casting, which is effective in up to 90% of patients, or long-term physical therapy, taping, and nocturnal splinting. The remaining patients require surgical intervention, such as releases of the ligaments and tendons. Although sometimes unavoidable, multiple surgeries can themselves lead to constriction of movement and persistent gait abnormalities.

(Pages 846-848, Chapter 213: Disorders of the Foot)

Answer 16-10. b

This case is a classic description of patellofemoral syndrome, which is caused by malalignment of the patella in the femoral groove. The pain is aggravated by exercise or prolonged flexion of the knees, such as by sitting in class or sitting in a car seat. Treatment is directed at symptomatic control and NSAIDs can be used judiciously for analgesia. This condition is unrelated to growth plate activity. Physical therapy targeted at quadriceps and hip girdle strengthening can be beneficial. Nerve stimulation through the use of a TENS unit has not been shown to be efficacious, nor is surgery typically required. Intra-articular corticosteroids would not be a treatment of choice, as this condition is not inflammatory in nature.

(Page 851, Chapter 214: Disorders of the Knee)

Answer 16-11. c

Developmental dysplasia of the hip is defined as an abnormal relationship between the femur and the acetabulum. Intrauterine conditions that place a strain on the hip and leg, such as breech presentation or oligohydramnios, predispose the fetus to DDH. Torticollis, or wryneck, can also be caused by this type of mechanism and children born with torticollis have a 14% to 20% incidence of DDH.

Patients with metatarsus adductus also have an increased risk of DDH due to the same mechanism; however, this mechanism is not associated with other causes of intoeing, such as tibial torsion or femoral anteversion. Teratologic hip dislocations can be due to conditions such as arthrogryposis. DDH is not specifically associated with congenital scoliosis, which is due to maldevelopment of vertebral bodies, or branchial cleft disorders.

(Pages 852-854, Chapter 215: Developmental Dysplasia of the Hip)

Answer 16-12. e

Developmental dysplasia of the hip, defined as an abnormal relationship of the proximal femur to the acetabulum, is not always diagnosed in infancy. If DDH is uncorrected, and the hip remains dislocated, the child will ambulate using only their hip girdle muscles, rather than relying on the articulation of the hip itself. The child may circumduct the leg and can frequently fall toward the affected side.

If the dislocation is bilateral, the child can have the appearance of generalized muscular weakness, such as that seen in a muscular dystrophy or in juvenile dermatomyositis, but the other findings presented are not consistent with those diagnoses. The description of the left knee being lower than the right is due to superior positioning of the dislocated femoral head and relative shortening of the thigh is called the Galeazzi test, which is sensitive for DDH. Legg-Calve-Perthes disease, which is caused by avascular necrosis of the femoral head, is rare in this age group. Physical examination would be more likely to demonstrate irritability of the hip in all directions and less of a leg length discrepancy. A positive Galeazzi sign would not be present. SCFE would be very rare in this age group and would demonstrate limited internal rotation on examination.

(Pages 852-856, Chapter 215: Developmental Dysplasia of the Hip)

Answer 16-13. d

Based on the symptoms, physical examination, and radiologic appearance of the hip, this patient has Legg-Calve-Perthes disease (LCPD) of the left hip. LCPD is an idiopathic condition that leads to avascular necrosis of the femoral head. It is more common in boys and occurs typically between the ages of 4 and 12. Bilateral disease is uncommon, occurring in less than 15% of patients, and is more likely secondary in nature, necessitating a workup for thyroid disease or hemoglobinopathies.

While patients can present with a painless limp, as the disease progresses, pain can develop and limit activities. Examination demonstrates loss of range of motion of the hip and surrounding muscle spasm. Radiographs may be negative initially, but as the avascular necrosis progresses, abnormalities become apparent as the femoral head fragments and heals. Once avascular necrosis becomes apparent on radiograph, there is no need for more specific radiologic tests, although MRI is more sensitive in detecting early avascular necrosis when radiographs are negative. LCPD is typically self-resolving within 12 to 18 months, after which children can return to their normal activities. The condition on healing of the femoral head is the best determinant of outcome for the patient; the

severely involved and irregular on resolution, the worse the result for the patient.

(Pages 854-855, Chapter 215: Developmental Dysplasia of the Hip)

Answer 16-14. c

This patient has a chronic slipped capital femoral epiphysis of the right hip. Outcomes following SCFE are determined by the extent of avascular necrosis of the femoral head, which is a result of compromised blood flow to the hip. Acute SCFEs are more highly associated with avascular necrosis, but chronic SCFEs can develop compromised blood flow at any point, which is why the patient should immediately become non–weight-bearing and should be transported via stretcher to the hospital. SCFEs require immediate surgical correction once identified, with subsequent modified weight-bearing and physical therapy. Unlike LCPD, SCFE is not self-resolving.

(Pages 855-856, Chapter 215: Developmental Dysplasia of the Hip)

Answer 16-15. a

Unlike chronic SCFE, acute SCFE presents as acute severe pain following a twisting injury or a minor fall. It can mimic an acute fracture, but typically the mechanism of injury is not sufficient to lead to a fracture of a long bone.

While both septic arthritis and gout are causes of severe joint pain, septic arthritis is typically associated with fever and limitation of range of motion in all directions. This is also true of gout, which would be rare in this age group and less likely to affect a hip. Acute testicular torsion can commonly cause referred pain to the groin, but the physical examination should provide clues to the diagnosis and would not cause limitation of range of motion in the hip itself.

(Pages 855-856, Chapter 215: Developmental Dysplasia of the Hip)

Answer 16-16. c

The differential diagnosis of acute hip pain with fever could include septic arthritis, osteomyelitis, transient synovitis of the hip, as well as other systemic infection. Both septic arthritis and transient synovitis may demonstrate a hip effusion on ultrasound and plain radiographs can be negative in both conditions early on. Even in the best of circumstances, the yield of blood cultures in septic arthritis is low. Diagnostic arthrocentesis with analysis of the synovial fluid is most likely to provide the diagnosis, in terms of both obtaining an organism on culture or Gram stain and determining the synovial fluid WBC count, as one would expect counts greater than 50,000/mm^3 with a predominance of neutrophils with septic arthritis and counts less than 15,000/mm^3 in transient synovitis.

(Page 856, Chapter 215: Developmental Dysplasia of the Hip)

Answer 16-17. c

The presentations of transient synovitis of the hip and septic arthritis of the hip can be very similar. Septic arthritis is more likely to be associated with a high fever and elevated inflammatory markers, which can be unremarkable in transient synovitis. On carefully eliciting the history, one may ascertain a recent viral infection, which commonly precedes the advent of transient synovitis. Both conditions can cause a hip effusion, which would be demonstrable on ultrasound of the hip. Because of the similarity of the 2 presentations, and the risk of missing the diagnosis of septic arthritis, it is not uncommon for patients with transient synovitis to undergo diagnostic arthrocentesis to exclude bacterial infection.

(Page 856, Chapter 215: Developmental Dysplasia of the Hip)

Answer 16-18. a

In congenital torticollis, the contracture of the SCM muscle leads to "overpull" and tilting of the head to the side of the contracture. This results in rotation of the chin to the contralateral side. While the muscle tightness may cause the inability to bring the chin to midline, congenital muscle torticollis is not the only disease to lead to this problem. In the absence of a palpable olive indicating SCM contracture, one must also consider other causes of torticollis, including congenital cervical vertebral abnormalities or rotatory subluxation of the atlantoaxial junction. Like other congenital contractures, torticollis is associated with a tight space in utero, such as is seen in breech presentations or with oligohydramnios. Cesarean section, while sometimes necessary with breech presentations, is not itself a cause of torticollis. Treatment includes stretching exercises and other strategies to encourage the infant to turn away from the affected side.

(Pages 856-857, Chapter 216: Disorders of the Neck and Spine)

Answer 16-19. b

This patient has Klippel-Feil syndrome, which is caused by abnormal development of the cervical spine. The triad of features includes a short, webbed neck, low posterior hair line, and limitation of range of motion of the cervical spine, typically due to fusion of cervical vertebrae. There can also be associated thoracic and lumbar vertebral abnormalities leading to scoliosis (30% of Klippel-Feil patients). Sprengel deformity, or elevation of the scapula, is seen in 50% of Klippel-Feil patients.

Recognition of this condition is important as the limitation of range of motion of the cervical spine can place the patient at risk for cervical spine injury during intubation for anesthesia or in the face of trauma. In addition, because intrauterine development of the vertebrae occurs at the same time as the genitourinary system, Klippel-Feil patients can have GU track abnormalities. The GU system should therefore be evaluated to confirm normal development.

(Page 857, Chapter 216: Disorders of the Neck and Spine)

Answer 16-20. b

Idiopathic scoliosis is the most common type of scoliosis and is found in approximately 2% of adolescents. It tends to be asymptomatic and is noted on screening physical examination or by others observing asymmetry of the shoulders, back, or waist. The Adam's forward bend test causes increased torque and therefore accentuates the curve. Pain on palpation of the spine is uncommon and should raise concern for other underlying abnormalities, such as fractures or malignancy. Tenderness on palpation of the spine requires further evaluation.

(Pages 857-860, Chapter 216: Disorders of the Neck and Spine)

Answer 16-21. c

There are 3 stages of treatment for idiopathic scoliosis. Initially, observation is appropriate as most patients with scoliosis do not progress sufficiently to require further intervention. Once a patient reaches a curve greater than 25°, bracing is used to prevent further progression of the curve by strengthening and realigning the surrounding musculature. If bracing is ineffective and the curve progresses above 45°, then surgery may be warranted. In an otherwise healthy girl, without underlying neuromuscular disease or weakness, bracing would be appropriate, as in this case. Physical therapy does not provide the same consistency as regular bracing and while providing a shoe lift may partially correct a secondary leg length discrepancy, it does not impact the scoliosis itself.

(Pages 857-860, Chapter 216: Disorders of the Neck and Spine)

Answer 16-22. d

There are multiple factors that contribute to course and prognosis in scoliosis. Patients who reach full skeletal maturity with curve of over 45° are likely to progress as adults. The younger the age of onset, the more time the curve has to progress; however, these patients can still be treated effectively with bracing. Patients with underlying neuromuscular or myopathic disease, however, respond poorly to bracing and are more likely to proceed to surgery.

(Pages 857-860, Chapter 216: Disorders of the Neck and Spine)

Answer 16-23. c

In a patient presenting with significant hyperkyphosis, the differential diagnosis includes postural hyperkyphosis (also known as benign roundback) and Scheuermann kyphosis. In postural kyphosis, the spine is flexible and there are no underlying skeletal abnormalities. This type of patient should be able to hyperextend his/her back without difficulty. Scheuermann kyphosis is a rigid process due to anterior wedging of multiple vertebrae, decreased disc spaces, and the presence of Schmorl nodes. In the absence of underlying metabolic bone disease and chronic corticosteroid use, compression fractures are very rare in the pediatric age group and would be unusual in an otherwise healthy male. Likewise it would be unusual to encounter a lytic lesion in the spine, which would be suspicious for malignancies such as multiple myeloma. Transitional lumbar vertebra can be a cause of lower back pain and low back stiffness, but would not account for this patient's upper back findings.

(Pages 860-861, Chapter 216: Disorders of the Neck and Spine)

Answer 16-24. a

Of the choices listed, a compartment syndrome is by far the most serious problem. Occurring following a fracture, compartment syndromes can occur as bleeding and swelling lead to compression of blood vessels within the muscular compartment leading to pain and subsequent ischemia. Pain in the immediate postoperative period is unlikely to be due to surgical site infection and is also too early for problems with persistent fracture displacement. A secondary fracture small enough to be missed on the primary evaluation is unlikely to cause this degree of pain. While children can have significant anxiety following a traumatic event, this anxiety is unlikely to be manifested in such a specific location with these types of symptoms.

(Page 863, Chapter 217: Disorders of the Upper Extremity)

Answer 16-25. c

This patient appears to have a ganglion cyst, a common benign cystic mass of the tendon sheath. Most ganglion cysts resolve spontaneously, so no treatment is necessary. There is a high recurrence rate following surgical intervention, so if the cyst is not impeding function of the wrist joint, conservative measures are appropriate. Ganglion cysts can be confused with juvenile idiopathic arthritis of the wrist, which would require regular anti-inflammatory therapy. The ultrasound finding of a cyst, and not synovitis, confirms the diagnosis.

(Pages 864-865, Chapter 217: Disorders of the Upper Extremity)

Answer 16-26. b

The history of an injury sustained to the left elbow from a fall from height as well as evidence of effusion on radiograph (fat pad sign) must raise suspicion for an occult fracture. Occult fractures are particularly common in young children and evidence on radiographs may only be apparent several weeks later as the fracture heals. Treatment should be immobilization with a cast or splint for several weeks until pain free. A sling is not sufficient to protect the joint and surgical fixation is not necessary. The joint effusion will resolve as the fracture heals and does not require aspiration and drainage. Occult elbow fractures need to be differentiated from subluxation of the radial head seen in nursemaid's elbow. Nursemaid's elbow should have a negative radiograph and can be reduced without sedation or anesthesia.

(Pages 865-866, Chapter 218: Injuries)

Answer 16-27. d

Toddler's fractures are occult or nondisplaced spiral fractures of the tibia that occur typically in the first 2 to 3 years of ambulation. Point tenderness in the area of the fracture can be present, although radiographs can be negative until the bone starts to heal.

While nonaccidental trauma should be considered in the context of any fracture, the absence of other signs of abuse would make this less likely. Rickets is a cause of persistent genu varum and worsens with weight-bearing, but should cause bilateral, rather than unilateral, symptoms. Osteomyelitis is most common in this age group, but should be accompanied by fever and signs of systemic inflammation. Growing pains are more common in the 5- to 12-year age group and are described as nonspecific leg pain that is typically bilateral and accompanied by a normal examination. The point tenderness found on this examination makes the diagnosis of growing pains less likely.

(Pages 866-867, Chapter 218: Injuries)

Answer 16-28. b

Sprains are classified based on the resulting degree of laxity, which in turn helps determine treatment.

Type I sprains have point tenderness along the ligament but no laxity compared with the unaffected side. Type II sprains have some associated laxity, while type III sprains have at least 10 mm of laxity compared with the contralateral side. Lower-grade sprains are treated with rest, ice, and elevation with relative rapid return to play as long as the patient is pain free. Type III sprains require much more significant intervention. While recurrent injury can lead to higher degrees of sprain, frequency is not part of the classification.

(Pages 868-869, Chapter 218: Injuries)

Answer 16-29. c

Epiphysitis, or inflammation of the bone leading to bone edema and physeal widening, is the result of chronic repetitive use. Medial epicondylitis of the elbow is an epiphysitis common to baseball pitchers. This condition is treated as an overuse injury, with rest and reduction in the number of pitches thrown.

Stress fractures are uncommon in the humerus, and, although they may cause point tenderness, they would not cause swelling at the epicondyle. Olecranon bursitis is very rare in the pediatric age group. Chronic arthritis of the elbow, such as that seen in juvenile idiopathic arthritis, could present similarly, but is usually accompanied by evidence of synovitis and limitation of range of motion. Mononeuritis multiplex is a sensory and motor peripheral neuropathy. In the absence of neurologic findings, mononeuritis multiplex would be unusual.

(Page 869, Chapter 218: Injuries)

Answer 16-30. b

This case is a classic presentation for a stress fracture, with pain occurring first with activity and then becoming persistent if the injury is not treated with rest, ice, compression, and elevation (RICE) measures. It is common that initial radiographs are negative, as the fracture may not become apparent for several weeks as the healing process occurs, but if the index of suspicion for fracture is high, then treatment for a stress fracture should be initiated. Once the fracture is healed, the patient should be able to return to her prior activities and does not need to give up her sport.

There is no evidence that having a stress fracture on one side predisposed the patient to a fracture on the contralateral side. Given the classic history for stress fracture and the negative radiograph, there is no need to pursue other diagnoses, unless measures to treat fracture do not resolve the patient's symptoms.

(Page 869, Chapter 218: Injuries)

Answer 16-31. a

This patient most likely has a solitary osteochondroma arising from the proximal humerus. Osteochondroma is the most common bone tumor and can be identified by recognition of a growing mass or as an incidental finding on a radiograph. While they do not spontaneously regress, such as is seen with nonossifying fibromas, definitive surgical excision is not necessary unless the mass is interfering with function or is cosmetically unacceptable.

The radiographic appearance of this benign tumor is much different from that seen in either osteosarcoma or Ewing sarcoma, but proper identification is important as all of these tumors are most common in adolescence.

(Page 870, Chapter 219: Tumors)

Answer 16-32. c

Nonossifying fibromas are due to disruption in normal bone growth in utero, leading to a fibrous-filled abnormality, typically in the metaphyseal region of long bones (Figure 219-2). Most nonossifying fibromas are asymptomatic and found incidentally. The radiographic appearance of a nonossifying fibroma, with a sharp, sclerotic border and radiolucent, multilobulated appearance arising from the metaphysis, is so distinctive that further workup is not necessary. Nonossifying fibromas typically resolve spontaneously. Unlike malignant bony tumors, they are not associated with radiation exposure (osteosarcoma) or periods of rapid growth. Metabolic conditions, such as rickets or hyperparathyroidism, are also not associated with this condition.

(Page 871, Chapter 219: Tumors)

Answer 16-33. a

While both types of bone cysts are most commonly located at the metaphysis, the expansion of unicameral bone cysts is symmetric, while aneurysmal bone cyst expansion is eccentric. In addition, both types of cysts extend to the growth plate, but aneurysmal bone cysts can, on occasion, extend through the growth plate to the epiphysis or into the diaphysis. Both types of bone cysts require treatment, particularly in younger children, in order to prevent pathologic fracture or disruption of the growth plate leading to growth disturbance. Treatments include curettage and grafting or corticosteroid injection, but, unfortunately, the recurrence rates following surgery are high for both types.

(Pages 871-872, Chapter 219: Tumors)

Answer 16-34. b

The patient described in this case has an osteoid osteoma of the left tibia. Osteoid osteomas are benign lesions of bone of unknown cause, found primarily in the pediatric population. These lesions can be self-limiting and resolve over time, but many patients have persistent pain during the course of the illness. While definitive therapy of an osteoid osteoma causing persistent discomfort is surgical excision, many patients find complete or temporary relief from NSAID therapy, which should be used as the initial treatment. Given the risk of Reye syndrome and the need to give aspirin therapy 4 times daily, the use of aspirin has not been studied in the treatment of osteoid osteoma. The lesion is highly reactive but not infectious in nature, and therefore antibiotic therapy would not be effective. There is no role for external beam radiation in the treatment of this benign lesion.

(Page 872, Chapter 219: Tumors)

Answer 16-35. d

The early treatment of toe walking in ambulatory cerebral palsy patients is critical to their ability to ambulate over time. Ankle–foot orthoses will provide stability, but do not alter the underlying spasticity, which is the reason that serial casting is ineffective. NSAID therapy may provide analgesia, but is not effective in reducing spasticity. Injection of botulinum toxin has become an effective strategy to deplete the neuromuscular junction, thereby reducing spasticity and improving range of motion.

Surgical procedures, such as gastrocnemius fascial lengthening and Achilles tendonotomy, are reserved for patients who have not responded to more conservative measures and continue to have functional impairment.

(Pages 872-873, Chapter 220: Neuromuscular Disorders)

Answer 16-36. e

The child sustained a Cozen fracture, which is a proximal tibial fracture that was slightly displaced. When this occurs in a young child, the leg can grow into a valgus position as the fracture heals. Like other causes of genu valgus, the deformity tends to correct over time; however, the condition requires regular follow-up.

(Page 875, Chapter 221: Common Orthopedic Misses)

Answer 16-37. b

Pes cavus, or an elevated horizontal arch, can occur in a variety of conditions. While pes cavus can be idiopathic, this is a diagnosis of exclusion and underlying, more serious illness must first be ruled out. The common causes of pes cavus are peripheral neuropathies such as Charcot-Marie-Tooth, or spinal cord abnormalities, such as a tethered cord or myelomeningocele. A detailed neurologic examination is mandatory to look for evidence of an underlying neurologic process, followed by EMGs and other diagnostic testing. Radiographs of the spine are not sufficiently sensitive to detect abnormalities and MRI is preferable. While some diseases that cause pes cavus, such as Friedreich ataxia, are genetically based, a karyotype would not be part of the initial diagnostic workup.

(Page 850, Chapter 213: Disorders of the Foot)

Answer 16-38. d

Hallux valgus, or bunions, is due to lateral deviation of the great toe to the point that the head of the first metatarsal becomes uncomfortable when bearing weight. The widening at the metatarsal joint, as well as overlapping of the great toe with the second and third toes, can also become a cosmetic issue for teenagers. Of the disorders listed, only pes planovalgus is associated with hallux valgus because the positioning of the foot places extra valgus pressure on the joint. Using an arch support can improve symptoms associated with both the pes planus and the hallux valgus. Surgical treatments of hallux valgus have low success rates and lead to impairment in range of motion of the joint and interference with physical activity and should be discouraged.

(Page 850)

Answer 16-39. c

Nursemaid's elbow, or subluxation of the annular ligament over the radial head, is typically caused by longitudinal traction on the arm. Once diagnosed, it is relatively easy to reduce, resulting in full return to function of the arm. Repetitive nursemaid's elbow, however, should raise flags for other causes of repetitive trauma to the arm. In this case, given the fact that the child has no other injuries that would occur from a fall from a height, and he cannot corroborate the story of the caregiver, child abuse must be considered. Loss of consciousness from a seizure or arrhythmia could lead to a fall, but the child should have other injuries or physical findings to explain this. Causes of hypermobility, such as Ehlers-Danlos syndrome or benign hypermobility, put the patient at higher risk for joint subluxation, but this hypermobility should be evident on examination.

(Page 866, Chapter 218: Injuries)

CHAPTER 17 | Infectious Disease

Dylan C. Kann, Duha Al-Zubeidi, Erica Pan,
Sunitha V. Kaiser, and Michael D. Cabana

17-1. A mother brings in her 4-month-old infant for a routine well-child check. She notes that the infant who usually takes her breast milk from a bottle has been having more difficulty feeding the past few days. In addition to fussiness with feedings, the mother has noticed white lesions inside the infant's mouth. Examination of the patient's mouth demonstrates white patches on both the tongue and buccal mucosa, which when scraped with a tongue blade have punctate bleeding and an erythematous base. You diagnose oral candidiasis.

You prescribe oral nystatin and do which of the following?

a. Initiate a basic immunodeficiency workup given the child's age at presentation.

b. Initiate a 14-day course of fluconazole to treat for esophageal candidiasis.

c. Recommend cleaning of the infants' bottle nipple and pacifier by boiling after every use.

d. Recommend temporary discontinuation of pumped breast milk.

e. Recommend no further therapeutic interventions.

17-2. A 14-year-old boy develops fevers, hypoxia requiring oxygen supplementation, and occasional hemoptysis. He is recovering from recent bone marrow transplantation and has profound neutropenia. He is started on broad-spectrum antibiotics and antifungals. Chest computed tomography shows a pulmonary nodule with a "halo sign" (ie, a haziness surrounding the nodule). No other focus for the patient's febrile neutropenia can be found.

What testing would be most helpful in confirming the diagnosis?

a. Bronchoalveolar lavage (BAL)

b. Direct sputum sample

c. Serologic complement fixation testing

d. Serologic assay to detect galactomannan

e. Lung biopsy

17-3. An overweight Filipino girl is brought into the neurology clinic for chronic headaches over the past 3 months with recent onset of intermittent double vision. She is visiting from California. She has had no bladder or bowel incontinence and the remainder of her physical examination is normal. On CT there are mild signs of increased intracranial pressure. An MRI is scheduled. An LP performed in clinic yields CSF with a lymphocytic pleocytosis, a glucose of 20 mg/dL, and a protein of 235 mg/dL. Opening pressure for the LP is normal.

Further questioning reveals that the patient had a red rash on her shin that recently resolved and a febrile illness several months ago. CSF is sent for culture and complement-fixing antibodies. Curative treatment for the patient's condition may include:

a. Intrathecal amphotericin B

b. Oral acetazolamide

c. Intravenous imidazole

d. Intravenous caspofungin

e. Referral to a weight loss program

17-4. Both histoplasmosis and blastomycosis are fungal infections that can occur in the United States. Both infections share many similarities. Which of the following statements helps distinguish the differences between their epidemiology, manifestations, and diagnosis?

a. Only *Histoplasma capsulatum* is found in the Ohio and Mississippi River basins.

b. Only *Blastomyces dermatitidis* is treated with amphotericin B.

c. Only *H. capsulatum* is a dimorphic fungus.

d. Only blastomycosis has skin manifestations.

e. Only *H. capsulatum* is commonly detected using serum antibody assays.

17-5. An ex–28-week-infant now on day of life 14 is noted to have a fever and an increased oxygen requirement. A chest radiograph demonstrates bilateral interstitial pulmonary infiltrates. A complete blood count shows an elevated white blood cell count and thrombocytopenia. The patient has blood cultures drawn from his central line through which he is receiving total parenteral nutrition (TPN) and intravenous lipids. Evaluation for necrotizing enterocolitis is negative. The patient has not received any blood products.

What should be the next step in the patient's clinical care?

a. Order a urinalysis.

b. Discontinue the intravenous lipid infusion.

c. Begin flucytosine.

d. Send off a skin culture for *Malassezia* species.

e. Discontinue the IV TPN.

17-6. An 8-year-old boy presents with a lesion on his hand. Six weeks ago, he sustained a laceration on the dorsum of his hand from a rose bush at the park. Over the past 6 weeks it has developed into a plaque-like, hyperpigmented lesion in the same area as his initial injury. He is given a course of cephalexin with no improvement in the lesion. Preliminary biopsy reveals pyogranulomatous inflammation. A wound culture is currently pending. He had a purified protein derivative test approximately 1 month ago that was negative. His mother is concerned that this may be a cancer. You reassure her that from the wound culture you most likely expect to see:

a. A monomorphic fungi

b. A dimorphic fungi

c. A spirochete

d. An acid-fast bacillus

e. A gram-negative bacterium

17-7. A 2-year-old girl with short gut syndrome is admitted for fever. Blood cultures are drawn from her peripherally inserted central catheter (PICC) through which she receives parenteral nutrition. Her urinalysis shows blood but no signs of infection. The patient is started on vancomycin and piperacillin–tazobactam, but she continues to have high spiking fevers and low blood pressures. A peripheral IV is placed to give her supplemental fluids. Her PICC culture returns at 12 hours with a gram-positive coccus yet to be identified and a yeast, which preliminarily appears to be a *Candida* species. Based on these findings you first:

a. Begin treatment with fluconazole through the PICC to treat the yeast.

b. Remove the PICC because it is growing a gram-positive coccus.

c. Remove the PICC because it is growing yeast.

d. Conclude the yeast is a contaminant and continue the current antibiotics.

e. Conclude that the gram-positive coccus is a contaminant and stop the antibiotics.

17-8. A 3-year-old girl presents with findings of encephalitis including fever, weakness, altered sensorium, and myoclonus. Evaluation also reveals flaccid paralysis. Her history is positive for several insect bites 2 weeks ago. Evaluation of her CSF is positive for a PCR test of West Nile virus (WNV). Her cerebrospinal fluid profile is most likely to reveal the following profile:

a. Eosinophilic pleocytosis, elevated protein, and low glucose

b. Neutrophilic pleocytosis, elevated protein, and normal glucose

c. Neutrophilic pleocytosis, elevated protein, and low glucose

d. Lymphocytic pleocytosis, elevated protein, and normal glucose

e. Lymphocytic pleocytosis, elevated protein, and low glucose

17-9. While caring for a 12-year-old boy undergoing chemotherapy for leukemia, he is noted to develop severe abdominal pain and profuse diarrhea and occasional vomiting. Tests for pancreatitis and bacterial causes are negative. A preliminary viral culture of the stool shows a non-polio enterovirus. This patient is most at risk for developing a chronic enteroviral infection because:

a. He has an acquired T-cell immunodeficiency.

b. He has an acquired B-cell immunodeficiency.

c. He has an acquired complement deficiency.

d. He has a central line for chemotherapy.

e. He has received cytarabine.

17-10. A concerned parent brings in their child to the urgent care clinic complaining of fever, rash, and refusal to eat. During examination of the child, the patient is noted to have lesions with the following appearance:

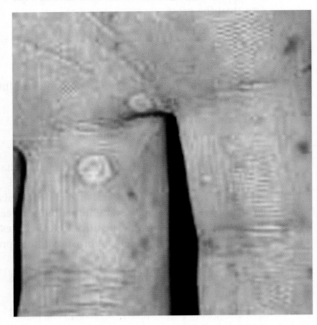

(Reproduced, with permission, from Wolff K, Johnson RA. *Fitzpatrick's Color Atlas and Synopsis of Clinical Dermatology.* 6th Ed. New York: McGraw-Hill, 2009.)

The most appropriate treatment for this child is:

a. Intravenous immune globulin

b. Intravenous doxycyline

c. Topical 1% permethrin

d. Topical 5% permethrin

e. Rest, antipyretics, and analgesics

17-11. A 10-month-old boy is being seen for reported hepatitis A exposure. The exposure is thought to be from contaminated strawberries that his family purchased. He has not received any hepatitis A vaccination. He is currently asymptomatic. All of his vaccinations are up-to-date. Exposure is estimated to have occurred less than 2 weeks ago. Appropriate therapy at this time would include:

a. Ribavirin

b. Alpha interferon

c. Hepatitis A vaccination

d. Hepatitis B vaccination

e. Intramuscular immune globulin

17-12. An 11-year-old boy is being seen for reported hepatitis A exposure. The exposure is from contaminated strawberries that his family purchased at a local market. He has not received any hepatitis A vaccination. He is currently asymptomatic. All of his other vaccinations are up-to-date. Exposure is estimated to have occurred less than 2 weeks ago. Appropriate therapy at this time would include:

a. Ribavirin

b. Alpha interferon

c. Hepatitis A vaccination

d. Hepatitis B vaccination

e. Intramuscular immune globulin

17-13. A 16-year-old unvaccinated homeless youth seeks evaluation approximately 3 weeks after exposure to hepatitis B from needle sharing with a known carrier. In addition to testing for other infectious diseases contracted by needle sharing, the following are the most likely laboratory findings indicating a hepatitis B infection if labs were taken the day of the visit:

a. HBV DNA negative, HBV core protein IgM negative, HBsAg negative

b. HBV DNA positive, HBV core protein IgM positive, HBsAg positive

c. HBV DNA positive, HBV core protein IgM positive, HBsAg negative

d. HBV DNA positive, HBV core protein IgM negative, HBsAg negative

e. HBV DNA positive, HBV core protein IgM negative, HBsAg positive

17-14. A mother with no prenatal care gives birth to a term infant with findings of IUGR, microcephaly, hepatosplenomegaly, thrombocytopenia, and during later testing sensorineural hearing loss and polymicrogyria. There is no history of cat exposure or raw meat exposure during pregnancy. This presentation is concerning for which congenital infection?

a. Cytomegalovirus (CMV)

b. Syphilis

c. Toxoplasmosis

d. Hepatitis B

e. *Neisseria gonorrhoeae*

17-15. A mother with no prenatal care gives birth to a term infant with findings of IUGR, microcephaly, hepatosplenomegaly, thrombocytopenia, and during later testing sensorineural hearing loss. You are concerned about cytomegalovirus (CMV). The most important diagnostic study for CMV evaluation for a newborn is:

a. Viral culture

b. Brain biopsy

c. Viral PCR

d. Rapid plasma reagin (RPR)

e. Antibody titers

17-16. A mother and daughter are in travel clinic, awaiting vaccination for yellow fever. The mother asks about symptoms of yellow fever. Which of the following findings is most commonly associated specifically with yellow fever infection?

a. Retro-orbital pain

b. Morbilliform rash

c. Bradycardia despite fever

d. Purulent pharyngitis, conjunctivitis, and edema

e. Swollen baby syndrome

17-17. A young man presents with symptoms of ongoing fever and sore throat for the past week along with mild headache and malaise. On examination of the oropharynx, he has reddened and enlarged tonsils without exudate with fine petechiae over the uvula and soft palate. There is bilateral cervical adenopathy present. Abdominal examination reveals an enlarged spleen. A rapid group A *Streptococcus* test from yesterday is negative. Hematologic tests from the day before show a slightly elevated white blood cell count and a mild thrombocytopenia of 120,000 platelets/μL. A blood smear is obtained.

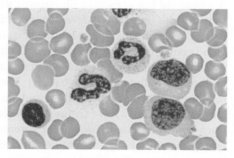

(Reproduced, with permission, from Lichtman MA, et al. *Wiliams Hematology.* 7th ed. New York: McGraw-Hill, 2006.)

The best treatment for the patient's condition is:

a. Acyclovir

b. Corticosteroids

c. Chemotherapy

d. Symptomatic treatment

e. Amoxicillin

17-18. A young girl who was born outside the United States is hospitalized for a rash with mild fever and itching, initially thought to be Stevens-Johnson syndrome. On further evaluation, however, the patient is diagnosed with chickenpox based on her now characteristic rash and immunofluorescent antibody staining of the vesicle's base. She is the only one in her family with the disease and is immunocompetent. The patient is placed in an isolated room, treated symptomatically for her fever and itching, with antipyretics and a histamine blocker, respectively, and observed. On day 4 of the exanthem, her rash seems to be worsening and is more painful. She continues to have high fevers. The next best course of action is to:

a. Start acyclovir.

b. Start antibiotics.

c. Start intravenous γ globulin.

d. Continue symptomatic treatment.

e. Start topical hydrocortisone.

17-19. An infant is born to an HIV-positive mother with low viral counts who is on antiretroviral therapy during the pregnancy, and who is delivered via caesarean section. The patient is initially started on zidovudine monotherapy. The optimal schedule for HIV testing in this newborn would be:

a. HIV antibody testing at birth, 14 to 21 days, 4 to 6 weeks, and 4 to 6 months of age.

b. HIV antibody testing at >1 month of age and >6 months of age.

c. HIV DNA/RNA assays at >1 month of age and >4 months of age.

d. HIV DNA/RNA assays 4 times during the first 4 to 6 months.

e. No testing can be completed until zidovudine is stopped.

17-20. Twelve children in a local Amish community have contracted a similar infection. They all present with a rising fever, conjunctivitis, cough and cold symptoms, and a maculopapular rash that appears on days 3 to 4 of fevers and that spreads from the hairline downward within a 24-hour span. All 12 children attend school together and 11 of the 12 are unvaccinated. One of the boys in the group is noted to have a few white lesions on his oral mucosa surrounded with red areolae. Which of the following is the most common complication of this disease process?

a. Subacute sclerosing panencephalitis

b. Corneal ulcers

c. Myocarditis

d. Spontaneous bleeding

e. Acute otitis media

17-21. A pregnant mother is picking up her child from day care when she is informed that there was a recent outbreak of parvovirus. She brings her child into the clinic the following day where her daughter is diagnosed with erythema infectiosum based on low-grade fever and a reticular, macular rash that appeared overnight. The mother is pregnant at 15 weeks and as such asks that her child be formally tested. The daughter is found to be IgM positive and IgG positive. Given concern for fetal effects the mother undergoes testing with the following results: IgM negative and IgG positive.

Based on these findings the best recommendation would be to:

a. Repeat the mother's antibody testing in 2 to 3 weeks.

b. Follow fetal ultrasounds weekly.

c. Tell the mother that no further testing is necessary.

d. Conduct parvovirus PCR testing from the mother's serum.

e. Conduct parvovirus IgM testing from fetal cordocentesis at 22 weeks.

17-22. A 12-year-old girl presents with abdominal pain, headache, and flu-like symptoms for 1 week. Several days later the patient begins experiencing increased headache and neck pain. She additionally has difficulty swallowing with increasing episodes of what are thought to be laryngeal spasms along with generalized weakness and progressive paralysis. She lives in a rural area.

Initial evaluation of the cerebral spinal fluid does not reveal any bacteria. Samples are sent for evaluation of different causes of encephalitis. Brain biopsy is undertaken given the patient's worsening condition and reveals Negri bodies.

The patient's current condition could have best been prevented by means of:

a. Passive and active immunization

b. Careful examination for ticks after exposures

c. Application of topical *N*, *N*-diethyl-*m*-toluamide (DEET)

d. Sodium stibogluconate

e. Albendazole

17-23. A 10-year-old girl presents at your primary care clinic with her parents for concerns about rabies.

Three days ago, she was on a school field trip where the class spent 2 nights in cabins in a rural area. On the last night it was noted that the inside, upper corner of the cabin roof was "infested" with several bats. The 3 bats later escaped. Of note, none of the 5 children or 2 adults recalled being bitten by the bats.

On examination, she is alert, calm, and cooperative. Temperature is 36.8°C axillary. Pulse is 95 bpm. Respiratory rate is 20 bpm. On examination of the skin, there were no lacerations or puncture wounds. Neurologic examination is nonfocal with a stable gait and station.

What is the appropriate recommendation for this patient?

a. Assume no rabies exposure as no bite marks are noted; no treatment is needed.

b. Assume rabies exposure; recommend immediate rabies immunization.

c. Assume rabies exposure; recommend immediate rabies immune globulin.

d. Assume rabies exposure; recommend immediate rabies immunization and immune globulin.

e. No bite marks noted; recommend nonurgent rabies immunization for future camping trips.

17-24. A father brings his 2 sons into the clinic with a primary complaint of perianal and perineal pruritus. He also states that on changing the diaper of the younger child a few days ago, he noted what looked like "white strings." A Scotch tape test is positive for pinworm ova in both children. In addition to a single dose of albendazole and a repeated dose 2 weeks later for the entire family, you should recommend:

a. Treatment with pyrantel pamoate for the parents

b. Shaking out the bed sheets prior to washing

c. Bathing well the morning after treatment

d. Discussing ways to improve the hygiene at the home

e. Installing nylon water filters

17-25. A 3-year-old boy presents with ongoing wheezing and rhonchi with intermittent fevers for several weeks. The patient's chest radiograph is nonspecific and a complete blood count reveals marked eosinophilia but otherwise no abnormalities. Further evaluation reveals an elevated erythrocyte sedimentation rate (ESR). The patient is tested for antihemagglutinin titers and has an elevated anti-B. He is from a low-income household. You also learn on further questioning of the parents that the family has several dogs. In addition, the patient has been seen eating dirt outside on occasion. The best treatment for this patient's condition should include:

a. Iron

b. Vitamin B_{12}

c. Praziquantel

d. Mebendazole

e. Albendazole

17-26. A mother and 2 children present several hours after eating sushi at a street fair with symptoms of severe stomach pain, nausea, and vomiting. On further history the mother relates that they all ate salmon and mackerel from the vendor that was "fresh caught." While waiting for further tests, one of the children vomits up a small worm that is identified as an anisakid larva. The next best step in therapy is:

a. Praziquantel

b. Albendazole

c. Supportive care

d. Endoscopic retrieval

e. Induction of vomiting

17-27. A 10-month-old girl is brought in by her parents because of concern over several small, white pieces in her stool that "look like rice" and are motile. They have been present for several weeks and the patient is otherwise asymptomatic. The small white bodies are submitted to the pathology lab that identifies them as gravid proglottids from *Dipylidium caninum*. This infection was most likely acquired from:

a. Ingestion of a dog or cat flea

b. Being bitten by a dog or cat flea

c. Ingestion of dog or cat feces

d. Arthropod bite

e. Larval penetration of the epidermis and dermis

17-28. A 14-year-old boy who recently emigrated from South America presents to the local emergency department after suffering a seizure. He has no family history or past history of seizures. His schoolmates report his right hand started shaking while the patient was in class and within a minute he lost consciousness, developing whole-body shaking, and subsequently stopped about 2 minutes later. An MRI done that day reveals the following image:

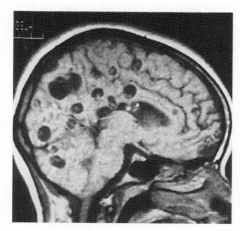

(Reproduced, with permission, from Rudolph CD, et al. *Rudolph's Pediatrics*. 22nd ed. New York: McGraw-Hill, 2011.)

Treatment for the patient's condition most likely includes:

a. Intravenous antibiotic medication

b. Intravenous antifungal medication

c. Intravenous antihelminth medication

d. Antiepileptic medication

e. Percutaneous drainage of cysts

17-29. An otherwise healthy 6-year-old boy is hospitalized for right upper quadrant abdominal pain, high fevers, and chills. Findings on liver ultrasonography are consistent with a liver abscess. He traveled with his parents to Mexico 4 months ago but has not traveled since that time. Blood cultures and stool samples are no growth after 2 days and serologic tests are pending. Liver abscess aspiration under CT guidance yields a yellow and gray paste-like material. A culture of the material reveals no growth. It is noted to be surprisingly odorless. The most likely diagnosis for this patient is a/an:

a. Hydatid liver cyst

b. Bacterial liver abscess

c. Amebic liver abscess

d. Fungal liver abscess

e. Malarial hypnozoite infection

17-30. A 6-year-old child presents with intermittent fevers up to 40°C for the past week including chills and sweats with occasional nausea. He recently visited his grandparents in southern New England during the summer. The area is endemic with deer ticks. The parents have been treating the child with antipyretics. The patient denies headache symptoms and during periods without fever says he feels much better. No rash is reported. In addition, no tick bite is reported. You recommend the following:

a. Supportive care with antipyretics.

b. Immediate treatment with amoxicillin.

c. Immediate treatment with doxycyline.

d. Testing for Lyme disease is clinically indicated.

e. Testing for babesiosis is clinically indicated.

17-31. A 4-year-old child is being seen for over a week of watery diarrhea, with several stools per day. The patient has had no fever, and no blood in the stool. Examination for ova and parasites is negative. An ELISA test is positive for *Cryptosporidium*. The patient is HIV negative. The most appropriate recommendation for this patient is:

a. Avoiding water that is nonchlorinated

b. Treatment with nitazoxanide

c. Treatment with paromomycin and azithromycin

d. Treatment with albendazole

e. Treatment with metronidazole

17-32. A teenage girl from the southeast United States presents to the emergency department complaining of fever, nausea, and headache. There are mild meningeal signs. The patient also notes a loss of smell. Further history from the patient's family details that she went swimming 4 days ago in a local river. CSF demonstrates large numbers of neutrophils, blood, hypoglycorrhachia, and elevated protein. Despite early treatment with amphotericin B and rifampin, the patient dies 7 days after presentation. Pathologic diagnosis is most likely to confirm that the patient suffered from:

a. *Naegleria fowleri* meningoencephalitis

b. Cryptococcal meningoencephalitis

c. Herpes encephalitis

d. *Baylisascaris* meningoencephalitis

e. Tick-borne encephalitis virus infection

17-33. The parents of a healthy 4-year-old girl who weighs 22 kg are planning to travel to India and want to get malaria prophylaxis prior to the journey. After discussion of their travels you determine they are going to an area with chloroquine-resistant *Plasmodium falciparum*. The best recommendation for a malaria prophylaxis agent for their daughter is:

a. Doxycyline

b. Atovaquone/proguanil

c. Quinine sulfate

d. Mefloquine

e. Clindamycin

17-34. A 5-year-old boy presents with foul-smelling diarrhea along with mild abdominal pain and loss of appetite for 2 weeks. He returned from a science camp over a week ago and he is now about to return to kindergarten. Evaluation of the patient's stool sample taken that day is positive for *Giardia lamblia* by EIA. The best treatment for the patient's condition would be:

a. Tinidazole

b. Metronidazole

c. Furazolidone

d. Nitazoxanide

e. Paromomycin

17-35. Your team is asked to consult on a teenage patient being treated with intensive antileukemic therapy. The patient now reports overnight onset of tachypnea and cough. He has no fever. The patient has also had decreased oxygen saturation since yesterday and is requiring supplemental oxygen. Review of the patient's chart reveals that he has not been receiving trimethoprim–sulfamethoxazole due to a pharmacy error. Chest radiograph reveals bilateral, diffuse alveolar disease with granular opacities. The preferred method for diagnosis of the patient's condition is:

a. Open lung biopsy

b. Bronchoalveolar lavage

c. DNA/RNA PCR

d. Gastric lavage

e. Hematoxylin and eosin staining

17-36. A 24-year-old female is diagnosed at 16 weeks of pregnancy via antibody titers as likely having contracted *Toxoplasma gondii* during gestation. She recently arrived from France to the United States. She is started on spiramycin and is scheduled for an ultrasound and an amniotic fluid PCR at 18 weeks with her new obstetrician. She is most likely to have acquired this infection by means of:

a. Blood transfusion

b. Food containing tissue cysts

c. Ingested house cat oocysts

d. Municipal water supply

e. Cat fleas containing larvae

17-37. A 4-year-old boy is brought into the emergency department with symptoms of fever, headache, a stiff neck, and altered mental status. On examination, he is also noted to have mild hypotension and sparse areas of petechiae. His family relates that the young boy has a history of severe anaphylactic reactions to amoxicillin and cephalexin. The best IV empiric therapy for the patient would be:

a. Cefotaxime

b. Ampicillin and gentamicin

c. Vancomycin and gentamicin

d. Vancomycin and chloramphenicol

e. Vancomycin and cefotaxime

17-38. A 2-year-old girl is hospitalized for a week with symptoms of altered mental status and headache. For the past 2 weeks, she has had an influenza-like illness. Her symptoms began in February. She has not had any seizures. Cerebrospinal fluid results showed a moderate mononuclear pleocytosis, with elevated protein and mild hypoglycorrhachia. Bacterial cultures are negative. The social worker, after speaking to the family, states that there is a rodent infestation in the family's house. The girl makes a full recovery after receiving supportive care and brief rehabilitation services. The most likely etiology is:

a. West Nile virus

b. Lymphocytic choriomeningitis virus (LCMV)

c. Herpes simplex virus-1

d. Mumps virus

e. Western equine encephalitis virus

17-39. A 15-year-old girl presents with symptoms of vaginal irritation, pruritus, and discharge. She is sexually active and uses condoms during sexual intercourse. She denies dysuria. A urine pregnancy test is negative. Tests are sent using the patient's urine for *Chlamydia* and gonorrhea. Examination reveals a normal-appearing cervix without motion tenderness and a nonspecific vaginal gray discharge with a pH >4.5 that has a slight fishy odor. Sodium chloride microscopy reveals a few PMNs but no trichomonads and possible stippling of some epithelial cells. The best presumptive treatment for the patient's condition would be:

a. Metronidazole 500 mg orally, twice daily, for 7 days

b. Metronidazole 2 g orally, once

c. Fluconazole 150 mg orally, once

d. Azithromycin 1 g orally, once, and ceftriaxone 250 mg IM, once

e. Tinidazole 2 g orally, once

17-40. A father brings in his 18-month-old son who is exhibiting symptoms of fever and refusal to walk. On examination, he is noted to be holding his right hip slightly flexed, abducted, and externally rotated and cries if the leg is passively manipulated. The patient has both an elevated ESR and CRP. Joint aspiration reveals a white blood cell count of 6000 WBC/mm^3. With this clinical information you are able to:

a. Exclude septic arthritis.

b. Exclude osteomyelitis.

c. Start empiric antibiotics.

d. Defer blood cultures.

e. Recommend arthrotomy.

17-41. You are rounding on a 14-year-old boy admitted to the pediatric ward yesterday for periorbital cellulitis of the right eye. On history his family reports that he frequently has sinus problems and seasonal allergies. The patient was started on oral clindamycin yesterday morning, but today shows signs of mild proptosis and chemosis that were not present at admission. The next best step is to:

a. Obtain an imaging of the orbit.

b. Change his antibiotic to IV vancomycin.

c. Change his antibiotic to IV cefotaxime.

d. Obtain an aspirate at the point of maximal periorbital skin inflammation.

e. Begin topical ophthalmic steroid therapy.

17-42. In the primary care clinic there are several patients whose parents have inquired about prophylaxis for dental procedures. Of the following patients, who best fits the recommendations for endocarditis prophylaxis when undergoing dental procedures?

a. A 6-year-old with a history of infective endocarditis (IE)

b. A 7-year-old with a history of rheumatic heart disease

c. A 12-year-old girl who had patch repair of her ventricular septal defect at age 3

d. A 5-year-old girl who has an unrepaired atrial septal defect

e. A 14-year-old boy with a bicuspid aortic valve

17-43. A 15-year-old boy presents with several days of worsening diarrhea and abdominal cramping. He and his parent describe his stool as very loose with ample mucous and reported blood. In clinic, the stool sample from the patient tests positive for blood with guaiac testing. The patient has no history of recent antibiotic use and no history of travel. He is not having fevers and is otherwise healthy. In addition to sending off a bacterial stool culture, the best additional test would be:

a. A blood culture

b. A stool enzyme immunoassay for *C. difficile* toxins

c. A stool sample for ova and parasite testing

d. A stool enzyme immunoassay for *Giardia*

e. A stool enzyme immunoassay for Shiga toxins

17-44. A 6-month-old infant who recently underwent a Kasai procedure (portoenterostomy) for biliary atresia presents to the pediatric emergency department with a fever. The patient's examination shows no clear source of the fever and urine laboratory results show no signs of infection. Blood laboratory results demonstrate a modest rise in the patient's bilirubin and white blood cell count. The most likely infectious etiology for the patient's condition is:

a. *Cytomegalovirus*

b. *Enterococcus*

c. *Entamoeba*

d. *Salmonella*

e. *Streptococcus*

17-45. A 12-day-old infant is found to have poor feeding, irritability, and prolonged jaundice. A urine catheterization is found to be positive for leukocyte esterase and urine culture returns a gram-positive organism to be further identified. He is started on appropriate antibiotics. This neonate was at higher risk for a urinary tract infection because:

a. He was term.

b. He was male.

c. He was circumcised.

d. He was exclusively breastfed.

e. He was blood type O.

17-46. While examining a young girl receiving total parenteral nutrition through a peripherally inserted central catheter, an area of induration along the catheter's subcutaneous path is noted. The patient reports it is mildly painful. There is no sign of redness or pain at the catheter exit site. She is otherwise feeling well without any fevers or systemic symptoms. Cultures taken from the catheter and peripherally are negative. The most appropriate next step would include:

a. A trial of topical antibiotics

b. Removal of the catheter

c. Treatment with IV vancomycin

d. Treatment with IV cefepime

e. Treatment with IV vancomycin and IV cefepime

17-47. An 11-year-old boy presents to the clinic with a neck mass. His mother reports that she noticed the mass several months ago, but in the last few weeks the mass has become hard. On physical examination, the boy is afebrile and has normal vital signs. The mass is on the angle of his jaw. He has no cervical lymphadenopathy. You perform an excisional biopsy. The Gram stain of

the tissue shows gram-positive filamentous, acid-fast negative organisms. After further questioning, the boy remembers having a molar tooth extracted several months before the mass developed.

What is the most likely etiology?

a. *Bartonella henselae*

b. *Actinomycosis israelii*

c. Mumps

d. *Moraxella catarrhalis*

e. Molluscum contagiosum

17-48. An 11-year-old boy is diagnosed with actinomycosis after presenting to the clinic with a neck mass. The diagnosis is confirmed after an excisional biopsy and a Gram stain of the tissue showed gram-positive filamentous, acid-fast negative organisms.

Which of the following is the preferred treatment for this infection?

a. Penicillin

b. Ceftriaxone

c. Vancomycin

d. Clindamycin

e. Bactrim

17-49. A 4-year-old boy presents to the emergency department with severe abdominal pain and watery diarrhea for the last 12 hours. Examination notes diffuse abdominal tenderness and an on-call surgeon is consulted to rule out an acute appendicitis. CT scan shows a normal appendix. While you are taking a careful history, his mother mentions that he woke up early yesterday morning and ate a leftover chicken burrito that his older teenage brother did not refrigerate the night before. You order a stool culture. Twenty-four hours later, the laboratory technician calls you and informs you that the Gram stain of the stool culture shows abundant, motile, comma-shaped, gram-negative bacilli.

Which of the following is the most likely organism causing this child's illness?

a. *Salmonella*

b. *Campylobacter*

c. *Shigella*

d. Shiga toxin–producing *E. coli* (STEC)

e. *Giardia*

17-50. A 14-year-old boy with pneumonia was just discharged from the hospital after being treated with broad-spectrum antibiotics for 2 weeks. He started having diarrhea on day 14 of illness. Stool testing revealed positive *Clostridium difficile* toxin by ELISA.

Which of the following is the best treatment option at this point?

a. Oral metronidazole.

b. Oral vancomycin.

c. IV vancomycin.

d. Rifampin.

e. No treatment is needed.

17-51. A 4-month-old male infant presents to your clinic for constipation and poor feeding. As you walk into the room, you notice that the baby has a weak cry with an expressionless face. On your physical examination, you notice poor suck with significant head lag. You also notice symmetric weakness of his upper extremities.

What is the most likely diagnosis?

a. Group B *Streptococcus*

b. *Shigella flexneri*

c. *Clostridium botulinum*

d. Hirschsprung disease

e. Down syndrome

17-52. You suspect infant botulism in a 14-week-old male infant who presents with constipation and poor feeding, as well as a weak cry, poor suck, an expressionless face, and significant head lag on examination.

What is the best next step in management of this patient?

a. Admit the baby to the hospital for supportive care.

b. Admit the baby to the hospital for supportive care and immediately administer human-derived Botulism Immune Globulin Intravenous (BIG-IV).

c. Admit the baby and start IV aminoglycosides.

d. Send a stool specimen for toxin assay to confirm diagnosis prior to hospital admission.

e. None of the above.

17-53. You suspect infant botulism in a 14-week-old male infant who presents with constipation and poor feeding, as well as a weak cry, poor suck, an expressionless face, and significant head lag on examination.

What is the best method to confirm the diagnosis?

a. Electromyographic (EMG) stimulation studies

b. A serum IgM level for *C. botulinum*

c. A serum toxin assay

d. A stool specimen for toxin assay

e. A stool culture for *C. botulinum*

17-54. A 16-year-old Hispanic male from California presents to the emergency department with fever for 3 weeks associated with night sweats. He complains of diffuse joint pain and malaise. On examination, you note hepatosplenomegaly, lymphadenopathy, and arthritis.

His mother reports that they just moved to California, and are living on a farm. On further questioning, the mother reports that they make their own goat cheese that he enjoys eating.

What is the most likely etiology?

a. *Naegleria fowleri*

b. *Bartonella henselae*

c. *Leptospira interrogans*

d. *Chlamydophila psittaci*

e. *Brucella abortus*

17-55. A 16-year-old Hispanic male from California presents with fever, hepatosplenomegaly, lymphadenopathy, and arthritis. The mother reports that they make their own goat cheese that he enjoys eating. Based on your history and examination, you suspect brucellosis.

Which of the following is the best treatment option?

a. Doxycycline for 6 weeks

b. Doxycycline for 45 days and gentamicin for 7 days

c. Rifampin for 4 to 6 weeks

d. Trimethoprim–sulfamethoxazole for 4 to 6 weeks

e. None of the above

17-56. A 16-year-old girl presents to your clinic with a round mass under her axillary area. She says that she first noticed this mass 2 weeks ago. There is no redness or tenderness overlying the right axilla. She was seen at an urgent care when it first started and was given a 7-day course of clindamycin with no improvement. Last night she noticed some purulent drainage oozing out of the lymph node that prompted her to come to your clinic. Past medical history is negative. She is not sexually active. She lives with her mother in Missouri, and was camping 2 months ago. She recently received a new kitten and a puppy for her birthday.

What is the most likely diagnosis?

a. Staphylococcal lymphadenitis

b. Streptococcal lymphadenitis

c. Cat scratch disease (CSD)

d. Human immunodeficiency virus (HIV)

e. Lymphoma

17-57. You have diagnosed a 16-year-old girl with cat scratch disease (CSD) after she presented with a right axillary mass. The mass has been present for 2 weeks. Her past medical history is negative.

What is the most accurate statement regarding treatment and prognosis?

a. Treatment of CSD is supportive.

b. Azithromycin is indicated.

c. Needle aspiration of lesions is curative.

d. She should avoid contact with immunocompromised patients.

e. She has a 35% chance of relapse of CSD.

17-58. While you are doing your rotation in a hospital in South Florida, you see a 17-year-old female in the ED complaining of extremely profuse watery diarrhea associated with crampy abdominal pain and generalized weakness. The diarrhea has become quite copious. It is pale gray in color with the appearance of "rice water."

She has just arrived from a mission after volunteering in Haiti after the earthquake. You send a stool specimen. Given her travel history, the diagnosis that you are mostly concerned about is:

a. Enterotoxigenic *Escherichia coli* traveler's diarrhea

b. Shigellosis

c. Rotavirus gastroenteritis

d. Toxigenic *V. cholera*

e. *Giardia* infection

17-59. You are treating a 17-year-old female for toxigenic *Vibrio cholera*. She is hospitalized and continues to have watery diarrhea, abdominal pain, and generalized weakness. What is the most common complication associated with this infection?

a. Thrombocytopenia

b. Shock

c. Intussusception

d. Gastrointestinal hemorrhage

e. Hemolytic anemia

17-60. A 12-year-old girl presents to your office with severe earache for 1 day. Yesterday she won several ribbons at a swimming meet. Initially the ear was pruritic, but has become more painful. On physical examination, she complains of severe pain when the auricle is pulled superiorly. You gently use your otoscope to try to see the tympanic membrane, but because of the edematous ear canal you are able to see only part of the canal. You are not able to visualize the tympanic membrane.

The most likely organism causing her symptoms is:

a. *Staphylococcus aureus*

b. *Haemophilus influenzae*

c. *Aspergillus niger*

d. *Pseudomonas aeruginosa*

e. *Moraxella catarrhalis*

17-61. You see a 13-year-old girl who has previously been treated for 2 episodes of otitis externa over the summer. She has been a very successful competitive swimmer and plans to continue swimming throughout the year. The parents ask you about different treatments that can be used to prevent another case of otitis externa.

Which of the following is the best strategy for the prevention of otitis externa for this patient?

a. Using ear plugs while swimming should be avoided because it will trap moisture and increase the likelihood of infection.

b. Using alcohol ear drops before and after swimming lowers the pH in the ear canal and helps prevent infection.

c. Taking low-dose oral antibiotics during the swimming season can help prevent infection.

d. Keeping the ear canal moist throughout the day will prevent fluctuations in moisture and decrease infections in the ear canal.

e. The patient should end her swimming career and consider other sports that do not involve water immersion.

17-62. You are treating a 17-year-old girl with otitis externa. There is no surrounding cellulitis or adenitis. Which of the following treatments is not appropriate for this case?

a. A combination polymyxin B/neomycin/hydrocortisone otic preparation

b. A combination ciprofloxacin and hydrocortisone otic preparation

c. Ciprofloxacin otic drops

d. Ofloxacin otic drops

e. Systemic antibiotics to cover *Pseudomonas aeruginosa*

17-63. A 14-year-old girl presented 2 days ago to the pediatric acute care clinic with sore throat. The rapid strep test was negative, but you sent for a throat culture.

The throat culture now shows colonies of gram-positive bacilli with a black opaque dot in the center of each colony. You call the patient to notify her of the results, and she informs you that she started to have a rash on her arms, especially on her extensor surfaces, but it is now fading.

The most likely organism causing her symptoms is:

a. *Arcanobacterium haemolyticum*

b. Group A β-hemolytic streptococci (GAS)

c. Epstein Barr Virus (EBV)

d. *Neisseria gonorrhoeae*

e. *Corynebacterium diphtheriae*

17-64. A 6-year-old previously healthy boy presented to the ED with fever, chills, and headache. Chest radiograph showed bilateral extensive interstitial infiltrates. In terms of pets at home, his older sister has a kitten and 1 macaw. Until recently, he had a parrot, which died recently from an unknown illness.

What is the most likely diagnosis?

a. Psittacosis

b. *Mycoplasma pneumoniae*

c. *Legionella pneumophila*

d. Community-acquired pneumonia

e. Influenza pneumonia

17-65. A 17-year-old girl presents with cough for 4 weeks. Examination shows diffuse rales and a chest radiograph notes a patchy infiltrate throughout. Immunizations are up-to-date. There is no history of travel or exposure to animals.

What are the most likely diagnoses?

a. *Chlamydia trachomatis*

b. *Chlamydophila psittaci* and *Mycoplasma pneumoniae*

c. *C. trachomatis* and *M. pneumoniae*

d. *Chlamydophila pneumoniae* and *M. pneumoniae*

e. *C. pneumoniae*, *C. trachomatis*, and *M. pneumoniae*

17-66. You are treating a 17-year-old girl who presents with cough for 4 weeks. She has pulmonary findings on examination and on her chest radiograph. In developing a treatment plan, you want to make sure you cover for atypical pneumonias, such as *Chlamydophila pneumoniae*. What is the drug of choice for the treatment of *C. pneumoniae*?

a. Azithromycin

b. Clindamycin

c. Bactrim

d. Amoxicillin

e. Levofloxacin

17-67. A 1-year-old infant presents with difficulty breathing and "fits" of coughing for the past 2 days. For the past few weeks he has had rhinorrhea and a mild cough; however, over the past 2 days, his parents have noted that his cough has continued to get worse. He has episodes of rapid coughing followed by an inspiratory sound as he catches his breath. This afternoon, he had an episode of nonbloody, nonbilious emesis after one of these coughing "fits." There is no past medical history; however, the child last had immunizations at 2 months of age. There is no history of fever. You begin a workup that includes a complete blood count (CBC).

What findings, associated with the child's diagnosis, would you expect on the CBC?

a. A macrocytic anemia (Hgb <8)

b. A thrombocytopenia (<100,000 platelets)

c. A bandemia (>10% bands)

d. An eosinophilia (>10% eosinophils)

e. A lymphocytosis (>10,000 lymphocytes/mm³)

17-68. You have diagnosed a 1-year-old infant with pertussis after he presents with difficulty breathing and "fits" of coughing for the past 2 days. Which of the following is the most common complication of pertussis?

a. Death

b. Rib fractures

c. Pneumonia

d. Seizures

e. Encephalopathy

17-69. You have diagnosed a 1-year-old infant with pertussis after he presents with difficulty breathing and "fits" of coughing for the past 2 days. Which of the following statements is correct about the treatment of pertussis?

a. Initiation of treatment with antibiotics once the paroxysmal phase has started will not have an effect on the patient's course of illness.

b. Trimethoprim–sulfamethoxazole is first-line antibiotic treatment.

c. Treatment with antibiotics is reserved only for confirmed cases of pertussis.

d. Treatment with cough expectorants and mucolytic agents is helpful for pertussis.

e. Supportive care for pertussis includes aggressive suctioning to remove mucus that may trigger paroxysms.

17-70. A 14-day-old infant presents with difficulty breathing and grunting. The diagnosis of pertussis is confirmed via polymerase chain reaction (PCR) testing on nasopharyngeal swab specimen.

What is the appropriate plan for prophylaxis?

a. Prophylaxis is given to unimmunized individuals only for 14 days after the last contact.

b. Household and day care contacts of confirmed pertussis patients should receive antibiotic prophylaxis for 14 days after the last contact.

c. Trimethoprim/sulfamethoxazole is the drug of choice for prophylaxis for 21 days after the last contact.

d. Prophylaxis for 21 days is needed only for the personnel who intubate the patient.

e. There is no prophylaxis needed, as pertussis is a self-limiting disease.

17-71. A 15-day-old infant presents with difficulty breathing and grunting. The diagnosis of pertussis is confirmed via polymerase chain reaction (PCR) testing on nasopharyngeal swab specimen. You decide to hospitalize the patient.

What is the best isolation plan for this patient?

a. No isolation

b. Contact isolation

c. Droplet isolation

d. Airborne isolation

e. Routine hand washing

17-72. A former 32-week-infant, who is now 13 days old in the NICU, presents with temperature instability, apnea, and increased residuals for nasogastric feedings. Blood culture at 24 hours is positive for enteroccocci species. The infant's bilirubin level peaked at 9 mg/dL at 5 days of age and he does not appear jaundiced.

What is the most likely underlying condition present in this patient?

a. Agammaglobulinemia

b. Galactosemia

c. Biliary atresia

d. Necrotizing enterocolitis

e. Breast milk jaundice

17-73. A 5-year-old previously healthy male is brought by his mother to the emergency department. She reports he was doing well, but since this morning he has had trouble breathing and is refusing to eat. In the ED, he is ill-appearing, and has temperature 38°C, RR 40, BP 90/50, and HR 100 bpm. He has bilateral chest retractions, and is leaning forward on the examination table and has also started drooling.

What is the next best step?

a. Obtain a lateral neck x-ray.

b. Start IV fluids.

c. Admit the patient for observation.

d. Immediately start IV ceftriaxone.

e. Consult the anesthesia service.

17-74. A 1-day-old infant is born prematurely. The birth was induced secondary to maternal hemodynamic instability and septic-like picture following a nonspecific flu-like illness and gastroenteritis.

The baby in the newborn nursery suddenly becomes septic. A full workup is performed including CSF analysis that shows: total cells 120, nucleated cells 100, 75% neutrophils, 13% lymphocytes, and 12% monocytes. CSF glucose is 39; CSF protein is 160 mg/dL. The mother reported a history of nonspecific flu-like illness around the time of delivery.

What is the most likely diagnosis?

a. Aseptic meningitis

b. Hypoglycemia

c. Listeriosis

d. Galactosemia

e. Necrotizing enterocolitis

17-75. You are concerned about the possibility of *Listeria monocytogenes* infection in a 1-day-old infant who born prematurely. The mother reported a history of nonspecific flu-like illness around the time of delivery.

Of the following, which is the best treatment for *L. monocytogenes*?

a. Ampicillin

b. Trimethoprim–sulfamethoxazole

c. Gentamicin

d. Cefazolin

e. Vancomycin

17-76. A 3-year-old female presents with an anterior cervical neck mass that developed over the past several days in the setting of a URI.

On physical examination, she is afebrile with a unilateral anterior cervical lymph node. The node is enlarged to 3 × 4 cm in diameter. It is tender, erythematous, and soft without fluctuance. Her past medical history is negative for prior similar episodes. There is no history of pet or animal exposure.

What is the most likely causative organism?

a. *Staphylococcus aureus*

b. *M. avium* complex (MAC)

c. Cat scratch disease

d. Group B *Streptococcus* (GABHS)

e. *Mycobacterium tuberculosis*

17-77. A 16-year-old healthy female presents with back pain and dysuria. Her urine culture is positive for *Staphylococcus*. Which of the following species is the most likely organism?

a. *S. epidermidis*

b. *S. hominis*

c. *S. aureus*

d. *Staphylococcus saprophyticus*

e. Methicillin-resistant *S. aureus* (MRSA)

17-78. A now 3-day-old neonate born at 25 3/7 weeks EGA is found to be bacteremic with *Staphylococcus aureus* after workup for sudden blood pressure instability. Despite appropriate antibiotic coverage, his blood cultures remain positive.

What is the next best step in management?

a. Remove his intravascular catheter as soon as possible.

b. Apply topical mupirocin in the nares as an adjunctive antibacterial therapy.

c. Add gentamicin.

d. Check CBC, CRP, and ESR daily to monitor response.

e. Start dialysis.

17-79. A healthy, term infant male is born to a 27-year-old woman with known untreated syphilis. Which of the following describes the best initial management strategy?

a. Full physical examination, RPR or VDRL serum testing, CSF testing, CBC, and long bone radiographs

b. Full physical examination, FTA-ABS serum testing, CBC, and long bone radiographs

c. Full physical examination and RPR or VDRL serum testing

d. RPR or VDRL serum testing

e. Full physical examination, FTA-ABS serum testing, CSF testing, CBC, and long bone radiographs

17-80. A full-term infant in the newborn nursery is born to a 19-year-old mother who is diagnosed with syphilis. What is the drug of choice for treatment of neonatal syphilis?

a. Tetracycline

b. Erythromycin

c. Penicillin G

d. Vancomycin

e. Azithromycin

17-81. A full-term infant in the newborn nursery is born to a 16-year-old mother who is diagnosed with syphilis. The mother reports severe allergic reaction to penicillin when she was treated for strep throat a year ago. You would like to treat the mother as well as the child. What is the drug of choice for treatment of syphilis in an adolescent patient with penicillin drug allergy?

a. Ceftriaxone

b. Tetracycline

c. Penicillin G

d. Vancomycin

e. Azithromycin

17-82. A 6-year-old male presents to the emergency department with large annular red macule on his arm with a targetoid pattern of central clearing after returning from a family trip in Connecticut. He additionally complains of tactile fevers, myalgias, and arthralgias of his lower limbs. The boy denies camping, but the mother reports removing a tick off him a week ago.

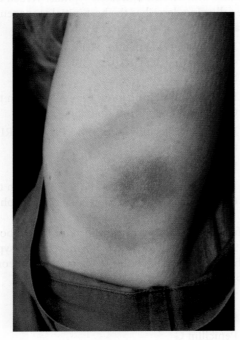

Based on this child's history and rash, what is the most likely diagnosis?

a. Tularemia

b. Lyme disease

c. Rocky mountain spotted fever

d. *Ehrlichia*

e. Kawasaki disease

17-83. A 10-year-old male presents to the emergency department with a large, erythematous targetoid lesion on his arm after returning from a family trip in Connecticut. You suspect Lyme disease.

What is the first-line treatment for Lyme disease?

a. Doxycycline

b. Trimethoprim–sulfamethoxazole

c. Ceftriaxone

d. Vancomycin

e. No need to treat, self-resolving illness

17-84. A 17-year-old college student presents to your clinic with a cough for 3 weeks and no other associated symptoms. Her 3-year-old nephew who lives in the same house had recently recovered from a similar illness of cough and posttussive emesis. Of note, there is a newborn infant in the house who is healthy. What is the most appropriate next step?

a. Obtain a chest radiograph to rule out bacterial pneumonia.

b. Obtain a NP swab for pertussis PCR, and consider giving Tdap booster to the patient and to the rest of unimmunized family members.

c. Start azithromycin for 14 days.

d. Give all household members trimethoprim/ sulfamethoxazole for chemoprophylaxis for 14 days.

e. Admit the newborn infant to the hospital for observation.

17-85. A 19-year-old female with paraplegia secondary to transverse myelitis now presents with a large swelling on the right buttock. The area of induration measures 7×7 cm in diameter. She is wheelchair bound and has a past medical history significant for recurrent urinary tract infections.

What is the next best step in management?

a. Incise and drain the lesion and send cultures to the lab for organism identification.

b. Admit the patient and start IV vancomycin after obtaining a blood culture.

c. Start linezolid; this patient has a history of multiple infections and is likely to harbor multidrug-resistant organisms.

d. Send the patient home on clindamycin po and follow up in 48 hours for response to therapy.

17-86. A 6-month-old infant boy was just admitted for a large perianal abscess, which was incised and drained and sent for culture. He has now been treated with IV vancomycin for several days with a slow recovery and his culture is growing MRSA. This is his second serious *Staphylococcus* infection that has required admission to the hospital. Which of the following tests is the most appropriate in diagnosing underlying immune dysfunction for this patient?

a. Total Ig levels

b. Neutrophil oxidase burst test

c. Lymphocyte subpopulation testing

d. Bone marrow biopsy

e. CBC with differential

17-87. A baby was diagnosed with neonatal *Streptococcus* meningitis 2 weeks ago. He completed a full course of therapy and presents to your clinic for follow-up. Which of the following is an important test to perform?

    a. Repeat CSF cultures

    b. Ig levels

    c. Hearing test

    d. Brain MRI

    e. Repeat blood cultures

17-88. You are asked to serve as the pediatric representative on an Infection Control Committee for a local hospital. The committee has limited resources and initially wants to address the most common reason for nosocomial infections for children.

Which of the following is the most common cause of nosocomial infection in a hospitalized child?

    a. Ventilator-associated pneumonia

    b. Catheter-related urinary tract infection

    c. Foodborne illnesses

    d. Viral infections

    e. Postsurgical skin and soft tissue infections

17-89. A 14-year-old female presents to the emergency department (ED) after a 2-day history of flu-like symptoms, fever, and vomiting. She had been seen 2 days earlier in outpatient clinic and diagnosed with viral syndrome. In the ED, her temperature is 40.1°C, HR is 160 to 168 bpm, respiratory rate is 22 bpm, and BP is 60 mm Hg/palpable. Her father reports that her mental status was fine when she went to bed last night, but he had difficulty awakening her this morning and she is unresponsive in the ED.

Your clinical examination today reveals that she has diffuse petechiae, with increased distribution on her extremities. An IV is placed immediately on arrival, and CBC and blood cultures are drawn. Lumbar puncture (LP) is also performed approximately 1 hour after arrival, and antibiotics are given immediately prior to the LP. Initial WBC is 2.9 and platelets are 55. Gram stain of her CSF reveals gram-negative diplococci.

Which of the following does this patient have?

    a. Systemic inflammatory response syndrome (SIRS)

    b. Sepsis

    c. Severe sepsis

    d. Septic shock

    e. All of the above

17-90. A 2-month-old former full-term infant presents to your clinic with a history of rhinorrhea, low-grade fevers, and poor feeding. The father reports that she has only taken 1 oz at a time every few hours over the last 24 hours. He does not remember the last time she had a wet diaper. You note on physical examination that her RR is 70 bpm, and she has significant grunting, flaring, and 2+ intercostal and abdominal retractions. Her oxygen saturation is 90% on room air, and on lung auscultation you hear diffuse rhonchi and intermittent wheezes, along with a "washing machine"–like sound diffusely. Her 2.5-year-old brother has also had a runny nose for 3 days.

Which of the following statements correctly describes the child's current condition?

    a. Appropriate immunizations at 2 months of age could have prevented this current infection.

    b. A maternal antibody-mediated response plays a significant role in response to this infection.

    c. The symptoms are due to an absence of any infant immune response to the infection.

    d. Prior infection with the same virus at 1 month of age would not have prevented the current infection.

    e. Immunoglobulin therapy to this specific viral infection was indicated at birth.

17-91. A mother who works in a day care brings in her full-term, 4-week-old infant to see you. She wants to know whether or not her son may have CMV infection. A coworker has a child who was just diagnosed with sensorineural deafness, and she read on the Internet that CMV is the most common cause. In addition, childcare workers, like herself, are at high risk for infection.

The child is now 4 weeks old. He was borderline SGA with borderline microcephaly (although both parents have small heads as well). The patient had one low blood sugar at a few hours of life that resolved, and has had an unremarkable course and physical examination. She passed her newborn hearing screen in the nursery.

What should you advise your patient's mother about CMV testing, diagnosis, and infection?

    a. Given the history and physical examination, it is appropriate to send a urine viral culture for CMV to assess for congenital CMV infection.

    b. Based on the current information you have, testing now will not be helpful.

    c. At this point, it is more appropriate to test the mother and the baby's CMV IgG and IgM levels.

    d. You should inform the mother that she should have received CMV vaccine during her pregnancy.

    e. Based on the history and physical examination, you should start IV ganciclovir treatment for the infant immediately.

17-92. A 5-year-old girl comes to you for her kindergarten entry physical examination. Her guardian tells you a detailed medical history for her. She is new to your practice, as she has just moved to your area from another state. Based on her history and a copy of her immunization records, her immunizations were kept up-to-date; however, she is due for most of her routine 4- to 5-year-old vaccines. Today she has a URI and her temperature is 100.5°F. Which of the following would be an absolute contraindication to giving one of the vaccines she is due for?

a. History of Guillain-Barré syndrome

b. Fever ≥105°F or hypotonic–hyporesponsive episode within 48 hours after a dose of a pertussis-containing vaccine

c. Encephalopathy within 7 days of a previous dose of a DTaP

d. Receipt of IVIG within the last month

e. Moderate illness with a fever

17-93. An 18-month-old toddler presents with a 1-day history of fever, severe fussiness, drooling, and poor oral intake. Her parents are extremely worried about her and report they cannot convince her to drink more than a teaspoon at a time. Her last wet diaper was over 10 hours ago. On examination she has a temperature of 101.0°F; HR is 160 to 168 bpm. She appears miserable, and cries with attempted examination. While she is crying, you are able to get a good look in her oropharynx and note several vesicular and ulcerative lesions on her upper and lower gum lines, buccal mucosa, tongue, and upper palate.

Along with adequate pain medication and hydration, which of the following is the most appropriate antiviral treatment?

a. Valacyclovir po

b. Foscarnet IV

c. Ganciclovir IV

d. Acyclovir IV

e. Acyclovir po

17-94. A 20-month-old toddler presents with a fever of 101.5°F, "ear tugging" of his right ear, and rhinorrhea. His father reports that he was seen by a different doctor about 1.5 weeks ago, diagnosed with an ear infection, and given a prescription for amoxicillin for 10 days. The 10 days are over, and the child still has a fever and does not seem to have improved significantly. Which of the following is *not* a reason the prior treatment may have failed?

a. β-Lactamase production

b. An active influx system importing too much antibiotic

c. Poor compliance with therapy

d. Decreased antibiotic uptake in the infected cells

e. Alteration in outer membrane proteins of the bacteria causing infection

17-95. A 7-year-old girl presents with a 2-week history of progressive scalp itchiness and irritation. She often likes to wear tight pigtails, and her mother just noted a couple of small bald patches at the back of her head. On examination, she is afebrile, and you note 2 scaly, bald areas with scattered "broken"-appearing hairs on her posterior upper scalp. You also note bilateral posterior cervical lymphadenopathy. What is the most appropriate first-line treatment of her condition?

a. Griseofulvin po for 6 weeks

b. Fluconazole po for 6 weeks

c. Griseofulvin po for 2 weeks

d. Topical clotrimazole

e. Seborrheic dermatitis shampoo only

17-96. A previously healthy 3-year-old girl presents with dysuria for 1 day, upper respiratory symptoms, and low-grade temperatures with a maximum of 100.0°F and no other symptoms. Her mother also reports she complains of some pain when bathing and cleaning her genital area. Her mother collects a clean-catch urine specimen. Urine dipstick shows normal specific gravity, 1+ esterase, and negative nitrites, and is otherwise negative. Culture is sent. You empirically prescribe cephalexin for 10 days.

Two days later the culture results are available and demonstrate 5000k enterococci, 10,000 *E. coli*, and 10,000k *Staphylococcus epidermidis*. You call the mother back, and her daughter's symptoms have resolved. The appropriate assessment and recommendation for the patient is:

a. Complete the 10-day course of cephalexin.

b. Add amoxicillin to her regimen.

c. Discontinue the cephalexin.

d. Change her antibiotic to ciprofloxacin.

e. Admit the patient for polymicrobial UTI and start IV antibiotics.

17-97. A 4-year-old boy presents with fever for 4 weeks. Specifically, he has been documented with an oral temperature ≥38.0°C (100.4°F) at least 5 times per week for the last 4 weeks. History is unremarkable. Physical examination is also noncontributory. After 1 week of outpatient investigation, no etiology for the fevers has been noted. He has no risk factors or evidence of immunodeficiency.

Which of the following is the most likely etiology?

a. *Bartonella henselae* infection (cat scratch disease).

b. Epstein-Barr virus infection.

c. *Borrelia burgdorferi* infection (Lyme disease).

d. Urinary tract infection.

e. No etiology will be identified.

17-98. A 15-year-old male with sickle cell disease presents with fevers of 102°F for 2 days and vague complaints of arthralgias. He has a history of multiple sickle cell crises and subsequent admissions. For which of the following infections is this patient at higher risk?

a. *Klebsiella* spp.

b. *Staphylococcus aureus*

c. *Streptococcus pneumoniae*

d. *E. coli*

e. *Enterococcus*

17-99. A 17-year-old previously healthy female presents to the ED with fever of 102°F, headache, photophobia, and stiff neck. She noted flu-like symptoms a couple of days ago, and now complains of increased headache. She and her parent have not noted any unusual rashes. There are no known ill contacts. Her immunizations are "up-to-date" according to her father. She recently returned from a "prospective freshman" visit with an overnight stay at a college. She has no known drug allergies. Vital signs in ED include HR of 150 bpm, RR 18 bpm, and BP 88/55 mm Hg. Her WBC is 18 with a left shift. Blood cultures have been sent, and LP was just performed with results pending.

The *best* option for empiric antibiotic therapy is:

a. Vancomycin and ceftriaxone

b. Ampicillin and gentamicin

c. Chloramphenicol

d. Vancomycin

e. Cefazolin

17-100. A 13-year-old boy with a history of tetralogy of Fallot presents with a rapidly progressive history of severe headaches, nausea, and vomiting. Today at school, he had an episode where he was described as "losing consciousness" for approximately 1 minute. He has had a low-grade fever, and no gastrointestinal symptoms. CT scan with contrast reveals a 3 cm ring-enhancing lesion in his left frontal lobe. Past medical history also includes multiple caries and recent dental procedure last week.

Empiric antimicrobial therapy for this patient should include:

a. Metronidazole

b. Ceftazidime

c. Vancomycin and ceftriaxone

d. Vancomycin, ceftriaxone, and metronidazole

e. Cefazolin

17-101. A 17-year-old girl presents with a headache for 1 day. Two days ago she developed a mild fever and sore throat. On the last day she has complained of a "9 out of 10" headache that is often severe. The pain decreases with ibuprofen. On examination, she complains of "neck pain" that is worsened by neck flexion. When you ask her to touch her chin to her chest, she opens the mouth to avoid flexing her neck.

The cerebrospinal fluid white blood cell (WBC) count is 74 WBC/mL with a predominance of neutrophils. Both the CSF glucose concentration and protein concentration are normal. Gram stain is negative. You are concerned about the possibility of viral meningitis. Which of the following statements is *correct* about acute viral meningitis?

a. Pleconaril is effective, available antiviral therapy.

b. HSV causes over 90% of cases.

c. CSF profile often shows a monocytic predominance early in the infection.

d. It occurs in approximately 90% of mumps cases.

e. It does not generally lead to long-term neurologic sequelae.

17-102. A 2.5-week-old former full-term infant presents with poor feeding, jitteriness, poor tone, and seizures.

The mother presented late to prenatal care late in her second trimester. Otherwise, prenatal and perinatal history is unremarkable. On examination, you note no jaundice, rash, or hepatosplenomegaly. Laboratory work shows normal liver function tests and no coagulopathy. Blood, urine, and CSF cultures are pending. A CT scan of the head shows diffuse, patchy abnormalities. Follow-up MRI, EEG results, and metabolic workup are pending. While you are awaiting these results, what is the best treatment strategy?

a. Start ampicillin and gentamicin.

b. Start fluconazole.

c. Send HSV PCR of CSF and start empiric acyclovir at neonatal CSF doses.

d. Send HSV PCR of CSF and start empiric ampicillin, gentamicin, and fluconazole.

e. Send HSV PCR of CSF and start empiric ampicillin, gentamicin, and acyclovir.

17-103. A 16-year-old sexually active male presents with dysuria and urethral discharge approximately 1 week after his last episode of unprotected sex. At first he reports 1 regular partner, but as you talk further with him about likely infection and treatment, he admits that he has had several other episodes of unprotected sex with different partners recently. You obtain a Gram stain of his urethral discharge and note >5 polymorphonuclear leukocytes, as well as gram-negative intracellular diplococci. The best next steps in management are:

a. Treat with cefixime or ceftriaxone alone.

b. Treat with azithromycin or doxycycline alone.

c. Treat with ciprofloxacin alone.

d. Ask him to identify all of his partners for the last year to be tested and treated appropriately.

e. Send gonococcal culture and treat with ceftriaxone and azithromycin.

17-104. A 10-year-old previously healthy female presents with a 4×4 cm, red, warm raised abscess with a surrounding cellulitis of about 0.5 cm beyond the abscess on her thigh. She has been afebrile, and is otherwise well appearing. When she first noted the lesion, her mother thought it was a spider bite. Among the following possible interventions, which therapeutic measure is *most* likely to improve her outcome?

a. Warm compresses to the area 3 to 4 times a day

b. Incision and drainage

c. Antibiotic therapy with cephalexin or oxacillin

d. Antibiotic therapy with clindamycin

e. Antibiotic therapy with trimethoprim–sulfamethoxazole (TMP-SMZ)

17-105. A 6-year-old male recently hospitalized for a complicated, ruptured appendicitis returns with fevers and severe right upper quadrant pain. He has had no recent travel, and no diarrhea. Abdominal ultrasound reveals a single lesion in his liver approximately 7×7 cm in diameter that looks consistent with a pyogenic abscess. His medical assessment and treatment should include the following:

a. Surgical aspiration and drainage

b. Catheter drainage for several weeks

c. IV antibiotics for 2 weeks

d. Aerobic culture only of his abscess drainage

e. Stool testing for ova and parasites (O&P)

17-106. When a catheter-related infection is suspected or diagnosed, in which of the following situations is immediate removal recommended?

a. Exit site infection without bacteremia

b. Bloodstream infection without signs of sepsis

c. *S. aureus* infection in a short-term catheter

d. *Candida* spp. infection

e. Coagulase-negative *Staphylococcus* spp. infection in 1 of 2 blood cultures obtained

17-107. You are asked on consult on a project to enhance the prevention of rotavirus diarrhea. Which of the following statements is *correct* about rotavirus?

a. Rotavirus tends to occur year-round in temperate climates.

b. Rotavirus is spread via a fecal–oral route.

c. Although rotavirus is a common etiology of diarrhea in the United States, it is uncommon worldwide.

d. Rotavirus usually occurs in adolescents and young adults.

e. Current vaccines have been proven ineffective in preventing rotavirus disease.

17-108 to 17-116. You are working in the pediatric urgent care center. You have admitted the patients listed below. Assign each patient to the appropriate types of hospital isolation recommended.

a. Standard precautions

b. Contact isolation precautions

c. Droplet precautions

d. Airborne isolation precautions

17-108. A 12-year-old boy with a cough and a pulmonary cavitary disease that is concerning for *Mycobacterium tuberculosis*.

17-109. A 6-year-old boy with a history of long-term antibiotic use who now has *C. difficile* diarrhea.

17-110. A 2-year-old boy with Kawasaki disease admitted for IVIg.

17-111. A 6-year-old girl with Lyme disease.

17-112. A 19-year-old with *Neisseria meningitides*.

17-113. A 17-year-old boy with *S. aureus* abscess and soft tissue infection.

17-114. An unimmunized 3-year-old girl with a maculopapular rash, cough, and coryza that is concerning for measles.

17-115. A 10-year-old with cat scratch disease.

17-116. A 6-month-old girl who is hypoxic with an RSV infection.

ANSWERS

Answer 17-1. c

This child is suffering from oropharyngeal candidiasis (thrush), which is almost always caused by *C. albicans*. This finding is common in infants less than 5 months of age. Immunodeficiency workups are generally reserved for recurrent or difficult-to-treat cases of thrush in children not receiving antibiotics or inhaled steroids. Treatment with fluconazole is used for cases that fail to respond to topical therapy (generally with nystatin or clotrimazole), in patients who are immunocompromised, or in patients complaining of symptoms (eg, dysphagia, odynophagia, nausea, vomiting) concerning for more diffuse GI tract involvement.

Addressing sites colonized with *Candida* is an important therapeutic component to eliminating the yeast. Rubber nipples and pacifiers should be boiled and skin in contact with the infant's mouth (fingers, the mother's nipple) should have nystatin applied. There is no indication for stopping breast milk.

(Page 1116, Section 17: Infectious Diseases, Chapter 297: *Candida*)

Answer 17-2. e

The patient's most likely diagnosis is invasive pulmonary aspergillosis. Aspergillosis is a fungal infection that most commonly affects the lungs. It occurs almost exclusively in patients with impaired host responses.

The CT finding of the "halo sign" or "air crescent" (ie, a haziness appearance surrounding the nodule) is more frequently noted in adults than in children with aspergillosis.

Lung biopsy remains the diagnostic gold standard. BAL and sputum samples may provide strong support but do not provide the confirmatory evidence of tissue invasion to establish a definitive diagnosis. Serologic complement fixation testing is not as useful in immunocompromised individuals.

Galactomannan is an *Aspergillus* antigen molecule found in the cell wall of the fungus. Detection of galactomannan,

especially when carried out via ELISA, provides additional supporting evidence of the diagnosis but not confirmation. It should be noted that galactomannan results can be affected by broad-spectrum antibiotics, such as piperacillin–tazobactam, which can cause false-positive results. Consumption of food products with galactomannan (eg, rice and pasta) can also give false-positive results. In addition, patients on antifungals can occasionally have false-negative results.

(Page 1114, Section 17: Infectious Diseases, Chapter 295: Aspergillosis)

Answer 17-3. a

Given the patient's residence in California and ethnicity, she is already at risk for coccidioidal disease. Other risk factors include older age, male sex, HIV infection, and pregnancy. Based on the clinical scenario she has likely contracted coccidioidal meningitis. Treatment is generally with a triazole (imidazole is a diazole) alone or often in combination with intrathecal amphotericin B. Both weight loss and acetazolamide are often used in treating pseudotumor cerebri. While acetazolamide may help with mild increases in intracranial pressure, if patients develop hydrocephalus in the setting of coccidioidal meningitis, they will often require a shunt.

Caspofungin is not a standard therapy for coccidioidal meningitis, although it has shown some promise in case reports.

(Page 1120, Section 17: Infectious Diseases, Chapter 298: Coccidioidomycosis)

Answer 17-4. e

These 2 fungal entities share many similarities including major areas of distribution throughout the United States, particularly in the Ohio and Mississippi River basins. Blastomyces does have endemic areas further north into Canada. Both can be treated with amphotericin B, although itraconazole is generally used as first-line treatment for milder disease. Both are dimorphic fungi. Both can cause skin manifestations in their disseminated forms. Histoplasma has several serum antibody tests used for diagnosis. Both complement fixation and immunodiffusion for the M and H bands are methods of evaluating for histoplasmosis and stage of the disease.

Culture can be used to diagnose both organisms. Blastomyces generally is not diagnosed using serum tests because of poor sensitivity and specificity, although newer EIA testing may change current options.

(Page 1115, Section 17: Infectious Diseases, Chapter 296: Blastomycosis; Page 1122, Chapter 300: Histoplamosis)

Answer 17-5. b

The infant has several concerning symptoms that point to sepsis. There is a characteristic syndrome associated with the organism *Malassezia furfur* in which patients (particularly neonates) receiving intravenous lipid infusion can present with *M. furfur* line infections with symptoms as described above (fever, bilateral pulmonary infiltrates, leukocytosis, and thrombocytopenia). While these findings are nonspecific, there are enough clinical data to discontinue the intravenous lipid infusion.

Lipid supplementation can worsen most *Malassezia* species infection. The line should be pulled shortly thereafter once IV access is established. A urinalysis, while helpful for evaluating the patient's renal status and hydration, does not further the patient's care.

Flucytosine is not effective for *M. furfur* infections. A skin culture is not helpful given that over 50% of premature infants will be colonized with *Malassezia* within the first 2 weeks of life. Almost all adults have colonization of their skin. Stopping the parenteral nutrition alone without stopping the intravenous lipid infusion does not hinder the *M. furfur* likely responsible for this infection.

(Page 1123, Section 17: Infectious Diseases, Chapter 301: *Malassezia furfur*)

Answer 17-6. b

The patient most likely has developed fixed cutaneous sporotrichosis. This type of sporotrichosis is one of the more common forms of the disease in children. It can present as an ulcer, plaque, or a maculopapular rash in the area of inoculation. *Sporothrix* is a dimorphic fungus.

The preferred treatment is itraconazole. An alternative treatment is oral potassium iodide that is much less costly.

Syphilis can cause skin ulcers and plaques, but this patient has no history that puts him at risk for syphilis. Nontuberculous mycobacteria can cause swollen lymph nodes and skin granulomas, but the former is usually found in the neck from inoculation in the mouth and the latter usually results in a positive PPD in addition to exposure from aquatic activities. There are few bacteria that present with a plaque-like lesion. If there were an ulcer, *Pseudomonas* should be

considered. *Nocardia*, a gram-positive bacterium, can present similarly to sporotrichosis.

(Page 1125, Section 17: Infectious Diseases, Chapter 303: Sporotrichosis)

Answer 17-7. c

Candidemia that is line related is a serious complication of central venous catheters. While every clinical situation is different, most experts recommend removing CVCs growing *Candida* immediately (along with lines growing *Staphylococcus aureus, Mycobacteria*, some gram-negative bacteria, as well as *Malassezia* and *B. cereus*).

Once the line is removed, treatment with fluconazole and potentially amphotericin B for added efficacy is recommended. The gram-positive cocci in this scenario have yet to be identified and so should not be concluded to be a contaminant (nor does their rate of growth in culture support them being a contaminant); however, most gram-positive cocci infections are treatable through the PICC line if medically necessary. Of note, this patient will require evaluation for systemic candidiasis once stabilized, especially in light of the hematuria.

(Page 1117, Section 17: Infectious Diseases, Chapter 297: *Candida*)

Answer 17-8. d

The patient in the clinical scenario has clinical signs of encephalitis from WNV. While only 1% of patients infected with WNV progress to meningitis and encephalitis, when CNS involvement occurs, patients tend to show a lymphocytic predominant pleocytosis, elevated protein, and normal glucose.

Profile A, while uncommon, could be consistent with a parasitic infection, such as those caused by *Baylisascaris procyonis*. Profile B could represent viral infections that present either with a polymorphonuclear pleocytosis in young patients (eg, Western equine encephalitis virus) or early in the course of illness (eg, Powassan virus). Profile C would be most consistent with bacterial meningitis. Profile E is most consistent with fungal or tubercular infections.

(Page 1130, Section 17: Infectious Diseases, Chapter 305: Arboviruses: West Nile Virus)

Answer 17-9. b

Chronic enteroviral infections can cause meningoencephalitis, pulmonary infections, and severe gastroenteritis in patients who have a lack or an impairment of antibody production. This scenario is most commonly seen with patients who have a congenital or acquired B-cell immunodeficiency. T-cell immunodeficiencies can be associated with enterovirus infections, but are more likely associated with human herpes viruses, adenoviruses, *Candida*, mycobacteria, and *Pneumocystis carinii*. A complement deficiency is a less likely side effect of chemotherapy and usually is associated with infections of encapsulated bacteria. A central line increases the risks of invasive infection but is not the primary reason for the patient's risk of an ongoing enteroviral infection. The chemotherapeutic agent cytarabine is not associated with chronic enteroviral infections; rather there is an association with streptococcal sepsis following use.

(Page 1137, Section 17: Infectious Diseases, Chapter 306: Enterovirus)

Answer 17-10. e

This patient has the rash and symptoms of hand, foot, and mouth disease that is most commonly associated with coxsackievirus A16, but may be associated with other group A coxsackieviruses as well as enterovirus 71. The illness usually lasts less than a week and is frequently complicated by poor enteral intake secondary to oral lesions. Treatment is generally supportive with rest, antipyretics, and analgesics. Immune globulin is occasionally used to help treat severe enteroviral infections in newborns and immunocompromised patients. Doxycycline is the primary treatment for Rocky Mountain spotted fever. Topical 1% permethrin is used to treat lice, and topical 5% permethrin is used to treat scabies.

(Page 1136, Section 17: Infectious Diseases, Chapter 306: Enterovirus)

Answer 17-11. e

The young patient in this scenario requires postexposure prophylaxis to hepatitis A. The 2 options for exposures less than 2 weeks prior include hepatitis A vaccination and intramuscular immune globulin. This patient is too young to receive hepatitis A vaccine and so should receive the intramuscular immune globulin. Ribavirin and alpha interferon are treatments for hepatitis C and are not used in postexposure prophylaxis for hepatitis A. Hepatitis B vaccination would be appropriate if the patient were behind on his other vaccinations.

(Page 1146, Section 17: Infectious Diseases, Chapter 308: Viral Hepatitis)

Answer 17-12. c

The patient requires postexposure prophylaxis to hepatitis A. Postexposure efficacies of HAV and IG are equivalent for children older than 12 months of age until 40 years of age. The exposure has to be within 14 days, as well. Given the recent time of exposure and the patient's age, HAV is recommended for this patient. If the exposure was more than 2 weeks ago, HAV may still be indicated if there is the potential for ongoing exposure.

(Page 1146, Section 17: Infectious Diseases, Chapter 308: Viral Hepatitis)

Answer 17-13. d

The early window period is the time during which HBsAg becomes undetectable but HBs antibody is being produced but is still undetectable. In the scenario above, the patient is

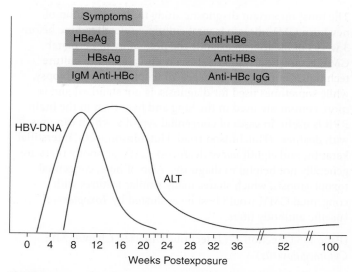

FIGURE 308-2. Time course of virologic, serologic, and clinical events during the course of acute hepatitis B infection. (Reproduced, with permission, from Rudolph CD, et al. *Rudolph's Pediatrics.* 22nd ed. New York: McGraw-Hill, 2011.)

still within the "early" window period during which tests for HBsAg are not yet positive, yet viral DNA from hepatitis B is detectable (See Figure 308-2). Generally, before 4 weeks there is no detectable core protein IgM, which is usually the basis for diagnosing acute hepatitis B infection, nor will there be detectable HBsAg or hepatitis B core-related antigen (HBeAg).

(Page 1145, Section 17: Infectious Diseases, Chapter 308: Viral Hepatitis)

Answer 17-14. a

The infant described in the clinical scenario is most consistent with congenital *cytomegalovirus* infection in its most severe form, cytomegalic inclusion disease. In addition to those findings mentioned above, these patients can have petechiae and purpura ("blueberry muffin" baby—which can also be classically seen in congenital rubella), ventriculomegaly, periventricular calcifications, cerebral atrophy, cortical dysplasia, and chorioretinitis.

Congenital syphilis can present with deafness (Hutchinson triad: Hutchinson teeth, interstitial keratitis, and eighth nerve deafness), as well as hepatosplenomegaly, snuffles, lymphadenopathy, pneumonia, rash, and hemolytic anemia within the first 2 months of age. Congenital toxoplasmosis shares many similar features with congenital CMV. Clinical manifestations include microcephaly, chorioretinitis, seizures, rash, hepatosplenomegaly, jaundice, and thrombocytopenia. The majority of infants with congenital hepatitis B infection are asymptomatic. Infants with newborn gonococcal infection usually present with conjunctivitis, bacteremia, arthritis, or meningitis.

(Page 1154, Section 17: Infectious Diseases, Chapter 310: *Cytomegalovirus*)

Answer 17-15. a

The most important diagnostic study in the evaluation of newborn CMV disease is viral culture, preferably done before 3 weeks of life to help exclude the possibility of perinatal CMV acquisition. Viral PCR is a useful adjunct to culture techniques but does not replace viral culture. Tissue biopsy, while sometimes used for diagnosis, is not standard and is more commonly used in the lung and liver than in the brain. RPR is useful in cases of congenital syphilis, which can present with deafness (Hutchinson triad: Hutchinson teeth, interstitial keratitis, and eighth nerve deafness). CMV antibody titers are generally not helpful in diagnosis. Also of note, congenital toxoplasmosis, which shares many similar features with congenital CMV, would best be evaluated by *Toxoplasma*-specific antibody titers.

(Page 1154, Section 17: Infectious Diseases, Chapter 310: *Cytomegalovirus*)

Answer 17-16. c

Yellow fever is endemic to much of South America and Africa. Classic symptoms of the infection period (which is followed by a remission period and in 15%-25% of patients an intoxication period) include fever, headache, malaise, musculoskeletal pain, nausea, conjunctival suffusion, flushing of skin, and relative bradycardia despite fever, known as Faget sign (although originally used to describe yellow fever, this sign can be seen in other illnesses). Retro-orbital pain, while present with many hemorrhagic fevers, is most associated with New World arenaviral fevers and dengue fever. Morbilliform rashes, at least among the hemorrhagic fevers, are most commonly seen in the filoviral (Marburg and Ebola) hemorrhagic fevers as well as dengue fever. Purulent pharyngitis, conjunctivitis, and edema (especially of the head and neck) are highly specific signs of Lassa fever. Swollen baby syndrome (widespread edema, abdominal distention, and bleeding) is also associated with Lassa fever.

(Page 1142, Section 17: Infectious Diseases, Chapter 307: Hemorrhagic Fevers)

Answer 17-17. d

This patient's symptoms and findings are all compatible with mononucleosis, generally treated with antipyretics. Acyclovir, while used for other herpes viruses, has not been generally effective in treating EBV. Corticosteroids are reserved for severe EBV disease (airway obstruction, neurologic complications, fulminant hepatitis, myocarditis, pericarditis, thrombocytopenic purpura, or hemolytic anemia). The patient's blood smear shows reactive lymphocytes, not cancerous cells, although a heterophil antibody test can help differentiate mononucleosis from oncologic problems. The patient is unlikely to have streptococcal pharyngitis and amoxicillin may additionally exacerbate the patient's condition by causing a morbilliform rash.

(Page 1157, Section 17: Infectious Diseases, Chapter 311: Epstein-Barr Virus [EBV])

Answer 17-18. b

The patient with chickenpox is expected to have some fevers during the prodrome and start of their exanthem, but past 48 hours, significant fever should be regarded as most likely a sign of secondary bacterial infection of the chickenpox lesions. Her additional report of worsening and more painful rash supports this. Usually, unless chickenpox lesions are on mucus membranes, they are not painful. Acyclovir is useful for patients at risk for severe disease such as secondary household contacts, older individuals, and those who are immunocompromised. Intravenous γ globulin is generally of use for postexposure prophylaxis, although vaccination and VariZIG are preferred methods depending on timing and clinical features. Symptomatic treatment can be continued, but it is not appropriate to ignore the continued fever and worsening/painful rash. Hydrocortisone therapy is not appropriate if there is a bacterial superinfection of the skin lesions, nor is it generally recommended for regular chickenpox lesions.

(Page 1163, Section 17: Infectious Diseases, Chapter 314: Varicella-zoster Virus Infections)

Answer 17-19. d

The infant in the above clinical scenario, despite prophylaxis measures, is still at risk of developing HIV. As such, testing per recommendations from the American Academy of Pediatrics (AAP) *Red Book* states that children, because of transplacentally acquired antibody to HIV-1, should be tested using HIV DNA or RNA PCR at birth, 14 to 21 days, 4 to 6 weeks, and 4 to 6 months. HIV antibody testing can be used after 6 months to help exclude HIV, but it is not part of the optimal testing schedule (although many still recommend an HIV-1 antibody test at 18 months), which is aimed at as early a diagnosis as possible. PCR testing should be done at least once before 1 month of age, and preferably before 14 days of life. A negative PCR test at >1 and >4 months, while not the preferred schedule for testing, would provide definitive exclusion of an HIV infection. Testing can be performed while zidovudine is being given.

(Page 1167, Section 17: Infectious Diseases, Chapter 315: HIV)

Answer 17-20. e

All of the answers listed can be complications of measles infection, which is the viral cause of the outbreak in the clinical scenario above. Unlike measles, rubella is generally without a cough and has a milder course. The oral lesions described in the case (Koplik spots) are pathognomonic for measles. Of the complications listed, otitis media (and more generally pyogenic bacterial infections) is relatively common following measles infection. Some sources argue for universal antibiotic prophylaxis following measles infection, although this has only been shown to decrease the incidence of pneumonia but not mortality. It must also be weighed against increasing microbial resistance.

Subacute sclerosing panencephalitis is quite rare with a case rate of 1:10,000 cases. Corneal ulcers following measles are uncommon in children who are not malnourished (particularly as regards vitamin A). Myocarditis is rare, although transient electrocardiographic abnormalities are common. Spontaneous bleeding is rare, although mild thrombocytopenia is not uncommon.

(Page 1173, Section 17: Infectious Diseases, Chapter 316: Measles)

Answer 17-21. c

The child in this case has had a recent infection with parvovirus B19, which, if acquired during pregnancy, can occasionally cause complications such as fetal wastage, fetal hydrops, and stillbirths, although in the majority of cases the fetus suffers no adverse effects. In the above case, despite the child having had a recent infection with human parvovirus, the mother's titers demonstrate that she is already immune, and thus requires no further testing or evaluation. If she were negative for both IgM and IgG, then retesting in 2 to 3 weeks is advised. If the mother's IgM were positive, regardless of her IgG, it is generally recommended that the fetal ultrasound be followed weekly to evaluate for possible complications. PCR testing of the mother's serum, while feasible, is generally more expensive and not as helpful as antibody titers. Cordocentesis for IgM is occasionally done for possible congenital rubella infections but is not used for parvovirus.

(Page 1177, Section 17: Infectious Diseases, Chapter 319: Parvovirus)

Answer 17-22. a

The patient in this clinical case has several symptoms and signs indicating encephalitis secondary to rabies virus. Most notable are the Negri bodies found on brain biopsy. Often laboratory isolation of the rabies virus can be difficult and other methods such as fluorescent antibody examination or mouse inoculations of brain tissue become necessary. Prevention is largely focused on animal control and vaccination measures, but postexposure prophylaxis includes passive and active immunization with rabies immune globulin and a 4- to 5-shot immunization series, respectively.

The clinical scenario is not consistent with tick-borne illnesses such as Lyme disease, babesiosis, or Rocky Mountain spotted fever and the time line is inconsistent for tick paralysis. DEET application is helpful in preventing arthropod infections but not rabies. Sodium stibogluconate is used in treating leishmaniasis. Albendazole is useful in treating most roundworm infections.

(Page 1181, Section 17: Infectious Diseases, Chapter 321: Rabies)

Answer 17-23. d

The decision to administer rabies immune globulin (Imogam® Rabies-HT) and rabies vaccine depends on the risk of exposure and whether or not the animal can be tested.

If a wound is noted, immediate and thorough local treatment of all wounds is a helpful preventive measure. The wound should be thoroughly and immediately cleansed with soap and water. Tetanus prophylaxis and measures to control bacterial infection should be given as indicated. It is always useful to consult with the Department of Public Health before rabies immune globulin is given. In general, rabies immune globulin is given promptly after exposure along with the first dose of vaccine.

If the animal can be captured and tested within 10 days, postexposure therapy can be delayed and averted if the animal tests negative. If not, it is recommended that *all* potential high-risk exposures consider postexposure therapy in consultation with experts.

Cases of bat exposure are unique, as it is not unusual that patients with bat bites are unaware of being bitten. Because bats have small teeth that may not leave easily seen marks, there may not be an obvious bite wound.

For this case, it is appropriate for all persons on the field trip to receive immune globulin and vaccine and the treatment was initiated immediately.

(Page 1181, Section 17: Infectious Diseases, Chapter 321: Rabies)

Answer 17-24. c

The 2 boys have pinworm (enterobiasis), which is a ubiquitous infection often seen in school-age children. Treatment consists of either mebendazole or albendazole as described above, and generally includes treatment of all the family members or at least individual examinations to include/exclude the condition. Treatment can be done with pyrantel pamoate as an alternative, but albendazole and mebendazole are not only effective but also less toxic and there is no need if treating with albendazole to also treat the adults in the family as with pyrantel pamoate. Shaking out sheets prior to washing is not recommended as this can disperse ova into the air. Bathing well the morning after treatment is highly recommended so as to remove remaining infective eggs. Pinworm infections are not a sign of poor hygiene or an unclean home; however, strict attention to hand washing, especially in the days after treatment, is helpful in preventing reinfection. Nylon water filters are used as a preventative measure for dracunculiasis, not pinworms.

(Page 1191, Section 17: Infectious Diseases, Chapter 327: Enterobiasis)

Answer 17-25. e

Toxocariasis (visceral larva migrans) is a nematode infection most commonly caused by the dog ascarid *Toxocara canis* and occasionally the cat ascarid *Toxocara cati*. Often these infections are subclinical, although as in this case, some children present with symptoms of asthma and wheezing.

Children are infected by ingestion of infective eggs of the parasite in soil. Children with exposure to dogs (and especially puppies) are at higher risk of infection. Children with pica have an increased likelihood of ingestion of the embryonated eggs and also an increased risk of toxocariasis. In terms of diagnosis, elevated antihemagglutinins are helpful indicators of infection. EIA testing is also available.

Iron deficiency has been related to pica, but no laboratory evidence in this clinical scenario supports iron supplementation presently. Further evaluation of the patient's iron status may be warranted however. Vitamin B_{12} deficiency is associated with *Diphyllobothrium latum*, not *Toxocara* infections. Praziquantel is used for tapeworm infections and generally not for roundworms. Albendazole is the preferred agent. Mebendazole can be used, but it has poor gastrointestinal absorption and may not reach therapeutic levels for tissue-dwelling larvae.

(Page 1197, Section 17: Infectious Diseases, Chapter 331: Toxocariasis)

Answer 17-26. d

Anisakiasis is a rare infection seen most often with raw or insufficiently cooked marine fish. Standard treatment is surgical or endoscopic removal of the organisms. No antihelminth agent has clearly been found to treat anisakiasis successfully, although albendazole has been reported to be successful in case reports. Praziquantel is used for tapeworm infections. Occasionally episodes of intestinal anisakiasis terminate with expulsion of the worms through coughing or defecation; however, for symptomatic patients, neither supportive care alone nor forced induction of vomiting is appropriate.

(Page 1200, Section 17: Infectious Diseases, Chapter 334: Anisakiasis)

Answer 17-27. a

The child in this clinical scenario has acquired an asymptomatic infection with *D. caninum*, more commonly known as the dog tapeworm. This infection occurs in both domesticated pets and humans by ingestion of adult fleas, which have acted as intermediate hosts for the tapeworm eggs.

Human infection is generally self-limited unless there is repeated exposure. A single dose of praziquantel is sufficient for treatment.

The infection cannot be acquired in humans from flea bites or the ingestion of dog or cat feces as the proglottid eggs require the flea larvae to mature and act as intermediate hosts for the tapeworm larvae to themselves mature.

Arthropod bites, while associated with several viral infections, malaria, and filariasis, are not associated with trematode infections. Larval penetration of the epidermis and dermis, such as that seen with hookworm, is not seen with dog tapeworm.

(Page 1204, Section 17: Infectious Diseases, Chapter 337: Dipylidiasis)

Answer 17-28. d

The patient in this clinical scenario has developed neurocysticercosis from ingestion of the eggs of *Taenia solium*.

Radiographic findings on CT or MRI often show multiple cysts, sometimes with visible scoleces or calcification. Focal seizures are not uncommon. Treatment consists of surgery, if necessary, oral antihelminth medications (albendazole and praziquantel have no IV forms), corticosteroids, and antiepileptic medication. Antibiotics and antifungals have no role in treatment. Surgery generally is for shunt placement or endoscopic removal and does not involve percutaneous drainage of cysts.

(Page 1209, Section 17: Infectious Diseases, Chapter 340: Taeniasis and Cysticercosis)

Answer 17-29. c

Most cases of amebic liver abscesses in the United States are in children who are originally from or have traveled to areas endemic with *Entamoeba histolytica*. In this clinical scenario, the serologic tests for antiamebic antibodies are likely to be positive, helping confirm the diagnosis, as well as antigen detection and PCR testing of the abscess fluid.

The absence of bacterial growth from both blood and abscess cultures as well as the appearance (lack of purulent material) and odorless aspirate does not fit the clinical picture of pyogenic bacteria that most commonly cause liver abscesses. Fungal abscesses general occur in those patients who are immunocompromised. Additionally *Candida*, the most common culprit of fungal abscesses, should grow when cultured. Certain species (*P. vivax* and *P. ovale*) of malaria can have dormant hypnozoites in the liver that can cause a reactivation and relapse but do not cause abscess formation. Hydatid liver disease caused by *Echinococcus* appears clinically different from liver abscesses caused by bacterial and amebic infections and can usually be differentiated on ultrasonography, CT, and MRI.

(Page 1210, Section 17: Infectious Diseases, Chapter 341: Amebiasis)

Answer 17-30. e

The patient has recently returned from an area endemic with both Lyme disease and babesiosis. Because of the absence of particular symptoms supporting Lyme disease such as rash, arthritis, and facial nerve palsy, there is a low pretest probability that the serologic tests will be of use. A much more likely diagnosis is that of babesiosis, a malaria-like illness transmitted by the ixodid tick (which is rarely recalled as being seen on history taking). Symptoms of intermittent fevers, along with chills, sweats, myalgia, arthralgia, nausea, and vomiting, support the diagnosis. Testing consists of Giemsa-stained thin blood smears or PCR and serology tests. Supportive care alone with antipyretics is not appropriate for this patient. Treatment for babesiosis is a combination of atovaquone and azithromycin.

Empiric treatment with amoxicillin is not recommended without a clear diagnosis but could be used to treat Lyme disease. Immediate treatment with doxycyline would be appropriate if Rocky Mountain spotted fever were high on the differential, but the fact that the patient has had a week of fevers without rash and he reports no headache makes the diagnosis less likely. Nonetheless, RMSF should be kept on the differential and treatment with doxycycline should be given if the patient's condition were to change or worsen.

(Page 1212, Section 17: Infectious Diseases, Chapter 342: Babesiosis)

Answer 17-31. b

This immunocompetent child has intestinal cryptosporidiosis that responds to therapy with nitazoxanide, although most cases in hosts with a normal immune system resolve on their own. Paromomycin in combination with azithromycin has been used in HIV-positive individuals with cryptosporidiosis with some effect. Nitazoxanide can also be used in these patients, although HAART is the primary means of treating the infection.

Albendazole is useful for roundworm infections but does not play a role in treating cryptosporidiosis. Metronidazole is used for anaerobic bacteria, amebiasis, and off-label for *Giardia* but has no role in the treatment of cryptosporidiosis. *Cryptosporidium* oocysts are unaffected by chlorination and only modestly affected by iodine tablets. However, boiling for >1 minute inactivates the parasite.

(Page 1215, Section 17: Infectious Diseases, Chapter 345: Cryptosporidiosis)

Answer 17-32. a

The patient in the clinical vignette was suffering from an infection with *N. fowleri* that causes primary amebic meningoencephalitis. The infection was likely acquired while swimming in fresh water several days before the symptoms began. Introduction of the amebas into the CNS is thought to occur through the nasal cribriform plate and nasal mucosa (hence the loss of smell). Treatment with amphotericin B and rifampin with or without use of miconazole and tetracycline is thought to be the best available treatment. Cryptococcal meningoencephalitis (lymphocyte predominance, mildly low glucose) is less likely given the patient's history and CSF findings. Herpes encephalitis, while usually having a similar time course and severity of illness, does not fit the clinical history or the CSF findings (generally lymphocyte predominant). *Baylisascaris* infections are from raccoon worms and generally cause an eosinophilia in the CSF. Tick-borne encephalitis virus also causes a lymphocytic pleocytosis on examination of the CSF and is not found in the United States.

(Page 1218, Section 17: Infectious Diseases, Chapter 348: Free-living Amebic Infections)

Answer 17-33. d

At the present time, mefloquine is the drug of choice for prophylaxis against chloroquine-resistant *P. falciparum*. While lack of a liquid suspension can make administration difficult, mixing with food and using the salt form in younger infants has proved successful. Contraindications include psychiatric

disorders and conduction abnormalities. Atovaquone/proguanil is a viable alternative but is taken daily as opposed to weekly and is therefore not the preferred agent. Doxycycline is another viable agent for malaria prophylaxis in children over the age of 8. Quinine, while used in the treatment, is no longer commonly used as a prophylactic agent given side effects (such as cinchonism, abnormal heart rhythms, and hypoglycemia). Clindamycin, while an adjunct to treatment regimens for malaria, is not used as a prophylactic medication.

(Page 1234, Section 17: Infectious Diseases, Chapter 352: Malaria)

Answer 17-34. a

There are multiple drugs to treat *Giardia*, although most individuals who are asymptomatic generally do not require treatment. However, in this case, given the patient's symptoms and potential to spread the infection to fellow classmates, treatment is advisable. Currently the most effective agent, and recommended by most as first-line therapy, is tinidazole, which can be given as a single dose and has an efficacy of 90% to 95%. It is FDA approved for those older than 3 years of age.

Metronidazole, while only slightly less effective (80%-95% efficacy), is taken for 5 to 7 days. It can be used in younger children, although it currently is unlicensed in the United States for treatment of *Giardia*. Furazolidone was the first agent approved for treatment of *Giardia* available in suspension and has an efficacy of 77% to 92%. As it is taken 4 times a day for 7 to 10 days, it is also not the best treatment of choice for this patient but is a viable alternative. Nitazoxanide is FDA approved to treat *Giardia* in adults and children and has an efficacy of 70% to 85%. Paromomycin (efficacy of 50%-70%) is used to treat symptomatic *Giardia* in pregnancy given its lack of systemic absorption.

(Page 1220, Section 17: Infectious Diseases, Chapter 349: Giardiasis)

Answer 17-35. b

The patient described above is at high risk for pneumocystis pneumonia (PCP) because of his immunocompromised state (which includes low CD4 T lymphocytes) compounded with lack of prophylaxis against *Pneumocystis carinii* pneumonia. Most recently the term *Pneumocystis jirovecii* has been used, instead of *P. carinii*.

The patient shows classic symptoms and signs of PCP such as hypoxia and chest radiograph with granular opacities. While lung biopsy remains the gold standard because it provides histology of the disease, bronchoalveolar lavage is the preferred method for diagnosis in children because of the possible complications from general anesthesia, pneumothorax, hemorrhage, and pneumomediastinum with biopsy.

Once a sample is obtained, it is stained with Gomori, toluidine blue O, calcofluor white, or Giemsa stains. Hematoxylin and eosin, while showing signs of PCP, does not stain the *Pneumocystis* itself. PCR can be used to supplement the diagnosis but has not been standardized or studied enough to replace current diagnostic standards of identification of *Pneumocystis* in fluid/tissue samples. Gastric lavage shows promise as a potential way to retrieve samples containing *Pneumocystis* but is not the preferred diagnostic method.

(Page 1235, Section 17: Infectious Diseases, Chapter 353: Pneumocystis Pneumonia)

Answer 17-36. b

The mother in this scenario most likely contracted *T. gondii* from the ingestion of undercooked meat that contained tissue cysts. It is estimated that in Europe and the United States 50% of toxoplasmosis cases are from foodborne sources. Other, less common means of contracting *T. gondii* include from cat oocysts in feces or mixed with dirt that are directly ingested. Even less common is from blood transfusions. There have been rare reports of surface water contamination of municipal water supplies, but this is also uncommon. Cat fleas containing larvae are a mode of transmission for *Dipylidium caninum*, the dog tapeworm, but not for toxoplasmosis.

(Page 1237, Section 17: Infectious Diseases, Chapter 354: Toxoplasmosis)

Answer 17-37. d

The patient in the clinical scenario presents with symptoms consistent with a bacterial meningitis. For patients who have severe β-lactam allergies, such as this young boy, a good alternative for gram-negative coverage would be chloramphenicol. Vancomycin, which is commonly used anyways in areas of high penicillin-resistant pneumococcal strains, would also be a good agent for patients with severe β-lactam allergies.

Cefotaxime and ampicillin cannot be used in this patient without desensitization, and in this patient who is on the verge of severe sepsis, antibiotic administration should not be delayed. Gentamicin, while commonly used in neonatal infections where GBS is a more common etiology, and also used for synergistic purposes in children with meningitis caused by gram-negative rods, should not be the primary agent for gram-negative coverage in older children.

(Page 915, Section 17: Infectious Diseases, Chapter 231: Bacterial Infections of the CNS)

Answer 17-38. b

Clinical differentiation of viral meningitis and encephalitis is often impossible. The patient above, however, has 2 key clinical findings supportive of an infection with LCMV. LCMV is often acquired through exposure to rodent urine and is one of the more common viral etiologies of meningitis/encephalitis during the winter season. Additionally, LCMV is known to have a biphasic course with an initial "influenza-like" illness with symptoms of fever, myalgia, headache, vomiting, photophobia, and pharyngitis that can last 1 to 3 weeks. West Nile virus and Western equine encephalitis virus can also have

a viral prodrome, although often not quite as lengthy. Mumps can cause an aseptic meningitis (in fact, the most common extrasalivary complication of mumps is a CSF pleocytosis), but the patient has no clinical signs of mumps. HSV-1 encephalitis is a more severe illness that does not usually self-resolve. HSV meningitis is usually caused by HSV-2. Like West Nile virus, Western equine encephalitis virus is a possible choice, but not the most likely, given that it usually has more severe neurologic sequelae and is additionally more common during the summer months.

(Page 919, Section 17: Infectious Diseases, Chapter 232: Viral Infections of the CNS)

Answer 17-39. a

This young women's most likely diagnosis is that of bacterial vaginosis (BV), which results from replacement of vaginal *Lactobacillus* with anaerobic bacteria. The patient's pH is >4.5 that makes a yeast infection unlikely, and as a result, fluconazole is not the correct choice for treatment. Both the microscopy using sodium chloride that supports the appearance of clue cells and the amine odor are supportive of BV rather than *Trichomonas*. The recommended treatment of BV is metronidazole 500 mg po BID × 7 days. A single treatment with 2 g is not as effective and is no longer recommended by the CDC. Treatment of trichomonal infections, however, still includes the use of a single 2 g of either metronidazole or tinidazole. The patient's symptoms are not indicative of cervicitis or infection with *Chlamydia* or gonorrhea; however, given that these infections can be asymptomatic, screening is advisable. As such, treatment of these 2 infections with azithromycin and ceftriaxone, unless other information is obtained, is not necessary at this time unless the patient fails to improve or the tests are positive.

(Page 931, Section 17: Infectious Diseases, Chapter 233: Sexually Transmitted Infections)

Answer 17-40. e

The patient in question likely has septic arthritis of the hip. While classically these types of infections on joint aspiration have WBC counts in the range of 50,000 cells/mm³, joint fluid can range widely from 2000 to 300,000 cells/mm³. As such, given the presentation, supportive labs, and joint aspiration findings, arthrotomy is recommended (with a decision of imaging the joint made in consultation with the orthopedic surgeon). Prior to arthrotomy and further imaging, exclusion of associated osteomyelitis may not be made based simply on the joint fluid. Blood cultures should always be obtained along with joint fluid, as they are positive in 30% to 40% of cases of septic arthritis. Antibiotics are best administered immediately after the patient's arthrotomy and blood cultures so as to improve the likelihood that a pathogen can be isolated and identified. To this end and the treatment benefit the patient receives from arthroscopy, surgery should not be delayed. Of note, recent literature lends support to the use of adjunctive glucocorticoid therapy in septic arthritis, although use is not standard practice currently.

(Page 938, Section 17: Infectious Diseases, Chapter 234: Bone, Joint, Soft Tissue Infections)

Answer 17-41. a

The boy in the clinical scenario likely has periorbital cellulitis secondary to contiguous structures, namely, his sinuses. Worsening while on antibiotic therapy and proptosis, in addition to ophthalmoplegia, decreased visual acuity, bilateral periorbital edema, and inability to evaluate the eye secondary to edema, are indications to image the orbit to evaluate for subperiosteal involvement, such as an abscess, which may not be responding to antibiotic therapy. If orbital involvement is discovered, emergent ophthalmologic consultation for drainage is necessary. It may become necessary to change his antibiotics to more broadly cover pathogens such as MRSA and gram-negative species; however, changing to vancomycin or cefotaxime alone may not offer sufficiently broad coverage. Topical ophthalmic steroid drops are not indicated at this time as the chemosis is likely secondary to the patient's infection. Aspirates of skin at the point of maximal inflammation are sometimes recommended for patients with cellulitis, but are rarely performed even in those cases.

(Page 939, Section 17: Infectious Diseases, Chapter 234: Bone, Joint, Soft Tissue Infections)

Answer 17-42. a

The American Heart Association made changes to its recommendations for IE prophylaxis in 2007. The guidelines recommend prophylaxis for prosthetic cardiac valves, previous IE, unrepaired cyanotic congenital heart disease (including palliative shunts and conduits), completely repaired congenital heart defect with prosthetic material or device during the first 6 months after the procedure (whether surgical or catheter intervention), repaired congenital heart disease with residual defects at the site or adjacent to the site of a prosthetic patch or prosthetic device, and cardiac transplantation recipients who develop cardiac valvulopathy. Of the patients above, only the patient in scenario A meets these criteria.

Conditions that were previously recommended for prophylaxis but are no longer recommended to receive antibiotics per AHA guidelines include mitral valve prolapse, rheumatic heart disease, bicuspid valve disease, VSDs and ASDs, and hypertrophic cardiomyopathy. Also of note, placement and removal of orthodontic hardware generally does not require any prophylaxis, regardless of the patient's condition.

(Page 941, Section 17: Infectious Diseases, Chapter 235: Cardiac Infections)

Answer 17-43. e

The patient in the clinical scenario has bloody diarrheal illness that fits the clinical presentation of Shiga toxin–producing *E. coli*. Because of its potential for more rapid identification and for public health concerns, bloody diarrhea specimens should be tested for Shiga toxins. The ELISA test is particularly helpful because while O157:H7 enterohemorrhagic *E. coli* can be grown on a sorbitol-MacConkey medium, other Shiga toxin–producing *E. coli* strains cannot. Stool culture assists in the identification of other bacteria that may cause inflammatory diarrhea. A blood culture may be indicated in febrile patients with diarrhea or for further testing purposes if bacteria are identified in the stool, but is unlikely to yield a positive result in the patient above, nor is it the next best test. The patient does not have risk factors for *C. difficile* colitis, such as recent antibiotic use. The patient is not immunocompromised and has no exposure history that would indicate a need for ova and parasite testing at this time. *Giardia* does not generally cause the appearance of blood or mucus in stools.

(Page 947, Section 17: Infectious Diseases, Chapter 236: Gastrointestinal Infections)

Answer 17-44. b

This child having undergone a Kasai procedure is at high risk for developing bacterial cholangitis given the abnormal anatomy of the bile ducts following surgery. Similar conditions that result in functional or mechanical obstruction of the bile ducts include gallstones, congenital hepatic fibrosis, choledochal cysts, and primary sclerosing cholangitis. The most common bacterial causes of cholangitis are *E. coli*, *Klebsiella*, *Enterobacter*, and *Enterococcus*. *Cytomegalovirus* can cause hepatitis, although this is more commonly seen in immunocompromised children such as those with liver transplantation. *Entamoeba histolytica*, along with other bacteria, is a cause of liver abscesses but not cholangitis. *Streptococcus* species and *Salmonella* can very rarely cause cholangitis but are more common causes of diffuse parenchymal liver disease. In developing countries, there are more likely to be parasitic causes of cholangitis, and etiologies include *Cryptosporidium*, *Ehrlichia*, and *Fasciola hepatica*.

(Page 948, Section 17: Infectious Diseases, Chapter 237: Infections of the Liver)

Answer 17-45. b

The infant in the clinical scenario above has a urinary tract infection that will need treatment with IV antibiotics. Of the risk factors listed, the only one conveying an increased risk of urinary tract infection in the neonatal age group was being male. This risk factor changes by 1 year of age so that females become the higher-risk group. Term infants are less likely to have urinary tract infections as compared with preterm infants. Similarly uncircumcised males are more likely to suffer from UTIs than are their circumcised counterparts (although possibility of a UTI is not an indication for a circumcision given the low frequency and usually mild nature of the disease in males). Breast-feeding has not been shown to increase one's risk of a urinary tract infection and, if anything, is likely protective. In older adults, blood type B or AB has been shown to predispose individuals to developing urinary tract infections.

(Page 951, Section 17: Infectious Diseases, Chapter 238: Urinary Tract Infections)

Answer 17-46. e

This young girl has a tunnel infection of her central venous catheter. However, she does not show signs of bacteremia, and, as such, would be a candidate for a trial of IV antibiotic therapy covering *S. aureus* and *Pseudomonas*. If no improvement was noted, or if she developed signs of systemic infection or bacteremia, the catheter should be removed and the tract cultured for more tailored antibiotic treatment. Treatment alone with either vancomycin or cefepime is not preferred. Topical antibiotics can be used for catheter exit site infections not associated with bacteremia.

(Page 958, Section 17: Infectious Diseases, Chapter 239: Catheter-Associated Infections)

Answer 17-47. b

This patient has cervicofacial disease secondary to actinomycosis. The most common form of actinomycosis is cervicofacial disease, which is characterized as a suppurative infection that progresses to a "woody" or lumpy mass. The lesion can also be complicated by fistula formation. "Sulfur granules" may be noted in the fistula drainage. The location is usually at the angle of the jaw, but can occur anywhere on the cheek, mandible, or anterior neck. The lesion is slowly progressive over several months; however, pain or fever is seldom prominent.

Actinomyces species are part of the normal flora of the human gastrointestinal tract. *A. israelii*, the species that most commonly produces human disease, is part of normal oral flora. Infection spreads by direct invasion from adjacent tissue. As a result, risk factors for actinomycosis include gingivitis, dental caries oral surgery, and local tissue damage. Mumps can cause swelling of the parotid glands; however, the causative organism is an RNA virus in the Paramyxoviridae family.

B. henselae (cat scratch disease) can manifest as a regional lymphadenopathy near the site of inoculation. *Bartonella* is unlikely in this case, as no lymphadenopathy was noted. Also, instead of the slow development of a "woody" or hard appearance, the lymphadenopathy develops over 1 to 2 weeks. In cat scratch disease, the overlying skin is more likely to be warm and erythematous. *M. catarrhalis* usually presents as otitis media or sinusitis. Molluscum contagiosum is a benign viral infection of the skin. The lesions are usually flesh-colored or "pearly" papules about 5 mm in diameter with central umbilication.

(Page 1017, Section 17: Infectious Diseases, Chapter 248: Actinomycosis)

Answer 17-48. a

Prolonged treatment with penicillin and surgery is the usual treatment for actinomycocsis. Initially, intravenous aqueous penicillin should be given for up to 4 weeks for cervicofacial disease followed by oral penicillin for up to 12 months. Patients allergic to penicillin may be treated with erythromycin, clindamycin, doxycycline, or tetracycline. Ceftriaxone, vancomycin, and clindamycin are all active against *Actinomyces* species but are not considered first-line therapy. Data regarding trimethoprim–sulfamethoxazole (Bactrim) activity are not available.

(Page 1017, Section 17: Infectious Diseases, Chapter 248: Actinomycosis)

Answer 17-49. b

C. jejuni and *C. coli* infection most commonly manifests as gastroenteritis. Symptoms include diarrhea, abdominal cramps, fever, headache, malaise, and myalgia. Abdominal pain can be severe and mistaken for appendicitis.

Diarrhea may initially be watery and profuse and later contain blood. Duration is usually less than 1 week; however, in 20% of cases, the disease may be prolonged or recur. Severe or persistent infection can mimic acute inflammatory bowel disease. Contaminated chicken is the most common source of *Campylobacter* infection. Other sources include unpasteurized milk and untreated water, as well as dogs, cats, hamsters, birds, and ferrets.

Salmonella is a gram-negative bacillus and is famous for producing hydrogen sulfide. It has been associated with foods such as fresh products and poultry. *Salmonella* gastroenteritis can present with watery diarrhea and severe abdominal pain. *Shigella* is a gram-negative bacillus that can cause bloody diarrhea. STEC, also known as enterohemorrhagic *E. coli*, are now the most frequent causes of acute renal failure in children in United States. The presentation usually begins with watery diarrhea that becomes bloody. *Giardia lamblia* is a protozoan parasite that can cause acute or chronic diarrhea.

(Page 1027, Section 17: Infectious Diseases, Chapter 255: *Campylobacter*)

Answer 17-50. a

C. difficile is a spore-forming, obligate anaerobic, gram-positive bacillus. Manifestations of *C. difficile*–associated disease (CDAD) include infection ranging from diarrhea to a pseudomembranous colitis. Risk factors include antimicrobial therapy, prolonged nasogastric tube placement, and repeated enemas. Treatment for *C. difficile* infection can be challenging.

Antibiotics or chemotherapeutic agents should be immediately discontinued if possible. In approximately 20% of immunocompetent patients, CDAD will resolve within 2 to 3 days of discontinuing the offending agent. Metronidazole for 7 to 10 days is the more cost-effective choice for the initial treatment of patients with CDAD. Although vancomycin is indicated for patients who do not respond initially to metronidazole or in cases of severe CDAD, vancomycin is only effective when given orally or by enema.

(Page 1021, Section 17: Infectious Diseases, Chapter 250: Clostridial Infections)

Answer 17-51. c

This infant's presentation (eg, constipation, poor feeding, weak cry, expressionless face, poor suck, hypotonia with associated head lag) is highly suspicious for infant botulism. Other potential presenting findings include ophthalmoplegia, a diminished gag reflex, and ptosis.

Infant botulism is the most common form of botulism reported in the United States. There is no gender predilection. The average age of the onset of symptoms is 13 weeks of age. Possible spore sources include foods, dust, and soil. A history of honey ingestion is present only in a minority of cases; however, in general, children younger than 12 months of age should not be fed honey.

Although Hirschsprung disease is associated with constipation, and Down syndrome is associated with hypotonia, these diagnoses would not explain the other symptoms. *S. flexneri* infection usually presents with bloody diarrhea, abdominal pain, and severe systemic symptoms. Late group B streptococcal infection is unlikely, as this condition more commonly occurs as bacteremia or meningitis around 1 month of age (not 4 months of age).

(Page 1022, Section 17: Infectious Diseases, Chapter 250: Clostridial Infections)

Answer 17-52. b

BIG-IV, currently marketed as BabyBIG®, is a human-derived botulism antitoxin that neutralizes botulinum toxin.

Treatment with BIG-IV should be instituted as soon as possible and should not be delayed for laboratory confirmation. BIG-IV immediately binds and neutralizes all circulating botulinum toxin and remains present in neutralizing amounts in the circulation for up to 6 months. This allows regeneration of nerve endings to proceed and leads to full recovery. Early treatment with BIG-IV within 0 to 3 days of admission shortens hospital stay by up to 1 week when compared with BIG-IV administered at 4 to 7 days of admission.

In infant botulism, supportive care is the mainstay of therapy. However, the early use of BIG-IV is now standard. Specific treatment with BIG-IV is highly effective, shortening hospital stays from 5.5 to 2.5 weeks, and reducing morbidity and mortality. It is not recommended in other forms of botulism.

(Page 1022, Section 17: Infectious Diseases, Chapter 250: Clostridial Infections)

Answer 17-53. d

Treatment with BIG-IV should be instituted as soon as possible and should not be delayed for laboratory confirmation.

Diagnosis can be confirmed by a stool specimen for toxin assay. Although serum toxin assay is possible, toxin is detected in serum in 1% of cases. Other potential samples that can be used for toxin assay include gastric aspirate or suspect foods.

Electromyelographic testing shows characteristic patterns of brief, small-amplitude motor action potentials (BSAPs); however, this finding is not a sensitive test for infants. Serum IgM levels are not a standard method used for diagnosis.

(Page 1022, Section 17: Infectious Diseases, Chapter 250: Clostridial Infections)

Answer 17-54. e

The patient has brucellosis. Risk factors for brucellosis include consumption of unpasteurized dairy products, such as milk or goat cheese. Between 100 and 200 cases occur each year in the United States. Most of these cases occur in immigrants or travelers with exposure from countries where *Brucella* is endemic. Although brucellosis can present with many nonspecific symptoms, the classic triad of brucellosis consists of fever, arthralgia or arthritis, and organomegaly. Fever is a common manifestation that can wax and wane.

C. psittaci presents a respiratory tract infection. The most common reservoir is birds, such as parakeets, parrots, macaws, pigeons, and turkeys. *L. interrogans* (leptospirosis) causes an acute illness associated with jaundice, vasculitis, and hemorrhagic pneumonitis. Infection occurs through exposure to an infected animal's urine. The most common reservoir hosts for leptospirosis are wild mammals, especially rodents. Cats, particularly kittens, are the natural reservoir for *B. henselae* (cat scratch disease), which manifests as a regional lymphadenopathy. Finally, *N. fowleri* presents as an amebic meningoencephalitis, which is not consistent with the presentation.

(Page 1025, Section 17: Infectious Diseases, Chapter 254: Brucellosis)

Answer 17-55. b

The commonly used treatment regimens consist of doxycycline for 45 days, in combination with gentamicin for 7 days; or doxycycline and rifampin for 45 days. Trimethoprim–sulfamethoxazole for 4 to 6 weeks in combination with rifampin is recommended for younger children. Monotherapy regimens are associated with a high failure rate.

(Page 1025, Section 17: Infectious Diseases, Chapter 254: Brucellosis)

Answer 17-56. c

Typical CSD is probably the most common cause of prolonged subacute regional lymphadenitis in children. CSD is caused primarily by *Bartonella henselae* and is typically transmitted after a cat's (frequently a kitten's) scratch or bite. In addition to the lymphadenitis, there may be an inoculation site papule. It is a self-limited infection. A few days to a few weeks after innoculation, a 2- to 5-mm erythematous, nonpainful papule appears at the inoculation site and persists for a few weeks. *B. henselae* can be found in these lesions. CSD rarely manifests as generalized adenopathy. Suppuration occurs in 10% to 20% and drainage of pus may persist for weeks.

Diagnosis is based on the indirect immunofluorescent antibody (IFA) test for serum antibodies to *Bartonella* antigens.

Staphylococcal lymphadenitis and streptococcal lymphadenitis are bacterial infections that will evolve in less than a week. This child's presentation is too long for an acute bacterial infection. There are no risk factors to suggest a diagnosis of HIV. Although less likely, HIV acute infection should be in the differential diagnosis for lymphadenopathy. Lymphadenopathy is a common presentation for lymphoma in this age, but the lack of fever, weight loss, or any other constitutional symptom points away from this diagnosis.

(Page 1029, Section 17: Infectious Diseases, Chapter 257: Cat Scratch Disease [*Bartonella henselae*])

Answer 17-57. a

Treatment of CSD is supportive, except for patients who are immunocompromised or have systemic disease. If treatment is warranted, macrolides, ciprofloxacin, trimethoprim, and rifampin have been effective. Duration of treatment is not known. Needle aspiration of lesions can help alleviate pain; however, incision and drainage should be avoided. Since humans play no role in transmission of *Bartonella henselae*, isolation precautions are not needed.

(Page 1029, Section 17: Infectious Diseases, Chapter 257: Cat Scratch Disease [*Bartonella henselae*])

Answer 17-58. d

Cholera is an acute life-threatening disease characterized by profuse diarrhea and vomiting. This waterborne disease has been responsible for global scourges for centuries; it is often seen in the wake of disaster situations, both man-made and natural.

The incubation period for cholera is short, ranging from 6 hours to 5 days, with most cases occurring between 1 and 3 days. Initially there is brownish fecal matter in the liquid stools, and then the diarrhea becomes more pale gray in color with mucus, giving it a "rice water" appearance. Anorexia and mild abdominal pain may precede diarrhea. In addition to oral rehydration therapy, treatment with doxycycline or tetracycline is indicated.

Shigella can begin with watery diarrhea but usually progresses to bloody diarrhea. Rotavirus gastroenteritis is more common for children less than 2 years of age. *Giardia lamblia* is a protozoan parasite that can cause acute or chronic diarrhea, but with the travel history to Haiti, cholera would be the most likely diagnosis.

(Page 1035, Section 17: Infectious Diseases, Chapter 260: Cholera)

Answer 17-59. b

Due to the massive amount of fluid and electrolyte loss, occasionally exceeding 1 L/h, severe dehydration and shock may develop within a few hours. In addition to signs of dehydration, a listless detached mental status is common. Other complications include seizures, hypoglycemia, and electrolyte abnormalities. Acute renal failure from protracted hypotension may develop if fluid resuscitation is not adequate.

Hemolysis, thrombocytopenia, and acute renal failure are characteristics of hemolytic uremic syndrome and associated with O157:H7 enterohemorrhagic *E. coli*. Intussusception and gastrointestinal hemorrhage are not associated with *V. cholera* infection.

(Page 1035, Section 17: Infectious Diseases, Chapter 260: Cholera)

Answer 17-60. d

This child has otitis externa or "swimmer's ear," which is an infection of the outer ear canal, as opposed to otitis media, an infection in the middle ear. The skin of the ear canal protects against infection. A layer of sebaceous and apocrine glands produces cerumen with an antimicrobial lysozyme. This lining is also slightly acidic (pH 6.9). Excessive moisture (from swimming, showering, or a humid environment) can change the acidic environment of the ear canal and increase the likelihood of bacterial or fungal infection. Trauma can also predispose to infection. A bacterial infection (90% of cases) is more likely than a fungal infection.

The differential diagnosis of otitis externa includes acute otitis media with perforation, mastoiditis, contact dermatitis, furunculosis, and foreign body. In this case there was tenderness when the auricle was manipulated. As a result, the diagnosis of acute otitis media with perforation is less likely.

Otitis externa is most commonly caused by *P. aeruginosa* followed by *S. aureus*. *S. aureus* also causes a variety of infections (eg, cellulitis, omphalitis, lymphadenitis, and infections associated with foreign bodies, such as catheters); however, it is not the most common cause of otitis externa. *H. influenzae* can cause both acute otitis media and conjunctivitis (usually on the same side of the ear infection). *A. niger* can cause ear infections but is most likely part of the normal ear flora. *M. catarrhalis* is associated with otitis media, not otitis externa.

(Page 1026, Section 17: Infectious Diseases, Chapter 255: *Burkholeria* and *Pseudomonas*)

Answer 17-61. b

There are several preventive measures that can be attempted and the child should be encouraged to continue swimming. Excessive moisture (from swimming, showering, or a humid environment) can change the acidic environment of the ear canal and increase the likelihood of bacterial or fungal infection. Keeping the ear canal as dry as possible can prevent otitis externa. This lining of the ear canal creates a slightly acidic (pH 6.9) environment. As a result, the use of alcohol ear drops before and after swimming lowers the pH in the ear canal and helps prevent infection. Prevention of otitis externa is not an indication for oral antibiotics.

Using ear plugs while swimming can help prevent moisture. Afterwards, drying the ear with a hair dryer on a low setting after swimming can also prevent moisture and maceration of the canal lining.

(Page 1026, Section 17: Infectious Diseases, Chapter 255: *Burkholeria* and *Pseudomonas*; Page 1315, Section 19: The Ear)

Answer 17-62. e

Topical antibiotics are sufficient to treat otitis externa. Systemic antibiotics can be used if there is a cellulitis or cervical adenitis. In addition, topical steroids can be helpful to relieve swelling and pain. If a fungal infection is suspected, topical steroids should not be used.

(Page 1026, Section 17: Infectious Diseases, Chapter 255: *Burkholeria* and *Pseudomonas*; Page 1315, Section 19: The Ear)

Answer 17-63. a

A. haemolyticum pharyngitis is similar in presentation to group A β-hemolytic streptococcal pharyngitis; however, palatal petechiae and strawberry tongue are usually absent. *A. haemolyticum* primarily affects adolescents and young adults and is estimated to be responsible for 0.5% to 3% of cases of bacterial pharyngitis. In up to 50% of cases, 1 to 4 days after symptoms of pharyngitis, a maculopapular or scarlatiniform rash develops. It begins peripherally on extensor surfaces of the extremities and spreads centrally, sparing the face, palms, and soles. Occasionally pruritic, the rash persists for over 2 days in the majority of patients. Although few studies are available, erythromycin is the treatment of choice.

EBV can cause a mononucleosis syndrome, also known as "kissing disease," that usually resolves with no treatment in several weeks. *N. gonorrhoeae* can cause pharyngitis and should be in the differential diagnosis in sexually active patients. *C. diphtheriae* is rare and presents with a grayish membrane on posterior pharynx and tonsils.

(Page 1024, Section 17: Infectious Diseases, Chapter 257)

Answer 17-64. a

Chlamydophila psittaci is an obligate intracellular gram-negative bacterium that causes an atypical pneumonia. The term psittacosis is used, as psittacine birds (eg, parrots, parakeets, macaws, and cockatiels) are major reservoirs of the disease; however, it is more appropriate to refer to the disease as an ornithosis, as *all* birds (eg, turkeys, ducks, chickens, and other fowl) can potentially be reservoirs. The disease is contracted from exposure to birds and inhalation of dried bird feces.

Symptoms are similar to an acute febrile respiratory tract infection and start 5 to 10 days after exposure. It is difficult to distinguish ornithosis (psittacosis) from other types of community-acquired pneumonias, such as *Legionella* or *Mycoplasma*. In general, ornithosis is rare in children.

Treatment is doxycycline or tetracycline for older children and adults. Macrolides are suggested for younger children.

M. pneumoniae is a common cause of pneumonia in this age, but the typical presentation is known as "walking pneumonia" indicating a less severe picture with the patient presenting with cough and some low-grade fever, with a chest x-ray that typically looks worse than the patient. *Legionella* can cause pneumonia and can be associated with diarrhea, neurologic findings such as confusion, and hematuria. The history of exposure to a sick parrot makes a diagnosis of ornithosis (psittacosis) most likely compared with other bacterial and viral etiologies.

(Page 1032, Section 17: Infectious Diseases, Chapter 259: *Chlamydia*)

Answer 17-65. d

C. pneumoniae (formerly *Chlamydia pneumoniae*) is a cause of community-acquired pneumonia in children and adults. The average incubation period is 21 days. Symptoms are nonspecific and may resemble influenza and include rhinitis, cough, sore throat, and fever. Examination may reveal pharyngitis, rales, rhonchi, or wheezing. Radiograph demonstrates a patchy infiltrate. Presentation is similar to *M. pneumoniae*.

M. pneumoniae is a common cause of pneumonia in this age. A typical presentation is known as "walking pneumonia" indicating a less severe picture with the patient presenting with cough and some low-grade fever. Chest radiograph is variable, but diffuse bilateral infiltrates are usually noted; focal abnormalities are less likely. Other examination findings may include otitis media, bullous myringitis, skin rash (in 10% of cases), and sinusitis.

C. trachomatis is a sexually transmitted infection as well as a perinatally transmitted infection. It is associated with a variety of infections, such as vaginitis, lymphogranuloma venereum, trachoma (a chronic follicular keratoconjuncitivis that is rare in the United States), and pneumonia. Unlike *C. pneumoniae* that presents in older children and adults, pneumonia due to *C. trachomatis* usually occurs during infancy, between 2 and 19 weeks of age.

C. psittaci can also cause an atypical pneumonia; however, this diagnosis is less likely in this case, as there is no history of exposure to birds associated with the disease. The disease is contracted from exposure to birds, especially psittacine birds (eg, parrots, parakeets, macaws, and cockatiels) and inhalation of dried bird feces.

(Page 1066, Section 17: Infectious Diseases, Chapter 273: *Mycoplasma* Infections; Page 1033, Section 17: Infectious Diseases, Chapter 259: *Chlamydia*)

Answer 17-66. a

C. pneumoniae (formerly *Chlamydia pneumoniae*) is a cause of community-acquired pneumonia in children and adults. Presentation is similar to *Mycoplasma pneumoniae*.

First-line treatment options include macrolides (erythromycin, azithromycin, and clarithromycin) and tetracycline (for children 8 years and older). Macrolides are also effective for the treatment of *M. pneumoniae*.

(Page 1033, Section 17: Infectious Diseases, Chapter 259: *Chlamydia*)

Answer 17-67. e

The child has pertussis, which can present with apnea, choking, or gasping in young infants. There are 3 phases: the catarrhal phase, the paroxysmal (or coughing) phase, and the convalescent phase.

The catarrhal stage is characterized by rhinorrhea and the symptoms resemble a common cold. The infant is infectious during this period. The paroxysmal phase can last from 1 to 6 weeks. It is marked by the characteristic episodes (paroxysms) of repeated coughing. At the end of a paroxysm of coughing, the infant inhales air quickly in through a partially closed glottis. This movement of air makes the characteristic inspiratory "whoop" of pertussis in toddlers and older children. Paroxysms of coughing may also end with posttussive emesis for infants and children of all ages. In the convalescent phase the coughing eventually lessens in frequency and severity.

Classic pertussis should be readily diagnosed based on clinical features. In addition, a CBC may be helpful, as the presence of absolute peripheral lymphocytosis (>10,000 lymphocytes/mm³) is supportive evidence for systemically active pertussis toxin. Pertussis is a clinical diagnosis. Although bacterial culture is considered the "gold standard" for diagnosis, polymerase chain reaction (PCR), direct fluorescent antibody (DFA) testing, and serology can also be used to assist in diagnosis.

(Page 1075, Section 17: Infectious Diseases, Chapter 278: Pertussis)

Answer 17-68. c

There are numerous complications associated with pertussis. The most common complications are pneumonia (22%) and otitis media. Seizures (2%) and encephalopathy (<1%) are uncommon. For infants less than 2 months of age, the fatality rate is 1%. Rib fractures secondary to violent fits of coughing have been reported in adults and adolescents with pertussis.

In general, pertussis is an afebrile condition. As a result, if a fever is noted, it is important to check for a secondary bacterial infection, such as otitis or pneumonia.

(Pages 1075-1076, Section 17: Infectious Diseases, Chapter 278: Pertussis)

Answer 17-69. a

Treatment for clinical pertussis is primarily supportive. Infants with pertussis who have demonstrated cyanosis or apnea should be hospitalized. Aggressive suctioning should be avoided, as this may trigger paroxysms.

Antibiotic therapy is helpful during the catarrhal phase; however, once the paroxysmal phase has started, antibiotics do not have a significant effect on the course of the illness. Despite this fact, treatment of *all* suspected and confirmed cases of pertussis is still recommended to prevent the spread of the disease. Macrolides are first-line treatment for pertussis. Trimethoprim–sulfamethoxazole is a second-line therapy for patients greater than months of age, who do not tolerate macrolides. Treatment with cough suppressants, expectorants, and mucolytic agents is not helpful for pertussis.

(Pages 1075-1076, Section 17: Infectious Diseases, Chapter 278: Pertussis)

Answer 17-70. b

Although bacterial culture is considered the "gold standard" for diagnosis, PCR testing on nasopharyngeal swab specimens for pertussis is becoming the most widely used diagnostic procedure.

Household and day care contacts of confirmed pertussis patients should receive antibiotic prophylaxis for 14 days after the last contact. Prophylaxis is indicated regardless of prior immunization status. Macrolides are the drugs of choice at the same dosages used for therapy.

(Page 1077, Section 17: Infectious Diseases, Chapter 278: Pertussis)

Answer 17-71. c

Contact transmission can be direct or indirect. Direct contact transmission occurs through direct body surface contact to body surface contact. Indirect contact transmission involves an intermediate object, such as a toy or instrument. Contact isolation precautions include gowns and gloves for providers.

Droplet transmission occurs when droplets containing the organisms are generated by the infected patient (eg, coughing or sneezing). Droplet isolation precautions include masks for providers. These relatively large droplets do not remain suspended in the air; as a result, special ventilation is not needed.

Airborne transmission occurs by spread of airborne droplet nuclei (particles ≤5 µm in size that remain suspended in air) or small particles containing spores that can be inhaled. As a result, airborne isolation precautions include single-patient rooms, special ventilation, and the use of personally fitted respirators, such as N95 respirators.

B. pertussis is highly contagious. The organism has been recovered from the nasopharynx of infected individuals after 5 days of macrolide therapy. As a result, hospitalized patients should be managed in respiratory isolation (droplet precautions) until 5 days after the initiation of macrolide therapy. A private room is preferred; however, multiple patients who are culture positive may be cohorted in the same area. Patients who are not being treated should remain in isolation until 3 weeks after the onset of paroxysms.

(Page 1077, Section 17: Infectious Diseases, Chapter 278: Pertussis; Page 887, Section 17: Infection Diseases, Chapter 225: Infection Control)

Answer 17-72. d

Enterococci normally inhabit the bowel and approximately half of newborn infants have acquired colonization by 1 week of age. Infections associated with enterococci include polymicrobial abdominal infections, urinary tract infection (UTI), device-associated infections, and bacteremia or sepsis. Intestinal perforation such as ruptured appendix or necrotizing enterocolitis may lead to enterococcal infection. The infant's history is consistent with normal physiologic jaundice and breast milk jaundice is not consistent with the examination. In addition, breast milk jaundice is not associated with enterococcal infection. Biliary atresia is unlikely without jaundice. Galactosemia is associated with *E. coli* infections.

(Page 1038, Section 17: Infectious Diseases, Chapter 262: *Enterococcus*)

Answer 17-73. e

This patient has epiglottitis, which is an acute upper airway obstruction caused by *Haemophilus influenzae* type B (Hib) infection of the epiglottis and supraglottic tissues. In this case, immediate consultation with the anesthesia service is needed for direct inspection of the epiglottis in the operating room or a similar controlled setting.

Epiglottitis may also be caused by a number of other bacterial, viral, and fungal pathogens like *H. influenzae* (types A, F, and nontypeable), streptococci, and *Staphylococcus aureus* including methicillin-resistant strains.

Routine immunization for Hib has led to a decrease in the incidence of epiglottitis; however, occasional cases still occur. Peak incidence of epiglottitis occurs for children 2 to 7 years of age. There is usually an abrupt onset with high fever and dysphagia. Classically, the patients present with progressive respiratory distress, tachypnea, stridor, cyanosis, and retractions. Patients with epiglottitis sit in a "tripod" position, leaning forward with the chin extended to maintain an open airway.

If epiglottitis is suspected, radiographic or diagnostic studies should not delay management, such as direct inspection of the epiglottis in the operating room and insertion of an endotracheal tube. The mortality rate is as high as 10% due to loss of the airway early in illness.

(Page 1040, Section 17: Infectious Diseases, Chapter 263: *Haemophilus influenzae*)

Answer 17-74. c

Listeria monocytogenes is primarily a foodborne pathogen that can affect neonates, pregnant women, the elderly, and the immunocompromised host.

Neonatal listeriosis is uncommon, but severe. There is an early and a late-onset presentation. Early onset disease usually presents at 1 to 2 days of age and typically exhibits a septic-like picture, although respiratory distress, pneumonia, and, rarely, meningitis and granulomatosis infantisepticum (diffuse granulomas in the liver, skin, and placenta as well as other organs) are described. Late-onset disease typically presents at 2 weeks of age, most commonly as meningitis. The case fatality rate in neonates is 20% to 30%.

Maternal listeriosis presents with a nonspecific illness (flu-like or gastrointestinal symptoms) and may progress to amnionitis, preterm labor, or septic abortion. Perinatal listeriosis results in neonatal death or stillbirth in 22% of the cases.

Group B *Streptococcus* and *E. coli* remain the most common causes of neonatal sepsis. The history of maternal flu-like illness points toward an infectious cause for this baby's decompensation. Galactosemia usually presents with jaundice and vomiting in the first few days of life after birth and initiation of breast milk or cows' milk–based formula feedings. NEC usually presents with change in feeding tolerance first, and then abdominal distention, and may progress into a sepsis-like picture if diagnosis is delayed.

(Page 1045, Section 17: Infectious Diseases, Chapter 266: Listeriosis)

Answer 17-75. a

First-line therapy is ampicillin. Although the combination of ampicillin and an aminoglycoside, such as gentamicin, is more effective, ampicillin alone is suitable for treatment. For penicillin-allergic patients, trimethoprim–sulfamethoxazole or vancomycin can be used. Cephalosporins are not effective for *L. monocytogenes*.

(Page 1045, Section 17: Infectious Diseases, Chapter 266: Listeriosis)

Answer 17-76. a

This vignette describes a classic presentation of cervical lymphadenitis. This infection often occurs within the setting of a URI and presents with a unilateral, tender, warm, enlarged lymph node. This most often occurs in the submandibular chain. The most common organisms causing this infection are *S. aureus* and group A *Streptococcus*, which together account for over 80% of infections. The presentation is acute over days and can progress to develop an area of fluctuance, which can indicate an underlying abscess. First-line therapy is oral antibiotics; however, children should be admitted for IV antibiotics if ill-appearing or needing surgical drainage of an underlying abscess. Ultrasound can be a helpful tool for assessing and guiding drainage of abscesses.

Lymphadenitis caused by MAC would be expected to have a more indolent course and can present with a draining sinus tract. Lymph node infection as a result of MAC is most common in young children because of their tendency to put objects contaminated with soil, dust, or standing

water into their mouths. *Bartonella* can cause generalized
lymphadenopathy but most commonly after exposure to a
kitten. GABHS can cause lymphadenitis in young infants as
part of late-onset GBS disease but is unlikely in this scenario.
M. tuberculosis also generally causes more indolent disease.

(Page 1338, Section 19: Disorders of the Ear, Nose, and Throat,
Chapter 373: Head and Neck Masses)

Answer 17-77. d

Urinary tract infections (UTIs) are common in girls,
with an overall incidence estimated at 8%. The gold
standard for diagnosing a UTI in an adolescent girl is
a clean-catch midstream specimen. The most common
organism to cause UTIs is *E. coli*, which causes over 70%
of infections. *S. saprophyticus* is the second most common
cause of uncomplicated UTIs in adolescent girls. Although
asymptomatic carriage of *S. saprophyticus* can occur,
the organism is generally detected in the presence of a
symptomatic UTI. Urine culture colony counts may be falsely
low with *S. saprophyticus*.

   S. epidermidis, S. hominis, S. aureus, and MRSA are not
known to cause UTIs.

(Page 1090, Section 17: Infectious Diseases, Chapter 284:
Staphylococcus Infections)

Answer 17-78. a

S. aureus is a common source of bacteremia and sepsis in
neonates with a central catheter in place, causing up to 20%
of bacteremias in neonatal intensive care units. It is infamous
for causing biofilms that help the organism adhere to a
foreign object such as the central line. The best approach
to management is to remove the central line to prevent
progression of the infection and metastatic complications.

   Topical antibiotics have been suggested for decolonization
but are not typically used for systemic infection. Performing
labs may be helpful but are not necessarily the next best step.
Treatment with gentamicin or dialysis is not indicated.

(Page 1092, Section 17: Infectious Diseases, Chapter 284:
Staphylococcus Infections)

Answer 17-79. a

All infants born to mothers with known syphilis that has
been inadequately treated should be evaluated for congenital
syphilis initially with a full physical examination and a
nontreponemal serum test, such as RPR or VDR. The titer
of the nontreponemal test needs to then be compared with
maternal titers. When the mother is inadequately treated, CSF
analysis, CBC, and long bone radiographs are also indicated.
Physical examination findings may include skin lesions, saddle
nose deformity, osteomyelitic lesions, jaundice, pneumonia,
splenomegaly, and lymphadenopathy.

(Page 1102, Section 17: Infectious Diseases, Chapter 288:
Syphilis)

Answer 17-80. c

Penicillin G is the treatment of choice for congenital syphilis
and neurosyphilis, and every effort should be made to treat
these infections with penicillin G. All infants should be
evaluated for CSF infection prior to initiation of treatment.
In children with neurosyphilis, CSF should be reexamined
at the end of therapy. All infants treated for syphilis should
also have vision testing, hearing testing, and developmental
evaluation.

   In penicillin-allergic individuals, tetracycline or
erythromycin given orally for 2 weeks provides an alternative.

(Page 1101, Section 17: Infectious Diseases, Chapter 288:
Syphilis)

Answer 17-81. b

Penicillin G is the treatment of choice for all forms of syphilis
including congenital, primary, secondary, tertiary, and
neurosyphilis. In penicillin-allergic individuals, tetracycline,
doxycycline, or erythromycin is used as an alternative. In
neonates, ceftriaxone can be used as an alternative if penicillin
G is unavailable. Regimen durations range from 2 to 4 weeks
depending on the particular infection.

(Page 1101, Section 17: Infectious Diseases, Chapter 288:
Syphilis)

Answer 17-82. b

The description above is consistent with erythema migrans,
the target lesion that is characteristic and diagnostic for Lyme
disease. Erythema migrans is the most common symptom
of Lyme disease and typically appears within 7 to 10 days at
the site of the tick bite. It begins as a red macule or papule
and expands to form a large, annular, erythematous lesion.
It may have central clearing or vesicular or necrotic areas
in the center. In Lyme disease, erythema migrans is often
accompanied by fevers, myalgias, arthralgias, headache, and
malaise. In early stages Lyme disease can be confused with
juvenile idiopathic arthritis. Travel to Connecticut is also a
clue since this area is endemic with Lyme disease along with
most of the northeastern, mid-Atlantic, and upper north
central regions of the United States. The other answer choices
are not diseases known to be associated with erythema
migrans.

(Page 1046, Section 17: Infectious Diseases, Chapter 267:
Lyme Disease)

Answer 17-83. a

Doxycycline is the drug of choice for treatment of early,
localized Lyme disease in children 8 years of age and older.
Treatment duration is for 14 days. For children under 8
years of age, amoxicillin is recommended. Precautions with
doxycycline include avoidance of exposure to the sun (eg, the
use of sunscreen) because a rash develops in sun-exposed areas
in about 20% of persons on the drug. Treatment in early stages

of Lyme, when only erythema migrans is present but systemic symptoms are lacking, almost always prevents later stages from occurring.

(Page 1047, Section 17: Infectious Diseases, Chapter 267: Lyme Disease)

Answer 17-84. b

Pertussis normally begins with a catarrhal stage with symptoms similar to the common cold, and then progresses to paroxysms of cough and posttussive emesis. The cough symptoms can last for weeks to months in the convalescent stage. Persistent cough in an adult or an adolescent should alert the physician to consider the diagnosis of pertussis, especially when there is a history of contact with a toddler in day care who recently had symptoms suggestive of pertussis. In the United States, Tdap booster vaccination is recommended to prevent infection in infants by removing a reservoir of infection.

Treatment with antibiotics is not indicated until a positive infection is confirmed. The newborn infant does not need admission to the hospital in the absence of confirmed infection or active symptoms.

(Page 1077, Section 17: Infectious Diseases, Chapter 278: Pertussis)

Answer 17-85. a

Since the mid-1990s, community-acquired methicillin-resistant *Staphylococcus aureus* (CA-MRSA) has become more widespread. CA-MRSA is a common cause of skin and soft tissue infections as well as severe invasive diseases such as necrotizing pneumonia, necrotizing fasciitis, and osteoarticular disease associated with deep vein thromboses. Soft tissue abscesses have emerged as a common presentation for CA-MRSA.

Lesions should be incised and the drainage sent for culture. In many circumstances, drainage and wound care will be sufficient for these lesions. However, antibiotics should be considered for more severe local disease or when disease has progressed in spite of incision and drainage.

(Page 1093, Section 17: Infectious Diseases, Chapter 284: *Staphylococcus* Infections)

Answer 17-86. b

Patients with chronic granulomatous disease typically experience recurrent infections caused by bacterial and fungal pathogens. Common manifestations include abscesses of the liver, spleen, lung, and perianal area. It is important to remember that recurrent staphylococcal infections may also be a sign of an underlying granulocyte dysfunction, notably chronic granulomatous disease. NOBT testing provides a

simple and rapid determination of neutrophil function and may guide the physician toward further evaluation.

(Page 1091, Section 17: Infectious Diseases, Chapter 284: *Staphylococcus* Infections)

Answer 17-87. c

Pneumococcal meningitis can be a complication of metastatic seeding in bacteremia. Asplenic patients are also particularly vulnerable to this encapsulated organism. Although the rates of invasive pneumococcal disease have rapidly declined with the introduction of the PCV-7 and PCV-14 vaccines, pneumococcal meningitis does continue to occur and has a case fatality rate of 5% to 10% in developed countries. Hearing loss is the most common neurologic sequela and can occur in up to 10% of infections; therefore, hearing evaluation is warranted. Repeat CSF culture, Ig levels, brain MRI, or repeat blood cultures are not routinely indicated after treatment.

(Page 1080, Section 17: Infectious Diseases, Chapter 280: Pneumococcal Infections)

Answer 17-88. d

Similar to outpatient infections, viral illnesses are still the most common hospital-acquired infection and can be transmitted from other patients, health care providers, as well as hospital visitors (family members, etc). While bacterial pneumonias, especially after prolonged ventilatory support, are also concerning and frequent nosocomial infections, they still occur less frequently than viral illnesses. Any indwelling catheter in the blood or urinary tract also increases the risk of infection, and risk increases with increased duration of catheterization. Intravascular infection risk varies with site of catheter as well, as femoral catheterizations pose much higher risk of infection than more peripheral sites or central venous access sites away from the groin area. Any interruption of host defenses including surgical incisions has the potential for infection, but postoperative wound infections are still less frequent than nosocomial viral infections.

(Page 885, Section 17: Infectious Diseases, Chapter 225: Infection Control)

Answer 17-89. e

This patient meets 3 of the 4 criteria for SIRS (hyperthermia, leukopenia, and tachycardia >2 SD above normal for age). She meets both of the first 2 essential criteria. She also meets the definition of sepsis because she has a proven infection as demonstrated by her positive CSF Gram stain. She meets the definition of severe sepsis because she has cardiovascular dysfunction. ARDS or multiorgan dysfunction would also be sufficient to meet the criteria for severe sepsis. Because she

TABLE 223-1. Criteria for Pediatric Systemic Inflammatory Response Syndrome[a]

| A. Leukopenia or leukocytosis (adjusted for age) |
| B. Core hyperthermia (>38.5°C) or hypothermia (<36°C) |
| C. Tachypnea: >2 SD above normal |
| D. Tachycardia: >2 SD above normal for age (or bradycardia if younger than 1 year) |

[a]Must meet 2 criteria, and one must be either A or B.

does clearly have cardiovascular dysfunction, she also meets the definition of septic shock (Table 223-1).

(Page 881, Section 17: Infectious Diseases, Chapter 223: Bacteremia, Sepsis, and Septic Shock)

Answer 17-90. d

This infant has respiratory syncytial virus (RSV) infection. Primary infection does not lead to immunity, as illustrated by children with recurrent RSV infections.

RSV virus manifestations are from a combination of actual viral cellular damage and injury caused by the host immune response. Since this infant was born at term, RSV immunoglobulin would not be indicated and there is currently no RSV vaccine available. Maternal antibodies are unlikely to play a significant role in protection since peak severe infections are noted in infants less than 6 months, when maternal antibody is still circulating.

(Page 884, Section 17: Infectious Diseases, Chapter 224: Viral Pathogenesis)

Answer 17-91. b

You should tell the mother that testing now cannot distinguish congenital versus horizontally acquired CMV infection. If CMV virus is detected in testing of urine (or saliva) done within the first 2 to 3 weeks of life, it is consistent with congenital infection. Beyond that it is not possible to distinguish between vertical and horizontal acquisition of CMV infection, so testing the baby's urine now will not be useful.

Approximately 1% of all infants in the United States have congenital CMV infection, but only 10% to 15% of those have any symptoms or manifestations.

Healthy infants and children who acquire CMV postnatally rarely have any symptoms or manifestations of infection. CMV is very ubiquitous, and 70% to 90% of adults are IgG positive, so testing the mother now for IgG (and the baby's IgG should simply reflect maternal antibodies) would not be useful. The presence of CMV IgM can signify several things, recent infection, reactivation, reexposure, or a false-positive, so it

also would not be very useful in this setting. Unfortunately, while CMV vaccine is needed and some trials are underway, vaccine is not currently available outside of clinical trials. Ganciclovir treatment has been shown to improve outcomes in infants with symptomatic congenital CMV infection involving the CNS, but there are no data to support the use of IV ganciclovir in asymptomatic and/or horizontally acquired CMV infections.

(Page 905, Section 17: Infectious Diseases, Chapter 230: Therapy for Perinatal and Neonatal Infections)

Answer 17-92. c

Encephalopathy within a week of a prior pertussis-containing vaccine is an absolute contraindication to giving another dose of DTaP. All of the other choices listed are precautions, but are not absolute contraindications. A history of Guillain-Barré syndrome would be concerning for a potential recurrence of Guillain-Barré syndrome, and would have to be weighed with current risk for exposure to the diseases prevented by the vaccine and/or the potential for severe complications from acquiring a vaccine-preventable disease. High fevers greater than 105°F, hypotonic episodes, or inconsolable crying within 48 hours after receiving a prior vaccine dose are reasons to take precautions and consider the risk of recurrence, but this would again need to be weighed with the risk of exposure and/or severe outcomes from vaccine-preventable disease. For example, if your community is in the midst of a pertussis outbreak and her mother is in her third trimester of pregnancy and works with young infants, you may strongly consider administering the vaccine and monitoring closely to avoid infant exposures and potential severe outcomes. Receipt of antibody-containing products such as IVIG are a precaution, and generally the duration of recommended delay until vaccination with live virus vaccines such as MMR or VZV depends on what antibody product was given and how much (see Table 244-4). For example, if this patient had been treated for Kawasaki disease within the last year at a dose of 2 g/kg IV, then you should wait 11 months prior to giving any live virus vaccine. Moderate to severe illness with fever is a precaution, but not a contraindication, and primarily you may consider delaying vaccines so that any ongoing illness and/or fever is not attributed to the vaccine inappropriately.

(Page 985, Section 17: Infectious Diseases, Chapter 244: Immunizations)

Answer 17-93. d

This patient is dehydrated based on history and tachycardia and clearly is not tolerating adequate oral fluid intake. Since her onset of symptoms is within the last 48 hours, anti-HSV therapy may shorten the duration of symptoms. Since she will need IV hydration, and she is not tolerating anything by mouth, she can also be treated with IV anti-HSV medication.

Valacyclovir is much more bioavailable orally than acyclovir; however, she is not tolerating oral feedings. Also, valacyclovir is not currently available in suspension preparation for pediatrics (although extemporaneous suspensions have been prepared with valacyclovir caplets). Foscarnet is typically reserved for acyclovir-resistant infections and has more significant side effects. Ganciclovir is antiviral therapy primarily for CMV infection, not first-line HSV treatment.

(Page 993, Section 17: Infectious Diseases, Chapter 245: Antiviral Therapy)

Answer 17-94. b

There are several mechanisms bacteria may use to develop resistance to antibiotics. These include enzyme production that inactivates the antibiotic (eg, β-lactamase production), active efflux systems that decrease uptake of the antibiotics into the infected cells, or changes in the outer membrane proteins of the bacteria blocking the entry of antibiotics. In addition, poor or difficult compliance is always a potential factor in any treatment failure.

(Page 1000, Section 17: Infectious Diseases, Chapter 246: Antibacterial Therapy)

Answer 17-95. a

Griseofulvin should be prescribed orally for at least 4 to 6 weeks, and often if symptoms have not resolved, refilled for longer. Tinea corporis involving only skin on the body (and not the scalp) can be treated with griseofulvin for shorter durations of 2 to 4 weeks. Fluconazole is used to treat *Candida* spp. infections, not dermatophytes such as *Trycophyton* spp. that typically cause tinea corporis and tinea capitis. Topical treatment alone is not sufficient for tinea capitis.

(Page 1015, Section 17: Infectious Diseases, Chapter 247: Antifungal Therapy)

Answer 17-96. c

Isolation of multiple organisms with low colony counts from a urine culture usually represents contamination. The positive leukocyte esterase can also be from a vaginal contaminant and this pattern of laboratory results likely represents normal vaginal flora and/or a mild vaginitis. Antibiotics should be discontinued. The parents should continue to ensure good perineal hygiene. If *Enterococcus* were thought to be a true pathogen, cephalexin would not be effective. If the *Enterococcus* was amoxicillin sensitive, the regimen would still not cover *S. epidermidis*. Finally, ciprofloxacin would not be effective for *Enterococcus* spp. or *S. epidermidis* and should be reserved for *Pseudomonas* or bacterial infections resistant to first-line therapies.

(Page 889, Section 17: Infectious Diseases, Chapter 226: Diagnostic Approaches for Infectious Diseases)

Answer 17-97. e

The patient fulfills the criteria for fever of unknown origin (FUO). The definition of FUO requires an immunologically normal host with oral or rectal temperature ≥38.0°C (100.4°F) at least twice a week for more than 3 weeks, a noncontributory history and physical examination, and 1 week of outpatient investigation.

More than two thirds of children with FUO resolve their fevers without determination of cause; thus, extensive workup in an otherwise well-appearing child may not need to be conducted until >3 to 6 weeks of fever have been sustained. Infectious etiologies account for approximately 40% of identified etiologies, and among those the most common sources are *B. henselae* infection, EBV infection, and UTIs.

(Page 896, Section 17: Infectious Diseases, Chapter 228: Fever of Unknown Origin)

Answer 17-98. c

Patients with splenic dysfunction, whether congenital or acquired, are at higher risk for infections with encapsulated organisms such as *S. pneumoniae, N. meningitidis, H. influenza* type b, and *Salmonella* spp. Empiric antibiotic coverage for these organisms should include coverage for these when treating a child with splenic dysfunction and fever. In addition, these patients should follow recommendations for vaccination for *S. pneumoniae, N. meningitidis,* and *H. influenza* type b, including polysaccharide 23-valent pneumococcal vaccine and early meningococcal vaccine as well as appropriate boosters.

The other organisms listed are not encapsulated and pose no higher risk in patients with splenic dysfunction than in the general population.

(Page 898, Section 17: Infectious Diseases, Chapter 229: Fever and Infection in the Immunocompromised Patient)

Answer 17-99. a

This patient has a presumed bacterial meningitis until proven otherwise. While viral meningitis is a possibility, her WBC and vital signs are very concerning for bacterial infection. Antimicrobial therapy should be started as soon as possible after appropriate blood cultures and CSF cultures are obtained. Therapy should be directed against the most likely pathogens based on her age, immunization status, and any other exposures. *S. pneumoniae* is a possibility, although less likely based on her presumed immunization status. Lack of petechiae or purpura does not rule out meningococcal disease, and her tachycardia and hypotension are very concerning for meningococcal sepsis and meningitis. Ceftriaxone alone would cover meningococcal infection; however, for a patient with this severity of illness, it is best to cover with vancomycin as well to cover *S. pneumoniae* with high-level resistance to third-generation cephalosporins. Ampicillin and gentamicin are more appropriate for the newborn age when group B *Streptococcus* and *Listeria* are in the differential diagnosis. Chloramphenicol may be considered for known, true allergies to β-lactams, but should only be used in those situations due to risks of severe blood dyscrasias and potential for irreversible bone marrow suppression. Cefazolin does not penetrate the CSF and would not be appropriate.

(Page 915, Section 17: Infectious Diseases, Chapter 231: Bacterial Infections of the Central Nervous System)

Answer 17-100. d

Depending on the size and location of the brain abscess, in an ideal situation, aspiration can be performed and appropriate aerobic and anaerobic cultures can be sent to direct appropriate therapy.

In the meantime, gram-positive cocci (both multiple *Streptococcus* spp. and *S. aureus*), aerobic gram-negative rods, and anaerobic odontogenic sources are all potential pathogens. As a result, broad therapy for all of the above is necessary until additional information is obtained. Intravenous antibiotic therapy may be necessary for several weeks. In addition, coverage may need to remain broad-spectrum if cultures cannot be obtained or remain negative with no pathogen identified.

(Page 917, Section 17: Infectious Diseases, Chapter 231: Bacterial Infections of the Central Nervous System)

Answer 17-101. e

While mild motor function abnormalities or other symptoms may take weeks to resolve, viral meningitis symptoms generally resolve completely and do not lead to long-term consequences. Pleconaril is an antiviral drug that did show some reduction of headache and other symptoms, but overall efficacy has not been established and it is not currently available in the United States. Enteroviruses (group B enteroviruses, polioviruses, and enterovirus 71) cause the vast majority of acute viral meningitis cases. Other causes of viral meningitis include mumps virus, lymphocytic choriomeningitis virus, herpes simplex virus, and the arthropod-borne viruses (eg, West Nile virus, St. Louis encephalitis virus). In the pre-mumps vaccine era, mumps was once a common cause of viral meningitis, and over half of clinically diagnosed mumps cases have CSF pleocytosis.

Viral meningitis CSF profiles when obtained within the first 1 to 2 days of onset often show a neutrophil predominance, which may make it hard to distinguish from bacterial meningitis; typically this shifts to a lymphocytic predominance when CSF is obtained later in the infection.

(Page 919, Section 17: Infectious Diseases, Chapter 231: Bacterial Infections of the Central Nervous System)

Answer 17-102. e

It is important to consider late-onset newborn bacterial sepsis and/or meningitis as well as HSV CNS disease and encephalitis in this 2-week-old neonate. Thus, ampicillin, gentamicin, and acyclovir are all recommended empiric therapy for this patient. In this full-term infant there is no current exposure or medical history concerning for fungal disease, so fluconazole

is not indicated. Although HSV typically causes temporal lobe findings in older patients, this finding is not the typical pattern in neonatal HSV encephalitis.

(Page 920, Section 17: Infectious Diseases, Chapter 232: Viral Infections of the Central Nervous System)

Answer 17-103. e

This patient should be treated presumptively for both gonococcal and chlamydial infections with ceftriaxone, as well as azithromycin or doxycycline.

Because 5% to 30% of males with gonorrhea are also coinfected with *Chlamydia*, presumptive treatment with a macrolide such as azithromycin or doxycycline for *Chlamydia* is recommended. He should be counseled and tested for other STIs as well, such as syphilis and HIV, especially with his reports of multiple partners and unprotected sex. Partner identification and treatment for all sexual partners within the last *60 days* is important to treat and prevent further infections among others. Reporting to your local health department may assist with this process, depending on local resources. While ciprofloxacin used to have good activity against *N. gonorrhoeae*, quinolone resistance had increased significantly. As a result, ciprofloxacin is no longer recommended.

(Page 928, Section 17: Infectious Diseases, Chapter 233: Sexually Transmitted Infections)

Answer 17-104. b

Incision and drainage is the most important therapy for purulent skin and soft tissue infections, and likely would resolve the infection alone. An increasing number of studies, although mostly in adults, have shown no difference in outcomes for patients treated with both incision and drainage and antibiotics compared with patients treated with incision and drainage alone.

Warm compresses will contribute to improvement, and may assist the abscess to drain on its own, but are likely not to be a definitive cure. Depending on local antibiotic susceptibilities and MRSA prevalence, first-generation cephalosporins such as cephalexin or antistaphylococcal penicillin such as oxacillin may be reasonable. However, with the high prevalence of MRSA across the country, it may not be adequate therapy. Clindamycin will be effective against both *S. aureus* and *S. pyogenes*, which are the 2 most likely pathogens, although *S. aureus* susceptibility to clindamycin varies in different geographic areas. TMP-SMZ has excellent antistaphylococcal activity; however, there is no activity against *S. pyogenes*.

(Page 939, Section 17: Infectious Diseases, Chapter 234: Bone, Joint, Soft Tissue Infections)

Answer 17-105. e

All of the following criteria are important in assessing appropriate treatment for liver abscesses: (1) single versus

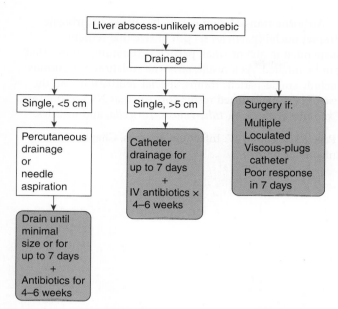

FIGURE 237-1. (Reproduced, with permission, from Rudolph CD, Rudolph AM, Lister GE, First LR, Gershon AA. *Rudolph's Pediatrics*. 22nd ed. New York: McGraw-Hill, 2011.)

multiple abscesses; (2) size <5 cm versus >5 cm, and (3) ongoing drainage of the abscess (vs loculated fluid or clogged drainage catheters).

Surgery is not necessarily indicated unless there are multiple loculated abscesses or the drainage catheter does not adequately drain the infection. Drains are normally in place for several days, not weeks. Drainage should be sent appropriately for both aerobic and anaerobic cultures and the patient should be treated with antibiotics for 4 to 6 weeks (See Figure 237-1). While this patient has no history of travel to countries where *Entamoeba histolytica* is endemic, it is reasonable to send stool for O&P while starting empiric antibiotic therapy. Treatment can be appropriately modified if amebic abscess is later diagnosed.

(Page 947, Section 17: Infectious Diseases, Chapter 237: Infections of the Liver)

Answer 17-106. d

See Table 239-2. Criteria considered when recommending immediate removal include severity of illness, underlying immune status, organism identified in blood cultures and usual response to antibacterial therapy and ability to make biofilms on catheters and virulence, role in commensal skin flora, and evidence of tunneled or exit site infection.

Infections with *Candida* spp., *S. aureus*, or atypical mycobacterium warrant immediate removal of long-term catheters. In short-term catheters, delayed removal can be considered for exit site infections without bacteremia or bloodstream infection without signs of sepsis. Coagulase-negative *Staphylococcus* are unfortunately both common skin flora and common sources of catheter-related bacteremia. They

generally do not lead to recommendations to remove a catheter immediately, especially if only 1 of multiple blood cultures grows the organism.

(Page 958, Section 17: Infectious Diseases, Chapter 239: Catheter-associated Infections)

Answer 17-107. b

Rotavirus is the most common pathogen causing acute gastroenteritis globally. Other etiologies include cholera, norovirus, adenovirus, and various enteric bacteria such as *Salmonella, Shigella, Campylobacter, Yersinia*, and *E. coli* spp. As use of rotavirus vaccine increases in the United States, Europe, and globally, hundreds of thousands of cases will be prevented.

Rotavirus is spread via a fecal–oral route. Although rotavirus tends to occur in the winter months in temperate climates, it is year-round in tropical areas. Rotavirus usually occurs in children 6 months to 2 years of age.

(Page 945, Section 17: Infectious Diseases, Chapter 236: Gastrointestinal Infections)

Answer 17-108. d (airborne precautions for *M. tuberculosis*)

Answer 17-109. b (contact precautions for *C. difficile* diarrhea)

Answer 17-110. a (standard precautions for Kawasaki disease)

Answer 17-111. a (standard precautions for Lyme disease)

Answer 17-112. c (droplet precautions for *N. meningitides* [until 24 hours of appropriate antibiotic therapy is completed])

Answer 17-113. b (contact precautions for *S. aureus*)

Answer 17-114. d (airborne precautions for measles)

Answer 17-115. a (standard precautions for cat scratch disease)

Answer 17-116. b and c (contact and droplet precautions are recommended for RSV infection)

Standard precautions refer to hand hygiene before and after all patient contacts. Gloves should be worn when touching body fluids or items contaminated with body fluids. Masks, eye protection, and face shields should be worn when there is the possibility that body fluids will be splashed or sprayed. Examples include cat scratch disease, Kawasaki disease, or Lyme disease.

Contact transmission can be direct or indirect. Direct contact transmission occurs through direct body surface contact to body surface contact. Indirect contact transmission involves an intermediate object, such as a toy or instrument. Contact isolation precautions include gowns and gloves for providers. Gowns should be used during contact with the patient, environmental surfaces, or any items in the patient room. Examples include *S. aureus* and other abscesses or draining wound infections, *C. difficile* diarrhea, or RSV (which also requires droplet precaution).

Droplet transmission occurs when droplets containing the organisms are generated by the infected patient (eg, coughing or sneezing). Droplet isolation precautions include masks for providers. These relatively large droplets do not remain suspended in the air; as a result, special ventilation is not needed. Examples include *N. meningitides, influenza*, and *RSV* (which also requires contact precautions).

Airborne transmission occurs by spread of airborne droplet nuclei (particles ≤5 μm in size that remain suspended in air) or small particles containing spores that can be inhaled. As a result, airborne isolation precautions include single-patient rooms, special ventilation, and the use of personally fitted respirators, such as N95 respirators. Examples include *M. tuberculosis, varicella*, and measles.

(Page 887, Section 17: Infection Diseases, Chapter 225: Infection Control)

CHAPTER 18 | Disorders of the Skin

Erin F.D. Mathes, Diana Camarillo, Ann L. Marqueling, Vikash Oza, Julie C. Philp, Deepti Gupta, and Barrett J. Zlotoff

18-1. Which of the following statements about the function of the skin is true?

   a. The stratum corneum is composed of dead skin cells with no purpose.

   b. Within the epidermis vitamin D_3 is converted to the active 1,25-dihydroxyvitamin D_3.

   c. Epidermal melanin potentiates transmission of ultraviolet rays.

   d. Langerhans cells in the skin provide immune surveillance, presenting antigen that activates lymphocytes.

   e. The skin contributes to thermoregulation via secretion of sweat from apocrine sweat glands.

18-2. Figure 356-3 demonstrates which of the following?

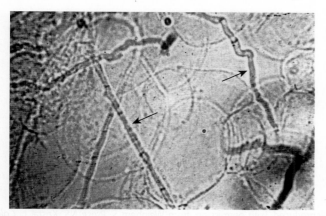

FIGURE 356-3. (Reproduced, with permission, from Rudolph CD, Rudolph AM, Lister GE, First LR, Gershon AA. *Rudolph's Pediatrics.* 22nd ed. New York: McGraw-Hill, 2011.)

   a. Multinucleate keratinocytes

   b. Normal keratinocytes

   c. Septate hyphae

   d. Budding yeast

   e. Crystallized potassium hydroxide (KOH) solution

18-3. A healthy, term, infant boy was noted to have a cleft lip and palate on prenatal ultrasound. His newborn examination is otherwise notable for a sharply demarcated, nontender, 1.5-cm bulla over the vertex scalp. What is the most likely diagnosis for the scalp lesion?

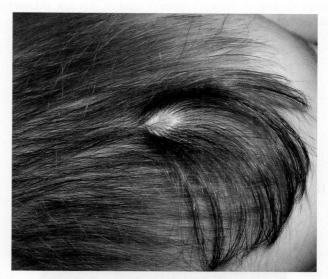

(Reproduced, with permission, from Rudolph CD, Rudolph AM, Lister GE, First LR, Gershon AA. *Rudolph's Pediatrics.* 22nd ed. New York: McGraw-Hill, 2011.)

   a. Herpes simplex

   b. Trauma from fetal scalp electrode

   c. Aplasia cutis congenita (ACC)

   d. Nevus sebaceous

   e. Congenital nevus

18-4. An otherwise healthy infant is noted to have a pedunculated, flesh-colored, firm papule on the preauricular cheek.

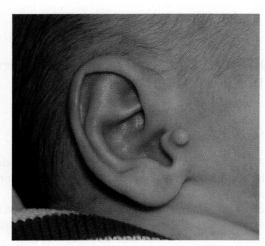

(Reproduced, with permission, from Rudolph CD, Rudolph AM, Lister GE, First LR, Gershon AA. *Rudolph's Pediatrics.* 22nd ed. New York: McGraw-Hill, 2011.)

What is the next step in management?

a. Referral to ENT for hearing evaluation

b. Renal ultrasound

c. Referral to surgery for removal

d. Referral to dermatology for removal

e. Ligation at the bedside with suture material

18-5. A 2-month-old infant in the cardiac ICU is noted to have clustered, 1-mm, noninflammatory vesicles in a linear array along the forehead. The vesicles rupture easily, contain clear fluid, and are nontender.

(Reproduced, with permission, from Rudolph CD, Rudolph AM, Lister GE, First LR, Gershon AA. *Rudolph's Pediatrics.* 22nd ed. <www.accesspediatrics.com>. Copyright © The McGraw-Hill Companies, Inc. All rights reserved.)

The bedside nurse remarks that the patient had a noninvasive cerebral perfusion monitor over the site postoperatively that was removed yesterday. The patient is otherwise stable. What is the most likely diagnosis?

a. Impetigo

b. Erythema toxicum neonatorum

c. Miliaria crystallina

d. Milia

e. Miliaria profunda

18-6. An otherwise healthy 4-week-old infant male is noted to have vesicles and pustules on his palms and soles. The patient's mother thinks the eruption may be pruritic because the infant is not sleeping well and is constantly rubbing his hands and feet. The mother describes the lesions as "coming in waves." Other members of the family are not itching. What is the most likely diagnosis?

a. Acropustulosis of infancy

b. Congenital syphilis

c. Scabies

d. Sucking blisters

e. Contact dermatitis

18-7. An otherwise healthy 2-day-old infant girl is noted to have small inflammatory pustules on the torso and extremities but sparing the palms and soles.

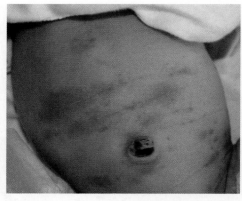

(Reproduced, with permission, from Weinberg S, Prose NS, Kristal L. *Color Atlas of Pediatric Dermatology.* 4th ed. New York: McGraw-Hill, 2007.)

A smear of the pustule contents is prepared. What would you expect to see on the smear?

a. Langerhans cells

b. Neutrophils

c. Cocci

d. Hyphae

e. Eosinophils

18-8. A 9-month-old infant boy is brought to your office by a frazzled mother. The mother reports that the patient has been constantly rubbing his feet together. It is affecting his sleeping and eating habits. On examination, the infant is noted to have a widespread polymorphous eruption with papules, nodules, vesicles, and crusted lesions. The palms and soles are involved, particularly the insteps. You notice that the mom is scratching her abdomen during the visit. What is the most likely diagnosis?

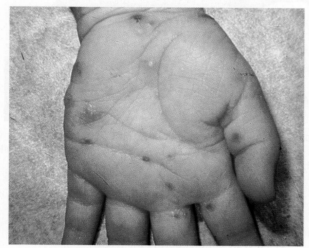

(Reproduced, with permission, from Weinberg S, Prose NS, Kristal L. *Color Atlas of Pediatric Dermatology.* 4th ed. New York: McGraw-Hill, 2007.)

a. Transient neonatal pustulosis

b. Impetigo

c. Atopic dermatitis

d. Scabies

e. Acropustulosis of infancy

18-9. A 3-month-old infant is noted to have failure to thrive, fussiness, and an erosive dermatitis around the mouth and in the diaper area. What is the most likely underlying cause of this constellation of symptoms?

a. Acrodermatitis enteropathica

b. Cystic fibrosis

c. Kwashiorkor

d. Maple syrup urine disease

e. Citrullinemia

18-10. An infant presents at 1 week of life with new painful skin with blisters, erythema, and erosions. He is febrile and irritable. You call for a stat dermatology consult and they perform a skin biopsy that is sent for frozen sections. The pathologist calls to tell you there is a split in the epidermis without full-thickness necrosis. Cultures were just sent, but the results are not back yet. What is the next best step in management?

a. Stop all medications and treat as a burn patient.

b. Wait for the cultures to come back before starting any medications.

c. Start treatment for staphylococcal scalded skin syndrome.

d. Ask the parents if the infant could have been sunburned.

e. Consult genetics to discuss the workup for epidermolysis bullosa.

18-11. A term newborn infant is born with scattered nonblanching purpuric lesions. Skin biopsy shows nucleated red blood cells and erythroid precursors. Which of the following is responsible for this finding?

a. Coxsackievirus

b. Varicella virus

c. Epstein-Barr virus

d. Congenital leukemia

e. Maternal vitamin deficiency

18-12. A newborn female infant is noted on the second day of life to have numerous vesicles in a linear array on her left arm. She is otherwise well appearing. In reading through the maternal history you note that the patient's mother had 3 spontaneous miscarriages of male fetuses. What diagnosis is suspected?

a. Thermal burn

b. Sucking blisters

c. Intrauterine varicella

d. Incontinentia pigmenti (IP)

e. Hypomelanosis of Ito

18-13. A 3-year-old child presents to your clinic. The mother states that they have run out of the creams prescribed for her son's eczema, and the child is itchy. She is concerned because there are some round blisters and open sores with crusting in the antecubital fossae, popliteal fossae, and face where the itching is worst.

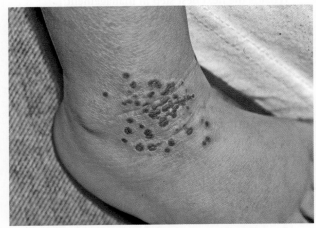

(Reproduced, with permission, from Rudolph CD, Rudolph AM, Lister GE, First LR, Gershon AA. *Rudolph's Pediatrics.* 22nd ed. New York: McGraw-Hill, 2011.)

Of the following, the *most* likely pathogen involved in this pattern of infection is:

a. Herpes simplex virus

b. Human papillomavirus

c. Molluscum contagiosum

d. Varicella-zoster virus

e. *Staphylococcus aureus*

18-14. A 12-month-old girl presents with a 3-month history of a pruritic rash that involves her cheeks, neck, anterior trunk, and antecubital and popliteal areas. The rash improves after use of an over-the-counter topical steroid cream, but still is present most days, and the infant often wakes up at night scratching. On physical examination, you observe a raised erythematous rash that has areas of lichenification.

In addition to prescribing low-medium–potency topical steroids, the most helpful intervention is to:

a. Eliminate fruit and acidic juices from the diet.

b. Eliminate milk, eggs, soy, and wheat from the diet.

c. Treat with topical mupirocin.

d. Prescribe a bedtime dose of oral hydroxyzine, 1 mg/kg/dose.

e. Prescribe a morning dose of oral cetirizine, 2.5 mg.

18-15. A 10-year-old boy presents to your office with a 2-day history of an intensely pruritic plaque studded with vesicles on his lower leg. He also has edema and erythema of his penis and scrotum. He returned from a camping trip in Northern California yesterday.

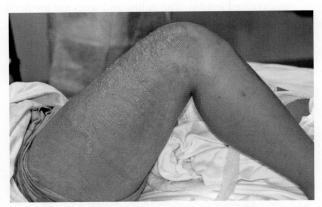

(Reproduced, with permission, from Rudolph CD, Rudolph AM, Lister GE, First LR, Gershon AA. *Rudolph's Pediatrics.* 22nd ed. New York: McGraw-Hill, 2011.)

The most likely diagnosis is:

a. Herpes simplex virus infection

b. Allergic contact dermatitis (ACD)

c. Atopic dermatitis

d. Candidal balanitis

e. Lichen striatus

18-16. A 15-year-old boy presents with the complaint of scalp scaling and mild itching for the last 6 months. He shampoos every other day. On examination, he has scaling throughout his scalp with minimal erythema. He has scaling and erythema in his alar grooves, and medial brows. He has no alopecia.

What is the most likely diagnosis?

a. Tinea capitis

b. Seborrheic dermatitis

c. Atopic dermatitis

d. Psoriasis

e. Contact dermatitis

18-17. A 6-month-old girl has been taking amoxicillin for an otitis media for the past 4 days. She has had 1 day of bright red papules and plaques in the diaper area. The inguinal folds are involved.

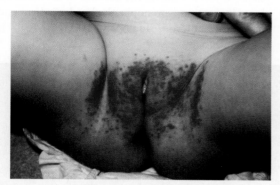

(Reproduced, with permission, from Rudolph CD, Rudolph AM, Lister GE, First LR, Gershon AA. *Rudolph's Pediatrics.* 22nd ed. New York: McGraw-Hill, 2011.)

Which of the following is the most appropriate treatment?

a. Clotrimazole cream

b. Triamcinolone ointment

c. Nystatin/triamcinolone cream

d. Terbinafine cream

e. Zinc oxide paste

18-18. The picture in eFigure 358-13 is most consistent with which of the following diagnosis?

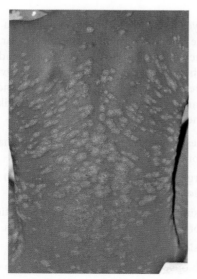

eFIGURE 358-13. (Reproduced, with permission, from Rudolph CD, Rudolph AM, Lister GE, First LR, Gershon AA. *Rudolph's Pediatrics.* 22nd ed. New York: McGraw-Hill, 2011.)

a. Atopic dermatitis

b. Seborrheic dermatitis

c. Pityriasis lichenoides chronica

d. Pityriasis rosea

e. Psoriasis

18-19. A 5-year-old African American girl presents to your office with a linear, hypopigmented, slightly scaly plaque on her anterior leg that has been present for 2 months. Her mother states that initially it was darker and violaceous. It is not itchy.

What is the most likely diagnosis?

a. Lichen striatus

b. Lichen nitidus

c. Lichen planus

d. Epidermal nevus

e. Contact dermatitis

18-20. A 9-year-old boy with a remote history of atopic dermatitis presents with a 1-month history of an intensely pruritic hand rash. He gets 1- to 2-mm deep-seated vesicles on his palms and the lateral aspects of his fingers. He has tried hydrocortisone 1% with no improvement.

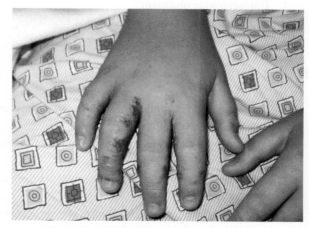

(Reproduced, with permission, from Kane KS, Lio PA, Stratigos AJ, Johnson RA. *Color Atlas & Synopsis of Pediatric Dermatology.* 2nd ed. New York: McGraw-Hill, 2010.)

What is the most appropriate treatment for him?

a. Hydrocortisone 2.5% ointment BID

b. Triamcinolone 0.025% ointment BID

c. Fluocinonide 0.05% ointment BID

d. Terbinafine cream BID

e. Oral prednisone for 7 days

18-21. The patient photographed in Figure 408-7 has had a 3-month history of a persistent rash around the mouth and in the groin. He/she is irritable.

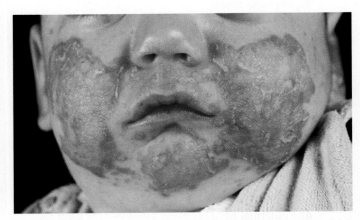

FIGURE 408-7. (Reproduced, with permission, from Rudolph CD, Rudolph AM, Lister GE, First LR, Gershon AA. *Rudolph's Pediatrics.* 22nd ed. New York: McGraw-Hill, 2011.)

Which of the following is the most appropriate therapy for this eruption?

a. Clotrimazole cream

b. Mupirocin ointment

c. Triamcinolone ointment

d. Cephalexin, by mouth

e. Zinc supplementation, by mouth

18-22. Which of the following statements about topical steroids is true?

a. Three times a day application is more effective than twice a day application.

b. For atopic dermatitis (AD), ointments are preferred over creams.

c. For hair-bearing areas such as the scalp, creams are the preferred vehicle.

d. The use of medium-potency topical steroids causes suppression of the hypothalamic–pituitary–adrenal axis.

e. For patients with hand eczema, superpotency or very-high-potency (Class I or II) steroids are always necessary.

18-23. An 8-year-old boy presents to urgent care. The mother states that for the past 3 weeks her son has an expanding "ring" on his hand. On examination, the boy's only skin finding is a 1 × 1 cm pink annular plaque without scale on the dorsum of his hand. On closer inspection, you notice the border is firm and consists of numerous small papules (Figure 359-1).

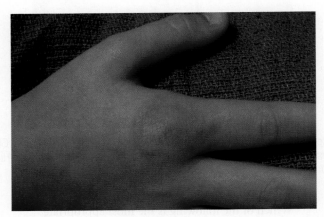

FIGURE 359-1. (Reproduced, with permission, from Rudolph CD, Rudolph AM, Lister GE, First LR, Gershon AA. *Rudolph's Pediatrics.* 22nd ed. New York: McGraw-Hill, 2011.)

Of the following, the *most* likely diagnosis is:

a. Nummular eczema

b. Psoriasis

c. Tinea corporis

d. Granuloma annulare

e. Erythema migrans

18-24. A 16-year-old girl presents to clinic with a brown, firm nodule extending from the helix of her ear. She claims to have first noticed a smooth rubbery nodule 2 years ago when she got a piercing at this site. Over time, this area has increased in pigmentation and become firm, and occasionally itches. She would like to discuss treatment options.

The best advice to give her regarding management of this condition is:

a. Surgical excision is highly successful in removing lesions.

b. A single treatment of intralesional corticosteroid is more efficacious than serial treatments.

c. Lesions will spontaneously resolve.

d. A biopsy should be performed prior to discussing treatment.

e. Avoidance of elective traumatic procedures such as piercings is critical in preventing future lesions.

18-25. A 15-year-old girl presents for a well-child visit. Her mother asks you about "stretch marks" that she has noticed on her daughter's abdomen over the past year. On examination, you note atrophic, red-violet linear plaques on her abdomen.

Which of the following diagnoses is most likely to be associated with the skin findings described above?

a. Marfan syndrome

b. Obesity

c. Bulemia

d. Topical steroid use

e. Hyperthyroidism

18-26. A 12-year-old girl presents with a complaint of painful tender nodules on her shins for the past 2 weeks. Her mother initially thought that they were insect bites but is questioning that diagnosis given their persistence. On examination, you note deep red, warm nodules in the pretibial area bilaterally that are extremely tender to palpation.

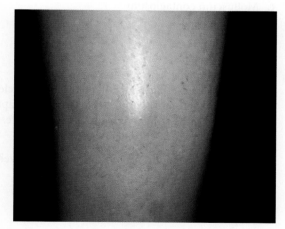

(Reproduced, with permission, from Weinberg S, Prose NS, Kristal L. *Color Atlas of Pediatric Dermatology.* 4th ed. New York: McGraw-Hill, 2007.)

Which test would help you identify the most common cause of this condition?

a. ASO

b. Colonoscopy

c. EBV serology

d. Incision and drainage with wound culture

e. *Bartonella henselae* serology

18-27. A 4-week-old ex-full-term infant presents for follow-up in your primary care clinic. The mother states that the infant was in the neonatal intensive care unit for 1 week. Discharge papers indicate the infant had low Apgars and was placed on a hypothermia cooling protocol for 24 hours after he was born for birth asphyxia. The paperwork also indicates that the infant developed tender, erythematous nodules and plaques on his back at day 4 of life. On examination today, the infant is well appearing, is gaining weight well, and has a normal cutaneous examination.

Which of the following conditions is this infant still at risk for?

a. Hypocalcemia

b. Hypercalcemia

c. Hyperglycemia

d. Thrombocytopenia

e. Hypothyrodism

18-28. A mother brings in her 14-year-old boy for evaluation of a rash that has progressed over the past 6 months. Initially, he had predominantly thin, white scale most prominent over the lower legs, but now has a very pruritic rash on the face, anterior trunk, and antecubital and popliteal areas. On physical examination, you also notice an increase in palmar markings on both hands.

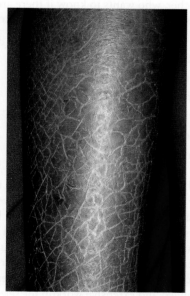

(Reproduced, with permission, from Rudolph CD, Rudolph AM, Lister GE, First LR, Gershon AA. *Rudolph's Pediatrics.* 22nd ed. New York: McGraw-Hill, 2011.)

In addition to atopic dermatitis, the presentation above is consistent with which of the following diagnoses?

a. Xerosis

b. Ichthyosis vulgaris

c. X-linked ichthyosis

d. Psoriasis

e. Pityriasis rosea

18-29. You are seeing an 18-month-old boy who is a new patient to your clinic. His mother states that his father has a diagnosis of neurofibromatosis type 1 (NF-1) and she is concerned that her son may have the condition.

In addition to a family history of NF in a first-degree relative, which other finding is diagnostic for NF type 1?

a. Three café au lait macules greater than 1.6 cm in diameter

b. Five café au lait macules greater than 0.5 cm in diameter

c. Six café au lait macules greater than 0.5 cm in diameter

d. Eight café au lait macules greater than 0.3 cm in diameter

e. Ten café au lait macules less than 0.5 cm in diameter

18-30. You are seeing a 12-year-old girl with neurofibromatosis type 1 (NF-1) in follow-up in your clinic. She was diagnosed with NF-1 at 3 years of age based on the presence of multiple café au lait macules and axillary freckling. She is followed regularly by ophthalmology for optic gliomas and has an individualized education plan (IEP) for learning difficulties. She is in clinic with her mother, who wants to know if there are any other features of NF-1 that she should be monitoring for.

Which of the following findings typically do not appear until after puberty in patients with NF-1?

a. Dermal neurofibromas

b. Plexiform neurofibromas

c. Lisch nodules

d. Sphenoid dysplasia

e. Central nervous system tumors

18-31. A mother brings her 1-month-old female infant in for her well-child check. She is growing well and her physical examination is normal; however, her mother appears very apprehensive and concerned despite this information. After further discussion, you find out that her mother has a friend whose 5-year-old child was recently diagnosed with tuberous sclerosis after a prolonged and extensive workup for seizures that developed during infancy. Her friend also told her that patients with tuberous sclerosis often have findings on the skin early in infancy that can aid in diagnosis.

Which cutaneous manifestation of tuberous sclerosis is the most consistent and often the earliest finding of the condition?

a. Adenoma sebaceum (angiofibromas)

b. Gingival fibromas

c. Periungual fibromas (Koenen tumors)

d. Shagreen patches (collagenomas)

e. Hypopigmented macules

18-32. A mother brings her 13-year-old son to your clinic requesting treatment for his acne. She says he has always had a few small red papules on his nose and cheeks since he was 6 years old, but over the past 2 years has developed many more of these in the same location. The papules are asymptomatic, but his mom says none of them ever resolve. She has never noticed any "blackheads" (open comedones) or pustules. Her son's past medical history is notable for developmental delay and seizures. On physical examination, you note numerous skin-colored to red papules on the central face, particularly the lower forehead, nose, and medial cheeks. There are no open or closed comedones or inflammatory pustules.

What is the diagnosis for his cutaneous findings?

a. Adenoma sebaceum

b. Acne vulgaris

c. Molluscum contagiosum

d. Shagreen patches

e. Keratosis pilaris

18-33. A 6-year-old boy who is new to your clinic has dysmorphic facies, sparse hair, hypoplastic nails, cleft palate, and hypodontia with teeth that are peg shaped. You also notice his father has a similar appearance. The patient otherwise has normal development.

What category of conditions does this patient have?

a. Ehlers-Danlos syndrome

b. Ichthyosis

c. Atopy

d. Ectodermal dysplasia

e. Neurocutaneous disorder

18-34. Which factor is the *most likely* cause of acquired melanocytic nevi in children?

a. Intense and intermittent sun exposure

b. Sun exposure in the late evening

c. Chemotherapy

d. Sunscreen

e. Chronic bullous pemphigoid

18-35. You are seeing a child for a regular well-child visit and find that shown in Figure 361-2D on her scalp. What is the most appropriate next step in management for this child?

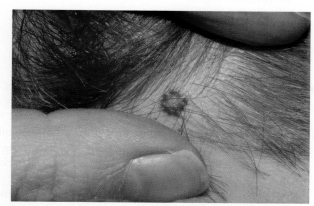

FIGURE 361-2D. (Reproduced, with permission, from Rudolph CD, Rudolph AM, Lister GE, First LR, Gershon AA. *Rudolph's Pediatrics.* 22nd ed. New York: McGraw-Hill, 2011.)

a. Observation

b. Urgent referral to pediatric dermatologist

c. Excisional skin biopsy

d. Genetic testing

e. Treatment with liquid nitrogen

18-36. Parents of a 2-year-old boy present to your office with concern regarding this lesion on their child's leg. They recently had a family friend pass away from melanoma. The lesion has been present since birth and has been increasing in size in proportion to the child's growth (Figure 361-3A).

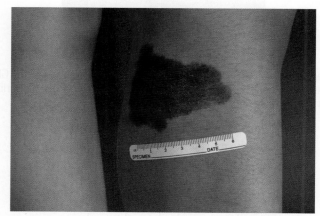

FIGURE 361-3A. (Reproduced, with permission, from Rudolph CD, Rudolph AM, Lister GE, First LR, Gershon AA. *Rudolph's Pediatrics.* 22nd ed. New York: McGraw-Hill, 2011.)

What is the best description of the lesion?

a. Large congenital melanocytic nevus (CMN)

b. Medium CMN

c. Melanoma

d. Nevus of Ota

e. Becker nevus

18-37. A 4-year-old child presents to the clinic with a 3-month history of an asymptomatic uniformly pink papule (Figure 361-2E) on her right cheek. It grew rapidly over the first 4 weeks and has since stabilized. Which of the following is the most likely diagnosis?

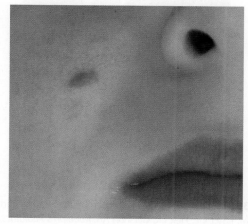

FIGURE 361-2E. (Reproduced, with permission, from Rudolph CD, Rudolph AM, Lister GE, First LR, Gershon AA. *Rudolph's Pediatrics.* 22nd ed. New York: McGraw-Hill, 2011.)

a. Dysplastic melanocytic nevus

b. Pyogenic granuloma

c. Cherry angioma

d. Spitz nevus

e. Acne vulgaris

18-38. Which of the following clinical features are associated with neurofibromatosis type 1?

a. Multiple lentigines, pulmonary stenosis, deafness, skeletal abnormalities

b. Generalized lentigines, atrial myxomas, blue nevi, psammomatous melanotic schwannomas

c. Axillary freckling, macrocephaly, optic glioma, sphenoid dysplasia

d. Café au lait macules, capillary and venous malformations, mental retardation, macrocephaly

e. Perioral lentigines, longitudinal melanonychia, multiple hamartomatous GI polyps, increased incidence of ovarian cancer

18-39. A 19-year-old boy presents to your clinic with a 4-month history of lightening of the skin on his leg as shown in Figure 361-4C. What is the etiology of this disorder?

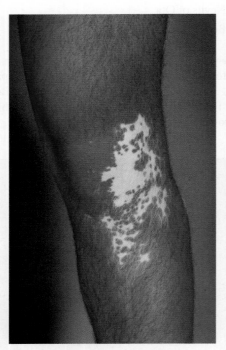

FIGURE 361-4C. (Reproduced, with permission, from Rudolph CD, Rudolph AM, Lister GE, First LR, Gershon AA. *Rudolph's Pediatrics.* 22nd ed. New York: McGraw-Hill, 2011.)

a. Autoimmune destruction of melanocytes in the epidermis and hair follicles

b. Primary adrenal insufficiency

c. Clone of cells with reduced melanogenic potential that arises during embryonic development

d. Protein deficiency

e. Copper deficiency

18-40. Which disorder can be associated with persistent extensive dermal melanocytosis (Mongolian spots) that affects the ventral and dorsal trunk, and can progress over time?

a. Tuberous sclerosis

b. Hurler syndrome

c. Menkes kinky hair syndrome

d. Neurofibromatosis type 1

e. Neonatal lupus erythematosus

18-41. An 18-year-old male presents to clinic with new onset of blue-gray discoloration within his acne lesions. Which medication was he prescribed for his acne?

a. Benzoyl peroxide gel

b. Tretinoin cream

c. Minocycline

d. Doxycycline

e. Clindamycin solution

18-42. A 5-year-old boy presents to the emergency room with a rash on his arms and legs that abruptly started 3 days ago. Other symptoms include the development of oral ulcers. On examination, you note an uncomfortable child with symmetrically distributed target lesions consisting of a dusky center surrounded by pale edema and a darker violaceous rim. The rash is located on the face and extremities with involvement of the palms and soles, and the rash spares the trunk. You also note blistering and hemorrhagic crusting of the lips and oral mucosa. The conjunctiva and genitalia are normal on examination.

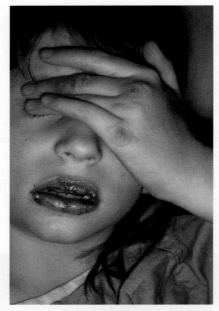

(Reproduced, with permission, from Rudolph CD, Rudolph AM, Lister GE, First LR, Gershon AA. *Rudolph's Pediatrics.* 22nd ed. New York: McGraw-Hill, 2011.)

What is the most common underlying etiology attributed for this rash?

a. *Mycoplasma pneumoniae*

b. Amoxicillin

c. Trimethoprim and sulfamethoxazole

d. HSV

e. Cefaclor

18-43. A 12-year-old presents to the emergency room with a chief complaint of fever and rash. The child has significant past medical history of poorly controlled epilepsy. He currently takes lamotrigine that was started 6 weeks ago. At the same time, he was tapered off valproic acid. On examination, you note a temperature of 39°C, heart rate of 130, respiratory rate of 28, and normal blood pressure. The child is lethargic and you note facial edema, enlarged bilateral cervical lymph nodes, and faint erythematous macular rash coalescing in patches and plaques and predominately involving the trunk. Labs are significant for a WBC 15,000 with 60% segmented neutrophils, 20% lymphocytes, and 10% eosinophils and a transaminitis AST 150, ALT 175 with normal bilirubin and alkaline phosphatase.

Which of the following is the best diagnosis?

a. Angioedema

b. Acute generalized exanthematous pustulosis (AGEP)

c. Acute urticaria

d. Stevens-Johnson syndrome

e. Drug hypersensitivity syndrome or drug reaction with eosinophilia and systemic symptoms (DRESS)

18-44. This 4-week-old infant presents to urgent care with a 2-day history of an asymptomatic rash (Figure 362-2). What is the most likely pathogenic factor in this child's disease?

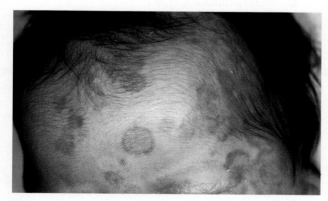

FIGURE 362-2. (Reproduced, with permission, from Rudolph CD, Rudolph AM, Lister GE, First LR, Gershon AA. *Rudolph's Pediatrics.* 22nd ed. New York: McGraw-Hill, 2011.)

a. Delayed hypersensitivity to baby shampoo

b. Hypersensitivity to *Malassezia furfur*

c. Inherited dry and sensitive skin

d. Inherited tendency toward psoriasis (HLA-CW6)

e. Transplacental transfer of anti-Ro antibodies

18-45. This girl has had 3 months of painful urination and defecation, and occasional pruritus. At the onset of symptoms she had a bruise on her labia minora and some swelling of the clitoral hood (Figure 362-4). She denies any sexual abuse. She had a negative urinalysis and urine culture.

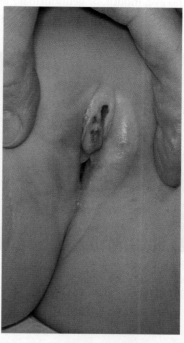

FIGURE 362-4. (Reproduced, with permission, from Rudolph CD, Rudolph AM, Lister GE, First LR, Gershon AA. *Rudolph's Pediatrics.* 22nd ed. <www.accesspediatrics.com>. Copyright © The McGraw-Hill Companies, Inc. All rights reserved.)

What is the best treatment for her?

a. Clotrimazole topical BID

b. Clobetasol ointment BID

c. Fluconazole PO for 5 days

d. Hydrocortisone 1% ointment BID

e. Zinc oxide paste topical BID

18-46. What is the most common type of skin disease in children with HIV?

a. Atopic dermatitis

b. Seborrheic dermatitis

c. Mucocutaneous candidiasis

d. Molluscum contagiosum

e. Verruca vulgaris

18-47. A 1-year-old boy is brought to urgent care for evaluation of abrupt-onset blisters on his face, abdomen, arms, and legs over the past 2 days. He is itchy and a little more fussy than usual. He is afebrile and eating and drinking normally. On examination, you note multiple clustered tense vesicles and bullae in a rosette pattern on his face, trunk, and extremities. He has no eye, mouth, or genitourinary lesions. He is generally well appearing with normal vital signs.

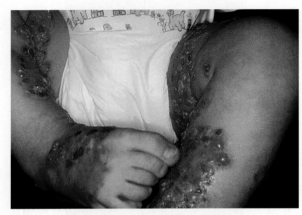

(Reproduced, with permission, from Kane KS, Lio PA, Stratigos AJ, Johnson RA. *Color Atlas & Synopsis of Pediatric Dermatology*. 2nd ed. New York: McGraw-Hill, 2010.)

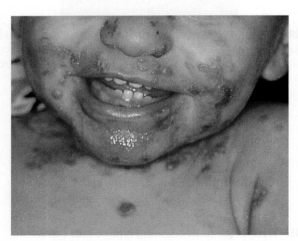

(Reproduced, with permission, from Kane KS, Lio PA, Stratigos AJ, Johnson RA. *Color Atlas & Synopsis of Pediatric Dermatology*. 2nd ed. New York: McGraw-Hill, 2010.)

What is the most likely diagnosis?

a. Bullous impetigo

b. Bullous pemphigoid

c. Erythema multiforme (EM)

d. Linear IgA bullous dermatosis (LABD)

e. Stevens-Johnson syndrome

18-48. A 2-month-old infant presents with a solitary 0.5 cm firm, dome-shaped, yellow-red papule on the left temple. The parents state that they did not notice the lesion at birth.

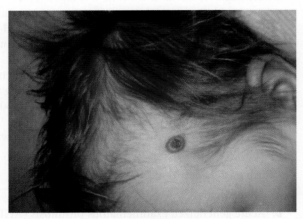

(Reproduced, with permission, from Kane KS, Lio PA, Stratigos AJ, Johnson RA. *Color Atlas & Synopsis of Pediatric Dermatology*. 2nd ed. New York: McGraw-Hill, 2010.)

The subset of patients with the above finding and which other condition have an increased incidence of myelogenous leukemia?

a. Down syndrome

b. Noonan syndrome

c. Neurofibromatosis type 1

d. Tuberous sclerosis

e. Ataxia telangiectasia

18-49. You are evaluating a 3-year-old boy who presents to the urgent care clinic with few scattered red-brown papules on his torso. His mother is concerned, because these lesions will occasionally be pruritic. When he scratches these spots or when he takes a warm bath, they will often flare up and become hive-like. What is the most likely diagnosis?

a. Urticaria pigmentosa

b. Dermatofibroma

c. Langerhans cell histiocytosis

d. Dermatitis herpetiformis

e. Erythema multiforme

18-50. A 2-month-old boy presents for a well-child visit. The infant is growing and developing well. On examination, you notice a total of 10 hemangiomas distributed on his scalp, back, and thighs. They are well circumscribed, not ulcerated, and on average 1.5 × 1.5 cm in size. The mother believes that these have been increasing in size for the past month.

The infant is at risk of developing which of the following conditions?

a. Kasabach-Merritt phenomenon (KMP)

b. Dandy-Walker malformation

c. Subglottic hemangioma

d. Hepatic hemangiomas

e. Congenital cardiac malformation

18-51. A 2.5-month-old male infant presents with a rapidly expanding vascular mass on the right upper eyelid. The mother states she noticed a deeply red vascular papule a couple weeks after he was born but this area has been increasing in size recently. On examination, the infant is well appearing but has a large, deeply red vascular tumor of the upper eyelid occluding approximately 75% of the visual field.

Which of the following is the most appropriate treatment?

a. Triamcinolone 0.1% ointment twice per day

b. Intralesional triamcinolone

c. Oral propranolol

d. Conservative watching

e. Referral for surgical debulking

18-52. The infant in Photo 364-1A is at risk for which of the following?

a. Cerebrovascular anomalies

b. Intracranial calcifications

c. Hepatic hemangiomas

d. Consumptive coagulopathy

e. Tethered cord

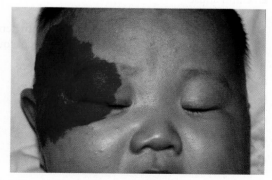

PHOTO 364-1A. (Reproduced, with permission, from Rudolph CD, et al. *Rudolph's Pediatrics*. 22nd ed. New York: McGraw-Hill, 2011.)

18-53. A 10-month-old infant presents to the emergency room in critical condition. The infant is lethargic and you notice a large, indurated purple mass on the thigh with an ecchymotic border. The mother states that the patient had a "birthmark" in this area that has rapidly increased in size in the last week. Labs reveal thrombocytopenia, hypofibrigonemia, and elevated D-dimer.

Which of the following vascular anomalies is associated with this condition?

a. Infantile hemangioma

b. Arteriovenous malformation

c. Rapidly involuting congenital hemangioma (RICH)

d. Tufted angioma

e. Angiokeratoma

18-54. The mother of a 4-year-old boy who you follow in your primary clinic has several questions as to whether her son requires further evaluation for a "birthmark" that he had as an infant. The mother states that her son had a faint pink patch on his midforehead that has faded over time. Pictures of the child as an infant reveal a pink patch affecting the midline forehead and glabella. On today's examination, no vascular stain is appreciated and he otherwise has a normal examination.

What is the most appropriate next step in the management of this patient?

a. Refer to neurology for developmental testing.

b. Refer to ophthalmology.

c. Reassurance that no further workup is needed.

d. CT head without contrast.

e. MRI of brain with and without contrast.

18-55. An infant is born with a large mass affecting the left neck. On examination, you note a large skin-colored mass that transilluminates and is compressible with palpation. A karyotype reveals an XO abnormality.

Which is the most likely diagnosis?

a. Infantile hemangioma

b. Thryoglossal duct cyst

c. Cystic hygroma

d. Venous malformation

e. Teratoma

18-56. What percentage of people aged 12 to 24 have acne?

a. 10%

b. 25%

c. 50%

d. 85%

e. 100%

18-57. Which of the following is involved in the pathogenesis of acne vulgaris?

a. Abnormal desquamation of follicular keratinocytes

b. Exaggerated host response to *Staphylococcus aureus*

c. Excessive intake of chocolate products

d. Exaggerated host response to *Pityrosporum*

e. Repeated trauma to the skin

18-58. A 14-year-old girl presents to your office with a few inflammatory papules and pustules and a moderate number of open comedones on her forehead. She has no scarring. She is quite bothered by her acne, and has tried only salicylic acid wash.

What is the most appropriate initial management plan for her?

a. Continue benzoyl peroxide 5% gel topical, twice a day.

b. Start benzoyl peroxide 5% and clindamycin 1% gel QAM, tretinoin cream 0.025% QHS.

c. Start tretinoin cream 0.025% topical, nightly.

d. Start minocycline 100 mg by mouth, twice a day.

e. Start doxycycline 100 mg by mouth, twice a day.

18-59. You see a 16-year-old boy in your office for his acne. He has been taking oral tetracycline for 3 months with no improvement. He is wearing a hooded sweatshirt that he is reluctant to take off because his acne is so severe. His face, chest, and back have large erythematous and fluctuant nodules and cysts, depressed scars, and many open comedones.

What is the best treatment for him?

a. Doxycycline

b. Minocycline

c. Trimethoprim/sulfamethoxazole

d. Cefadroxil

e. Isotretinoin

18-60. A mother brings her 5-year-old girl in for an urgent appointment. She has noticed that her daughter has had a bald patch on her scalp for the last week. Her scalp is not itchy. She is otherwise well. On examination, you notice a round, quarter-sized area of alopecia with a light peach color on the parietal scalp. There is no scale. There are no broken hairs.

What is the most likely diagnosis?

a. Alopecia areata

b. Congenital triangular alopecia

c. Telogen effluvium

d. Tinea capitis

e. Trichotillomania

18-61. A 7-year-old boy presents to your office for evaluation of a lump on his upper arm that has been growing slowly over the past 5 months. On examination, he has a 1-cm bluish, firm, subcutaneous nodule on his upper arm. It appears tethered to the overlying dermis and when you press down on one side, the other side elevates, like a teeter-totter.

What is the most likely diagnosis?

a. Acne cyst

b. Epidermal inclusion cyst

c. Granuloma annulare (GA)

d. Abscess

e. Pilomatricoma

18-62. A mother is concerned for her 2-year-old son because he looks pale and is constantly found eating sand from the sand box in the park. He is very picky eater and is only taking a limited number of solids. You perform a CBC with differential and discover the child has iron deficiency anemia. What nail abnormality is most likely associated with iron deficiency anemia?

a. Koilonychia

b. Onycholysis

c. Melanonychia striata

d. Nail pitting

e. Subungual debris

18-63. A 1-year-old child comes in for his well-child check. On physical examination, you see 1- to 2-mm, transverse, white bands on the fingernails. What should you screen for?

a. Asthma

b. Seasonal allergies

c. Lead poisoning

d. Milk protein intolerance

e. Child abuse

18-64. You are seeing a 16-year-old boy in clinic with acne and plan to start him on minocycline. What effects could the medication have on the child's nails?

a. Nail pitting

b. Blue discoloration of lunulae

c. Thickening of nails

d. Leuconychia

e. Brown or black discoloration of nails

18-65. A 6-month-old female infant is brought to urgent care for a blistering diaper rash. The mother reports a 4-day history of blisters that easily rupture. The rash is limited to the diaper area. On examination, the child is afebrile and well appearing. In the diaper area, there are scattered flaccid bullae and moist superficial erosions, some with a collarette of scale (Figure 3-3). The remainder of the skin examination is normal.

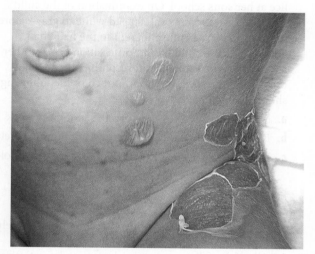

FIGURE 3-3. (Reproduced, with permission, from Weinberg S, Prose NS, Kristal L. *Color Atlas of Pediatric Dermatology*. 4th ed. New York: McGraw-Hill, 2007.)

Which of the following is the most likely diagnosis?
a. Epidermolysis bullosa
b. Friction blisters
c. Bullous impetigo
d. HSV
e. Staphylococcal scalded skin syndrome

18-66. A 5-year-old boy with a history of atopic dermatitis presents to the emergency department with redness and swelling of his left lower leg. On physical examination, the child is non–toxic-appearing and febrile to 38.5°C. His left lower leg shows bright red ill-defined erythema that is warm to the touch and somewhat painful. There is groin lymphadenopathy. A CBC reveals an elevated WBC of 15 with neutrophil predominance. Which of the following is the most likely diagnosis?
a. Impetigo
b. Erysipelas
c. Cellulitis
d. Necrotizing fasciitis
e. Atopic dermatitis flare

18-67. What percentage of common warts (verruca vulgaris) will spontaneously resolve within 2 years?
a. 10%
b. 25%
c. 50%
d. 85%
e. 95%

18-68. A 7-year-old girl presents to her pediatrician for a new-onset itchy rash. Her mother notes that she had many skin-colored bumps that have recently become red and intensely itchy. On physical examination, the child is well appearing and has scattered skin-colored 2 to 4 mm, dome-shaped, umbilicated papules surrounded by erythematous scaly patches of the abdomen and inner thighs. Which of the following is the most appropriate next step in management?
a. Cantharidin topical application in the office
b. Cryotherapy
c. Topical corticosteroids
d. Watchful waiting
e. Imiquimod 5% cream

18-69. A 2-year-old boy presents to the emergency department with fever, poor appetite, decreased energy, and rash. He has also been complaining of ear pain for the past week. His mother states the rash started yesterday with generalized redness. On examination, an ill-appearing child is lying in bed with generalized tender erythema most marked in the axillae and inguinal folds. There are many scattered large erosions with collarettes of scale and few intact flaccid bullae. Nikolsky sign is positive. Crusting and fissuring is present periorally and periorbitally. Mucous membranes are spared. In addition to supportive care, which of the following is the most appropriate antibiotic choice?
a. Ceftriaxone
b. Vancomycin
c. Clindamycin
d. Zosyn
e. Acyclovir

18-70. A 10-year-old healthy girl presents to her pediatrician for her annual well-child visit. Her mother reports concern that her child has been scratching her scalp recently. On examination of her scalp, you see patchy areas of scaling erythema and associated broken hairs with few scattered pustules. Suboccipital lymphadenopathy is present. Which of the following is the best treatment option?

   a. Cephalexin oral antibiotic for 2-week course

   b. Triamcinolone 0.1% ointment BID until condition resolved

   c. Counseling the patient to stop pulling her hair

   d. Clotrimazole cream BID for 2 weeks

   e. Griseofulvin for 6-week course

18-71. A 10-year-old boy presents to the emergency department with intense pain in his left foot that has been worsening acutely over the past few hours. His parents report he has had fever since yesterday. On examination, the child is febrile and appears uncomfortable. There is diffuse swelling of his left foot with overlying ill-defined erythema and ecchymosis. Crepitus is noted on deep palpation. The child also cries out in pain when the foot is palpated. Distal pulses are intact. Which of the following is the most crucial next step?

   a. Start intravenous antibiotics.

   b. Obtain an MRI of the foot.

   c. Consult surgery.

   d. Order CBC with differential and ESR.

   e. Consult dermatology.

18-72. Which of the following is the most likely diagnosis (Figure 367-3)?

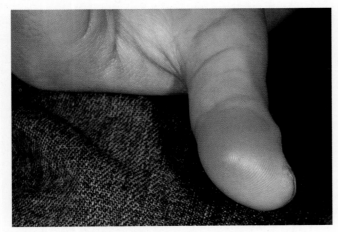

FIGURE 367-3. (Reproduced, with permission, from Rudolph CD, Rudolph AM, Lister GE, First LR, Gershon AA. *Rudolph's Pediatrics.* 22nd ed. New York: McGraw-Hill, 2011.)

   a. Herpetic whitlow

   b. Varicella

   c. Friction blister

   d. Blistering dactylitis

   e. Bullous impetigo

18-73. A 7-year-old boy is brought to pediatric urgent care by his mother because she was told there is an outbreak of lice at her son's school. On examination of the child's scalp, there are many oval-shaped white to gray-colored capsules that are firmly adherent to the hair shaft. You suspect the child has lice infestation. The mother asks you what treatment you recommend and when the child can return to school. Which of the following should you tell her?

   a. Malathion lotion 0.5%, return to school in 1 week

   b. Ivermectin 200 μg/kg, return to school immediately

   c. Permethrin 1% cream rinse (Nix), return to school immediately

   d. Pyrethrin shampoo (Rid-A), return to school in 1 week

   e. Hot air device to hair, return to school immediately

18-74. Which of the following is true about papular urticaria (insect bite–induced hypersensitivity)?

   a. The eruption is asymmetric.

   b. Course is progressive with worsening over time.

   c. Children less than 2 years old are often affected.

   d. Fleas, mosquitoes, and bed bug bites are commonly implicated.

   e. Treatment with oral steroids is often necessary.

18-75. A 10-year-old girl is brought to urgent care by her mother for a new skin rash that started 3 weeks ago. The rash is intensely itchy. Topical over-the-counter hydrocortisone has not improved the rash. On examination, she is well appearing with an eruption consisting of many excoriations, erythematous papules, a few vesicles, and 2 fine linear plaques between her fingers. Which of the following is the most likely diagnosis?

   a. Papular urticaria

   b. Atopic dermatitis

   c. Scabies infestation

   d. Viral exanthem

   e. Tinea corporis

ANSWERS

Answer 18-1. d

The skin is a vital organ with many important functions. The outermost skin layer, the stratum corneum, prevents desiccation of a primarily aqueous body in a dry atmosphere. It also contains moisturizing factors and components of the innate immune system. Langerhans cells in the epidermis provide immune surveillance, presenting antigen that activates lymphocytes. In atopic dermatitis immune function in skin is dysfunctional and the risk of infection is increased. The skin is also the body's major interface with UV light. Within the epidermis, UVB light isomerizes provitamin D to vitamin D_3, which is them converted to the active form (1,25-dihydroxyvitamin D_3) in the kidney. Epidermal melanin absorbs UV light, thereby protecting the keratinocytes from DNA damage induced by UV radiation. Sweat secreted from eccrine ducts in the skin helps with thermoregulation.

(Page 1249, Chapter 356: Functional Overview)

Answer 18-2. c

Figure 356-3 shows a photograph of a KOH preparation of scale with septate hyphae—most commonly seen in dermatophyte infections. The hyphae are thicker and more refractile than the keratinocyte borders, have parallel cell walls, and traverse multiple cell boundaries. Yeasts are round structures that occasionally demonstrate budding. Multinucleate keratinocytes are best seen when stained with methylene blue, toluidine blue, and Wright or Giemsa stains. Cytopathic viruses (eg, herpes simplex, herpes zoster, vaccinia) induce formation of multinucleate giant cells with enlarged nuclei and prominent nuclear inclusions. Crystallized KOH solution is an artifact seen when KOH dries out resulting in geometric crystals on the slide.

(Pages 1251-1252, Chapter 356: Functional Overview)

Answer 18-3. c

This patient has ACC (eFigure 357-1). The bulla is too large for herpes simplex or a fetal scalp electrode injury. Nevus sebaceous and congenital nevi do not blister.

ACC is a congenital absence of the skin that is often seen on the vertex scalp. It can present as a bulla, ulcer, or scar-like lesion. Most cases are sporadic, but autosomal dominant and autosomal recessive inheritance has been reported. It is characterized by an absent epidermis. In full-thickness lesions, all skin layers may be absent. It can be associated with underlying skull defects extending to the dura or meninges. Midline lesions (such as those over the vertex scalp) should be imaged to rule out connections to underlying structures.

ACC has been associated with various syndromes and anomalies, including cleft lip and palate, limb anomalies, cutaneous organoid nevi, and epidermolysis bullosa.

(Page 1252, Chapter 357: Neonatal Dermatology)

Answer 18-4. c

This infant has an accessory tragus. Accessory tragi can occur anywhere from the preauricular cheek to the angle of the mouth, and can be bilateral or multiple (eFigure 357-4). Their association with deafness and renal anomalies is controversial and screening for these anomalies is only recommended if there are concerning signs or symptoms. Since most lesions contain cartilage, they may have a connection to the external ear canal and therefore should only be removed by experienced surgeons.

(Page 1253, Chapter 357: Neonatal Dermatology)

Answer 18-5. c

The infant has miliaria crystallina (eFigure 357-7). Impetigo can be bullous but usually causes more inflammation and has a characteristic honey crust. Erythema toxicum neonatorum usually occurs in the first 2 days of life, typically presenting as scattered erythematous macules, wheals, and vesiculopustules. Milia are tiny cysts, rather than vesicles. Miliaria profunda causes deep edematous papules rather than vesicles.

Miliaria is also called "prickly heat." There are 3 variants: crystallina, rubra, and profunda. Miliaria crystallina is the most superficial of the variants and causes superficial subcorneal vesicles. Miliaria occurs when the ostia of eccrine ducts are incompletely canalized or obstructed, causing the accumulation of sweat droplets in the skin. Miliaria can be caused by excessive heat, bundling, or occlusion (as was the case with this patient). It is self-limited.

(Page 1254, Chapter 357: Neonatal Dermatology)

Answer 18-6. a

The infant has acropustulosis of infancy. Acropustulosis of infancy is a very pruritic eruption on the palms, soles, and lower extremities (eFigure 357-9).

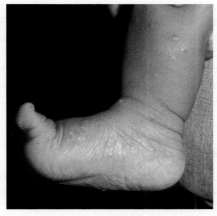

eFIGURE 357-9. (Reproduced, with permission, from Rudolph CD, Rudolph AM, Lister GE, First LR, Gershon AA. *Rudolph's Pediatrics.* 22nd ed. New York: McGraw-Hill, 2011.)

It is most commonly seen in African American males. Skin biopsy reveals intraepidermal vesicles with eosinophils or neutrophils. Treatment is with high-potency topical steroids and antihistamines to relieve the severe pruritus.

Congenital syphilis can cause lesions on the palms and soles, but patients usually have other stigmata (such as snuffles and multisystem disease) as well. Scabies should be included in the differential diagnosis, but it is likely that other family member would be itching as well. In addition, scabies usually causes a generalized eruption, not one localized to the hands and feet. Sucking blisters are present at birth, are not found on the feet, and are not pruritic. Contact dermatitis is extremely rare in neonates and the distribution is not consistent with contact dermatitis.

(Page 1254, Chapter 357: Neonatal Dermatology)

Answer 18-7. e

The infant has erythema toxicum neonatorum (eFigure 357-8). This common newborn eruption typically spares the palms, soles, and perioral region and this distribution of lesions can be used to differentiate erythema toxicum neonatorum from transient neonatal pustulosis. Smears of pustule contents typically show eosinophils. Smears from the pustules of transient neonatal pustulosis typically show neutrophils. Cocci would be seen in bacterial infection and hyphae in cutaneous candidiasis.

(Page 1254, Chapter 357: Neonatal Dermatology)

Answer 18-8. d

The infant has scabies. Scabies classically presents with a polymorphic eruption and severe pruritus. The distribution in infant can be generalized, but tends to involve the palms, insteps of feet, and axillae most prominently. Usually there are other family members who are itchy as well. The diagnosis can be made from a skin scraping that tends to be positive for mites, feces, or eggs. It is important to remember to treat infant with 5% permethrin from head to toe and then to repeat the treatment a week later. Other family members must be treated as well and decontamination procedures should be employed.

This infant is too old for transient neonatal pustulosis that is usually present at birth or appears within the first 24 hours of life. Impetigo does not generally cause severe pruritus. Atopic dermatitis can certainly cause severe pruritus, but the eruption is usually less polymorphous than that of scabetic dermatitis. Acropustulosis of infancy can also cause pruritic pustules, but these tend to be confined to the hands and feet.

(Page 1255, Chapter 357: Neonatal Dermatology)

Answer 18-9. b

This vignette describes an infant with a nutritional or metabolic deficiency. Any infant with an erosive, periorificial dermatitis should prompt a metabolic investigation. These skin manifestations are not specific for a unique deficiency; as such, all of the listed conditions can cause these findings; however, cystic fibrosis is the most common cause. Additional workup may include HIV screening, plasma zinc levels, and amino acid and organic acid profiles. Note that in the case of acrodermatitis enteropathica (or inherited zinc deficiency), improvement in symptoms and skin eruption occurs within days of starting zinc replacement therapy.

(Page 1254, 1257, Chapter 357: Neonatal Dermatology; Page 1261, Chapter 358: Disorders of the Epidermis)

Answer 18-10. c

The differential for painful skin with blisters and erosions in a neonate includes staphylococcal scalded skin syndrome, toxic epidermal necrolysis, and epidermolysis bullosa. In this case, the pathology is consistent with staphylococcal scalded skin syndrome and the patient should be treated before the cultures are back. Empiric antibiotics for *Staphylococcus aureus* are the treatment of choice. Cultures of the bullae and erosions will be negative, but the infection can often be found at a remote location (conjunctiva, nares, urine, umbilicus, etc).

Infants with epidermolysis bullosa usually present at birth and are not febrile. Toxic epidermal necrolysis shows full-thickness necrosis on biopsy and is associated with medications, graft-versus-host disease, and *Klebsiella* sepsis.

(Page 1256, Chapter 357: Neonatal Dermatology)

Answer 18-11. a

The rash described in this vignette is characteristic of extramedullary hematopoiesis or "blueberry muffin baby" phenotype. Skin biopsy of these lesions is an important part of making the diagnosis and shows nucleated red blood cells and erythroid or myeloid precursors. Extramedullary hematopoiesis can be caused by various congenital infections including syphilis, rubella, cytomegalovirus, coxsackievirus, parvovirus B19, and toxoplasmosis. Noninfectious causes include twin transfusion syndrome and intrauterine anemia resulting from Rh or ABO incompatibility.

Congenital leukemia can cause purpuric nodules in the newborn but skin biopsies show a neoplastic infiltrate. Maternal vitamin deficiency does not cause extramedullary hematopoiesis.

(Page 1257, Chapter 357: Neonatal Dermatology)

Answer 18-12. d

The patient most likely has IP, an X-linked dominant genodermatosis (eFigures 357-10 and 357-11). It results from a mutation in the NEMO gene. This condition is usually lethal in males, explaining the history of miscarriage in the mother. The skin findings in IP are characterized by 4 stages that often overlap. The earliest findings are usually vesicles that follow the lines of Blaschko. The other stages are verrucous, hyperpigmented, and hypopigmented/atrophic. The diagnosis is made via skin biopsy that shows eosinophilic spongiosis and dyskeratosis. There is no treatment and IP patients can have associated dental, CNS, and bone abnormalities.

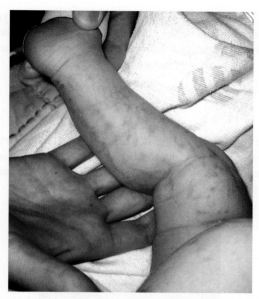

eFIGURE 357-10. Linear erythematous papules and vesicles following the lines of Blaschko in the vesicular stage of incontinentia pigmenti. (Reproduced, with permission, from Rudolph CD, Rudolph AM, Lister GE, First LR, Gershon AA. *Rudolph's Pediatrics.* 22nd ed. New York: McGraw-Hill, 2011.)

There was no history of thermal burn in this patient. Sucking blisters are usually not numerous. Patients with intrauterine varicella usually have widespread lesions and can have limb hypoplasia. Hypomelanosis of Ito is characterized by hypopigmented patches that follow the lines of Blaschko, but there is no preceding bullous or verrucous stage.

(Page 1254, Chapter 357: Neonatal Dermatology; Page 1267, Chapter 360: Genetic Disorders of the Skin)

Answer 18-13. a

Patients with atopic dermatitis are at risk for cutaneous infection with molluscum contagiosum and herpes simplex (eczema herpeticum). Eczema herpeticum presents as multiple vesicles or punched-out erosions that may be grouped or dispersed and are found on both normal and eczematized skin, as seen in the photo above. Children with primary eczema herpeticum often have a low-grade fever and malaise at the beginning of their illness. They are also often itchy and uncomfortable. Eczema herpeticum can often be treated with oral acyclovir. However, IV acyclovir should be used if the eczema herpeticum is widespread, the child is less than 3 months, or the child is ill-appearing.

The differential diagnosis also includes infections with group A *Streptococcus* infection, varicella, and *S. aureus.* Group A *Streptococcus* and *S. aureus* commonly infect children with atopic dermatitis, but do not cause vesicles, nor such monomorphous erosions. Molluscum contagiosum presents with shiny, flesh-colored, domed papules. VZV infection presents with diffuse vesicles on an erythematous base.

(Pages 1258-1259, Chapter 358: Disorders of the Epidermis)

Answer 18-14. d

The age of the patient, duration of the symptoms, and the itching combined with erythematous, scaly plaques make atopic dermatitis (AD) the most likely diagnosis. AD in infants younger than 2 years old often involves the extensor surfaces of the extremities in addition to the cheeks. Older children have the classic distribution of antecubital and popliteal fossae. The most significant aspect of preventive therapy is decreasing skin dryness with emollients and by avoidance of strongly alkaline soaps. Topical corticosteroids are the first-line therapy for management of disease exacerbations. For most patients, AD can be controlled with low- and medium-potency topical corticosteroids.

Oral antihistamines are useful adjuncts to therapy for control of pruritus. By scratching at night this child is creating more plaques of eczema and more openings in her epidermal barrier. A single nighttime dose of a sedating antihistamine will help break the "itch–scratch cycle" that is making her AD worse. In acute flares, doses may need to be increased until sedation is achieved. With milder disease, a single nighttime dose is given to reduce scratching during the night. Nonsedating antihistamines (such as cetirizine) are not particularly effective.

Allergy testing may be appropriate if the history suggests a specific food allergen trigger, but most children respond to standard dermatologic therapy and do not require investigation of dietary triggers or food avoidance. Topical mupirocin is usually not helpful in the treatment of AD because children with AD carry *Staphylococcus aureus* on uninvolved and involved skin.

(Page 1258, Chapter 358: Disorders of the Epidermis)

Answer 18-15. b

This patient is suffering from acute ACD most likely to a plant from the genus *Toxicodendron* (formerly *Rhus*—poison oak, ivy, or sumac) that he encountered on his camping trip (eFigure 358-6). Acute ACD is characterized by intense pruritus, erythema, and vesiculation. The eruption begins 7 to 14 days after exposure in primary sensitization reactions and after 1 to 4 days in subsequent exposures. Transfer of antigen to areas of sensitive skin (eg, face and eyelids, penis, and scrotum) may result in marked dermal edema and swelling.

Nickel allergy is the most common cause of chronic ACD. Chronic ACD is scaly rather than vesicular (Figure 358-3). HSV would present with clustered vesicles that are painful rather than itchy. Atopic dermatitis usually involves flexor surfaces of the extremities, and does not involve the genitalia. Balanitis involves only the scrotum and would not affect the leg. Lichen striatus presents with a linear scaly plaque, does not involve the genitalia, and is not intensely pruritic.

(Page 1260, Chapter 358: Disorders of the Epidermis)

Answer 18-16. b

This is a description of adolescent seborrheic dermatitis. In adolescents, seborrheic dermatitis usually presents as dandruff, or diffuse scalp scaling, which is often itchy and may be accompanied by midfacial erythema and scaling, particularly in the alar grooves and eyebrows. Seborrheic dermatitis is a chronic condition that may be caused by elevated hormone levels (in early infancy and adolescence). The yeast *Pityrosporum ovale* may play a role in seborrheic dermatitis.

Tinea capitis is very itchy and usually presents as a localized patch of scale or crust, commonly with associated hair loss, although there is a diffuse variant that appears similar to seborrheic dermatitis. Tinea capitis is more common in younger children. Atopic dermatitis of the scalp can be hard to distinguish from seborrheic dermatitis, but the patient will usually have evidence of atopic dermatitis elsewhere. Psoriasis has more of a silvery scale and is more erythematous than seborrheic dermatitis. Patients may or may not have plaques of psoriasis elsewhere. Contact dermatitis of the scalp is usually inflammatory and has a more acute onset than seborrheic dermatitis.

(Page 1260, Chapter 358: Disorders of the Epidermis)

Answer 18-17. a

The presence of satellite pustules, intense erythema, or involvement of the folds suggests *Candida* dermatitis. *Candida albicans* commonly infects the diaper area, particularly if the irritant rash has been present for a few days or if the patient is being administered oral antibiotic therapy. In contrast, irritant diaper dermatitis typically presents with erythema that is most prominent on the lower abdomen, inner thighs, and the buttocks, and tends to spare the folds.

The appropriate treatment for candidal diaper dermatitis is a topical antifungal such as clotrimazole or nystatin in addition to frequent diaper changes, use of superabsorbent diapers, avoidance of aggressive cleaning, and application of a barrier cream. Low-potency topical steroids are sometimes necessary to clear severe diaper dermatitis, but stronger steroids such as triamcinolone, alone, or in combination, should be avoided. Terbinafine treats dermatophyte infection, but is not effective for *Candida* infections.

(Pages 1260-1261, Chapter 358: Disorders of the Epidermis)

Answer 18-18. e

This photograph is a classic example of guttate psoriasis. The prototypic lesion of psoriasis is a uniform erythematous papule or plaque, sharply delineated from the surrounding normal skin, and covered with *tightly* adherent, silvery scale. Guttate psoriasis is particularly common in childhood and is characterized by the rapid development of numerous small, scaly papules and plaques on the trunk, face, and proximal extremities, as seen in the picture provided. Streptococcal infections of the upper respiratory tract and perianal skin have been implicated as provocative factors for guttate psoriasis, and marked improvement in the skin is often seen with appropriate antibiotic therapy.

Atopic dermatitis is less uniform and less well demarcated from the surrounding skin. Seborrheic dermatitis is often less erythematous and has less scale. The plaques of pityriasis rosea are oval shaped, less pink, and less well demarcated. In pityriasis lichenoides chronica the scaly plaques are more variable than psoriatic plaques.

(Page 1262, Chapter 358: Disorders of the Epidermis)

Answer 18-19. a

This is a classic description of lichen striatus. Lichen striatus is a relatively common childhood skin disease, characterized by a linear array of small, violaceous, flesh-colored, erythematous, or hypopigmented papules (eFigure 358-19).

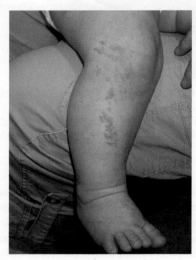

eFIGURE 358-19. (Reproduced, with permission, from Rudolph CD, Rudolph AM, Lister GE, First LR, Gershon AA. *Rudolph's Pediatrics.* 22nd ed. New York: McGraw-Hill, 2011.)

It is most common on the arms and legs, but can be seen elsewhere. Lichen striatus resolves over several months to a year without treatment. A mild topical corticosteroid is useful for symptomatic patients, but treatment is not required for most patients. It typically results in postinflammatory hypopigmentation, but this eventually disappears.

Lichen nitidus presents as tiny papules that can be clustered or widespread, often in areas of prior trauma, such as a scratch (this is known as a Koebner phenomenon). Lichen planus is uncommon in children. It presents with flat-topped, polygonal, violaceous plaques that are very itchy. It does not cause hypopigmentation. An epidermal nevus would have been noted earlier in life. Contact dermatitis can be linear, but can be distinguished by associated pruritus.

(Pages 1262-1263, Chapter 358: Disorders of the Epidermis)

Answer 18-20. c

This is a description of dyshidrotic eczema or pompholyx—a recurrent, acute eczematous eruption involving the hands and, less commonly, the feet. This child has the characteristic small, firm vesicles on the lateral borders of the finger. The disorder is intensely pruritic, and subsequent fissuring of the fingers and palms may be painful.

The accompanying photograph shows an example of atopic dermatitis, dyshidrotic type. The case is severe and notable for fissuring, scaling, and eroded patches after widespread vesiculation.

The appropriate treatment for dyshidrotic eczema is potent topical corticosteroids. Table 358-1 shows the different corticosteroid potency levels. Potent topical steroids are necessary because of the intense inflammation and the thickness of acral skin. Fluocinonide is a potent (Class II) steroid. Hydrocortisone 2.5% is low potency (Class VII). Triamcinolone 0.025% is medium (Class V). Terbinafine would treat tinea manuum, but while this is very itchy, it does not present with small vesicles. Prednisone is reserved for the most severe, disabling forms of dyshidrotic eczema.

(Page 1260, Chapter 358: Disorders of the Epidermis)

Answer 18-21. e

Zinc deficiency results in a periorificial and acral dermatitis. Lesions are typically sharply marginated, eroded, and crusted plaques but may be psoriasiform in nature. Dermatitis, diarrhea, alopecia, and irritability are signs of zinc deficiency. Zinc deficiency may occur as an acquired or as an inherited disorder, acrodermatitis enteropathica. Acquired zinc deficiency is most common during prolonged total parenteral nutrition with inadequate zinc supplements, malabsorption syndromes, chelation therapy, in premature infants, and in patients with restricted diets. The diagnosis is established by a low plasma zinc concentration. A trial of zinc therapy is indicated in all infants with a suggestive clinical phenotype. Response to zinc therapy is rapid (eg, 2-4 days) and dramatic.

While this patient may have candidal or even bacterial superinfection in the diaper area, clotrimazole, mupirocin, and cephalexin will not address the underlying cause. Triamcinolone ointment is a mid-potency topical steroid and is rarely used in the diaper area.

(Page 1261, Chapter 358: Disorders of the Epidermis)

Answer 18-22. b

Topical corticosteroids are the first-line therapy for management of AD and many other inflammatory skin conditions. Because of their better emolliency and greater potency, ointments are generally preferred over creams for AD. More liquid vehicles such as oil, solution, foam, and lotion are better for hair-bearing areas. For most patients, AD can be adequately and safely controlled with low- and medium-potency topical corticosteroids (Table 358-1). Twice-daily application is sufficient; there is no evidence that more frequent application enhances efficacy. In general, the mildest corticosteroid that will be effective should be chosen. With appropriate use, topical corticosteroids are not associated with significant adverse effects (eg, suppression of the hypothalamic–pituitary–adrenal axis or growth). For thicker,

TABLE 358-1. Topical Corticosteroid Therapy

Vehicle	Comments
Creams	Generally less effective than ointments May contain irritants or sensitizers
Ointments	Best for chronic dermatoses and palmoplantar eruption Generally most effective formulation Greasy quality may be undesirable Excellent emolliency Less likely to sting on application
Gels	Best for hairy or greasy sites Generally effective formulations May sting on application Poor emolliency
Solutions	Good for scalp May sting on application
Foams	Good for scalp May sting on application (for alcohol-based preparations)

Potency of Ointment Vehicle (Cream Vehicle Generally 1-2 Classes Lower)

Potency	Class	Topical Corticosteroid
Super[a]	Class I	Clobetasol propionate 0.05 Flurandrenolide tape Betamethasone dipropionate 0.05 (augmented) Halobetasol propionate 0.05
Very high	Class II	Mometasone furoate 0.05 Diflorasone diacetate 0.05 Betamethasone dipropionate 0.05 (nonaugmented) Fluocinonide 0.05 Desoximetasone 0.25 Halcinonide 0.5
High	Class III	Triamcinolone acetonide 0.5 Betamethasone valerate 0.1 Fluticasone propionate 0.005
Medium-high	Class IV	Triamcinolone acetonide 0.1 Flurandrenolide 0.05 Fluocinolone 0.025 Hydrocortisone valerate 0.2[b]
Medium	Class V	Triamcinolone acetonide 0.025 Desonide 0.05 Alclometasone dipropionate 0.05[b] Hydrocortisone butyrate 0.1[b] Fluocinolone acetonide 0.01
Low		Hydrocortisone 1, 2.5[b]

[a]Rarely indicated in children; high potential for local atrophy and systemic effects. Best prescribed by a dermatologist.

[b]Nonhalogenated; less potential for atrophy and other local effects.

acral lesions sometimes high-potency steroids are needed, but this is not always the case and steroid potency should be tailored to each specific patient and lesion. Class I or II steroids are typically prescribed only by dermatologists.

(Pages 1258-1259, Chapter 358: Disorders of the Epidermis)

Answer 18-23. d

Granuloma annulare is a common benign inflammatory disorder that is often misdiagnosed as tinea corporis since both conditions often result in solitary, expanding annular lesions. Granuloma annulare is characterized by asymptomatic, flesh-colored to pink to violaceous annular plaques most often occurring on the dorsa of the hands and feet. It can occur at any age but most often affects school-age children. A key distinguishing feature from tinea corporis is the firm smooth border and the lack of scale. Common treatments for granuloma annulare are topical and intralesional corticosteroids; however, these treatments do not often lead to dramatic responses. Granuloma annulare typically disappears spontaneously without sequelae in months to years.

Nummular eczema consists of "coin-like" lesions composed of minute papules and vesicles on a background of xerotic skin. Psoriasis is distinguished from granuloma annulare by the thick, adherent silver scale. Erythema migrans is the distinguishing feature of early, localized Lyme disease. It presents as an expanding red patch at the site of the tick bite. While it also lacks scale, erythema migrans can be distinguished by granuloma annulare as it is erythematous, a flat patch, has central clearing, and is often accompanied by systemic symptoms such as fevers, myalgias, and malaise.

(Page 1263, Chapter 359: Disorders of the Dermis and Subcutaneous Tissue)

Answer 18-24. e

The clinical vignette describes a patient with a keloid. Keloids are benign dermal tumors characterized by the growth of fibroblasts and increased synthesis of collagen. They occur most often in dark-pigmented individuals and occur at sites of trauma, either exogenous (piercings, surgery, trauma, tattoos) or endogenous (acne, varicella). Keloids are distinguished from hypertrophic scars in that they tend to overgrow the boundary of the wound and recur after excision.

Keloids are difficult to treat and any discussion of treatment should also focus on preventing future lesions by avoiding elective traumatic procedures. Patients are often motivated to treat keloids since they can cause cosmetic disfigurement and can be symptomatic causing pain and pruritus. A biopsy prior to treatment is often not necessary as this entity is easily diagnosed by history and clinical features. A common first-line treatment is intralesional corticosteroids; however, multiple injections are often needed to flatten lesions. Surgical excision is associated with high rates of recurrence (45%-100%). Other less common treatments include carbon dioxide laser, pulsed dye laser, silicon occlusive sheeting, cryotherapy, and intralesional interferon.

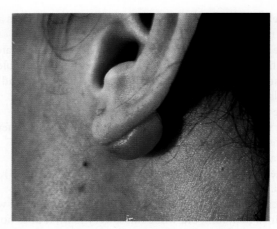

FIGURE 17-36. (Reproduced, with permission, from Weinberg S, Prose NS, Kristal L. *Color Atlas of Pediatric Dermatology*. 4th ed. New York: McGraw-Hill, 2007.)

Figure 17-36 shows a keloid that was caused by ear piercing.

(Page 1263, Chapter 359: Disorders of the Dermis and Subcutaneous Tissue)

Answer 18-25. b

The patient described in this vignette most likely has evidence of striae (stretch marks). These are linear depressions of the skin that are initially pink-purple and over time can become more flesh-colored and atrophic. They often affect areas subject to stretching and found most often on the abdomen, inner thighs, and breasts in girls and outer aspect of thighs and lumbosacral area in boys.

Common causes of striae include rapid growth as seen in adolescence, obesity, pregnancy, and cortisol excess (Cushing syndrome or prolonged systemic or topical corticosteroid). Connective tissue disorders, such as Ehlers-Danlos and Marfan syndromes, may cause striae, but are not a common cause. Anorexia nervosa is associated with striae due to abrupt weight changes; however, bulimia is not typically associated with significant weight gain or weight loss. Cutaneous manifestations that can be seen in hyperthyroidism include pretibial myxedema, thinning of hair, palmar erythema, increased sweating, and nail changes.

(Page 1264, Chapter 359: Disorders of the Dermis and Subcutaneous Tissue)

Answer 18-26. a

β-Hemolytic streptococcal infections are the most common cause of erythema nodosum in children; therefore, an ASO should be part of the initial workup. Erythema nodosum is a hypersensitivity reaction causing inflammation of underlying subcutaneous fat. Patients present with warm, tender, red nodules most often affecting the extensor surface of the lower legs. Lesions can last 3 to 6 weeks and can be accompanied by systemic symptoms of fever, malaise, and arthralgias.

Less common causes include viral infections such as EBV, *Mycoplasma*, tuberculosis, and coccidiomycosis in endemic areas. *B. henselae* infection has rarely been associated with erythema nodosum. Inflammatory conditions such as inflammatory bowel disease, sarcoidosis, and Behçets have all been associated with erythema nodosum. Medications commonly associated with erythema nodosum include oral contraceptives, sulfonamides, and penicillins. Lastly, pregnancy is also associated with the development of erythema nodosum and therefore a urine pregnancy should be performed in postpubertal females. There is no role for incision and drainage as erythema nodosum reflects a hypersensitivity reaction and not a direct supportive infection.

(Page 1264, Chapter 359: Disorders of the Dermis and Subcutaneous Tissue)

Answer 18-27. b

The clinical vignette describes a case of subcutaneous fat necrosis of the newborn (SCFN). SCFN is a form of panniculitis that affects full-term infants. Birth asphyxia and hypothermia are the most commonly associated risk factors for development of SCFN. The condition is characterized by the development of firm, mobile, circumscribed nodules and plaques most often affecting the back. These typically develop in the first week of life.

Hypercalcemia is the most often cited metabolic derangement and can occur up to 6 months after the diagnosis of the SCFN. Therefore, these infants should be monitored for hypercalcemia even after discharge from the NICU. Hypercalcemia is believed to be caused by extrarenal production of 1,25-dihydroxyvitamin D_3 from underlying granulomatous inflammation in the subcutaneous adipose tissue. Less common complications seen in patients with SCFN include hypoglycemia, hypertriglyceridemia, and thrombocytopenia. Treatment for SCFN is usually not needed beyond treating the complications.

(Page 1264, Chapter 359: Disorders of the Dermis and Subcutaneous Tissue)

Answer 18-28. b

Ichthyosis vulgaris is the most common form of ichthyosis and is due to a mutation in the gene encoding filaggrin. This gene has also been implicated in atopic dermatitis, and as such the risk of atopic dermatitis is increased in patients with ichthyosis vulgaris. It presents typically after 3 months of age as fine white scale with minimal to no erythema that is most prominent on the extensor extremities, particularly the lower legs (Figure 360-1). Often the appearance of ichthyosis vulgaris becomes more prominent during childhood or at puberty. An associated finding is hyperlinear palms, in which there is an increase in prominence of the markings on the palms; this can also be seen on the soles.

X-linked ichthyosis is another form of inherited ichthyosis, although it is much less common. It presents with more pronounced, larger, and darker scale on the neck, trunk, and extremities, often sparing the antecubital and popliteal fossa.

X-linked ichthyosis is due to a mutation in steroid sulfatase; other associated findings include asymptomatic minute corneal opacities and cryptorchidism. Xerosis is another term for dry skin; while patients with atopic dermatitis often have xerosis, the additional features of prominent fine white scale on the lower legs and hyperlinear palms are more consistent with ichthyosis vulgaris. Psoriasis is an inflammatory condition that presents with well-demarcated erythematous plaques with silvery scale. It is not associated with atopic dermatitis or hyperlinear palms. Pityriasis rosea is a transient eruption that presents with a pink scaly patch, the so-called herald patch, followed by multiple pink scaly papules on the trunk, often following skin tension lines on the back in a "Christmas tree" distribution.

(Pages 1264-1265, Chapter 360: Genetic Disorders of the Skin)

Answer 18-29. c

Diagnosis of NF-1 requires at least 2 of 7 major criteria. Of these, the most common is the presence of café au lait macules, which are seen in greater than 99% of patients with this diagnosis. To meet diagnostic criteria, a patient needs to have 6 or more café-au-macules that are greater than 0.5 cm in diameter in prepubertal children and greater than 1.5 cm in diameter in postpubertal children. The additional diagnostic criteria include NF-1 in a first-degree relative, axillary or inguinal freckling (Crowe sign), neurofibromas (2 or more dermal neurofibromas, or 1 plexiform neurofibroma), optic gliomas, Lisch nodules (pigmented iris hamartomas), and specific osseous findings such as sphenoid dysplasia. The patient in the vignette would meet criteria for NF-1 based on having a first-degree relative with NF-1 and having 6 café au lait macules greater than 0.5 cm in diameter (Figure 7-10).

There are many additional findings that may be seen in patients in NF-1. About one third of patients have associated

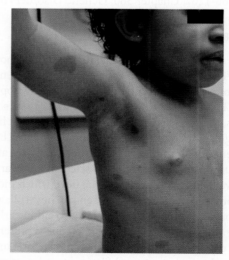

FIGURE 7-10. Four-year-old female with neurofibromatosis demonstrating characteristic smooth-bordered ("coast-of-California") café au lait spots, axillary freckles, and Tanner stage 3 breast development. (Reproduced, with permission, from Kappy MS, Allen DB, Geffner ME. *Pediatric Practice: Endocrinology.* New York: McGraw-Hill, 2010.)

speech and learning difficulties. There is an increased risk of malignancy, including central nervous system tumors and nonlymphocytic leukemia during childhood, as well as malignant peripheral nerve sheath tumors in adulthood. Patients with NF-1 should have their blood pressure checked regularly during well-child visits, as rarely hypertension may occur due to renal artery stenosis or even less commonly pheochromocytoma.

(Pages 1266-1267, Chapter 360: Genetic Disorders of the Skin)

Answer 18-30. a

Diagnosis of NF-1 requires the presence of at least 2 of 7 major criteria: 6 of more café au lait macules greater than 0.5 cm in diameter in prepubertal children and greater than 1.5 cm in diameter in postpubertal children, axillary or inguinal freckling (Crowe sign), neurofibromas (2 or more dermal neurofibromas, or 1 plexiform neurofibroma), optic gliomas, Lisch nodules (pigmented iris hamartomas), specific osseous findings such as sphenoid dysplasia, and a first-degree relative with NF-1. While the majority of these findings present in early childhood, dermal neurofibromas usually first appear after puberty.

Dermal neurofibromas present as soft sessile or pedunculated papules or nodules. They first are apparent typically after puberty and patients with NF-1 will have increasing numbers of neurofibromas with age. Plexiform neurofibromas, on the other hand, typically appear during infancy and early childhood as large irregular café au lait macules with overlying hypertrichosis. Over time, they progressively increase in bulk and can be difficult to manage. Patients with NF-1 are at increased risk for the development of central nervous system tumors and nonlymphocytic leukemia, but these typically develop in childhood.

(Pages 1266-1267, Chapter 360: Genetic Disorders of the Skin)

Answer 18-31. e

Tuberous sclerosis is an autosomal dominant neurocutaneous disorder. The most common cutaneous finding, seen in the vast majority of patients with tuberous sclerosis, is hypopigmented macules. These are 1- to 4-cm macules that can be shaped like ash leaves, the so-called ash-leaf spots, but also can be round, oval, irregular, or confetti-like in their appearance (Figure B). The presence of 3 or more hypomelanotic macules at birth should raise suspicion for tuberous sclerosis and warrants further evaluation. Connective tissue nevi, which includes a fibrous forehead plaque and shagreen patches (collagenomas, a type of connective tissue nevus), may also aid in early diagnosis, especially when the fibrous forehead plaque is present at birth.

Other cutaneous findings of tuberous sclerosis include adenoma sebaceum, periungal fibromas, and gingival fibromas. Adenoma sebaceum is composed of numerous angiofibromas (skin-colored to red papules) over the central face. The angiofibromas begin to appear during childhood and continue to increase in size and number with age. Periungual fibromas,

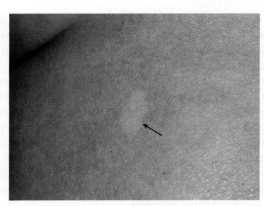

FIGURE B. Ash-leaf spot. (Reproduced, with permission, from Lueder GT. *Pediatric Practice Ophthalmology.* New York: McGraw-Hill, 2011.)

also called Koenen tumors, and gingival fibromas tend to appear in puberty or adulthood.

(Page 1267, Chapter 360: Genetic Disorders of the Skin)

Answer 18-32. a

The patient in this vignette most likely has tuberous sclerosis with adenoma sebaceum. Adenoma sebaceum is the term used to describe the numerous angiofibromas that appear on the central face in most patients with tuberous sclerosis (Figure 360-4). Individually, angiofibromas are small skin-colored to red papules, and in tuberous sclerosis these begin to appear during childhood, persist in their appearance, and continue to increase in size and number with age. As a result, adenoma sebaceum in late adolescence and adulthood can be quite disfiguring.

In patients with tuberous sclerosis, adenoma sebaceum can be initially mistaken for acne vulgaris as it becomes much more prominent in early adolescence and the papules may be of similar size and color. Key differences are that the first angiofibromas typically present earlier in childhood, with patients often having at least 1 angiofibroma by 4 to 6 years of age, and the papules are persistent as opposed to the transient papules and pustules

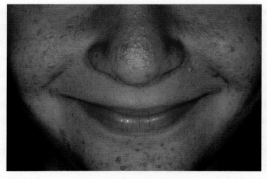

FIGURE 360-4. Tuberous sclerosis. Hallmarks include flesh- to pink-colored papules and nodules appearing on the central face (adenoma sebaceum). (Reproduced, with permission, from Rudolph CD, Rudolph AM, Lister GE, First LR, Gershon AA. *Rudolph's Pediatrics.* 22nd ed. New York: McGraw-Hill, 2011.)

of acne vulgaris. In addition, the hallmark of acne vulgaris is the presence of comedones, which this patient does not have.

Molluscum contagiosum presents as umbilicated papules with a central white core. It is caused by a virus and the lesions are transient in nature. They can be anywhere on the body and typically do not cluster on the central face. Keratosis pilaris is characterized by folliculocentric papules with a central keratotic core, most commonly on the lateral upper arms, but can occur on the anterior upper legs, trunks, and cheeks, where it typically is more lateral than medial.

(Page 1267, Chapter 360: Genetic Disorders of the Skin)

Answer 18-33. d

The ectodermal dysplasias are a collection of disorders characterized by the absence or underdevelopment of 2 or more ectodermally derived structures. Ectodermally derived structures include hair, nails, sweat glands, sebaceous glands, and teeth. The patient described likely has a type of ectodermal dysplasia associated with clefting as seen in mutations in p63 (Rapp-Hodgkin syndrome, Hay-Wells syndrome, and ectrodactyly, ectodermal dysplasia, and clefting [EEC]). Other types of ectodermal dysplasia include hypohidrotic ectodermal dysplasia, an X-linked recessive condition characterized by dysmorphic facies, partial anodontia, sparse hair, and diminished or absent sweating leading to frequent fevers and overheating, as well as hidrotic ectodermal dysplasia, which has hair and nail hypoplasia and a palmoplantar keratoderma.

Ehlers-Danlos syndrome is a group of disorders with easy bruising, poor wound healing, and hyperextensibility of joints and skin. The ichthyoses are a group of disorders with abnormal development and maturation of the skin. Neurocutaneous disorders include conditions such as neurofibromatosis and tuberous sclerosis. Atopy includes the atopic triad of atopic dermatitis, asthma, and hay fever.

(Page 1269, Chapter 360: Genetic Disorders of the Skin)

Answer 18-34. a

Acquired melanocytic nevi often appear after the first 6 months of life. During childhood and adolescence they continue to increase in number, reaching a peak number during the third decade, and then slowly regress with age. Both environmental and genetic factors play a role in the development of acquired melanocytic nevi. Sun exposure, especially intense and intermittent sun exposure, is the primary environmental influence. There are a variety of other factors that can contribute to the development of acquired melanocytic nevi including chemotherapy and chronic blistering disorders, although the most likely cause is intense and intermittent sun exposure. Sunscreen use can decrease the development of acquired melanocytic nevi. Sun exposure in the late evening can cause acquired melanocytic nevi, but they are still more common with intense and intermittent sun exposure. (Multiple other causes are listed in Table 361-1.)

(Page 1271, Chapter 361: Melanocytic Lesions and Disorders of Pigmentation)

TABLE 361-1. Environmental Triggers for the Development and Growth of Melanocytic Nevi in Children and Adolescents

Light Exposure

Sun exposure leading to multiple or severe sunburns[a]

Intermittent intense sun exposure (eg, on sunny holidays)

Chronic moderate sun exposure (eg, residence at lower latitudes)

Neonatal phototherapy

Cutaneous injury

Blistering Processes (Other than Severe Sunburns)

Toxic epidermal necrolysis/Stevens-Johnson syndrome[a]

Epidermolysis bullosa: junctional (particularly generalized atrophic benign) > recessive dystrophic > recessive simplex[a]

Childhood bullous pemphigoid

Scarring Processes

Lichen sclerosus[b]

Systemic immunosuppression

Chemotherapy, particularly for childhood hematologic malignancies[a,b,c]

Allogeneic hematopoietic stem cell transplantation[c]

Solid-organ transplantation, particularly renal[a,c]

Human immunodeficiency viral infection/acquired immunodeficiency syndrome[a]

Antitumor necrosis factor therapy (eg, infliximab, etanercept)[a,c]

Increased hormone levels

Growth hormone (increased size, not number, of nevi)

Addison disease[a]

Thyroid hormone[a]

Pregnancy[a,d]

Other

Atopic dermatitis[e]

Postoperative fever[a]

[a]Eruptive nevi have been reported.

[b]An increased number of atypical nevi may also be seen.

[c]Nevi have a predilection for the palms and soles.

[d]Relative immunosuppression may also play a role; based on case reports, an increase in the size or number of nevi has not been clearly demonstrated for pregnant women in general.

[e]Some studies have found a decreased nevus density in children with atopic dermatitis.

Adapted from Schaffer JV. Pigmented lesions in children: when to worry. *Curr Opin Pediatr.* 2007;19(4):430–440.

Answer 18-35. a

Nevi on the scalp of children often have a tan center and stellate brown rim, often referred to as a "fried egg" appearance. The nevus above is symmetric, has regular borders, and is well circumscribed making it less concerning for melanoma. Therefore, urgent referral to a pediatric dermatologist or excisional biopsy is not warranted.

Scalp nevi during childhood can represent an early indicator of an individual who may develop many nevi or atypical mole syndrome in those at risk due to their family history. However, genetic testing is not routinely performed for this syndrome. Scalp nevi have a tendency to involute over time. Gradual lightening and regression has been observed for various types of scalp nevi, ranging from eclipse nevi (common acquired lesions with a tan center and stellate brown rim) to congenital melanocytic nevi.

Treatment with liquid nitrogen is used in actinic keratosis, precancerous lesions, warts, and inflamed seborrheic keratosis, which this lesion does not represent.

(Page 1272, Chapter 361: Melanocytic Lesions and Disorders of Pigmentation)

Answer 18-36. b

CMN are classically defined as melanocytic nevi present at birth or within the first few months of life. The lesions are categorized on the basis of final size into 3 major groups: small (<1.5 cm), medium (1.5-20 cm), and large (>20 cm; in a neonate, >9 cm on the head and >6 cm on the body). CMN enlarge in proportion to the child's growth. The color of CMN ranges from tan to black, and the borders are often geographic and irregular. Many CMN have an increased density of dark, coarse hairs. Many of these features are represented above and the size of the lesion is 6 cm, making it a medium CMN. The risk for the development of cutaneous melanoma within small- and medium-sized CMN is controversial and is thought to be 1% or less over a lifetime.

Becker nevi are a cutaneous hamartoma, often located on the shoulder or upper trunk, as a large tan or brown patch that breaks up into smaller islands at the periphery. Nevus of Ota presents as speckled grayish brown to blue-black patches involving the skin, conjunctiva, sclera, tympanic membrane, and/or oral and nasal mucosa in areas innervated by the first and second divisions of the trigeminal nerve.

(Pages 1273-1274, Chapter 361: Melanocytic Lesions and Disorders of Pigmentation)

Answer 18-37. d

Spitz nevi are benign, usually acquired, proliferations of melanocytes with histopathologic features that sometimes overlap with those of melanoma. Most Spitz nevi appear during childhood, often with a rapid initial growth phase. The face and lower extremities are the most common locations. Lesions classically appear as uniformly pink, tan, red, or red-brown, solitary, dome-shaped papules. They are usually symmetric, well circumscribed, and less than 1 cm in diameter. The surface may be smooth or verrucous; darkly pigmented lesions are occasionally observed.

Pyogenic granulomas often grow rapidly, but are associated with a history of easy bleeding. Cherry angiomas are usually smaller in size and do not have a history of rapid growth. Dysplastic nevi often appear after puberty and on the trunk, and are less likely to appear as a solitary lesion. Acne vulgaris, though possible in a 4-year-old child, is less likely and also does not present as a solitary lesion.

(Pages 1272-1273, Chapter 361: Melanocytic Lesions and Disorders of Pigmentation)

Answer 18-38. c

Neurofibromatosis type 1 is an autosomal dominant disorder categorized by a mutation in the NF1 (neurofibromin) gene. Diagnostic criteria for neurofibromatosis type 1 include at least 2 of the following: 6 café au lait macules that measure 0.5 cm or more before puberty and 1.5 cm or more in diameter in adults, freckling of the axillary and/or inguinal areas, a plexiform neurofibroma or 2 or more dermal neurofibromas, 2 or more Lisch nodules (iris hamartomas), optic nerve glioma, skeletal dysplasia (ie, tibial or sphenoid wing dysplasia), and affected first-degree relative. NF1 is also associated with macrocephaly and learning disabilities.

Leopard (multiple lentigines) syndrome presents as multiple lentigines, pulmonary stenosis, deafness, and skeletal abnormalities. Carney complex (also known as NAME or LAMB) syndrome is characterized by generalized lentigines, atrial myxomas, blue nevi, and psammomatous melanotic schwannomas. Bannayan-Riley-Ruvalcaba syndrome is associated with café au lait macules, capillary and venous malformations, mental retardation, and macrocephaly. Children with Peutz-Jeghers syndrome can have perioral lentigines, longitudinal melanonychia, multiple hamartomatous GI polyps, and an increased incidence of ovarian cancer.

(Page 1275, Chapter 361: Melanocytic Lesions and Disorders of Pigmentation)

Answer 18-39. a

The above photograph depicts vitiligo. Vitiligo is a benign disorder characterized by complete loss of pigmentation (depigmentation) within well-demarcated areas of skin. It is an autoimmune process with destruction of melanocytes in the epidermis and less often hair follicles. It is a common acquired disorder affecting approximately 1% of the population. In 50% of the cases onset is prior to 20 years of age. Although it is a benign disorder, the disfigurement of childhood vitiligo may lead to considerable psychologic distress, decreased self-esteem, and social isolation.

Primary adrenal insufficiency, Addison disease, causes hyperpigmentation. Protein and copper deficiency cause pigmentary dilution, but not depigmentation or complete loss of melanocytes. A nevus depigmentosus is a clone of cells with reduced melanogenic potential that arises during embryonic development. Despite its name, a nevus depigmentosus is a hypopigmented patch, not depigmented.

(Pages 1276-1277, Chapter 361: Melanocytic Lesions and Disorders of Pigmentation)

Answer 18-40. b

Congenital dermal melanocytosis are ill-defined, homogeneous, gray-blue patches, most often in the sacral and buttocks areas, that are present at birth (Figure 361-3E). The bluish discoloration is a result of active melanocytes in the middle to lower dermis. These patches are quite common, present in nearly 85% to 100% of Asian neonates, more than 60% of African American neonates, and almost 10% of Caucasian neonates. They can also be seen in extrasacral sites such as the upper back, shoulders, arms, and legs, though less commonly. Usually by 6 to 10 years of age the bluish discoloration will disappear, but in approximately 5% of individuals they can have persistence into adulthood, especially with patches located on the distal extremities.

Extensive persistent dermal melanocytosis that affects the ventral and dorsal trunk, and enlarges over time can be a sign of a lysosomal storage disease (eg, Hurler syndrome or GM1 gangliosidosis).

Tuberous sclerosis, Menkes kinky hair syndrome, neurofibromatosis type 1, and neonatal lupus erythematous are not associated with persistent and progressive dermal melanocytosis.

(Page 1275, Chapter 361: Melanocytic Lesions and Disorders of Pigmentation)

Answer 18-41. c

Minocycline can cause a blue-gray discoloration often localized to the anterior shins or sites of inflammation. It can occasionally be a generalized "muddy brown" hyperpigmentation located in sun-exposed areas. Pigmentation deposition can occur years after treatment. None of the answer choices are associated with this side effect.

(Page 1277, Chapter 361: Melanocytic Lesions and Disorders of Pigmentation)

Answer 18-42. d

The clinical vignette is a description of erythema multiforme (Figure 362-1). Erythema multiforme is an acute, self-limited hypersensitivity reaction. The most common cause of erythema multiforme is a recent HSV infection. As highlighted by the description, a cardinal feature of erythema multiforme is the development of target lesions. The rash usually starts as an erythematous, edematous papule that then rapidly progresses to a target lesion that can range from 1 to 3 cm in size. A target lesion is defined by 3 zones: dusky, vesicular, or purpuric center; a pale, edematous surrounding ring; and an erythematous or violaceous outer ring. Features that help distinguish erythema multiforme from Stevens-Johnson syndrome (SJS) include distribution (erythema multiforme is often distributed acrally where SJS is more often on the trunk), lesion morphology (skin lesions in SJS are often atypical targets with only 2 rings), and mucosal involvement (by definition SJS involves more than 1 mucosal surface).

As mentioned, HSV is the most common cause of erythema multiforme. Multiple medications, and bacterial and viral infections have been implicated in cases of erythema multiforme, yet, by far, the most common underlying cause is HSV. *M. pneumoniae* and trimethoprim and sulfamethoxazole are 2 of the most common causes of SJS. Cefaclor is classically associated with serum-like sickness.

(Pages 1278-1279, Chapter 362: Immunologic Diseases)

Answer 18-43. e

Important considerations when assessing any patient with a potential drug eruption include the timing of the rash compared with when the medication was started, morphology, distribution of the rash, and associated systemic symptoms. The patient described above has the defining features of DRESS. The most commonly described cutaneous findings in DRESS are facial edema and a morbilliform rash. The systemic symptoms associated with DRESS include fever, lymphadenopathy, hepatitis, and signs of systemic inflammatory response syndrome such as hematodynamic instability. Lab abnormalities often associated with DRESS include transaminitis, eosinophilia or elevated atypical lymphocyte count, and the development of hypothyroidism that can occur months after DRESS has resolved. The most common treatment of DRESS is systemic steroids and patients are often on prednisone for weeks and tapered very slowly to prevent recurrence.

It is most important to be able to distinguish DRESS from a simple or morbilliform drug eruption by the presence of facial edema, lab abnormalities, and signs of systemic illness. The alternative answer choices in this question can be distinguished by skin morphology.

Angioedema presents as swelling in the deep dermis and subcutaneous tissue often associated with allergic causes (drugs, food, latex, venom) and lacks the same systemic findings and laboratory findings of DRESS.

Urticaria presents as edema in the upper dermis and is mediated by IgE as a type I hypersensitivity.

AGEP presents with generalized erythroderma and widespread superficial pustules and has been associated with β-lactam antibiotics being one of the most common causes. Lastly, Stevens-Johnson syndrome has cardinal features of atypical target lesions with more than 1 mucosal site involvement with ulcerations effecting oral mucosa, conductive, or genitalia.

(Pages 1278-1279, Chapter 362: Immunologic Diseases)

Answer 18-44. e

This child has a rash characteristic of neonatal lupus erythematosus (NLE) with annular, erythematous patches or plaques over the head and neck. NLE may also present with diffuse facial erythema, particularly in a periorbital distribution referred to as "raccoon eyes," or telangiectatic lesions. Extracutaneous manifestations of NLE include permanent congenital heart block, thrombocytopenia, leukopenia, hemolytic anemia, hepatitis, pulmonary disease, and central nervous system involvement. NLE is caused by transplacental passage of maternal anti-Ro (SSA), or less commonly anti-La (SSB), or anti-U1RNP antibodies from mother to fetus.

Atopic dermatitis (inherited dry and sensitive skin) and contact dermatitis (delayed hypersensitivity to baby shampoo) are usually not annular, polycyclic, or well demarcated. Psoriasis rarely presents with facial lesions in early infancy. Neonatal cephalopustulosis (hypersensitivity to *M. furfur*) is more papular and not so brightly erythematous.

(Page 1279, Chapter 362: Immunologic Diseases)

Answer 18-45. b

This child has lichen sclerosus. The correct treatment is high-potency topical steroids. Lichen sclerosus is an inflammatory disorder of unknown etiology that most often affects the anogenital area of prepubertal girls. Symptoms are chronic vulvar pruritus, dysuria, and painful defecation. The typical clinical appearance is a white discoloration with atrophy of the vulva and perianal area in a "figure-of-8" pattern. Clitoral hood edema is also common. The presence of purpura, telangiectasia, or erosions of the vulva or perianal skin may lead to a mistaken diagnosis of sexual abuse. Chronic lichen sclerosus may cause adhesions and effacement of the labia minora and sometimes scarring.

Topical steroids are the most effective treatment for vulvar and perianal disease. A high-potency topical steroid is usually required. Children should be followed long term for scarring and adhesions.

The other answer choices are not effective treatment for lichen sclerosus.

(Page 1279, Chapter 362: Immunologic Diseases)

Answer 18-46. c

Mucocutaneous infection is the most common type of skin disease associated with HIV. Persistent oral candidiasis and/or candidal diaper dermatitis occur in more than 65% of children with HIV infection. Other fungal infections include unusual and severe patterns of tinea corporis, tinea capitis, and onychomycosis. Cutaneous viral infections such as molluscum and verruca vulgaris can be particularly severe in children with HIV, but are less common. Cutaneous inflammatory disorders such as seborrheic dermatitis, eczema, and psoriasis are exacerbated by HIV infection.

(Page 1281, Chapter 362: Immunologic Diseases)

Answer 18-47. d

This is a description of LABD, also known as chronic bullous dermatosis of childhood. LABD usually has its onset during the first decade of life after 1 year of age. Typically, there is a sudden eruption of tense bullae and vesicles with clustering into annular or rosetted arrays. The scalp, face, perineum, abdomen, buttocks, and thighs are the most commonly affected sites, but the distal extremities may also be involved. Some patients have mucous membrane involvement. Scarring does not occur, but postinflammatory pigmentary changes may be pronounced. Pruritus is a variable symptom.

LABD is often initially misdiagnosed as bullous impetigo or bullous EM. Bullous impetigo usually has a less generalized distribution and the vesicles and bullae are flaccid or ruptured. Bullous EM should still have target lesions with a bullous center, edematous ring, and peripheral erythema. Patients with Stevens-Johnson syndrome must have involvement of at least 2 mucous membranes. Bullous pemphigoid is less common than LABD in childhood and does not have the classic rosettes of bullae, but biopsy is necessary to distinguish these 2 entities.

(Page 1281, Chapter 362: Immunologic Diseases)

Answer 18-48. c

The infant described in the above vignette is presenting with a juvenile xanthogranuloma (JXG), which is characterized by an infiltration of histiocytes into the skin. They commonly present within the first year of life, and are on the head and neck most often. Infants who present with JXG should be evaluated for neurofibromatosis type 1 with a thorough clinical examination, as this subset is at increased risk for developing myelogenous leukemia.

Patients with JXG and Down syndrome, Noonan, ataxia telangiectasia, or tuberous sclerosis are not at any increased risk for myelogenous leukemia.

(Page 1282, Chapter 363: Neoplastic and Proliferative Disorders)

Answer 18-49. a

The boy in the vignette is exhibiting signs of urticaria pigmentosa, the most common form of cutaneous mastocystosis in children. It presents with varying numbers of red to brown macules, papules, or plaques on any part of the body. They often produce a cobblestone-like appearance to the skin. These lesions can cause a wheal and flare reaction, known as Darier sign, when stroked (see Figure 19-5).

Some medications, such as aspirin, alcohol, morphine, codeine, thiamine, scopolamine, and polymyxin B, can cause mast cell

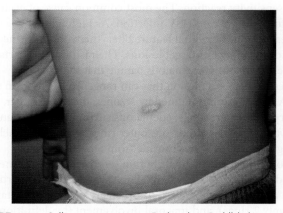

FIGURE 19-5. Solitary mastocytoma, Darier sign. Reddish brown macule that urticates with mild trauma. (Reproduced, with permission, from Kane KS, Lio PA, Stratigos AJ, Johnson RA. *Color Atlas & Synopsis of Pediatric Dermatology*. 2nd ed. New York: McGraw-Hill, 2010.)

degranulation and thereby cause a reaction. Also physical stimuli such as hot or cold baths or swimming pools can induce acute mast cell granulation. Most children with urticarial pigmentosa follow a benign, self-limited course with improvement or spontaneous resolution within the first decade of life.

Dermatofibroma is usually a solitary, firm, light brown papule. Langerhans cell histiocytosis can present with varying morphologies, but most commonly flat-topped, scaly papules in the scalp. Dermatitis herpetiformis presents with very itchy vesicles and papules. Erythema multiforme presents with target lesions.

(Page 1282, Chapter 363: Neoplastic and Proliferative Disorders)

Answer 18-50. d

Infants with 5 or more infantile hemangiomas are at increased risk of extracutaneous hemangiomas. The most common extracutaneous hemangiomas noted in these patients are hepatic hemangiomas. Therefore, infants with more than 5 hemangiomas should undergo at minimum an abdominal ultrasound to rule out visceral hemangiomas. Infants with hepatic hemangiomas are at risk of developing high-output cardiac failure and hypothyroidism.

Both Dandy-Walker malformation and congenital cardiac malformations are features of PHACE disorder. PHACE is classically associated with a large, segmental facial hemangioma and not multiple localized hemangiomas. Subglottic hemangiomas are most often associated with hemangiomas involving the mandibular area, that is, "beard" hemangiomas; therefore, patients with hemangiomas in this distribution should be referred to otolaryngology to rule out airway hemangiomas.

KMP is associated with kaposiform hemangioendothelioma or tufted angiomas and is characterized by a consumptive coagulopathy. KMP is not associated with infantile hemangiomas.

(Page 1284, Chapter 364: Vascular Tumors and Malformations)

Answer 18-51. c

The majority of infantile hemangiomas do not require medical therapy as the natural time line of hemangiomas involves spontaneous involution. The typical growth phase of infantile hemangiomas is 4 to 6 months (deep or segmental hemangiomas can continue to grow up to 1 year of age) and then they start to slowly involute. However, certain hemangiomas are life or disease threatening and require early aggressive medical therapy.

Periorbital hemangiomas place infants at risk of astigmatism and as they grow, they can obstruct the visual axis causing amblyopia. The first-line treatment for disease threatening hemangiomas would be either oral corticosteroid or oral propranolol.

Since 2008, the efficacy of oral propranolol has been shown in multiple case reports and case series and it is currently being used instead of oral corticosteroids as a first-line agent in many institutions. The mechanism by which propranolol acts to rapidly arrest the growth phase of hemangiomas and promote

involution is unknown but could be related to vasoconstriction or suppression angiogenesis factors such as basic fibroblast growth factor (bFGF) and vascular endothelial growth factor (VEGF). Topical or intraregional corticosteroids have inferior efficacy compared with oral corticosteroids or oral propranolol when the desired effect is to quickly arrest hemangioma growth and promote involution. Given the response of infantile hemangiomas to medical therapy or pulsed dye laser therapy, surgical debulking is rarely used as first-line therapy.

Other types of hemangiomas that would necessitate referral and expedited treatment include life-threatening hemangiomas (high-output cardiac failure or airway occlusion), nasal tip hemangiomas (risk of splaying ala cartilage), extensive ear involvement (risk of permanent disfigurement), hepatic hemangiomas, airway hemangioma, and hemangiomas complicated by large ulcerations.

(Pages 1284-1285, Chapter 364: Vascular Tumors and Malformations)

Answer 18-52. a

The infant depicted in the photo has a large, segmental facial hemangioma. Segmental facial hemangiomas are the cutaneous marker of PHACE disorder. This disorder is characterized by the following features: P (posterior fossa abnormalities), H (hemangioma—segmental type), A (arterial anomalies—most often cerebrovascular), C (cardiac malformations including tetralogy of Fallot, VSD, ASD, PDA, and aortic coarctation), and E (eye abnormalities including cataract, optic atrophy, microphthalmia, and others). When midline sternal defects or supraumbilical raphe are present, an S is added to denote PHACES syndrome. Large segmental hemangiomas in the lumbosacral areas are associated with underlying spinal dysraphism and genitourinary anomalies.

Cortical calcifications are a feature of Sturge-Weber syndrome and occur in a setting of cortical atrophy and pial angiomatosis ipsilateral to the side of the port wine stain. On close inspection of the photograph, one can distinguish the more brightly red raised plaque distinguishing this lesion as a hemangioma. Port wine stains are violaceous, flat patches that do not have a growth phase and occur in a V1 distribution when associated with Sturge-Weber syndrome.

Hepatic hemangiomas are associated with multiple (>5) hemangiomas. Consumptive coagulopathy (Kasabach-Merritt phenomenon) is associated with kaposiform hemangioendothelioma or tufted angiomas. Tethered cord can be associated with lumbosacral hemangiomas.

(Pages 1284-1285, Chapter 364: Vascular Tumors and Malformations)

Answer 18-53. d

The clinical vignette describes an infant with Kassabach-Merritt phenomenon (KMP). KMP is characterized by thrombocytopenia from platelet trapping and coagulopathy from consumption of coagulation factors in the vascular tumor.

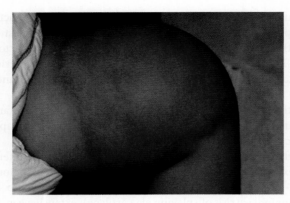

FIGURE 364-1D. Tufted angioma in a patient with Kasabach-Merritt phenomenon; note associated hypertrichosis. (Reproduced, with permission, from Rudolph CD, et al. *Rudolph's Pediatrics*. 22nd ed. New York: McGraw-Hill, 2011.)

Kaposiform hemangioendothelioma and tufted angioma are the vascular tumors associated with KMP—infantile hemangiomas are not associated with KMP. Tufted angiomas can be present at birth or develop shortly after and can present as either violaceous plaque or firm cutaneous nodule (Figure 364-1D). Hypertrichosis is commonly found overlying tufted angiomas.

RICH is present at birth and is GLUT-1 negative (Figure 364-1C). Unlike infantile hemangiomas, RICH have no growth phase and demonstrate accelerated spontaneous involution often leaving skin atrophy. RICH is not associated with KMP. Arteriovenous malformations are high-flow vascular malformations that can lead to serious sequelae such as high-output cardiac failure, bony erosion, or catastrophic bleeding but are not associated with thrombocytopenia and coagulopathy. Angiokeratomas are benign vascular malformation of capillaries with overlying hyperkeratosis.

(Page 1285, Chapter 364: Vascular Tumors and Malformations)

Answer 18-54. c

The clinical vignette describes an infant with a nevus simplex, commonly referred to as a salmon patch. A nevus simplex is a common type of capillary malformation that affects the glabella, eyelids, perinasal area, upper lip, and nape. It commonly fades by age 2; however, lesions on the nape can persist much longer. Nevus simplex is not associated with underlying pathology and does not require further referrals or testing.

It can be quite difficult to distinguish nevus simplex from a port wine stain particularly in the young infant. Nevus simplex that involves the forehead tends to have a V-shaped distribution in the middle of the forehead as opposed to following a trigeminal distribution. Furthermore, port wine stains persist throughout the patient's life. Port wine stains grow proportionally with child's overall growth and tend to darken overtime from a pink-red to a deep purple hue.

Sturge-Weber syndrome is a neurocutaneous syndrome characterized by a port wine stain in a V1 distribution, ipsilateral cerebral vascular malformations (cerebral atrophy, cortical calcifications, and leptomeningeal vascular malformations), and ophthalmic abnormalities (glaucoma, increased retinal vascularity). Patients with an isolated V2 or V3 distributed port wine stain are not at increased risk for Sturge-Weber syndrome.

(Page 1285, Chapter 364: Vascular Tumors and Malformations)

Answer 18-55. c

Macrocystic lymphatic malformations, also known as a cystic hygroma, are caused by aberrant lymphatic channels and are often present at birth. They commonly affect the head, neck, chest, and axilla. A characteristic feature is that these lesions will enhance with transillumination and this helps distinguish this lesion from other vascular anomalies and tumors. Furthermore, cystic hygromas are associated with karyotype abnormalities, most often Turner syndrome but also Down syndrome, Noonan syndrome, and trisomy 18 and 13. Cystic hygromas can be so large that they can be detected by in utero ultrasound and can lead to life-threatening airway pathology requiring tracheostomy. Diagnosis can be confirmed through imaging such as MRI. The most common treatment is sclerotherapy.

Infantile hemangioma, venous malformation, and teratoma would not transilluminate. A thyroglossal duct cyst is midline, rather than lateral neck.

(Page 1286, Chapter 364: Vascular Tumors and Malformations)

Answer 18-56. d

Acne vulgaris is one of the most common skin disorders and occurs in more than 85% of individuals between the ages of 12 and 24 years. The onset of clinical disease usually occurs between the ages of 12 and 14 years, but mild disease may develop as early as 7 to 8 years of age and tends to occur somewhat earlier in girls than in boys. Even though it is common, acne can cause psychologic distress during critical years of social and sexual development. Treatment should be tailored to the severity of disease, the types of lesions, and the patient's motivation.

(Page 1287, Chapter 365: Acne and Other Disorders of the Pilosebaceous Unit)

Answer 18-57. a

Acne is a multifactorial disease, involving excessive or increased sebum production, abnormal epithelial cell proliferation and desquamation, microbial proliferation, and inflammation. The primary pathogenic step is believed to be abnormal desquamation of follicular keratinocytes that results in comedone or microcomedone formation. The primary bacterium involved is *P. acnes*. *Pityrosporum* and *S. aureus* are not involved in the pathogenesis of acne, although both can cause pustules. Repeated trauma to the skin (picking) is a sequela of acne and can lead to scarring. Eating chocolate does not cause acne.

(Page 1287, Chapter 365: Acne and Other Disorders of the Pilosebaceous Unit)

Answer 18-58. b

The patient in the vignette has mild inflammatory and comedonal acne. Because she has no scarring and only a few inflammatory lesions, it is reasonable to start with topical therapy. The majority of patients with acne can be treated with topical medications of 3 types: benzoyl peroxide products, antibiotics, and retinoids. Each has distinct advantages, and combination therapy is more effective than monotherapy.

Topical retinoids treat the comedonal component of this patient's acne by normalizing keratinocyte differentiation and decreasing the "stickiness" of the epidermal cells lining the follicular lumen. Topical clindamycin treats the inflammatory component by decreasing *P. acnes* proliferation and inflammation. Benzoyl peroxide has both bactericidal and mild comedolytic activities. Frequent use of benzoyl peroxide inhibits the development of bacterial resistance.

(Page 1287, Chapter 365: Acne and Other Disorders of the Pilosebaceous Unit)

Answer 18-59. e

Oral isotretinoin is a vitamin A derivative that is a highly effective treatment for acne. It is FDA approved for the treatment of nodulocystic, scarring, and recalcitrant acne. Because it is teratogenic, all patients and prescribing providers must register with the iPLEDGE system. (See www.ipledgeprogram.com for more information.) Because it is expensive and has a risk of severe, but transient side effects, its use is limited to patients with severe acne such as the patient described in the vignette. All of the antibiotics listed in the question will help his acne, but may not control his scarring and large cysts, especially given that he has failed treatment with tetracycline. He should be referred to a provider who is registered with the iPLEDGE program and can prescribe isotretinoin.

(Page 1287, Chapter 365: Acne and Other Disorders of the Pilosebaceous Unit)

Answer 18-60. a

The patient in this vignette has a classic history for alopecia areata. Alopecia areata is a common, idiopathic disorder characterized by the sudden appearance of round or oval patches of hair loss on the scalp and other body sites. The typical lesion of alopecia areata is a smooth, shiny, hairless, round patch of the scalp that appears suddenly over the course of several days. Two clinical forms of alopecia areata occur: patchy alopecia areata (as in the patient in the vignette) and alopecia totalis or universalis. In the former, a few or many patches of hair are lost and the prognosis for regrowth, either spontaneously or with treatment, is good. Children with alopecia totalis or universalis have a poorer prognosis and even if some of the hair regrows with treatment, there is a risk of recurrent episodes.

Congenital temporal triangular alopecia is characterized by a nonscarred circumscribed area of hypotrichosis in the frontotemporal scalp (Figure 365-3). In this condition there remain fine, vellus hairs within the patch. Telogen effluvium is a form of diffuse nonscarring hair loss that occurs after severe stress to the body; the hair typically regrows within 2 to 3 months. Tinea capitis often presents with an itchy, erythematous, scaly plaque on the scalp with broken hairs. Trichotillomania is characterized by compulsive pulling, twisting, or breaking of hair. In contrast to alopecia areata, affected areas of the scalp demonstrate irregularly shaped areas of partial alopecia with broken hairs of varying lengths, giving the scalp a "moth-eaten" appearance.

(Pages 1288-1289, Chapter 365: Acne and Other Disorders of the Pilosebaceous Unit)

Answer 18-61. e

Pilomatricomas are benign cysts that most frequently appear before 10 years of age and present as deep-seated nodules fixed to the overlying tissue, with a faint blue or purple discoloration. The most common locations are the face, arms, and legs.

Multiple pilomatricomas may be associated with several conditions, including myotonic dystrophy, Gardner syndrome, Turner syndrome, and Rubenstein-Taybi syndrome. The treatment of pilomatricomas is surgical excision.

Epidermal inclusion cysts and acne cysts are rare before puberty. GA is most commonly an annular dermal plaque without a subcutaneous component. The deep, subcutaneous variant of GA is uncommon and is not blue colored. An abscess would be painful and fluctuant with overlying erythema.

(Page 1290, Chapter 365: Acne and Other Disorders of the Pilosebaceous Unit)

Answer 18-62. a

Koilonychia can be seen in a variety of conditions including iron deficiency anemia, hypothyroidism, hemochromatosis, and lichen planus, or can be an autosomal dominant trait (eFigure 366-2).

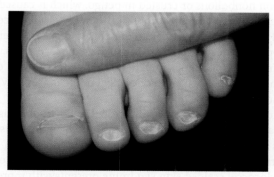

eFIGURE 366-2. (Reproduced, with permission, from Rudolph CD, Rudolph AM, Lister GE, First LR, Gershon AA. *Rudolph's Pediatrics.* 22nd ed. New York: McGraw-Hill, 2011.)

It can present in infancy and if it is an isolated finding in infancy, it resolves spontaneously over time. Onycholysis is the separation of nail plate from nail bed and can be caused by trauma, psoriasis, fungal or yeast infections, or certain medications. Melanonychia striata are longitudinal brown or black bands that can be present in melanocytic nevi or a lentigo in the nail matrix. Nail pitting can be a normal variant or can be seen in psoriasis, alopecia areata, or eczema. Subungual debris can be seen in onychomycosis, but is not seen with iron deficiency anemia.

(Page 1291, Chapter 366: Disorders of Nails)

Answer 18-63. c

The child in the vignette is presenting with Mees lines, 1 to 2 mm transverse white bands on the nails. These can often be seen with lead, arsenic, or thallium poisoning. Seasonal allergies, asthma, milk protein intolerance, and child abuse are not associated with Mees lines.

(Page 1291, Chapter 366: Disorders of Nails)

Answer 18-64. e

Minocycline can cause brown or black discoloration of the nails, but can also cause discoloration of the teeth, skin, lips, tongue, and gums. Nail pitting can be a normal variant or seen in patients with psoriasis, eczema, or alopecia areata. Blue discoloration of lunulae can be seen in Wilson disease or with zidovudine. Nail thickening is often seen with onychomycosis and accompanied by subungual debris and yellow discoloration of the nails. Leuconychia are white discolorations of the nail that can be seen with trauma.

(Page 1291, Chapter 366: Disorders of Nails)

Answer 18-65. c

Bullous impetigo is caused by toxin-producing *S. aureus* strains that cause blister formation in the epidermis just below the stratum corneum, producing superficial flaccid bullae. Infants are most commonly affected. There is a predilection for involvement of intertriginous areas such as the diaper area, axillae, and neck folds. This is in contrast to the more common nonbullous or crusted impetigo, which is caused by *S. aureus* or less frequently group A β-hemolytic streptococci (GABHS). Nonbullous impetigo presents in older children and typically affects exposed areas such as the face, arms, and legs. Treatment of bullous impetigo is with either topical or oral antistaphylococcal antibiotics, depending on severity of infection.

Epidermolysis bullosa usually presents at birth in areas of trauma and friction. Friction blisters would be quite unusual in this location and in this age group. HSV presents with clusters of small monomorphous, round vesicles or erosions. Staphylococcal scalded skin syndrome presents with more generalized erythema and painful skin.

(Page 1292, Chapter 367: Skin Infections and Exanthems)

Answer 18-66. c

Cellulitis is an infection of the deep dermis and subcutaneous fat that is commonly caused by group A β-hemolytic streptococci (GABHS) or *S. aureus*. Fever and leukocytosis are often seen. Erysipelas is an infection of the more superficial dermis most often caused by GABHS, which presents with more raised, well-demarcated erythema. Necrotizing fasciitis is a life-threatening, often polymicrobial infection of the superficial fascia that requires urgent surgical intervention. Early on, it may appear similar to cellulitis, but pain is often out of proportion to examination. Later, more overt signs of skin necrosis such as bullae, dusky erythema, and crepitus predominate.

(Page 1293, Chapter 367: Skin Infections and Exanthems)

Answer 18-67. d

Approximately 85% of common warts will spontaneously resolve within 2 years. For this reason, overly aggressive treatment is not indicated. Especially in younger patients, watchful waiting may be the most appropriate option. Common treatment modalities include cryotherapy and topical salicylic acid preparations.

(Page 1294, Chapter 367: Skin Infections and Exanthems)

Answer 18-68. c

This clinical vignette describes a patient with molluscum contagiosum and an associated eczematous dermatitis or so-called molluscum dermatitis. This is thought to represent an inflammatory reaction to molluscum that often heralds spontaneous regression. Children who are symptomatic with pruritus should be treated with mid-potency topical corticosteroids. In children without associated dermatitis, treatment options include watchful waiting, cantharidin application in office, curettage, cryotherapy, and imiquimod cream.

(Page 1295, Chapter 367: Skin Infections and Exanthems)

Answer 18-69. c

Based on the history and physical examination, this child is most likely suffering from staphylococcal scalded skin syndrome (SSSS), which is caused by exfoliative toxin-producing strains of *Staphylococcus aureus* (Figure 367-8). Clindamycin is the most appropriate antibiotic choice as it has the added benefit of inhibiting *S. aureus* toxin production. SSSS is caused by hematogenous spread of the exfoliative toxin from a primary infection site such as the middle ear, mucous membranes, or umbilicus. Patients are ill-appearing with fever and generalized skin pain. Erythema is accentuated in the skin folds and perioral and periorbital areas and progresses within 24 hours to flaccid bullae and erosions. Lateral pressure applied to the skin will produce separation (positive Nikolsky sign). Eventual generalized superficial desquamation occurs. Supportive care with wound care and intravenous fluids in addition to antimicrobial therapy is critical.

(Page 1297, Chapter 367: Skin Infections and Exanthems)

Answer 18-70. e

The constellation of clinical findings presented in this vignette is most consistent with a diagnosis of tinea capitis. Clinical manifestations of tinea capitis vary. Some children may present with isolated scaling and minimal erythema, making the diagnosis more difficult. In more severe cases, a kerion may develop, manifested by a crusted boggy plaque with associated alopecia. Because tinea capitis is caused by dermatophyte infection of the hair follicle, topical antifungals are ineffective as they do not penetrate deep enough. Systemic therapy is indicated with oral antifungals such as griseofulvin or terbinafine for a course of 6 to 8 weeks.

(Page 1299, Chapter 367: Skin Infections and Exanthems)

Answer 18-71. c

The child in this vignette has necrotizing fasciitis, which is a true surgical emergency. It is a life-threatening infection of the superficial fascia that may also affect the overlying dermis. The underlying muscle is rarely involved. Infection is typically polymicrobial with organisms such as group A *Streptococcus* and *Clostridium*. The course is rapidly progressive with mortality of up to 70%. Prompt surgical exploration and debridement is essential. Intravenous antibiotics should also be administered as an adjunct to surgery. The crepitus on examination is concerning for cutaneous gangrene and therefore raises the clinical suspicion for necrotizing fasciitis.

(Page 1293, Chapter 367: Skin Infections and Exanthems)

Answer 18-72. d

Blistering dactylitis is a superficial skin infection caused by either group A β-hemolytic streptococcus or *S. aureus*. A tense bullae with surrounding erythema of the distal volar fat pad is the classic presentation. Multiple fingers are typically involved. Blisters are caused by local production of an exfoliative exotoxin.

Herpetic whitlow presents with multiple small vesicles on the tip of the finger. Varicella infection causes disseminated vesicles on an erythematous base. A blister from friction would have less surrounding erythema. Bullous impetigo would be flaccid rather than tense bullae, and does not usually involve the fingertips.

(Page 1293, Chapter 367: Skin Infections and Exanthems)

Answer 18-73. c

First-line treatment for head lice is permethrin 1% cream rinse (Nix) that is an over-the-counter formulation. Parents should be instructed to wash the hair with a normal shampoo, towel dry, and then apply the permethrin cream rinse and leave in for at least 10 minutes. The hair is then rinsed and the treatment is repeated in 10 days. Other initial treatment of choice is pyrethrin or malathion. For resistant case, oral ivermectin can

be used. Nit removal with a comb is a good adjunctive therapy because none of the above medications are 100% ovicidal.

Although it is best to start treatment promptly, children can return to school immediately. In describing management on the day of diagnosis, the most recent American Academy of Pediatrics (AAP) statement states, "because a child with an active head lice infestation likely has had the infestation for 1 month or more by the time it is discovered and poses little risk to others from the infestation, he or she should remain in class but be discouraged from close direct head contact with others." The statement emphasizes that "no healthy child should be excluded from or allowed to miss school time because of head lice" (Frankowski, 2010).

(Page 1302, Chapter 368: Infestations)

Frankowski BL, Bocchini JA, the Council on School Health and Committee on Infectious Diseases. Head lice. *Pediatrics*. 2010;126:392–403.

Answer 18-74. d

Papular urticaria is a chronic and recurrent exaggerated response to insect bites including fleas, mosquitoes, and bed bugs. Cat fleas are most commonly implicated. Papular urticaria typically begins after age 2 and resolves by age 10.

The eruption is characterized by grouped urticarial papules distributed symmetrically over the exposed areas of the extremities in addition to the torso and may be seen along the sock and waist lines. Lesions often have a central punctum and are arranged in a linear so-called breakfast, lunch, and dinner configuration. Children eventually develop tolerance and the condition resolves with time. Treatment is supportive with antihistamines and topical corticosteroids. It is important to treat household pets for flea eradication and apply insect repellant to children when prolonged outdoor activity is expected.

(Page 1303, Chapter 368: Infestations)

Answer 18-75. c

This child's clinical description is most consistent with the presentation of scabies. The multiple different morphologies (papules, excoriation, and burrows) are characteristic of scabies. Older children have the classic distribution that can be generalized with accentuation in the folds, umbilicus, and genitalia, and between the fingers. In older children, the head and neck should be spared. Diagnosis is confirmed by demonstration of a mite, egg, or scybala (feces) microscopically from skin scrapings. First-line treatment is with permethrin 5% cream that is approved in infants 2 months and older. Treatment should be repeated about 1 week later. All household contact should be treated. Mite control precautions should be taken.

Papular urticaria, atopic dermatitis, tinea, and viral exanthems can all be itchy, but do not have the same polymorphous appearance, nor do they have burrows (fine linear plaques).

(Page 1301, Chapter 368: Infestations)

CHAPTER 19 | Disorders of the Ear, Nose, and Throat

Anna K. Meyer and Kristina W. Rosbe

19-1. A 3-week-old baby is brought to clinic with her first-time mother because of very painful breast-feeding. The baby nurses for 40 minutes on each side and the nipple is compressed when she finishes. The baby was slow to regain her birth weight. She has worked with several lactation consultants, but the pain and difficulty with breast-feeding persist. Physical examination reveals anterior tethering of the tip of the tongue and the tongue does not protrude from the mouth. What do you recommend for management?

  a. Refer to an otolaryngologist for evaluation for frenotomy.

  b. Advise her that this is normal and she should return to a lactation consultant for additional guidance.

  c. Consider supplementation with formula and discontinuing breast-feeding.

  d. Advise to switch to pumping and exclusive bottle-feeding.

  e. Advise her that breast-feeding is often painful at first and the mother will become accustomed to the pain.

19-2. An 8-year-old child presents with hearing loss in the left ear of an unclear length of time. He recently failed hearing screening at school on the left side. He has had intermittent otorrhea and a history of pressure equalization tubes at 3 years of age for chronic otitis media with effusion. Physical examination reveals a translucent tympanic membrane that moves well on pneumatoscopy, a light reflex, and with a small area of tympanosclerosis in the anterior-inferior portion of the drum and an area of yellow-brown crust superior to the malleus. What is the most likely cause of the hearing loss?

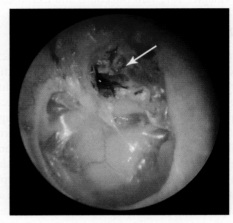

(Reproduced, with permission, from Knoop KJ, Stack LB, Storrow AB, Thurman RJ. *Atlas of Emergency Medicine*. 3rd ed. New York: McGraw-Hill, 2010.)

  a. Damage to the ossicles from his previous history of chronic otitis media with effusion

  b. Impaired function of the tympanic membrane from the tympanosclerosis

  c. Erosion of the ossicles by cholesteatoma in the superior portion of the tympanic membrane

  d. Damage to the tympanic membrane from the previous myringotomy and pressure equalization tube

  e. Ongoing Eustachian tube dysfunction resulting in abnormal middle ear pressure

19-3. A 7-month-old infant transfers to your clinic for her pediatric care. She was the product of an uncomplicated pregnancy and a normal spontaneous vaginal delivery. She has had normal growth and development. She has no identifiable risk factors for hearing loss and there is no family history of hearing loss. She responds to her name, is babbling vowel sounds, and her parents are not concerned about her hearing. You review her records and notice that she did not complete universal newborn hearing screening. Screening her for hearing loss is:

a. Important because congenital hearing loss is relatively common compared with other diseases screened in the newborn period

b. Not essential because her parents' report of her responses to sound is reassuring and she is demonstrating normal auditory development

c. Important for recognizing severe to profound hearing loss early, but is not as essential for mild forms of hearing loss

d. Not essential because she has no identifiable risk factors for hearing loss

e. Important because children with significant hearing loss require early introduction to sign language in order to communicate

19-4. A 10-year-old child presents with sudden vertigo. He has had a runny nose and cough for 3 days prior to presentation and awoke this morning with severe dizziness and nausea that is present all of the time and does not worsen with head movement. He does not complain of any hearing loss or tinnitus. Examination reveals an afebrile child without middle ear effusions. What is the most likely cause of the vertigo?

a. Benign paroxysmal vertigo of childhood

b. Bacterial labyrinthitis

c. Benign paroxysmal positional vertigo

d. Viral labyrinthitis

e. Serous labyrinthitis

19-5. A 13-year-old girl presents with a smooth mass in her midline neck. The area became acutely swollen over the past 2 days. On examination, she has a tender, 2-cm anterior neck mass just right of midline overlying the cricoid that moves with swallowing. The overlying skin is mildly erythematous (see Figure 372-2).

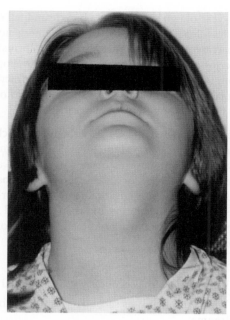

FIGURE 372-2. (Reproduced, with permission, from Rudolph CD, Rudolph AM, Lister GE, First LR, Gershon AA. *Rudolph's Pediatrics.* 22nd ed. New York: McGraw-Hill, 2011.)

You treat her with amoxicillin, and when she returns to clinic a week later, you can no longer feel the mass. What should be her future management?

a. Observation, as this is likely a case of lymphadenitis that has resolved.

b. Further evaluation with imaging, and if no lesion is identified, then watchful waiting is acceptable.

c. Watchful waiting, and if the lesion recurs, referral for surgical resection.

d. Referral to an otolaryngologist for surgical resection.

e. Further imaging, and if a cystic area is identified, needle aspiration.

19-6. What is the most important physical examination finding in diagnosing otitis media with effusion?

a. Dull tympanic membrane

b. Absent light reflex

c. Decreased tympanic membrane mobility

d. Obscured ossicles

e. Air bubbles behind the tympanic membrane

19-7. A 6-year-old girl was riding a bicycle and fell onto the handlebars. She presented to the emergency department with tachypnea, stridor, and bruising of her anterior neck. She was taken urgently to the operating room for an evaluation of her airway. No fracture or displacement of her laryngeal structures was observed, but there was significant laryngeal edema.

She was intubated and CT was obtained, which confirmed no laryngeal fractures. She subsequently developed a ventilator-associated pneumonia and remained intubated for a week. She was extubated and initially had no signs of airway distress or stridor. She was discharged home and then presented 2 weeks later with increased work of breathing and worsening biphasic stridor.

What is the most likely cause of her stridor?

a. Laryngeal edema secondary to the original trauma

b. Vocal cord paralysis secondary to the original trauma

c. An unidentified laryngeal fracture

d. Stenosis secondary to endotracheal intubation

e. Laryngomalacia

19-8. A 2.5-year-old boy presents with a 1-month history of a slow growing, nontender mass beneath the right mandible. The overlying skin is erythematous, and 2 days ago it began to spontaneously produce purulent drainage.

What is the most effective treatment for this child?

a. Oral antibiotics

b. Incision and drainage of abscess

c. Curettage

d. Needle aspiration

e. Surgical excision

19-9. A 1.5-year-old child returns to clinic 6 weeks after undergoing myringotomies and tube placement for recurrent otitis media. Examination of the ear reveals small blue tympanostomy tubes in each ear drum; however, you cannot see down the lumen of the one on the right and are therefore not sure if it is patent. The family gives you their note from audiology, who performed hearing testing this morning. The report says that the tympanometry showed patent tubes bilaterally.

Which tympanometry report corresponds with this conclusion?

a. Type A (normal peak), normal volume (of ear canal)

b. Type A (normal peak), large volume (of ear canal)

c. Type B (flat, no peak), normal volume (of ear canal)

d. Type C (retracted peak), normal volume (of ear canal)

e. Type B (flat, no peak), large volume (of ear canal)

19-10. A 4-year-old child has had a lifelong history of intermittent wet cough and 2 pneumonias. He is also small for his age (fifth percentile). He has a normal voice. After his most recent pneumonia, a modified barium swallow study was obtained that showed aspiration of thin liquids. He was placed on thickened liquids, but still has intermittent wheezing not improved by albuterol.

What is an important cause of aspiration that is often missed at this age?

a. Type 1 posterior laryngeal cleft

b. Bilateral vocal cord paralysis

c. Unilateral vocal cord paralysis

d. Laryngomalacia

e. Tracheomalacia

19-11. A full-term newborn product of an uncomplicated pregnancy and delivery has stertor (sound of partial obstruction at the nasal level) without respiratory distress at birth. Both nasal cavities are suctioned. An 8 Fr catheter does not pass down the left side. What is the next most appropriate step?

a. Try a 6 Fr catheter.

b. Flexible nasopharyngoscopy.

c. MRI.

d. CT scan.

e. Genetics consultation.

19-12. A 3-year-old presents to your office with 24 hours of unilateral malodorous rhinorrhea. Her mother is concerned because the battery from a greeting card she received is missing. After you suction the nose, you see crusting on the septum.

What should you do next?

a. Try to pick off the crusts.

b. Pass a suction catheter farther into the nose.

c. Get a radiograph of the nose.

d. Pediatric otolaryngology consultation.

e. Prescribe nasal saline and Vaseline and make a follow-up for 1 week.

19-13. A 6-week-old presents to your office with progressive stridor and intermittent respiratory distress. An awake flexible fiber-optic laryngoscopy suggests a subglottic mass. The infant is then taken to the OR for laryngoscopy and bronchoscopy. The figure below demonstrates the findings. You recommend starting propranolol. Which of the following statements is true?

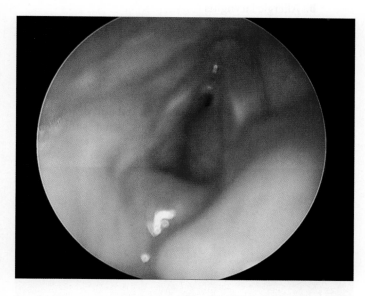

a. The child will need to be admitted to the hospital for the entire course of treatment.

b. The child can be sent home and treated as an outpatient.

c. The child needs a cardiology consult, EKG, and echocardiogram prior to starting treatment.

d. Pulse rate can be used to guide dosing.

e. The child should be fed every 2 hours while on propranolol due to the risk of hypoglycemia.

19-14. A submucous cleft palate could be associated with all of the following except:

a. A chromosome 22 abnormality

b. Velocardiofacial syndrome (VCFS)

c. Pierre Robin sequence

d. Velopharyngeal insufficiency (VPI)

e. Medialization of the carotid arteries

19-15. A 10-month-old child presents to your office with increasing feeding difficulties and intermittent episodes of respiratory distress, especially when laying flat. On physical examination, you note a cystic mass at the tongue base. The rest of the physical examination is normal.

The most likely diagnoses on your differential include all of the following except:

a. Branchial cleft cyst

b. Teratoma

c. Dermoid

d. Thyroglossal duct cyst

e. Lingual thyroid

19-16. A 4-year-old developmentally delayed wheelchair-bound child presents to you with excessive drooling. He goes through 8 bibs a day. Physical examination reveals 1+ tonsils and maceration of his oral commissure skin and chin.

Your initial treatment recommendation would be:

a. Bilateral submandibular and parotid duct ligation

b. Intensive oromotor therapy

c. Glycopyrrolate (Robinul)

d. Botulinum toxin injections to his submandibular and parotid glands

e. Bilateral submandibular and parotid gland excision

19-17. A 3-year-old developmentally delayed child presents to you with excessive drooling. Physical examination reveals 1+ tonsils and maceration of his oral commissure skin and chin. He has been undergoing oromotor therapy and using Robinul for 3 months without any improvement in his drooling.

What would you recommend next?

a. Unilateral submandibular and parotid duct ligation

b. Bilateral submandibular gland duct ligation

c. Botulinum toxin (eg, Botox, Dysport) injections of the submandibular glands only

d. Botulinum toxin (eg, Botox, Dysport) injections of the submandibular and parotid glands

e. Bilateral parotid gland duct ligation

19-18. A 6-year-old presents to your office with intermittent high fevers, sore throat, lymphadenopathy, and sores in her mouth. Her throat has been cultured several times and has never grown group A β-hemolytic *Streptococcus*.

Your most likely diagnosis is:

a. Kikuchi disease

b. PFAPA syndrome (periodic fever, aphthous stomatitis, pharyngitis, adenitis)

c. Lymphoma

d. Kawasaki disease

e. Viral pharyngitis

19-19. Which of the following treatments has been shown effective for patients with PFAPA (periodic fever, aphthous stomatitis, pharyngitis, adenitis)?

a. Tonsillectomy

b. Oral steroids

c. IVIG

d. Antibiotics

e. Methotrexate

19-20. A 4-year-old child presents to your practice with complaints of restless sleep, snoring, and mild difficulties with attention and concentration at preschool. You order a sleep study and results are significant for an apnea hypopnea index (AHI) of 4 and a minimum oxygen saturation of 90%. What would be your next step?

a. Reassure and explain to the parents that the child will grow out of this.

b. Refer to a pediatric otolaryngologist for adenotonsillectomy.

c. Place the child on nasal steroids and schedule a follow-up in several months.

d. Order another sleep study to be done in 3 months.

e. Refer to a sleep medicine specialist.

19-21. You are called to the emergency department to see a 3-year-old child with a 1-day history of high fever and drooling. His parents state he will no longer take anything by mouth and does not want to move his neck. He is most comfortable sitting upright. His parents state that he has not had vaccinations because they do not believe in them. You order a lateral neck x-ray and this reveals a thickened epiglottis.

What do you do next?

a. Order an MRI for more detail of the airway.

b. Call a pediatric otolaryngologist to assess the patient.

c. Intubate the patient.

d. Give dexamethasone.

e. Give racemic epinephrine.

19-22. A 7-year-old presents to your office with a hoarse voice for over a year. He has no signs of respiratory distress or shortness of breath. He had gastroesophageal reflux disease (GERD) as an infant and was treated with ranitidine until he was 6 months old. There is also a strong family history of seasonal allergies and he takes an antihistamine in the fall and spring when he has itchy eyes and sneezing. He has 2 older brothers and loves to play "Star Wars," which involves using light sabers and loud yelling. His dad recently took him to a baseball game and he was more hoarse the next day.

What is the most likely diagnosis?

a. Recurrent respiratory papillomatosis (RRP)

b. Allergic laryngitis

c. Vocal fold nodules

d. GERD

e. Vocal cord paralysis

19-23. An 18-month-old toddler presents with a preauricular mass that has been red and draining intermittently for several months. What is the most likely diagnosis?

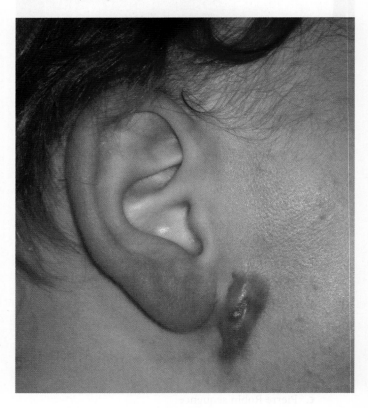

a. Infected preauricular sinus

b. Atypical mycobacteria (ATB)

c. Pilomatrixoma

d. Mucoepidermoid carcinoma of the parotid gland

e. First branchial cleft cyst/sinus (BCC)

ANSWERS

Answer 19-1. a

Infants with ankyloglossia who have significant trouble latching on or maternal pain with breast-feeding could benefit from frenotomy. This is especially true for those who have already been evaluated by a lactation consultant or have poor weight gain. It is not correct to advise a breast-feeding mother that long-term pain with breast-feeding is "normal." Because of the clear benefits of breast-feeding, in children with ankyloglossia, frenotomy is preferred to discontinuation of breast-feeding and conversion to formula. Switching to pumping and bottle-feeding may possibly lead to nipple confusion and refusal of the breast. Frenotomy is a simple, fast, low-risk procedure that can be done in the office without anesthesia.

(Page 1327, Section 19: Disorders of the Ear, Nose, and Throat, Chapter 371: The Pharynx and Upper Airway)

Answer 19-2. c

The normal tympanic membrane is composed of 3 layers, except for the superior portion, the pars flaccida, which has only 2 layers. This makes it susceptible to the effects of chronic negative middle ear pressure and is more likely to develop retraction pockets and a cholesteatoma (keratinizing squamous epithelium in the middle ear or mastoid process).

Desquamated debris accumulates in these pockets and becomes moist and infected. The debris can weep and cause otorrhea or can crust over and look like cerumen adherent to the tympanic membrane. Children with cholesteatoma often present with hearing loss or otorrhea. Inflammatory factors from the cholesteatoma and growth of the lesion lead to erosion of the ossicles and, in severe cases, can erode into the facial nerve, inner ear, or brain. Acquired cholesteatoma occurs most commonly in the superior portion of the drum. It can often be missed if care is not taken to examine this area. This particularly happens when examiners focus on the anterior-inferior quadrant and identification of the light reflex or cone of light. The light reflex is not a reliable diagnostic tool and should not be used to assess for the presence of fluid.

Tympanosclerosis, which is a white scar of the tympanic membrane from previous episodes of otitis media, rarely causes hearing loss. While a history of chronic otitis media with effusion, myringotomies, and Eustachian tube dysfunction can all be causes of hearing loss, the presence of a crust on the superior portion of the drum and good movement of the drum on pneumatoscopy (the most reliable tool to assess for otitis media with effusion) in this patient makes cholesteatoma the most likely cause of hearing loss in this patient.

(Page 1314, Section 19: Disorders of the Ear, Nose, and Throat, Chapter 369: The Ear)

Answer 19-3. a

Congenital hearing loss occurs in 1 to 3 per 1000 births and is one of the more common diseases detected in the newborn period with proper screening. Parental report of hearing is unreliable and milder forms of hearing loss can easily be missed when observation of hearing behaviors is the only modality used to assess hearing. Universal newborn hearing is important for recognizing hearing loss from mild to profound in order to develop early intervention and referral to programs for the hearing impaired.

For children whose families desire their children to develop oral language, early introduction of hearing aids and evaluation for candidacy for cochlear implantation in those with severe to profound hearing loss is essential. Other families, especially those who identify with the deaf culture and the use of sign language, will also benefit from early identification and providing of appropriate manual communication resources.

(Page 1309, Section 19: Disorders of the Ear, Nose, and Throat, Chapter 369: The Ear)

Answer 19-4. d

Viral labyrinthitis typically presents with acute-onset vertigo and nausea that does not go away with lying completely still and is not affected by head movement. It is often preceded by an upper respiratory infection. It differs from bacterial labyrinthitis, as the latter has a more severe presentation, often with associated meningitis and sensorineural hearing loss. Serous labyrinthitis is typically less severe and associated with either an acute or a chronic otitis media. Benign paroxysmal vertigo of childhood presents as intermittent bouts of vertigo, often has a family history of migraine, and is associated with a risk of migraine later in life. Benign paroxysmal positional vertigo presents as intermittent vertigo associated with head movement and symptoms desist when lying completely still.

(Page 1313, Section 19: Disorders of the Ear, Nose, and Throat, Chapter 369: The Ear)

Answer 19-5. d

This presentation is classic for thryoglossal duct cyst, although the differential includes dermoid and lymph node. It is difficult to differentiate between these entities presurgically. Because of the propensity for continued growth, potential impingement on vital aerodigestive tract structures, risk of secondary infection, cosmetic deformation, higher risk for surgical complications in a previously infected field, and rare reports of malignancy associated with untreated lesions, early surgical resection is recommended. Imaging is most helpful in determining the presence of a thyroid gland, as these can sometimes be associated with hypodevelopment of the thyroid gland and removal can result in hypothyroidism. A lack of identification of a cyst or mass on imaging, with the presentation in this case, does not rule out the continued presence of a thryoglossal duct cyst.

(Page 1336, Section 19: Disorders of the Ear, Nose, and Throat, Chapter 372: The Head, Face, and Neck)

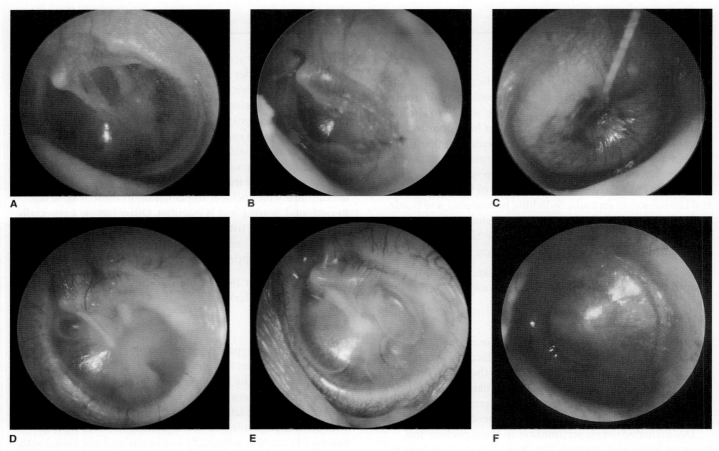

FIGURE 243-1. (**A**) Normal tympanic membrane. (**B**) Early acute otitis media (AOM). A mildly erythematous tympanic membrane is seen with a small purulent effusion in the middle ear. (**C**) AOM. The middle ear is filled with purulent material behind an erythematous bulging tympanic membrane. (**D**) Otitis media with effusion (OME). A clear amber-colored effusion with a single air–fluid level is seen in the middle ear behind an otherwise normal tympanic membrane. (**E**) OME. A clear amber-colored effusion with multiple air–fluid levels is seen in the middle ear behind an otherwise normal tympanic membrane. (**F**) Bullous myringitis. A large fluid-filled bulla is seen distorting the surface of the tympanic membrane. This can result from viral or bacterial infections and usually resolves spontaneously. (Reproduced, with permission, from Knoop KJ, Stack LB, Storrow AB, Thurman RJ. *Atlas of Emergency Medicine*. 3rd ed. New York: McGraw-Hill, 2010.)

Answer 19-6. c

The American Academy of Pediatrics strongly recommends the use of pneumatic otoscopy in order to assess the mobility of the tympanic membrane as the most reliable method for determining whether otitis media with effusion is present. The color of the tympanic membrane and the presence or absence of the light reflex are not reliable examination findings in diagnosing otitis media with effusion. In a well-aerated middle ear, one may be able to see all 3 ossicles, but this is not a reliable measure of whether fluid is present. As noted in Figure 243-1, some effusions have air bubbles, but many do not.

(Page 975, Section 17: Infectious Diseases, Chapter 243: Infections of the Ear)

Answer 19-7. d

The most common cause of laryngeal trauma is not external trauma, but endotracheal intubation, especially prolonged intubation. This child underwent thorough evaluation for laryngeal injury and initially did well post extubation and therefore is unlikely to have developed stridor secondary to the original external trauma or an unidentified fracture. Vocal cord paralysis can occur from prolonged intubation, but stridor is usually only present in bilateral paralysis and would be present immediately after extubation. Progressive stridor after intubation is a hallmark sign of stenosis secondary to intubation injury. In younger children, this most commonly occurs in the subglottis, whereas in older children and adults, the glottis is the area of highest risk for scar formation. Laryngomalacia can be acquired, but is usually secondary to neurologic insult rather than direct laryngeal trauma.

(Page 1338, Section 19: Disorders of the Ear, Nose, and Throat, Chapter 372: The Head, Face, and Neck)

Answer 19-8. e

This description is a classic presentation of atypical mycobacterium. The diagnosis is typically clinical; however, a weakly positive PPD or culture of specimen from excision can be confirmatory. Oral antibiotics alone are not effective, but sometimes are used for residual disease after incomplete resection. Needle aspiration and incision and drainage are not effective and can lead to fistula formation. Curettage can be used in areas that are difficult to resect, but outcomes are not as good as with surgical excision.

(Page 1340, Section 19: Disorders of the Ear, Nose, and Throat, Chapter 373: Head and Neck Masses)

Answer 19-9. e

Tympanometry is essentially an objective, quantitative method of pneumatic otoscopy. Air is insufflated into the ear canal and the volume of air and required pressure to move to ear drum are measured. When there is a perforation or a patent tympanostomy tube (the tube is in a surgically made perforation), the tympanic membrane will not move because the forced air does not displace it, but rather goes through the hole into the middle ear. Therefore, a patent tube would not have either a Type A (normal peak) or a Type C (retracted peak, where the drum is retracted, but still mobile), but would have a Type B (flat, no peak) tympanometry tracing. When the tympanic membrane is intact, the volume of air measured is of just the external ear canal lateral to the intact drum. When the tympanic membrane has a perforation or patent tube, the volume measured is of the external ear canal and the middle ear. Therefore, a Type B (flat), large volume tympanometry reading would correlate to a patent tube. A Type B, normal volume would indicate a tympanic membrane that is not mobile, but is intact, which most commonly occurs in the case of acute otitis media or otitis media with effusion.

Answer 19-10. a

Type 1 posterior laryngeal cleft, in which the interarytenoid notch is deeper (to the level of the vocal cords), is an increasingly diagnosed cause of long-term subtle aspiration in young children (see eFigure 371-1).

These children may be misdiagnosed with primary lung disorders. They usually do not have stridor or vocal changes, but have had frequent pneumonias, prolonged "chest colds," chronic cough, or poorly controlled "asthma." Direct laryngoscopy with palpation is the definitive method for diagnosis, as flexible laryngoscopy will not allow adequate visualization of the interarytenoid notch in this mildest form of laryngeal cleft. Many children respond to thickening of liquids and in those who do not, surgical closure of the defect can be accomplished endoscopically.

Bilateral vocal cord paralysis typically is associated with stridor, although voice often is normal. Unilateral vocal cord paralysis is usually associated with a hoarse or airy voice, although in neonates and infants, stridor can also be present. Laryngomalacia can be associated with aspiration and failure to thrive, but classically presents with inspiratory stridor, and tracheomalacia most typically presents with expiratory stridor that can be difficult to differentiate from wheezing, especially in young children.

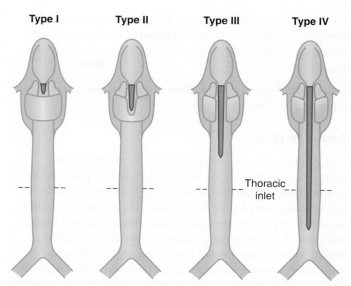

eFIGURE 371-1. Classification of posterior laryngeal clefts. Type I: interarytenoid cleft–superior to the glottis. Type II: partial cricoid cleft–extends inferior to the glottis and partially through the posterior lamina of the cricoid. Type III: total cricoid cleft, with or without extension into the cervical tracheoesophageal wall. Type IV: laryngotracheoesophageal cleft extending beyond the thoracic inlet. (Reproduced, with permission, from Rudolph CD, Rudolph AM, Lister GE, First LR, Gershon AA. *Rudolph's Pediatrics.* 22nd ed. New York: McGraw-Hill, 2011.)

(Page 1331, Section 19: Disorders of the Ear, Nose, and Throat, Chapter 371: The Pharynx and Upper Airway; Chapter 371: Larynx: Congenital Malformations)

Answer 19-11. b

Flexible nasopharyngoscopy by a pediatric otolaryngologist should be the next diagnostic procedure performed to confirm a diagnosis of unilateral choanal atresia or stenosis. This procedure can confirm patency by direct visualization. In contrast, the inability to pass a 6 Fr catheter still does not provide a definitive diagnosis.

Unilateral choanal atresia does not necessarily require urgent repair if the child does not exhibit respiratory distress or develop failure to thrive. A CT scan is the imaging study of choice to visualize the bony structures of the nasopharynx. Choanal atresia can be associated with CHARGE syndrome, so a genetics evaluation is generally warranted.

(Page 1319, Section 19: Disorders of the Ear, Nose, and Throat, Chapter 370: Nose and Sinus)

Answer 19-12. d

Disc batteries require urgent removal or they can erode through mucosa and cartilage. This child is at risk for a septal perforation. This child requires nasal endoscopy with removal of the battery under general anesthesia by a pediatric otolaryngologist. A radiograph may help localize the battery. Extremely anterior nasal foreign bodies can be removed in the office safely. Nasal foreign bodies that cannot be fully visualized or are farther back in the nasal cavity are at risk of being pushed posteriorly and aspirated if attempts are made to remove without complete control of the foreign body and the airway.

(Page 1320, Section 19: Disorders of the Ear, Nose, and Throat, Chapter 370: Nose and Sinus)

Answer 19-13. d

The child has an airway hemangioma. Close monitoring with inpatient observation is recommended for patients with symptomatic airway disease or infants less than 3 months of age who are treated with propranolol. Those who do not have severe airway symptoms and are older than 3 months of age are given slowly increasing doses of propranolol beginning with 0.3 mg/kg/day divided every 8 hours with increases every 3 days at 0.3 mg/kg increments to a target dose of 2 mg/kg/day. In those managed as inpatients, more rapid increases in dosing can be used with initial dosing at 1 mg/kg/day and increased to 2 mg/kg/day a few days later. Patients less than 6 months of age can be fed every 3 to 4 hours to avoid drug-induced hypoglycemia. Heart rates are monitored either at home or by the primary care physician every few days to assure that bradycardia does not develop. Some patients have reported sleep disturbances, a known, though infrequently reported side effect of the medication. There is currently not a consensus about appropriate cardiac evaluation in infant starting propranolol for airway hemangioma.

(Page 1334, Section 19: Disorders of the Ear, Nose, and Throat, Chapter 371: The Pharynx and Upper Airway)

Answer 19-14. c

Pierre Robin sequence generally involves the triad of a complete cleft palate involving both the muscle and the mucosa, micrognathia, and glossoptosis.

VCFS involves a mutation on chromosome 22 and can be associated with VPI and medialization of the carotid arteries. It is generally recommended that children with VCFS undergo imaging prior to adenoidectomy to assess the position of the carotid arteries and that a superior adenoidectomy only be performed to reduce the chance of postoperative VPI.

(Page 705, Section 12: Clinical Genetics and Dysmorphology, Chapter 176: Syndromes of Multiple Congenital Anomalies/ Dysplasias)

Answer 19-15. a

Branchial cleft cysts, sinuses, and fistulae occur laterally, not in the midline. Teratoma, dermoid, thyroglossal duct cyst, and lingual thyroid can all occur in the midline. MRI would be the next best step in workup of this mass. MRI with gadolinium would provide the anatomic detail and enhancing characteristics to best identify the diagnosis. MRI can also demonstrate whether thyroid tissue is present in the normal

anatomic location. If not, the family will need to be counseled that after removal of the mass, the child may require lifelong thyroid hormone supplementation.

(Page 1339, Section 19: Disorders of the Ear, Nose, and Throat, Chapter 373: Head and Neck Masses)

Answer 19-16. b

The approach to the drooling child should start with the least invasive intervention. Drooling can be normal in a neurologic intact child up to age 5. Tonsil size should always be examined as tonsillar hypertrophy can contribute to ineffective swallowing of saliva and secretions. If oromotor therapy is unsuccessful, medical therapy should be considered before surgical intervention. Glycopyrrolate is an anticholinergic medication that decreases secretions; however, side effects include constipation, confusion, visual problems, headaches, and difficulty falling asleep, among others.

(Page 1326, Section 19: Disorders of the Ear, Nose, and Throat, Chapter 371: The Pharynx and Upper Airway)

Answer 19-17. d

Botulinum toxin (eg, Botox, Dysport) temporarily blocks the parasympathetic input to the salivary glands. The submandibular glands are responsible for baseline saliva production and the parotid glands are responsible for stimulated saliva production in response to eating. In the chronic drooling child, all 4 glands are injected; however, this procedure does not eliminate all saliva. The effects generally wear off in 3 to 6 months and may need to be repeated. The injections are usually done under general anesthesia with ultrasound localization of the glands. Salivary duct ligations and/or excision are reserved for severe drooling refractory to conservative measures due to their associated morbidities including risks of ranula formation, scar, facial nerve injury, or lingual nerve injury.

(Page 1326, Section 19: Disorders of the Ear, Nose, and Throat, Chapter 371: The Pharynx and Upper Airway)

Answer 19-18. b

PFAPA syndrome involves periodic fevers, adenitis, pharyngitis, and aphthous ulcers. There is no specific treatment for PFAPA syndrome. The syndrome seems to self-resolve by the time affected children reach 10 years of age. Kikuchi disease or histiocytic necrotizing lymphadenopathy involves large painful lymph nodes, rash, joint pain, leukopenia, and anemia and average age of presentation is 30 years. Lymphoma can present in a multitude of ways, so if there is a high index of suspicion, tissue should be obtained and sent for flow cytometry. Kawasaki disease or mucocutaneous lymph node syndrome is considered an autoimmune disease causing vasculitis. Other signs include strawberry tongue and palmar erythema, and children can develop coronary artery aneurysms. Aspirin and IVIG are used to treat Kawasaki disease and children should also undergo an echocardiogram.

(Page 1327, Section 19: Disorders of the Ear, Nose, and Throat, Chapter 371: The Pharynx and Upper Airway)

Answer 19-19. a

PFAPA syndrome involves periodic fevers, adenitis, pharyngitis, and aphthous ulcers. There is no specific treatment for PFAPA syndrome. The syndrome seems to self-resolve by the time affected children reach 10 years of age. Oral steroids may relieve the acute symptoms but have no impact on frequency of episodes or prevention of future episodes. Both tonsillectomy and cimetidine have been shown to decrease the chance of further episodes of PFAPA.

(Page 837, Section 15: Rheumatology, Chapter 209: Autoinflammatory Disorders)

Answer 19-20. c

The AHI describes the severity of sleep apnea. The AHI includes the number of apneic or hypopenic events divided by the number of hours of sleep.

An AHI <1 is generally considered normal for children on polysomnography. An AHI of 1 to 5 is scored as mild sleep-disordered breathing (SDB). Nasal steroids have been shown to be effective treatment for mild SDB and to shrink adenoid tissue. Length of treatment varies but can be as short as 3 months. Sustained improvement in symptoms has been demonstrated even when treatment is stopped.

(Section 27: Disorders of the Respiratory System, Chapter 508: Disorders of Respiratory Control and Sleep-Disordered Breathing)

Answer 19-21. b

This child's history and examination are consistent with acute epiglottitis. The most common infectious etiology is *Haemophilus influenza* type B (Hib). Since the use of the Hib vaccine routinely in children, the incidence of acute epiglottitis has dramatically decreased. These children generally do not want to be touched or manipulated. A pediatric otolaryngologist will likely alert the operating room and plan a direct laryngoscopy and intubation in a controlled setting with a pediatric anesthesiologist. Once the child is intubated, antibiotics and steroids can be given and most children can be extubated within several days.

Laryngotracheobronchitis, or croup, generally presents with a more indolent course in younger children and will demonstrate the "steeple sign" on plain radiograph, which is narrowing of the subglottic airway. These children often will respond to oral corticosteroids and racemic epinephrine and will not require intubation.

(Page 1333, Section 19: Disorders of the Ear, Nose, and Throat, Chapter 371: The Pharynx and Upper Airway)

Answer 19-22. c

Although this child may have allergic laryngitis and GERD contributing to his symptoms, the most likely diagnosis in his age is vocal fold nodules. These form due to vocal strain and overuse. They are tiny calluses on the anterior third of the vocal fold. The best next step in evaluation is laryngoscopy. The child's larynx should be visualized to confirm the diagnosis. Vocal hygiene can also be reinforced. The natural history of vocal fold nodules is that the majority will resolve without surgical intervention once the child is no longer performing the behaviors that are strenuous for the vocal folds.

RRP generally presents at an earlier age and can progress to respiratory distress. RRP is associated with human papillomavirus (HPV) and is found more commonly in firstborn children of mothers with active vaginal papillomas during delivery. Spread of RRP is felt to be hematogenous, however, because rates are similar in babies delivered vaginally and in those delivered by cesarean section.

Unilateral vocal cord paralysis could present with hoarseness but is extremely unusual without risks factors in the history such as traumatic delivery requiring forceps or vacuum extraction with possible shoulder dystocia (thought to be a stretch injury on the nerve, which would likely resolve by age 7 years), and prior neck or cardiac surgery.

(Page 1334, Section 19: Disorders of the Ear, Nose, and Throat, Chapter 371: The Pharynx and Upper Airway)

Answer 19-23. e

This is the classic history and location for a first BCC. Type I BCC is a duplication of the external auditory canal (EAC) and can sometimes have an opening in the EAC. Embryologically, this involves only ectoderm. Type II BCC follows the course of the facial nerve and involves mesoderm and ectoderm.

Preauricular sinuses are related to abnormal development of the axon hillocks and occur superior to the root of the helix. The other diagnoses can occur in this location but are less likely. A PPD should be placed, and if it demonstrated intermediate reactivity, this finding would be consistent with ATB. A pilomatrixoma is a benign, appendageal, pediatric tumor that originates from the hair follicle matrix, and is usually very firm to palpation due to the calcium. Malignancies of the parotid gland are rare in children and would be more likely to present as a palpable mass without skin involvement.

(Page 1334, Section 19: Disorders of the Ear, Nose, and Throat, Chapter 372: The Head, Face, and Neck)

CHAPTER 20 | Disorders of the Oral Cavity

Susan Fisher-Owens and Michael D. Cabana

20-1. A 2-week-old infant presents for follow-up after discharge from the nursery after an uneventful prenatal course. Her weight is 1% below birth weight. She is awake at least 4 times a night fussing. She breast-feeds 7 to 10 times a day and she is making 4 to 6 yellow diapers. On physical examination, she is fussy but consolable, sucks hard on your finger, and is noted to have a thick white plaque covering her cheeks and dorsum of the tongue. The best treatment would be:

   a. Discontinue breast-feeding and switch to bottle-feeding.

   b. Initiate oral antiretroviral therapy.

   c. Reassure the parents.

   d. Prescribe oral nystatin.

   e. Admit the infant for an immune status workup.

20-2. Your next patient is a 22-month-old male whose father is upset because he has white lacy spots on the tips of his teeth "and I didn't want him to get cavities like his Mom." The father reports that the child's mother had poor oral health. As a result, the child's father has been careful to make sure the child brushes his teeth twice a day with pea-sized amount of toothpaste. In addition, the patient's father had asked the last pediatrician to put his son on fluoride supplements, since they have well water.

   Your next step should be:

   a. Increasing dose in fluoride supplement

   b. Encouraging the urgent removal of teeth

   c. Increasing amount of toothpaste used

   d. Recommending the use of a new, firmer toothbrush for cleaning

   e. Recommending the use of a smear of toothpaste

20-3. As you evaluate an 18-month-old male for his well-child check, you see brown lesions near the gumline of the top teeth. You ask the mother about his eating habits, and she says he never took a bottle. He uses a sippy cup. On one occasion, she saw him sucking on his brother's tube of toothpaste. Your best advice to her is:

   a. This is from excess fluoride, so the parent should keep him away from toothpaste and only give him water that is not fluoridated.

   b. The rates of this condition are increasing in the United States.

   c. These teeth will fall out, so the parent does not need to worry about them.

   d. This is a slowly progressing disease, so the parent has time to wait until age 3 years to have the child seen by a dentist.

   e. The cause of this lesion was spread by the mother, so she needs to go to the doctor.

20-4. A previously healthy 3-year-old female with chronic constipation has come to urgent care for refusing to eat and drooling. The symptoms were of sudden onset. Mom denies that the patient was left with any inappropriate providers. She has urinated twice already today, but she has not had a stool. On examination, her temperature is 38.7°C. The heart rate is 88 beats/min. She is sitting up in her chair without distress but is refusing mom's efforts to convince her to drink. She has no rash. Examination of her mouth reveals 2- to 3-mm ulcerations on the soft palate, uvula, and posterior pharynx. Immunizations are up-to-date.

   Which treatment is best for this patient?

   a. Antibiotics to cover for *H. influenzae*

   b. Diphenhydramine–Maalox–lidocaine swish

   c. Analgesics and oral fluids

   d. Admission for intravenous fluids

   e. Acyclovir for HSV

20-5. A 16-year-old female presents with severe headache and ear pain on her right side, which she reports is limiting her being able to open her mouth. She reports a tactile temperature the night before, and said she had difficulty sleeping because of the pain. She has had this pain before. On examination, both tympanic membranes are mobile and unremarkable.

Which of the following would *not* be recommended as part of therapy?

a. Amoxicillin

b. Splint therapy

c. Stress relief

d. Soft diet

e. NSAIDs

20-6. When a 3-day-old infant is seen for his nursery follow-up visit, you notice his tongue is only able to extend to his lip.

The most appropriate way to counsel the parent is that this condition:

a. Is more common in females

b. Must be treated to prevent speech problems

c. Can be treated with laser frenectomy

d. Must be treated to prevent failure to thrive

e. Frequently causes poor breast-feeding and neonatal dehydration

20-7. A 2-year-old male is brought in by his mother for his well-child visit. He was the full-term product of a normal pregnancy, and has had a normal postnatal course with no hospitalizations. He drinks tap water supplied by your city. He eats a balanced diet including daily fruits, vegetables, and meat and without abnormal eating patterns. He does not take any supplements except a multivitamin. He is growing well and has a normal physical examination, only notable for black staining on the teeth.

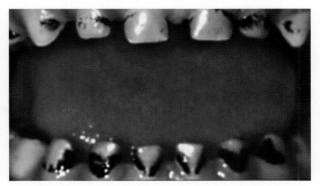

eFIGURE 378-3. (Reproduced, with permission, from Rudolph CD, Rudolph AM, Lister GE, First LR, Gershon AA. *Rudolph's Pediatrics.* 22nd ed. New York: McGraw-Hill, 2011.)

The most likely cause of this is:

a. Tetracycline use during his gestation

b. Iron staining

c. Excessive fluoride

d. Hyperbilirubinemia

e. Inadequate teeth brushing

20-8. A 3.4-kg newborn girl presents with an oral lesion seen below (see Figure 378-3). There is a pedunculated, soft tissue mass attached to the alveolar ridge by a broad base.

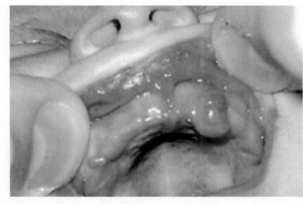

FIGURE 378-3. (Reproduced, with permission, from Rudolph CD, Rudolph AM, Lister GE, First LR, Gershon AA. *Rudolph's Pediatrics.* 22nd ed. New York: McGraw-Hill, 2011.)

What is the diagnosis?

a. Eruption hematoma

b. Ankyloglossia

c. Congenital epulis

d. Neonatal cyst

e. Fibroma

20-9. Your advice nurse is called by a father whose 14-year-old son had a tooth knocked out when roughhousing with some friends. He reports that the tooth socket appears very bloody.

Which of the following statements is correct?

a. The father should hold the tooth by the root to keep the periodontal ligament warm.

b. The child's tooth does not need to be reimplanted, since it is not a primary tooth.

c. The tooth should be placed in a cold, ice-water bath.

d. The child does not need a tetanus vaccine since he did not come in contact with a "dirty" source.

e. The child should receive antibiotics.

20-10. Your 16-year-old patient, who has always been responsible, returns to clinic outraged and requests a referral to a new dentist. She complains that the dental hygienist said she has gingival disease. She states that she knows that gingival disease is a disease of the elderly because she completed a project on the topic in science class last year.

Your best response is to:

a. Tell her that she is absolutely correct and refer her to a new dental office.

b. Explain that adolescents can have gingival and periodontal disease.

c. Reassure her that she cannot have gingival disease since she is Asian.

d. Warn her that gingivitis that is severe in adolescence tends to be even more severe in older age groups.

e. Explain that gingival disease is only caused by *Streptococcus mutans*, the bacterium that causes dental caries.

20-11. The family of a 22-month-old boy presents to your practice for the first time. They have recently moved from out of state to an area supplied by well water. The well water was recently tested and found to have a fluoride ion level in drinking water of 0.8 ppm. What is the appropriate supplementation to prescribe for this 22-month-old patient?

a. 0.25 mg/day

b. 0.50 mg/day

c. 1.00 mg/day

d. 2.50 mg/day

e. None of the above

20-12. A 9-year-old female who is new to your practice presents to the office with concerns about canker sores. She returns twice more in the coming year, reporting that some of the episodes last as much as a month.

The best advice you can give her is:

a. This condition is caused by HSV.

b. There is a definitive treatment.

c. This condition will go away when she grows up.

d. This condition will not scar.

e. This condition can be caused by stress.

20-13. A 6-year-old patient is brought in by his new foster mom, who was concerned when she brushed his teeth last night. She noticed that his tongue was red in certain distinct patterns (see Figure 378-5). He has otherwise not been ill.

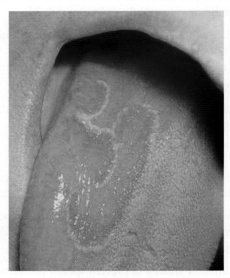

FIGURE 378-5. (Reproduced, with permission, from Rudolph CD, Rudolph AM, Lister GE, First LR, Gershon AA. *Rudolph's Pediatrics.* 22nd ed. New York: McGraw-Hill, 2011.)

The most likely diagnosis he has is:

a. Kawasaki disease

b. Pyogenic granuloma of the tongue

c. Geographic tongue

d. Hairy tongue

e. *Candida*

20-14. Your next patient is a 10-year-old male with a mild fever, red cheeks, and cheek pain. The pain occurs with meal time and then dissipates after several hours. He has no other medical history. Immunizations are up-to-date.

What statement reflects the patient's diagnosis?

a. This condition is most commonly caused by blockage of the parotid duct.

b. This swelling can last days.

c. The condition could require surgery.

d. He is likely to develop bilateral orchitis.

e. He should avoid foods that would stimulate salivary flow.

20-15. An 18-month-old girl is in your clinic with her parents. They are concerned about the fact that she does not have any teeth yet.

All of the following are possible causes, except:

a. Vitamin D–resistant rickets

b. Radiation

c. Apert syndrome

d. Ankyloglossia

e. Down syndrome

20-16. A 9-year-old female presents to clinic with the complaint that her mouth feels full; however, she denies pain. On examination, you notice her tongue is displaced by a smooth, bluish swelling; it is not warmer than the rest of her mouth.

The most likely cause is:

a. Genetic

b. Trauma

c. Blocked salivary duct

d. Surgery

e. Bleeding disorder

20-17. The family of several children lives in an area supplied by well water. The well water was tested and found to have a fluoride ion level in drinking water of less than 3 ppm. The parents have children who are 5 months old, 5 years old, and 15 years old. Which of the 3 children should be prescribed fluoride supplementation?

a. All of the children

b. The 5-year-old and the 15-year-old

c. The 5-month-old and the 5-year-old

d. Only the 5-month-old

e. Only the 15-year-old

20-18. The mother of an 8-year-old boy calls your clinic. The child was playing with friends earlier this afternoon when he was struck in the mouth by another child who was swinging a baseball bat. The boy was fortunate not to have any teeth dislodged, but at least 1 tooth was hit and displaced (see Figure 375-7). He has not lost all his teeth yet.

The best way to advise the mother is:

a. The mother should extract the tooth that was struck.

b. The child should be referred to an emergency department for tooth extraction.

c. The child should be referred for assessment and reduction of the displaced tooth.

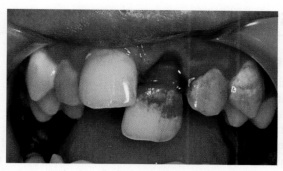

FIGURE 375-7. (Reproduced, with permission, from Rudolph CD, Rudolph AM, Lister GE, First LR, Gershon AA. *Rudolph's Pediatrics.* 22nd ed. New York: McGraw-Hill, 2011.)

d. You should call Child Protective Services (CPS).

e. The permanent teeth will not be affected by any injury to the primary teeth.

20-19. You are approached by the parent of a 7-year-old patient, who was told by an orthodontist that she will need orthodontia. She is worried that this is a trend for children to receive intervention at younger and younger ages.

After reviewing your knowledge of malocclusion, you provide her with the following advice:

a. Early correction is just for aesthetics.

b. Dental crowding is not an issue at this age.

c. Treatment can improve some speech problems.

d. Early correction will result in longer treatment needs.

e. Few children benefit from early correction of malocclusion.

20-20. You are seeing a 20-month-old child in clinic. As you walk in the room, you notice the child using a bottle filled with whole milk. The mother states that he uses a bottle and rarely uses a "sippy cup." In addition, he sometimes falls asleep with the baby bottle in his mouth. Based on your observations and history, what oral pathology are you most likely to note during your examination of this child?

a. Crowding of the maxillary teeth

b. Erythema and thin scaling formation of the lips

c. Localized atrophy of the filiform papillae on the tongue

d. Tooth decay on the maxillary incisors

e. A mucous retention cyst on the floor of the mouth

ANSWERS

Answer 20-1. d

The child in this vignette has candidiasis or thrush. The condition is normal in a newborn infant and can be also associated with several conditions. Fungi thrive in warm, moist environments, and few places on the body are a better environment for *Candida* than the mouth of a newborn, who is taking frequent meals. Nystatin solution should be applied to the cheeks and tongue 4 times daily until after the infection resolves.

Although oral candidiasis is one of the most common manifestations of HIV in children, this case is still more likely to be due to frequent feeding. As a result, antiretrovirals do not need to be initiated, nor does the child need to be admitted for an immune status workup.

There is no indication to cease breast-feeding, although the pediatrician should counsel the mother on care of her breast so as not to develop a candidal mastitis. Nystatin or clotrimazole can be applied to the mother's breasts. In addition, any item that comes in contact with the child's mouth (eg, pacifier, sheets) should be boiled or washed in hot water. Reassurance alone is not adequate.

(Page 1357, Section 20: Disorders of the Oral Cavity, Chapter 378: Oral Pathology)

Answer 20-2. e

It is appropriate that the father was concerned about child's oral hygiene, given mother's status; however, it is likely that the patient has been exposed to excess fluoride and has fluorosis.

It is not clear if the well water was tested for the natural fluoride level. Well water should be tested before supplements are started, as there can be naturally high levels of fluoride in well water. Even a pea-sized amount of toothpaste is an excessive amount of toothpaste for a child of this age. He should have a "smear" of toothpaste on the toothbrush. Children frequently apply too much toothpaste to their toothbrush. Children's toothbrushes should be soft unless instructed otherwise by the dentist. Given that his enamel is weakened, a soft brush should be recommended. Although these teeth have slightly weakened enamel, they do not need to be removed.

(Page 1345, Section 20: Disorders of the Oral Cavity, Chapter 374: Dental Caries)

Answer 20-3. b

Caries are most commonly caused by *Streptococcus mutans*. Early childhood caries, affecting primary teeth, are a particularly virulent form. While caries rates for all other age groups have decreased, rates continue to increase in young children. Having untreated caries in the primary teeth is a strong predictor for caries in secondary teeth.

Fluorosis typically is white and lacy, and presents on the distal portion of the tooth. While children should not be allowed to eat fluoridated toothpaste, all children should brush with fluoridated toothpaste twice daily and should be encouraged to drink fluoridated tap water. While the bacterial exposure may be traced to the mother, it can also be spread from other caregivers or horizontally. She should be seen by a dentist regardless of her status.

(Page 1343, Section 20: Disorders of the Oral Cavity, Chapter 374: Dental Caries)

Answer 20-4. c

The diagnosis is most likely herpangina. Herpangina is associated with coxsackievirus infection and evolves from small vesicles to shallow ulcers on the soft palate, tonsillar pillars, tonsils, uvula, and posterior pharynx. Hand, foot, and mouth disease is also associated with coxsackievirus. Lesions can occur on the hands, feet, and mouth.

Given the mild presentation and a complete immunization history, the case is not consistent with *H. influenzae*. HSV presents as vesicular lesions that progress to ulceration. These lesions tend to coalesce. In addition, HSV frequently involves the gingiva.

Children typically are able to take sufficient oral fluids at home, but adequate pain control is needed. A 3-year-old child is too young for a swish with lidocaine.

(Page 1360, Section 20: Disorders of the Oral Cavity, Chapter 378: Oral Pathology)

Answer 20-5. a

This is most likely temporomandibular joint (TMJ) pain. These disorders are not common in children; however, the incidence increases with age. Because of the age, otitis media is unlikely, and thus amoxicillin is not necessary.

Pain control is needed. TMJ pain is associated with anxiety, so stress relief can be helpful. Moving the patient to a soft diet, and eliminating any foods/snacks that require excessive mastication, such as gum or popcorn, is recommended. Some patients improve when given a splint or bite plate. Some patients may need to wear a splint or bite plate almost 24 hours a day to relieve the pain, and then be weaned off.

(Page 1362, Section 20: Disorders of the Oral Cavity, Chapter 379: Temporomandibular Joint Disorders)

Auvenshine RC. Temporomandibular disorders: associated features. *Dent Clin North Am.* 2007;51:105–127.

Answer 20-6. c

Ankyloglossia, also known as "tongue tie," is a congenital condition where the lingual frenulum is short, tight, and/or anteriorly inserted. It is accepted that the sign on examination is of a tongue that cannot extend beyond the alveolar ridge, or has a "heart shape" with a divot in the tongue midline when extended.

Frenectomy is performed for ankyloglossia associated with poor weight gain, pain with breast-feeding, or neonatal dehydration. The condition is more common in males, with a ratio of 2.6:1. Literature now suggests less pain and shorter recovery time for patients treated with lasers instead of surgery.

(Page 1356, Section 20: Disorders of the Oral Cavity, Chapter 378: Oral Pathology)

Answer 20-7. b

Staining of the teeth can be intrinsic or extrinsic. Examples of intrinsic include hereditary conditions (of enamel formation or systemic illnesses or metabolic diseases) or tetracycline use during pregnancy or while the teeth are forming. Extrinsic causes include iron supplements, poor oral hygiene leading to caries (usually white stains early on and brown stains later), or abnormal food habits. eFigure 378-3 shows a case of black extrinsic staining, which is the result of vitamins containing iron.

Minocycline can also cause staining of the teeth post eruption. It would be difficult to develop fluorosis from municipal water without also having a habit of eating toothpaste or taking fluoride supplements. One third of the US population does not have access to fluoridated public water.

(Page 1361, Section 20: Disorders of the Oral Cavity, Chapter 378: Oral Pathology)

Answer 20-8. c

The infant has congenital epulis, which is rare, but more common in females than in males (8:1). It is a flesh-toned gingival granular cell tumor growing off the maxillary anterior alveolus. Treatment is excision of the lesion.

An eruption hematoma typically comes up on the gumline at that point where the crown of the tooth is about to break through; it is usually blue, because of the bleeding into the cysts. Ankyloglossia (tongue tie) is caused by a short and/or anteriorly displaced frenulum. A fibroma is a pedunculated or sessile growth that occurs secondary to irritation. The buccal mucosa and interdental gingiva are the most common sites (as opposed to the alveolus). Neonatal cysts are remnants of epithelia tissue (Epstein pearls) or mucus gland tissue (Bohn nodules). These cysts can be white, gray, or yellow in appearance. Surgery for neonatal cysts is not indicated, as spontaneous resolution is common.

(Page 1357, Section 20: Disorders of the Oral Cavity, Chapter 378: Oral Pathology)

Answer 20-9. e

The avulsed tooth is dealt with differently when it is a primary tooth versus a secondary tooth. Primary teeth generally start exfoliating around 6 years old, with the last ones falling out about 12 years, so it is unlikely that this is a primary tooth. Primary teeth do not need to be reimplanted. Adult or permanent teeth should be reimplanted immediately. The tooth should always be held by the crown and not the root. The tooth should be put back into the space if clean and if the patient can tolerate the procedure. Otherwise the tooth can be placed into Hank's balanced salt solution, milk, saline, or saliva (including the patient's own cheek, if able) until seen by a dentist. The patent should be referred to a hospital emergency room with dental coverage, or a dental office for immediate splitting. The child will need antibiotics and tetanus booster, unless he already received it at his 11-year-old visit.

(Page 1348, Section 20: Disorders of the Oral Cavity, Chapter 375: Dental Emergency Care)

Answer 20-10. b

While periodontal disease is the more severe form of gingival disease, either is possible in teenagers. In fact, gingival disease may be worse in adolescence. Rates of localized, aggressive periodontitis are higher in African American children; however, no racial or ethnic group is immune. Young teens have a prevalence of gingival disease of almost 50%. While gingival and periodontal disease is more common in children with uncontrolled caries, it can also be caused by fungi, medication, allergies, or systemic issues. Gingivitis can be found in children under 10 years old, but it gets more severe in adolescence and then tends to improve in adulthood.

(Page 1354, Section 20: Disorders of the Oral Cavity, Chapter 377: Periodontal and Gingival Health and Diseases)

Answer 20-11. e

Appropriate fluoride supplementation depends on patient's age and the fluoride content of water. Table 13-2 lists the daily recommended dietary fluoride supplementation, based on recommendations from the American Dental Association, the American Academy of Pediatrics, and the American Academy of Pediatric Dentistry. Since the fluoride ion level is greater than 0.6 ppm, no supplementation is required.

(Page 1345, Section 20: Disorders of the Oral Cavity, Chapter 374: Dental Caries)

TABLE 13-2. Daily Recommended Dietary Fluoride Supplementation Depending on Drinking Water Content

Age	<0.3 ppm	0.3-0.6 ppm	>0.6 ppm
Birth to 6 months	0	0	0
6 months to 3 years	0.25 mg	0	0
3-6 years	0.50 mg	0.25 mg	0
6 years up to at least 16 years	1.00 mg	0.50 mg	0

Adapted from American Academy of Pediatric Dentistry (http://www.aapd.org/media/Policies_Guidelines/G_FluorideTherapy.pdf).

Answer 20-12. e

Recurrent aphthous stomatitis is common. The disorder comes in 3 forms: minor, major, and herpetiform. There is no definitive treatment and it generally does continue into adulthood, with no clear preference by age, sex, race, or geography.

This patient appears to have the major form, also known as Sutton disease, based on the time needed for healing, which can take from a week to a month. These lesions can scar. Herpetiform recurrent aphthous stomatitis clinically resembles recurrent herpes, but does not last as long as major form.

Stress can be a precipitating factor, but there is a wide differential that can also be associated with recurrent aphthous stomatitis. In severe cases, possible systemic conditions should be ruled out. These include anemia, nutritional deficiencies, diabetes mellitus, immunosuppression, and inflammatory bowel disease.

(Page 1359, Section 20: Disorders of the Oral Cavity, Chapter 378: Oral Pathology)

Answer 20-13. c

Geographic tongue can have a changing appearance, hence its alternative description, erythema migrans. It involves atrophy of the filiform papillae, usually on the dorsum of the tongue. It is harmless and common.

Hairy tongue is usually dark colored; it is caused by excess keratin and hypertrophy and elongation of the filiform papillae. Usually these patients are asymptomatic. Patients with Kawasaki traditionally have "strawberry tongue," where the tongue is red and slightly swollen and the papillae appear white as a contrast. These patients are generally quite ill, with high fevers for several days and other symptoms. Pyogenic granulomas can grow on the tongue, although they would be more commonly found on the gingiva, as they are caused by the body's reaction to irritation. It is a painless mass that can be red, blue, or purple. *Candida* usually causes a white adherent plaque on the tongue, and the child may complain of burning pain or feeling like the mouth contains cotton.

(Page 1358, Section 20: Disorders of the Oral Cavity, Chapter 378: Oral Pathology)

Answer 20-14. c

Obstructive sialadenitis is most commonly caused by blockage of submandibular duct. Swelling can last several hours. Cases of recurrent obstructive sialadenitis can require surgery. Mumps parotitis is less likely to cause orchitis in prepubertal males. In addition, this condition is less common now due to improved immunization rates for mumps. Salivary flow should be stimulated, and heat applied, as adjunctive therapies to antibiotic treatment of obstructive sialadenitis.

(Page 1359, Section 20: Disorders of the Oral Cavity, Chapter 378: Oral Pathology)

Answer 20-15. d

Delayed tooth eruption can be caused by local or systemic reasons. Local reasons more commonly cause delayed secondary teeth, and include crowding, ectopic teeth, supernumerary teeth, early loss of primary teeth, odontoma, gingival hyperplasia, and primary tooth ankylosis. Systemic factors and conditions include endocrine disorders, radiation or chemotherapy, nutritional deficiencies, Down syndrome, Apert syndrome, or cleidocranial dysplasia. Delayed tooth eruption has been linked with vitamin D–resistant but not vitamin D–deficient rickets.

Ankyloglossia (tongue tie) is caused by a short and/or anteriorly displaced frenulum. It is not associated with delayed tooth eruption.

(Page 1350, Section 20: Disorders of the Oral Cavity, Chapter 376: Dental Occlusion and Its Management)

Answer 20-16. b

The patient has a ranula, a mucous retention cyst. This condition most commonly occurs under the tongue, off the lingual frenulum. It is more commonly associated with the sublingual gland than the submandibular gland. Ranulas can be congenital, but they are more commonly associated with trauma. Treatment is excision. A blood-filled cyst under the tongue would be a very unusual presentation of a bleeding disorder.

(Page 1359, Section 20: Disorders of the Oral Cavity, Chapter 378: Oral Pathology)

Answer 20-17. b

Water fluoridation has been an effective method at preventing dental caries. For children who do not have access to adequately fluoridated water, supplementation may be necessary, depending on the child's age and the level of fluoridation.

Table 13-2 lists the daily recommended dietary fluoride supplementation, based on recommendations from the American Dental Association, the American Academy of

TABLE 13-2. Daily Recommended Dietary Fluoride Supplementation Depending on Drinking Water Content			
Age	**<0.3 ppm**	**0.3-0.6 ppm**	**>0.6 ppm**
Birth to 6 months	0	0	0
6 months to 3 years	0.25 mg	0	0
3-6 years	0.50 mg	0.25 mg	0
6 years up to at least 16 years	1.00 mg	0.50 mg	0

Adapted from American Academy of Pediatric Dentistry (http://www.aapd.org/media/Policies_Guidelines/G_FluorideTherapy.pdf).

Pediatrics, and the American Academy of Pediatric Dentistry. If the fluoride ion level is less than 0.3 ppm, supplementation is required from age 6 months to 16 years of age. The amount of fluoride supplementation will vary, based on the age of the child.

(Page 1345, Section 20: Disorders of the Oral Cavity, Chapter 374: Dental Caries)

Answer 20-18. c

Displacement injuries are treated with reduction. The goal of treatment is normal reattachment of the periodontal ligament to both the tooth and the alveolar bone. After reduction, the tooth is stabilized for up to 4 weeks. Prognosis can be difficult to assess until 3 months after the initial trauma.

Prophylactic extractions are not necessarily recommended, especially without an examination. To prematurely remove a tooth also makes the others more likely to grow in crooked and unevenly. Similarly, trauma to a tooth can cause hypoplasia to the crown, root deformities, and eruption problems, from accelerated to delayed eruption, as well as ectopic eruption.

While it is never wrong for a practitioner to have a high index of suspicion for nonaccidental trauma, contacting CPS at this point may be premature. He, at minimum, would need to be brought into clinic for examination and assessment.

(Page 1346, Section 20: Disorders of the Oral Cavity, Chapter 375: Dental Emergency Care)

Answer 20-19. c

Early correction of orthodontic problems may improve aesthetics and self-esteem of a child, but that is not the sole reason for it to be done at this point. Correction can lead to helping with some speech problems, correct some poor oral health habits, and can reduce the amount of time a child later will need for treatment. Dental crowding in the primary or mixed dentition can impair the eruption, placement, and risk of impaction of permanent teeth.

(Page 1352, Section 20: Disorders of the Oral Cavity, Chapter 376: Dental Occlusion and Its Management)

Answer 20-20. d

Developmentally, the child should be transitioned from a baby bottle to a sippy cup. In addition, the child should not fall asleep with a bottle in his mouth. As a result of these behaviors, the child is at risk for early childhood caries or "baby bottle tooth decay." Typically, the tooth decay occurs on the maxillary incisors and then spreads to the maxillary and mandibular molars. See Figure 374-1.

Crowding is due to multiple factors, including tooth/jaw size discrepancies, premature loss of primary teeth, or ectopic eruption of teeth.

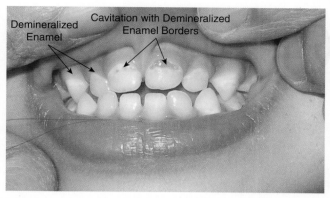

FIGURE 374-1. Demineralization and early cavitation. (Reproduced, with permission, from Rudolph CD, Rudolph AM, Lister GE, First LR, Gershon AA. *Rudolph's Pediatrics.* 22nd ed. New York: McGraw-Hill, 2011.)

Erythema and thin scaling formation, as well as mild edema, are features of cheilitis. Cheilitis can be due to chronic lip licking or mechanical irritation of the lips. See Figure 378-2.

Localized atrophy of the filiform papillae is a description of geographic tongue or erthyema migrans. See Figure 378-5. The etiology is unknown. It is not associated with prolonged bottle use.

A mucous retention cyst on the floor of the mouth is a description of a ranula. A ranula can be congenital or associated with recent trauma. It presents as dome-shaped, painless, fluctuant swelling. It is not associated with prolonged bottle use.

(Page 1344, Section 20: Disorders of the Oral Cavity, Chapter 374: Dental Caries)

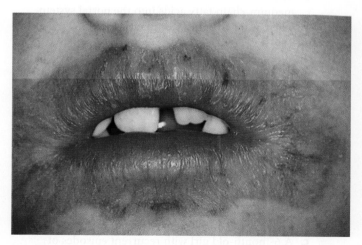

FIGURE 378-2. Cheilitis. The habit of chronic lip licking can result in significant inflammation of the perioral tissues. Severe cases typically respond well to topical steroids. (Reproduced, with permission, from Rudolph CD, Rudolph AM, Lister GE, First LR, Gershon AA. *Rudolph's Pediatrics.* 22nd ed. New York: McGraw-Hill, 2011.)

CHAPTER 21 | Disorders of the GI Tract

Kristin L. Van Buren, Haley C. Neef, and Eric H. Chiou

21-1. Two healthy siblings are followed in a primary pediatric care clinic. The younger sibling was breastfed until 10 months of age; the older sibling was exclusively formula-fed from birth.

Which of the following statements about the siblings during their infancy is true?

a. The breastfed infant had significantly higher lactase activity compared with the formula-fed infant.

b. The breastfed infant absorbed significantly more dietary lipid than the formula-fed infant.

c. Both the breastfed infant and the formula-fed infant secreted pancreatic lipase and bile salt to a greater degree than their adult parent.

d. The formula-fed infant absorbed significantly less dietary protein when compared with the breastfed infant.

e. The breastfed infant was able to directly absorb medium-chain fatty acids into the portal system, whereas the formula-fed infant was not.

21-2. Vomiting is a common presenting symptom in general pediatrics. In addition, cyclic vomiting syndrome (CVS) has an estimated prevalence of 2%. Which of the following scenarios is consistent with a child with the diagnosis of CVS?

a. A 5-year-old boy with recurrent episodes of nonbilious vomiting that occur after he sleeps in during the weekend or after a high-protein meal

b. A 6-year-old girl with recurrent episodes of "fast"-paced vomiting (up to 4 emeses/h) every 3 weeks that begin in the morning and last about 24 hours

c. A 6-month-old girl with recurrent episodes of bilious vomiting and abdominal pain every 4 to 6 hours

d. A 5-year-old girl with recurrent episodes of nonbilious vomiting every 4 hours, occipital headache, and mild ataxia

e. A 6-week-old girl with recurrent episodes of nonbilious vomiting after every feed

21-3. A 7-year-old girl presents to the emergency department (ED) after vomiting 15 times over the past 8 hours. The vomiting began suddenly on awakening that morning. After examining her medical record, you note that she has had similar 24-hour episodes of vomiting, approximately every 4 weeks for the past 3 months. All the episodes required intravenous fluid rehydration. Aside from the 24-hour vomiting episodes, she has been otherwise healthy.

She has a heart rate of 130 bpm, blood pressure of 105/76 mm Hg, and appears listless, but is able to answer your questions appropriately. She has urinated once earlier today. Physical examination reveals tacky mucous membranes. There are no focal neurologic findings or symptoms. She takes sips of water in the emergency room, but 10 minutes later, she has an episode of nonbloody, nonbilious emesis.

You suspect cyclic vomiting syndrome (CVS). What would be the next appropriate step in management of this patient?

a. Administer intravenous fluid rehydration.

b. Send blood for electrolytes, glucose, blood urea nitrogen, and creatinine.

c. Order an abdominal radiograph.

d. Administer an intravenous proton pump inhibitor.

e. Order head CT.

21-4. An 11-year-old boy presents to clinic with a complaint of 1 to 2 episodes of vomiting at least 1 time per week over the past 3 months. He reports that vomiting consists of nonbloody, nonbilious food material and is preceded by several minutes of burning substernal pain. His body mass index is in the 80th percentile for age.

What is the next most appropriate step in the management of this patient?

a. A 2-week trial of H_2-receptor antagonist.

b. Referral to pediatric gastroenterology clinic.

c. Send blood for CBC, AST, ALT, and pancreatic lipase.

d. Obtain upper gastrointestinal contrast study.

e. A 2-week trial of odansetron as needed for nausea.

21-5. A 12-year-old female is admitted to the hospital with elevated lipase and suspected pancreatitis based on initial evaluation completed in the emergency room. She is tearful and complaining of pain in her lower neck and shoulders.

What is the reason for the location of her pain?

a. Inflammation of the pancreas in direct contact with pleural surface

b. Direct activation of the visceral efferent nervous system

c. Irritation of the parietal peritoneum surrounding the inflamed pancreas

d. Convergence of activated visceral afferent nerves with somatic afferent nerves in the spinal cord

e. Unreliable reporting of symptoms due to patient distress

21-6. You are examining a 9-year-old boy in the emergency department who complains of severe abdominal pain for the past 6 hours. He said the pain started in the umbilical area and now seems to be "lower down" toward his right side. His temperature is 38.5°C.

During your physical examination, which of the following signs is associated with acute appendicitis?

a. A bluish discoloration of the flank.

b. When the patient is lying down, the right hip and knee are flexed; pain is elicited when the ankle is rotated away from the body, while the knee is rotated inward.

c. When palpating below the right costal margin, pain is elicited with deep inspiration.

d. When the thigh is bent at the hip and the knee, pain is elicited with subsequent extension of the knee.

e. When the knee is bent slightly, the ipsilateral ankle is dorsiflexed abruptly; pain is elicited in the popliteal area.

21-7. A 10-year-old obese child is seen in follow-up at clinic for chronic functional abdominal pain. This patient is most likely to have what other concomitant characteristic?

a. Major depressive disorder

b. Female gender

c. Pain with application of pressure by examiner to point of maximal abdominal tenderness when patient assumes a partial sitting position

d. Anxiety

e. Resolution of symptoms with antispasmodic medication

21-8. A 15-year-old female complains of daily periumbilical abdominal pain without identifiable trigger for the past 12 months. Review of growth records indicates she has been between the 50th and 75th percentiles for body mass index over the past several years. Physical examination is unremarkable.

What additional finding suggests an organic cause for her pain rather than a functional etiology?

a. Pain severe enough to cause significant school absenteeism

b. History of irritable bowel syndrome in first-degree relative

c. Sensation of incomplete evacuation after passage of stool

d. Complaint of fatigue and headache in addition to abdominal pain

e. Awakening from sleep to pass loose stool at night

21-9. A 30-month-old previously healthy child presents to urgent care clinic in the winter with a 24-hour history of profuse diarrhea. There have been streaks of bloody mucous intermittently mixed in with the stool over the past 8 hours. On examination, the patient has moist mucous membranes, is alert, and is drinking grape juice from a sippy cup. His mother states he is acting hungry, but she is concerned about "how fast everything is going through him," so she has not offered him food. Which of the following statements about this patient is true?

a. Solid foods should be deferred in favor of clear fluids until the diarrhea has resolved.

b. Loperamide is an appropriate treatment for the child's diarrheal illness.

c. Stool cultures are not necessary as long as the child is able to maintain adequate hydration with oral intake.

d. Stool culture should be sent.

e. The most likely etiology of this child's illness is rotavirus infection.

21-10. A 20-month-old female is seen in clinic with a 4-month history of 3 to 5 watery stools per day. She is in the 60th percentile for weight and 75th percentile for height. Her mother describes her as a playful child and has no concerns other than the diarrhea. Dietary history reveals that the girl eats 3 meals and at least 2 small snacks and drinks 2 to 3 cups of apple juice in addition to 12 oz of cow's milk each day.

Which of the following is the next appropriate step in management of this patient?

  a. Determination of stool electrolytes and osmolality

  b. Determination of stool pH and reducing substances

  c. Stool culture

  d. Two-week trial of lactose-free diet

  e. Two-week trial of juice-free diet

21-11. A 32-month-old girl presents to clinic for evaluation of constipation. Which of the following findings in the child's medical history suggests an organic cause of constipation rather than functional cause?

  a. Daily fecal soiling in undergarments

  b. Two urinary tract infections within the last 6 months

  c. Large-caliber stools that sometimes clog the toilet

  d. Small-caliber, thin-appearing stools

  e. Episodes of posturing during which the child crosses legs and screams

21-12. A 4-month-old breastfed infant is seen in clinic for a well-child examination. His mother describes him as a generally happy baby, but expresses concern that he is constipated because he only passes stool every 3 to 5 days. She explains that when he does have a bowel movement, he will briefly become red in the face and fuss, and then pass a large, soft, yellow stool that sometimes spills out of his diaper. His physical examination is unremarkable and his weight gain and growth have been excellent.

The most appropriate response to this mother's concern about the infant's stooling pattern is:

  a. The infant is constipated and she should offer 2 oz of diluted apple juice daily.

  b. The infant is constipated and she should give lactulose 1 mL/kg/day divided BID.

  c. The infant is constipated and should undergo barium enema to evaluate for possible Hirschsprung disease.

  d. The infant is not constipated and this may be a normal stooling pattern for a healthy breastfed baby.

  e. The infant is not constipated and is displaying behavior consistent with colic.

21-13. A previously healthy 8-year-old boy presents to the emergency room with a history of passing 3 large bloody stools in the last 6 hours. Initial vital signs show a heart rate of 140, blood pressure of 76/40, oxygen saturation of 98% on room air, and respiratory rate of 24. He appears pale and sleepy.

What is the next most appropriate step in management of this patient?

  a. Obtain a complete medical history from his parents.

  b. Obtain venous access and infuse normal saline bolus.

  c. Consult pediatric gastroenterology for emergent endoscopy.

  d. Consult pediatric surgery for emergent surgical exploration.

  e. Send for immediate angiography.

21-14. Which of the following is a cause of painless lower gastrointestinal bleeding in an infant?

  a. Intestinal duplication

  b. Infectious colitis

  c. Malrotation with volvulus

  d. Anal fissure

  e. Intussusception

21-15. On examination of a 4-day-old infant male in the newborn nursery, you palpate a nonmobile abdominal mass in the right flank; the examination is otherwise unremarkable. What is the most likely cause of the mass?

  a. Constipation

  b. Neuroblastoma

  c. Hepatomegaly

  d. Hydronephrosis

  e. Sacrococcygeal teratoma

21-16. You are performing a pelvic examination on a 16-year-old female who is not sexually active and are able to palpate a left-sided, round, well-circumscribed pelvic mass estimated at approximately 9 cm diameter. It is nontender to palpation. Ultrasound demonstrates that the mass is solid and ovarian in origin.

Which of the following statements is true about this palpable pelvic mass?

a. The patient should be referred for prompt surgical evaluation to correct ovarian torsion.

b. The mass should be monitored by ultrasound every 3 months; if there is an increase in size after 6 months, surgical consultation is warranted.

c. The patient should be referred to a gynecologist for an ovarian cyst.

d. The patient should be referred for prompt surgical evaluation for evaluation of possible neoplasm.

e. Ovarian masses in children are neoplastic in less than 50% of cases.

21-17. A 2-week-old term breastfed infant presents to the emergency department with a 6-hour history of bilious emesis. His father states he had been feeding well and passing soft, yellow bowel movements several times a day up until the onset of emesis. Examination reveals a nondistended abdomen; however, the infant cries when you attempt to palpate the abdomen and is somewhat difficult to console afterwards. Vital signs are within age-appropriate norms and the infant has brisk distal capillary refill.

The radiologic study with the highest diagnostic yield for this patient is:

a. Abdominal ultrasound

b. Plain abdominal film

c. CT scan

d. Contrast enema

e. Upper GI contrast study

21-18. A 1-day-old infant in the newborn nursery vomits with each attempt at breast-feeding. You are unable to pass a nasogastric tube to the stomach. This child is most likely to have what other coexisting condition?

a. Trisomy 21

b. Prematurity

c. Cystic fibrosis

d. Low birth weight

e. Congenital cardiac anomaly

21-19. A 10-year-old male with a history of Fontan procedure for hypoplastic left heart syndrome is admitted with a 4-kg weight gain, peripheral edema, and diarrhea. An echocardiogram done 3 months ago demonstrated elevated right atrial pressures. You suspect protein-losing enteropathy and decide to send fecal α_1-antitrypsin as part of the diagnostic workup.

Which of the following statements is true?

a. Fecal α_1-antitrypsin assay is unreliable if sample is contaminated with urine.

b. Fecal α_1-antitrypsin assay is reliable for detection of esophageal and gastric protein loss.

c. Fecal α_1-antitrypsin is stable at room temperature allowing for ease of specimen transport and storage.

d. Fecal α_1-antitrypsin assay is preferable to radioisotopic techniques for the diagnosis of protein-losing enteropathy.

e. Fecal α_1-antitrypsin assay is not affected by meconium and the test can be used in newborn infants.

21-20. Which of the following laboratory findings is most consistent with a diagnosis of Crohn disease?

a. Hypoalbuminemia

b. Elevated blood urea nitrogen

c. Elevated MCV

d. Hyperbilirubinemia

e. Hypophosphatemia

21-21. You are caring for a 15-year-old patient with Crohn disease who has required complete duodenal resection and bypass due to stenosis and gastric outlet obstruction from her disease. She has developed dumping syndrome characterized by severe diarrhea after eating as a result.

The absence of which of the following histologic entities may be contributing to her diarrhea?

a. Enterochromaffin cells

b. Peyer patches

c. Crypts of Lieberkuhn

d. Brunner glands

e. Chief cells

21-22. A 3-year-old boy with Down syndrome presents with abdominal pain, intermittent abdominal distension, and nonbloody, watery diarrhea for the past 3 months. His mother is concerned that he has not gained any significant weight in the last 6 months. On examination, his vital signs are within normal limits for age and he is afebrile. His examination is notable for Down facies and short stature, but is otherwise unremarkable. No rash is present.

What test would you order next?

a. HLA-DQ2/DQ8 genetic typing for celiac disease

b. Esophagogastroduodenoscopy (EGD)

c. Sweat chloride test

d. Anti–tissue transglutaminase (TTG) IgA and serum IgA levels

e. Stool rotavirus assay

21-23. Which of the following statements regarding small intestinal bacterial overgrowth (SIBO) is correct?

a. SIBO is diagnosed when bacterial counts exceed 1000 organisms/mL on a quantitative culture from a jejunal aspirate.

b. Anatomic abnormalities, such as intestinal duplications, bowel dilation, or small intestinal atresias, are not associated with increased development of SIBO.

c. Symptoms of excessive gas formation and abdominal distension are associated with metabolism of carbohydrates by intraluminal bacteria.

d. A late rise in breath hydrogen levels on glucose breath hydrogen testing is diagnostic of SIBO.

e. Acid-suppressing medications can be used as empiric treatment of SIBO in children.

21-24. An 11-month-old infant with a history of multiple small bowel atresias has been maintained on total parental nutrition (TPN) via a central venous catheter since birth. He was recently started on trophic enteral feeds via a gastrostomy tube and was discharged from the neonatal intensive care unit 1 week ago. He now presents to your office with a 1-day history of lethargy, fever, and vomiting. Serum chemistries reveal chronic, mild elevation of hepatic transaminases and alkaline phosphatase, but are otherwise normal.

The *most* likely cause of this infant's findings is which of the following?

a. Cholelithiasis

b. Fulminant hepatic failure

c. Intrahepatic cholestasis

d. Infection of the central venous catheter

e. D-Lactic acidosis

21-25. A 3-month-old infant has had diarrhea since the first week of life. The stool is watery and nonbloody. The patient has been exclusively breastfed and he has not yet started any solid foods. When enteral feeds are held, the diarrhea decreases but does not completely resolve. Findings on physical examination include weight at less than 5th percentile and length at the 10th percentile for age; cachexia; a protuberant abdomen; stool for reducing substances 2+; stool culture negative for enteric pathogens; and sweat chloride, 10 mEq/L. The patient undergoes an esophagogastroduodenoscopy and biopsies of the small intestine reveal diffuse villous atrophy.

These findings are *most* consistent with which of the following diagnoses?

a. Celiac disease

b. Cystic fibrosis

c. Congenital chloride diarrhea

d. Acrodermatitis enteropathica

e. Microvillus inclusion disease

21-26. A 14-year-old female adolescent who has severe juvenile rheumatoid arthritis presents to your office with epigastric abdominal pain. Six weeks earlier she began taking a nonsteroidal anti-inflammatory drug (NSAID) because of worsening joint complaints.

The most appropriate *initial* management of her symptoms would be which of the following?

a. Administration of an antibiotic effective against *Helicobacter pylori*

b. Administration of a proton pump inhibitor

c. Dietary modification

d. Substitution of salicylate for NSAID

e. Upper endoscopy and gastric biopsy for gastric adenocarcinoma

21-27. A 17-year-old male presents with a several-week history of progressive abdominal pain, nausea, and 1 episode of coffee-ground emesis. He localizes the pain primarily to the epigastrium, and describes the pain as "burning" in character. The pain occurs 2 to 3 hours after meals and is relieved by antacids. He denies taking any nonsteroidal anti-inflammatory medications.

Of the following, the most appropriate *initial* step in the evaluation and management of suspected *Helicobacter pylori* infection is:

a. Begin an empiric 2-week course of amoxicillin therapy.

b. Begin a trial of omeprazole therapy.

c. Refer for urea breath testing.

d. Obtain blood sample for *H. pylori* antibody testing.

e. Refer for endoscopy and gastric biopsy.

21-28. A 2-day-old term infant presents with feeding intolerance and bilious emesis in the newborn nursery. The abdominal examination is notable for distension and a "doughy" character on palpation. The infant has not yet passed meconium. The rectal examination reveals a small amount of white mucous in the vault, but is otherwise normal without explosive passage of stool. The plain abdominal radiograph shows multiple fluid-filled loops of bowel, which have a "ground-glass" appearance. An upper gastrointestinal tract contrast study is normal, without evidence of malrotation. Retrograde contrast enema is then performed and is significant for a small-caliber colon, or microcolon of normal length. Contrast fills the colon and is refluxed into the terminal ileum that appears to be filled with pellet-like masses. A 24-hour postevacuation radiograph is obtained and shows complete clearance of contrast.

Of the following, these findings are *most* consistent with:

a. Hirschsprung disease (HD)

b. Cystic fibrosis (CF)

c. Cow's milk protein allergy

d. Duodenal atresia

e. Congenital anal stenosis

21-29. A 16-year-old male with a history of cystic fibrosis (CF) presents to the emergency department with a complaint of acute-onset, crampy, right lower quadrant abdominal pain, abdominal distension, vomiting, and no bowel movements for the past 3 days. A plain abdominal film is obtained that shows a large amount of stool in the distal ileum. After the patient is admitted, a nasogastric tube is placed for decompression. The patient receives several retrograde enemas with water-soluble contrast as well as oral osmotic laxatives and is successfully disimpacted.

Of the following, which would be the *most* important in preventing a recurrence of this patient's symptoms?

a. Increased dietary fiber intake

b. Daily use of high-dose stimulant laxatives

c. Daily use of rectal glycerin suppository

d. Optimization of fat-soluble vitamin supplementation

e. Optimization of pancreatic enzyme supplementation

21-30. A 14-year-old female presents to your office with the chief complaint of abdominal pain for 4 months. On further questioning, she admits to very poor appetite and she has lost 10 lb since her last visit with you. She reports to occasional loose stool, but no hematochezia. On rectal examination, she is hemoccult positive and you notice 2 moderate skin tags. The labs that you sent show a hemoglobin of 8.8 g/dL and an albumen of 3.2 g/dL. You're concerned she most likely has which condition?

a. Chronic *Giardia* infection

b. Crohn disease

c. Celiac disease

d. Anorexia nervosa

e. Irritable bowel syndrome

21-31. A 15-year-old male presents to your office for his yearly well-child examination. Four weeks ago he had been diagnosed with ulcerative colitis and is currently being induced into remission with oral prednisone. The patient's mother is concerned about the consequences of him taking this medication.

What side effects of corticosteroids will you discuss with the patient's mother?

a. Adrenal insufficiency, hypertension, bone demineralization, and hyperglycemia

b. Adrenal insufficiency, weight loss, acne, and hypertension

c. Hyperglycemia, hypertension, muscle redistribution, and hirsutism

d. Acne, bone demineralization, cataracts, and leucopenia

e. Emotional disturbances, bone demineralization, vitamin D deficiency, and adrenal insufficiency

21-32. A 10-year-old male presents to your office with 12 days of bloody diarrhea, abdominal pain, and weight loss. He has been afebrile. His mom has a history of ulcerative colitis and she is very concerned her son has now developed this condition.

What enteric pathogens should be ruled out prior to referral to gastroenterology?

a. *Giardia, Yersinia, Salmonella*, and *E. coli 0157/H7*

b. *Yersinia, Salmonella, C. difficile*, and *Cryptosporidium*

c. *C. difficile, Salmonella, Giardia*, and *Campylobacter*

d. *C. difficile, Salmonella, Shigella*, and *E. coli 0157/H7*

e. *Cryptosporidium, Giardia, C. difficile*, and *E. coli 0157/H7*

21-33. A 7-year-old male presents to your office for the first time with his mother for a routine well-child check. You notice bluish brown macules on his lips and buccal mucosa (Figure 414-1).

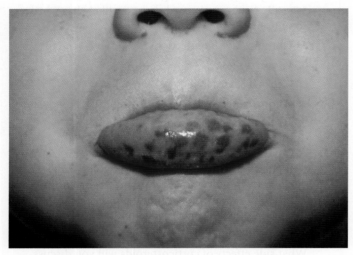

FIGURE 414-1. (Reproduced, with permission, from Rudolph CD, Rudolph AM, Lister GE, First LR, Gershon AA. *Rudolph's Pediatrics.* 22nd ed. New York: McGraw-Hill, 2011.)

You ask his mother if there is any family history of which of the following conditions?

a. Tuberous sclerosis

b. Peutz-Jeghers syndrome

c. Neurofibromatosis

d. Familial adenomatous polyposis syndrome

e. Juvenile polyposis syndrome

21-34. A 2-month-old male presents to your office with his mother for a routine well-child check. During the family history you elicit a strong family history of familial adenomatous polyposis (FAP) syndrome. There has been no gene mutation identified in this family on testing affected members. At what time should you refer the patient for screening?

a. Now to determine if this infant carries an APC mutation.

b. Only on the development of symptoms such as hematochezia.

c. During his late teens for an evaluation for colectomy due to the high risk of colorectal cancer.

d. No referral is necessary given the fact that no gene mutation has been identified.

e. At 12 years of age or with the development of symptoms for screening colonoscopy.

21-35. A 3-year-old female presents to your office for follow-up of her rectal bleeding. You had previously referred her to pediatric gastroenterology for painless rectal bleeding. She was found to have 3 polyps on her colonoscopy that were identified as juvenile polyps on histology. There is no history of juvenile polyps in the family.

Which of the following statements is the most appropriate in counseling the parents?

a. Juvenile polyps are common in this age group and she does not need any further follow-up and she is not at increased risk of cancer.

b. The patient's siblings should be screened for polyps with colonoscopy given her new diagnosis of juvenile polyposis syndrome (JPS).

c. The patient should now receive yearly colonoscopy screening to evaluate for recurrence of polyps.

d. This patient now has close to a 50% lifetime risk of developing colorectal cancer.

e. She should be screened for germline mutations of *SMAD4* and *BMPR1A* to determine if she has JPS.

21-36. A 17-year-old female presents with a 3-week history of recurrent nausea, vomiting, anorexia, and abdominal pain. This is the first time she has had these types of symptoms. She denies dieting or intentional weight loss, but her mother thinks she has lost about 15 lb in the last 3 weeks. She has not had any significant diarrhea or constipation. On examination, her BMI is now <5th percentile for age. She has some mild abdominal distension and epigastric tenderness on abdominal examination. Her physical examination is otherwise unremarkable. Serum markers for inflammation (sedimentation rate, C-reactive protein), complete blood cell count, serum albumin, and serum lipase levels are all normal. An upper gastrointestinal contrast study is obtained and demonstrates a dilated stomach and duodenum with abrupt cutoff of the duodenum at the level of the third lumbar vertebra.

Of the following, these findings are *most* consistent with:

a. Superior mesenteric artery syndrome (SMAS)

b. Crohn disease

c. Duodenal stenosis

d. Chronic pancreatitis

e. Celiac disease

21-37. An 18-month-old boy presents to the emergency department with a 4-hour history of colicky abdominal pain and vomiting. During the episodes of pain, the child is observed to have flexed hips and knees. The child appears calm but lethargic and pale in between episodes. Physical examination is notable for the absence of palpable bowel in the right lower quadrant. Of the following, the *most* appropriate diagnostic test is:

a. Abdominal ultrasonography

b. Plain film radiograph of the abdomen

c. Air contrast enema

d. Technetium-99m pertechnetate scan

e. Upper gastrointestinal tract contrast study with small bowel follow-through

21-38. Which of the following scenarios would be *most* concerning for a diagnosis of infantile hypertophic pyloric stenosis (IHPS)?

a. A 4-month-old baby boy with postprandial vomiting and weight maintained at the 50th percentile for age

b. A 3-week-old baby girl with recurrent regurgitation, frequent gagging while feeding, and lack of interest in feeding

c. A 3-day-old baby boy with trisomy 21 and postprandial, bilious emesis

d. A 6-week-old baby boy with jaundice and hypochloremic, hypokalemic alkalosis, but appears hungry and eager to feed

e. A 3-month-old baby girl with 3 days of severe vomiting, now with profuse diarrhea, and found to have hypernatremic, metabolic acidosis

21-39. A 6-week-old male infant presents with a history of progressive, postprandial vomiting. The infant's parents report forceful, projectile vomiting after every feeding. On examination, the patient appears dehydrated and peristaltic waves across a dilated, upper abdomen are visible. The patient undergoes abdominal ultrasonography that demonstrates a pyloric channel with a thickness of 4 cm and a length of 3 cm.

Of the following, which is the *best initial* step in the management of this patient?

a. Placement of nasogastric tube for administration of fluids and nutrition

b. Consult for emergent surgical pyloromyotomy

c. Initiation of treatment with a gastric motility prokinetic agent such as erythromycin

d. Endoscopic balloon dilation of the pyloric channel

e. Intravenous fluids and correction of any electrolyte imbalances

21-40. An 18-month-old female infant presents for a well-child visit. On examination, she has pallor and mild generalized edema. Her mother reports that these findings have been very gradual in onset. She otherwise appears well and does not exhibit any signs of lethargy or tachycardia. She has not been exposed to any sick contacts. The patient's diet consists of 36 to 40 oz of whole cow's milk daily and some fruits. She does not like eating vegetables or meats. Patient has 1 to 2 nondiarrheal stools daily. She is sent for laboratory studies that are significant for hemoglobin 6.2 g/dL, mean corpuscular volume 65 fL, and albumin 2.1 g/dL. Both white blood cell count and differential are within normal limits for age. A stool guaiac test for blood is negative.

Of the following, which is the *most* likely diagnosis?

a. Cow's milk protein–induced proctocolitis

b. Iron-deficiency anemia and protein-losing enteropathy

c. Food protein–induced enterocolitis syndrome (FPIES)

d. Eosinophilic gastroenteritis

e. Early-onset Crohn disease

21-41. A 3-week-old male infant presents due to several episodes of painless hematochezia. The stool is described as liquid mixed with mucus and flecks of blood. The infant has otherwise been feeding and growing well. He is primarily breastfed. Physical examination, including perirectal examination, is normal. Family history is notable for several family members with asthma and eczema, and an older brother with peanut and tree nut allergy. Of the following, which is the *best* initial step in the diagnosis and management of this condition?

a. Maternal dietary restriction of peanuts and tree nuts.

b. Switch to a soy-based formula.

c. Obtain hemoglobin level and submit stool sample for bacterial culture.

d. Referral for flexible sigmoidoscopy.

e. Switch to a cow's milk protein hydrolysate formula.

21-42. A 4-week-old male infant presents with a mass in the right inguinal region, just superior to the scrotum. His past medical history is significant for premature delivery at 31 weeks' gestation. His mother reports that the mass appears most visible when the patient is crying, while at other times, it is not very noticeable. The patient does not have any symptoms of irritability or pain, and has been tolerating feeds well. On examination, a smooth, firm mass is palpable in the right inguinal area. The mass reduces spontaneously when the infant stops crying. Both testes are descended and the overlying skin appears normal.

Of the following, which is the best *next* step in the evaluation and management of this condition?

a. Admission to the hospital for urgent repair of an incarcerated inguinal hernia

b. Referral to a pediatric surgeon for elective inguinal hernia repair within the next month

c. Referral to a pediatric surgeon for elective inguinal hernia repair, only if the hernia persists beyond 1 year of age

d. Referral to the emergency department for an urgent ultrasound for suspected testicular torsion

e. Referral to interventional radiology for diagnostic aspiration of the groin mass

21-43. Which of the following conditions or complications is *more* likely to be associated with an infant born with gastroschisis than with an infant with omphalocele?

a. Intestinal dysmotility

b. Beckwith-Weidemann syndrome (BWS)

c. Congenital heart defect

d. Trisomy 21

e. Intestinal malrotation

21-44. A preterm infant born with gastroschisis undergoes primary fascial and skin closure at approximately 24 hours of life. At 12 hours postoperatively, the neonatal intensive care unit nurse first notes increasing abdominal distension. An hour later, there is loss of urine output and decreased pedal pulses. A capillary blood gas is significant for an elevated carbon dioxide level. Of the following, which is the *best* option for the management of this patient?

a. Placement of a nasogastric tube to low intermittent wall suction for gastric decompression

b. Initiation of intravenous antibiotics for empiric coverage of suspected gram-negative bacterial sepsis

c. Prompt evisceration of the bowel and placement of a protective silo

d. Increased ventilator respiratory rate settings to maximize ventilation

e. Abdominal ultrasound with Doppler for evaluation of a vascular thrombus

21-45. An expectant mother undergoes a routine prenatal ultrasound and severe polyhydramnios is diagnosed. The differential diagnosis of polyhydramnios includes congenital anomalies such as esophageal atresia (EA).

Of the following types of EA, which is the most common?

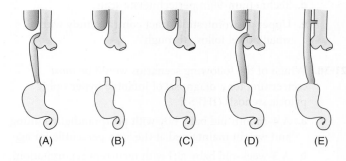

(A)   (B)   (C)   (D)   (E)

a. Proximal EA with distal tracheoesophageal fistula (TEF)

b. True EA without TEF

c. EA with proximal TEF

d. EA with proximal and distal TEF

e. Isolated TEF

21-46. A 7-year-old girl with a history of esophageal atresia and distal tracheoesophageal fistula repaired in infancy presents with progressive dysphagia for solid foods. She reports having a previous episode of food impaction while eating a hot dog. She has symptoms of heartburn and acid regurgitation approximately twice weekly. Her parents deny any history of chronic cough or recurrent respiratory tract infections. Of the following, which is the best *next* step in the management of this patient?

a. Maximization of the dosage of proton pump inhibitor medication for treatment of gastroesophageal reflux disease

b. Combined esophagoscopy and bronchoscopy to evaluate for recurrent tracheoesophageal fistula

c. Barium swallow examination to evaluate for anastomotic stricture formation

d. Trial of calcium channel blocker medication to help with lower esophageal sphincter relaxation

e. Providing reassurance, since underlying abnormal peristalsis of the lower esophageal segment is common in the natural history of esophageal atresia, even after surgical correction

21-47. A 5-week-old boy presents with symptoms of frequent regurgitation following feeds. His mother reports that he "spits up" 4 or 5 times per day. The volume of regurgitated milk varies, but it occurs effortlessly and the patient does not appear to be uncomfortable. He is exclusively breastfed and continues to nurse every 2 to 3 hours. Since regaining his birth weight at 2 weeks of age, he has exhibited appropriate weight gain for age. There is no history of bilious vomiting, abdominal distension, fever, diarrhea or bloody stools, or respiratory symptoms.

Of the following, which is the *best* option for management of this patient?

a. Obtain an upper gastrointestinal (UGI) contrast study.

b. Start patient on empiric proton pump inhibitor therapy.

c. Start a prokinetic agent to enhance gastric emptying.

d. Switch to a high-calorie formula to compensate for the loss of calories from frequent regurgitation.

e. Provide parental reassurance and education.

21-48. A 15-year-old boy with a history of asthma presents with symptoms of dysphagia, especially with solid foods. He has experienced food impactions that resolved spontaneously on 2 separate occasions. An upper gastrointestinal contrast study is obtained and is normal. He is started on twice-daily proton pump inhibitor therapy for 6 weeks. Due to continued symptoms of dysphagia, he then undergoes esophagogastroduodenoscopy that reveals linear furrowing and small, white adherent plaques throughout the entire esophagus. Biopsies from the proximal and distal esophagus show increased eosinophils (>15 eosinophils/high-powered field) in superficial clusters near the epithelium.

Of the following, which is the *best* option for treatment of this condition?

a. Pneumatic balloon dilation of the lower esophageal sphincter

b. Referral for allergy testing to identify likely allergic triggers

c. Addition of histamine-2-receptor blocker medication to current proton pump inhibitor therapy

d. A 2-week course of oral fluconazole

e. A 2-week course or oral acyclovir

21-49. A 2-year-old girl presents to the emergency department after a witnessed ingestion of a bottle containing liquid oven cleaner. At approximately 1 hour after the time of ingestion, the patient appears irritable, but in no acute distress. She is breathing comfortably. There are no visible oral lesions and the patient is not drooling, but currently refuses to drink. Of the following, which is the *best* option for managing this patient?

a. Administration of an emetic agent.

b. Placement of a nasogastric tube for decompression.

c. Immediate endoscopic evaluation to assess extent of injury.

d. Admit for observation and intravenous hydration.

e. No further treatment is necessary since stomach acid will neutralize the alkali.

21-50. Which of the following scenarios is most suspicious for a diagnosis of achalasia?

a. A 17-year-old girl with symptoms of dysphagia and chest pain, dilated esophagus with distal narrowing on barium swallow, and a nonrelaxing lower esophageal sphincter with complete lack of esophageal peristalsis on esophageal manometry

b. A 15-year-old boy with episodic chest pain, normal barium swallow, and evidence of nonperistaltic, prolonged, high-amplitude contractions on esophageal manometry

c. A 16-year-old girl with dysphagia, Raynaud phenomenon, normal barium swallow, and abnormally low-amplitude peristaltic contractions and hypotensive lower esophageal sphincter on esophageal manometry

d. A 10-year-old boy with symptoms of chest pain and heartburn, normal barium swallow, and normal peristalsis on esophageal manometry

e. A 9-month-old girl with gagging and choking on solid consistency foods and evidence of a short, circumferential narrowing at the level of the cervical esophagus

21-51. Which of the following statements regarding congenital imperforate anus is correct?

a. Congenital anorectal anomalies usually occur in isolation and are not associated with increased incidence of other lesions.

b. Children with "high" anorectal defects are more likely to successfully achieve continence than those with "low" lesions.

c. The most common congenital anomaly of the anorectum in males is an imperforate anus with a fistula between the distal anorectum and the urethra.

d. All patients with anorectal malformations require a staged repair, including placement of a temporary diverting colostomy.

e. Long-term problems with fecal incontinence or constipation are rare.

21-52. A 6-month-old girl presents with a history of episodic back arching and rigid posturing, mainly involving the neck, back, and upper extremities. These episodes are generally brief, lasting only 1 to 2 minutes, but occur on a daily basis, usually after feeding. On occasion, the patient's parents have observed visible regurgitation into the mouth during an episode. The patient usually cries after the episode, but does not appear to be sleepy or lethargic after the episode. Of the following, which diagnostic test would be best in identifying the cause of these abnormal movements?

a. Electroencephalogram

b. Upper gastrointestinal radiography

c. Upper endoscopy with biopsy of the esophagus

d. Nuclear scintigraphy

e. 24-Hour esophageal pH–impedance monitoring

21-53. A 3-year-old female presents to your office secondary to vomiting. You had seen her in your office 3 weeks ago for mononucleosis. Mom reports that since her illness she has not had much of an appetite. She will often vomit in the evening and mom has noticed that the emesis included food she had eaten from breakfast earlier in the day. She has not lost any weight. You suspect she has developed a postinfectious gastroparesis related to her recent infection with the Epstein-Barr virus. You confirm this diagnosis with a scintigraphic gastric emptying study.

Your first treatment approach would include which of the following?

a. Recommend small, high-fat meals to make sure she meets her caloric needs.

b. Refer to gastroenterology for endoscopic pyloric Botox injections.

c. Recommend small, frequent liquid meals low in fat to aid in transit.

d. Initiate a trial of domperidone, a promotility agent.

e. Initiate nasojejunal feeds until the gastric emptying improves.

21-54. A 7-day-old male with trisomy 21 presents to your office for his first hospital follow-up and weight check. Mom mentions to you that he passed meconium at 72 hours of life after rectal stimulation with a thermometer. He has not had another bowel movement and mom is concerned that his abdomen appears more distended. He has been spitting up after feeds. Your examination demonstrates a distended but soft abdomen with appropriate bowel sounds. Your rectal examination demonstrates a normally placed anus with a tight anal canal.

You are most concerned about which of the following conditions?

a. A duodenal web

b. Hirschsprung disease

c. Milk protein intolerance

d. Cystic fibrosis

e. Functional constipation

21-55. A 6-week-old former 29-week premature infant presents to your office with feeding intolerance. She was discharged last week from the hospital and is establishing care with your practice. She had a relatively uncomplicated neonatal course with the exception of some feeding intolerance that included large-volume vomiting when fed via nasogastric bolus feeds. Prior to discharge she was transitioned to nasogastric drip feeds. Mom feels this is an inconvenience and asks if you can prescribe a medication to help her infant better tolerate the bolus feeds.

You discuss the possibility of starting erythromycin, to increase gastric emptying, but you are most concerned about which of the following potential adverse events?

a. Dumping syndrome

b. Duodenal web

c. Dystonic reaction

d. Tardive dyskinesia

e. Pyloric stenosis

21-56. A 3-year-old female presents to your office with bloody diarrhea. Her symptoms began with fever, abdominal pain, and diarrhea about 1 week ago. The stools subsequently became bloody and mom is concerned about her dehydrated and pale appearance. Her brother had similar symptoms; however, his condition resolved without complication. You decide to obtain a stool sample of culture and a complete blood count and chemistry. Her CBC shows a hemoglobin of 8.0 g/dL and platelets of 30,000 cells/L. Her creatinine is 2.8 mg/dL. Her stool culture remains pending. What do you advise mom to do next?

a. Have the patient drink plenty of fluids and repeat labs in 2 days after her hydration improves.

b. Monitor the patient closely as an outpatient until her infectious colitis resolves.

c. Prescribe a course of oral antibiotics to shorten the course of her infectious colitis.

d. Admit the patient to the hospital for supportive treatment of presumed hemolytic-uremic syndrome (HUS).

e. Admit the patient to the hospital for workup for ulcerative colitis given her protracted course of bloody diarrhea.

21-57. A 4-year-old female presents to your office with 2 weeks of intermittent abdominal pain. Her mother reports that the patient has been having occasional blood in her stool and 2 episodes of vomiting. The last 2 days she has noticed dark purple-blue lesions on her buttocks and thighs that seem to resemble bruises. Mom reports over that past 2 hours she has been having episodes of severe abdominal pain where she will draw her legs up and scream. She appears exhausted from the episodes. She had a bowel movement in your waiting room that was loose with more blood than mom has recently observed.

What is your next step in management?

a. Refer her to the local hospital to rule out intussusception.

b. Refer her to the local hospital to rule out malrotation with volvulus.

c. Start a course of oral steroids and have her return to clinic tomorrow to monitor progress.

d. Recommend ibuprofen treatment for abdominal pain and reassure the mother.

e. Send a stool culture to evaluate for an infectious colitis.

21-58. You round on a 12-hour-old male infant for his routine newborn examination. The maternal history is significant for a cystic lesion noted in the newborn's abdomen on a routine prenatal ultrasound at 20 weeks' gestation. It was reported to be consistent with a duplication cyst of the small bowel.

What is your recommendation to the family?

a. This is an incidental finding and given the benign nature no further action is warranted unless symptoms develop.

b. Surgical consultation is needed to evaluate for resection of the cyst given the increased risk of obstruction, intussusception, and bleeding.

c. The cyst will need to be monitored every 6 months via ultrasound to monitor for any changes.

d. Obtain a CT scan, as surgical intervention is only necessary if the cyst is involving other structures such as the urinary system or spine.

e. Obtain a biopsy of the cyst and surgically remove if there are concerning histologic features of malignancy.

21-59. A 4-year-old male presents to your office secondary to the presence of blood with stooling. You have been following him regularly for chronic constipation, but he

has not been taking his stool softener as recommended. He is otherwise healthy. Mom is concerned that there has been bright red blood found on the toilet paper when he stools for the past 2 days. His stools have been large, hard, and difficult to pass. On your examination, you see a small purple mass at the anal verge. It is not painful. The remainder of his rectal examination is normal.

What would you recommend?

a. Have him be seen by a surgeon for incision and evacuation of the hemorrhoid to prevent further bleeding.

b. Restart his stool softener, and titrate it to daily soft stools.

c. Refer him to gastroenterology to evaluate for chronic liver disease.

d. Make a referral to Child Protective Services for concern of sexual abuse.

e. Refer him to gastroenterology for colonoscopy to rule out other vascular lesions of the colon.

21-60. A mother brings her 1-year-old infant to your office secondary to a protrusion from his anus. This occurred 30 minutes ago after he passed a hard, large stool. On your examination, you see a red-purple, cylindrical mass from his anus.

Your next step is which of the following?

a. Ask mom to keep the area moist and proceed to the emergency room for reduction.

b. Inform mom that the prolapse will spontaneously reduce without further intervention.

c. Send the patient for an emergent surgical evaluation for surgical reduction.

d. Prescribe a stool softener to allow the prolapse to spontaneously reduce over the next few days.

e. Apply gentle pressure to the prolapsed mucosa to manually reduce.

21-61. A 2-year-old presents to your office with severe diaper rash. On examination, it appears bright red, well demarcated, and has impetiginous vesicles and honey-colored crusting.

What is the most appropriate treatment for this rash?

a. Oral penicillin

b. Topical nystatin

c. Topical antibiotics

d. Oral nystatin

e. Topical cholestyramine

21-62. A 9-month-old female with Down syndrome presents to your office for chronic vomiting. You obtain a plain film abdominal radiograph for further evaluation. You are able to view the film prior to the radiologist's interpretation and you see a "double bubble" in the region of the stomach and first portion of the small intestine (Figure 399-1).

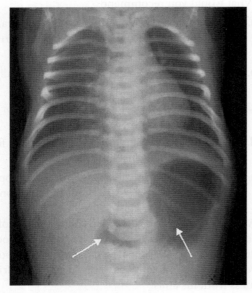

FIGURE 399-1. (Reproduced, with permission, from Rudolph CD, Rudolph AM, Lister GE, First LR, Gershon AA. *Rudolph's Pediatrics.* 22nd ed. New York: McGraw-Hill, 2011.)

This patient most likely has which diagnosis?

a. Pyloric stenosis

b. Hirschsprung disease

c. Annular pancreas

d. Antral web

e. Choledochal cyst

21-63. An 11-year-old male with a history of epilepsy controlled by valproic acid is admitted to your inpatient hospital service with epigastric abdominal pain and vomiting. His labs including a complete blood cell count, electrolytes, and liver function tests were unremarkable.

His serum lipase was 3 times the upper limits of normal. He had an abdominal ultrasound that showed an enlarged pancreas, but otherwise normal. He plays football but denies any recent abdominal trauma. He has had no other infectious symptomatology including fever and, other than his seizure disorder, is healthy.

What is the most likely etiology of the patient's acute pancreatitis?

a. Choledocholithiasis

b. Systemic disease

c. Viral induced

d. Medication induced

e. Remote blunt abdominal trauma

21-64. You get called to the bedside of a 6-hour-old infant secondary to abdominal distension. The infant had meconium aspiration at birth requiring endotracheal suctioning and bag mask ventilation. Over the course of the last few hours she has developed more abdominal distension and lethargy, and has fed poorly on 2 attempts. The patient has no respiratory distress and currently has normal blood pressure and heart rate. You obtain an abdominal radiograph and find a large pneumoperitoneum (Figure 400-2).

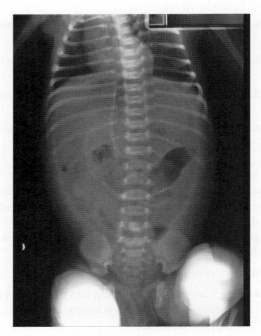

FIGURE 400-2. (Reproduced, with permission, from Rudolph CD, Rudolph AM, Lister GE, First LR, Gershon AA. *Rudolph's Pediatrics.* 22nd ed. New York: McGraw-Hill, 2011.)

What is your next step in management?

a. Transfer to the neonatal intensive care unit (NICU) for nasogastric decompression prior to refeeding.

b. Transfer to the NICU for nasogastric decompression and sepsis workup.

c. Transfer to the NICU for nasogastric decompression with a follow-up abdominal radiograph to evaluate for improvement.

d. Transfer to the NICU for nasogastric decompression, administration of antibiotics, and an operative evaluation and management.

e. Transfer to the NICU for nasogastric decompression and paracentesis.

21-65. A previously healthy 21-day-old male presents to the emergency department with lethargy, bilious vomiting, and abdominal distension that has developed over the morning. The upper gastrointestinal contrast study is shown (Figure 397-2A).

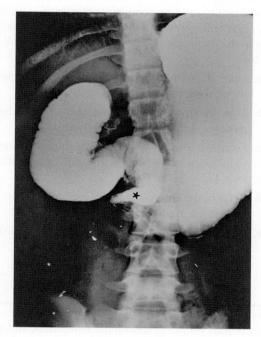

FIGURE 397-2A. (Reproduced, with permission, from Rudolph CD, Rudolph AM, Lister GE, First LR, Gershon AA. *Rudolph's Pediatrics.* 22nd ed. New York: McGraw-Hill, 2011.)

What is the most likely diagnosis?

a. Pyloric stenosis

b. Duodenal atresia

c. Jejunal atresia

d. Antral web

e. Malrotation with midgut volvulus

21-66. You are called by the newborn nursery nurse secondary to see a 1-day-old infant vomiting with every feed. The patient takes the formula well, but vomits large amounts soon after his feed. The emesis is nonbilious. The only significant history is polyhydramnios during his mother's pregnancy. You obtain an abdominal radiograph and find a large, dilated stomach.

What is the most likely diagnosis?

a. Pyloric stenosis

b. Duodenal web

c. Jejunoileal atresia

d. Pyloric atresia

e. Duodenal atresia

21-67. A neonate is diagnosed with colonic atresia soon after birth. What other congenital anomalies may also be associated with this condition?

a. Colonic aganglionosis, abdominal wall defects, and small bowel atresias

b. Colonic aganglionosis, hearing impairment, and skeletal abnormalities

c. Hearing impairment, ophthalmologic defects, and cardiac defects

d. Abdominal wall defects, cardiac defects, and asplenia

e. Hearing impairment, asplenia, and cardiac abnormalities

21-68. An 11-year-old presents to your office with fever and abdominal pain. Mom reports he was in his usual state of good health last night when he went to bed. He awoke at 3 AM with a fever of 101°F and periumbilical abdominal pain. He has associated symptoms of anorexia and 1 episode of nonbloody nonbilious vomiting. On your examination, he has pain in the right lower quadrant when you palpate either the right or the left lower abdomen. You obtain a complete blood count and find an elevated white blood cell count and mild bandemia.

What is your next step?

a. Obtain stool studies as the patient has likely developed an acute infectious gastroenteritis.

b. Refer him to the emergency department for concern of a small bowel obstruction.

c. Refer the patient to the emergency department to seek a surgical evaluation for appendicitis.

d. Discuss with mom that he likely has mesenteric adenitis given the right lower quadrant pain and ask him to return tomorrow for close monitoring.

e. Obtain an ultrasound of the gallbladder to evaluate for cholelithiasis and acute cholecystitis.

21-69. You admit a 3-year-old boy who has been passing large amounts of blood per rectum since last night. His hemoglobin in the emergency room was 6 g/dL. He has had no preceding symptoms (eg, no fever, vomiting, diarrhea, or abdominal pain).

What is the next most appropriate diagnostic step?

a. Technetium-99m pertechnetate scintigraphy scan

b. Magnetic resonance scan of the abdomen

c. Colonoscopy with biopsies

d. Esophagogastroduodenoscopy with biopsies

e. Stool studies for stool culture and *Clostridium difficile* toxin

21-70. A 4-year-old female presents to your office secondary to recurrent abdominal pain and drainage at her umbilicus. Mom reports that the patient will intermittently complain of abdominal pain. Around these episodes mom will notice some yellow discharge and crusting at her umbilicus and her pain appears to be relieved until the next episode. She does not have any fever. You confirm your suspicion of an omphalomesenteric sinus and cyst via a fistulogram.

What is your next step in treatment?

a. Long-term antibiotics to clear bacterial contamination of the sinus and cyst.

b. Recurrent excision and drainage of the cyst at the time of initial onset of abdominal pain.

c. Surgical excision of the omphalomesenteric sinus and cyst.

d. No further treatment is necessary given spontaneous drainage.

e. Suture placement at the opening of the fistula in the umbilicus to prevent further drainage.

21-71. A 3-year-old male presents to your office after his mother witnessed him swallowing a button battery earlier that morning.

He has normal vital signs. He is asymptomatic including no respiratory distress, no dysphagia, no drooling, and no complaints of pain. You obtain a chest radiograph and discover the button battery is in the esophagus. What is the next appropriate step?

a. Since given no symptomatology, provide mom reassurance that it will pass spontaneously.

b. Observe for symptoms and obtain a repeat chest radiograph weekly to verify progression.

c. Set up an urgent appointment with gastroenterology to have removal of the battery performed within the next 48 hours.

d. Refer to the emergency room now for urgent endoscopic removal.

e. Observe for symptoms and obtain repeat chest radiograph within 6 hours to verify passage.

ANSWERS

Answer 21-1. b

Breastfed infants absorb significantly more dietary lipid when compared with formula-fed infants because they ingest a unique breast milk lipase that assists in the majority (up to two thirds) of lipid hydrolysis.

Breastfed and formula-fed infants have comparable levels of lactase activity, which peaks at birth and then declines to about 25% of term levels by 1 year of age. Both breastfed and formula-fed newborn infants have relatively lower pancreatic lipase and bile salt secretion overall when compared with adults, with formula-fed infants malabsorbing 10% to 15% of dietary lipids. All infants have efficient protein digestion and absorption; there is no difference between breastfed and formula-fed infants. Both breastfed and formula-fed infants are able to absorb medium-chain fatty acids directly into the portal system, whereas long-chain fatty acids require transport proteins for absorption.

(Pages 1368-1369, Chapter 381: Normal Structure and Function of the Gastrointestinal System)

Answer 21-2. b

The typical patient with CVS presents with recurrent, stereotypic episodes of frequent emesis every 2 to 4 weeks that begin suddenly and last 24 to 48 hours. There is a return to periods of baseline health between episodes. The vomiting cannot be attributed to another disorder. A thorough history and physical examination is important, as specific conditions and symptoms suggest that the diagnosis is not consistent *with* CVS. These conditions are (1) presentation at less than 2 years of age; (2) bilious vomiting, abdominal tenderness, and/or severe abdominal pain; (3) attacks associated with intercurrent illness, fasting, and/or a high-protein meal; (4) abnormalities on neurologic examination; or (5) progressively worsening episodes or a conversion to a continuous or chronic pattern.

The patient in scenario A had nonbilious emesis that occurs after a period of fasting or a high-protein meal. These symptoms suggest a partial urea cycle enzyme deficiency, which can occur after such situations. The patient in scenario C has bilious emesis and abdominal pain. Although CVS can present with similar symptoms, it is important to rule out a surgical condition, such as volvulus or malrotation, as well as pancreatitis. In addition, this child does not have a 3-week cycle with a return to baseline. The patient in scenario D has neurologic symptoms, which is concerning for increased intracranial pressure or a metabolic disorder. The patient in scenario E has symptoms consistent with pyloric stenosis.

(Pages 1373-1375, Chapter 382: Approach to the Child With Acute, Chronic, or Cyclic Vomiting)

Answer 21-3. b

A child who presents with acute vomiting should first be evaluated for the degree of dehydration; if severe (5%-10%) dehydration is present, immediate intravenous access and fluids should be provided. However, this child is not severely dehydrated.

In addition, there is a high suspicion for CVS. If CVS is suspected in a child without other "alarm" symptoms such as severe dehydration, shock, abnormal neurologic examination, or severe abdominal pain, it is appropriate to check labs prior to initiation of intravenous fluids. Serum electrolytes can help assess for the possibility of a metabolic, renal, or endocrine disorder. They can also demonstrate abnormalities such as hypoglycemia or elevated BUN/creatinine that would assist in deciding on appropriate fluid resuscitation.

Abdominal radiograph may be useful in patients with suspected intestinal obstruction; head CT may be useful in patients with focal neurologic findings on examination suggesting increased intracranial pressure as a cause for vomiting. Intravenous proton pump inhibitors are unlikely to be helpful in the immediate treatment of acute recurrent nonbloody, nonbilious vomiting.

(Pages 1373-1375, Chapter 382: Approach to the Child With Acute, Chronic, or Cyclic Vomiting)

Answer 21-4. a

This patient has chronic recurrent vomiting, with at least 3 episodes of mild but frequent emesis over a 3-month period. Among the most frequent causes of vomiting in the school-age child and adolescent are gastroesophageal reflux disease, which may occur after meals and is not typically associated with weight loss. In a child with chronic vomiting without alarm symptoms or other concerning examination findings, the most likely diagnosis is an acid-peptic disorder such as gastroesophageal reflux disease or gastritis that should be initially treated with empiric 2- to 4-week trial of H_2-receptor antagonist or proton pump inhibitor for acid suppression.

If there is no symptomatic improvement after a time-limited trial of these medications, it may then be appropriate to proceed with laboratory testing, imaging, or consultation with pediatric gastroenterology. Odansetron may be useful for symptomatic improvement in the setting of acute, rather than chronic, vomiting.

(Pages 1372-1375, Chapter 382: Approach to the Child With Acute, Chronic, or Cyclic Vomiting)

Answer 21-5. d

Pain secondary to pancreatitis localized to the neck and shoulders occurs when the inflamed pancreas causes irritation of the diaphragm, which is in close proximity to the pancreas. Diaphragmatic irritation activates the visceral afferent nerves, which converge in the spinal cord with somatic afferent nerves, leading to well-localized somatic pain. This type of pain is commonly called referred pain.

The pancreas is not in direct contact with the pleural surface; however, pleural irritation due to pneumonia can cause poorly localized lower abdominal pain due to the convergence of pleural somatic afferent nerves with visceral afferent nerves converging in the spine. Parietal peritoneal irritation typically is well localized to the abdomen. There is no reason to believe this patient is a poor historian given that there is a reasonable physiologic explanation for the location of her pain.

(Page 1375, Chapter 383: Acute Abdominal Pain)

Answer 21-6. b

Several physical examination signs are associated with acute appendicitis. Choice B describes the obturator sign. When the maneuver is performed, the obturator internus muscle can irritate the appendix causing right lower quadrant pain. Other maneuvers associated with acute appendicitis include the Rovsing sign (left lower quadrant palpation to elicit right lower quadrant pain), as well as the iliopsoas sign (pain on passive extension of the right hip).

The tenderness from appendicitis eventually migrates to McBurney point (located two thirds of the way lateral on a line from the umbilicus to the anterior superior iliac spine) as peritoneal irritation increases. Abdominal ultrasound may demonstrate inflammation of the appendix and also support the diagnosis. Surgical consultation is appropriate if suspicion for acute appendicitis is high; however, it is appropriate to pursue complete examination and imaging first if possible to support the diagnosis.

Choice A describes Grey Turner sign, which is associated with retroperitoneal bleeding. Choice C describes Murphy sign, which is associated with acute cholecystitis. Choice D describes Kernig sign, which is associated with meningitis. Finally, choice E describes Homan sign, which is associated with venous thrombosis in the lower extremity.

(Page 1377, Chapter 383: Acute Abdominal Pain)

Answer 21-7. d

Up to 80% of children with functional abdominal pain have some form of anxiety; approximately 40% will have a depressive disorder.

Gender has not been shown to be a distinguishing factor for patient with functional versus organic abdominal pain. The examination technique known as the Carnett test, in which the examiner applies pressure to the point of maximal abdominal tenderness and then instructs the patient to assume a partial sitting position, may suggest an organic abdominal wall disorder rather than functional etiology if there is greater tenderness on palpation in partial sitting position compared with relaxed supine position. Antispasmodic medications, such as hyoscyamine, are commonly used in clinical practice to treat functional bowel disorders, but efficacy is controversial.

(Page 1378, Chapter 384: Chronic Abdominal Pain)

Answer 21-8. e

Abdominal pain that awakens a child from sleep and/or nocturnal diarrhea should raise the degree of suspicion for an organic etiology of the pain, such as inflammatory bowel disease, and warrant further investigation with laboratory testing and possibly imaging and/or endoscopy.

Children with functional pain frequently miss school due to their discomfort, and once the diagnosis of functional pain is certain, one of the physician's main goals should be to reinstate regular school attendance. Irritable bowel syndrome is one type of functional abdominal pain, and it is known that there is a high frequency of functional disorders among family members. Therefore, history of irritable bowel syndrome in a first-degree relative should support this patient's diagnosis of functional pain rather than refute it. One possible symptom of irritable bowel syndrome is the sensation of incomplete evacuation after passage of stool. Associated symptoms of headache, pallor, and/or fatigue are present in greater than 50% of patients with functional abdominal pain.

(Page 1378, Chapter 384: Chronic Abdominal Pain)

Answer 21-9. d

A stool culture should be performed in every child with bloody diarrhea because bacterial pathogens have been implicated in up to 20% of such cases. It is important to determine which bacterial pathogen is present, because infection with *Shigella* and cholera warrant antibiotic therapy, whereas antibiotic therapy for enterohemorrhagic *E. coli* may increase the risk of subsequently developing hemolytic-uremic syndrome and should be deferred. Stool cultures in children with nonbloody diarrhea are not necessary as they will be unlikely to alter the appropriate therapy.

Patients with acute diarrhea who are able to maintain adequate hydration with oral intake should be offered small, frequent volumes of oral rehydration therapy (ORT) solution; there is no contraindication to offering breast milk, formula, or solid feeds in addition to ORT while diarrhea is ongoing. Loperamide is an opiate antimotility agent that is not recommended for management of acute diarrhea in children because it may cause ileus, nausea, and sedation. Rotavirus is a common cause of watery diarrhea in the winter months but typically does not cause bloody diarrhea, and so is a less likely cause of this patient's diarrhea.

(Page 1383, Chapter 385: Diarrhea)

Answer 21-10. e

This patient most likely has chronic nonspecific diarrhea of childhood, also called toddler's diarrhea. She is well grown, has no other symptoms other than diarrhea, and has significant intake of apple juice daily, which has a high fructose-to-glucose ratio and is often implicated in toddler's diarrhea. Toddler's diarrhea is thought to be caused by mild carbohydrate malabsorption and hypermotility; a reasonable first step in treatment of suspected toddler's diarrhea is elimination of juice from the diet with reevaluation.

Determination of stool electrolytes and osmolality can be helpful in distinguishing between osmotic and secretory diarrhea. Stool pH and reducing substances may help in screening for malabsorptive causes of diarrhea. Stool cultures may help identify infectious causes of chronic diarrhea such as protozoal or bacterial infection. However, in an otherwise healthy, well-grown child who has a history consistent with toddler's diarrhea, empiric elimination of juice from the diet is a more reasonable first step in management rather than pursuing laboratory evaluation for less likely causes. Although

lactose intolerance/lactase deficiency may be another cause of chronic diarrhea in childhood, excessive juice intake is more likely and should be pursued as a cause prior to trying a lactose-free diet.

(Page 1385, Chapter 385: Diarrhea)

Answer 21-11. d

It is important to distinguish between the common problem of functional constipation and less common organic causes of constipation, including Hirschsprung disease. A diagnosis of Hirschsprung disease is suggested by small-caliber soft stool, episodes of explosive soft stool preceded by a lack of stool passage and abdominal distension, and history of delayed meconium passage in the first few days of life. If Hirschsprung disease is suspected, suction rectal biopsy should be considered as the next step in evaluation.

Children with functional constipation may have fecal incontinence (encopresis) with soiling of the undergarments due to seepage of liquid stool around impacted rectal fecal mass. Urinary tract infections may also occur due to partial urethral obstruction by pressure from fecal mass in the colon or by ascending infection from soiled undergarments. Many children with functional constipation have a history of large-caliber stools and stool retentive posturing in an attempt to avoid uncomfortable passage of large and/or hard stools.

(Pages 1387-1388, Chapter 386: Constipation and Fecal Incontinence)

Answer 21-12. d

Breastfed infants often pass stools infrequently, up to every 5 days, which may be completely normal if the stool is soft and passage is not painful. It is not unusual for an infant to strain briefly with stooling but this does not necessarily reflect pain. This child is not constipated and no specific intervention is required; reassurance should be offered to the mother.

An infant younger than 6 months who is having hard, infrequent stools may be constipated and can be offered 2 to 4 oz diluted fruit juice initially as treatment. In infants over 6 months of age, lactulose or polyethylene glycol 400 can also be used to treat constipation. There is no reason to believe this otherwise healthy child with no constipation has Hirschsprung disease, so imaging with barium enema is not warranted. Colic is a behavioral diagnosis characterized by frequent inconsolable crying in infants that has not been correlated with a specific gastrointestinal etiology.

(Page 1386, Chapter 386: Constipation and Fecal Incontinence)

Answer 21-13. b

This child is having acute lower gastrointestinal bleeding and is tachycardic and hypotensive, indicative of hemodynamic instability. The most appropriate initial intervention is rapid intravascular volume expansion with crystalloid solution such as normal saline, followed by replacement of blood.

Although it is important to obtain this patient's complete medical history at some point to try to determine what the source of the gastrointestinal bleeding may be, it is more important to stabilize the patient with fluid resuscitation as soon as possible. Performing endoscopy or proceeding with surgical exploration prior to obtaining venous access and addressing this patient's hemodynamic instability initially would be dangerous; once the patient is stabilized, it is more appropriate to consider surgical exploration for lower GI bleeding. Angiography is an imaging study that is sensitive with hemorrhage of at least 0.5 mL/min and may also allow embolization of vascular lesions by interventional radiologists; however, it would be unsafe to send this hemodynamically unstable patient for imaging initially.

(Page 1390, Chapter 387: Upper and Lower Gastrointestinal Bleeding)

Answer 21-14. a

Painless lower gastrointestinal bleeding in an infant may be caused by Meckel diverticulum, intestinal duplication, or lymphonodular hyperplasia. Other causes of lower gastrointestinal bleeding in infants who typically present with apparent abdominal pain include infectious colitis, malrotation with volvulus, anal fissure, and intussusception.

(Page 1390, Chapter 387: Upper and Lower Gastrointestinal Bleeding)

Answer 21-15. d

Over 50% of abdominal masses detected by physical examination of infants or children are actually cases of organomegaly. Among neonates, the most common cause of flank mass is an enlarged kidney due to hydronephrosis or multicystic dysplastic kidney. Among neonates, hydronephrosis and multicystic dysplastic kidney occur in equal frequency and comprise 75% of abdominal masses.

Constipation would be unusual in a neonate but is a common cause of palpable abdominal mass in children. Neuroblastoma and hepatomegaly are other possible causes of palpable neonatal abdominal mass that are less common. Sacrococcygeal teratoma is the most common abdominal neoplasm in neonates, but is not the most common cause of abdominal mass in neonates.

(Page 1391, Chapter 388: Abdominal Masses)

Answer 21-16. d

Pelvic masses in females should prompt vaginal examination and initial imaging with ultrasound. If a mass is solid or mixed consistency, prompt surgical consultation should be obtained, as ovarian masses in children are neoplastic 64% of the time, with the differential diagnosis including both germ cell and epithelial tumors.

It is not appropriate to monitor this mass with serial ultrasounds. Simple ovarian cysts in children under 1 year

of age may be monitored with ultrasound every 3 months; if there is failure of regression by 6 months of age, or complex or necrotic cysts, surgical referral should be made. Patients with pelvic mass secondary to ovarian torsion typically have severe pain and warrant prompt surgical referral, but torsion would not appear as a solid painless ovarian mass on ultrasound as in this case.

(Page 1393, Chapter 388: Abdominal Masses)

Answer 21-17. e

This infant most likely has volvulus with intestinal malrotation, which most commonly presents in the first week of life but can occur at any age. An infant with volvulus typically has progressive bilious emesis and pain out of proportion to the examination without initial abdominal distension; if the volvulus is not detected and addressed, the patient may later develop abdominal distension and hemodynamic instability. In this hemodynamically stable infant with suspected volvulus, an emergent upper GI contrast study should be obtained and is diagnostic if malrotation with volvulus is present.

Abdominal ultrasound is diagnostic for hypertrophic pyloric stenosis. Plain abdominal film can help diagnose various causes of neonatal intestinal obstruction, including necrotizing enterocolitis, meconium ileus, congenital duodenal obstruction, or distal intestinal obstruction. Contrast enema can help diagnose intussusception, Hirschsprung disease, or intestinal stricture. CT scan is rarely useful in initial diagnosis of causes of neonatal intestinal obstruction and will expose the infant to harmful ionizing radiation.

(Page 1395, Chapter 389: Gastrointestinal Obstruction)

Answer 21-18. e

A newborn with early feeding intolerance in which the examiner cannot pass a nasogastric tube is suggestive of esophageal atresia. Neonates with gastrointestinal obstruction due to esophageal atresia or anorectal malformations may have these anomalies as part of VACTERL syndrome, which is characterized by multiple associated congenital anomalies that can affect the vertebrae, anus, heart, trachea, esophagus, and/or limbs.

Children with trisomy 21 are more likely to have intestinal obstruction due to Hirschsprung disease or congenital duodenal obstruction. Premature or very-low-birth-weight infants are at risk for developing necrotizing enterocolitis. Cystic fibrosis is associated with intestinal obstruction due to meconium ileus.

(Page 1394, Chapter 389: Gastrointestinal Obstruction)

Answer 21-19. d

Fecal α_1-antitrypsin excretion in the stool has largely replaced radioisotopic techniques for diagnosis and evaluation of protein-losing enteropathy.

Among the many advantages of this assay are that it remains reliable even if the sample is contaminated with urine and it is stable at room temperature. One disadvantage of the assay is that α_1-antitrypsin is digested in gastric juice, so the reliability of fecal α_1-antitrypsin in detecting esophageal or gastric protein loss is questionable. In addition, meconium contains large amounts of α_1-antitrypsin. As a result, the test is not valid until after 1 week of age.

(Page 1397, Chapter 390: Protein-losing Enteropathy)

Answer 21-20. a

Fifty percent to 60% of children with Crohn disease have mild to pronounced hypoalbuminemia.

Elevated blood urea nitrogen, hyperbilirubinemia, and hypophosphatemia are not associated with Crohn disease. MCV may be low in patients with Crohn disease, as a microcytic anemia may be present due to chronic gastrointestinal blood loss with associated iron deficiency.

(Page 1397, Chapter 390: Protein-losing Enteropathy)

Answer 21-21. d

Brunner glands are found in the submucosal layer of the duodenum only, and secrete bicarbonate to neutralize acidic gastric contents as they enter into the small intestine. In patients lacking Brunner glands (like this patient, who has had a duodenal resection), acidic gastric contents are not properly neutralized prior to entering the remaining small intestine and may precipitate osmotic fluid shift into the intestine, leading to postprandial diarrhea known as dumping syndrome.

Enterochromaffin cells are specialized hormone-secreting cells that are found in the gastric antrum. Peyer patches are a type of lymphoid aggregate that appear in high numbers in the ileum. Throughout the small intestine, crypts of Lieberkuhn appear at the bases of villi and house epithelial stem cells. Chief cells, also called oxyntic cells, secrete pepsinogen and are located mainly in the gastric body.

(Pages 1365-1366, Chapter 381: Normal Structure and Function of the Gastrointestinal System)

Answer 21-22. d

Based on the history and physical examination, this child most likely has celiac disease, an immune-mediated enteropathy secondary to ingestion of gluten. Serologic screening with anti-TTG antibody test is highly sensitive and specific for celiac disease and would be the appropriate lab test to order. This patient's history of Down syndrome places him in a high-risk group for development of celiac disease. Other conditions associated with celiac disease include other autoimmune conditions, type 1 diabetes, Turner syndrome, and Williams syndrome.

The anti–endomysium antibody (EMA) test is also used routinely for screening for celiac disease. A serum IgA level is recommended at the time of testing to identify those who are IgA deficient, and who would need IgG-based tests for EMA or TTG.

Celiac disease can present in early or late childhood, adolescence, or even adulthood. Gastrointestinal symptoms such as diarrhea, abdominal pain, distension, and bloating are common in the initial presentation of celiac disease. Nongastrointestinal manifestations include decrease in linear growth velocity, delayed onset of puberty, dermatitis herpetiformis rash (see Figure 408-1), and dental enamel hypoplasia.

Histopathologic evidence of celiac disease in the small intestine, such as increased intraepithelial lymphocytes and villous blunting (Figure 408-4), is needed to definitively confirm the diagnosis of celiac disease. An EGD to perform small intestinal biopsy, however, is usually recommended only after screening tests such as TTG and EMA are found to be positive. Although the presence of genetic markers HLA-DQ2 and/or DQ8 is strongly associated with celiac disease, they are also found in 30% of the general population. Therefore, HLA-DQ2/DQ8 testing is usually not useful in the initial screening evaluation for celiac disease. Given this patient's presentation of chronic diarrhea (symptoms lasting longer than 2 weeks), it is unlikely he has an acute viral gastroenteritis, such as rotavirus infection. A sweat chloride test can be obtained in the evaluation of suspected cystic fibrosis, which can also present with poor growth in early childhood, but is usually characterized by steatorrhea, or fatty foul-smelling stools, as well as pulmonary manifestations.

(Section 21: Disorders of the Gastrointestinal System, Chapter 408: Disorders of Digestion and Absorption)

Answer 21-23. c

SIBO is characterized by an increased number and/or type of bacteria in the upper gastrointestinal tract. One of the primary mechanisms believed to result in the development of gastrointestinal symptoms such as excessive gas or abdominal distension is metabolism of ingested carbohydrates by intraluminal bacteria. Other processes related to the overgrowth of intestinal bacteria include deconjugation of bile acids leading to secretory diarrhea, fat malabsorption, and direct mucosal injury. The gold standard for diagnosis of bacterial overgrowth is quantitative culture from a jejunal aspirate. A bacterial concentration greater than 10^5 organisms/mL fluid is considered diagnostic. A bacterial count of 1000 organisms/mL is considered within normal for the small intestine. A practical alternative to jejunal culture is breath hydrogen analysis. When a patient ingests a test dose of carbohydrate, such as glucose or lactulose, there is an early peak in breath hydrogen level, which corresponds to early metabolism of the carbohydrate by intestinal bacteria. Empiric treatment of SIBO when the index of suspicion is high has been advocated. Antibiotics, such as metronidazole, amoxicillin–clavulanic acid, and trimethoprim–sulfamethoxazole, are the mainstay of therapy. Acid blockade, which results in hypochlorhydria in the stomach, has been associated with increased bacterial counts in the stomach.

(Section 21: Disorders of the Gastrointestinal System, Chapter 408: Disorders of Digestion and Absorption)

Answer 21-24. d

Complications associated with short bowel syndrome (SBS) in children are commonly associated with the use of a central venous catheter as well as TPN. Central line infections are among the most frequent and serious complications. The rate of infection is approximately between 1 and 6 infections per 1000 days of parental nutrition, and varies with the indication for intravenous nutrition. Patients who present with fever, jaundice, and lethargy, such as the infant in the vignette, should be evaluated carefully and blood and site cultures obtained. In those with suspected catheter-related infections, empiric antibiotic therapy should be initiated to treat coagulase-negative staphylococci, the most common cause of infections, as well as gram-negative enteric organisms. Because there are limited sites available for placement of central catheters, potential line infections are treated aggressively. However, in some patients who have fungal infection, endocarditis, or persistent positive blood cultures or signs of infection, the central venous catheter must be removed. Thrombotic and thromboembolic catheter problems can also occur. Chronic use of parental nutrition can lead to cholestasis and hepatocellular injury that can develop into chronic liver disease and liver failure. Cholelithiasis occurs in 10% to 40% of children receiving parental nutrition and is thought to result from stasis and biochemical imbalance in the composition of bile. Jaundice and abdominal pain may occur, but fever and lethargy are unlikely. In some children, cholelithiasis is an incidental finding without symptoms. Cholestasis and bile duct proliferation can often occur in those receiving TPN for more than 2 weeks, but life-threatening hepatic cirrhosis rarely presents acute fulminant hepatic failure. Elevation of serum transminase and alkaline phosphatase activities without jaundice can result from fatty infiltration of the liver as a result of excessive calories. D-Lactic acidosis is another potential complication related to SBS, characterized by recurrent episodes of lethargy and ataxia and metabolic acidosis. In this condition, carbohydrates are metabolized by bacterial overgrowth in the colon into D-lactic acid, which then results in recurrent episodes of encephalopathy. Patients usually do not have acute fever.

(Section 21: Disorders of the Gastrointestinal System, Chapter 408: Disorders of Digestion and Absorption)

Answer 21-25. e

Given the young age of onset of chronic diarrhea with evidence of villous atrophy on small intestinal biopsy, this clinical scenario is highly suspicious for a congenital enteropathy, such as microvillus inclusion disease. Congenital microvillus inclusion disease is characterized by watery, secretory diarrhea, usually with onset in the first days after birth. Histologically, the small intestine demonstrates diffuse villous atrophy, while electron microscopy reveals mucosal surface enterocytes that lack microvilli altogether or show involutions of the apical membrane containing microvilli.

Other conditions that present with early-onset severe diarrhea and evidence of villous atrophy include tufting enteropathy and IPEX syndrome (immune dysregulation, polyendocrinopathy, enteropathy, and x-linkage). Villous atrophy on histologic examination is a nonspecific finding. Although villous atrophy is also classically found in celiac disease, the young age of the patient and lack of exposure to gluten protein in the diet makes celiac disease unlikely to be the diagnosis. Patients with cystic fibrosis can present with chronic diarrhea secondary to pancreatic insufficiency, but this patient has had a normal result on sweat chloride testing. Both congenital chloride diarrhea and congenital sodium diarrhea are caused by defects in intestinal transport of electrolytes. They are characterized by large-volume watery stools at the time of birth, which persistent even when the infant is given nothing via the enteral route. Both conditions can result in severe dehydration, but congenital chloride diarrhea is associated with metabolic alkalosis, while congenital sodium diarrhea is associated with development of metabolic acidosis. Acrodermatitis enteropathica is an autosomal recessive disorder of zinc absorption. Symptoms of zinc deficiency develop in infancy after discontinuation of breast-feeding. Clinical manifestations include dermatitis with bullous and pustular lesions (typically distributed around the mouth), alopecia, diarrhea, and growth retardation. The infant in this clinical vignette is still being breastfed and does not have the characteristic skin findings, which makes acrodermatitis enteropathica unlikely.

(Section 21: Disorders of the Gastrointestinal System, Chapter 408: Disorders of Digestion and Absorption)

Answer 21-26. b

Acute and chronic ingestion of NSAIDs has been associated with gastritis and mucosal ulceration that can result in upper gastrointestinal blood loss. The toxic consequences of NSAID use are the result of both direct topical injury and systemic effects, resulting in an imbalance of the gastric mucosal aggressive and protective mechanisms (Figure 409-1). As potent inhibitors of prostaglandin synthesis, NSAIDs decrease mucosal bicarbonate and mucus production, reduce mucosal blood flow, interfere with neutrophil adherence, and inhibit gastric acid production. Enterohepatic recirculation of NSAIDs also may be important in the development of mucosal injury. The effects of NSAIDs on platelet aggregation further potentiate bleeding and may interfere with the normal healing process of the upper gastrointestinal tract.

There appears to be no relationship between the development of NSAID-induced ulceration and infection with *H. pylori*, so administration of an antibiotic against this pathogen would not be helpful. Aspirin is as toxic as NSAIDs in promoting gastroduodenal inflammation, so substitution of salicylate would not be appropriate. Dyspeptic symptoms are quite common in patients receiving NSAID therapy. However, there are no clinical indicators to differentiate patients who only have dyspepsia from those who have ulcerations. Indeed, patients who have NSAID-associated ulcers are less likely to be symptomatic than patients who have ulcers and have not received NSAID therapy.

Given the efficacy of pharmacologic therapy for peptic ulcer disease, there is little reason to rely on dietary modification as the primary intervention in such patients. A proton pump inhibitor that affords greater suppression of gastric acid—in comparison to an H_2 blocker—may be more effective in healing gastric ulcers in patients who must continue NSAIDs. Sucralfate is a mucosal protective agent that is effective in the treatment of gastric ulcers, but does not appear to be particularly effective in healing ulcers when the NSAID is continued. The extremely low incidence of gastric malignancy in the pediatric population obviates the need for endoscopy in the initial management of a child suspected of having a gastric ulcer. Endoscopic evaluation of the stomach is reserved for those who fail to respond to an initial course of acid suppression. If endoscopy is performed, assessment for the presence of *H. pylori* should be undertaken.

(Section 21: Disorders of the Gastrointestinal System, Chapter 409: Inflammatory Disorders of the Stomach)

Answer 21-27. c

H. pylori is an S-shaped, flagellated, gram-negative rod that colonizes the mucus layer of the stomach and produces urea. The organism's production of urease contributes to its ability to survive in the hostile gastric environment and to penetrate the mucosa of the gastric enterocyte. The pathogenesis of *H. pylori* infection remains unclear, but it is likely to include direct penetration through the mucus layer that disrupts the gastric enterocyte and permits back-diffusion of gastric acid. Almost all individuals infected with *H. pylori* have some degree of gastritis, but the degree of inflammation and association with complications such as peptic ulcer disease are variable. The most prevalent pattern of gastritis in children in the Western world is an antral-predominant gastritis, with little or no involvement of the body of the stomach. Recent studies have shown an association between long-term infection with *H. pylori* and the development of gastric cancer as well as lymphoma arising from mucosa-associated lymphoid tissue (MALT). The incidence of gastric malignancy in the pediatric population, however, is extremely low.

The presence of *H. pylori* should be confirmed prior to starting antibiotic therapy. Testing should be reserved for children and adolescents who are most likely to benefit from treatment, such as those with suspected peptic ulcer disease. Noninvasive testing includes urea breath testing and stool antigen testing. Urea breath testing relies on the ability of urease from *H. pylori* to split C13- or C14-labeled urea into isotope-labeled carbon dioxide. The breath is sampled for labeled carbon dioxide using gas chromatography. Urease breath testing is not yet widely available in all areas for children. A reasonable alternative to urea breath testing is monoclonal stool antigen testing. Antibody testing using blood, serum, or saliva is not recommended in children for clinical use. Antibody tests can remain positive for years after eradication or resolution of infection. A positive antibody test therefore does not indicate the presence of an active infection with *H. pylori*. Endoscopy with biopsies provides the most accurate approach for definitive diagnosis of *H. pylori* infection, as well as gastritis and peptic ulcer disease, but is invasive. Biopsies of the gastric mucosa (not gastric fluid) can be cultured, stained, and assessed for urease activity. Culture and sensitivity analysis of *H. pylori* can be helpful in refractory cases where antibiotic resistance is suspected. The presence of spiral organisms on the surface of the gastric mucosa or within the mucus layer confirms the diagnosis of *H. pylori*. It is important to note that results of biopsy staining, urease detection, and culture as well as urea breath testing can be affected by prior use of antibiotics, bismuth subsalicylate, H_2-receptor antagonists, antacids, and topical anesthetic agents.

(Section 21: Disorders of the Gastrointestinal System, Chapter 409: Inflammatory Disorders of the Stomach)

Answer 21-28. b

Approximately 10% to 20% of newborn infants with CF will present with meconium ileus. The mechanical intestinal obstruction is created by abnormally thick, viscous meconium that results from the relative deficiency of pancreatic proteinases in infants with CF. Patients can present with abdominal distension, feeding intolerance with or without bilious emesis, and failure to pass meconium. The intestinal obstruction associated with meconium ileus is typically located at the level of the terminal ileum. Plain abdominal radiographs are the initial diagnostic test of choice in the setting of most cases of suspected bowel obstruction. In infants with meconium ileus, the inspissated, thick meconium mixed with gas can have a "soap-bubble" or "ground-glass" appearance in the bowel loops, in addition to evidence of obstruction with proximally dilated loops of bowel. Retrograde contrast enema may be therapeutic as well as diagnostic, showing a patent, unused microcolon with evidence of obstructing meconium in the terminal ileum. Use of hyperosmolar contrast agents or mucolytic agents for the retrograde enema can help mobilize the impacted meconium with the goal of relieving the intestinal obstruction. In patients with persistent obstruction despite retrograde enemas, or those with intestinal perforation or pseudocyst formation, operative exploration may be necessary.

HD, or congenital aganglionic megacolon, can also present with features of intestinal obstruction in the neonatal period. Failure to pass meconium within the first 48 hours of life is a common feature. Evidence of a cone-shaped transition zone or caliber change in the rectosigmoid area on barium enema examination is highly suspicious for HD. In the very early newborn period, or in infants with total colonic involvement, however, a transition zone may be absent. In contrast to infants with meconium ileus, however, infants with HD will characteristically show significant amounts of retained barium on a 24-hour postevacuation film.

Infants with cow's milk protein allergy or intolerance are typically healthy in appearance, but present with blood-tinged stools. Infants with duodenal atresia, as well as other types of intestinal atresias, also commonly present with abdominal distension and vomiting within the first 48 hours of life. Affected infants may or may not pass meconium. There is often a prenatal history of polyhydramnios. Plain film radiography may reveal a "double-bubble" sign suggesting duodenal atresia, but an upper GI contrast study is usually necessary to make the diagnosis and establish the level of obstruction. Malformations of the anorectum, including anal stenosis, can present with abdominal distension and abnormal passage of meconium and stools early in life. These conditions are generally able to be diagnosed on physical examination. Anorectal malformations are often associated with other congenital malformations as well.

(Section 21: Disorders of the Gastrointestinal System, Chapter 403: Meconium Diseases of Infancy and Distal Intestinal Obstruction Syndrome)

Answer 21-29. e

Distal intestinal obstruction syndrome (DIOS), formerly known as "meconium ileus equivalent," is characterized by an acute complete or partial obstruction of the ileocecum by intestinal contents. By contrast, constipation in patients with CF is characterized by gradual onset of fecal impaction of the total colon. DIOS can occur at any age, but it is more common in older patients and those with pancreatic insufficiency. The most common manifestation of DIOS is crampy abdominal pain, which generally is located in the right lower quadrant. The onset of symptoms usually is acute, and the symptoms tend to become progressively severe over time. Other features include decreased or absent bowel movements, abdominal distension, weight loss, and poor appetite. On examination, a mass may be palpated in the right lower quadrant. Plain abdominal x-rays typically show stool in the distal ileum and proximal colon; signs of small bowel obstruction with air–fluid levels on upright films are also common. DIOS should be distinguished from chronic constipation, in which the onset of symptoms is more gradual and the stool is distributed more evenly throughout the colon. Patients with incomplete (impending) DIOS usually respond to oral rehydration and osmotic laxatives. Those with complete DIOS or signs of peritonitis may require surgery.

Initial management should be aimed at correcting fluid and electrolyte abnormalities. Once electrolyte abnormalities have been corrected, treatment should be aimed at removal of the inspissated plug. This can be attempted using a combination of enemas and laxatives until normal stooling patterns are established. Once the inspissated plug has been eliminated, it is important to initiate or optimize appropriate pancreatic enzyme replacement.

Traditional strategies aimed at treating constipation, such as increased fiber supplementation, rectal suppositories, or stimulant laxatives, may have some benefit, but they do not address the underlying pathophysiology of DIOS. Similarly, although fat-soluble vitamin deficiency is also associated with pancreatic insufficiency, treatment with fat-soluble vitamins will not likely reduce the risk of DIOS recurrence.

(Section 21: Disorders of the Gastrointestinal System, Chapter 403: Meconium Diseases of Infancy and Distal Intestinal Obstruction Syndrome)

Answer 21-30. b

Based on the constellation of symptoms of anorexia, loose stools, abdominal pain, weight loss, anemia, hypoalbuminemia, and occult blood in stools, and skin tags, the most likely diagnosis is Crohn disease. Presenting symptoms in pediatric Crohn disease include abdominal pain (62%-95%), diarrhea (66%-77%), weight loss (80%-92%), rectal bleeding (14%-60%), growth impairment (30%-33%), perirectal disease (25%), and extraintestinal manifestation (15%-25%). *Giardia* is unlikely given the hemoccult positive stools, lab abnormalities, and skin tags. While celiac can result in abdominal pain, anemia, hypoalbuminemia, diarrhea, and weight loss, it would be unusual to have hemoccult positive stools or skin tags. Anorexia nervosa is unlikely given the other clinical symptoms besides poor appetite and weight loss. Irritable bowel would not have skin tags, anemia, hypoalbuminemia, weight loss, or hemoccult positive stools.

(Section 21: Disorders of the Gastrointestinal System, Chapter 410: Inflammatory Bowel Disease)

Answer 21-31. a

Side effects of corticosteroids include bone demineralization, adrenal insufficiency, fluid retention, weight gain, striae, acne, fat redistribution, hirsutism, hypertension, hyperglycemia, cataracts, osteonecrosis, myopathy, emotional disturbances, and benign intracranial hypertension. Corticosteroids result in weight gain, not weight loss. They can also result in fat redistribution and muscle mass loss but not muscle redistribution. Corticosteroids can cause leucocytosis, not leucopenia. They do not cause vitamin D deficiency.

(Section 21: Disorders of the Gastrointestinal System, Chapter 410: Inflammatory Bowel Disease)

Answer 21-32. d

Salmonella, *Shigella*, *Campylobacter*, *Yersinia*, *E. coli 0157/H7*, and *C. difficile* can all cause bloody diarrhea and should be excluded before a diagnosis of inflammatory bowel disease can be made. *Giardia* and *Cryptosporidium* can cause chronic diarrhea; however, it is watery and not bloody diarrhea.

(Section 21: Disorders of the Gastrointestinal System, Chapter 410: Inflammatory Bowel Disease)

Answer 21-33. b

Peutz-Jeghers syndrome is associated with hamartomas of the small bowel, stomach, and colon. Another characteristic finding is blue-brown macules on the vermillion border of the lips and buccal mucosa. Tuberous sclerosis is associated with hypomelanotic macules of the skin, facial angiofibromas, shagreen patches, and fibrous facial plaques. Neurofibromatosis is associated with café au lait spots and freckling of the axilla and inguinal area. There are no unique skin findings for familial adenomatous polyposis syndrome or juvenile polyposis syndrome.

(Section 21: Disorders of the Gastrointestinal System, Chapter 414: Polyps and Tumors of the Gastrointestinal Tract. Hereditary Hamartomatous Polyposis Syndromes)

Answer 21-34. e

The patient should begin screening endoscopy by 12 years of age or sooner at the onset of symptoms such as hematochezia, diarrhea, or abdominal pain. If polyps are detected, then they should undergo yearly screening endoscopies. If the affected family members have been screened for an APC gene mutation and none was found, negative genetic testing does not rule out FAP in this patient. The timing of colectomy is determined on a case-by-case basis. It would not be considered in a patient without a diagnosis of FAP. The timing of colectomy is determined based on polyp burden, presence of increasing adenoma dysplasia or adenocarcinoma, and the maturity of the patient. Ten percent of patients with FAP have no identifiable APC gene mutation. Family members still require screening as negative testing does not exclude the possibility of them having FAP.

(Section 21: Disorders of the Gastrointestinal System, Chapter 414: Polyps and Tumors of the Gastrointestinal Tract. Hereditary Hamartomatous Polyposis Syndromes)

Answer 21-35. a

Juvenile polyps are a common gastrointestinal disorder. Up to 2% of children under the age of 10 years may have juvenile polyps. JPS is diagnosed when there are 5 or more colonic juvenile polyps, there is a presence of juvenile polyps in the stomach or small intestine, or there is a presence of any juvenile polyp with a family history of JPS.

This patient does not meet criteria for JPS; therefore, she is not at increased risk of cancer, nor does she or her family need to undergo yearly surveillance or genetic testing. Patients with JPS may have germline deletions in either *SMAD4* or *BMPR1A*. Once a patient is found to have 5 or more juvenile polyps, genetic testing may prove helpful when counseling family members of their risk. Findings of juvenile polyps do not increase the risk of colorectal cancer; however, 5 or more polyps suggestive of JPS increase your lifetime risk of colorectal cancer to close to 50%.

(Section 21: Disorders of the Gastrointestinal System, Chapter 414: Polyps and Tumors of the Gastrointestinal Tract. Hereditary Hamartomatous Polyposis Syndromes)

Answer 21-36. a

SMAS is characterized by gastrointestinal obstruction resulting from compression of the duodenum between the abdominal aorta posteriorly and the superior mesenteric artery anteriorly (Figure 406-1).

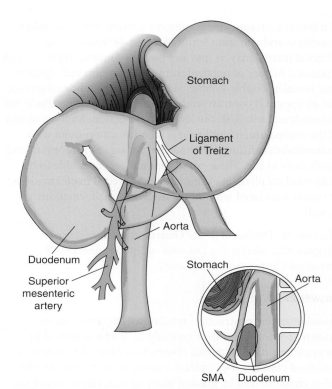

FIGURE 406-1. Anterior–posterior and lateral illustration of the anatomic location of the stomach and duodenum in relation to the aorta and the superior mesenteric artery (SMA). (Reproduced, with permission, from Rudolph CD, Rudolph AM, Lister GE, First LR, Gershon AA. *Rudolph's Pediatrics.* 22nd ed. New York: McGraw-Hill, 2011.)

SMAS is more common in females than in males and is associated with acute weight loss. Acute weight loss is thought to result in loss or reduction in size of the anterior mesenteric fat pad that contributes to the angle between the superior mesenteric artery and the aorta, which usually is between 45° and 60°. In individuals with SMAS, this angle can be significantly reduced. Symptoms of SMAS may be acute or chronic, and can include vomiting, nausea, anorexia, abdominal distension, abdominal pain, early satiety, and weight loss. The diagnosis of SMAS is commonly made by upper gastrointestinal contrast radiography that shows a dilation of the stomach and proximal duodenum, with abrupt cutoff or narrowing of the small bowel at the level of third vertebra just proximal to the ligament of Treitz. Retrograde peristalsis of contrast is sometimes observed in the proximal dilated segment of small bowel. The diagnosis can also be made by computerized tomography or at laparotomy. Treatment of SMAS is primarily aimed at bowel decompression, fluid stabilization, and nutritional support. Small, frequent meals may be helpful; in more severe cases, postpyloric feeds with a nasojejunal tube or parenteral nutrition may be necessary.

Crohn disease can also present with nonspecific symptoms of abdominal pain, anorexia, and weight loss as well. Development of a small bowel stenosis is possible, but is usually secondary to chronic inflammation and fibrosis.

The patient in this clinical vignette also lacks evidence of systemic inflammation, hypoalbuminemia, and symptoms of diarrhea, which would be more typical in the setting of chronic intestinal inflammation secondary to Crohn disease. Intestinal stenosis and atresia are relatively common congenital anomalies that can affect the duodenum. It would be highly unusual, however, to have a delayed presentation beyond the neonatal period without any other history of intestinal obstruction. Chronic pancreatitis can present with recurrent episodes of acute pancreatitis or with gradual onset of chronic abdominal pain. Radiographic findings, such as calcifications within the pancreas on plain film or computerized tomography, are suggestive of chronic pancreatitis. Obstruction of the duodenum, however, is not a commonly associated finding. Finally, celiac disease is also characterized by involvement of the duodenum resulting in symptoms of abdominal pain and weight loss; however, duodenal inflammation in celiac disease does not typically result in obstruction.

(Section 21: Disorders of the Gastrointestinal System, Chapter 406: Superior Mesenteric Artery Syndrome)

Answer 21-37. c

Intussusception is characterized by the telescoping of a segment of intestine (intussusceptum) into the lumen of the adjacent bowel (intussuscipiens).

Lymphatic and venous drainage can be compromised by the prolapse, leading to edema, ischemia, and ultimately necrosis of the involved intestine. Intussusception is the most common cause of intestinal obstruction in children under 2 years of age, with a peak incidence between 4 and 10 months, and with a male predominance (see Figure 404-2).

Intussusception is idiopathic in 90% of pediatric cases, with the vast majority of these cases being the ileocolic type. Only 10% of cases can be attributed to gross pathologic lead point, such as Meckel diverticulum (most common), intestinal polyp (eg, Peutz-Jegher syndrome), and tumor (lymphoma). Both hemolytic-uremic syndrome and Henoch-Schönlein purpura are vasculitic syndromes that can present with intussusceptions.

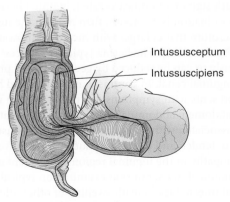

Intussusceptum
Intussuscipiens

FIGURE 404-2. Ileocolic intussusception. (Reproduced, with permission, from Ziegler M, Azizkhan R, Weber T, eds. *Operative Pediatric Surgery*. 3rd ed. New York: McGraw-Hill, 2003.)

The presenting signs and symptoms of intussusceptions include colicky abdominal pain, vomiting and bloody (currant jelly) stools, and an abdominal mass. Between episodes of pain, the child is usually comfortable. Lethargy may be the only presenting complaint in some young children. Initial abdominal examination usually reveals no tenderness, but a sausage-like mass may be present in the right upper quadrant or midabdomen. Stools may be normal or diarrhea-like in the beginning, but as ischemia progresses, they may become bloody.

In children suspected of having an intussusception, abdominal radiography may reveal an intestinal mass, evidence of small bowel obstruction, or intraperitoneal air when the bowel perforates. Radiographic findings can be normal, however, and do not rule out the presence of an intussusception. Abdominal ultrasonography can reveal a "target" sign with concentric layers of serosa and mucosa, but again a normal study does not exclude intussusceptions. Radiographic contrast enemas (air or hydrostatic) have the advantage of being diagnostic and potentially therapeutic. Air contrast enemas are safer than barium or gastrograffin enemas in the event of perforation and are generally more successful in reducing the intussusception. Failure to reduce the intussusceptions radiographically should result in surgical consultation and management.

Technetium pertechnetate radionuclide scans can identify Meckel diverticulum, but they have no role in the diagnosis or management of patients who have suspected intussusception. An upper gastrointestinal contrast study with small bowel follow-through may be helpful in the evaluation of suspected small bowel obstruction. In cases of suspected intussusceptions, however, they are not the first diagnostic test of choice.

(Section 21: Disorders of the Gastrointestinal System, Chapter 404: Intussusception)

Answer 21-38. d

IHPS is the most common surgical cause of nonbilious vomiting in infants. The pyloric muscle is not usually hypertrophied at birth, but appears to hypertrophy after birth, leading to gastric outlet obstruction. The typical age of presentation of IHPS is between 3 and 8 weeks old, with the incidence in males being 4 to 6 times higher than in females. Typical symptoms include postprandial, projectile, nonbilious vomiting. Despite the persistent vomiting, the infant often remains hungry and appears very eager to feed. In later stages or when the diagnosis is delayed, dehydration, weight loss, and development of a hypochloremic, hypokalemic alkalosis can result.

Symptoms of frequent gagging, choking, or coughing with feeds are concerning for possible aspiration. This is often associated with oral aversion and feeding refusal. A history of trisomy 21 and bilious emesis in early infancy should raise suspicions for duodenal atresia or stenosis. Finally, dehydration can occur in infants with severe vomiting and diarrhea secondary to a viral gastroenteritis. The dehydration usually leads to a metabolic acidosis, rather than alkalosis that is seen in IHPS secondary to loss of secreted hydrogen ion from the stomach.

(Section 21: Disorders of the Gastrointestinal System, Chapter 392: Infantile Hypertrophic Pyloric Stenosis)

Answer 21-39. e

Infants with infantile hypertrophic pyloric stenosis (IHPS) commonly present with dehydration and electrolyte abnormalities secondary to persistent vomiting. In the initial phase of management, appropriate fluid/electrolyte resuscitation remains the priority. Placement of a nasogastric tube for feeding or hydration is unnecessary. Pyloromyotomy is the gold standard for treatment, but is nonemergent and should be performed only after the patient is stabilized and alkalosis and hypokalemia are corrected. Surgical therapy provides safe and effective treatment, with prompt relief of symptoms. Endoscopic dilation of the pylorus is not an effective, long-term therapy for IHPS. Enhancement of gastric motility with erythromycin is not beneficial for patients with IHPS. In fact, early exposure to erythromycin in infancy has been linked to the development of IHPS.

(Section 21: Disorders of the Gastrointestinal System, Chapter 392: Infantile Hypertrophic Pyloric Stenosis)

Answer 21-40. b

Cow's milk protein–induced anemia can present in children between the ages of 1 and 3 years, as a result of iron-deficiency anemia and protein-losing enteropathy. Key characteristics include a history of excess cow's milk intake (typically greater than 32 oz of whole milk daily), profound microcytic anemia (hemoglobin 6-8 g/dL), and hypoalbuminemia. Because of the gradual development of anemia and hypoalbuminemia, the child does not develop orthostatic hypotension of symptoms. Stool studies are notable for elevated α_1-antitrypsin excretion indicating a protein-losing enteropathy. However, stool guaiac test for blood is negative, which is an important distinction from patients with cow's milk protein–induced proctocolitis or allergic colitis. The mechanism by which cow's milk induces anemia is not completely understood, but is likely related to iron deficiency (secondary to excess milk intake) or mucosal toxicity rather than from hypersensitivity to cow's milk protein.

Cow's milk protein–induced proctocolitis typically presents at 4 to 12 weeks of age with symptoms of painless hematochezia mixed with mucus and occasional diarrhea. FPIES is a non–IgE-mediated process that is associated with an anaphylactic-like reaction with rapid onset of symptoms of vomiting and diarrhea as well as systemic manifestations of pallor, hypotension, and shock. Eosinophilic gastroenteritis is characterized by dense eosinophilic inflammation of the gastrointestinal mucosa. Typical symptoms include abdominal pain, vomiting, diarrhea, and growth failure. In more severe cases, iron-deficiency anemia and protein-losing enteropathy can develop, but are associated with eosinophilia and increased

serum IgE. It is rare for Crohn disease to present at this stage in early childhood, but the presenting symptoms include diarrhea and growth failure. With this degree of iron-deficiency anemia, history of diarrhea, and hematochezia, blood loss would be more likely.

(Section 21: Disorders of the Gastrointestinal System, Chapter 411: Allergic and Eosinophilic Gastroenteropathies)

Answer 21-41. e

The diagnosis of cow's milk protein–induced eosinophilic proctocolitis, also referred to as "allergic colitis" or cow's milk protein hypersensitivity, is made based on the typical symptom presentation and response to removal of the offending antigen. Eosinophilic proctocolitis typically begins at 4 to 12 weeks of age and presents with painless hematochezia mixed with mucus and flecks of blood. Anemia is uncommon at the time of presentation, unless untreated for long periods. The most common protein sensitivities are to either cow's milk or soy proteins; therefore, switching to a soy-based formula is not recommended. Maternal restriction of cow's milk is effective in over 80% of breastfed cases. In infants with mild symptoms, a cow's milk protein hydrolysate or elemental (amino acid) formula should be used for at least 1 month to allow adequate time for mucosal healing. At 1 year, 45% to 50% of infants become fully tolerant to cow's milk protein.

Elimination of peanuts and tree nuts from the mother's diet is less likely to result in symptom resolution than elimination of cow's milk protein. In patients with typical symptom presentation, further testing is usually not necessary. However, if symptoms persist or do not respond to appropriate dietary management, a full evaluation including hemoglobin, stool cultures, and flexible sigmoidoscopy should be strongly considered.

(Section 21: Disorders of the Gastrointestinal System, Chapter 411: Allergic and Eosinophilic Gastroenteropathies)

Answer 21-42. b

The hallmark sign of a nonincarcerated, inguinal hernia on physical examination is a smooth, firm mass in the inguinal region or scrotum that enlarges with increased intra-abdominal pressure (Figure 405-1). The hernia typically reduces spontaneously or can be reduced by gentle, manual pressure along the inguinal canal. In contrast, an incarcerated hernia generally presents with symptoms of irritability, pain in the groin and abdomen, abdominal distension, and vomiting. The mass associated with an incarcerated hernia is usually well defined, tender, and does not reduce. Suppurative lymphadenopathy in the inguinal region can present as a persistent inguinal mass, but skin examination typically reveals a superficial infected lesion with swelling of other affected nodes in the area. Testicular torsion usually presents as a tender, erythematous mass in the groin, with absence of a gonad in the scrotum of the same side.

Inguinal hernias in infants less than 1 year of age are unlikely to resolve spontaneously. Due to the high risk of incarceration in the first 6 to 12 months of life, referral to a pediatric surgeon and repair should proceed promptly. In children older than 1 year, the risk of incarceration is less and repair is less urgent. In the case of an incarcerated hernia, failure to treat can lead to strangulation and infarction of the hernia contents. In a patient with prolonged history of incarceration (>12 hours), signs of peritonitis, or small bowel obstruction, the mass should not be manually reduced and surgical consultation should be obtained emergently. Aspiration of a groin mass is discouraged because of the risk of injury to the hernia sac. Ultrasonography can differentiate hernia, hydrocele, and lymphadenitis, as well as identify the presence of testicular torsion. However, as in the case above, physical examination generally suggests a diagnosis of inguinal hernia and additional diagnostic studies are not typically required.

(Section 21: Disorders of the Gastrointestinal System, Chapter 405: Inguinal and Other Hernias)

Answer 21-43. a

Gastroschisis is a congenital abdominal wall defect through which intraperitoneal contents protrude. The defect typically occurs to the right of the umbilical cord and can range in size from 2 to 5 cm. In contrast, omphalocele is a congenital defect of the midline anterior abdominal wall, where the extruded abdominal organs are covered by a protective membrane.

Intestinal dysmotility is very common in infants with gastroschisis. Many infants have a prolonged ileus after closure of the abdominal wall resulting in delayed achievement of full enteral feeds. In a smaller proportion of gastroschisis infants, intestinal dysmotility can be prolonged for years into childhood. Infants with gastroschisis are also associated with premature delivery, intestinal atresia, and higher risk of developing necrotizing enterocolitis.

Unlike gastroschisis, omphalocele is associated with additional abnormalities, such as structural defects of the heart, kidneys, limbs, and face, in up to 60% of infants. Omphaloceles have been associated with trisomies 13, 14, 15, 18, and 21 as well as other genetic syndromes, such as BWS. BWS is associated with macrosomia, macroglossia, hypertrophy of solid organs, and a predisposition for childhood cancers, as well. Unlike gastroschisis, infants born with omphaloceles are relatively protected from heat and fluid loss by the intact membrane covering the viscera, and usually do not have impaired gastrointestinal function when the sac remains intact. Omphalocele is associated with variable rotational anomalies of the intestine.

(Section 21: Disorders of the Gastrointestinal System, Chapter 396: Abdominal Wall Defects)

Answer 21-44. c

Primary fascial and skin closure of a gastroschisis abdominal wall defect is possible in one half to two thirds of infants.

Closure of the abdomen may be complicated by abdominal compartment syndrome. After returning the viscera to the abdominal cavity, patients should be monitored for signs of tightness around the viscera. These include evidence of decreased ventilation, loss of pedal pulses, loss of urine output, and discoloration of the intestine. If abdominal compartment syndrome is suspected, immediate evisceration and placement of a protective silo over the intestine is performed. In infants in whom primary closure is not possible, a staged approach may be employed.

Placement of a nasogastric tube for decompression, intravenous fluid resuscitation, and initiation of antibiotics are all potentially helpful in supporting and stabilizing a patient with abdominal compartment syndrome. However, none of these strategies address the underlying problem. Likewise, both alterations of ventilator settings and ultrasound evaluation are inappropriate options in the management of this emergent complication.

(Section 21: Disorders of the Gastrointestinal System, Chapter 396: Abdominal Wall Defects)

Answer 21-45. a

Congenital atresia of the esophagus and TEF are relatively common congenital anomalies, occurring in 1 of every 2500 to 3000 live births. EA has been classified into 5 types based on whether the esophagus is present and the location of fistula to the trachea.

The vast majority (85%) of infants born with EA have atresia of the esophagus with a distal TEF. Also known as Type C EA, the esophageal fistula typically originates just proximal to the carina in the posterior trachea. The next most common type is a pure esophageal atresia without TEF (10%). Once the diagnosis of esophageal atresia is made, a search for associated anomalies is required, including VACTERL association, which includes anomalies of the vertebrae, intestinal atresia, cardiac malformations, TEF, renal anomalies, and limb anomalies (see Figure 392-1).

(Section 21: Disorders of the Gastrointestinal System, Chapter 392: Anatomic Disorders of the Esophagus)

Answer 21-46. c

A patient with a history of surgical repair for esophageal atresia and symptoms of isolated dysphagia should be evaluated for stricture formation at the site of the esophageal anastomosis. Strictures have been reported to develop in 30% to 40% of patients. Early complications following surgical repair include anastomotic leak, anastomotic stricture, and recurrent fistula. Late stricture development, as in this clinical vignette, is typically attributed to gastroesophageal reflux. Evaluation for stricture formation is performed with a barium swallow esophagram. Anastomotic strictures are usually treated via dilation with a balloon dilator or by progressive bougienage dilation. Refractory strictures may require steroid injection at the time of dilation or surgery.

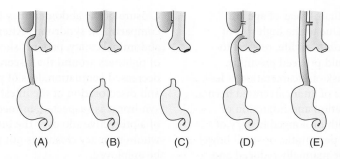

	A	B	C	D	E
Description	Proximal EA distal TEF	True EA without fistula	Proximal TEF	Proximal and distal fistula	Isolated TEF (H or N fistula)
Abnormal X-ray	Distal gas	Gasless abdomen	Gasless abdomen	Distal gas	Distal gas
Incidence	85%	6%	3%	1%	6%
Gross classification	C	A	B	D	E

FIGURE 392-1. Various types of esophageal atresia along with their incidence (%), anatomic findings, and Gross/Vogt classifications. **(A)** Esophageal atresia with distal tracheoesophageal fistula. **(B)** Esophageal atresia alone. **(C)** Esophageal atresia with proximal tracheoesophageal fistula. **(D)** Esophageal atresia with double fistula. **(E)** Isolated tracheoesophageal fistula. EA, esophageal atresia; TEF, tracheoesophageal fistula. (Reproduced, with permission, from Oldham KT, et al, eds. *Principles and Practice of Pediatric Surgery*. Philadelphia: Lippincott Williams & Wilkins; 2005:1040.)

Although gastroesophageal reflux is exceedingly common in EA patients following repair, and is likely a causative factor in the formation of an anastomotic stricture, treatment with proton pump inhibitors alone will unlikely lead to resolution of a significant stricture. Patients with severe reflux may require antireflux surgery and should be monitored long term due to the risk of developing Barrett esophagus and esophageal cancer. Recurrent tracheoesophageal fistula is a rare complication following TEF repair, but typically presents with symptoms of coughing, choking, apnea, and recurrent pulmonary infections, rather than dysphagia. A calcium channel blocker medication such as nifedipine enhances lower esophageal sphincter relaxation, and may provide some benefit for patients with dysphagia secondary to esophageal achalasia, but not for patients with a mechanical obstruction secondary to anastomotic stricture. Finally, although the majority of patients with esophageal atresia have some degree of dysmotility or abnormal peristalsis in the lower esophageal segment, even after surgical repair, the presence of an anastomotic stricture must be ruled out first.

(Section 21: Disorders of the Gastrointestinal System, Chapter 392: Anatomic Disorders of the Esophagus)

Answer 21-47. e

A thorough history and physical examination is generally sufficient to make a diagnosis of uncomplicated or physiologic gastroesophageal reflux (GER) in infancy. Additional diagnostic testing is usually unnecessary unless there are warning signs, such as forceful or bilious vomiting, abdominal tenderness or distension, gastrointestinal bleeding, diarrhea, constipation, fever, hepatosplenomegaly, seizures, macrocephaly or microcephaly, or onset of vomiting after 6 months of age.

An UGI contrast study is useful for diagnosing anatomic abnormalities that present with recurrent vomiting. The UGI is not useful for diagnosis of GER because reflux of ingested contrast occurs in healthy individuals.

In uncomplicated GER, characterized by the lack of warning signs or potential complications, such as weight loss, inadequate weight gain, excessive irritability, feeding difficulties, or recurrent respiratory distress, reassurance of the parents is usually sufficient for management. A diagnosis of gastroesophageal reflux disease (GERD) is considered when there are significant complications from GER. Nonpharmacologic options for treatment of GER may be considered for symptomatic infants, including a trial of a hypoallergenic formula or thickening of formula with rice cereal. A high-calorie formula is not indicated for an infant with appropriate growth. Proton pump inhibitor therapy is highly effective for treatment of esophagitis; however, for an infant with uncomplicated GER, acid suppression is unlikely to result in any significant clinical benefit. There are currently no available motility or prokinetic agents that have been proven clearly effective for GERD.

(Section 21: Disorders of the Gastrointestinal System, Chapter 394: Gastroesophageal Reflux and Other Causes of Esophageal Inflammation)

Answer 21-48. b

The clinical presentation of eosinophilic esophagitis (EE) varies depending on the age of the patient. Symptoms include feeding refusal in infants, gagging and solid food aversion in preschool children, and dysphagia and food impaction in adolescents. EE is a clinicopathologic diagnosis, which requires histologic evaluation of esophageal biopsies. It is characterized by an intense eosinophilic infiltrate of the esophageal wall, with evidence of ≥15 eosinophils/high-power field (HPF), and involvement of the entire proximal to distal esophagus. This finding is in contrast with gastroesophageal reflux disease (GERD), in which eosinophilic involvement is typically less intense (<7 eosinophils/HPF) and limited to the distal esophagus. Endoscopy usually reveals a combination of characteristic features: edema, linear furrowing, ringed appearance (tracheralization), and white adherent plaques. EE patients commonly have a personal and family history of atopy. Food allergies may be triggers of EE. Therefore, allergy testing may identify likely causes of EE and guide management of the condition with an elimination diet.

Since the patient in the clinical vignette has already received 6 weeks of high-dose proton pump inhibitor therapy, it is unlikely that the inflammation seen on endoscopy is secondary to GERD. Therefore, further escalation of acid suppression therapy with the addition of a histamine-2-receptor blocker is not indicated. Pneumatic balloon dilation of the lower esophageal sphincter is an appropriate option for treatment of achalasia, not EE. Infections of the esophagus are rare, except in the immunocompromised host. The typical presenting symptoms of esophageal infection are dysphagia and odynophagia. *Candida albicans* is the usual cause of *Candida* esophagitis, and is characterized by evidence of white plaques on endoscopy. Budding yeast and hyphae forms are usually present on histology. *Candida* esophagitis usually responds to treatment with fluconazole. Herpes simplex virus can cause esophagitis in both the immunocompromised and immunocompetent hosts. Endoscopically, the infection is usually characterized by discrete ulcers with a surrounding raised edge. If herpes simplex virus is suspected, treatment with acyclovir may shorten the disease course.

(Section 21: Disorders of the Gastrointestinal System, Chapter 394: Gastroesophageal Reflux and Other Causes of Esophageal Inflammation)

Answer 21-49. d

Ingestion of strong caustic agents can result in injury to the esophagus and stomach. Acids cause coagulation necrosis of the mucosa and formation of an eschar, while alkali substances produce liquefactive necrosis with intense inflammation of the surrounding tissue.

The acid produced by the stomach has limited neutralizing capacity compared with the alkalinity of even small volumes of strong alkalis. Symptoms following caustic ingestion include oral pain, ulcerations, drooling, dysphagia, vomiting, and abdominal pain. Concurrent airway damage is also possible. Symptoms can develop rapidly or be delayed for several hours. Clinical manifestations, such as the presence or absence of oral cavity burns, are generally poor predictors of esophageal injury. Young children with symptoms or an inability to tolerate clear liquids should be admitted for observation and intravenous hydration.

Emetics and buffers should not be given because of the risk of vomiting and subsequent aspiration. Nasogastric tubes should not be passed in the acute setting because they may perforate a damaged esophagus or stomach. Endoscopic evaluation is recommended between 12 and 36 hours after ingestion to allow evaluation of the degree of esophageal injury. Earlier endoscopy may miss the full extent of injury, since injury may evolve over the first 12 hours. Esophagoscopy after 48 hours is associated with increased risk of perforation.

(Section 21: Disorders of the Gastrointestinal System, Chapter 394: Gastroesophageal Reflux and Other Causes of Esophageal Inflammation)

Answer 21-50. a

Achalasia is a motor disorder of the esophagus with characteristic radiographic features on barium swallow (dilated esophagus with "bird's beak" appearance secondary to a narrowed gastroesophageal junction) and manometric findings of incomplete relaxation of the lower esophageal sphincter and lack of normal esophageal peristalsis.

Presenting symptoms include dysphagia, regurgitation of undigested food, recurrent pneumonia, weight loss, and chest pain. Diffuse esophageal spasm is rare in childhood, but is associated with symptoms of chest pain and evidence of nonperistaltic, prolonged, high-amplitude contractions on esophageal manometry. Patients with systemic scleroderma may present with skin findings, such as Raynaud phenomenon, as well as esophageal manifestations. The manometric findings in scleroderma include low-amplitude peristaltic contractions with abnormally low pressures in the lower esophageal sphincter. Gastroesophageal reflux disease (GERD) can also be a cause of a secondary motility disorder. Manometric findings are usually nonspecific, including prolonged esophageal contraction, aperistaltic contractions, and multiple peaked contractions. Mechanical obstruction, such as from an esophageal web or stricture, should always be considered in the evaluation of a patient who presents with dysphagia. Congenital defects are most likely to present when infants are transitioned to solid consistency foods.

(Section 21: Disorders of the Gastrointestinal System, Chapter 393: Disorders of Esophageal Motility)

Answer 21-51. c

The spectrum of anorectal malformations ranges from lesions such as anal stenosis to persistent cloaca. Many of these conditions share a common finding of imperforate anus, or lack of a visible normal anal opening onto the perineum. The most common defect is an imperforate anus with a fistula between the distal anorectum and urethra in boys, or the vestibule in girls.

The terms "high" and "low" are used to describe the location of the distal rectum and anal canal, respectively, relative to the perineum. In high lesions, the rectum ends above the levator muscle. In low lesions, the rectal pouch completely crosses the levator musculature and a fistula is usually evident on the skin. Congenital anorectal anomalies often coexist with other lesions. Newborns should undergo evaluation for other congenital lesions such as vertebral and sacral anomalies and genitourinary abnormalities. In terms of repair, the newborn infant with anal stenosis, perineal fistula, or an anteriorly displaced anus can usually undergo a primary, single-stage procedure without a colostomy. Patients with more complex anorectal malformations, meconium-stained urine, or other life-threatening anomalies require an initial colostomy, as the first part of a 3-stage reconstruction. The most common postoperative complications seen in children with anorectal malformations include constipation, soiling, and incontinence. Patients with "low" lesions and a normal sacrum usually have the best prognosis with regards to continence.

(Section 21: Disorders of the Gastrointestinal System, Chapter 415: Congenital Anomalies of the Anorectum)

Answer 21-52. e

In patients with suspected gastroesophageal reflux–associated Sandifer syndrome, esophageal pH–impedance monitoring (typically performed over 24 hours) is useful in demonstrating gastroesophageal reflux and in clarifying any temporal association of reflux and posturing.

Other diagnostic tests commonly performed in association with evaluation of gastroesophageal reflux disease, such as upper gastrointestinal radiography, nuclear scintigraphy, and upper endoscopy with esophageal biopsies, may be helpful in documenting the presence of gastroesophageal reflux, but are not able to temporally correlate reflux events with symptoms.

Sandifer syndrome involves spasmodic torsional dystonia with arching of the back and rigid posturing, mainly involving the neck, back, and upper extremities, associated with symptomatic gastroesophageal reflux. Spasms are commonly mistaken for seizures, although most patients do not have a clonic component to the movements. An electroencephalogram is usually normal for patients with suspected Sandifer syndrome, and therefore of little benefit unless the clinical presentation is unclear. A relationship with feeding may suggest a diagnosis of Sandifer syndrome, which commonly occurs after feeding. Typically, Sandifer syndrome is observed from infancy to early childhood. Peak prevalence is in individuals younger than 24 months. Children with mental impairment or spasticity may experience Sandifer syndrome into adolescence.

(Section 21: Disorders of the Gastrointestinal System, Chapter 394: Gastroesophageal Reflux and Other Causes of Esophageal Inflammation)

Answer 21-53. c

Children may develop delayed gastric emptying after an infection with certain organisms, such as rotavirus, Norwalk virus, herpes zoster virus, or infectious mononucleosis. The symptoms often resolve in time. The gastroparesis can result in symptoms or early satiety, nausea, vomiting, or abdominal discomfort. Children may vomit food hours or even days later.

The goals of treatment are to maintain adequate nutrition and hydration while attempting to control symptoms. With a child with mild postinfectious gastroparesis such as the one presented in this question, conservative initial treatment makes most sense. This strategy would include introducing small, low-fat meals. Meals lower in fat have a shorter gastric emptying time. Liquid meals also have a shorter emptying time. Meals high in fat will further delay her gastric emptying.

Pyloric injections of Botox would only be considered if she failed medical management including altering her diet and failure of promotility drugs.

Domperidone is a prokinetic medication; however, it is not approved for use in the United States by the Food and Drug Administration and it is not readily available for use. Other promotility drugs such as metoclopramide and erythromycin are available for use and could be given to this patient if altering her diet is not effective. Metoclopramide, however, does have a risk of tardive dyskinesia making its use less popular than erythromycin.

Initiation of nasojejunal feeds may need to be considered in patients with significant delayed gastric emptying and weight loss who have failed more conservative therapy; however, this strategy would not be a first line of treatment.

(Chapter 407: Delayed Gastric Emptying)

Answer 21-54. b

Hirschsprung disease occurs in 1 in 5000 live births. Up to 10% of children with Down syndrome have Hirschsprung disease. Hirschsprung disease is a result of aberrant migration of neural crest cells during colonic development. Ninety-four percent of neonates with Hirschsprung do not pass meconium within 24 hours of birth. Other symptoms at presentation may include vomiting, abdominal distension, and enterocolitis. The clues in this case making Hirschsprung disease most likely are his diagnosis of trisomy 21, delayed passage of meconium, and a tight anal canal.

Patients with trisomy 21 are at higher risk of duodenal web. However, while vomiting would be a key symptom related to a web, the patient should not have a tight anal canal or delayed passage of meconium. Milk protein intolerance can be associated with vomiting and constipation in infants; however, one would not expect delayed passage of meconium and the rectal examination should demonstrate normal tone. Infants with cystic fibrosis may present with constipation or even a small bowel obstruction from meconium ileus; however, again, they should not have an abnormal rectal examination.

Given this patient's history of trisomy 21, delayed passage of meconium, and tight anal canal on rectal examination, functional constipation should not be an initial consideration.

(Chapter 407: Hirschsprung Disease)

Answer 21-55. e

Erythromycin is a motilin receptor agonist used to accelerate gastric emptying. There is a caution in using this drug in young infants due to the increased risk of the development of hypertrophic pyloric stenosis. While erythromycin accelerated gastric emptying, it has not been associated with dumping syndrome. In addition, erythromycin has not been associated with duodenal webs. Both tardive dyskinesia and dystonic reactions are side effects of metoclopramide that is also a prokinetic medication used in delayed gastric emptying.

(Chapter 407: Delayed Gastric Emptying)

Answer 21-56. d

With the patient's constellation of signs including anemia, thrombocytopenia, elevated creatinine, and history of likely infectious colitis, her most likely diagnosis is HUS. HUS is often preceded by an infection such as *Escherichia coli 0157:H7*, *Shigella*, *Campylobacter*, *Yersinia*, or *Salmonella*. Given her anemia and elevated creatinine, this patient needs to be admitted for supportive care. Although most cases of infectious colitis resolve, given her development of the complication of HUS, it is not appropriate to monitor her as an outpatient.

A course of oral antibiotics will not change the outcome of her HUS, and potentially could increase risk for HUS if given during a course of *E. coli 0157:H7*, *Shigella*, *Campylobacter*, *Yersinia*, or *Salmonella*.

With the patient's symptoms occurring for only 1 week, the history of a sick contact, and now the development of HUS, ulcerative colitis is unlikely.

(Chapter 412: Hemolytic Uremic Syndrome)

Answer 21-57. a

This patient is most likely presenting with *Henoch-Schönlein purpura* (HSP). Ten percent of children with HSP and abdominal pain will have intussusception. This patient will need to be evaluated in the emergency department for diagnosis and decompression with a water-soluble enema or surgery.

Her symptoms of abdominal pain and bloody stools could represent malrotation with volvulus; however, the abdominal pain would unlikely come in intermittent waves as it does with intussusception. Also, the purpuric lesions on her legs are not consistent with malrotation with volvulus.

Steroids and ibuprofen can be used in patients with abdominal pain and HUS; however, this patient is presenting with symptoms suggestive of intussusception that requires emergent evaluation and treatment to avoid complications.

Given the description of purpuric lesions, an infectious colitis would be much less likely the source of her bloody

stools. HSP is a systemic vasculitic disease that results in bowel ischemia, not infection.

(Chapter 412: Systemic Vasculitic Disease)

Answer 21-58. b

Intestinal duplications are rare congenital anomalies. An enteric duplication is defined by: (1) the presence of smooth muscle coat, (2) an intimate association with the alimentary tract, and (3) an inner lining of intestinal epithelium. The treatment for duplication cysts is surgical resection due to the risk of complications such as obstruction and bleeding.

A CT scan may be needed if there is concern that the cyst is involving other organs; however, this test would not determine whether or not surgery is warranted. Duplication cysts are benign lesions and do not require biopsy to determine surgical resection.

(Chapter 401: Duplications and Cysts)

Answer 21-59. b

This patient has an external hemorrhoid. They are generally associated with chronic constipation. Symptoms generally improve with the treatment of the underlying constipation. Incision and evacuation by a surgeon would be considered if the hemorrhoid was thrombosed. Anorectal varices may occur with chronic liver disease; however, in a child with a normal examination and chronic constipation, chronic liver disease would not likely be the etiology. Hemorrhoids may be a sign of sexual abuse; however, with a history of chronic constipation and no other signs of perianal trauma, this diagnosis would not be the most likely etiology. The patient does not need a colonoscopy, as hemorrhoids are not associated with other intestinal vascular lesions.

(Chapter 416: Hemorrhoids and Anorectal Varices)

Answer 21-60. e

This patient has a rectal prolapse, likely from his constipation and straining with stooling. Most cases spontaneously resolve. However, in situations where the mucosa does not spontaneously resolve, gentle pressure may be applied to manually reduce the prolapse. This may be done in the home or office setting. If the mucosa does not reduce with gentle pressure, then surgical reduction may be warranted. A stool softener may be needed to treat the underlying condition; however, this treatment would only prevent future prolapses and would not result in resolution of the current prolapse.

(Chapter 416: Other Anorectal Disorders)

Answer 21-61. a

This rash is classic for perianal streptococcal infection. Oral penicillin, as opposed to topical antibiotics, is usually effective in treatment. Candidal diaper rash usually has more erythematous plaques with satellite lesions and would be treated with topical nystatin. Topical cholestyramine may be used to bind bile acids in children with a diaper dermatitis related to diarrhea. Neither nystatin nor cholestyramine would be used for a bacterial infection.

(Chapter 416: Other Anorectal Disorders)

Answer 21-62. c

Annular pancreas presents with symptoms of a high obstruction including vomiting. It arises from incomplete rotation of the ventral bud off the duodenum during embryonic pancreatic development. It is often associated with a duodenal diaphragm or stenosis.

Pyloric stenosis and antral web are obstructive processes at the gastric outlet. On abdominal radiograph, one would not see the area of duodenal dilation. Hirschsprung disease would present with a more distal obstructive symptomatology such as constipation and infrequent stooling. You may find a lack of air in the rectum on abdominal radiograph with dilated loops of bowel proximal to the effected segment of aganglionosis. A choledochal cyst is found in the hepatobiliary ducts and is seen on other radiologic modalities such as ultrasound, CT scan, or magnetic resonance imaging.

(Chapter 417: Congenital Anomalies of the Pancreas)

Answer 21-63. d

The patient is taking a chronic medication, valproic acid, which is known to cause pancreatitis. L-Asparaginase, azathioprine, and 6-mercaptopurine are also associated with pancreatitis. All the other conditions are also associated with acute pancreatitis; however, his abdominal ultrasound did not indicate gallstone disease. Epilepsy within itself is not associated with acute pancreatitis and he did not have any other signs or symptoms of a systemic condition or viral illness. Blunt trauma is associated with acute pancreatitis; however, it would be recent and not a remote event.

(Chapter 417: Acute Pancreatitis)

Answer 21-64. d

This neonate has likely experienced a gastric perforation due to trauma from esophageal intubation and bag mask ventilation. The pneumoperitoneum is confirmed by an abdominal radiograph. Symptoms include poor feeding, lethargy, and abdominal distension. Treatment includes nasogastric decompression, antibiotics, and surgical management.

Refeeding would not occur until surgical repair has occurred. A sepsis workup would not be the first course of action prior to surgical repair. Monitoring with repeated radiographs would not be appropriate, as the diagnosis has already been confirmed. A paracentesis would be the appropriate step preoperatively if the patient is experiencing hemodynamic instability or respiratory compromise, which this patient does not demonstrate.

(Chapter 400: Gastric Perforation)

Answer 21-65. e

The image shows a complete duodenal obstruction with tapering to the typical "bird's beak" appearance at the site of the volvulus in a patient with malrotation and midgut volvulus. Seventy-five percent of patients with malrotation and midgut volvulus will present in the first week to month of life.

In pyloric stenosis and antral web, the obstruction would be at the gastric outlet and the patient would not present with bilious vomiting. A patient with obstruction due to duodenal or jejunal atresia would not be healthy and tolerating feeds for 3 weeks prior to an acute onset of symptoms as the obstruction is present at birth.

(Chapter 397: Malrotation and Volvulus)

Answer 21-66. d

Neonates with pyloric atresia will present with early onset of vomiting that is nonbilious, as well as a dilated stomach at birth. The mother may also have polyhydramnios during her pregnancy.

Pyloric stenosis is an acquired condition and would not present on the first day of life, nor would it be associated with a large stomach at birth and polyhydramnios. Duodenal webs and atresias would likely present with bilious vomiting. Jejunoileal atresias would also likely present with bilious vomiting and abdominal distension.

(Chapter 399: Congenital Atresias, Stenosis, and Webs)

Answer 21-67. a

Infants with colonic atresia may also have associated abnormalities such as aganglionosis, abdominal wall defects, skeletal defects, cardiac defects, ophthalmologic defects, and other small bowel atresias. It is not associated with hearing impairment or asplenia.

(Chapter 399: Congenital Atresias, Stenosis, and Webs)

Answer 21-68. c

This patient has the classic presentation of appendicitis including fever, anorexia, leukocytosis, and periumbilical abdominal pain evolving to right lower quadrant pain. This patient is also experiencing the Rovsing sign where palpation of the left lower quadrant results in more pain in the right lower quadrant. A surgical evaluation in the emergency room is most appropriate to make the diagnosis, administer antibiotics, and obtain surgical intervention.

This patient could have acute infectious gastroenteritis that may be mimicking appendicitis. *Yersinia* is a classic example of this. However, the diagnosis of an infectious gastroenteritis would be considered only after the exclusion of appendicitis. A small bowel obstruction would likely present with bilious vomiting and abdominal distension. Patients presenting with infectious symptoms and right lower quadrant pain may have mesenteric adenitis; however, appendicitis must be ruled out first. Often right lower quadrant lymph nodes are present in the face of a normal-appearing appendix on ultrasound or CT scan imaging. Acute cholecystitis may present with fever, leukocytosis, and pain; however, the pain is typically right upper quadrant in location and character as opposed to a periumbilical pain evolving to a right lower quadrant pain.

(Chapter 413: Acute Appendicitis)

Answer 21-69. a

The most common cause of massive lower gastrointestinal bleeding in children less than 4 years of age is a Meckel diverticulum. It is most commonly located 2 ft from the ileocecal valve and presents when the gastric mucosa found in the diverticulum causes ulceration of the adjacent mucosa with subsequent bleeding. The Meckel scan, technetium-99m pertechnetate scintigraphy scan, identifies the gastric mucosa in the diverticulum by concentrating the radiolabeled pertechnetate in gastric epithelium. The test is 85% sensitive and 95% specific in diagnosing a Meckel diverticulum.

Magnetic resonance scan is not the imaging of choice to identify Meckel diverticulum. A colonoscopy or upper endoscopy would not be of benefit as the diverticulum is located 2 ft from the ileocecal valve in the small bowel and is not within range of scoping. Given that this patient has no diarrhea, abdominal pain, or fever and has had a significant acute bleeding event, an infectious etiology would be unlikely.

(Chapter 402: Meckel Diverticulum)

Answer 21-70. c

The treatment of choice for omphalomesenteric sinuses and cysts is surgical excision or the patient will continue to experience recurrence of symptoms. Long-term antibiotics are unnecessary given the cyst has drained and the patient has no fever or other signs of infection. Recurrent drainage of the cyst will only treat recurrent symptoms and will not result in resolution of the underlying cyst. Despite the cyst spontaneously draining, the patient is at risk for recurrence of symptoms. Suture placement at the umbilicus opening of the sinus tract will only result in accumulation of fluid with no ability for the cyst to spontaneously drain.

(Chapter 402: Omphalomesenteric Duct Remnants)

Answer 21-71. d

Twenty percent of foreign body impactions occur within the esophagus. Children may present with a choking episode, respiratory symptoms, coughing, drooling, refusing oral intake, dysphagia, or chest pain. If the child is symptomatic, it warrants urgent endoscopy. Other reasons for an urgent endoscopy include an esophageal impaction with a button battery or sharp object. It is not appropriate to delay removal of a button battery in the esophagus as a button battery may cause a low-voltage burn and corrosive injury of the esophageal mucosa. This injury may occur as early as 4 hours after impaction.

(Chapter 395: Foreign Body Ingestion)

CHAPTER 22 | Disorders of the Liver

Sarah Shrager Lusman and Haley C. Neef

22-1. Zone 1 of the liver acinus contains portal and periportal cells, whereas zone 3 contains centrilobular cells.

Which of the following statements about zone 1 versus zone 3 cells is true?

a. Zone 1 cells receive less oxygenated blood than zone 3 cells.

b. Zone 1 cells are more prone to viral injury than zone 3 cells.

c. There is a higher concentration of Kupffer cells in zone 1 than in zone 3.

d. Zone 1 cells are farther away from the terminal hepatic venules than zone 3 cells.

e. Zone 1 cells are more prone to anoxic injury than zone 3 cells.

22-2. A 3-month-old infant is admitted to the intensive care unit with idiopathic severe acute liver failure. Which of the following metabolic processes would most likely be impaired in this patient?

a. Gluconeogenesis

b. Protein catabolism

c. Transformation of potentially hepatotoxic hydrophilic compounds to hydrophobic form for excretion into bile

d. Direct secretion of cholesterol in LDL form

e. Insulin secretion

22-3. Which of the following statements about bile is true?

a. The rate of bilirubin formation in healthy infants is lower than the rate of bilirubin formation in adults.

b. Bilirubin is a hydrophilic molecule.

c. Bilirubin is formed in part from the degradation of cytochromes and muscle myoglobin.

d. Contraceptive steroids and anticonvulsants can increase UDG-GT activity, leading to an increase in bilirubin conjugation.

e. Bilirubin secretion is inhibited by phenobarbital and enhanced by estrogens and anabolic steroids.

22-4. A 10-year-old child with severe acute liver failure is being cared for in the intensive care unit. Which of the following laboratory findings best reflects worsening liver function in this patient?

a. Uptrending AST

b. Uptrending ALT

c. Hyperglycemia

d. Uptrending total bilirubin

e. Uptrending factor VII

22-5. A 7-year-old girl is admitted with new-onset elevated serum aminotransferases and jaundice; gallstones within the gallbladder and dilation of the common bile duct are visualized on initial right upper quadrant ultrasound, as well as single stone within the common bile duct. Which is the next most appropriate evaluation of the hepatobiliary system to pursue?

a. Computed tomography (CT)

b. Liver biopsy

c. Percutaneous transhepatic cholangiography (PTC)

d. Hepatobiliary iminodiacetate (HIDA) scan

e. Endoscopic retrograde cholangiopancreatography (ERCP)

22-6. A 2-week-old term infant girl is brought to the emergency room because her parents noticed that her eyes and skin have "looked yellow" for the past 2 days and she has been somewhat fussy on the day of presentation. Laboratory evaluation reveals a total bilirubin of 8.2 mg/dL and a direct bilirubin of 6.5 mg/dL. Rectal temperature is 38.4°C. On examination, the child is well nourished, has moist mucous membranes, is crying but easily consolable with feeds, and appears jaundiced from head to toe with scleral icterus present. Which of the following is the next most appropriate laboratory test to send?

a. Catheterized urinalysis and culture

b. Epstein-Barr virus PCR

c. Serum ammonia

d. Total and free carnitine

e. Factors V and VII

22-7. A previously healthy 9-year-old male presents to the ER with asymptomatic jaundice and is found to have a total bilirubin of 11 mg/dL with a direct component of 8.5 mg/dL. Which of the following tests is the most useful indicator of hepatic synthetic function?

a. Cortisol

b. Total and free carnitine and acylcarnitine

c. Complete blood count with platelets

d. Prothrombin time (PT)

e. Antinuclear antibody

22-8. A 4-week-old infant male presents to clinic for routine well-child examination. Liver edge is palpable 2 cm below the right costal margin, but is not palpable below the xiphoid process. His physical examination is otherwise unremarkable and he has been growing and gaining weight well. What is the next most appropriate step?

a. Order nonurgent abdominal ultrasound.

b. Send viral hepatitis panel.

c. Obtain complete blood count with platelets and comprehensive metabolic panel including AST, ALT, and bilirubin fractions.

d. Obtain urine succinylacetone.

e. Reexamine liver carefully at next routine well-child examination for change.

22-9. A 7-year-old female is admitted to the pediatric general care floor with jaundice and fatigue. Laboratory evaluation reveals elevated AST, ALT, bilirubin, prolonged INR, IgA deficiency, and a positive anti–liver kidney microsomal type 1 (LKM-1)

antibody titer. Which of the following is the most likely diagnosis?

a. Primary sclerosing cholangitis

b. Lupus

c. Type I autoimmune hepatitis (AIH)

d. Type II AIH

e. Intrahepatic cystic biliary dilation (Caroli disease)

22-10. Treatment options are considered for a 14-year-old female with newly diagnosed type I autoimmune hepatitis who has not yet started on any therapy. Which of the following is the best choice for initial treatment in this patient?

a. Prednisone

b. Cyclosporine

c. Mycophenolate

d. Tacrolimus

e. Azathioprine

22-11. A 20-day-old breastfed girl presents to the emergency department with jaundice, vomiting, lethargy, and rectal temperature of 39.0°C. Physical examination is significant for hepatomegaly. Catheterized urinalysis demonstrates reducing substances and white blood cells. Urine Gram stain shows gram-negative rods. What is the most likely diagnosis?

a. Hereditary fructose intolerance

b. Hereditary tyrosinemia

c. Type I glycogen storage disease

d. Type IV glycogen storage disease

e. Galactosemia

22-12. A 6-week-old infant with hepatomegaly on physical examination is diagnosed with hereditary tyrosinemia. Which of the following statements about this infant is true if he is left untreated?

a. The infant is likely to acquire cataracts.

b. The infant will have markedly low serum tyrosine and methionine concentrations.

c. The infant is likely to develop disease of the skeletal and cardiac muscle.

d. The infant is at risk for developing renal tubular dysfunction.

e. The infant is likely to have giant cell hepatitis on liver histology.

22-13. A 4-week-old girl presents to the emergency department with a 2-day history of upper respiratory congestion and cough followed by progressive feeding intolerance and lethargy. The infant is seizing at time of presentation. Laboratory evaluation shows a blood glucose of 20 mg/dL, AST of 500 U/L, and ALT of 600 U/L. Urinalysis is negative for ketones.

Which of the following is the most likely underlying disease?

a. Mitochondrial disorder

b. Galactosemia

c. Fatty acid oxidation disorder

d. Tyrosinemia

e. Glycogen storage disease

22-14. A 12-week-old infant with indirect hyperbilirubinemia is found to have homozygous deficiency of the protein inhibitor ZZ (PiZZ) phenotype. Which of the following is also likely to be true about this patient?

a. Liver biopsy is likely to show microsteatosis.

b. Liver disease is secondary to decreased proteolytic activity of α_1-antitrypsin within the hepatocytes.

c. The patient is at risk for developing renal disease in young adulthood.

d. The PiZZ defect is due to a single amino acid substitution mutation.

e. Liver transplantation is a futile intervention for patients with PiZZ phenotype who progress to end-stage liver disease.

22-15. A 14-year-old boy seen in your clinic has a history of Wilson disease. Which of the following tissues may accumulate excessive copper if the disease is left inadequately treated?

a. Skeletal system

b. Pancreas

c. Ovaries

d. Brain

e. Salivary glands

22-16. Which of the following statements about neonatal iron storage disease (also known as neonatal hemochromatosis) is true?

a. It is caused by the same genetic mutation that causes hereditary hemochromatosis.

b. Untreated mortality rate is low.

c. It can be diagnosed by MRI of the pancreas and/or heart.

d. It is inherited in an autosomal recessive pattern.

e. The disease may recur following liver transplantation.

22-17. You send genetic testing on a 16-year-old patient with a history of weakness, fatigue, arthralgias, recent onset of diabetes, and hepatomegaly who you suspect may have a disorder of metal metabolism.

Which of the following genes is likely to carry a mutation?

a. *ATP7B* associated with Wilson disease

b. *HFE* associated with hereditary hemochromatosis

c. *UGT1A1* associated with Gilbert syndrome

d. *cMOAT/MRP2* associated with Dubin-Johnson syndrome

e. *ABCB11* associated with progressive family intrahepatic cholestasis

22-18. Which of the following statements regarding the structure of the liver is correct?

a. The cystic duct joins the common hepatic duct to form the common bile duct.

b. The hepatic artery supplies 75% of the blood flow to the liver.

c. The portal vein carries blood from the liver to the inferior vena cava.

d. The hepatocytes in zone 1 of the acinus are the most prone to ischemic injury.

e. Each portal tract contains branches of the hepatic artery, bile ductule, and central vein.

22-19. Which of the following statements regarding hepatic function in infants is correct?

a. At birth, hepatic glycogen concentration is significantly lower compared with that found in the adult liver.

b. Albumin production does not begin until several days after birth.

c. Serum α-fetoprotein levels increase dramatically during the first year of life.

d. At birth, an infant's bile acid pool is comparable in size to that of an adult.

e. Neonates lack the bacteria *Clostridium ramosum* and *Escherichia coli* and are thus more likely to reabsorb bilirubin from the intestine.

22-20. A 3-year-old girl presents to the emergency room after her mother discovered her on the bathroom floor with an open, mostly empty bottle of acetaminophen tablets. *N*-Acetylcysteine is administered and she is admitted to the intensive care unit for observation. Although each of the following might be considered appropriate investigations during the course of her illness, which is most useful for monitoring the synthetic function of this patient's liver?

a. Serum alanine aminotransferase

b. Prothrombin time (PT)

c. Ultrasound of the abdomen

d. Serum alkaline phosphatase

e. Acetaminophen level

22-21. A 6-week-old boy presents to the pediatrician's office for evaluation of "yellow eyes." His parents report that they noticed this 2 days ago. They state that he is otherwise well. He has gained 1 lb since his last visit 2 weeks ago. Physical examination reveals an alert, afebrile, well-appearing infant with icteric sclerae. His liver edge is palpable 1 cm below the right costal margin. There is no stool in the diaper. The pediatrician orders blood work, which reveals a total bilirubin of 9.6 mg/dL, conjugated bilirubin of 3.2 mg/dL, and a GGT of 412 U/L. Which of the following is the most appropriate next step in evaluation?

a. Blood and urine cultures

b. Liver biopsy

c. Endoscopic retrograde cholangiopancreatography

d. Abdominal ultrasound

e. Serum β-carotene level

22-22. A 14-year-old girl presents with jaundice and fatigue. Her physical examination is notable for icteric sclerae, a softly distended abdomen, and splenomegaly. Laboratory testing shows the following: aspartate aminotransferase 285 U/L, alanine aminotransferase 347 U/L, total bilirubin 4.5 mg/dL, serum IgG 1295 mg/dL, and anti–smooth muscle antibody titer of 1:40. Liver biopsy shows an infiltrate of plasma cells with piecemeal necrosis. Which of the following is a correct statement regarding this patient's condition?

a. The condition occurs with equal frequency in males and females.

b. Patients with this condition are unlikely to have associated autoimmune diseases.

c. This patient's symptoms are expected to improve with immunosuppressive treatment.

d. This patient is presenting with acute hepatitis.

e. Liver transplantation is a curative treatment for this condition.

22-23. A 13-year-old boy with ulcerative colitis presents for a routine follow-up visit. He is receiving infliximab infusions every 8 weeks. The last infusion was 5 weeks ago. He reports that he is having 1 to 2 formed bowel movements per day with no visible blood. Physical examination reveals excoriated areas on his arms, legs, and the back of his neck. On further questioning, he admits that he has been itchy for the past 4 weeks and has been scratching these areas. His physical examination is also notable for a yellowish discoloration under his tongue and hepatomegaly.

What is the most likely diagnosis?

a. Atopic dermatitis

b. Allergic reaction to infliximab

c. α_1-Antitrypsin deficiency

d. Primary sclerosing cholangitis (PSC)

e. Scabies

22-24. A 7-month-old boy is brought to the pediatrician's office for evaluation of vomiting that began 3 weeks prior. He has not gained any weight since his last visit 4 weeks ago. Since that visit, he was weaned from breast milk to cow's milk–based formula and pureed fruits and vegetables were introduced. Physical examination reveals a jaundiced, irritable infant. The liver edge is palpable 3 cm below the right costal margin.

What is the most likely diagnosis?

a. Hypothyroidism

b. Galactosemia

c. Hereditary fructose intolerance

d. Milk protein intolerance

e. Glycogen storage disease type I

22-25. An 18-year-old female with a history of attention deficit-hyperactivity disorder returns from her first semester at college and presents for evaluation of fatigue. She reports that she has had difficulty keeping up with her studies due to falling asleep in class and trouble focusing on her work. She denies fever, rash, upper respiratory symptoms, and sore throat. Physical examination reveals a well-nourished female who is mildly jaundiced. Her liver is enlarged and firm. Which of the following tests is most likely to lead to a definitive diagnosis of this patient's liver disease?

a. Liver biopsy for copper content

b. Serum alkaline phosphatase

c. Serum ceruloplasmin

d. Heterophile antibodies to Epstein-Barr virus

e. Urinalysis

22-26. A female infant born at 38 weeks' gestation becomes ill appearing 6 hours after birth. An evaluation for sepsis is begun. Laboratory evaluation reveals the following abnormalities: white blood cell count 17,100, platelets 37,000, international normalized ratio 6.8, alanine aminotransferase 121 U/L, total bilirubin 18.1 mg/dL, direct bilirubin 9.0 mg/dL, and serum ferritin 8000. The following day the infant's physical examination is notable for jaundice, abdominal distension, and a large bruise at the site of her intravenous catheter. The neonatologist correctly suspects neonatal hemochromatosis.

Which of the following statements regarding this condition is correct?

a. It is caused by a mutation in the same gene that is implicated in hereditary hemochromatosis.

b. This infant's future siblings will not have an increased risk of having the disease.

c. Liver biopsy reveals increased iron deposition and findings consistent with acute hepatitis.

d. Ninety percent of infants with this condition will recover spontaneously with supportive care.

e. This condition results from a gestational alloimmune response.

22-27. A 4-month-old boy presents for evaluation of jaundice that started 1 week prior to the visit. He is exclusively breastfed. He has 8 to 10 loose stools per day. His length is at the 10th percentile for age; weight is at the 5th percentile for age. His physical examination is notable for icteric sclerae, a firm liver edge palpable 2 cm below the right costal margin, and excoriated areas on his face. Laboratory evaluation reveals aspartate aminotransferase of 92 U/L, alanine aminotransferase of 104 U/L, alkaline phosphatase of 425 U/L, γ-glutamyl transferase of 12 U/L, and elevated serum bile acid levels.

What is the most likely diagnosis?

a. Dubin-Johnson syndrome

b. Progressive familial intrahepatic cholestasis (PFIC) type 1

c. Benign recurrent intrahepatic cholestasis

d. PFIC type 3

e. Breast milk jaundice

22-28. A female infant is born at 28 weeks' gestation and weighs 600 g at birth. She remains in the neonatal intensive care unit for 4 months. She is intubated at birth due to respiratory distress and then weaned to continuous positive airway pressure and finally to supplemental oxygen via nasal cannula. Her hospital course is complicated by an episode of necrotizing enterocolitis, leading to the resection of 10 cm of small bowel, creation of an ileostomy, and subsequent bowel reanastomosis. She also develops multiple episodes of sepsis. During this time she requires total parenteral nutrition (TPN). She is discharged to home on a combination regimen of parenteral nutrition and enteral tube feedings.

Which of the following is a true statement regarding this infant's prognosis?

a. It is expected that she will require parenteral nutrition for life.

b. Her prematurity is protective against the development of cholestatic liver disease.

c. Enteral feeding may help to stimulate bile flow and lessen cholestasis.

d. She is unlikely to develop significant liver disease.

e. Administration of a lipid emulsion as a component of parenteral nutrition will decrease her risk of liver disease.

22-29. Which of the following is *not* a true statement regarding cystic fibrosis–associated liver disease?

a. In many cases the course is benign and does not contribute significantly to morbidity or mortality.

b. This condition is more commonly seen in females.

c. The genetic defect in cystic fibrosis results in the production of thick, viscous secretions in the hepatobiliary system.

d. Patients with cystic fibrosis have an increased risk of gallstones.

e. Therapy with ursodeoxycholic acid has been associated with improvement in clinical liver disease as well as biochemical parameters.

22-30. An 11-year-old boy presents to the emergency department for evaluation of abdominal pain and nausea. His parents report that he was in his usual good state of health until 3 days ago, when he began complaining of abdominal pain. They became more concerned today because his abdomen appeared swollen and his eyes were yellow. Physical examination is notable for icteric sclerae, abdominal distension with a fluid wave, and hepatomegaly. He is awake, alert, and oriented to time, place, and person. Laboratory evaluation reveals aspartate aminotransferase 435 U/L, alanine aminotransferase 527 U/L, total bilirubin 8.3 mg/dL, prothrombin time 28.2, and international normalized ratio (INR) 3.5. The boy is admitted to the pediatric intensive care unit for observation and further testing.

Which of the following is a correct statement about this patient's condition?

a. There are multiple known etiologies of this condition in children that vary by age.

b. This patient has normal hepatic synthetic function.

c. This patient cannot be in acute liver failure because his mental status is normal.

d. This patient will most likely require liver transplantation regardless of the cause of his symptoms.

e. The presence of hyperbilirubinemia indicates that this patient has an underlying chronic liver disease.

22-31. A previously healthy 16-year-old girl presents with the acute onset of jaundice, hepatomegaly, and altered mental status. She is found to be in acute liver failure, with an international normalized ratio of 4.6. Further evaluation includes an ophthalmologic examination that reveals Kayser-Fleischer rings, 24-hour urinary copper that is elevated, and serum ceruloplasmin that is low. She is diagnosed with Wilson disease and placed on the waiting list for liver transplantation.

Which of the following might be considered an appropriate intervention while she is waiting for an available donor organ?

a. Aggressive intravenous hydration with 100% to 125% of maintenance fluids

b. Sedation with benzodiazepines to prevent self-injury

c. Parenteral nutrition support with a solution of 10% dextrose and 3 g/kg of protein per day

d. Cultures of blood and urine

e. Treatment with loperamide to prevent dehydration from diarrhea

22-32. Which of the following is an *incorrect* statement about portal hypertension?

a. Thrombotic events are rarely the cause of portal hypertension in children.

b. Portal hypertension is defined as a portal pressure gradient of above 10 to 12 mm Hg.

c. An enlarged spleen found on physical examination is consistent with a diagnosis of portal hypertension.

d. Imaging tests are indicated to confirm the diagnosis of portal hypertension.

e. Children with portal hypertension may require an upper endoscopy to evaluate for esophageal varices.

22-33. A 7-year-old boy presents to the emergency department after multiple episodes of frank bloody emesis. The attending physician observes that he is pale and listless. His heart rate is 140 bpm, and blood pressure is 80/35 mm Hg. His physical examination is notable for a firm liver edge and an enlarged spleen. Laboratory evaluation reveals hemoglobin 6 mg/dL, platelets 60,000, and international normalized ratio 1.4.

Which of the following is the most appropriate immediate next step in management?

a. Emergent endoscopic evaluation to determine the source of bleeding

b. Placement of a Sengstaken-Blakemore tube

c. Insertion of a large-bore intravenous cannula followed by the administration of packed red blood cells

d. Placement of a transjugular intrahepatic portosystemic shunt

e. Placement of a nasogastric tube for lavage of the stomach

22-34. A 16-year-old girl presents for follow-up of autoimmune hepatitis. She states that she was feeling well until a few weeks ago, when she began to experience bloating. Her physical examination reveals a distended abdomen that is dull to percussion. A fluid wave is detected on palpation. Abdominal ultrasound reveals significant ascites.

Which of the following is a true statement regarding this patient's condition?

a. The development of ascites is a sign of liver regeneration.

b. Vitamin K should be administered before this patient undergoes a diagnostic paracentesis.

c. This patient is predisposed to infection of the ascitic fluid by anaerobic bacteria from the intestine.

d. The composition of the ascitic fluid in this patient is likely similar to that found in patients with heart failure.

e. This patient should be instructed to limit her sodium intake to 0.5 g/day.

22-35. A 17-year-old Hispanic male presents for a health supervision visit. His only complaint is occasional right upper quadrant pain that usually occurs after eating. His body mass index is 32 kg/m², above the 95th percentile for age. Physical examination reveals a morbidly obese teenager in no acute distress. He reports mild tenderness on deep palpation of the abdomen in the right upper quadrant. Laboratory evaluation is notable for aspartate aminotransferase of 65 U/L, alanine aminotransferase of 59 U/L, and international normalized ratio of 1.1.

Which of the following is a correct statement regarding further evaluation and management of this patient?

a. Given his normal international normalized ratio, this patient's elevated transaminases are of no concern and he does not require further evaluation.

b. This patient should be referred for a liver biopsy to confirm the likely diagnosis of nonalcoholic fatty liver disease (NAFLD).

c. An ultrasound of the abdomen is sufficient to diagnose this patient with NAFLD.

d. This patient's liver disease is unlikely to result in significant liver dysfunction and no treatment is necessary.

e. It is not necessary to exclude other causes of liver disease because this patient is morbidly obese.

22-36. A 2-year-old girl presents for evaluation of increasing abdominal distension. Her parents report that she was born at 32 weeks' gestation. She spent 5 weeks in the neonatal intensive care unit. During that time she required continuous positive airway support and received fluids and medications via an umbilical vein catheter. She is otherwise healthy and developing normally.

Physical examination is notable for a firm liver edge, prominent vasculature visible over her central abdomen, and an enlarged spleen. Abdominal ultrasound with Doppler examination reveals multiple periportal collateral vessels.

What is this patient's most likely diagnosis?

a. Extrahepatic biliary atresia

b. Total parenteral nutrition–related cholestasis

c. Congestive heart failure

d. Cavernous transformation of the portal vein

e. Choledochal cyst

22-37. A 6-month-old girl presents to the emergency room due to 2 weeks of persistent emesis. On physical examination, she is noted to have mildly icteric sclerae and a palpable mass in the right upper quadrant of the abdomen. Abdominal ultrasound reveals cystic dilation of the common bile duct measuring 6 cm.

Which of the following is a correct statement regarding this patient's condition?

a. It is recommended that the cystic portion of the bile duct as well as the gallbladder be excised due to the risk of malignant transformation.

b. This condition occurs more commonly in males.

c. Elevation of serum amylase and lipase is rarely seen in patients with this condition.

d. Endoscopic retrograde cholangiopancreatography with biopsy of the bile duct is necessary to confirm the diagnosis.

e. Diagnosis of this condition after the age of 2 months is associated with poor survival.

22-38. Which of the following conditions is depicted in this percutaneous transhepatic cholangiogram (Figure 427-1)?

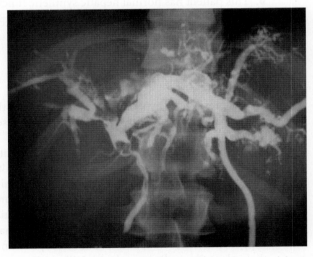

FIGURE 427-1. (Reproduced, with permission, from Lendoire J, et al. Bile duct cyst type V (Caroli's disease): surgical strategy and results. *HPB (Oxford)*. 2007;9(4):281–284.)

a. Extrahepatic biliary atresia

b. Budd-Chiari syndrome

c. Choledochal cyst

d. Caroli disease

e. Alagille syndrome

22-39. A 2-month-old boy is being evaluated for jaundice and failure to thrive. He undergoes a percutaneous liver biopsy that shows a paucity of bile ducts. Which of the following would *not* be considered an appropriate investigation in the course of his disease evaluation?

a. Skin biopsy

b. Echocardiogram

c. Ophthalmologic examination

d. Chest radiograph

e. Renal ultrasound

22-40. A 5-week-old African American infant who is exclusively breastfed is brought to the pediatrician because he "looks yellow." She notes that his stools changed from bright yellow to gray in the last 2 weeks. Physical examination reveals a well-nourished infant with icteric sclerae, and a liver edge palpable 4 cm below the right costal margin. Laboratory evaluation is notable for a total bilirubin of 7.3 mg/dL, direct bilirubin of 3.1 mg/dL, alanine aminotransferase of 127 U/L, and γ-glutamyl transpeptidase of 800 U/L. An abdominal ultrasound is obtained that is normal except for nonvisualization of the gallbladder.

Of the following, the *most* appropriate next step is:

a. Echocardiogram

b. Hemoglobin electrophoresis

c. Hepatobiliary scintigraphy

d. Measurement of urine-reducing substances

e. Sweat chloride testing

22-41. A 10-year-old boy with sickle cell anemia complains of right upper quadrant pain that is worse after eating. He reports that the pain lasts for approximately 30 minutes at a time. He feels nauseated but has not vomited. On physical examination, he is thin with icteric sclerae and has tenderness in the right upper quadrant with voluntary guarding. Laboratory evaluation is notable for hemoglobin of 8.1 g/dL, alanine aminotransferase of 161 U/L, total bilirubin of 3.4 mg/dL, and direct bilirubin of 0.6 mg/dL. Abdominal ultrasound reveals multiple stones within the gallbladder and dilation of the common bile duct.

Which of the following is a true statement regarding this patient's condition?

a. His sickle cell anemia confers an increased risk of cholesterol gallstones.

b. Cholecystectomy is recommended for relief of his symptoms.

c. Treatment with ursodeoxycholic acid should be started immediately to prevent the formation of more gallstones.

d. This patient is not a candidate for endoscopic retrograde cholangiopancreatography.

e. The finding of a dilated common bile duct does not affect management of this patient's gallstones.

ANSWERS

Answer 22-1. d

The functional unit of the liver is the acinus, which is divided into 3 zones (see Figure 418-1). Zone 1 cells are located in the periportal area surrounding the bile duct and terminal branches of the hepatic artery and portal vein, which carry oxygenated blood to the liver. Zone 1 cells are farthest away from the terminal hepatic venules, around which zone 3 cells are clustered. Zone 3 cells are centrilobular in location and receive the least amount of oxygenated blood; therefore, they are more prone to toxic, viral, or anoxic injury than zone 1 cells. The highest concentration of Kupffer cells (hepatic macrophages) is found in zone 1 within the sinusoidal wall.

(Page 1492, Chapter 418: Structure and Function of the Liver)

Answer 22-2. a

The liver plays an important role in carbohydrate metabolism, specifically in the uptake and storage of glucose as glycogen in addition to gluconeogenesis, which is the process in which glucose is synthesized from lactate, amino acids, or other small molecules. In a patient with severe liver failure, glucose storage and gluconeogenesis may be impaired, leading to hypoglycemia.

The liver plays a major role in protein synthesis, but not in protein catabolism. Detoxification of potentially hepatotoxic compounds is performed in the liver, but these compounds are typically transformed from hydrophobic form to hydrophilic form for easier excretion into the bile or urine. The liver typically exports cholesterol to the tissues in VLDL and HDL particles; it is uncommon for direct secretion of LDL cholesterol from the liver to occur except in pathologic states such as familial hypercholesterolemia. Insulin secretion occurs from the pancreas, not the liver.

(Page 1493, Chapter 418: Structure and Function of the Liver)

Answer 22-3. d

UDP-GT is the enzyme that conjugates glucuronic acid with bilirubin within the hepatocyte. Narcotics, anticonvulsants, contraceptive steroids, and bilirubin itself can increase UDP-GT activity.

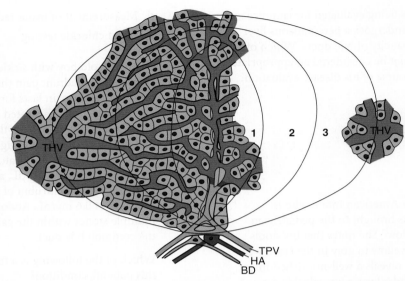

FIGURE 418-1. Diagram of the liver acinar unit as described by Rappaport. Terminal extensions of a portal venule (TPV), hepatic arteriole (HA), terminal hepatic venules (THV), and bile ductule (BD). The zones of the liver include zone 1 adjacent to the portal area, zone 2 in the middle of the acinus, and zone 3 around the terminal hepatic venule. (Reproduced, with permission, from Arias I, et al. *The Liver: Biology and Pathobiology.* New York: Raven Press; 1982:647–661.)

Healthy term infants form bilirubin at a rate of 6 to 8 mg/kg/day compared with healthy adults, who form bilirubin at a rate of 3 to 4 mg/kg/day; the higher rate in infants is attributable to increased red blood cell mass and shorter red blood cell life span compared with adults. Bilirubin is a lipophilic, nonpolar, hydrophobic molecule. It is formed from the degradation of heme products including hemoglobin, cytochromes, catalases, tryptophan pyrrolate, and muscle myoglobin. Conjugated bilirubin secretion is enhanced by phenobarbital and inhibited by estrogens and anabolic steroids.

(Pages 1494-1495, Chapter 418: Structure and Function of the Liver)

Answer 22-4. d

A rising total bilirubin in the setting of acute liver failure with loss of hepatic function is an ominous sign that is likely multifactorial in nature. This may be due to reduced hepatic uptake, decreased bile conjugation, and/or decreased biliary excretion as hepatocyte death progresses.

Serum aminotransferase elevation is usually secondary to hepatocellular injury due to inflammation, toxin, or passive congestion, although there are extrahepatic causes of elevated transaminases as well. Aminotransferases levels may remain stable or trend downward even as bilirubin rises as liver failure and hepatocellular dealt progress, so uptrending AST/ALT do not necessarily reflect loss of hepatic function. Hypoglycemia, not hyperglycemia, may occur as hepatic dysfunction progresses due to loss of glycogen stores and gluconeogenesis within the liver. Factor VII is a clotting protein synthesized in the liver that, when levels decline to less than 12% of normal, may predict fulminant hepatic failure.

(Page 1496, Chapter 419: Evaluation of the Infant and Child With Liver Disease)

Answer 22-5. e

In a child with cholestasis due to extrahepatic biliary obstruction by gallstones clearly visualized on ultrasound, it is most appropriate to pursue evaluation with ERCP, which not only provides excellent images of the intrahepatic and extrahepatic biliary tree but also allows for endoscopic interventions including stone removal.

CT is useful for 3-dimensional imaging of the hepatobiliary tree but exposes the patient to ionizing radiation and does not offer the therapeutic opportunity that ERCP does. A liver biopsy is useful for evaluation of microscopic hepatic structure and would not be useful for this patient with biliary obstruction of known cause. PTC allows visualization of the biliary tract by transhepatic injection of contrast into the ductal system and is useful especially for visualization of ducts not accessible by ERCP; it does not offer therapeutic intervention as ERCP does. HIDA scan is useful in evaluating infants with cholestatic liver disease or gallbladder structure and function in older individuals.

(Page 1497, Chapter 419: Evaluation of the Infant and Child With Liver Disease)

Answer 22-6. a

Other than fever and fussiness, this infant with direct hyperbilirubinemia is well appearing. Urine culture to rule out urinary tract infection and/or urosepsis as a cause of direct hyperbilirubinemia is an appropriate first-tier diagnostic study to order in this case. In the ill-appearing infant or the well-appearing infant with normal first-tier diagnostic studies, additional studies such as Epstein-Barr virus PCR, serum ammonia, total and free carnitine, and factors V and VII levels may be appropriate.

(Page 1498, Chapter 419: Evaluation of the Infant and Child With Liver Disease)

Answer 22-7. d

The most useful indicator of this child's hepatic synthetic function is the PT, which will be prolonged if the liver fails to synthesize clotting factors.

Cortisol level, total and free carnitine and acylcarnitine, and antinuclear antibody are second-tier diagnostic tests that should be sent for the well-appearing or ill-appearing child in which the etiology of direct hyperbilirubinemia remains unestablished after first-tier tests return with normal results. Complete blood count with platelets is an appropriate first-tier test to send in a child with direct hyperbilirubinemia, but abnormalities in this test do not necessarily indicate hepatic synthetic dysfunction.

(Page 1499, Chapter 419: Evaluation of the Infant and Child With Liver Disease)

Answer 22-8. e

A liver palpable 2 cm below the right costal margin is considered normal during infancy. It is reasonable to document this finding and reexamine the liver at the next routine examination for any changes. If the liver edge is palpated beyond 2 cm in an infant and/or is palpable below the xiphoid, an ultrasound is warranted to evaluate for hepatomegaly.

A viral hepatitis panel and/or urine succinylacetone to screen for tyrosinemia are tests that may reveal the underlying etiology of existing hepatomegaly, but are not warranted in this patient because the liver is normal in size. Complete blood count and comprehensive metabolic panel are an important part in the workup of an infant with direct hyperbilirubinemia and/or hepatomegaly, but also are not warranted in this patient.

(Page 1500, Chapter 419: Evaluation of the Infant and Child With Liver Disease)

Answer 22-9. d

This patient most likely has type II AIH, which is characterized by positive anti-LKM-1 antibody and/or anti-liver cytosol-1 antibody. Compared with patients with type I AIH, patients with type II AIH tend to present at a younger age and to have a higher incidence of partial IgA deficiency and acute liver failure at presentation (which is suggested by this patient's coagulopathy).

Type I AIH is more common than type II AIH and is characterized by positivity for antinuclear antibody (ANA), anti–smooth muscle antibody (SMA), or anti–F-actin antibodies. Primary sclerosing cholangitis is an autoimmune inflammatory condition targeting the extrahepatic bile ducts

that may be associated with other autoimmune disorders such as AIH, inflammatory bowel disease, or thyroiditis. Patients with primary sclerosing cholangitis are usually ANA, SMA, and LKM-1 negative, although these values are occasionally positive in patients with overlap syndrome, in which AIH and PSC occur together. Patients with lupus may have an elevated ANA titer, which is also seen in patients with AIH, but typically do not present with positive LKM-1 and acute liver failure. Caroli disease is a disease that presents with hyperbilirubinemia that is not associated with positive LKM-1 or IgA deficiency.

(Page 1501, Chapter 420: Autoimmune Disorders of the Liver)

Answer 22-10. a

Autoimmune hepatitis responds very well to steroid therapy. The recommended initial therapy for AIH is 2 mg/kg/day of prednisone. Once transaminases are below 100, prednisone can be weaned to low dose. Once bilirubin levels have normalized, azathioprine may be started as maintenance therapy, preferably in concert with low-dose steroids to prevent initial relapse. In patients who are intolerant of both corticosteroids and azathioprine, cyclosporine, tacrolimus, or mycophenolate may be considered.

(Page 1502, Chapter 420: Autoimmune Disorders of the Liver)

Answer 22-11. e

Galactosemia is a disorder of carbohydrate metabolism in which early ingestion of galactose, found in breast milk and cow's milk formula, leads to jaundice, lethargy, vomiting, acidosis, cataracts, failure to thrive, and bleeding; lab abnormalities may include indirect hyperbilirubinemia and coagulopathy, and urinalysis with reducing substances present but negative glucose on dipstick. Infants with galactosemia commonly present with gram-negative rod UTI or urosepsis, such as in this patient.

Hereditary fructose intolerance is another disorder of carbohydrate metabolism caused by genetic deficiency of fructose-1,6-bisphosphate aldolase, leading to depletion of tissue ATP. The disease typically presents in infants after they are first exposed to fructose-containing foods (ie, after the introduction of baby food), either with acute onset of vomiting, hypoglycemia, and hypophosphatemia or with subacute development of failure to thrive, irritability, poor feeding, and chronic emesis with eventual development of hepatomegaly, steatosis, jaundice, and ascites. Hereditary tyrosinemia is a protein metabolism disorder characterized by deficiency of an enzyme in the tyrosine degradation pathway that leads to accumulation of toxic metabolites of tyrosine. It may present either acutely in infancy with severe liver dysfunction (jaundice, hepatosplenomegaly, ascites, coagulopathy) or chronically in older children (cirrhosis, renal tubular dysfunction, rickets, and/or hepatocellular carcinoma). It is not associated with gram-negative rod urinary tract infections. Glycogen storage diseases are disorders of carbohydrate metabolism characterized by the inability to utilize glycogen stores within the liver or other tissues. Glycogen overload causes hepatomegaly in type

I and IV GSD; type IV GSD is associated with progressive liver disease that may lead to portal hypertension in early childhood. Both type I and IV GSD can present with hepatomegaly and hypoglycemia but are not associated with urinary tract infection or acute onset of infantile symptoms.

(Page 1504, Chapter 421: Metabolic and Genetic Disorders of the Liver)

Answer 22-12. d

This infant with hereditary tyrosinemia is at risk for renal tubular dysfunction producing a Fanconi syndrome. Serum tyrosine and methionine are characteristically markedly elevated in infants with untreated tyrosinemia.

Cataract development is associated with galactosemia. Individuals with glycogen storage diseases are at risk for developing disease of skeletal and cardiac muscle due to glycogen overaccumulation. Liver histology of tyrosinemia usually shows fatty infiltration, iron deposition, hepatocyte necrosis, pseudoacinar formation, and/or cirrhosis with fibrosis and regenerative nodules. One metabolic cause of giant cell hepatitis in the neonate is not tyrosinemia, but rather α_1-antitrypsin deficiency.

(Page 1505, Chapter 421: Metabolic and Genetic Disorders of the Liver)

Answer 22-13. c

One of the hallmark features of fatty acid oxidation disorders is nonketotic hypoglycemia, as in this patient. Fatty acid oxidation disorders can present with symptomatic hypoglycemia, which may cause seizures and lethargy, presenting after decreased PO intake, such as during a URI.

Mitochondrial disorder, galactosemia, and tyrosinemia can all present acutely in infants with feeding intolerance, lethargy, transaminitis, and hypoglycemia; however, infants with these disorders are able to synthesize ketones in context of fasting hypoglycemia, whereas those with fatty acid oxidation disorders cannot. Children with glycogen storage disease often present with fasting hypoglycemia because they are unable to utilize glycogen stores to produce glucose; however, they, too, are able to mount a ketotic response.

(Page 1506, Chapter 421: Metabolic and Genetic Disorders of the Liver)

Answer 22-14. d

The PiZZ phenotype is the most common defect to cause α_1-antitrypsin deficiency, a disorder with varying clinical manifestations, including liver and/or lung disease. The PiZZ defect is caused by single amino acid substitution of lysine for glutamate, which leads to misfolding of the protein and retention in the endoplasmic reticulum.

Accumulation of the misfolded protein within the hepatocytes leads to liver injury in patients with α_1-antitrypsin deficiency. In addition, patients are at risk for developing

lung disease (specifically early emphysema), due to decreased proteolytic activity of the enzyme in the lungs. They are not at risk for developing renal disease.

Giant cell hepatitis is a typical histologic finding in neonates with α_1-antitrypsin deficiency; microsteatosis is not a typical finding. Liver transplantation is curative for patients progressing to end-stage liver disease because the recipient assumes the Pi type of the donor organ.

(Page 1507, Chapter 421: Metabolic and Genetic Disorders of the Liver)

Answer 22-15. d

Wilson disease is a metal metabolism disorder characterized by excessive copper deposition in the liver, brain, kidneys, and eyes.

Patients with Wilson disease may suffer from arthralgias and osteoarthritis but do not typically develop copper deposition in the bones, pancreas, ovaries, or salivary glands. Infants with neonatal iron storage disease typically have excessive iron deposition in the liver, heart, pancreas, and salivary glands. Patients with hereditary hemochromatosis may present with amenorrhea but do not have excessive iron deposition in the ovaries.

(Page 1507, Chapter 421: Metabolic and Genetic Disorders of the Liver)

Answer 22-16. c

Neonatal iron storage disease is diagnosed by demonstration of hepatic insufficiency and findings of extrahepatic siderosis, by either salivary gland biopsy or MRI of the pancreas and/or heart. It is not caused by the same genetic mutation as hereditary hemochromatosis. The current theory is that it is caused by a gestational alloimmune response rather than a primary abnormality in iron metabolism. There is no clear pattern of inheritance, although the rate of occurrence in subsequent newborns to the same parents is 60% to 80%. Untreated mortality rate is extremely high. The disease is not known to recur following liver transplantation.

(Page 1509, Chapter 421: Metabolic and Genetic Disorders of the Liver)

Answer 22-17. b

This patient has symptoms consistent with hereditary hemochromatosis, which is most commonly caused by homozygosity for the C28Y mutation in the *HFE* gene. A mutation in the *ATP7B* gene may cause Wilson disease, which is a disorder of copper metabolism. Both Gilbert syndrome and Dubin-Johnson syndrome are disorders of bilirubin metabolism, associated, respectively, with mutations in the *UGT1A1* and *cMOAT/MRP2* genes. Progressive family intrahepatic cholestasis type II is an inherited disorder of bile formation associated with a defect in the *ABCB11* gene.

(Page 1509, Chapter 421: Metabolic and Genetic Disorders of the Liver)

Answer 22-18. a

At the porta hepatis, the right and left hepatic ducts coalesce to form a common hepatic duct, which is joined by the cystic duct to create the common bile duct. The liver has a dual blood supply. Seventy-five percent of the blood is supplied by the portal vein, which carries nutrients from the gastrointestinal tract. The remainder of the blood is supplied by the hepatic artery and is highly oxygenated. The hepatic veins drain blood from the liver and connect to the inferior vena cava. Microscopically, the functional unit of the liver is the acinus, with the most highly oxygenated blood located closest to the portal tracts. Each portal tract contains branches of the hepatic artery, bile ductule, and portal vein. Zone 1 hepatocytes are located closest to the portal tracts and are the last to die and the first to regenerate. Zone 3 hepatocytes, which are farthest from the blood supply, are the most prone to toxic, viral, or anoxic injury.

(Section 22: Disorders of the Liver and Biliary Tract)

Answer 22-19. e

Throughout gestation the fetus actively stores some glucose as glycogen, so that at birth hepatic glycogen is about twice the adult concentration at 40 to 60 mg/g of liver. The majority of this stored glycogen is utilized in the immediate postnatal period. Hepatic protein synthesis begins during fetal life, although albumin concentration in fetal plasma is low and does not reach adult levels until several months after birth. During this period there is a corresponding decrease in serum concentrations of α-fetoprotein. Bile acid synthesis also begins prenatally; however, infants have a considerably smaller bile acid pool compared with adults.

Bilirubin is formed from the degradation of heme products, taken up by hepatocytes and conjugated with glucuronic acids within the endoplasmic reticulum of the hepatocytes. Once conjugated, it is secreted in bile into the intestinal lumen, where bacteria, such as *C. ramosum* and *E. coli*, convert it to urobilinogens that are excreted. Conjugated bilirubin that is not converted to urobilinogens is reabsorbed by the enterohepatic circulation. Neonates lack the gut bacteria *C. ramosum* and *E. coli* and are thus more likely to absorb bilirubin from the intestine.

(Section 22: Disorders of the Liver and Biliary Tract)

Answer 22-20. b

Although commonly referred to as "liver function tests," the majority of serum tests measure the enzymes that are produced within the hepatocytes or biliary system but are not measures of physiologic function.

Serum alanine aminotransferase is a marker of hepatocellular injury and may be markedly elevated after exposure to hepatotoxins such as acetaminophen. Serum alkaline phosphatase may be elevated in cholestasis and also in conditions unrelated to hepatic function such as bone injury or growth. Ultrasound of the liver is useful for detecting changes in echotexture that may be due to infiltrative diseases, as well as cystic or solid tumors. It is not useful for evaluating hepatic function.

Conjugated bilirubin, glucose, ammonia, albumin, PT/international normalization ratio (INR), factor V, factor VII, and fibrinogen are all markers of hepatic synthetic function. Prolonged PT and INR may be seen in both acute and chronic liver injury and, when present, suggest liver dysfunction.

(Section 22: Disorders of the Liver and Biliary Tract)

Answer 22-21. d

This infant has jaundice, and a conjugated bilirubin level that is greater than 2 mg/dL or greater than 20% of the total bilirubin, consistent with a direct hyperbilirubinemia.

An abdominal ultrasound is useful to exclude a choledochal cyst or other anatomic abnormalities and should be performed in all infants presenting with direct hyperbilirubinemia. A liver biopsy may be performed if other less invasive screening methods do not identify an etiology for the jaundice. Endoscopic retrograde cholangiopancreatography provides detailed imaging of the biliary tree, but is invasive and technically difficult in young infants. There are limited data to support its use in the diagnosis of extrahepatic biliary atresia.

Sepsis is a common cause of direct hyperbilirubinemia in sick-appearing infants. As this infant is afebrile and well appearing, the clinical suspicion for sepsis is low. Carotinemia, a condition often seen in children taking a pureed diet containing yellow, carotene-containing vegetables, presents with yellow discoloration of the skin and clear sclera. Infants with carotinemia have normal serum bilirubin levels.

(Section 22: Disorders of the Liver and Biliary Tract)

Answer 22-22. c

This patient's most likely diagnosis is autoimmune hepatitis. Autoimmune hepatitis is more common in females than in males. Twenty percent of patients have other autoimmune conditions such as thyroiditis, diabetes mellitus, or inflammatory bowel disease. This condition may present in a variety of ways. Some patients are asymptomatic, others present with acute hepatitis or with jaundice and fatigue, and still others present with fulminant liver failure. This particular patient has splenomegaly, likely due to cirrhosis and portal hypertension, which indicates chronic liver disease. Immunosuppressives such as prednisone and azathioprine are the mainstays of treatment. Despite treatment, approximately 10% of patients progress to end-stage liver disease and require liver transplantation. Although liver transplantation has been shown to improve survival, recurrence of disease in the graft is common.

(Section 22: Disorders of the Liver and Biliary Tract, Chapter 420: Autoimmune Disorders of the Liver)

Answer 22-23. d

PSC is a chronic inflammatory condition targeting primarily the extrahepatic bile ducts. In children it is a rare disorder that is most often associated with inflammatory bowel disease, especially ulcerative colitis. The most common presenting symptoms are jaundice, hepatomegaly, and pruritus. Atopic dermatitis and scabies could cause pruritus but would not explain the other findings on physical examination. Allergic reactions to infliximab occur most often during an infusion and may present with symptoms of anaphylaxis. α_1-Antitrypsin deficiency is a disorder that results in damage to the liver due to increased deposition of α_1-antitrypsin. It may present with jaundice but is not associated with inflammatory bowel disease.

(Section 22: Disorders of the Liver and Biliary Tract)

Answer 22-24. c

Hereditary fructose intolerance is an autosomal recessive disorder caused by a deficiency of the enzyme fructose-1,6-bisphosphate aldolase. The classical presentation occurs in infants on the initial presentation of fructose-containing foods with the acute onset of vomiting, hypoglycemia, and hypophosphatemia followed by the development of hepatomegaly with steatosis, jaundice, and ascites. Chronic exposure to fructose causes poor feeding, failure to thrive, vomiting, irritability, and poor growth. Treatment involves strict avoidance of fructose, sorbitol, and sucrose.

Galactosemia usually presents in the first few weeks of life following ingestion of galactose (contained in breast milk and cow's milk formula). Clinical features of galactosemia include jaundice, lethargy, vomiting, acidosis, cataracts, failure to thrive, and bleeding. Milk protein intolerance may present with vomiting and failure to thrive but does not cause jaundice or hepatomegaly. Glycogen storage disease type I generally presents with fasting hypoglycemia and may lead to hepatomegaly, but jaundice usually does not occur until there is chronic liver disease. Clinical features of congenital hypothyroidism include jaundice, hepatomegaly, and feeding difficulties. These infants may have other abnormalities on physical examination. In the United States, the vast majority of infants with congenital hypothyroidism are identified by newborn screening.

(Section 22: Disorders of the Liver and Biliary Tract, Chapter 421: Metabolic and Genetic Disorders of the Liver)

Answer 22-25. a

This patient most likely has Wilson disease (hepatolenticular degeneration), an autosomal recessively inherited disorder of copper metabolism. Wilson disease should be considered in any child with an unexplained hepatic, neurologic, or psychiatric illness. Patients with Wilson disease have variable elevation in serum aminotransferase values and in the conjugated and unconjugated serum bilirubin concentrations. Serum alkaline phosphatase levels tend to be normal or even low, but this is not diagnostic of the disease. Serum ceruloplasmin, a protein involved in copper transport, is typically low, although it may also be reduced in other liver diseases. Hepatic copper content remains the gold standard for the diagnosis of Wilson disease. The typical diagnostic concentration is more than 250 g per gram dry weight of liver, commonly more than 1000 g/g. Copper toxicity in the kidneys

may lead to nephrocalcinosis, hematuria, and aminoaciduria, but urinalysis is not diagnostic of the underlying disorder. Infectious mononucleosis due to Epstein-Barr virus may manifest with fatigue and hepatomegaly but generally does not cause jaundice. This patient has no other signs of infection and her psychiatric symptoms predate the current illness.

(Section 22: Disorders of the Liver and Biliary Tract)

Answer 22-26. e

Neonatal hemochromatosis is a form of neonatal liver failure characterized by an in utero onset of hepatic and extrahepatic iron deposition. It is unrelated to the iron accumulation caused by hereditary hemochromatosis that is seen in adults. Neonatal hemochromatosis results from a gestational alloimmune response to a fetal liver antigen that crosses the placenta. The occurrence of severe neonatal iron storage disease in at-risk pregnancies can be significantly reduced by treatment with high-dose intravenous immunoglobulin during gestation. The rate of recurrence in subsequent newborns after the index case is 60% to 80%. Liver biopsy in these patients reveals changes consistent with chronic liver disease. Extrahepatic siderosis can be demonstrated by either biopsy of a minor salivary gland or magnetic resonance imaging of the pancreas and/or heart. Infants with neonatal hemochromatosis have an expected mortality of more than 90% unless prompt treatment and/or liver transplantation is undertaken.

(Section 22: Disorders of the Liver and Biliary Tract)

Answer 22-27. b

The term *PFIC* denotes a group of inherited disorders of bile formation, often presenting in infancy and associated with progression at a variable rate to end-stage liver disease. Type 1 commonly presents in the first year of life with pruritus and jaundice. Patients with this type may also have extrahepatic manifestations such as malabsorption and pancreatitis. Type 3 may present at any age and generally progresses more slowly. The pruritus is usually less severe in type 3. Types 1 and 2 exhibit low or normal γ-glutamyl transferase, while this is elevated in type 3. Benign recurrent intrahepatic cholestasis is characterized by attacks of jaundice and pruritus separated by symptom-free intervals. Progression to cirrhosis and long-term complications of chronic liver disease do not occur. Dubin-Johnson syndrome is a disorder of conjugated hyperbilirubinemia due to defective transport of organic anions. It may present with jaundice, in the absence of pruritus, and follows a relapsing course. Breast milk jaundice develops rapidly and presents as unconjugated hyperbilirubinemia in the second week of life, usually resolving by 1 to 3 months of life. It does not cause pruritus.

(Section 22: Disorders of the Liver and Biliary Tract)

Answer 22-28. c

Administration of TPN is associated with liver disease. TPN-associated cholestasis is defined as a conjugated bilirubin greater than 2 mg/dL in an individual receiving

TPN who has no evidence of another underlying primary liver disease. Risk factors for TPN-associated liver disease include low birth weight, prematurity, sepsis, and longer length of time receiving TPN. TPN-associated cholestasis has been reported to occur in as many as 90% of children who receive intravenous nutrition for more than 3 months. TPN-associated liver disease may progress to liver failure and cirrhosis. It is reasonable to expect that this patient who had just 10 cm of bowel resected would tolerate full enteral nutrition over time. Enteral feedings, even in small amounts, have been shown to stimulate bile flow and lessen the degree of cholestasis. Various components of TPN and lipids have been implicated in the pathogenesis of TPN-induced liver disease including dextrose, manganese, lipids, phytosterols, and others.

(Section 22: Disorders of the Liver and Biliary Tract, Chapter 422: Drug, Toxin, and TPN Liver Disease)

Answer 22-29. b

Cystic fibrosis is a multisystem disease that results from a genetic defect in the cystic fibrosis transmembrane conductance regulator, a chloride channel found in the respiratory, intestinal, and biliary epithelium. This defect leads to the accumulation of thick mucus in these organs. Liver disease in cystic fibrosis occurs in several different forms and affects up to 50% of patients. In most cases, the course is benign and does not progress to end-stage liver disease. However, a minority of patients may develop biliary cirrhosis and associated complications. They may also develop complications of the biliary system such as gallstones and sludge in the gallbladder.

This condition is seen more commonly in males by a ratio of 3:1. Ursodeoxycholic acid decreases the viscosity of bile and displaces hepatotoxic bile acids, and has been shown to be beneficial in cystic fibrosis–associated liver disease.

(Section 22: Disorders of the Liver and Biliary Tract, Chapter 423: The Liver in Systemic Disease)

Answer 22-30. a

Acute liver failure in adults has been defined as the presence of hepatic encephalopathy and uncorrectable coagulopathy within 8 weeks of the development of clinical jaundice, in the absence of known preexisting chronic liver disease. The definition of acute liver failure in pediatrics differs from that used in adults, in part because of the difficulty of detecting hepatic encephalopathy, particularly the earlier stages, in infants and small children.

The criteria for acute liver failure in pediatrics are: (1) no known evidence of chronic liver disease, (2) biochemical evidence of acute liver injury, and (3) hepatic-based uncorrectable coagulopathy defined as an INR greater than or equal to 1.5 in the presence of clinical hepatic encephalopathy or (3a) an INR ≥2.0 without hepatic encephalopathy.

This patient is in acute liver failure of unknown etiology. Possible etiologies in his age group include infection, toxins,

ischemia, metabolic, and immune conditions. His synthetic function is abnormal as shown by his elevated bilirubin and INR. Hyperbilirubinemia can be seen in both acute and chronic liver disease. Some patients with acute liver failure do require transplantation. The cause of acute liver failure is an important factor in determining whether transplantation therapy should be utilized.

(Section 22: Disorders of the Liver and Biliary Tract, Chapter 424: Acute Liver Failure)

Answer 22-31. d

Complications of acute liver failure can involve every organ system. Death is usually attributable to cerebral edema with or without herniation, massive hemorrhage of the upper intestinal tract from stress injury, sepsis, or multisystem organ failure. The child with acute liver failure should be cared for in a pediatric intensive care unit that allows close serial observation with surveillance for potential life-threatening complications, yet provides a quiet environment with minimal stimulation to prevent increases in intracranial pressure.

Susceptibility to infection is common and a result of poor host defenses. Blood and urine cultures should be obtained with any significant changes in clinical condition. Empiric antibiotics may be warranted if sepsis is suspected.

Careful attention to fluid status is required to prevent overhydration that may lead to cerebral edema. Fluid requirements may be in the range of 85% to 100% of maintenance fluids. Sedation usually is not needed, and the use of benzodiazepines should be avoided. Hypoglycemia and renal dysfunction are common. While patients may require intravenous dextrose, protein intake should be limited to 1 g/kg/day to decrease the risk of nephrotoxicity. Hyperammonemia is associated with the development of encephalopathy that may respond to lactulose that precipitates loose stools. Constipation, on the other hand, may lead to increased intracranial pressure and may worsen hepatic encephalopathy. Loperamide is an opioid receptor agonist that has a primary effect in the large intestine, with no central nervous system effects. Loperamide slows transit time in the intestine, as well as suppresses the gastrocolic reflex. Because of its effect on constipation, loperamide should be avoided in patients with acute liver failure.

(Section 22: Disorders of the Liver and Biliary Tract)

Answer 22-32. a

Portal hypertension is defined as a portal pressure gradient (portal vein to hepatic vein gradient) of above 10 to 12 mm Hg. The mechanism leading to portal hypertension is increased resistance to blood flow from the visceral or splanchnic portal circulation to the right atrium. In children, the location of this increased resistance and hence obstruction of portal flow can be at the prehepatic/presinusoidal, intrahepatic/sinusoidal, or postsinusoidal level. Thrombosis of the portal or hepatic veins is a common cause of portal hypertension in children.

Physical examination findings suggesting underlying liver disease such as ascites, hypersplenism, spider angiomas, clubbing, and bruising are often present. Imaging tests to confirm the presence of portal hypertension and define the portal venous anatomy include ultrasonography with Doppler examination, magnetic resonance angiography or contrast-enhanced computed topography, and ultimately mesenteric angiography. An upper endoscopy is often performed to determine a patient's risk of bleeding from esophageal varices.

(Section 22: Disorders of the Liver and Biliary Tract, Chapter 425: End-stage Liver Disease)

Answer 22-33. c

This patient has physical examination findings compatible with end-stage liver disease and is likely having a variceal upper gastrointestinal bleed. Placement of a nasogastric tube may puncture a varix and is relatively contraindicated when a variceal bleed is suspected.

The first step in management is hemodynamic stabilization via the administration of isotonic crystalloid or packed red blood cells. Concurrently, an intravenous infusion of octreotide may be started to reduce splanchnic blood flow. Once this is achieved, endoscopic evaluation is indicated to determine the source of bleeding and to perform therapeutic intervention.

Endoscopic band ligation is the method of choice in larger children; in those under 10 kg sclerotherapy is generally performed. Surgical management such as placement of a transjugular intrahepatic portosystemic shunt or splenic embolization is indicated for recurrent or uncontrollable bleeding. Placement of a Sengstaken-Blakemore tube, designed to balloon tamponade gastroesophageal variceal bleeding, is a temporizing measure used for uncontrollable bleeding.

(Section 22: Disorders of the Liver and Biliary Tract, Chapter 425: End-stage Liver Disease)

Answer 22-34. e

Development of ascites is a poor prognostic sign in children with chronic liver disease. Because sodium retention is one of the main mechanisms in the formation of ascites, restriction of sodium intake is an essential part of management.

A diagnostic paracentesis in which 10 to 20 mL of ascitic fluid is withdrawn can be safely performed even in patients with coagulopathy. Ascitic fluid should be inspected visually, and then sent for cell count, Gram stain and direct inoculation in blood culture media at the bedside, glucose, LDH, triglycerides, albumin, total protein, and amylase. Patients with ascites are predisposed to spontaneous bacterial peritonitis, but the most frequent organisms are gram-negative enteric flora and gram-positive cocci. Anaerobic infections are rare.

In liver disease, the ascitic fluid is a transudate that develops as a result of an increased portal venous pressure. The serum-to-ascites albumin gradient (SAAG) accurately identifies the presence of portal hypertension and is easily calculated by subtracting the ascitic fluid albumin value from the serum albumin value. A gradient greater than 1.1 g/dL is consistent

with portal hypertension. Patients with heart failure have ascites with a high protein concentration and thus a gradient less than 1.1 g/dL.

(Section 22: Disorders of the Liver and Biliary Tract, Chapter 425: End-stage Liver Disease)

Answer 22-35. b

NAFLD is the most common reason for unexplained abnormal liver tests in the pediatric population. Nonalcoholic steatohepatitis (NASH) is a subtype of NAFLD that includes steatosis, ballooning degeneration, and inflammation. NASH-related cirrhosis has been reported in children and thus early detection and referral is important for this serious disease. The majority of pediatric patients with NAFLD are obese, and many are clinically asymptomatic. Other etiologies of chronic liver disease must be excluded. The diagnosis of NAFLD is a histologic one, and liver biopsy is the gold standard to confirm the diagnosis. Ultrasonography is not completely diagnostic of NAFLD, potentially demonstrating hyperechoic tissue that may be fibrosis, rather than fatty infiltration or missing fatty infiltration all together. Lifestyle modification, including dietary changes and exercise, is the mainstay of treatment for NAFLD and NASH.

(Section 22: Disorder of the Liver and Biliary Tract, Chapter 426: Other Disorders of the Liver)

Answer 22-36. d

The presence of multiple serpiginous collateral veins surrounding a small or thrombosed portal vein is referred to as cavernous transformation of the portal vein. It leads to elevated portal resistance and portal hypertension. It is the result of the body's effort to maintain hepatopetal portal flow to a normal liver in the face of thrombotic occlusion of the extrahepatic portal vein. Umbilical catheter placement is a known cause of portal vein thrombosis.

Extrahepatic biliary atresia and choledochal cysts are abnormalities of the biliary system. While patients with these disorders may develop portal hypertension later in life, they would not have collateral vessels visible on ultrasound. This patient has no jaundice to suggest TPN-related liver disease. Congestive heart failure may lead to passive congestion of the liver but would not cause the development of periportal collateral vessels.

(Section 22: Disorders of the Liver and Biliary Tract, Chapter 426: Other Disorders of the Liver)

Answer 22-37. a

This patient most likely has a choledochal cyst, a malformation of the common bile duct that most commonly presents with jaundice, abdominal pain, and a right upper quadrant mass. Patients may also present with fever due to cholangitis, nausea and vomiting, and associated pancreatitis. The etiology of cyst formation is unclear, although there is growing evidence that the dilation results from an anomalous junction of the common bile duct and the pancreatic duct that may allow for the reflux of pancreatic proteases into the extrahepatic biliary tree, resulting in cholangitis and stenosis.

Eighty percent of patients with choledochal cysts are females, and most present during the first decade of life. These patients may have abnormal serum aminotransferase, bilirubin, and pancreatic enzyme levels. The abnormality is most easily visualized on ultrasound. Endoscopic retrograde cholangiopancreatography may provide better delineation of the anatomy, but a biopsy is not required to make the diagnosis. Early treatment is required to prevent hepatic complications including fibrosis. The most worrisome complication of choledochal cyst is the high incidence of associated malignancy. This has led to the recommendation that cysts be completely excised with concurrent removal of the gallbladder.

(Section 22: Disorders of the Liver and Biliary Tract, Chapter 427: The Biliary Tract)

Answer 22-38. d

This cholangiogram depicts the saccular and cystic dilation of the intrahepatic bile ducts and enlargement of the major intrahepatic and extrahepatic biliary passages seen in Caroli disease, a congenital ductal plate disorder. When this lesion is combined with the changes of congenital hepatic fibrosis, as is typically the case, the disorder is termed Caroli syndrome.

In extrahepatic biliary atresia, the extrahepatic bile ducts are not seen. In Alagille syndrome, there is commonly a paucity of the intrahepatic bile ducts. Budd-Chiari syndrome is a disorder of the hepatic veins, not the biliary system. A choledochal cyst appears as a singular cystic dilation at the level of the common bile duct.

(Section 22: Disorders of the Liver and Biliary Tract, Chapter 427: The Biliary Tract)

Answer 22-39. a

The finding of bile duct paucity on liver biopsy, in the setting of poor growth, is characteristic of Alagille syndrome, a multisystem, inherited disorder with highly variable clinical features. A paucity of bile ducts is considered the most important and constant feature of this disease. In addition to bile duct paucity, 3 other features including cholestasis, cardiac defects, skeletal abnormalities, characteristic facies, or ophthalmologic abnormalities are required for diagnosis.

Evaluation includes an echocardiogram to evaluate for cardiac anomalies and peripheral pulmonic stenosis, AP and lateral chest radiographs to allow evaluation for the presence of butterfly vertebrae, ophthalmologic examination to identify anterior chamber involvement, renal ultrasound and renal function testing to identify renal complications, and screening for early identification of any developmental delays. A skin biopsy is unlikely to be useful in evaluating the cause of this patient's liver disease.

(Section 22: Disorders of the Liver and Biliary Tract, Chapter 427: The Biliary Tract)

Answer 22-40. c

This infant's presentation with cholestasis and acholic stools is concerning for extrahepatic biliary atresia, a fibro-obliterative cholangiopathy resulting in obstruction of the common bile duct as its central component. In infants with possible biliary atresia it is important to make a diagnosis promptly since the success of surgical intervention decreases with age. Diagnosis and surgical treatment before 45 days of age is considered optimal.

Ultrasound is important for ruling out other anatomic causes of cholestasis such as a choledochal cyst, but nonvisualization of the gallbladder is not specific for biliary atresia. Hepatobiliary scintigraphy has traditionally been used to demonstrate an absence of bile secretion into the intestinal lumen. As this infant is only 5 weeks old and there is some time to make the diagnosis, this noninvasive test is the next step. If the infant were older, a percutaneous liver biopsy would likely be performed immediately. Liver biopsy, when interpreted by an experienced pathologist, can be valuable for differentiating between biliary atresia and other causes of neonatal cholestasis. However, there are no pathognomonic findings on biopsy, and the gold standard for diagnosis is an intraoperative cholangiogram. Cardiac abnormalities may be seen in syndromic forms of biliary atresia, but an echocardiogram is not immediately helpful in making the diagnosis. Hemoglobinopathies and galactosemia (diagnosed with elevated urine-reducing substances) usually result in an indirect hyperbilirubinemia. Infants with cystic fibrosis, diagnosed by sweat chloride testing, may present with liver disease, but because biliary atresia is a time-sensitive diagnosis, sweat testing would not be the next step.

(Section 22: Disorders of the Liver and Biliary Tract, Chapter 427: The Biliary Tract)

Answer 22-41. b

Cholelithiasis refers to the presence of gallstones within the gallbladder or bile ducts, whereas choledocholithiasis is the presence of gallstones in the common bile duct. The 3 most common types of stones include cholesterol stones, black pigmented stones, and brown pigmented stones. Hemolytic disease such as sickle cell anemia is associated with an increased risk of black pigmented stones that are composed of calcium salts and bilirubin.

Ursodeoxycholic acid is a mainstay of conservative management for cholesterol stones but is not effective for pigmented stones. The dilation of the common bile duct on this patient's ultrasound is concerning for choledocholithiasis. Thus, cholecystectomy combined with an intraoperative cholangiogram is indicated. Endoscopic retrograde cholangiopancreatography may also be done preoperatively or postoperatively for retained stones or if the cholangiogram does not demonstrate stone clearance.

(Section 22: Disorders of the Liver and Biliary Tract, Chapter 427: The Biliary Tract)

CHAPTER 23 | Disorders of the Blood

James Huang and Tannie Huang

23-1. The mother of a 4-year-old patient calls to report that she noticed he has developed red spots and purplish bruises on both of his legs, some of which are firm and palpable, even though he denies any history of trauma. Moreover, he told his mother that his most recent stool appeared bloody. You ask that they go to the ED where a CBC reveals that his platelet count is 397×10^9/L. You suspect Henoch-Schönlein purpura (HSP). Which of the following findings would be consistent with your diagnosis?

   a. Decreased factor VIII level

   b. Wet purpura (purpura in the oral mucosa)

   c. Elevated blood pressure

   d. Hypofibrinogenemia

   e. Prolonged prothrombin time

23-2. You are asked to evaluate a 5-year-old with persistently elevated hemoglobin. The p50 (the partial pressure of oxygen at which the patient's hemoglobin is 50% saturated with oxygen) is 20 mm Hg (normal is 26 mm Hg) and his hemoglobin saturation curve is left shifted. This suggests that his polycythemia is due to which of the following?

   a. Chuvash polycythemia

   b. Presence of a *JAK2* mutation

   c. Living at high altitude

   d. Cyanotic cardiac disease

   e. Higher-affinity hemoglobin

23-3. A neonate's blood differs from that of older children and adults in many respects. Which of the following correctly describes a characteristic that is particular to the neonate?

   a. The RBC of the neonate has a low MCV that increases as the patient ages.

   b. Newborns have a high hemoglobin concentration that declines over the first 2 days of life.

   c. Neonatal RBCs contain primarily embryonic hemoglobin.

   d. Newborn blood has higher oxygen affinity than that of a 1-year-old.

   e. The neonate has higher levels of protein C than a 1-year-old.

23-4. You are counseling a family about iron supplementation after their son was found to have iron-deficiency anemia on routine screening at his 1-year well-child visit. Which of the following is true about supplementation for iron deficiency?

   a. All iron supplementation, regardless of formulation, should be taken with milk.

   b. Proton pump inhibitors can improve the absorption of iron supplementation.

   c. To avoid gastrointestinal pain, iron should always be taken with food.

   d. The hemoglobin begins to rise within 1 week of starting iron supplementation.

   e. Taking iron supplementation with orange juice can improve absorption.

23-5. Which of the following correctly orders the sequence with which the laboratory findings of iron deficiency become evident?

   a. Decreased iron stores and decreased ferritin > decreased transferrin saturation, increased zinc protoporphyrin > anemia, microcytosis

   b. Decreased transferrin saturation, increased zinc protoporphyrin to heme ratio > decreased iron stores and decreased ferritin > anemia, microcytosis

   c. Decreased iron stores and decreased ferritin > anemia, microcytosis > decreased transferrin saturation, increased zinc protoporphyrin to heme ratio

   d. Increased iron stores and increased ferritin > decreased transferrin saturation, increased zinc protoporphyrin to heme ratio > anemia, microcytosis

   e. Decreased iron stores and decreased ferritin > decreased transferrin saturation, decreased zinc protoporphyrin to heme ratio > anemia, microcytosis

23-6. A patient with juvenile rheumatoid arthritis is found to be mildly anemic, with a hemoglobin of 10.5 g/dL. His iron studies show normal transferrin saturation and an elevated ferritin level. You suspect that he has anemia of chronic disease. Which of the following is likely to have contributed to his anemia?

   a. Decreased hepcidin levels

   b. Increased ferroportin expression

   c. Decreased intestinal iron absorption

   d. Enhanced release of iron from macrophages

   e. Increased renal iron excretion

23-7. A 2-year-old boy presents to your office with pallor and fatigue. His mother tells you that he is a picky eater who drinks at least 32 oz of milk each day. His laboratory studies reveal a hemoglobin of 4.8 g/dL and a MCV of 51 fL. You suspect iron-deficiency anemia. In counseling the mother, you tell her that:

   a. The patient should drink milk when taking the iron you are prescribing.

   b. The patient should continue to drink milk as it is a good source of iron.

   c. Milk should be avoided because it contains phytates that chelate iron.

   d. Milk proteins can irritate the GI tract and lead to microscopic blood loss.

   e. The patient will require iron therapy for 1 month.

23-8. A 4-year-old girl presented to your office with fever and dysuria 1 week ago. Her urinalysis is positive for leukocyte esterase and nitrites. Her urine culture eventually grew out >100,000 *E. coli*. You started her on a course of trimethroprim–sulfamethoxazole. Her fever and dysuria resolved completely, but the mother returns to the clinic today for the development of a rash. On examination, she is well appearing, but there are multiple punctate nonblanching macular purplish spots on her arms, legs, and trunks. You obtain a CBC that shows a white blood cell count of 1.7×10^9/L, hemoglobin of 7 g/dL, and platelets of 25×10^9/L. What is the *most* likely cause of her laboratory findings?

   a. Acute lymphoblastic leukemia

   b. Drug effect

   c. Viral suppression

   d. Congenital bone marrow failure syndrome

   e. Aplastic anemia

23-9. A 3-year-old male comes to your clinic to establish care. He is well appearing and does not have abnormal physical examination findings. His growth and development have been excellent. However, his mother tells you that he has been diagnosed with Fanconi anemia after a brother died of complications of chemotherapy for treatment of infant acute myeloid leukemia. Which of the following is true regarding his diagnosis?

   a. No additional follow-up is needed other than genetic counseling when he is older, unless he develops symptoms.

   b. Diagnostic testing for Fanconi anemia includes measurement of telomere length.

   c. He may need frequent electrolyte replacement therapy to make up for his urinary losses.

   d. Patients with bone marrow failure can undergo treatment with oxymetholone, but many patients eventually become resistant to androgen therapy.

   e. Once he undergoes stem cell transplant, his risk of cancer will decrease to that of the normal population.

23-10. A 9-month-old previously healthy male is brought to your office by his mother for decreasing activity levels. He has not had any fevers or complaints of pain. He has marked pallor, but the rest of his examination, including an abdominal examination, is normal. The mother tells you that he drinks 10 oz of milk a day and is not a picky eater. You obtain a CBC that shows a white blood cell count of 12×10^9/L, hemoglobin of 5 g/dL, and platelets of 273×10^9/L. His differential is normal, with no blasts. His MCV is 86 fL, and his reticulocyte count is <1%. A test for parvovirus is negative. Of the following, which test will likely be helpful in rendering a diagnosis?

   a. Serum iron level

   b. Hemoglobin electrophoresis

   c. Erythrocyte adenosine deaminase

   d. G6PD enzyme levels

   e. Lead level

23-11. You are seeing a 15-year-old patient with Fanconi anemia for her well-child visit and sports physical. Her blood counts have been stable with persistence of a mild macrocytic anemia and thrombocytopenia. On physical examination, you notice that she has a painless ulceration on the lateral aspect of her tongue. She denies knowledge of any antecedent trauma to the tongue. You suspect that this is:

   a. Due to an enteroviral infection and will self-resolve

   b. Due to a herpes virus and prescribe acyclovir

   c. Squamous cell cancer and refer to an otolaryngologist

   d. Leukoplakia that is commonly seen in FA patients

   e. Oral candidiasis and prescribe nystatin

23-12. You are seeing a 3-year-old patient new to your practice who has had long-standing mild pancytopenia and macrocytosis. You entertain the diagnosis of an inherited bone marrow failure syndrome that is associated with pancytopenia. Your leading considerations are congenital amegakaryocytic thrombocytopenia, Diamond-Blackfan anemia (DBA), dyskeratosis congenita, Fanconi anemia (FA), and Shwachman-Diamond syndrome. These syndromes also have in common what other feature?

a. Increased risk of malignancy

b. Absent thumb

c. Pancreatic insufficiency

d. Mutation in cMPL, the TPO receptor

e. Elevated erythrocyte adenosine deaminase (eADA) activity

23-13. You are seeing a 2-year-old boy whose family has recently moved to your area for his initial visit. His past medical history is notable for bilateral pollicization surgeries (surgery to create thumbs from fingers) for his congenitally absent thumbs. The parents also report that at the time of surgery, he was found to have a slightly low platelet count, but he did not need a transfusion before the surgery. In addition to repeating the CBC, you decide to order an abdominal ultrasound. Which of the following tests will confirm the diagnosis that you suspect?

a. Bone marrow aspirate and biopsy

b. Radiographs of forearms

c. Telomere length assays for leukocyte subsets

d. Chromosome fragility test with diepoxybutane (DEB)

e. Erythrocyte adenosine deaminase levels

23-14. A newborn female develops jaundice at 12 hours of life. Her indirect bilirubin is 21.2 mg/dL. His mother's blood type is AB+; her blood type is A+. Her direct Coombs test is negative. Her CBC is as follows:

WBC: 15.2×10^9/L
Hgb: 10 g/dL
Hct: 30%
MCV: 98 fL
MCHC: 37 g/dL
Platelets: 275×10^9/L
What is the next best step?

a. G6PD enzyme activity in erythrocytes

b. Hemoglobin electrophoresis

c. UGT1A1 activity

d. Osmotic fragility

e. Abdominal ultrasound

23-15. A 2-year-old girl is being evaluated for persistent anemia. She was a term newborn who was found to be jaundiced on the first day of life. Blood type of both the mother and the patient is O+. The father has had mild anemia all of his life, and he reports that his father (the paternal grandfather) had a splenectomy for an unspecified blood disorder. The patient's current labs show a hemoglobin of 10.9 g/dL, MCHC of 38 g/dL (31-36), reticulocyte count of 300×10^9/L, a total bilirubin of 1.8 mg/dL, and the following peripheral blood smear (Figure 433-2A):

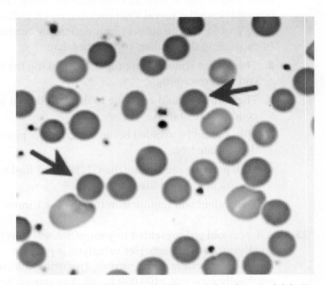

FIGURE 433-2A. (Reproduced, with permission, from Rudolph CD, et al. *Rudolph's Pediatrics*. 22nd ed. New York: McGraw-Hill, 2011.)

You tell the parents that:

a. The patient has normal blood because she is not anemic.

b. The patient's condition will improve after treatment with steroids.

c. The patient needs iron supplementation.

d. The patient likely has a defect in the RBC membrane–cytoskeletal complex.

e. The patient likely has an autosomal recessively inherited hemolytic anemia.

23-16. A 15-month-old male is brought to your office with a fever. He is well appearing without any localizing signs. You order a urinalysis that is positive for leukocyte esterase and nitrites. You start him on trimethroprim–sulfamethoxazole. The urine culture eventually grows out 100,000 colonies of *E. coli*. Two days later, his mother returns to your office. She reports that he has been irritable and his eyes have turned a yellow color. She also reports that his urine has turned a dark brown color. His urinalysis is positive for blood, although there are only a few red blood cells on microscopic analysis. You check his hemoglobin and find that it is 8.5 g/dL. What is the best test to diagnose the etiology of this patient's illness?

   a. Parvovirus antibody

   b. Glucose-6-phosphate dehydrogenase (G6PD) enzyme testing

   c. Allergy testing

   d. CK levels

   e. Serum creatinine

23-17. A 5-year-old with a history of hereditary spherocytosis presents with pallor and fatigue. One week ago, he was seen by his primary care doctor for a fever and runny nose. He was diagnosed with an upper respiratory tract infection at that time. His mother reports that his fevers and runny nose resolved, but over the past several days he has developed progressive fatigue and pallor. His vital signs are as follows: temperature 36.7, heart rate 160, RR 26, and BP 110/54. On examination, you note an extremely pale child. A complete blood count reveals:

   White blood cell count: 13×10^9/L
   Hemoglobin: 5.4 g/dL
   Hematocrit: 16.2%
   Platelets: 164×10^9/L
   Reticulocyte count: <1%

   What test will likely reveal an underlying etiology?

   a. Parvovirus B19 PCR

   b. Direct antibody testing

   c. Stool blood testing

   d. PTT

   e. Bone marrow biopsy

23-18. A 5-year-old male presents with pallor and fatigue. Two weeks ago, he was seen by his primary care doctor for a fever and runny nose. He was diagnosed with an upper respiratory tract infection at that time. His mother reports that his fevers and runny nose resolved, but over the past several days he has developed progressive fatigue and pallor. On examination, you note an extremely pale child. Temperature 36.7, heart rate 160, RR 26, and BP 110/54. A complete blood count reveals:

   White blood cell count: 13×10^9/L
   Hemoglobin: 5.4 g/dL
   Hematocrit: 16.2%
   Platelets: 134×10^9/L
   Reticulocyte count: 210×10^9/L
   Direct antiglobulin test positive for IgG

   What is the best treatment for this patient?

   a. Plasmapheresis

   b. Corticosteroids

   c. IVIG

   d. Splenectomy

   e. Antithymocyte antiglobulin

23-19. A 14-year-old male presents with sudden onset of left upper quadrant abdominal pain. Doppler ultrasound reveals a hepatic vein thrombosis. His past medical history is significant for aplastic anemia, which was diagnosed at age 10. He was treated with antithymocyte antiglobulin and cyclosporine, with good recovery of his counts. His current blood counts are all within normal ranges.

   What laboratory test will be likely to reveal an etiology for his thrombosis?

   a. Protein C

   b. Factor V Leiden

   c. Bone marrow biopsy

   d. Homocysteine levels

   e. Flow cytometry

23-20. A 16-year-old female with a history of systemic lupus erythematosus presents with a temperature of 38.8. Her heart rate is 125, blood pressure is 145/85, respiratory rate 16, and oxygen saturations 100% on room air. When you examine her, she is uncooperative and combative. Her cardiovascular examination is notable for a systolic murmur heard best at the left lower sternal border. Her lungs are clear to auscultation bilaterally. Her abdomen is soft and nontender; she has no hepatosplenomegaly.

Her laboratory results are as follows:

White blood cell count: 16.5×10^9/L
Hemoglobin: 7 g/dL
Hematocrit: 21%
Platelets: 72×10^9/L
Smear notable for schistocytes

Na: 135 mmol/L
K: 4.1 mmol/L
Cl: 108 mmol/L
CO_3: 25 mmol/L
BUN: 35 mg/dL
Cr: 2.25 mg/dL

What is the best diagnostic test for this patient?

a. ADAMTS13 levels
b. Stool culture for *Escherichia coli* O157:H7
c. Bone marrow biopsy
d. Direct Coombs test
e. Blood culture

23-21. A 4-year-old presents with petechiae after a diarrheal illness and is found to have thrombocytopenia and hypertension. His stool studies are positive for *E. coli* 0157: H7. Which of these lab results would be expected?

a. Normal RBCs
b. Positive direct Coombs test
c. High haptoglobin
d. Low LDH
e. Elevated creatinine

23-22. A newborn whose mother is known to have sickle cell trait, and whose father has β-thalassemia trait, has a newborn screen from day of life 1 that reveals the presence (in alphabetical order) of hemoglobin A, hemoglobin F, and hemoglobin S. You can conclude that:

a. The patient has sickle cell anemia.
b. The patient has hereditary persistence of fetal hemoglobin.
c. The patient has 1 normal β-globin gene.
d. The patient has sickle cell trait.
e. The patient has β-thalassemia trait.

23-23. Although sickle hemoglobin is present only in red blood cells, patients with sickle cell anemia are at risk of having multiple organs damaged as a consequence of either hemolysis or vaso-occlusion arising from sickled RBCs. Which of the following studies is routinely performed to assess the likelihood of damage to a target organ?

a. Audiology examination to assess the risk of hearing loss
b. Renal ultrasound to assess the risk of hyposthenuria
c. Bone density scan to assess bone damage from vaso-occlusive crises
d. Chest radiograph to assess the risk of pulmonary hypertension
e. Transcranial Doppler ultrasound to assess the risk of stroke

23-24. A 5-year-old female with a history of sickle cell anemia comes to the emergency room with fever and a cough. She looks otherwise well, but her chest x-ray shows a right lower lobe pneumonia. Which of the following would be the best antibiotic regimen for this patient?

a. Amoxicillin and clavulanic acid
b. Amoxicillin and clindamycin
c. Ceftriaxone and azithromycin
d. Ceftriaxone and vancomycin
e. Ciprofloxacin monotherapy

23-25. Which of the following are completed yearly as part of the comprehensive care of a pediatric patient with sickle cell disease?

a. Chest radiographs
b. Transcranial Dopplers
c. Biliary ultrasounds
d. Pulmonary ventilation–perfusion scans
e. Glomerular filtration rate

23-26. A 5-year-old African American boy with HIV is taking dapsone for PCP prophylaxis due to a sulfa allergy. He presents with tachypnea and fatigue, and appears cyanotic, but his oxygen saturation does not improve with supplemental oxygen. You suspect pseudocyanosis from methemoglobinemia as a complication of dapsone therapy. Before you treat him with methylene blue, you ask about the family history or personal history of which of the following disorders?

a. Cyanotic heart disease
b. Glucose-6-phosphate dehydrogenase (G6PD) deficiency
c. Pyruvate kinase deficiency
d. Scott syndrome
e. Hereditary spherocytosis

23-27. Which of the following is frequently observed in patients with sickle cell *trait*?

   a. Microcytic anemia

   b. Priapism

   c. Hematuria

   d. Stroke

   e. Normal hemoglobin electrophoresis

23-28. You are seeing a 15-month-old patient who has microcytosis (MCV 55), mild anemia (Hgb 10 g/dL), and normal serum iron. You recall that his newborn screen showed a small amount of abnormal hemoglobin (hemoglobin Barts), so you order a repeat hemoglobin electrophoresis. The results are normal. You suspect he has the following:

   a. Silent carrier for α-thalassemia

   b. α-Thalassemia trait

   c. β-Thalassemia trait

   d. Hemoglobin H disease

   e. α-Thalassemia major

23-29. A baby is born to parents who are both known to have β-thalassemia minor due to heterozygosity for β^0 mutations. The baby is found to have a normal hematocrit at birth. You conclude that:

   a. The patient does not have thalassemia major.

   b. A diagnosis for thalassemia cannot be made until 6 months of age.

   c. Hemoglobin electrophoresis should be done now.

   d. The patient has a 25% chance of having thalassemia trait.

   e. The patient has a 50% chance of having thalassemia major.

23-30. You are seeing a 3-year-old Vietnamese female for the first time. The mother reports that she has a history of iron-deficiency anemia, which was originally diagnosed around 1 year of age when routine screening revealed a hemoglobin of 10.5 g/dL. The mother admits that it is often difficult to get her daughter to take the iron regularly, and that it often gives her constipation. You send more blood work that shows:

   White blood cell count: 6.8×10^9/L
   Hemoglobin of 10.6 g/dL
   Platelets of 302×10^9/L
   Mean corpuscular volume is 59 fL
   Red blood cell count: 5.41×10^{12}/L
   Ferritin: 45 (normal: 12-160 ng/mL)
   Transferrin saturation: 35 (normal: 20%-50%)
   Serum iron: 35 (normal: 26-170 µg/dL)

A hemoglobin electrophoresis shows Hgb A 98%, hemoglobin A2 2%, and no Hgb S or F
Smear: Many hypochromic microcytic cells noted. Multiple target cells noted

Given these lab findings, what is the most likely diagnosis?

   a. Iron deficiency

   b. β-Thalassemia major

   c. α-Thalassemia trait

   d. Intestinal malabsorption

   e. β-Thalassemia intermedia

23-31. You are counseling a father about the treatment options for his child with β-thalassemia major. In addition to the increased risk of infection, splenectomized patients are at an increased risk of which of the following?

   a. Aplastic anemia

   b. Increased bleeding

   c. Cancer

   d. Renal failure

   e. Thrombosis

23-32. Based on a screening transcranial Doppler, it is determined that your patient with sickle cell disease is at high risk for stroke. You are counseling the family on starting chronic transfusion therapy. After hearing of the risk of iron overload, the parents ask you to anticipate when he will need to start chelation therapy. You tell them chelation will start:

   a. Only if he has the mutations for hereditary hemochromatosis

   b. As soon as he starts the transfusions

   c. Only if he shows symptoms of iron overload

   d. After he has received approximately 200 mL/kg of PRBCs

   e. As soon as his ferritin is above the normal range

23-33. A healthy newborn is circumcised in the nursery prior to discharge. After the circumcision, his wound continues to ooze blood despite pressure and bandaging. His laboratory studies reveal the following: PT is 15.9 seconds (12.2-15.8 seconds) and his PTT is 80 seconds (25-60 seconds), and his platelet count is 200×10^9/L (145-450×10^9/L). Factor VII is 35% (40%-150%), factor VIII 12% (43%-168%), factor IX 30% (60%-160%), and vWF antigen 150 (42%-190%). You conclude that the patient likely has:

   a. Factor VII deficiency

   b. Hemophilia A

   c. Hemophilia B

   d. von Willebrand disease type III

   e. A platelet defect

23-34. You are evaluating a patient with hereditary hemorrhagic telangiectasia (HHT), and you note multiple punctate telangiectasias on his lips and tongue. Which of the following is true regarding this patient's disorder?

   a. Although this syndrome is characterized by telangiectasias, these are benign entities that do not need to be investigated further.

   b. The most common presenting symptom is frequent epistaxis.

   c. Telangiectasias only form on the viscera.

   d. Bleeding into the joints is common, leading to arthritis and limited mobility.

   e. Patients frequently have soft tissue hypertrophy of 1 extremity.

23-35. Deficiency of which of the following vitamins is associated with increased risk of thrombosis?

   a. Vitamin A

   b. Vitamin D

   c. Vitamin C

   d. Vitamin K

   e. Vitamin E

23-36. You are counseling a mother on nutrition for her children. She is very interested in the roles that vitamins play in health. Which of the following is appropriate advice?

   a. Vitamin C deficiency can lead to mucosal bleeding.

   b. Vitamin K is only important in the synthesis of procoagulants.

   c. Vitamin E deficiency leads to decreased clot generation.

   d. Vitamin B_{12} deficiency is common in infants.

   e. Folic acid (vitamin B_9) has no role in blood production.

23-37. A 2-year-old boy is being evaluated for easy bruising and epistaxis. His family history is notable for his mother who had heavy menstrual periods as a teenager, but has not had any formal evaluation. On examination, his skin is doughy and elastic, and he has increased joint mobility. There are no telangiectasias in his nares or on his skin. His laboratory studies reveal a normal PT/PTT, and CBC, his ristocetin cofactor level is 98%, his von Willebrand antigen level is 110%, and his factor VIII level is 90%. You suspect that he has:

   a. A mutation in the endoglin gene (*HHT1*)

   b. vWD type I

   c. vWD type II

   d. vWD type III

   e. Ehlers-Danlos syndrome

23-38. You are counseling a 17-year-old boy with mild hemophilia A and his parents about the use of desmopressin (DDAVP) prior to his upcoming wisdom teeth extraction. In discussing the possible complications associated with DDAVP, you tell them that DDAVP may lead to:

   a. Hypernatremia

   b. Flushing

   c. Thrombocytopenia

   d. Inhibitor development

   e. Diuresis

23-39. You are evaluating a boy who has frequent nose bleeds and a prolonged aPTT. His family history is notable for a maternal uncle and a first cousin (the son of mom's sister) who have been diagnosed with "hemophilia." You find that he has a factor VIII level of 120%. You suspect he most likely has:

   a. Type 2N vWD

   b. Type 3 vWD

   c. Type 1 vWD

   d. Hemophilia A

   e. Hemophilia B

23-40. You are evaluating a 15-year-old from the Aland Islands, an autonomously governed Swedish-speaking part of Finland, for her menorrhagia. She has had heavy periods since the onset of her menses, and reports that she also bruises easily, has frequent nosebleeds, and had prolonged bleeding after a tooth extraction. There is a history of menorrhagia for many of the women on her maternal side, beginning with her great grandmother who was diagnosed with "pseudohemophilia" by Dr Erick von Willebrand. Her mother tells you that the family's diagnosis has since been reclassified as von Willebrand disease. Her laboratory studies show: platelet count, 180×10^9/L; von Willebrand factor activity (vW:RCof), 40%; von Willebrand antigen (vW:Ag), 35%; normal distribution of vWF multimers; factor VIII activity of 70%. You conclude that she has type 1 von Willebrand disease. The most important criterion used in establishing this diagnosis is:

   a. Clinical history and family history

   b. Ristocetin cofactor level

   c. von Willebrand antigen level

   d. Factor VIII level

   e. vWF multimer

23-41. You are evaluating an 8-year-old, premenarchal girl with a history of easy bruising. Her mother is concerned about the possibility of the patient having von Willebrand disease because the mother has been diagnosed with von Willebrand disease type 2B. The patient has no prior surgeries, and no history of frequent nosebleeds. Which of the following set of labs would be most consistent with the patient having the same diagnosis as her mother?

   a. Platelet count, 180×10^9/L; von Willebrand factor activity (vW:RCof), 28%; von Willebrand antigen (vW:Ag), 30%; factor VIII activity, 50%; slightly decreased, but normal distribution of vWF multimers; no platelet aggregation in response to low-dose ristocetin

   b. Platelet count, 200×10^9/L; von Willebrand factor activity (vW:RCof), 10%; von Willebrand antigen (vW:Ag), 32%; factor VIII activity, 50%; absent high- and intermediate-sized vWF multimers; no platelet aggregation in response to low-dose ristocetin

   c. Platelet count, 0×10^9/L; von Willebrand factor activity (vW:RCof), 40%; von Willebrand antigen (vW:Ag), 45%; factor VIII activity, 80%; absent high-molecular-weight multimers; platelets do aggregate in response to low-dose ristocetin

   d. Platelet count, 200×10^9/L; von Willebrand factor activity (vW:RCof), 10%; von Willebrand antigen (vW:Ag), 32%; factor VIII activity, 50%; slightly decreased, but normal distribution of vWF multimers; no platelet aggregation in response to low-dose ristocetin

   e. Platelet count, 180×10^9/L; von Willebrand factor activity (vW:RCof), 40%; von Willebrand antigen (vW:Ag), 45%; factor VIII activity, 8%; slightly decreased, but normal distribution of vWF multimers; no platelet aggregation in response to low-dose ristocetin

23-42. A 4-year-old boy presents with a history of epistaxis and easy bruising. His mother reports that she has been diagnosed with von Willebrand disease type 2M. The patient's von Willebrand panel results are as follows: von Willebrand activity (ristocetin cofactor, von Willebrand factor [vWF]:RCo) 15% (>50%), von Willebrand antigen (vWF:Ag) 30% (>50%), factor VIII activity 55% (>50%), and absence of large and intermediate-sized vWF multimers. Based on these results, you tell the mother that the patient:

   a. Has type 2M vWD

   b. Has type 2A vWD

   c. Does not have vWD

   d. Likely can be treated with DDAVP

   e. Has type 1 vWD

23-43. A 14-year-old girl is being seen for menorrhagia. She has always bruised easily and has a past history of frequent nosebleeds that have since resolved. Her mother reports that she also has heavy periods, and her mother, the patient's grandmother, is reported to have had a hysterectomy because of heavy periods. The patient's laboratory studies are as follows: hemoglobin 10.5 g/dL, platelet 300×10^9/L, normal PT and PTT, von Willebrand activity (ristocetin cofactor, vWF:RCo) 28% (>50%), von Willebrand antigen (vWF:Ag) 30% (>50%), factor VIII activity 55% (>50%), and normal distribution, but slightly diminished amounts of vWF multimers. You conclude that the patient has:

   a. von Willebrand disease type 1

   b. von Willebrand disease type 2A

   c. von Willebrand disease type 2M

   d. von Willebrand disease type 2N

   e. von Willebrand disease type 3

23-44. A 2-year-old boy with severe hemophilia A, who has not had any hemarthroses since starting prophylaxis 1 year ago, begins to have knee bleeds that are refractory to his usual treatment dose of recombinant factor VIII. Laboratory studies reveal an inhibitor of 11 Bethesda units (BU). You inform his parents that:

   a. Inhibitors occur in 90% of severe hemophilia A patients.

   b. It is not possible to eradicate the inhibitor.

   c. His titer of 11 BU is considered a low-titer inhibitor.

   d. Immune tolerance therapy may eradicate the inhibitor.

   e. The inhibitor is likely to spontaneously resolve.

23-45. A 3-year-old boy presents with prolonged bleeding from a torn frenulum that occurred when he fell against the coffee table. Parents report that both he and his 5-year-old sister tend to bruise easily, but there is no known bleeding disorder in the family. His laboratory studies reveal a normal platelet count and PT, a PTT of 60 seconds (23-34), von Willebrand activity (ristocetin cofactor, vWF:RCo) 45% (>50%), von Willebrand antigen (vWF:Ag) 48% (>50%), factor VIII activity 6% (>50%), and normally distributed, but slightly diminished amounts of vWF multimers. His sister also has a prolonged PTT, with a factor VIII activity of 9%. You suspect that this patient and his sister have:

   a. Mild hemophilia A

   b. von Willebrand disease type 1

   c. von Willebrand disease type 2A

   d. von Willebrand disease type 2N

   e. von Willebrand disease type 3

23-46. An 18-year-old patient with type 1 von Willebrand disease is planning to undergo wisdom teeth extraction. Because he has previously been shown to respond well to intranasal desmopressin (DDAVP), he will be using DDAVP and aminocaproic acid (an antifibrinolytic) as coverage for his procedure. You remind him that:

a. DDAVP may result in retention of free water.

b. He should use DDAVP daily for 7 days.

c. He should increase his daily intake of fluids.

d. DDAVP will decrease factor VIII levels.

e. DDAVP should be used 4 times a day.

23-47. A newborn baby is noted to have profuse bleeding after circumcision, requiring urological intervention. On further questioning, the mother reports that she has a history of heavy periods, and that she recalls an aunt who needed a transfusion after childbirth. You send off some preliminary lab work that shows a white blood cell count of 12×10^9/L, hemoglobin of 9 g/dL, and platelets of 372×10^9/L. PTT 37 seconds, PT 13.1 seconds, and fibrinogen 202 mg/dL. Factor VIII activity is 9%, and factor IX activity 35%. Of the following choices, what is the *most* likely diagnosis?

a. von Willebrand disease

b. Disseminated intravascular coagulation

c. Hemophilia B

d. Afibrinogenemia

e. Vitamin K deficiency

23-48. A 12-year-old girl presents with menorrhagia and a history of significant bleeding 4 days after a tonsillectomy. Her family history is notable for her having a brother who had an intracranial hemorrhage in the newborn period as a full-term newborn, and for her mother having had 3 miscarriages. Her PT, PTT, platelet count, and peripheral smear are all normal, as is her von Willebrand panel. You suspect the following:

a. Decreased clot solubility

b. Increased clot solubility

c. Elevated factor XIII level

d. Decreased factor V level

e. Increased protein C level

23-49. A 2-year-old is brought to the ED after being found playing with a rodenticide. His INR is 3.5 and you suspect that he has ingested a vitamin K antagonist commonly used in rodenticides. Which of the following factors is expected to be normal?

a. Factor II

b. Factor V

c. Factor VII

d. Factor IX

e. Factor X

23-50. A 1-week-old presents to your office with bruising and coffee ground emesis. She was a term baby who was born at home, and is now exclusively breastfed. Her PT is >100 seconds, and her PTT is 160 seconds. This patient has:

a. Low factor VIII level

b. Low factor V level

c. Factor V Leiden

d. Low factor VII level

e. Cystic fibrosis

23-51. Which of the following is associated with an increased risk of thrombosis?

a. Thrombocytopenia

b. Prothrombin gene mutation

c. Factor V deficiency

d. Nephritic syndrome

e. Homocysteine deficiency

23-52. A 16-year-old girl was started on oral contraceptive pills for acne 2 months ago. She presents with a swollen and painful left leg. Doppler ultrasound reveals a thrombus in her left iliac and femoral veins. She is placed on anticoagulation with subsequent resolution of her clot. You obtain studies after stopping anticoagulation 6 months after her presentation. Which one suggests that she has a higher risk of thrombosis than the normal population?

a. Protein C activity of 165% (76-146)

b. Antithrombin activity of 102% (79-120)

c. Factor VIII activity level of 97% (43-168)

d. Factor V that is resistant to cleavage by activated protein C (APC)

e. Plasma homocysteine level of 7 μmol/L (4-14)

23-53. A 6-year-old male is brought into your clinic because his mother has noticed increased bruising. She reports that he has been otherwise doing well with no fevers and normal appetite and activity levels. He is well appearing, but you note multiple bruises on his trunk and legs. The rest of his examination is unremarkable. You obtain labs that show:

WBC: 8.4×10^9/L
Hgb: 13 g/dL
Platelets: 15×10^9/L

You suspect immune thrombocytopenic purpura (ITP). Which of the following is true about this disease?

a. The diagnosis must be confirmed by a bone marrow biopsy.

b. He should be given platelet transfusions to minimize his bleeding risk.

c. Laboratory testing for platelet autoantibodies should be performed by the blood bank.

d. Most patients will have resolution of their symptoms within 3 months.

e. Once this episode resolves, the patient will be at an increased risk to develop leukemia.

23-54. You are asked to evaluate a term newborn, born to a healthy G1P1 mother after an uncomplicated pregnancy and delivery, who is noted to have petechiae and prolonged oozing after a heel stick for the newborn screen. Aside from petechiae over his face and chest, he is a well-appearing newborn. Of note, he has normal thumbs and forearms, and no hepatosplenomegaly. A CBC is obtained from his cord blood that is normal except for a platelet count of 12×10^9/L. His mother has a normal platelet count. In addition to a head ultrasound to evaluate for the possibility of intracranial hemorrhage, which of the following is the most appropriate next step?

a. Transfusion of maternal platelets since the patient may have neonatal alloimmune thrombocytopenia (NAIT)

b. Abdominal ultrasound to evaluate for renal anomalies since Fanconi anemia is in the differential

c. IVIG because the patient may have maternally derived neonatal autoimmune thrombocytopenia

d. TORCH titers to evaluate for the possibility that his symptoms are due to CMV infection during the pregnancy

e. Platelet aggregation studies to rule out the possibility of Glanzmann thrombasthenia

23-55. A full-term infant is admitted to the nursery after an uncomplicated delivery to a G1P1 mother. He is noted to have multiple bruises. A complete blood count shows a white blood cell count of 17×10^9/L, hemoglobin of 15 g/dL, and platelets of 24×10^9/L. The mother's platelet count is normal, and the infant's HPA-1a testing is positive. You diagnose neonatal alloimmune thrombocytopenia (NAIT). What is the next best course of action?

a. Transfusion of maternal platelets

b. Transfusion of random donor platelets

c. Observation

d. IVIG

e. Steroids

23-56. You are asked to evaluate an otherwise well term newborn baby boy who presented with petechiae at birth and was found to have a platelet count of 70×10^9/L. His physical examination is normal and no infectious source is identified. His family history is notable for his mother and a maternal aunt and uncle with hearing loss and easy bruising. Additionally, his uncle is on dialysis for renal failure. Which test would you order next?

a. X-rays of his forearms

b. Diepoxybutane chromosome breakage test

c. Examination of his peripheral blood smear

d. Bone marrow aspirate and biopsy

e. Platelet aggregation studies

23-57. A 17-year-old girl on the varsity cross-country team presents with menorrhagia for her last 2 periods. Prior to this, she has had normal periods since menarche at age 12. There is no family history of bleeding symptoms or a bleeding disorder. She does report frequent use of ibuprofen following long training runs. Laboratory studies show: hemoglobin 11.5 g/dL, platelet count 170×10^9/L, a peripheral smear that is normal in appearance, normal PT and PTT, and a normal von Willebrand panel with von Willebrand activity (ristocetin cofactor, vWF:RCo) 55%, von Willebrand antigen (vWF:Ag) 60%, factor VIII activity 76%, and normal vWF multimers. You suspect that the patient has:

a. von Willebrand disease type 1

b. Acquired cyclooxygenase deficiency

c. May Hegglin (a MYH9-related disorder)

d. Factor VII deficiency

e. Immune thrombocytopenia (ITP)

23-58. You are seeing a 1-year-old boy for a well-child visit. In reviewing his history, you note that he has had 4 episodes of otitis media and 1 hospitalization for pneumonia, and has had eczema since 4 months of age. You obtain a screening CBC and note that he has Hgb of 11 g/dL, WBC of 6×10^9/L, and a platelet count of 47×10^9/L. The pathologist notes that the platelets appear small. You suspect that this patient has:

a. Thrombocytopenia absent radius

b. Wiskott-Aldrich syndrome (WAS)

c. Fanconi anemia

d. Congenital amegakaryocytic thrombocytopenia

e. Hyper-IgE syndrome

23-59. A 1-year-old female is brought to the emergency room by her mother with fever and irritability for 1 day. On examination, you find a toxic-appearing infant, with a temperature of 39.5, HR of 168, BP 108/68, and a RR of 34. She has no abnormal lymphadenopathy. You hear clear breath sounds in both lung fields, and she is tachycardic with a systolic flow murmur. Her abdomen is nontender with no hepatosplenomegaly. You do not note any rashes. You obtain labs, including a complete blood count, and blood and urine cultures. A complete blood count shows a white blood cell count of 17×10^9/L, hemoglobin of 13 g/dL, and platelets of 1105×10^9/L. Her blood culture eventually grows out *Streptococcus pneumoniae*. She is admitted and treated with antibiotics. What is the most likely cause of her high platelet count?

a. Familial thrombocytosis

b. Essential thrombocytosis

c. Iron-deficiency anemia

d. Reactive thrombocytosis

e. Kawasaki disease

23-60. A 4-year-old boy presents with epistaxis and a history of easy bruising. There is no family history of bleeding problems. The patient's laboratory studies are as follows: normal PT, PTT; normal von Willebrand panel with von Willebrand activity (ristocetin cofactor, vWF:RCo) 85%, von Willebrand antigen (vWF:Ag) 90%, factor VIII activity 105%, and normal vWF multimers. A CBC showed Hgb of 12 g/dL, WBC 6.5 × 10^9/L, and platelet count of 140×10^9/L, and large platelets were noted on the smear. Platelet aggregation studies showed a lack of response to ristocetin. The most likely diagnosis is:

a. Bernard-Soulier syndrome

b. Glanzmann thrombasthenia

c. Shwachman-Diamond syndrome

d. Kostmann disease

e. Pearson syndrome

23-61. A 3-year-old boy presents with prolonged epistaxis and a history of easy bruising. There is no family history of bleeding problems. The patient's laboratory studies show a normal CBC and smear, normal von Willebrand panel, and normal PT and PTT, but platelet aggregation showed no response to adenosine diphosphate (ADP), thrombin, and epinephrine, and platelets were found to lack GpIIb/IIIa. The most likely diagnosis is:

a. Bernard-Soulier syndrome

b. Glanzmann thrombasthenia

c. Shwachman-Diamond syndrome

d. Kostmann disease

e. Pearson syndrome

23-62. You are counseling the family of a 6-year-old girl with severe hereditary spherocytosis who is considering splenectomy regarding the complications following the procedure. You explain that after splenectomy, she is likely to have an elevated platelet count because:

a. She may have undiagnosed subclinical ITP that improves with splenectomy.

b. Splenectomy increases the risk of essential thrombocythemia.

c. This is a lab artifact from the machine misreading unfiltered RBC fragments.

d. Approximately 30% of the platelet mass normally resides in the spleen.

e. She will be in a constant inflammatory state due to infections after splenectomy.

23-63. A newborn with cardiac anomalies and heterotaxy is being evaluated for Ivemark syndrome. Additionally, he is found to have an elevated platelet count. You suspect that this may be due to his underlying syndrome. Which of the following would confirm your hypothesis?

a. Presence of Howell-Jolly bodies on the smear

b. Positive test for a mutation in JAK2

c. Elevated erythrocyte sedimentation rate

d. Decreased number of RBC pits

e. Low serum iron levels

23-64. A 13-year-old African American female comes to your clinic. A routine blood count done to screen for iron deficiency revealed an absolute neutrophil count of 900×10^6/L. The rest of her blood count was normal. She has been healthy all her life, with no hospitalizations or serious infections. She denies any mouth ulcers or gingivitis. She is not on any medications. As far as the family knows, there is no history of inherited bone disorders or children who died at young ages. Which of the following is the *most* likely diagnosis?

a. Myelokathexis

b. Reticular dysgenesis

c. Kostmann syndrome

d. Ethnic pseudoneutropenia

e. Glycogen storage disease type 1b

23-65. An 18-month-old male presents to your clinic to establish care. His mother reports that he has been hospitalized multiple times. He was hospitalized at 2 months of age for *E. coli* urosepsis. He was hospitalized again at 9 months of age for pneumonia. She reports that since then, he seems to have fevers on a monthly basis, but has not needed to be hospitalized. She reports that he occasionally has "cold sores" around the time of his febrile episodes, but otherwise has been doing well.

On physical examination, his vital signs are T 37.6, HR 110, RR 16, and BP 90/58; weight is 10 kg. He is well appearing, and active in your office. His head is normocephalic, pupils are reactive, and tympanic membranes are well visualized with a good light reflex. Cardiac examination reveals no heart murmurs. Lungs are clear to auscultation bilaterally. Abdomen is soft, nontender with no hepatosplenomegaly. He has normal tone and bulk.

You obtain a CBC that shows a white blood count of 5.4×10^9/L, a hemoglobin of 13 g/dL, and platelets of 350×10^9/L. His absolute neutrophil count is 3500 cells/μL. What further evaluation would be needed to establish a diagnosis?

a. Complete blood counts 3 times a week

b. Quantitative immunoglobulin levels

c. Bone marrow biopsy

d. HIV testing

e. No further testing needed

23-66. You are asked to see an 8-month-old infant who is hospitalized for pneumonia and failure to thrive. The child has a history of steatorrhea and pancreatic insufficiency. His laboratory studies show a WBC of 4.1×10^9/L with an ANC of 900×10^6/L, Hgb 10.5 g/dL, MCV 92 fL, and platelet 102×10^9/L. His sweat test is normal. You suspect that he has a mutation in:

a. *TERT* associated with dyskeratosis congenita

b. *CFTR* associated with cystic fibrosis

c. *RMRP* associated with cartilage-hair hypoplasia

d. *SBDS* associated with Shwachman-Diamond syndrome (SDS)

e. All of the above

23-67. Shwachman-Diamond syndrome, Chediak-Higashi syndrome, severe congenital neutropenia, cyclic neutropenia, and cartilage-hair hypoplasia all have which of the following in common?

a. Increased risk of malignancy

b. ELA2 mutations

c. Ribosome dysfunction

d. Neutropenia

e. Platelet dysfunction

23-68. A 6-year-old female is admitted for fever and pneumonia. The mother reports that she has been admitted several times for various bacterial infections. On physical examination, her vital signs are T 40.2, HR 190, RR 50, and BP 70/38; oxygen saturation level is 92% on room air. She is ill-appearing. Her heart rate is tachycardic, and a systolic murmur is appreciated. Her abdomen is soft, nontender. Please see figure below for further clinical findings. Of the following options, which is mostly likely to be true regarding this patient?

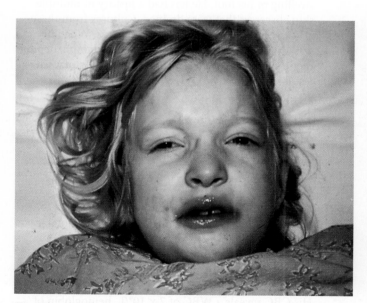

(Reproduced, with permission, from Weinberg S, Prose NS, Kristal L. *Color Atlas of Pediatric Dermatology*. 4th ed. New York: McGraw-Hill, 2007.)

a. She has pancreatic insufficiency.

b. She has nail dystrophy.

c. She has triphalangeal thumbs.

d. She has peripheral neuropathy.

e. She has elevated IgE levels.

23-69. A 3-month-old male is admitted for pneumonia after presenting with a 1-day history of fever and increased work of breathing. In taking his history, his mother notes that his umbilical cord did not fall off until about a month of age. On physical examination, his vital signs are T 40.2, HR 180, RR 50, BP 70/38, and oxygen saturations 92% on 1 L of oxygen. He is sleepy and ill-appearing. His head is normocephalic, his pupils are reactive, and his tympanic membranes are well visualized with a good light reflex. His heart rate is tachycardic, and a systolic murmur is appreciated. He is tachypneic with crackles and decreased breath sounds on the right side. His abdomen is soft, nontender with no hepatosplenomegaly. He has normal tone and bulk. You obtain labs and start him on antibiotics. His CBC shows a white blood cell count of $32,000 \times 10^6$/L, a hemoglobin of 12.5 g/dL, and platelets of 550×10^9/L. His absolute neutrophil count is $29,000 \times 10^6$/L. What is the most likely diagnosis?

a. Leukemoid reaction

b. Acute leukemia

c. Leukocyte adhesion deficiency-1 (LAD-1)

d. Drug reaction

e. Myeloproliferative disease

23-70. A 10-year-old male is admitted for osteomyelitis of his right fourth metatarsal after presenting with pain and swelling of his foot. He has had a history of multiple skin abscesses that were drained. Cultures from these abscesses grew out *Staphylococcus aureus*. When he was 5 years old, he also had 1 episode of lymphadenitis requiring antibiotics. Given this patient's history, what test is mostly likely to reveal a diagnosis?

a. Bone marrow biopsy

b. Dihydrorhodamine test

c. IgE levels

d. Skin biopsy

e. Lymphocyte subsets

23-71. You are evaluating a 3-year-old boy who has an eczematous rash. His past medical history is notable for a hospitalization at 8 months of age for pneumonia and 15 episodes of otitis media in the first year of life. His physical examination is unremarkable except for a pruritic, papular rash on his face and extremities. His CBC reveals a WBC of 7×10^9/L, hemoglobin of 11 g/dL, and platelet count of 150×10^9/L. His serum IgG level is 600 IU/mL and IgE level 3000 IU/mL. You conclude that he has:

a. Wiskott-Aldrich syndrome

b. Hyper-IgE syndrome

c. Thrombocytopenia absent radii (TAR)

d. Leukocyte adhesion defect

e. Milk protein allergy

23-72. A 10-year-old male was involved in car accident and is brought to the emergency department. He has multiple fractures and lacerations. His initial vital signs show a heart rate of 135 beats/min and a blood pressure 80/40 mm Hg. He is intubated; a chest tube is placed for a pneumothorax, and he is taken to the operating room where he is found to have a splenic rupture. His initial CBC shows a hemoglobin of 5.4 g/dL and a hematocrit of 16.2%. He requires 12 U of PRBCs before his vital signs and hemoglobin stabilize. His fractures are repaired in the operating room. You are checking labs on him later in the night and notice the following laboratory findings:

Na: 135 mmol/L
Cl: 105 mmol/L
K: 5.1 mmol/L
CO_3: 31 mmol/L
BUN: 25 mg/dL
Cr: 0.7 mg/dL
Ca: 7.6 mmol/L
Mg: 2.1 mmol/L
PO_4: 4.5 mmol/L
Amylase: 10 U/L
Lipase: 16 U/L

The most likely cause of this patient's laboratory abnormalities is:

a. Acute renal failure

b. Postoperative SIADH

c. Citrate toxicity

d. Sepsis

e. Traumatic pancreatitis

23-73. A 16-year-old female with menorrhagia presents to the emergency room with fatigue and is found to have a hemoglobin level of 6.2 g/dL. She is transfused 2 U of packed red blood cells. This episode is her first transfusion. Within minutes of starting the transfusion, she develops shortness of breath, her oxygen saturation drops to 80%, and her blood pressure is 70/30. Her temperature is 37°C. The transfusion is immediately stopped and she is given diphenhydramine, hydrocortisone, and epinephrine. What test should be included in the evaluation of her transfusion reaction?

a. Chest x-ray

b. IgE levels

c. IgA levels

d. Skin allergy testing

e. Early morning cortisol level

23-74. A 12-year-old male who is undergoing chemotherapy for acute lymphoblastic leukemia has chemotherapy-induced pancytopenia, for which he receives a blood transfusion. After the transfusion starts, he develops vomiting, fever, and chills. He does not have any rash or shortness of breath. His blood transfusion is stopped, with rapid resolution of his symptoms. Shortly afterwards, his urine turns dark colored and cloudy. What other findings are consistent with the patient's clinical picture?

    a. New infiltrate on chest x-ray

    b. Metabolic alkalosis

    c. Hypocalcemia

    d. Low haptoglobin

    e. Polycythemia

23-75. One of your patients is going to the operating room tomorrow for cardiac surgery. The surgeon asks you to get consent from the family for possible blood transfusion. Which of the following is not routinely screened at the blood bank?

    a. Hepatitis A

    b. Hepatitis B

    c. Hepatitis C

    d. Human immunodeficiency virus

    e. Human T-lymphotrophic virus-1 (HTLV-1)

ANSWERS

Answer 23-1. c

Patients with HSP may have renal involvement, which may lead to hypertension. Therefore, evaluation of patients suspected of HSP should include careful attention to vital signs for evidence of renal involvement, including close attention to evidence of hypertension. The petechiae and purpura associated with HSP are characteristically in the lower extremities rather than mucosal. Although patients have petechiae and purpura, the lesions arise from vasculitis and are not due to coagulopathy, so fibrinogen and clotting factor levels and prothrombin time are normal.

(Page 1537, Section 23: Disorders of the Blood, Part 1: Principles of Blood Disorders, Chapter 428)

Answer 23-2. e

A leftward-shifted oxygen dissociation curve and a lower-than-normal p50 are consistent with an increased hemoglobin oxygen affinity. This results in less oxygen release to the tissues, and thus a compensatory increase in hemoglobin. Figure 434-4 shows a graphic display of effects of pH, 2,3-BPG, and temperature on oxygen affinity. Chuvash polycythemia is due to mutations in the von Hippel-Lindau gene, which is part of the oxygen sensing apparatus. *JAK2* mutations are associated with polycythemia vera. Patients living at high altitude and with cyanotic cardiac disease have increased red blood cell mass due to chronic hypoxia, but have normal hemoglobin oxygen affinity.

(Page 1537, Section 23: Disorders of the Blood, Part 1: Principles of Blood of Disorders, Chapter 428; Pages 1561-1562, Part 2: Disorders of Red Blood Cells and Anemia, Chapter 434)

Answer 23-3. d

Fetal hemoglobin has higher oxygen affinity than hemoglobin A. Newborn RBCs have high levels of fetal hemoglobin ($\alpha2\gamma2$)—approaching 70%. After birth, the percentage of fetal hemoglobin decreases after synthesis of γ-globin is replaced by β-globin synthesis. At 4 months of age fetal hemoglobin accounts for 40% of the total hemoglobin, and by 1 year of age, hemoglobin A ($\alpha2\beta2$) is predominant—98%. The higher oxygen affinity of fetal hemoglobin is due to its relative decrease in affinity for 2,3-bisphosphogylcerate (2,3-BPG) compared with HbA. The RBC of the neonate has a high MCV (on average 107 fL) that decreases in the first year of life, and then rises with age. Newborns have a high hemoglobin level that then rises in the first 2 days of life as plasma volume initially decreases postnatally. Protein C levels are low at birth and rise with age, reaching adult levels by adolescence.

(Pages 1539-1541, Section 23: Disorders of the Blood, Part 1: Principles of Blood Disorders, Chapter 429)

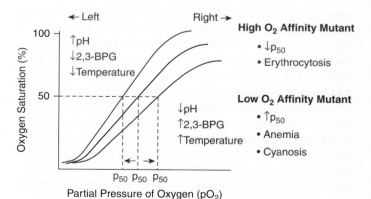

FIGURE 434-4. Oxyhemoglobin dissociation curve and its physiologic modulation and pathophysiologic perturbations. BPG, bisphosphoglycerate. (Reproduced, with permission, from Rudolph CD, et al. *Rudolph's Pediatrics.* 22nd ed. New York: McGraw-Hill, 2011.)

Answer 23-4. e

Iron deficiency is the most common global nutritional deficiency, and iron-deficiency anemia is the most common hematologic disease of infancy and childhood. Nonheme dietary iron comes primarily in the ferric state (Fe^{3+}) and is reduced to the ferrous state (Fe^{2+}) in an acidic environment. Ascorbic acid can therefore improve the absorption of iron. Iron supplementation should never be taken with milk, food, or proton pump inhibitors as these all inhibit the absorption of iron. Hemoglobin is one of the last indices to improve, although reticulocytosis can be seen within 1 week of starting iron supplementation.

(Pages 1546-1547, Section 23: Disorders of the Blood, Part 2: Disorders of Red Blood Cells and Anemia, Chapter 431)

Answer 23-5. a

Anemia and microcytosis are late findings in iron deficiency. First, in the pre–latent phase, iron stores are depleted and ferritin levels are typically low. Importantly, ferritin levels can remain normal or elevated if there is concurrent inflammation. This is followed by latent iron deficiency, which is evident in a decrease in transferrin saturation. The final step of heme formation is the incorporation of an iron molecule into the porphyrin ring. As the amount of iron being transported in the plasma decreases, there is less iron available to be incorporated into the porphyrin ring and a resulting rise in the ratio of zinc protoporphyrin to heme. Finally, with overt iron-deficiency anemia, there is a diminution in red blood cell volume and quantity. See Table 431-1 for laboratory values associated with different stages of iron deficiency.

(Pages 1546-1548, Section 23: Disorders of the Blood, Part 2: Disorders of Red Blood Cells and Anemia, Chapter 431)

Answer 23-6. c

Anemia of chronic disease is multifactorial and likely due to impaired iron mobilization and decreased intestinal absorption of iron. As in this vignette, the anemia is usually mild to moderate, normocytic, and normochromic. Serum iron levels are low, but transferrin saturation is normal and serum ferritin is typically elevated due to the inflammatory state. Additionally, in anemia of chronic inflammation, production of hepcidin, a peptide hormone synthesized by the liver, is increased. Hepcidin acts as a negative regulator of iron release by acting to decrease ferroportin expression. As ferroportin is required for both intestinal transport of iron and macrophage release of iron, the decrease in ferroportin leads to decreased iron absorption and decreased release of iron from macrophage stores. Humans do not have a mechanism of active iron excretion.

(Pages 1546-1548, Section 23: Disorders of the Blood, Part 1: Principles of Blood Disorders, Chapter 431)

Answer 23-7. d

Milk can contribute to the development of iron deficiency in multiple ways. It is a poor source of iron, so toddlers who rely primarily on milk for nutrition have insufficient iron intake. Milk contains proteins that can irritate the gastrointestinal tract of some patients and lead to microscopic blood loss, and milk inhibits the absorption of iron. Phytates are compounds found in plants; they can chelate iron and inhibit its absorption. Typical therapy for iron-deficiency anemia continues for several months after the anemia is corrected in order to replenish iron stores.

(Pages 1546-1548, Section 23: Disorders of the Blood, Part 2: Disorders of Red Blood Cells and Anemia, Chapter 431)

Answer 23-8. b

The patient developed pancytopenia after a course of TMP-SMX, which is known to cause bone marrow suppression. Other than the petechiae, she is well appearing with no fevers, hepatosplenomegaly, or pain that would point toward an underlying leukemia. The patient had a bacterial UTI, with no other signs of a concurrent viral infection. While this could be the first presentation of an acquired aplastic anemia or congenital bone marrow failure syndrome, these are relatively rare diseases, and drug effect is more likely.

(Page 1549, Section 23: Disorders of the Blood, Part 2: Disorders of Red Blood Cells and Anemia, Chapter 432)

Answer 23-9. d

Fanconi anemia is a result of defective double-strand DNA repair mechanisms. Up to 25% of patients have no physical abnormalities, but since marrow failure usually starts in the first decade of life, these patients should have quarterly blood counts and periodic bone marrow biopsies. Oral androgen treatment with oxymetholone would be an appropriate therapy. Androgen therapy yields an increase in RBCs in approximately half of patients in the first 2 months; it may take up to year for platelet counts and white blood cell counts to rise. Most patients lose the response to androgens as the bone marrow failure progresses.

Diagnostic testing is made by looking at chromosome breakage in peripheral blood lymphocytes cultured with mitomycin C or diepoxybutane. Telomere length testing is done to look for the diagnosis of dyskeratosis congenita. The only curative treatment for bone marrow failure due to Fanconi is hematopoietic stem cell transplant, although patients continue to have an increased risk for other solid tumors such as breast cancer and squamous cell carcinoma. Fanconi syndrome, a defect of the proximal tubules leading to loss of sodium, glucose, calcium, and phosphates, is unrelated to Fanconi anemia, although both of them were first described by the same physician, Swiss pediatrician Guido Fanconi.

(Page 1550, Section 23: Disorders of the Blood, Part 2: Disorders of Red Blood Cells and Anemia, Chapter 432)

Answer 23-10. c

The patient has anemia with a low reticulocyte count, indicating that the anemia resulted from a production failure. Erythrocyte adenosine deaminase levels help distinguish between Diamond-Blackfan anemia and transient erythrocytopenia of childhood (TEC), both of which can present with pure red cell aplasia. Diamond-Blackfan anemia is a bone marrow failure syndrome that results from a defect in ribosome biosynthesis, causing red blood cells to be sensitive to death by apoptosis. Patients have elevated levels of erythrocyte adenosine deaminase. Most patients can be treated with steroids, but some will need chronic transfusions. TEC is a diagnosis of exclusion that describes the temporary and spontaneous cessation of erythropoiesis. Patients are managed with supportive care and eventually recover.

Anemia in hemoglobinopathies and red cell enzyme mutations results from increased red cell turnover of the abnormal cells. They typically have high reticulocyte counts. Although the anemia seen in lead toxicity or iron deficiency is also from ineffective erythropoiesis, and patients can also have a low reticulocyte count, it is typically a microcytic anemia.

(Pages 1550-1551, Section 23: Disorders of the Blood, Part 2: Disorders of Red Blood Cells and Anemia, Chapter 432)

Answer 23-11. c

Fanconi anemia is an autosomal recessive syndrome of defective double-strand DNA repair. Patients with Fanconi anemia are at increased risk of squamous cell carcinoma as well as aplastic anemia, myelodysplastic syndrome, and acute myelogenous leukemia. In some patients, squamous cell carcinoma may be the initial manifestation of the disease. Congenital anomalies are common, presenting in more than half the patients—these include anomalies of the thumb and radius, as well as of the kidneys, esophagus, genitals, and head and neck.

The other answer choices are not associated with Fanconi anemia. Of note, leukoplakia is commonly seen in patients with dyskeratosis congenita, another bone marrow failure syndrome that also predisposes to squamous cells carcinoma as well as bone marrow failure.

(Pages 1550-1552, Section 23: Disorders of the Blood, Part 2: Disorders of Red Blood Cells and Anemia, Chapter 432)

Answer 23-12. a

Many inherited bone marrow failure syndromes are classically associated with a defect in one cell line; however, many progress to pancytopenia and aplastic anemia. Congenital amegakaryocytic thrombocytopenia, DBA, dyskeratosis congenita, FA, and Shwachman-Diamond syndrome all are associated with an increased risk of malignancy. Additionally, patients with thrombocytopenia absent radii (TAR), which is not bone marrow failure syndrome, have an increased risk of leukemia, although aplastic anemia has not been reported. TAR

patients may have hypoplastic or misplaced thumbs, but not the absent thumbs that are associated only with FA patients. Pancreatic insufficiency is a feature of Shwachman-Diamond syndrome as well as Pearson syndrome, which is another bone marrow failure syndrome, and which arises from mitochondrial DNA deletion. Mutations in cMPL are specific to CAMT, and elevated eADA is a diagnostic test for DBA.

(Pages 1550-1552, Section 23: Disorders of the Blood, Part 2: Disorders of Red Blood Cells and Anemia, Chapter 432)

Answer 23-13. d

The patient's thumb abnormalities and thrombocytopenia are symptoms frequently seen in patients with Fanconi anemia. While patients with thrombocytopenia absent radii (TAR) may have misplaced or hypoplastic thumbs, they are distinguished from Fanconi anemia patients who may have absent thumbs. Although the bone marrow of Fanconi anemia patients is often abnormal, the diagnostic test is confirmation of increased chromosomal fragility in the presence of DNA cross-linking agents such as DEB or mitomycin C.

Telomere length assays are useful in the diagnosis of dyskeratosis congenita, which is classically characterized by a triad of lacy pigmentation, oral leukoplakia, and dysplastic nails. Erythrocyte adenosine deaminase levels are elevated in Diamond-Blackfan anemia patients. Although patients with Diamond-Blackfan anemia may have hypoplastic thumbs, the hallmark of the disease is RBC aplasia, not thrombocytopenia.

(Pages 1550-1552, Section 23: Disorders of the Blood, Part 2: Disorders of Red Blood Cells and Anemia, Chapter 432)

Answer 23-14. d

The patient has hereditary spherocytosis, which can be confirmed by osmotic fragility testing. This patient's jaundice is not consistent with physiologic jaundice given the elevated bilirubin level within the first 24 hours of life. In this setting, with an MCHC of greater than 36 g/dL, the most likely diagnosis is hereditary spherocytosis in the newborn period. Outside the newborn period this typically presents as intermittent jaundice and palpable splenomegaly.

Neonates with G6PD deficiency can also present with nonphysiologic jaundice; however, G6PD deficiency is X-linked and this patient is a female. In addition, the MCHC is normal in patients with G6PD. Hemoglobin electrophoresis would delineate the type of hemoglobin present (ie, HbA, S, C). UGT1A1 activity is useful in the diagnosis of Gilbert syndrome and an abdominal ultrasound would not be clinically useful at this time.

(Pages 1553-1554, Section 23: Disorders of the Blood, Part 2: Disorders of Red Blood Cells and Anemia, Chapter 433)

Answer 23-15. d

The patient's elevated reticulocyte count indicates that her RBC turnover is increased, even though her anemia is mild. Further,

her increased MCHC, the presence of spherocytes on her smear, and elevated total bilirubin level all indicate a hemolytic anemia. While patients with autoimmune hemolytic anemia can also have spherocytes, the family history is suggestive of an autosomal dominantly inherited hemolytic anemia such as hereditary spherocytosis. Hereditary spherocytosis is a defect in the erythrocyte membrane that decreases the ability of the cell to deform and it becomes trapped in the sinusoids of the spleen, resulting in extravascular hemolysis. In iron-deficiency anemia, the RBCs are microcytic and hypochromic with a low MCHC. Autoimmune-mediated hemolytic anemia can be treated with corticosteroids. The treatment for hereditary spherocytosis is primarily supportive.

(Pages 1552-1556, Section 23: Disorders of the Blood, Part 2: Disorders of Red Blood Cells and Anemia, Chapter 433; Pages 1543-1545, Chapter 430)

Answer 23-16. b

This patient has signs of intravascular hemolysis with a low hemoglobin and hemoglobinuria. In the setting of a recent exposure to a sulfa-based antibiotic, the patient likely has G6PD deficiency. G6PD is an X-linked disorder. Although many patients are asymptomatic, they can present with intravascular hemolysis after exposure to certain triggers including infections, sulfa drugs, fava beans, or mothballs. Although parvovirus can lead to anemia, this is due to acute aplasia from destruction of early red blood cell precursors in the bone marrow. It does not lead to jaundice and hemoglobinuria. The reaction to sulfa drugs in patients with G6PD deficiency is not an IgE-mediated allergy. CK and creatinine levels would not be helpful in diagnosing the underlying etiology of this patient's hemolysis.

(Pages 1553-1554, Section 23: Disorders of the Blood, Part 2: Disorders of Red Blood Cells and Anemia, Chapter 433)

Answer 23-17. a

In patients with high rates of RBC turnover, such as patients with hemoglobinopathies, enzymopathies, hemolytic anemias, or erythrocyte membrane defects, infections with parvovirus B19 cause a low hemoglobin with a low reticulocyte count. The infection destroys early red blood cell precursors and causes red blood cell aplasia for about a week. Because red blood cells last approximately 120 days, most children are able to maintain adequate hemoglobin levels and are asymptomatic. However, patients who have higher rates of red blood cell turnover may not be able to maintain their levels and can develop severe anemia. Direct antibody testing and stool blood testing would be negative as this patient's anemia is due to decreased production of red blood cells. His PTT should be normal. A bone marrow biopsy would reveal decreased erythrocyte precursors; however, this would not reveal the underlying etiology.

(Page 1553, Section 23: Disorders of the Blood, Part 1: Principles of Blood Disorders, Chapter 433; Page 1559, Chapter 434)

Answer 23-18. b

Given the presence of IgG on the RBCs, this patient has warm-reactive autoimmune hemolytic anemia (AIHA). The IgG autoantibodies bind to red cell antigens; these opsonized cells are then cleared by the spleen, leading to the anemia and clinical symptoms described in this vignette. Warm-reactive AIHA is responsive to corticosteroids.

Splenectomy is used to treat refractory AIHA; it is only used after other treatment options have been exhausted since postsplenectomy patients are at an increased risk for infection. Plasmapheresis is only effective in cold-reactive AIHA, where circulating IgM antibodies can be cleared. IVIG and antithymocyte antiglobulin have not been shown to be effective.

(Page 1555, Section 23: Disorders of the Blood, Part 2: Disorders of Red Blood Cells and Anemia, Chapter 433)

Answer 23-19. e

Idiopathic thrombosis in males is extremely rare. The differential diagnosis includes underlying genetic thrombophilias and drug effects, but should also include paroxysmal nocturnal hemoglobinuria (PNH), a clonal disease characterized by chronic intravascular hemolysis and recurrent thrombosis. This patient most likely has PNH. Only about 25% of patients present with classic nocturnal hemoglobinuria. Patients with aplastic anemia and thromboses involving unusual sites should all be screened for PNH. In particular, PNH has been shown to develop more commonly in patients successfully treated with an antithymocyte antiglobulin and cyclosporine. Diagnosis has traditionally been made with a Ham acid test, which detects complement-mediated hemolysis. However, flow cytometry has become the standard for diagnosis.

Protein C, factor V Leiden, and homocysteine levels are associated with prothrombotic states; however, given this patient's history of aplastic anemia, PNH is the more likely diagnosis.

(Page 1556, Section 23: Disorders of the Blood, Part 2: Disorders of Red Blood Cells and Anemia, Chapter 433)

Answer 23-20. a

The patient has anemia, thrombocytopenia, and schistocytes that indicate a microangiopathic hemolytic anemia. The pentad of fever, microangiopathic hemolytic anemia, thrombocytopenia, renal disease, and neurologic disease is diagnostic of thrombotic thrombocytopenic purpura (TTP). Endothelial cells typically release large vWF multimers; these multimers are cleaved by a metalloproteinase, ADAMTS13. However, in patients with TTP, this metalloproteinase is absent, often because an antibody binds to ADAMTS13, rendering it inactive. The increased number of circulating vWF multimers promotes the formation of microthrombi, consuming platelets. Patients with autoimmune disorders, such as SLE, can develop a specific autoantibody inhibitor to ADAMTS13. More rarely, this can be caused by a germline genetic mutation in the ADAMTS13 gene.

The differential diagnosis for microangiopathic hemolytic anemia includes hemolytic uremic syndrome, as seen with infection from *E. coli* O157:H7, but these patients often present with bloody diarrhea and do not typically have neurologic changes. A bone marrow biopsy would not be useful in the diagnosis of TTP. A direct Coombs test would be helpful in patients with autoimmune hemolytic anemia; however, this does not present with schistocytes, and patients do not develop neurologic changes or renal dysfunction. ADAMTS13 levels would be more specific than blood cultures in making the diagnosis of TTP.

(Page 1556, Section 23: Disorders of the Blood, Part 2: Disorders of Red Blood Cells and Anemia, Chapter 433)

Answer 23-21. e

This child has hemolytic uremic syndrome (HUS) secondary to enterotoxic *E. coli*. Children will present with abdominal pain and fever. HUS is characterized by the triad of microangiopathic hemolytic anemia, thrombocytopenia, and acute renal failure. Given this patient's hypertension, it is likely he has laboratory evidence of acute renal injury as seen with an elevated creatinine. HUS leads to intravascular hemolysis; therefore, the red blood count is expected to be low and RBC fragments (schistocytes) are often seen on a blood smear. The hemolysis often leads to low haptoglobin as it is bound with hemoglobin from hemolyzed cells and an elevated LDH due to the cell lysis. The direct Coombs test, however, would be negative as patients with HUS do not have an antibody-mediated hemolysis.

(Page 1556, Section 23: Disorders of the Blood, Part 2: Disorders of Red Blood Cells and Anemia, Chapter 433)

Answer 23-22. d

The presence of hemoglobin A and hemoglobin S allows us to infer that the patient synthesizes both normal β-globin and $β^S$-globin chains. This indicates that one of her β-globin alleles makes wild-type β-globin, and the other β-globin allele makes sickle β-globin. Hence, the patient has sickle cell trait and not sickle cell anemia, where both β-globin alleles are $β^S$. Without information on the relative abundance of the HgbA versus HgbS, there is insufficient information to know whether the allele making β-globin is a wild-type allele or an allele that has diminished β-globin synthesis (a $β^+$), so no conclusion can be drawn as to whether the patient has a normal β-globin gene or has β-thalassemia. The major form of hemoglobin present in all newborns (except those with γ-chain mutations) is fetal hemoglobin, so no conclusion can be drawn as to whether the patient has persistence of fetal hemoglobin from a newborn screen done on day of life 1.

(Pages 1557-1558, Section 23: Disorders of the Blood, Part 1: Principles of Blood Disorders, Chapter 434)

Answer 23-23. e

Hemolysis and vaso-occlusion are the 2 main causes of complications from sickle cell disease (SCD) (see Figure 434-1). Transcranial Doppler ultrasounds are used to screen for sickle cell patients who are at increased risk of stroke. Clinical strokes occur in 11% of patients with SCD by the age of 18 years if they do not receive primary stroke prophylaxis and of those patients who have a clinically overt stroke, 50% to 90% have an additional stroke. Transcranial Dopplers are used to detect stenosis in the major cerebral arteries. Children with stenosis begin chronic transfusions to maintain their HbS concentration at less than 30% to decrease their stroke risk.

While sickle cell patients are at risk for renal dysfunction and pulmonary hypertension, and can have vaso-occlusive crises that cause bone damage, renal ultrasound, chest radiograph, and bone density scanning are not used to screen for these disorders, respectively. Screening for hearing loss is typically only used in sickle cell patients who are being chelated due to iron overload, as hearing loss is not linked directly to SCD.

(Pages 1557-1561, Section 23: Disorders of the Blood, Part 2: Disorders of Red Blood Cells and Anemia, Chapter 434)

Answer 23-24. c

This patient meets the criteria for acute chest syndrome, defined as fever and changes on chest x-ray. Acute chest syndrome is the leading cause of mortality for patients with sickle cell disease. There are many causes of acute chest syndrome, including infarction, atelectasis, pulmonary edema, bronchospasm, and infection. Although an infectious agent is often not identified, empiric antibiotic therapy with ceftriaxone and azithromycin is necessary to cover the usual respiratory pathogens, such as pneumococcus, as well as atypical bacteria such as *Mycoplasma* and *Chlamydia pneumoniae*. Supplemental oxygen and hydration are also mainstays of treatment.

(Pages 1559-1560, Section 23: Disorders of the Blood, Part 1: Principles of Blood Disorders, Chapter 434)

Answer 23-25. b

Without transfusion prophylaxis, symptomatic strokes occur in about 11% of sickle cell patients. Even asymptomatic children often have nonspecific white matter changes on MRI. Given the high rate of cerebrovascular disease, children with sickle cell disease should be screened yearly with a transcranial Doppler ultrasound of their major cerebral arteries. Those patients with abnormal ultrasounds should be started on a transfusion prophylaxis schedule. Although renal damage is common in patients with sickle cell disease, screening with a urinalysis and BUN and creatinine is sufficient. Similarly, although chronic lung damage is common in patients with sickle cell disease, chest radiographs and ventilation–perfusion scans are not necessary. Cholelithiasis, from chronic hemolytic anemia, is common even in young children; however, biliary ultrasounds do not need to be completed unless patients are symptomatic.

(Page 1560, Section 23: Disorders of the Blood, Part 2: Disorders of Red Blood Cells and Anemia, Chapter 434)

Answer 23-26. b

Methemoglobin is created when the iron component of hemoglobin is in the ferric state (Fe^{3+}), which cannot bind oxygen. This occurs throughout the RBC life cycle, but is typically reduced through an intracellular cytochrome b_5 reductase enzyme. There are congenital and acquired causes of methemoglobinemia, which occurs when the intracellular reductase pathways are overwhelmed or dysfunctional. In acquired methemoglobinemia, methylene blue is the treatment of choice. Methylene blue reduces methemoglobin via an alternative NADPH–flavin pathway. Importantly, the NADPH–flavin pathway requires G6PD to generate glutathione. In patients with G6PD deficiency, methylene blue is ineffective, and may cause hemolysis.

Patients with cyanotic heart disease are not pseudocyanotic. Both pyruvate kinase deficiency and hereditary spherocytosis are hemolytic anemias that do not affect the use of methylene blue. Scott syndrome is a qualitative platelet defect.

(Pages 1562-1563, Section 23: Disorders of the Blood, Part 2: Disorders of Red Blood Cells and Anemia, Chapter 434; Pages 1554-1555, Chapter 433)

Answer 23-27. c

Hematuria is often seen in patients with sickle cell trait. Sickle cell trait is the heterozygous state for the β^s gene. It is relatively common, affecting 1 in 12 African Americans. Although the red blood cells do not typically sickle, sickling can be observed in the renal medulla, which is a relatively acidic and hypertonic environment. This can lead to renal papillary necrosis and intermittent episodes of gross hematuria. Patients with sickle cell trait typically have about 30% to 40% hemoglobin S, which can be seen in hemoglobin electrophoresis. These patients otherwise have normal red blood cell indices, and do not typically suffer the vaso-occlusive complications of sickle cell disease.

(Pages 1560-1561, Section 23: Disorders of the Blood, Part 1: Principles of Blood Disorders, Chapter 434)

Answer 23-28. b

Hemoglobin Barts is a tetramer of 4 γ-globin chains. The presence of hemoglobin Barts in the neonatal period indicates that there is an excess of γ-globin chains relative to α-globin chains. (Remember, fetal hemoglobin is made up of $\alpha_2 \gamma_2$.) Once γ-chain synthesis is turned off and replaced by β-globin chains, a similar excess of β-globin would result in the formation of hemoglobin H (a tetramer of 4 β-globin chains). Since the repeat hemoglobin electrophoresis does not show the presence of hemoglobin H, the decrease in the amount of

α-globin is not as severe as that seen in hemoglobin H disease (3 α-globin gene mutations), but since the patient is slightly anemic and microcytic, the patient is not a silent carrier (single α-globin gene mutation). Hence, the patient likely has α-thalassemia trait (2 α-globin gene mutations). Patients with β-thalassemia trait have a relative excess of α-globin chains compared with β-globin chains.

(Page 1563, Section 23: Disorders of the Blood, Part 2: Disorders of Red Blood Cells and Anemia, Chapter 434)

Answer 23-29. c

β-Thalassemia is caused by mutations in the β-globin gene. Heterozygosity for the β-thalassemia gene results in a mild reduction of β-globin synthesis and a mild reduction in HbA production. Children born to parents who are both heterozygous for β-globin thalassemic mutations have a 50% chance of inheriting 1 mutant thalassemic allele and a 25% chance of inheriting both mutated alleles. Depending on the degree of compromise in synthesis of β-globin chains associated with the mutated alleles, these children may exhibit either the thalassemia intermedia or thalassemia major phenotype. However, because fetal hemoglobin ($\alpha_2 \gamma_2$) is the major hemoglobin at birth, patients who have no functioning β-globin alleles can have normal hematocrits at birth and do not become anemic until γ-globin chain synthesis is turned off. A hemoglobin electrophoresis should be done at birth. The hemoglobin electrophoresis will identify β-thalassemia major patients who synthesize no β-globin chains because it would show only the presence of hemoglobin F, without any hemoglobin A.

(Pages 1563-1566, Section 23: Disorders of the Blood, Part 2: Disorders of Red Blood Cells and Anemia, Chapter 434)

Answer 23-30. c

Microcytic anemia that is "refractory" to iron supplementation is most often caused by poor compliance. However, other causes must be considered, and in this patient, microcytic anemia with normal iron indices is most likely caused by an underlying thalassemia. This patient has a Mentzer index (MCV/RBC) of less than 13, which is indicative of an underlying thalassemia. A patient with β-thalassemia major or intermedia would have increased HgbA2 percentage. There are 4 α-globin genes. Patients with deletion of a single gene are asymptomatic "silent carriers" with no abnormal hematologic indices. Patients with a 2-gene deletion often have an asymptomatic microcytic anemia, as this patient does. Patients with 3 genes deleted have hemoglobin H disease and patients with a 4-gene deletion have hydrops fetalis.

(Pages 1563-1564, Section 23: Disorders of the Blood, Part 2: Disorders of Red Blood Cells and Anemia, Chapter 434)

Answer 23-31. e

Splenomegaly can be a complication of chronic transfusions, which is the mainstay of treatment for thalassemia major.

Chronic transfusions can decrease extramedullary hematopoiesis and prolong and improve quality of life. However, patients who develop splenomegaly have an increased transfusion requirement due to the associated hypersplenism and increased RBC clearance. As a result, splenectomy can be recommended. It is well known that asplenic patients are at higher risk of infection from encapsulated organisms, and should be immunized prior to splenectomy. However, these patients are also at higher risk for thrombosis and pulmonary hypertension. There is no known association between splenectomy and renal failure, malignancy, aplastic anemia, or increased bleeding.

(Page 1566, Section 23: Disorders of the Blood, Part 1: Principles of Blood Disorders, Chapter 434)

Answer 23-32. d

Because there is no physiologic mechanism for iron excretion, patients on chronic transfusion regimens inevitably develop iron overload, whether or not they have a genetic predisposition. However, chelation starts only after sufficient chelatable iron has accumulated, which usually occurs after approximately 200 mL/kg of PRBCs. The goal of chelation is to prevent the organ damage that gives rise to the symptoms of iron overload. These include endocrinopathies, cardiac dysfunction, and liver dysfunction. While ferritin is used to monitor the iron stores, it is not a precise measure as it fluctuates with inflammation as well. Hence, while it is useful to monitor trends, it should only be used in conjunction with more precise quantitation by liver biopsy or radiologic imaging methods.

(Page 1566, Section 23: Disorders of the Blood, Part 1: Principles of Blood Disorders, Chapter 434)

Answer 23-33. b

The levels of a number of procoagulant and antithrombotic factors are different in the neonate when compared with adult values. Notably, the vitamin K–dependent coagulation factors (II, VII, IX, X) are approximately half the adult values in the healthy newborn and rise to 80% by 6 months of age. Therefore, the factor VII and IX levels in this clinical scenario are normal for age. Factor VIII levels, however, are comparable to adult values in the healthy newborn. Thus, this patient's factor VIII level is abnormally low, even for a newborn. While low factor VIII levels can be seen in von Willebrand disease, von Willebrand antigen is absent in type III vWD patients. A qualitative platelet disorder is not ruled out by a normal platelet count; however, the presence of a low factor VIII in this patient makes hemophilia A (mild) the most likely diagnosis.

(Pages 1567-1568, Section 23: Disorders of the Blood, Part 3: Disorders of Coagulation and Platelets, Chapter 435; Pages 1570-1573, Chapter 436)

Answer 23-34. b

HHT, also known as Osler-Weber-Rendu syndrome, is most frequently present with epistaxis, and any patient presenting with frequent nosebleeds should be examined for mucosal telangiectasias leading to their symptoms. HHT is characterized by the cutaneous and visceral vasculopathies, including telangiectasias and arteriovenous malformations, which can lead to potentially life-threatening bleeding. This genetic disorder has been associated with mutation of the endoglin gene (*HHT1*) or of the activin receptor-like kinase 1 (alk1) gene (*HHT2*). Although synovial hemangiomas have been described in this syndrome, they are quite rare, and HHT patients generally do not have problems with joint bleeding and motility. Port wine stains, varicose veins, and soft tissue hypertrophy of 1 extremity are characteristic of Klippel-Trenaunay-Weber syndrome.

(Page 1568, Section 23: Disorders of the Blood, Part 3: Disorders of Coagulation and Platelets, Chapter 435)

Answer 23-35. e

Deficiency in vitamin E is associated with an increased risk of thrombosis, particularly in neonates, due to its role in platelet aggregation. Vitamin K deficiency leads to hemorrhagic disorders, since vitamin K is essential in the production of coagulation factors II, VII, IX, X, and proteins C and S. Increased bruising can be seen in vitamin C deficiency due to an inability to synthesize collagen. Vitamins A and D are not associated with either an increased bleeding or thrombosis risk.

(Page 1569, Section 23: Disorders of the Blood, Part 3: Disorders of Coagulation and Platelets, Chapter 435)

Answer 23-36. a

Vitamin C deficiency (scurvy) impairs collagen synthesis and can lead to mucosal bleeding, easy bruising, and poor wound healing. Vitamin K is required for production of both procoagulant and anticoagulant proteins. Vitamin E deficiency has been associated with the hypercoagulability in infants. B_{12} deficiency occurs rarely in infants, but can present in exclusively breastfed infants of vegan mothers. Folate is required for rapidly dividing cells, and thus is often supplemented in hemolytic anemias.

(Page 1569, Section 23: Disorders of the Blood, Part 3: Disorder of Coagulation and Platelets, Chapter 435; Page 1574, Chapter 437; Page 1543, Part 2: Disorders of Red Blood Cells and Anemia, Chapter 430)

Answer 23-37. e

As collagen is an integral component of blood vessels, collagen disorders can also present with bleeding symptoms. This patient's elastic skin and hypermobility is suggestive of Ehlers-Danlos syndrome. The endoglin gene is mutated in hereditary hemorrhagic telangiectasia (Osler-Weber-Rendu syndrome), which is characterized by the presence of skin and mucosal telangiectasias. His von Willebrand activity and antigen levels are well matched and within the normal range, making type

II and III vWD unlikely. Although these levels may be seen in vWD type I patients under certain circumstances, the lack of a clear family history and the presence of other clinical signs consistent with a collagen defect favor Ehlers-Danlos syndrome.

(Pages 1568-1569, Section 23: Disorders of the Blood, Part 3: Disorders of Coagulation and Platelets, Chapter 435; Pages 1571-1573, Chapter 436)

Answer 23-38. b

Flushing is a common side effect from DDAVP. DDAVP is a synthetic form of vasopressin (antidiuretic hormone). It can cause retention of free water, leading to hyponatremia and oliguria. In type 2B von Willebrand disease patients, DDAVP can cause thrombocytopenia because the defective von Willebrand factor (vWF) has an increased affinity for platelet GpIb/IX/V binding site. This leads to an apparent thrombocytopenia as the platelets are now bound to vWF. Inhibitor formation is most likely in severe hemophilia A patients who are exposed to exogenous factor. As DDAVP causes release of endogenous factor VIII and vWF from storage pools, there is no exposure to exogenous factor.

(Pages 1570-1571, Section 23: Disorders of the Blood Part 3: Disorder of Coagulation and Platelet, Chapter 436)

Answer 23-39. e

Hemophilia B, also known as Christmas disease, is an X-linked recessive trait that results in the congenital deficiency of factor IX. This patient's prolonged aPTT along with his family history, which is consistent with an X-linked disorder, points to hemophilia B as the most likely diagnosis. Type 2N and type 3 vWD, as well as hemophilia A patients, would all have low factor VIII levels, hence are incorrect. While type I vWD patients can have normal factor VIII levels, the aPTT would also be normal.

(Pages 1570-1574, Section 23: Disorders of the Blood, Part 3: Disorders of Coagulation and Platelets, Chapter 436)

Answer 23-40. a

The diagnosis for von Willebrand disease rests on a combination of personal and family bleeding history, along with supportive laboratory studies. Her von Willebrand activity and antigen levels are in a range that does not clearly distinguish between type 1 patients and healthy controls, as many factors can modulate vW factor levels. Most individuals have antigen, ristocetin cofactor, and factor VIII activity above 50%. However, levels between 30% and 50% can be normal as blood type, thyroid state, and other factors can modulate these lab values. Therefore, personal bleeding history and family history are critical to diagnosing von Willebrand disease.

(Pages 1571-1572, Section 23: Disorders of the Blood, Part 3: Disorders of Coagulation and Platelets, Chapter 436)

Answer 23-41. c

Patients with type 2B vWD have increased affinity of the abnormal vWF for platelet GpIb. Hence, they have a positive response in low-dose ristocetin-induced platelet aggregation and have diminished high-molecular-weight vWF multimers and thrombocytopenia because of clearance of the vWF-bound platelets. Answer A is the expected finding in a patient with type 1 vWD. Answer B is findings in type 2A vWD, as the activity to antigen ratio is decreased and high and intermediate multimers are absent. Answer D represents type 2M since the activity to antigen ratio is decreased, but the multimer distribution is normal. Answer E suggests either type 2N vWD or mild hemophilia A (in a female patient, this may occur due to extreme lyonization, Turner syndrome, or, rarely, coinheritance of 2 mutated factor VIII alleles).

(Pages 1571-1573, Section 23: Disorders of the Blood, Part 3: Disorders of Coagulation and Platelets, Chapter 436)

Answer 23-42. b

Type 2 von Willebrand disease is characterized by a qualitative defect in vWF; therefore, this patient's disproportionately low vWF activity level, relative to vWF antigen, indicates a type 2 defect. However, the absence of intermediate and large multimers distinguishes his subtype from type 2M, which has normal multimer appearance. Type 2A is an autosomal dominant disorder. These patients typically respond poorly to DDAVP treatment. Type 1 is a quantitative vWF deficiency with a proportional decrease in vWF activity and antigen. See Figure 436-1 for a summary of the von Willebrand disease types.

(Pages 1571-1573, Section 23: Disorders of the Blood, Part 3: Disorders of Coagulation and Platelets, Chapter 436)

Answer 23-43. a

Her proportionally low vW activity and antigen levels, and the appearance of her multimers, as well as her family history and personal bleeding history, are all consistent with type 1 von Willebrand disease. More than 75% of patients with von Willebrand disease have type 1. Type 2A is ruled out by the normal activity to antigen ratio and the presence of normal distribution of multimers. Type 2M is ruled out by the activity to antigen ratio. Type 2N is characterized by low factor VIII levels due to a mutation that selectively inactivates the factor VIII–binding site on the vWF; therefore, type 2N is ruled out by the normal factor VIII level. The patient's vWF activity and antigen levels are too high to be type 3, which is characterized by complete absence of vWF.

(Pages 1571-1573, Section 23: Disorders of the Blood, Part 3: Disorders of Coagulation and Platelets, Chapter 436)

Answer 23-44. d

Inhibitors occur in approximately 30% of patients with severe hemophilia A, usually within the first 20 exposures; however, they can occur at any age. Inhibitors can be eradicated with repeated exposure to factor VIII concentrate (immune tolerance therapy); however, this may take months to years. If a patient with a known inhibitor is actively bleeding, treatment with recombinant FVIIa or a prothrombin complex concentrate may be needed. Inhibitor titers ≤5 BU are considered low titers and more likely to be transient. Given the patient in this vignette has a titer >5, it is not likely to spontaneously resolve.

(Pages 1570-1571, Section 23: Disorders of the Blood, Part 3: Disorder of Coagulation and Platelet, Chapter 436)

Answer 23-45. d

While factor VIII activity levels of 6% and 9% are consistent with mild hemophilia A, the presence of similar levels and symptoms in his older sister suggests an autosomal recessively inherited trait rather than an X-linked trait. Hence, vWD type 2N is more likely. The factor VIII level is not consistent with vWD types 1 and 2A, while the multimers and vWF activity and antigen levels do not reflect those seen in types 2A and 3. See Figure 436-1 for a summary of the von Willebrand disease types.

(Pages 1572-1573, Section 23: Disorders of the Blood, Part 3: Disorder of Coagulation and Platelet, Chapter 436)

Answer 23-46. a

DDAVP (a synthetic form of vasopressin, or antidiuretic hormone) use can lead to fluid retention and hyponatremia. Patients should therefore limit fluid intake and serum sodium needs to be monitored. As tachyphylaxis occurs, the dosing is typically daily to every 2 days, and treatment is generally limited to 3 consecutive days. Factor VIII levels rise with the release of von Willebrand factor that results from DDAVP use.

(Pages 1570-1573, Section 23: Disorders of the Blood, Part 3: Disorder of Coagulation and Platelet, Chapter 436)

Answer 23-47. a

This patient's bleeding history, family history, and laboratory evaluation are most consistent with von Willebrand disease type 2N. In type 2N factor VIII is low due to an autosomal recessive mutation that selectively inactivates the factor VIII–binding site on vWF. A low factor VIII level could also be indicative of hemophilia A; however, a deficiency of factor VIII is caused by mutations on the X chromosome, and, in general, females are unaffected carriers. Therefore, this patient's family history is not consistent with hemophilia A. Moreover, it is not an answer choice. Patients with von Willebrand disease type 2N are often misdiagnosed as having hemophilia A.

Hemophilia B is a bleeding disorder caused by a low factor IX levels, and this patient's levels are within normal range for age. The patient has a normal fibrinogen level and normal platelets, which is not consistent with disseminated intravascular coagulation or afibrinogenemia. Vitamin K deficiency would lead to abnormal coagulation studies.

(Page 1573, Section 23: Disorders of the Blood, Part 3: Disorder of Coagulation and Platelet, Chapter 436)

Answer 23-48. b

Factor XIII deficiency is an autosomal recessive disorder associated with excessive bruising, muscle and joint bleeding, menorrhagia, delayed postsurgical bleeding, umbilical stump bleeding, and intracranial hemorrhage. In its activated form factor XIII is responsible for cross-linking the fibrin clot. Therefore, in a factor XIII–deficient patient, clot solubility is increased. Increased factor XIII would result in decreased clot solubility. The normal PT makes factor V deficiency unlikely, and increased protein C level does not cause increased bleeding symptoms.

(Page 1574, Section 23: Disorders of the Blood, Part 3: Disorder of Coagulation and Platelet, Chapter 436)

Answer 23-49. b

Synthesis of factors II, VII, IX, and X requires vitamin K as a cofactor. Factor V is a liver synthesized factor that is not vitamin K dependent. It is, therefore, useful in distinguishing liver failure from vitamin K deficiency.

(Page 1574, Section 23: Disorders of the Blood, Part 3: Disorder of Coagulation and Platelet, Chapter 437)

Answer 23-50. d

Classical vitamin K deficiency bleeding in newborns presents in the first week of life. Typical symptoms include easy bruising, mucus membrane bleeding, and hematemesis. Risk factors include babies who have not been given vitamin K treatment, are breastfed, or are poor feeders. Such patients will have low levels of vitamin K–dependent factors: II, VII, IX, and X. Factor V and VIII levels are unaffected. Factor V Leiden is a prothrombotic mutated factor V that is resistant to degradation by activated protein C. While neonates with pancreatic disease such as cystic fibrosis are at risk for vitamin K deficiency bleeding due to poor absorption of fat-soluble vitamins, this is an unlikely presentation of CF during the first week of life. Of note, early onset vitamin K deficiency bleeding occurs in the first 24 hours of life due to placental transfer of antibodies that interfere with vitamin K. Late-onset vitamin K deficiency bleeding presents at 2 weeks to 6 months.

(Pages 1574-1575, Section 23: Disorders of the Blood, Part 3: Disorders of Coagulation and Platelets, Chapter 437; Pages 1579-1580, Chapter 438)

Answer 23-51. b

Prothrombin G20210A mutation occurs in approximately 3% of the general population, and increases the risk for thrombosis mainly by causing excess prothrombin production. Factor V deficiency is associated with increased bleeding, not with increased thrombosis. (Factor V Leiden is the most common inherited thrombophilia and the mutation causes a resistance of factor V to inactivation by activated proteins C and S.) Patients with nephrotic syndrome, not nephritic syndrome, are at an increased risk of thrombosis due to loss of clotting factors in the urine. Hyperhomocysteinemia is a risk factor of stroke in children. Table 438-3 provides a differential diagnosis for thrombophilia.

(Pages 1579-1580, Section 23: Disorders of the Blood, Part 3: Disorders of Coagulation and Platelets, Chapter 438)

Answer 23-52. d

Factor V resistance to cleavage by APC is known as factor V Leiden. Cleavage of factor V inactivates this clotting factor; therefore, in factor V Leiden, factor V is unable to be inactivated by APC. Heterozygotes for this mutation have a 5- to 8-fold increase in thromboembolic disease, and homozygotes have an 80-fold increase in lifetime risk. Protein C is an anticoagulant; therefore, a slightly elevated level would not increase her risk of thrombosis. The antithrombin, factor VIII, and plasma homocysteine levels are normal.

(Pages 1579-1580, Section 23: Disorders of the Blood, Part 3: Disorders of Coagulation and Platelets, Chapter 438)

Answer 23-53. d

Isolated thrombocytopenia in a well-appearing child points toward ITP, an autoimmune-mediated process leading to increased destruction of platelets. While patients have circulating autoantibodies, there is no standardized laboratory test to identify these antibodies and in otherwise healthy-appearing children with no other concerning findings (eg, fevers, hepatosplenomegaly, red or white cell abnormalities on the smear), a bone marrow biopsy is not needed. Over 75% of patients will have resolution of their symptoms within 3 months with no further sequelae. Many patients can be observed without treatment, but those with active bleeding and platelet counts below 10,000 can be treated with steroids, IVIG, or anti-D immunoglobulin (in Rh+ patients). Platelet transfusions are not indicated except in cases of severe or life-threatening bleeding, as the circulating antibodies will also destroy transfused platelets.

(Pages 1582-1583, Section 23: Disorders of the Blood, Part 3: Disorders of Coagulation and Platelets, Chapter 439)

Answer 23-54. a

NAIT arises from a mismatch between maternal and paternal platelet antigens, most often HPA1. Maternal IgG antibodies against HPA1 cause peripheral platelet destruction in the newborn. Unlike Rh incompatibility, NAIT can present in the firstborn child and presents typically with petechiae, purpura, or mucosal bleeding immediately after birth. Treatment is to transfuse maternal platelets. However, it is acceptable to transfuse random platelets as well. Intracranial hemorrhage can occur in 10% to 20% of infants.

The normal maternal platelet count rules out maternally derived neonatal autoimmune thrombocytopenia. While IVIG may also provide some benefit in NAIT, it is not first choice for treatment. The uncomplicated pregnancy with a well-appearing newborn makes a TORCH infection unlikely. Glanzmann thrombasthenia is a functional platelet disorder and is not associated with thrombocytopenia. Other causes of thrombocytopenia to be considered in a neonate including Fanconi anemia, thrombocytopenia absent radii (TAR), and congenital amegakaryocytic thrombocytopenia (CAMT) are also in the differential, but given the patient's low counts, transfusion should be prioritized over additional diagnostic testing.

(Pages 1583-1587, Section 23: Disorders of the Blood, Part 3: Disorders of Coagulation and Platelets, Chapter 439)

Answer 23-55. a

While NAIT is self-limited with resolution within 2 to 6 weeks, 10% to 20% of patients have intracranial hemorrhage while the platelet count is low. Treatment is a temporizing measure aimed at raising the platelet count to reduce the risk of intracranial hemorrhage. The *best* choice for transfusion is maternal platelets that lack HPA-1a, and therefore will not be cleared by the circulating alloantibodies. Often, these platelets are not available, and a random donor unit will be used instead. IVIG can also be used, but takes 24 to 72 hours to take effect, and should be given in conjunction with platelet support. Steroids have not been shown to be beneficial and observation is unacceptable given the high rate of intracranial hemorrhage (10%-20%).

(Page 1583, Section 23: Disorders of the Blood, Part 3: Disorders of Coagulation and Platelets, Chapter 439)

Answer 23-56. c

The vignette describes a classic autosomal dominant pattern of inheritance. The thrombocytopenia, and family history of easy bruising associated with hearing loss and renal disease, suggests a MYH9-related disorder. MYH9-related disorders are caused by mutation in the nonmuscle myosin heavy chain II leading to pathognomonic Dohle-like bodies in neutrophils that can be seen on light microscopy. Examination of the peripheral blood smear would show macrothrombocytopenia.

X-ray of the forearms is useful in diagnosing thrombocytopenia absent radii (TAR). The diagnosis of Fanconi anemia is made with the diepoxybutane chromosome breakage test. A bone marrow biopsy would show congenital amegakaryotic thrombocytopenia. Bernard-Soulier syndrome is associated with macrothrombocytopenia; however, it is an inherited disorder of platelet function and not associated with hearing loss and renal failure.

(Page 1585, Section 23: Disorders of the Blood, Part 3: Disorders of Coagulation and Platelets, Chapter 439; Page 1550, Part 2: Disorders of Red Blood Cells and Anemia, Chapter 432)

Answer 23-57. b

Nonsteroidal anti-inflammatory drugs such as ibuprofen inhibit cyclooxygenase activity, leading to platelet dysfunction that can manifest as increased mucosal bleeding or menorrhagia. Although patients with type 1 vWD can present with relatively normal von Willebrand activity and antigen levels, the lack of a family history and the recent onset of her symptoms suggest that vWD is unlikely. Since she has a normal smear, a MYH9-related disorder is also unlikely, as this is an autosomal dominant macrothrombocytopenia. Given this patient's normal PT, factor VII deficiency is also unlikely. Her normal platelet count also eliminates ITP from consideration.

(Pages 1585-1586, Section 23: Disorders of the Blood, Part 3: Disorders of Coagulation and Platelets, Chapter 439)

Answer 23-58. b

WAS, and the related entity X-linked thrombocytopenia (XLT), should be suspected in any male patient with thrombocytopenia and small platelets. WAS differs from XLT in that patients with WAS have impaired immunity and are at risk for infections and lymphoreticular malignancies. Patients typically present to medical attention due to bleeding during infancy.

While thrombocytopenia absent radius, Fanconi anemia, and congenital amegakaryocytic thrombocytopenia are all associated with thrombocytopenia, the presence of small platelets and frequent infections in this patient is more suggestive of WAS. Patients with hyper-IgE syndrome are also likely to have infections and eczema, but do not have small and decreased numbers of platelets.

(Page 1585, Section 23: Disorders of the Blood, Part 3: Disorder of Coagulation and Platelet, Chapter 439; Page 1594, Part 4: Disorders of the Spleen and Lymph Nodes, Chapter 441; Page 1550, Part 2: Disorders of Red Blood Cell and Anemia, Chapter 432)

Answer 23-59. d

Thrombocytosis in children is almost always reactive to an underlying condition; in this patient's case, the elevated platelet count is a response to the patient's bacteremia. Importantly, thrombocytosis under these circumstances is not associated with an increased risk of thrombosis. Essential thrombocythemia, a clonal disorder, and familial thrombocytosis are extremely rare, and would not be the most likely diagnoses. Reactive thrombocytosis is more common, with 1 series reporting it in 15% of hospitalized patients. The patient does not meet any of the other criteria for Kawasaki disease.

(Page 1585, Section 23: Disorders of the Blood, Part 3: Disorders of Coagulation and Platelets, Chapter 439)

Answer 23-60. a

Glycoprotein Ib/IX/V is defective or deficient in patients with Bernard-Soulier syndrome. Because it is the platelet receptor

for von Willebrand factor, the patient's platelet is unable to aggregate in response to ristocetin. The von Willebrand activity, antigen, and multimer are normal. See eFigure 439-4 for a schematic representation of other inherited platelet function disorders.

Patients with Glanzmann thrombasthenia lack glycoprotein IIb/IIIa, which is required for bridging platelets. Unlike those of patients with Bernard-Soulier syndrome, platelets from patients with Glanzmann thrombasthenia do respond to ristocetin. Shwachman-Diamond syndrome is a congenital neutropenia syndrome arising from mutations in the SBDS gene. Pearson syndrome is a similar disorder arising from deletions of mitochondrial DNA. Kostmann disease is an autosomal recessive form of severe congenital neutropenia.

(Pages 1586-1587, Section 23: Disorders of the Blood, Part 3: Disorders of Coagulation and Platelets, Chapter 439; Page 1567, Chapter 435; Page 1572, Chapter 436)

Answer 23-61. b

Patients with Glanzmann thrombasthenia lack glycoprotein IIb/IIIa, which is required for bridging platelets. Platelets are activated by ADP, serotonin, and thromboxane A2.

GpIIb/IIIa activation follows platelet activation from these agonists. Platelets lacking GpIIb/IIIa do not aggregate in response to these agonists. Platelets of patients with Bernard-Soulier syndrome are only defective in response to ristocetin, as they lack GpIb/IX/V, the von Willebrand factor receptor. Shwachman-Diamond syndrome is a congenital neutropenia syndrome arising from mutations in the SBDS gene. Pearson syndrome is a similar disorder arising from deletions of mitochondrial DNA. Kostmann disease is an autosomal recessive form of severe congenital neutropenia.

(Pages 1586-1587, Section 23: Disorders of the Blood, Part 3: Disorders of Coagulation and Platelets, Chapter 439; Page 1567, Chapter 435; Pages 1590-1593, Part 4: Disorders of the Spleen and Lymph Nodes, Chapter 441)

Answer 23-62. d

Thrombocytosis is defined as a platelet count $>500 \times 10^3/$mm^3 and is usually secondary to another condition, for example, postsplenectomy. See Table 439-2 for a complete list of the primary and secondary causes of thrombocytosis. Postsplenectomy, patients have thrombocytosis due to the fact that the spleen is normally the reservoir for 30% of the platelet mass.

(Pages 1585-1587, Section 23: Disorders of the Blood, Part 4: Disorders of the Spleen and Lymph Nodes, Chapter 440)

Answer 23-63. a

Howell-Jolly bodies are seen in asplenia, and Ivemark syndrome is associated with congenital absence of the spleen in addition to cyanotic congenital heart defects, dextrocardia or

TABLE 439-2. Causes of Thrombocytosis
Primary
Familial thrombocytosis
Myeloproliferative disorders
Essential thrombocythemia
Polycythemia vera
Chronic myelogenous leukemia
Secondary (Reactive)
Infectious/inflammatory state
Tissue damage (trauma/surgery/burns)
Postsplenectomy
Iron deficiency
Kawasaki disease
Malignancy
Hepatoblastoma
Neuroblastoma
Lymphoma
Renal disease
Hemolytic anemia
Autoimmune disease
Blood loss
Drugs
Epinephrine
Corticosteroids
Vinca alkaloids
Other causes
Low birth weight
Allergies
Metabolic diseases
Myopathies
Neurofibromatosis
Rebound thrombocytosis

mesocardia, abdominal heterotaxy, and symmetrically trilobed lungs.

Mutations in JAK2 are associated with polycythemia vera and essential thrombocytosis. Platelet counts can be elevated with inflammation, which is also associated with elevated ESR, but is not a hallmark of Ivemark syndrome. Similarly, the platelet count may also be increased with iron-deficiency anemia. Lack of splenic function, not asplenia, would lead to increased number of RBC pits.

(Pages 1587-1589, Section 23: Disorders of the Blood, Part 4: Disorders of the Spleen and Lymph Nodes, Chapter 440; Pages 1585-1586, Part 3: Disorders of Coagulation and Platelets, Chapter 439; Pages 1537-1538, Part 1: Principles of Blood Disorders, Chapter 428)

Answer 23-64. d

Persons of African ancestry may have lower normal range for neutrophil counts. The mechanism of this phenomenon is still unclear.

Patients with myelokathexis, reticular dysgenesis, and Kostmann syndrome would all have had a history of infections. Patients with glycogen storage disease type 1b have other associated problems, including hypoglycemia, growth delay, and hyperlipidemia. In this otherwise healthy patient, ethnic pseudoneutropenia is the best answer.

(Page 1590, Section 23: Disorders of the Blood, Part 5: Disorders of White Blood Cells, Chapter 441)

Answer 23-65. a

The history of serious recurrent infections as well as cyclic fevers is concerning for cyclic neutropenia. Cyclic neutropenia is caused by a mutation in *ELA2*, the gene encoding for neutrophil elastase, and is inherited in an autosomal dominant pattern. Patients with cyclic neutropenia have nadir neutrophil counts that can be below 200 cells/μL approximately every 3 weeks.

During these nadirs, patients may have aphthous ulcers, gastroenteritis, and cervical lymphadenopathy. Patients will also be susceptible to life-threatening infections from *Clostridium perfringens* and gram-negative organisms. In between episodes, patients will have normal neutrophil counts and normal examinations. Therefore, a single normal neutrophil count is not sufficient to rule out cyclic neutropenia. The diagnosis is made by monitoring neutrophil counts 3 times a week over 6 to 8 weeks. Quantitative immunoglobulin levels and bone marrow biopsy would not be useful in the diagnosis of cyclic neutropenia. This recurrent, cyclic pattern of illness is not consistent with HIV infection.

(Pages 1590-1591, Section 23: Disorders of the Blood, Part 5: Disorders of White Blood Cells, Chapter 441)

Answer 23-66. d

The differential for neutropenia with concurrent pancreatic insufficiency is SDS and Pearson syndrome. SDS is an autosomal recessive disorder; the vast majority of patients have mutations in SBDS gene on chromosome 7. SDS patients may also have anemia and thrombocytopenia and usually present like the child in vignette with failure to thrive and steatorrhea. Patients with Pearson syndrome have mitochondrial DNA mutations (not a choice given here). They also present with lactic acidosis and sideroblastic anemia.

CFTR mutations are seen in cystic fibrosis patients. Interestingly, one of the first cohorts of identified SDS patients was found in cystic fibrosis clinics because they also had pancreatic insufficiency and pulmonary infections (due to their neutropenia).

TERT mutations are seen in some patients with dyskeratosis congenita, and RMRP mutations are found in cartilage-hair hypoplasia patients. While both of these disorders are associated with neutropenia, neither is associated with pancreatic insufficiency.

(Pages 1591-1592, Section 23: Disorders of the Blood, Part 5: Disorders of White Blood Cells, Chapter 441)

Answer 23-67. d

All of these disorders share the finding of neutropenia. Most, but not all, also have an increased risk of malignancy. Cartilage-hair hypoplasia, a rare autosomal recessive disorder characterized by dwarfism, fine hair, and immunodeficiency, has an increased risk of cancer, particularly non-Hodgkin lymphoma and basal cell carcinoma. Patients with Chediak-Higashi syndrome are at an increased risk of developing lymphomas while patients with severe congenital neutropenia and Shwachman-Diamond syndrome have an increased risk of developing myelodysplastic syndrome and acute myeloid leukemia. However, patients with cyclic neutropenia do not have an increased risk of cancer despite having mutations on the same gene (ELA2) as patients with severe congenital neutropenia. Among this group, only Shwachman-Diamond syndrome has been associated with ribosomal defects and Chediak-Higashi syndrome with platelet defects.

(Pages 1591-1592, Section 23: Disorders of the Blood, Part 5: Disorders of White Blood Cells, Chapter 441)

Answer 23-68. d

This patient has Chediak-Higashi syndrome. Patients with Chediak-Higashi syndrome have partial oculocutaneous albinism and silvery hair. They are also at risk for recurrent bacterial infections due to neutrophil dysfunction. They also have peripheral neuropathy and prolonged bleeding times. Chediak-Higashi syndrome is caused by a defect in granule formation, leading to the formation of giant granules with impaired chemotactic activity and intracellular killing. This picture depicts an ill-appearing child with light skin and silvery hair associated with the disease.

Pancreatic insufficiency is seen in Shwachman-Diamond syndrome, which is not associated with oculocutaneous albinism. Nail dystrophy is a characteristic of patients with dyskeratosis congenita, along with lacy reticulated pigmentation, dysplastic nails, and oral leukoplakia.

Triphalangeal thumbs are seen in a number of genetic disorders including Diamond-Blackfan syndrome, Fanconi syndrome, and Holt-Oram syndrome, but are not typically found in patients with Chediak-Higashi syndrome. Elevated IgE levels are found in hyper-IgE syndrome, which is associated with coarse facial features and hyperextensible joints.

(Page 1592, Section 23: Disorders of the Blood, Part 5: Disorders of White Blood Cells, Chapter 441)

Answer 23-69. c

While both acute leukemia and leukemoid reactions can present with high white counts, the patient's overall picture is more consistent with leukocyte adhesion deficiency. LAD-1 is a rare autosomal recessive congenital immunodeficiency caused by a deficiency of the β_2 subunit of the leukocyte adhesion molecule. As a result, neutrophils are produced, but cannot migrate to sites of infection. LAD-1 is characterized by recurrent infections, marked leukocytosis, and delayed umbilical cord separation. Older patients have recurrent episodes of periodontitis.

In leukemoid reactions, high leukocyte counts are seen in response to severe bacterial infections, and are usually marked by increased numbers of myelocytes, metamyelocytes, and bands (not seen in this patient). More immature precursors are seen in acute leukemias. There are drugs that can cause leukocytosis—for example, steroids are known to cause a transient increase in the white blood cell count due to demargination of the neutrophils—but this response would not be the best answer in a patient with severe infection and a history of delayed cord separation. Myeloproliferative disease can also present with leukocytosis, but again does not present with a history of delayed cord separation. See Figure 441-2 for an approach to leukocytosis.

(Pages 1593-1595, Section 23: Disorders of the Blood, Part 5: Disorders of White Blood Cells, Chapter 441)

Answer 23-70. b

This patient's history is consistent with chronic granulomatous disease (CGD), a defect in phagocytes that renders them unable to kill microbes with the reactive oxygen species. Patients with CGD do not produce H and as a result, patients often get recurrent infections with catalase-positive organisms (eg, *S. aureus*, *Klebsiella*, *Salmonella*) as well as fungi. Specifically, patients with a history of recurrent bacterial infections with catalase-positive organisms, or who have osteomyelitis at multiple sites or in the small bones of the hands or feet (as in this patient), should be evaluated for CGD. The classic test for CGD is the nitroblue tetrazolium dye test. Patients with CGD are unable to activate the NADPH oxidase system; therefore, the neutrophils cannot reduce the yellow water-soluble tetrazolium dye to an insoluble blue formazan pigment. Newer diagnostic methods include the dihydrorhodamine test, which is a flow cytometric approach that measures the conversion of DHR to rhodamine on neutrophil activation.

Patients with hyper-IgE also have recurrent *Staphylococcus* infections, but have other clinical features including chronic eczema, retention of primary dentition, and a coarse facial appearance. Bone marrow biopsy, skin biopsy, and lymphocyte subsets would not be helpful in the diagnosis of GCD.

(Pages 1594-1596, Section 23: Disorders of the Blood, Part 5: Disorders of White Blood Cells, Chapter 441)

Answer 23-71. b

This patient's history of infection, eczematoid rash, and increased IgE levels is most consistent with hyper-IgE syndrome. By school age, patients have history of recurrent skin abscesses, pneumonias, and chronic otitis media. Although patients with Wiskott-Aldrich syndrome or milk protein allergy also may have eczema, neither of these is associated with the degree of elevation in IgE in this vignette. Patients with hyper-IgE syndrome typically have IgE levels exceeding 2500 IU/mL. Patients with TAR have a high frequency of cow's milk allergy, but do not have elevated IgE levels. Patients with leukocyte adhesion defect may have similar infections as this patient, but have an elevated WBC count.

(Page 1594, Section 23: Disorders of the Blood, Part 5: Disorders of White Blood Cells, Chapter 441; Page 1585, Part 3: Disorders of the Coagulation and Platelets, Chapter 439)

Answer 23-72. c

Massive transfusion is defined as transfusion of a volume of blood greater than a patient's total blood volume in 24 hours, or more than half the patient's blood volume in 1 hour. Metabolic complications of massive transfusion include metabolic alkalosis, hypocalcemia, and hyperkalemia. Many of the metabolic disturbances are primarily due to citrate toxicity, which is used as an anticoagulant in blood units. Each adult unit of packed red blood cells contains about 3 g of citrate. Citrate is metabolized to bicarbonate, leading to metabolic alkalosis, and can bind calcium, leading to hypocalcemia. Hyperkalemia results in lysis of red blood cells as the stored units age—this is not usually a problem unless a large number of units are transfused. Patients can also develop dilutional thrombocytopenia and coagulopathy as a result of massive transfusion.

(Page 1597, Section 23: Disorders of the Blood, Part 6: Principles of Transfusion, Chapter 442)

Answer 23-73. c

Anaphylaxis is a dramatic but extremely rare adverse reaction to blood products. However, patients with IgA deficiency are at risk of an anaphylactic reaction during the first blood transfusion due to the presence of circulating anti-IgA antibodies. IgA deficiency is one of the most common immunodeficiencies, affecting approximately 1 in 600 individuals. Many of these patients are asymptomatic, often diagnosed during routine blood donation. Future transfusions should be with units donated by other IgA-deficient individuals.

Routine testing for transfusion reactions involves a clerical review of the unit and computer records, and posttransfusion direct antibody testing as well as bilirubin, haptoglobin, and urinalysis if hemolysis is suspected.

A chest x-ray is not required in a patient whose respiratory symptoms have resolved. While anaphylaxis is generally caused by IgE-mediated mast cell degranulation, anaphylaxis in blood transfusion is usually due to IgG anti-IgA antibodies circulating in an IgA-deficient patient. Early morning cortisol levels are used to check for adrenal insufficiency after long-term steroids, and are not necessary for doses given during an anaphylactic episode.

(Page 1601, Section 23: Disorders of the Blood, Part 6: Principles of Transfusion, eTable 442-9)

Answer 23-74. d

The patient is having an acute hemolytic reaction. This is a noninfectious reaction that results from the transfusion of ABO-incompatible red cells. These patients have signs of intravascular hemolysis with evidence of hemoglobin in their urine.

A low serum haptoglobin is also indicative of intravascular hemolysis as the release of free hemoglobin binds to haptoglobin causing a drop in serum haptoglobin levels. Additionally, due to active hemolysis, patients will have lower-than-expected rise in posttransfusion hemoglobin levels. Occasionally, these patients may develop renal failure, shock, and disseminated intravascular coagulation if a large volume is transfused.

Transfusion-related acute lung injury is another noninfectious complication of transfusion, and is confirmed by chest x-ray findings, but is not consistent with this patient's clinical picture. Hypocalcemia and metabolic alkalosis are often signs of citrate toxicity, which is a complication of massive transfusion (defined as greater than the patient's

eTABLE 442-9. Noninfectious Complications of Transfusion

Hemolysis
Incompatible recipient or donor isohemagglutinins that react with transfused RBCs or recipient RBCs, respectively
Osmotic, thermal, or mechanical lysis of cells before infusion
Nonhemolytic Febrile Reactions
Leukocyte cytokines in cellular blood products
Bacteria in any type of blood component
Allergic/Anaphylactic
Recipient sensitivity to plasma proteins in any type of blood product
Anti-IgA (in IgA-deficient recipient)
Pulmonary Reactions
Volume overload
Anti-WBC and anti-HLA antibodies in blood product or recipient

blood volume in 24 hours). See eTable 442-9 for additional noninfectious complications of transfusions.

(Page 1601, Section 23: Disorders of the Blood, Part 6: Principles of Transfusion, Chapter 442)

Answer 23-75. a

Hepatitis A is not tested routinely in blood banks in the United States, and is rarely transmitted through blood products. It is most often transmitted through the fecal–oral route. All blood products undergo testing for hepatitis B surface antigen (HBsAg), hepatitis B core antibody (HBcAb), hepatitis C antibody (HepCAb), and HIV antibody. Improved testing for HIV has reduced the risk of transmission to 1 in 3 million. HTLV-1 is a retrovirus that is implicated in causing T-cell leukemia, and has been screened by blood banks since the late 1980s.

(Page 1601, Section 23: Disorders of the Blood, Part 6: Principles of Transfusion, Chapter 442, eTable 44-2)

CHAPTER 24 | Neoplastic Disorders

Ashley Ward and Robert Goldsby

24-1. A 6-month-old girl is found to have bilateral leukocoria on her well-child exam. After referral to a pediatric ophthalmologist and appropriate imaging studies, she is diagnosed with bilateral retinoblastoma. Which of the following tumors is she also at high risk for?

a. Hepatoblastoma

b. Neuroblastoma

c. Hodgkin lymphoma

d. Osteosarcoma

e. Medulloblastoma

24-2. You are examining a newborn term boy in your clinic and notice several unusual features. He appears to lack irises and has mild hypospadias. You question the parents, and there is no family history of either aniridia or genitourinary abnormalities. You explain that you will need to follow this patient with serial abdominal ultrasounds. Which of the following statements about this baby is also true?

a. This patient also has hemihypertrophy

b. This patient will eventually develop a Wilms tumor (nephroblastoma)

c. This patient will eventually develop a hepatoblastoma

d. This patient has a deletion of the *PAX6* gene

e. This patient has a deletion of chromosome 11p15

24-3. A 17-year-old girl presents with a painful mass involving her right fourth rib. Biopsy reveals small round blue cells. Identification of which of the following translocations by FISH would confirm the diagnosis of Ewing sarcoma?

a. t(2;13)

b. t(X;18)

c. t(2;5)

d. t(9;22)

e. t(11;22)

24-4. A 10-year-old boy has just been diagnosed with osteosarcoma of the left distal tibia. On further enquiry about his history, it is revealed that his mother recently died from breast cancer at age 34, and his maternal grandfather survived a diagnosis of leukemia in his early 40s only to be diagnosed with colon cancer at age 65. Which of the following would you expect to find in this patient?

a. Amplification of *NMYC*

b. Mutation of p53

c. Loss of heterozygosity at 11p15

d. Mutation of *MEN1*

e. Mutation of *VHL*

24-5. Which of the following chemotherapeutic agents is classified as an alkylating agent?

a. Cyclophosphamide

b. 6-mercaptopurine

c. Etoposide

d. Methotrexate

e. Doxorubicin

24-6. A 13-year-old girl presented to the emergency room with a 1-week history of diffuse bruising, pallor, and fatigue. Complete blood counts reveal a white blood cell count of $54,000 \times 10^9/L$ with 95% blasts, platelets of $13 \times 10^9/L$, and a hemoglobin of 7.2 g/dL. After examination of her peripheral smear and flow cytometric analysis of her blast cells, she is diagnosed with acute myelogenous leukemia and started on chemotherapy. She responds well to her therapy, and rapidly goes into remission. Two years after completion of chemotherapy, she returns to the clinic for routine follow-up complaining of swollen ankles and a night-time cough. You get an echocardiogram, which shows an ejection fraction of 30% (normal 50–70%). Which of her chemotherapeutic agents is most likely to blame?

a. Daunorubicin

b. Cytarabine

c. Etoposide

d. Vincristine

e. Topotecan

24-7. A 15-year-old girl is admitted to the hospital for her fourth course of chemotherapy for relapsed rhabdomyosarcoma with cyclophosphamide and doxorubicin. She tolerates the chemotherapy well and her nausea is well-controlled. On the day of discharge, she develops dysuria, urinary frequency, and blood-tinged urine. She is afebrile. The most appropriate next action is

a. start broad-spectrum antibiotics

b. increase hydration

c. restart mesna

d. consult urology to place a foley catheter

e. discharge the patient home

24-8. Which of the following statements about phase III clinical trials is correct?

a. They are designed to identify the appropriate dose and schedule of a novel chemotherapeutic agent

b. They are designed to confirm the results of a smaller trial that demonstrated significant superiority of a novel chemotherapeutic agent over standard therapy

c. They are designed to define the toxicities of a novel chemotherapeutic agent at multiple dosing levels

d. They are designed to compare the current best available therapy to a novel treatment approach, typically in a randomized fashion

e. They are designed to determine whether or not a novel chemotherapeutic agent can produce an objective response against a cancer of interest

24-9. A baby boy is born at term after a pregnancy complicated by a lack of prenatal care. He does well in the immediate newborn period, nursing well and making 10–12 wet diapers per day, and is discharged home. At his 2-week well-child examination, he is well-appearing. His pulse is 110 and blood pressure 107/72. On examination, his pediatrician palpates an abdominal mass. She orders an abdominal ultrasound, which reveals a large solid mass involving the left kidney. What is the most likely diagnosis?

a. Hemangioma

b. Nephroblastoma

c. Rhabdoid tumor

d. Renal cell carcinoma

e. Mesoblastic nephroma

24-10. The most common childhood malignancy is:

a. Acute myelogenous leukemia

b. Acute lymphoblastic leukemia

c. Neuroblastoma

d. Brain tumors

e. Hepatoblastoma

24-11. A 4-year-old boy with a 2-week history of fatigue, anorexia, and bruising has a WBC count of $35 \times 10^9/L$ with evidence of blast cells on his peripheral blood smear. He undergoes bone marrow aspiration and biopsy. It reveals 95% blast cells, consistent with the diagnosis of leukemia. A sample of marrow is sent for flow cytometry. The blast cells express CD19, CD22, and CD10, but no immunoglobulin and no CD3. What type of acute lymphoblastic leukemia does this child have?

a. Mature B-cell

b. Mature T-cell

c. Common (early pre) B-cell

d. Pro B-cell

e. Pre T- cell

24-12. An 18-year-old college student presents to her health center with fatigue, cough, fevers, and swollen lymph nodes in her neck and groin for the past 2 weeks. A monospot test is negative. The doctor orders a complete blood count, which demonstrates a WBC of 2×10^9/L, a hemoglobin of 8.5 g/dL, and a platelet count of 51×10^9/L. Which of the following tests or procedures is most important to do before the patient undergoes anesthesia for a diagnostic bone marrow biopsy?

a. Chest X-ray

b. Creatinine

c. Needle biopsy of lymph node

d. Platelet transfusion

e. PT and PTT

24-13. A child presents to the emergency room with intermittent fever for 10 days, fatigue, and extensive bruising. Physical exam reveals pallor, diffuse petechiae, and a spleen palpable 10 cm below the left costal margin. You order a peripheral blood smear, which demonstrates abundant large blast cells with scant cytoplasm and a uniform appearance.

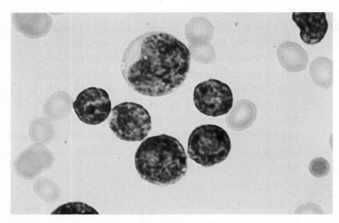

(Reproduced, with permission, from Longo et al, eds. *Harrison's Principles of Internal Medicine*. 18th ed. New York: McGraw-Hill, 2012.)

Flow cytometry confirms B-cell acute lymphoblastic leukemia. Which patient with B-cell acute lymphoblastic leukemia has the worst prognosis?

a. A 5-year-old boy whose cytogenetics demonstrate hyperdiploidy

b. A 5-year-old girl whose cytogenetics demonstrate t(12;21), the *TEL–AML* translocation

c. An 11-year-old boy whose cytogenetics demonstrate hyperdiploidy

d. A 6-month-old girl whose cytogenetics demonstrate t(4;11), the *MLL* translocation

e. A 3-year-old boy whose cytogenetics demonstrate t(1;19), the *TCF3–PBX1* translocation

24-14. An 11-year-old boy presents with a 3-week history of increasing back and leg pain and a 2-day history of increasing shortness of breath. His temperature is 38.3°C. His heart rate is 110 and his respiratory rate is 20. His blood pressure is 126/78. He is awake, alert, and cooperative. His lungs are clear bilaterally. He has diffuse lymphadenopathy. His spleen is 2 cm below the left costal margin. His CBC shows a white count of 52,000/µL, hemoglobin of 7.5 g/dL, and a platelet count of 45,000/µL. The most appropriate initial step in his evaluation is to:

a. Transfuse blood products

b. Perform a bone marrow aspirate and biopsy

c. Obtain a chest X-ray, blood culture, and chemistries

d. Administer a dose of steroids

e. Give him a large bolus of IV fluids

24-15. For children with acute lymphoblastic leukemia, the term remission is best defined as

a. A state where there is no need for additional therapy

b. A state where there is macroscopic residual disease

c. A state where there is no clinical or laboratory evidence of disease

d. A state where disease can be identified by flow cytometry only

e. A state where there are no adverse effects from disease treatment

24-16. An 8-year-old girl who has just been diagnosed with pre B-cell acute lymphoblastic leukemia has a white blood cell count of 64,000/µL. Which of the following chemotherapy agents should be added to her induction regimen?

a. IV methotrexate

b. IV daunomycin

c. PO 6-mercaptopurine

d. IV cytoxan

e. SQ Ara-C

24-17. Approximately, 15% of children with ALL relapse. Of those who relapse, which of the following scenarios is associated with the worst prognosis?

a. Central nervous system relapse occurring in less than 36 months of initial diagnosis

b. Central nervous system relapse occurring in more than 36 months of initial diagnosis

c. Testicular relapse

d. Isolated bone marrow relapse occurring in less than 36 months of initial diagnosis

e. Isolated bone marrow relapse occurring in more than 36 months of initial diagnosis

24-18. A 16-year-old girl in the middle of the delayed intensification therapy for her acute lymphoblastic leukemia presents with new fever and cough of 1 day duration. On examination, her lungs are clear, but her heart rate is 125, her respiratory rate 32, and her oxygen saturation 88% on room air. Chest X-ray reveals bilateral "lacy" interstitial pneumonia. Upon further questioning, she admits that she has not taken her trimethoprim-sulfamethoxazole in months. Which organism are you most concerned about?

   a. *Haemophilus influenzae*

   b. Aspergillus

   c. *Mycoplasma pneumoniae*

   d. *Pneumocystis carinii*

   e. *Streptococcus pneumoniae*

24-19. A newborn boy with features of Down Syndrome has complete blood count showing a WBC of 25,000/ μL with blasts noted on peripheral smear. He has no respiratory distress, lymphadenopathy, or hepatomegaly. Which of the following is the most appropriate management?

   a. Start alkylating fluids and allopurinol in anticipation of starting high-dose chemotherapy

   b. Consult BMT as this patient is likely to need a bone marrow transplant

   c. Start prednisone and monitor for tumor lysis syndrome

   d. Evaluation of liver function and close observation

   e. Order leukopheresis to bring down his white blood cell count

24-20. A young man was diagnosed with localized Ewing sarcoma of the right proximal femur at age 15. He completed the standard treatment regimen, including chemotherapy and resection 2 years ago. Since that time, he has been followed every 3 months in the outpatient clinic with X-rays, blood counts, and a physical exam. At his most recent visit, he felt well, but his CBC revealed a white blood cell count of 23,000/μL, a hemoglobin of 9.0 g/dL, and a platelet count of 41,000/μL. Which of the following chemotherapy agents that he received for treatment of his Ewing sarcoma is likely to be responsible for these findings?

   a. Ifosfamide

   b. Etoposide

   c. Vincristine

   d. Doxorubicin

   e. Cyclophosphamide

24-21. A 14-year-old girl presents to the emergency room with intermittent fevers for 2 weeks, fatigue, and bruising. Multiple leukemic blasts are noted on her peripheral smear, and the diagnosis of acute promyelocytic leukemia (APL) is made. Which cytogenetic abnormality would you expect to find on analysis of her leukemia cells?

   a. t(8;21)

   b. inv(16)

   c. t(9;22)

   d. t(9;11)

   e. t(15;17)

24-22. A 12-year-old girl has just been diagnosed with acute myeloid leukemia. Which of the following cytogenetic abnormalities or molecular alterations would portend the best prognosis?

   a. Monosomy 5

   b. Monosomy 7

   c. *FLT3* ITD with high allelic ratio

   d. *PML–RARα* translocation

   e. Balanced *MLL* translocation

24-23. A 15-month-old boy is seen by his primary pediatrician for a well-child exam. She notes that the infant looks thinner than he did when she last saw him, though his abdomen is very protruberant and firm, and his overall weight is unchanged. She also notices that he is much quieter than she remembers from his last visit, and does not engage in her attempts to play with him. In addition, his lower legs are covered with bruises, which the mother attributes to his recent attempts to walk. The pediatrician sends off a CBC, which shows a white blood cell count of 42,000/μL with 50% monocytes, and a fetal hemoglobin level, which is abnormally high. What treatment is this child likely to require?

   a. ATRA and arsenic

   b. Dexamethasone, vincristine, and asparaginase

   c. Hematopoietic stem-cell transplant

   d. Daunorubicin and cytarabine

   e. Leukopheresis

24-24. A 4-year-old girl from Kenya presents with fevers, weight loss and a large, firm, nontender, nonfluctuant swelling beneath her right mandible. Biopsy reveals an infiltration of small monomorphic cells with a thin rim of basophilic cytoplasm and very high mitotic rate, which stain positive for CD19 and CD20. Which of the following viruses is likely to have caused her disease?

a. CMV

b. HIV

c. HHV-6

d. EBV

e. HSV

24-25. A young woman is referred to a pediatric oncologist by her pediatrician for evaluation of a large abdominal mass palpable on physical exam. Abdominal CT scan reveals a large mass encasing portions of her bowel as well as multiple enlarged para-aortic lymph nodes. All of these areas appear bright on PET scan. The rest of her staging workup, including lumbar puncture and bone marrow biopsy, is negative for disease. She is sent to a pediatric surgeon, who is unable to remove the entire tumor. A biopsy of the primary mass reveals lymphoblastic lymphoma. How would you describe her disease stage?

a. Stage I lymphoma

b. Stage II lymphoma

c. Stage III lymphoma

d. Stage IV lymphoma

e. Leukemia

24-26. A 20-year-old college sophomore presents to his school health clinic with 2 weeks of intermittent fevers, weight loss, decreased energy, and swollen lymph nodes in his neck. On exam, he has multiple firm, large, nontender lymph nodes palpable in his anterior and posterior cervical chains and axillae bilaterally. Chest X-ray reveals mediastinal lymphadenopathy as well. He is sent for fine needle biopsy of one of the nodes, which reveals prominent Reed–Sternberg cells. History of which of the following symptoms would give him a worse prognosis?

a. Alcohol-induced pain

b. Pruritis

c. Malaise

d. Anorexia

e. Drenching night sweats

24-27. A 15-year-old boy presents to his pediatrician for left elbow pain for the last 2 months. He has had pain in that elbow, but he is in the middle of baseball season. He assumed it was due to sports-related overuse, though he does not remember a specific injury.

Over the past few days, the elbow has become more painful and swollen, despite rest, ice, and elevation at the recommendation of his coach. On exam, he is unable to fully extend the elbow without significant pain, but distal strength and sensation are intact, and his skin has normal coloration. X-ray of the elbow reveals a lytic lesion in the distal humerus, with ossification of the surrounding soft tissue in a "sunburst" pattern. Biopsy demonstrates malignant cells with abundant osteoid formation. The distal humerus is a moderately unusual location for this type of tumor. Where is this tumor most commonly found?

a. Distal femur

b. Proximal radius

c. Jaw

d. Ribs

e. Pelvic bones

24-28. You are completing the staging workup for a 17-year-old girl with newly diagnosed osteosarcoma of the distal femur. Which of the following is the best way to assess for metastasis to the lungs?

a. Chest X-ray

b. Bone scan

c. PET scan

d. Chest CT

e. Chest MRI

24-29. A 10-year-old girl with localized osteosarcoma of the proximal tibia is treated with 10 weeks of high-dose methotrexate, doxorubicin, and cisplatin chemotherapy. She then undergoes limb-sparing surgical resection followed by additional adjuvant chemotherapy. Without knowing her Huvos grade (percent tumor necrosis), you estimate her 5-year survival to be which of the following?

a. 10%

b. 30%

c. 50%

d. 70%

e. 90%

24-30. A 17-year-old Caucasian girl has noticed a nagging pain in the middle of her back for about 8 months that occasionally wakes her up out of sleep. More recently, she has developed a cough, as well as some weakness in her legs and an occasional loss of urinary continence. Her pediatrician orders a spinal MRI, which shows a lytic lesion of her T7 vertebra with swelling of the surrounding soft tissue and some cord compression. Biopsy of the vertebra reveals small round blue cells positive for CD99 expression but not osteoid, and harboring a translocation involving chromosome 22. Follow-up chest X-ray reveals multiple round nodules varying in size from 0.5 to 3.0 cm throughout both lung fields. What is the most likely diagnosis?

- **a.** Lymphoma
- **b.** Rhabdomyosarcoma
- **c.** Osteosarcoma
- **d.** Neuroblastoma
- **e.** Ewing sarcoma

24-31. Which of the following is a reason to opt for local control of Ewing sarcoma with radiation instead of surgery?

- **a.** Decreased risk of secondary malignancies
- **b.** Improved likelihood of survival
- **c.** Anticipate better cosmetic or functional outcome
- **d.** Tumor is small and peripherally located
- **e.** Using radiation as local control means no chemotherapy is required

24-32. A 12-year-old girl who was treated for embryonal rhabdomyosarcoma as a toddler is referred to your clinic for evaluation of a painful swelling of her left proximal tibia. You order an X-ray, which demonstrates a lytic lesion, and biopsy confirms your suspicion of osteosarcoma. Which genetic mutation best explains this cancer pattern?

- **a.** Germline *HRAS* mutation
- **b.** Germline *NF1* mutation
- **c.** Germline *RB1* mutation
- **d.** Germline *p53* mutation
- **e.** Germline *CREBBP* mutation

24-33. You are seeing a 14-year-old boy in your clinic who complains of difficulty urinating for the last 2 weeks. He states that he feels the urge to urinate, but has trouble getting a stream to start and feels like he is not fully emptying his bladder. He denies dysuria or hematuria. He denies history of back pain or injury, as well as constipation or other changes in his bowel habits. His neurologic exam is completely normal. A urine dip shows trace heme but is otherwise normal. You refer him to an urologist, who gets a pelvic MRI, which reveals a large mass in the lower pelvis compressing his bladder and urethra. Biopsy reveals neoplastic cells of variable cellularity within a loose, myxoid stroma. Many of the cells are elongated and eosinophilic with cross striations and stain positive for desmin. Further workup reveals no metastatic disease. Which of the following is true?

- **a.** This patient is likely to be cured with surgical resection of the tumor alone
- **b.** If his tumor cannot be fully resected, his chance of long-term survival is 30–40%
- **c.** The site of this tumor is considered favorable
- **d.** This patient falls into the high-risk group
- **e.** If his tumor cannot be fully resected, he will require radiation therapy

24-34. You are conducting a routine pre-op workup on a 3-year-old boy with Wilms tumor scheduled for resection and note that his PTT is prolonged. Your colleague asks you why this might be. You respond:

- **a.** He probably has acquired the von Willebrand disease
- **b.** He probably has an inherited factor VIII deficiency
- **c.** He probably has an inherited factor VII deficiency
- **d.** He probably has a consumptive coagulopathy
- **e.** It is probably a lab error

24-35. A 3-year-old girl has just been diagnosed with Stage II, favorable histology Wilms tumor. According to Children's Oncology Group criteria, which of the following will influence her treatment regimen?

- **a.** *MYCN* amplification
- **b.** Loss of heterozygosity for 16q
- **c.** Loss of heterozygosity for 11q
- **d.** *PHOX2B* mutation
- **e.** *PAX6* deletion

24-36. A 2-year-old girl is brought into your clinic by her parents because they have noticed that over the last few weeks, she has been progressively unsteady on her feet and bumping into walls. They have also noticed some occasional twitching movements of her arms and legs over that same time period that they do not recall seeing before. On physical exam, you notice that she has difficulty maintaining her gaze on an object, and you palpate a mass in her abdomen. What kind of tumor do you suspect?

- **a.** Wilms tumor
- **b.** Hepatoblastoma
- **c.** Pheochromocytoma
- **d.** Metastatic brain tumor
- **e.** Neuroblastoma

24-37. A 19-month-old girl has newly diagnosed neuroblastoma. Presence of which of the following in her tumor correlates with favorable prognosis?

   a. Near-triploid DNA content

   b. Near-tetraploid DNA content

   c. *MYCN* amplification

   d. Deletion of chromosome 1p

   e. Gain of chromosome 17q

24-38. A patient with high-risk neuroblastoma has recently completed multiagent chemotherapy followed by 1 autologous stem cell transplantation and radiation to the primary tumor site, and is in complete remission. The tumor was completely resected, and most recent MIBG scan and bone marrow biopsy were negative for disease. The patient should now receive:

   a. No further therapy

   b. 13-*cis*-retinoic acid for 6 months

   c. All-*trans*-retinoic acid for 6 months

   d. Allogeneic stem cell transplant

   e. ^{131}I-MIBG therapy

24-39. A 6-year-old girl who emigrated from China 2 years ago presents to your office with 2 weeks of nausea and vomiting. On exam, she appears cachectic, and you palpate a right upper quadrant mass, which is confirmed to be a tumor in the right lobe of the liver by ultrasound. Upon review of her records, you note that she has a history of hepatitis B infection, and that she weighs only 1 pound more than she did at her last well-child check a year ago. What type of tumor does this child most likely have?

   a. Hepatoblastoma

   b. Hemangioendothelioma

   c. Undifferentiated embryonal sarcoma

   d. Hepatocellular carcinoma

   e. Cholangiocarcinoma

24-40. A 3-year-old otherwise healthy girl is diagnosed with hepatoblastoma after presenting to her pediatrician with a painless abdominal mass. Family history reveals a maternal grandfather who died from colon cancer at age 42. Screening for a mutation in which gene would you recommend?

   a. *GPC3*

   b. *ABCB11*

   c. *APC*

   d. *NOTCH2*

   e. *FAH*

24-41. A 14-month-old boy presents with an enlarged abdomen and a palpable right upper quadrant mass. Ultrasound reveals a large mass in the left lobe of the liver. Hepatoblastoma is suspected. Which of the following represents a good prognostic factor in this disease?

   a. Low alpha-fetoprotein levels

   b. Pure fetal histology

   c. Small-cell undifferentiated histology

   d. History of prematurity

   e. Presence of hemihypertrophy

24-42. A teenage girl presents to the emergency room complaining of worsening abdominal pain for the last 8 hours, and recent onset of nonbloody, non-bilious vomiting without diarrhea. She is tachycardic, but afebrile, with normal blood pressure. Abdominal exam reveals a large mass in the right lower quadrant. Ultrasound reveals a solid mass originates from the ovary, which has no apparent blood flow by doppler. She is taken to the operating room, where a 15-cm tumor arising from a torsed and necrotic ovary is identified and removed. Pathology reveals a germ cell tumor, with strong staining for alkaline phosphatase but negative staining for AFP, B-HCG and CD30. This girl most likely has a:

   a. Mature teratoma

   b. Yolk sac tumor

   c. Dysgerminoma

   d. Embryonal carcinoma

   e. Choriocarcinoma

24-43. You are asked to see a newborn baby boy who was noted to have a prominent sacral mass at birth. He is otherwise well-appearing. You recommend checking a serum alpha-fetoprotein level, which comes back elevated for age. Biopsy shows abundant cells with Schiller–Duval bodies. What treatment recommendations would you give?

   a. No treatment required; the mass will resolve on its own with time

   b. Surgical resection only

   c. Chemotherapy only

   d. Surgical resection and chemotherapy

   e. Surgical resection and radiation

24-44. A 6-year-old child is noted to have 7 café au lait spots as well as axillary freckling, but is otherwise healthy. There is no other family history of genetic disorders. You send blood for DNA testing to support your clinical diagnosis. What is the other intervention you would recommend?

  a. Annual physical exams only

  b. Brain MRI

  c. Examination by an ophthalmologist

  d. Echocardiogram

  e. Renal function testing

24-45. A 7-year-old boy presents with headaches and ataxia. On physical exam, he has difficulty with finger-nose-finger testing and you note a left cranial nerve VI nerve palsy. You send him for an MRI, which reveals a large cystic area surrounded by a ring of enhancing solid tumor with a mural nodule. A pediatric neurosurgeon is able to completely resect the lesion, which is confirmed by postoperative MRI. What is the next step in his treatment?

  a. MRI of the spine and lumbar puncture to complete a staging workup

  b. Radiation to the site of the original tumor

  c. Radiation to the entire brain and spine

  d. Chemotherapy

  e. Observation with periodic MRIs

24-46. A 7-month-old baby is brought to your attention because she has been losing milestones. She was formerly able to roll over and sit with support, but now she can do neither. She also is no longer reaching for things with her right hand, according to her father. On your exam, you note that her head circumference has increased from the 35th percentile at her 4-month well-child check to the 95th percentile now. MRI of the brain reveals a large mass in the left cerebral hemisphere. Neurosurgeons are able to resect the tumor, which demonstrates deletion of *INI1*. What type of brain tumor does this child have?

  a. Medulloblastoma

  b. Atypical teratoid/rhabdoid tumor

  c. Ependymoma

  d. Low-grade fibrillary astrocytoma

  e. Gliobastoma multiforme

24-47. The parents of a 4-year-old girl who was treated for unilateral retinoblastoma at the age of 2 are newly pregnant with their second child, and are worried that this child will develop retinoblastoma too. Both parents are healthy, and there is no other history of retinoblastoma or other cancers in the family. You tell them that their chances of having another child with retinoblastoma are:

  a. <10%

  b. 25%

  c. 50%

  d. 75%

  e. 100%

24-48. You are caring for a patient with a 15 cm Kaposiform hemangioendothelioma of her left chest wall. You have been following her with serial physical exams and measurements of the tumor, and bloodwork to screen for Kasabach–Merritt phenomenon. At this visit, she complains that the tumor has started to ooze periodically. CBC, fibrinogen, fibrin split products, and PT/PTT are all normal. You decide that therapy is warranted to try to help control the traumatic bleeding. The most effective therapy for this tumor is:

  a. Steroids

  b. Vincristine

  c. α-interferon

  d. Surgical resection

  e. Radiation

24-49. A 2-year-old boy is brought to his pediatrician with 2 weeks of intermittent low-grade fevers, generalized malaise, weight loss, and a scaly, reddish-brown papular rash scattered over about 10% of his body. A skin biopsy reveals proliferative cells with rod-shaped granules that stain positive for CD1a. In addition to blood counts, skeletal survey, and liver function tests, which of the following is an essential part of this child's subsequent workup?

  a. Brain CT

  b. Evaluation for diabetes insipidus

  c. Chest CT

  d. Bone marrow biopsy

  e. Nothing else

24-50. A 10-month-old girl presents to the emergency room with 1 week of high fevers, decreased appetite, lethargy, and weight loss. On physical exam, her spleen is palpable 5 cm below her left costal margin, and her liver is enlarged as well. Preliminary laboratory testing reveals a ferritin of 14,000 μg/L and a fibrinogen level of 42 mg/dL. Which of the following additional results would allow you to make the diagnosis of hemophagocytic lymphohistiocytosis?

  a. Elevated soluble IL-2 receptor levels

  b. Elevated natural killer cell activity

  c. Elevated WBC count

  d. Elevated transaminases

  e. Elevated erythrocyte sedimentation rate

ANSWERS

Answer 24-1. d

The child in this vignette most likely has inherited a germline mutation in one copy of the tumor suppressor gene *RB1*. Hereditary RB mutations are more likely to present bilaterally and at a younger age (younger than 11 months). The RB1 gene has been localized to chromosome 13. The loss of the retinoblastoma protein, pRB, allows unregulated growth and proliferation, thereby contributing to tumorgenesis. The patient in the vignette is at risk for developing new retinoblastoma tumors during early childhood, and for developing osteosarcoma at any age. There is a dramatically increased risk of osteosarcoma in the radiation field; this is one reason why chemotherapy or localized cryotherapy is preferred over radiation for the treatment of these tumors.

Hepatoblastoma, neuroblastoma, Hodgkin lymphoma, and medulloblastoma have not been specifically identified as RB dependent tumors.

(Section 24: Neoplastic Disorders; Part 1: Principles of Oncology, Chapter 443, pp 1603–1605)

Answer 24-2. d

This patient has WAGR syndrome (Wilms tumor, aniridia, genitourinary abnormalities, and mental retardation), which is a contiguous gene syndrome involving the loss of chromosome 11p13, which contains both the *PAX6* gene (causing aniridia and mental retardation) and the *WT1* gene (predisposing the patient to Wilms tumor and genitourinary abnormalities). However, as the WT1 gene is a classic tumor suppressor gene, Wilms tumors only develop in ~30% of the patients who develop a "second hit" to their wild-type copy. All patients with WAGR should be screened every 3–4 months from birth until age 5 with abdominal ultrasound.

WAGR syndrome is not associated with hemihypertrophy. Loss of chromosome 11p15 causes the Beckwith–Wiedemann syndrome, which is associated with hemihypertrophy and increased risk of Wilms tumor, hepatoblastoma, and other malignancies.

(Section 24: Neoplastic Disorders; Part 1: Principles of Oncology, Chapter 443, p 1604)

Answer 24-3. e

The t(11;22) translocation is found in more than 90% of cases of Ewing sarcoma, and results in the formation of the *EWS–FLI1* fusion protein. In most of the remaining cases, *EWS* is fused with other partners. Translocation t(2;13) is characteristic of alveolar rhabdomyosarcoma. This translocation results in the fusion of the DNA-binding domain of *PAX3* to the transactivation domain of the transcription factor *FOXO1A*. t(X;18) is seen in synovial sarcoma. t(2;5) fuses nucleophosmin (NPM) on chromosome 2 with the receptor kinase *ALK* on chromosome 5 and is found in anaplastic large cell lymphoma.

t(9;22), also known as the "Philadelphia chromosome," results in the generation of the *BCR–ABL* fusion protein and is found in almost all cases of chronic myelogenous leukemia and sometimes in other forms of leukemia.

(Section 24: Neoplastic Disorders; Part 1: Principles of Oncology, Chapter 443, p 1604)

Answer 24-4. b

This boy's family meets all 3 clinical diagnostic criteria for Li Fraumeni syndrome, which include (1) the patient is diagnosed with a sarcoma before the age of 45, (2) a first-degree relative has been diagnosed with any cancer before the age of 45, and (3) another fist-degree or a second-degree relative has been diagnosed with any cancer before the age of 45 or a sarcoma at any age. Li Fraumeni syndrome is caused by a germline mutation in 1 copy of the p53 tumor suppressor gene. According to the Knudsen two-hit model, a cancer develops when the second copy of p53 in a cell develops a sporadic mutation. The normal function of p53 is to assist in repair or destruction of damaged DNA before allowing the cell to grow and divide, so the loss of p53 causes the damaged cells to grow in an uncontrolled manner resulting in cancer.

Amplification of *NMYC* is seen in high-risk neuroblastoma. Loss of heterozygosity at 11p15 is a hallmark of embryonal rhabdomyosarcoma. Mutation of *MEN1* causes the familial cancer syndrome multiple endocrine neoplasia, which is associated with tumors of the pancreas, pituitary, and thyroid. Mutation of *VHL* causes the Von Hippel–Lindau syndrome, in which patients frequently develop frequent and numerous retinal and CNS hemangioblastomas, along with occasional pheochromocytomas or renal cell carcinomas.

(Section 24: Neoplastic Disorders; Part 1: Principles of Oncology, Chapter 443, p 1605)

Answer 24-5. a

Alkylating agents cross-link guanine nucleotides in DNA, which prevents the strands from uncoiling, thereby preventing DNA replication. Since cancer cells grow and divide much faster than normal cells, they replicate DNA more quickly and are thus more susceptible to replication errors. Therefore, cancer cells are particularly vulnerable to chemotherapeutic agents that interfere with DNA replication or induce DNA damage. DNA damage triggers a cell to undergo apoptosis. The relevant class of alkylating agents includes cyclophosphamide, ifosfamide, cisplatin, and carboplatin, which are used to treat a variety of tumors including sarcomas. It also includes melphalan and busulfan, which are used primarily in the transplant setting, and temozolomide and procarbazine, which are used to treat brain tumors.

Methotrexate and 6-mercaptopurine are antimetabolites. Methorexate inhibits the enzyme dihydrofolate reductase, which decreases folic acid stores and prevents synthesis of the purines required for synthesis of new RNA or DNA molecules. Etoposide and doxorubicin are topoisomerase inhibitors, which cause single- and double-strand DNA breaks.

(Section 24: Neoplastic Disorders; Part 1: Principles of Oncology, Chapter 445, pp 1609–1610)

Answer 24-6. a

Anthracyclines, including doxorubicin and daunorubicin, are valuable agents in the treatment of childhood cancers. However, their use can lead to long-term cardiac complications, including arrhythmias, heart failure due to cardiomyopathy, and death. Cardiotoxicity from anthracyclines occurs in a dose-dependent fashion. While the risk of clinically evident cardiac damage rises steeply after a cumulative dose of 700 mg/m^2 of daunorubicin, acute or chronic cardiac disease can occur after any dose, probably in combination with other risk factors such as malnutrition, age, or concomitant radiation therapy. The cardiotoxic effects of anthracyclines can be somewhat reduced by administering them along with dexrazoxane, a chelator that decreases the formation of superoxide radicals, although there is some debate over whether this may decrease the antitumor efficacy of anthracyclines. Cytarabine, etoposide, vincristine, and topotecan are not known to cause significant cardiotoxicity.

(Section 24: Neoplastic Disorders; Part 1: Principles of Oncology, Chapter 445, p 1611)

Answer 24-7. b

The patient has most likely developed hemorrhagic cystitis secondary to cyclophosphamide. Cyclophosphamide is broken down in the liver to the urotoxic metabolite acrolein. As acrolein collects in the bladder awaiting urination, the bladder tends to be more severely affected than other urothelial tissues. Every effort is made to prevent the development of hemorrhagic cystitis in patients receiving a high dose cyclophosphamide or ifosfamide by giving aggressive IV hydration and scheduled therapy with mesna (2-mercaptoethane sulfonate), which binds to acrolein and reduces its toxicity. If hemorrhagic cystitis develops, the initial treatment of choice is to increase hydration and encourage frequent urination, which flushes the bladder and helps prevent clot formation.

While mesna helps prevent the development of hemorrhagic cystitis, it is ineffective after the bladder damage occurs. It is important to work the patient up for other possible causes of her symptoms by sending a CBC, a urinalysis, urine culture, and urinary viral studies. However, broad-spectrum antibiotics should not be initiated unless the patient is febrile or there is evidence of infection on the urinalysis. If the urethra becomes obstructed by a blood clot, urology should be consulted to assist with a large-bore urethral catheter placement or clot extraction to restore the flow of urine out of the bladder; otherwise it is not necessary to place a foley catheter. The patient should not be discharged home until she is urinating without difficulty and she is no longer passing bloody urine.

(Section 24: Neoplastic Disorders; Part 1: Principles of Oncology, Chapter 445, p 1611)

Answer 24-8. d

Phase III clinical trials compare the current best available therapy to a new treatment approach for which there is a body of evidence supporting potential superiority. These trials enroll large numbers of patients and typically compare the efficacy of 2 or more therapeutic regimens at promoting tumor response or prolonging event-free or overall survival.

Phase I clinical trials are designed to identify the appropriate dose and schedule of a novel chemotherapeutic agent as well as define the toxicities of a novel chemotherapeutic agent at multiple dosing levels. Phase II trials attempt to determine whether or not a novel chemotherapeutic agent can produce an objective response against the tumor. Answer choice B is incorrect, because for ethical reasons, it is not appropriate to randomize patients to a therapeutic regimen that has been shown to be inferior to another regimen.

(Section 24: Neoplastic Disorders; Part 1: Principles of Oncology, Chapter 446, p 1613)

Answer 24-9. e

The most common cause of a solid renal mass in a newborn is congenital mesoblastic nephroma (CMN). CMN is a solitary hamartoma that originates from the mesenchymal tissue in the embryonic kidney and is frequently associated with the translocation t(12;15), which results in generation of the fusion protein *ETV6–NTRK3*. CMN is often detected before birth by prenatal ultrasound, and can be associated with polyhydramnios and pre-term labor as well as hematuria, hypercalcemia, and hypertension in the newborn. Treatment is with surgical resection alone, as this type of tumor rarely metastasizes.

It is impossible to distinguish CMN from nephroblastoma (Wilms tumor) by ultrasound, but nephroblastoma is rare in the neonatal period, as are renal cell carcinomas and rhabdoid tumors. Hemangiomas are common in the first few months of life, but are rarely seen in the kidneys. The majority of renal masses palpated in the newborn are non-neoplastic, including hydronephrosis and renal cysts.

(Section 24: Neoplastic Disorders; Part 1: Principles of Oncology, Chapter 447, p 1615)

Answer 24-10. b

Acute lymphoblastic leukemia is the most common childhood malignancy. It represents more than 25% of all childhood malignancies with approximately 2400 new cases annually in the United States. Acute lymphoblastic leukemia represents approximately 85% of childhood leukemia with acute myelogenous leukemia representing approximately 15% of childhood leukemias. The peak incidence acute lymphoblastic leukemia is in the 2- to 6-year-old age group.

Neuroblastoma is the most common childhood malignancy in children under 2 years of age. There are approximately 650 new cases annually in the United States. Brain tumors represent the most common solid tumor in childhood cancers and are second to acute lymphoblastic leukemia as the most common childhood cancer.

(Section 24: Neoplastic Disorders; Part 2: Hematologic Malignancies, Chapter 449, p 1620)

Answer 24-11. c

Expression of cell surface markers on leukemia cells can be used to determine the lineage (B, T, or myeloid) as well as the maturation stage (pro-cell, pre-cell, mature cell, etc) of the blasts cells, providing prognostic information and guiding therapy options. For this reason, flow cytometry has become a critical part of the initial workup for leukemia. The B-cell markers CD19 and CD22 are present on most B lineage lymphoid cells, regardless of the maturation stage. The common ALL antigen (CALLA, CD10), is present on early pre ("common") and many pre B-cells, but disappears by the mature B-cell stage. Immunoglobulin first appears in the cytoplasm of pre B-cells, and then on the surface of mature B-cells. Since this patient's blast cells express CD19 and CD22, they are of B lineage, and since they express CD10 but not immunoglobulin, they are early pre, or common B-cell precursors. Expression of CD3 would suggest that the cells are of T-cell lineage.

(Section 24: Neoplastic Disorders; Part 2: Hematologic Malignancies, Chapter 449, p 1620)

Answer 24-12. a

This patient has lymphadenopathy, fever, and pancytopenia, which raises suspicion that the patient has a hematopoietic malignancy (ie, leukemia or lymphoma). Although a needle biopsy of the lymph node is one possible mechanism of confirming the diagnosis, most physicians would proceed directly to bone marrow biopsy since it is a required part of the staging workup for a hematopoietic malignancy anyway. Patients with lymphoma or T-cell leukemia may present with a mediastinal mass. This patient has a cough, but many patients with mediastinal masses are asymptomatic. As general anesthesia relaxes the muscles that help keep the chest open, patients with an anterior mediastinal mass are at risk of life-threatening upper airway obstruction. It is therefore critical to get a 2-view chest X-ray on every patient with a suspected hematopoietic malignancy prior to allowing them to undergo general anesthesia.

Although this patient has thrombocytopenia, it is not severe enough to require transfusion prior to the procedure. A bone marrow biopsy is generally considered a safe procedure at any platelet count and INR as any post-procedure bleeding is external and can be monitored and treated as needed. If a lumbar puncture is also planned, most practitioners use a platelet count cutoff of between 30 and 50×10^9/L, although there is little evidence that doing a lumbar puncture at lower platelet counts increases the risk of spinal cord compression from an acute bleed. Although hematopoietic malignancies can present with renal compromise due to toxic tumor breakdown products, it does not usually have any additional consequences for a patient undergoing a short procedure.

(Section 24: Neoplastic Disorders; Part 2: Hematologic Malignancies, Chapter 449, p 1621)

Answer 24-13. d

Age is an important prognostic factor. Patients diagnosed with acute lymphoblastic leukemia between the ages of 1 and 9 years generally have the best prognosis. Biological features influence the prognosis. The most common genetic alterations in B-cell acute lymphoblastic leukemias are hyperdiploidy (>51 chromosomes) and a translocation between chromosomes 12 and 21. Both of these findings are associated with a better prognosis, as is the less common translocation between chromosomes 1 and 19. Infants under 1 year of age, particularly those under 6 months of age, commonly have a translocation between chromosomes 4 and 11. These infants have a poor prognosis with a 5-year event-free survival of approximately 40%.

(Section 24: Neoplastic Disorders; Part 2: Hematologic Malignancies, Chapter 449, p 1621)

Answer 24-14. c

Since patients with newly diagnosed leukemia or lymphoma can present with mediastinal involvement it is important to monitor carefully for respiratory compromise. In this case, a chest X-ray should be done prior to proceeding with a bone marrow aspirate and biopsy to assess airway status. If this patient demonstrated a significant mediastinal mass, the diagnosis of leukemia could be obtained by microscopic, flow cytometric and cytogenetic evaluation of peripheral blood. Patients with newly diagnosed leukemia can present with infections and metabolic disorders therefore blood cultures and chemistries would be an important part of the initial evaluation in this patient.

While this patient will likely need blood products, he does not have active bleeding or hemodynamic instability that would warrant emergent transfusions. Administration of IV fluids will ultimately be necessary, but should be given with caution in a patient with compensated anemia to avoid congestive heart failure. Steroids should be given after making a definitive bone marrow diagnosis unless required for urgent airway or CNS compromise.

(Section 24: Neoplastic Disorders; Part 2: Hematologic Malignancies, Chapter 449, p 1623)

Answer 24-15. c

The term *remission* was coined to define a state in which there was no clinical or laboratory evidence of residual disease.

The initial therapy for ALL is called induction and the goal of this therapy is to *induce* remission. Post-remission therapy is required to consolidate and maintain remission. Flow cytometry is used to define the subtype of leukemia and to monitor minimal residual disease.

(Section 24: Neoplastic Disorders; Part 2: Hematologic Malignancies, Chapter 449, p 1623)

Answer 24-16. b

Patients with ALL are defined as standard risk if they are between the ages of 1 and 9, have a white blood cell count of less than 50,000/μL, and have no CNS or testicular disease. These patients receive a standard 3-drug induction phase of chemotherapy with vincristine, steroid, and L-asparaginase. All other patients have high risk disease. Four-drug induction with vincristine, steroid, L-asparaginase, and daunomycin has been demonstrated to be superior to the 3-drug induction in patients with high risk ALL. Given the patient in the vignette has a WBC above 50,000/μL, this patient should receive daunomycin. Methotrexate, 6-mercaptopurine, cytoxan, and ara-c are all effective in the treatment of ALL, but are typically given in later rounds of therapy, after the completion of the induction phase.

(Section 24: Neoplastic Disorders; Part 2: Hematologic Malignancies, Chapter 449, p 1624)

Answer 24-17. d

Early bone marrow relapse, occurring within 36 months of diagnosis, is associated with the worst prognosis. Treatment usually consists of reinduction followed by an allogenic bone barrow transplant from a matching sibling or matched unrelated donor. Relapse at isolated extramedullary sites, such as the CNS or the testicles, tends to be associated with a more favorable outcome than bone marrow relapse. Patients relapsing late, more than 36 months from the initial diagnosis, tend to have a more favorable outcome. Late isolated extramedullary relapse is usually treated with chemotherapy and local therapy directed at the site affected.

(Section 24: Neoplastic Disorders; Part 2: Hematologic Malignancies, Chapter 449, p 1625)

Answer 24-18. d

All patients who receive chemotherapy that puts them at risk for low lymphocyte counts must receive prophylaxis for *Pneumocystis carinii* pneumonia (PCP). Patients with acute lymphoblastic leukemia are particularly at risk. Although the causative organism has been renamed *Pneumocystis jiroveci*, many practitioners continue to refer to the older name. Although the disease often has an indolent course in HIV patients, PCP carries a mortality rate of 30–50% in patients who do not have HIV. Trimethoprim-sulfamethoxazole and pentamidine are both effective at preventing *Pneumocystis carinii* infection.

Haemophilus influenzae and *Streptococcus pneumoniae* are more likely to produce a focal consolidation visible on X-ray. Aspergillus pneumonia typically appears as numerous round fungal lesions surrounded by a "halo." *Mycoplasma pneumoniae* is certainly possible in this patient, but is less likely to have such an acute and severe presentation.

(Section 24: Neoplastic Disorders; Part 2: Hematologic Malignancies, Chapter 449, p 1625)

Answer 24-19. d

This newborn has transient myeloproliferative disorder (TMD). Children with Down syndrome are at a greater risk for developing TMD, and have an overall greater than 15-fold increased risk of leukemia. As the name TMD implies, this is usually a transient process. Newborns with Down Syndrome (DS) and TMD who have evidence of liver dysfunction and markedly elevated WBC (>50,000/μL) may benefit from low-dose chemotherapy, as sicker infants with TMD are at risk of developing liver and/or multiorgan failure. In most cases, however, TMD resolves spontaneously over several weeks, so close follow-up is warranted. Infants with DS who exhibit TMD are at an even higher risk for developing acute leukemia later in life, therefore ongoing follow-up is indicated. Leukopheresis is not indicated unless WBC count is greater than 100,000 and there is concern for organ damage from hyperleukocytosis.

(Section 24: Neoplastic Disorders; Part 2: Hematologic Malignancies, Chapter 450, p 1626)

Answer 24-20. b

This patient most likely has a secondary, therapy-related acute myeloid leukemia (tAML) caused by etoposide. Alkylating agents and topoisomerase-II inhibitors, like etoposide, have been linked to secondary AML. The percentage of patients who receive etoposide who go on to develop tAML ranges from 1 to 20% depending on the cumulative dose and dosing schedule, with higher cumulative doses and prolonged or more frequent exposure leading to higher risk. Etoposide-induced tAML tends to occur 2–4 years after initial therapy with the agent and is characteristically marked by a translocation involving the *MLL* gene on chromosome 11. Cyclophosphamide and ifosfamide are both alkylating agents, which also carry a high risk of inducing secondary AML. However, leukemias induced by alkylating agents tend to occur 4–10 years after the initial therapy and are often associated with monosomy of chromosomes 5 or 7. Vincristine and doxorubicin are not strongly associated with the development of secondary malignancies.

(Section 24: Neoplastic Disorders; Part 2: Hematologic Malignancies, Chapter 450, p 1626)

Answer 24-21. e

The translocation t(15;17), which results in generation of the fusion protein *PML–RARα*, is pathognomonic for APL anemia. t(9;22) results in generation of the fusion protein *BCR–ABL*, which is ubiquitous in chronic myelogenous leukemia but also detected in some acute myeloid and acute lymphoid leukemias. Translocations involving the *MLL* gene (eg t(9;11)), inversion(16) and t(8;21), which result in the formation of the fusion protein *CBFA–ETO,* are among the most common translocations seen in nonpromyelocytic acute myelogenous leukemia.

(Section 24: Neoplastic Disorders; Part 2: Hematologic Malignancies, Chapter 450, p 1628)

Answer 24-22. d

The *PML–RARα* translocation is characteristic of the APL subtype of AML and the resultant fusion protein causes maturation arrest of myeloid cells in the promyelocyte stage. Although the mechanism of action is uncertain, all-trans retinoic acid (ATRA) causes these cells to once again proceed normally through maturation, which, in combination with arsenic and traditional chemotherapy, results in a very high cure rate for APL of 70–90%. Interestingly, a "differentiation syndrome" occurs in about 25% of patients with APL who receive ATRA (it can also be induced by arsenic). This syndrome is characterized by fever, respiratory distress, hypotension, and organ failure caused by the release of inflammatory cytokines from the promyelocytes. This syndrome is specific to APL and is not seen if ATRA or arsenic is used to treat other myeloid malignancies (which is uncommon). In addition, it is specific to the induction phase of therapy, and is dependent on neither the dose nor starting WBC count. Treatment consists of supportive care, steroids, and temporarily holding chemotherapy if necessary.

Monosomy 5, monosomy 7, *FLT3* internal tandeum duplicates with high allelic ratio and any translocations involving the *MLL* gene all result in poor prognosis.

(Section 24: Neoplastic Disorders; Part 2: Hematologic Malignancies, Chapter 450, p 1629)

Answer 24-23. c

This child probably has juvenile myelomonocytic leukemia (JMML). Suggestive clinical features of JMML include hepatosplenomegaly, lymphadenopathy, pallor, fever, and/or skin rash. The diagnosis of JMML requires a persistent peripheral blood monocytosis ($>1 \times 10^9$/L) with no evidence of the *BCR–ABL* fusion gene (the presence of the Philadelphia chromosome would suggest chronic myeloid leukemia) and <20% blasts in the bone marrow (a higher percentage of blasts would indicate acute myeloid leukemia). In addition, at least 2 of the following criteria must be met: increased hemoglobin F, immature myeloid precursors on the peripheral smear, peripheral white blood cell count greater than 10×10^9/L,

clonal cytogenetic abnormalities, or GM-CSF hypersensitivity of myeloid progenitors. Although some cases of JMML spontaneously remit for reasons that are not currently known, JMML cannot otherwise be cured except with hematopoietic stem cell transplant.

ATRA and arsenic form the standard induction therapy for APL leukemia. Dexamethasone, vincristine, and asparaginase form the standard induction therapy for acute lymphoid leukemia. Daunorubicin and cytarabine are part of the standard induction therapy for non-APL acute myeloid leukemia. Leukopheresis is rarely used for patients with white blood cell counts $<100 \times 10^9$/L.

(Section 24: Neoplastic Disorders; Part 2: Hematologic Malignancies, Chapter 450, pp 1629–1630)

Answer 24-24. d

This child has evidence of a mature B-cell lymphoma. She probably has endemic Burkitt lymphoma, in which EBV infection is necessary, but not sufficient, to cause disease. Endemic Burkitt lymphoma is the form typically seen in children in equatorial Africa, and there is some recent evidence to suggest that co-infection with EBV and malaria may help promote the development of the disease. Nonendemic forms of Burkitt lymphoma, found in North America and Europe, appear pathologically identical to endemic Burkitt lymphoma, but are not always associated with EBV infection. The endemic form typically presents in children in the head and neck, particularly with jaw involvement. CMV, HIV, HHV-6, and HSV have no association with Burkitt lymphoma.

(Section 24: Neoplastic Disorders; Part 2: Hematologic Malignancies, Chapter 451, p 1631)

Answer 24-25. c

Pediatric non-Hodgkin lymphomas are classified according to the St. Jude staging system. This is different from the Ann Arbor staging system used to stage adult non-Hodgkin lymphomas, because children tend to have higher rates of extranodal involvement and metastatic spread that make the Ann Arbor staging system of limited predictive value for children in regards to outcome. According to the St. Jude staging system, Stage I disease is disease in only 1 location, either as a single extra-nodal tumor, or involving lymph nodes in only 1 part of the body. Lymphomas in the chest and abdomen are never classified as Stage I. To be classified as Stage II, a lymphoma must meet 1 of the following criteria: (a) single extra-nodal tumor plus nearby lymph nodes, (b) 2 or more nodal areas on the same side of the diaphragm, (c) 2 extra-nodal tumors with or without regional node involvement on the same side of the diaphragm, or (d) a primary GI tract tumor +/− associated mesenteric nodes that can be completely resected. Lymphomas in the chest are never classified as Stage II. The following tumors are classified as Stage III: (a) 2 extra-nodal tumors on opposite sides of the diaphragm, (b) 2 or more nodal areas above and below the diaphragm, (c) any intrathoracic tumor, (d) unresectable intra-abdominal disease, and (e) all paraspinal or epidural tumors. If there is CNS or bone marrow involvement, the disease is classified as Stage IV. If bone marrow involvement exceeds 25%, the disease is classified as leukemia. The patient in the vignette has intra-abdominal disease that cannot be resected, but no CNS or bone marrow involvement, so she has Stage III disease.

(Section 24: Neoplastic Disorders; Part 2: Hematologic Malignancies, Chapter 451, p 1631 (eTable 451.1))

Answer 24-26. e

The presence of Reed–Sternberg cells on lymph node biopsy is pathognomonic for Hodgkin lymphoma. The presence of "B symptoms," which include (1) drenching night sweats (typically requiring changing of clothing or bedding during the night), (2) >10% unexplained weight loss over preceding 6 months, and/or (3) fever >38°C for at least 3 consecutive days, are present in about one third of patients with Hodgkin disease and are associated with a worse prognosis. Other symptoms, including alcohol-induced pain, itching, malaise, and anorexia are frequently reported in patients with Hodgkin disease, but have not been shown to be useful prognostic indicators. Alcohol-induced pain of involved nodal areas, which frequently occurs minutes after alcohol consumption, and generalized pruritis are curious symptoms that are fairly specific to Hodgkin lymphoma. It is not known why these symptoms develop; however, they resolve with treatment of the malignancy.

(Section 24: Neoplastic Disorders; Part 2: Hematologic Malignancies, Chapter 452, p 1634)

Answer 24-27. a

The presence of osteoid formation in a lytic bone tumor is pathognomonic for osteosarcoma. The vast majority of osteosarcomas arise near the ends one of the long bones (femur, tibia, fibula, humerus, radius, or ulna), with almost 50% found in either the distal femur or the proximal tibia and another 10–20% found in the arm, most often the proximal humerus. These tumors are more rarely found in the axial skeleton, short bones, or bones of the face and skull. These locations are in contrast to Ewing sarcoma, which most frequently arises in the flat bones of the axial skeleton (eg, ribs, pelvis), and when it does arise in long bones, typically is found in the midshaft or diaphysis.

(Section 24: Neoplastic Disorders; Part 3: Solid Tumors, Chapter 453, p 1637)

Answer 24-28. d

Approximately 20% of patients with osteosarcoma will have evidence of metastatic disease at diagnosis. The lungs are the most frequent site of metastasis, followed by "skip lesions" in the same bone as the primary tumor and other bony

metastases. A radionuclide bone scan is routinely preformed at the time of diagnosis to define the extent of the primary tumor and detect skip lesions. Although a chest X-ray, PET scan, or chest MRI might pick up metastases to the lungs, chest CT is the most sensitive and is the imaging procedure of choice to rule out lung metastases.

(Section 24: Neoplastic Disorders; Part 3: Solid Tumors, Chapter 453, p 1638)

Answer 24-29. d

Localized osteosarcoma treated with modern protocols that include neoadjuvant chemotherapy consisting of methotrexate, doxorubicin and cisplatin as well as definitive local control by surgical resection followed by additional chemotherapy is associated with a 70% 5-year overall survival.

Chemotherapy is typically given prior to surgical resection to make surgery easier and to yield predictive information about prognosis based on histologic response of the tumor, although timing of surgery in relation to chemotherapy most likely does not affect the risk of tumor relapse. Percent tumor necrosis after 10 weeks of neo-adjuvant therapy is thought to have significant prognostic value, with unfavorable response (<90% or <98% necrosis, depending on the study) lowering the 5-year survival estimates to nearly 50% and favorable response increasing them to 80–90%. Unfortunately, intensification of chemotherapy in patients with an unfavorable response has not been shown to improve outcomes.

(Section 24: Neoplastic Disorders; Part 3: Solid Tumors, Chapter 453, pp 1638–1639)

Answer 24-30. e

This patient most likely has Ewing sarcoma. Ewing sarcoma is the second most common bone tumor in children and adolescents after osteosarcoma. It has been reported to be found in almost every bone, but most commonly arises in flat bones, like vertebrae. Many patients present with a history of chronic pain for many months before diagnosis.

All of the tumors listed can appear as small, round, blue cells on histologic examination, but osteoid expression must be present to diagnose small round cell osteosarcoma, and only lymphoma, rhabdomyosarcoma, and Ewing sarcoma express CD99. Lymphoma would be more likely to appear as enlarged mediastinal lymph nodes than as intrapulmonary masses. While Ewing sarcoma and rhabdommyosarcoma both frequently present with metastases to the lung, only Ewing sarcoma has a characteristic *EWS* translocation involving the *EWS* gene on chromosome 22. The most common fusion partner is *FLI1* on chromosome 11, although other translocation partners for *EWS* can include the *ETS* family members *ERG*, *FEV*, *ETV1*, or *E1AF*. The alveolar subtype of rhabdomyosarcoma is typically characterized by a t(2;13) translocation, while the embryonal subtype is frequently associated with loss of heterozygosity of 11p15.

(Section 24: Neoplastic Disorders; Part 3: Solid Tumors, Chapter 454, pp 1640–1641)

Answer 24-31. c

The most common reason to opt for local control of Ewing sarcoma with radiation therapy instead of surgery is a tumor that is large, centrally located, or otherwise not amenable to surgery without significant cosmetic or functional consequences. Most physicians would recommend surgical resection for small and peripherally located tumors because patients who receive radiation as the local control have a worse overall survival than those whose tumors undergo complete resection. However, Ewing sarcomas appear to be very sensitive to radiation, and it is possible that much of this difference is caused by characteristics of the tumor itself (eg, size). Radiation therapy is associated with a higher risk of secondary malignancies in the radiation field, and should probably be avoided in patients with genetic predispositions to cancer, such as Li Fraumeni syndrome. As only a small fraction of patients with localized Ewing sarcoma will be cured with local control alone, aggressive chemotherapy is required in all cases to treat presumed micrometastases at diagnosis.

(Section 24: Neoplastic Disorders; Part 3: Solid Tumors, Chapter 454, p 1641)

Answer 24-32. d

Osteosarcoma and rhabdomyosarcoma are both associated with the Li Fraumeni familial cancer syndrome, characterized by germline mutations of the *p53* tumor suppressor gene. Other malignancies frequently seen in this syndrome include other soft tissue sarcomas, breast cancer, brain tumors, and acute leukemia.

Germline *HRAS* mutations are associated with Costello syndrome, which is characterized by developmental delay, mental retardation, facial dysmorphisms, and other congenital defects in addition to an increased risk of benign skin papillomas and rhabdoyosarcomas. Germline *NF1* mutations cause neurofibromatosis type 1 (NF-1), which is associated with characteristic physical findings including axillary freckling, café au lait spots, Lisch nodules in the iris of the eye, and sometimes mild cognitive impairment. Patients with NF-1 are at increased risk of benign skin tumors called neurofibromas (plexiform or nodular), as well as optic pathway gliomas, malignant peripheral nerve sheath tumors, and pheochromocytomas. Mutations in the tumor suppressor *RB1* are associated with retinoblastoma and secondary sarcomas, particularly in or near the radiation field following radiation therapy to the primary retinoblastoma. These secondary sarcomas are most commonly osteosarcomas, but can also be rhabdomyosarcomas or other cancers. Germline *CREBBP* mutations cause Rubinstein–Taybi syndrome, a rare syndrome clinically characterized by broadening of the thumbs and big toes, dysmorphic facies, short stature, hirsutism, developmental delay, mental retardation and, albeit rarely, rhabdomyosarcoma.

(Section 24: Neoplastic Disorders; Part 3: Solid Tumors, Chapter 455, p 1642)

Answer 24-33. e

A positive stain for desmin in the context of cells with myogenic appearance is highly suggestive of rhabdomyosarcoma. This patient has the embryonal variant, which can be distinguished from the alveolar variant by its mixed cellularity, loose, myxoid stroma, and cytogenetics demonstrating 11p15.5. By contrast, the alveolar variant has small cells with round nuclei and scant cytoplasm that are gathered into clusters divided by fibrovascular septae and spaces that give the tissue an "alveolar" appearance and typically has a *PAX3–FOXO1* or *PAX7–FOXO1* translocation. All rhabdomyosarcomas require systemic chemotherapy to treat presumptive micrometastatic disease. Favorable sites of RMS are limited to the orbit, superficial head and neck, paratesticular, vagina, uterus, and biliary tract. This patient has a tumor involving the bladder, which is an unfavorable site. This patient does not have metastatic disease, so he does not fall into the high-risk group, which would have a long-term survival estimate of 30%. If his tumor can be grossly resected, he would fall into the low-risk group, which has an 85–95% estimated long-term survival. If it is not grossly resected, he would fall into the intermediate risk group, which is associated with a 60–70% long-term survival. Although embryonal sarcoma has a better prognosis than it's alveolar counterpart, and can often be treated with less chemotherapy, definitive local control is required. If the tumor cannot be fully resected, it must be radiated.

(Section 24: Neoplastic Disorders; Part 3: Solid Tumors, Chapter 455, p 1643)

Answer 24-34. a

Approximately 8% of patients with Wilms tumor develop an acquired von Willebrand disease, although the pathophysiology of this relationship remains unknown. In the literature, cases of both type I and type III acquired von Willebrand disease have been reported. Although most patients with Wilms tumor and acquired von Willebrand disease do not experience any clinically significant bleeding, there have been some instances of severe hemorrhage, so the standard of care is to screen all newly diagnosed Wilms tumor patients for a coagulopathy, and then to correct any abnormalities detected prior to surgery. DDAVP should be attempted first, regardless of the type of von Willebrand disease, because if patients respond to DDAVP, it is possible that administration of blood products can be avoided.

(Section 24: Neoplastic Disorders; Part 3: Solid Tumors, Chapter 455, p 1645)

Answer 24-35. b

Loss of heterozygosity (LOH) of chromosomes 1p or 16q is associated with a worse prognosis for patients with favorable histology Wilms tumor, and require augmentation of therapy regardless of tumor stage, with the exception of children under the age of 2 with Stage I disease and tumor weight <550 g, who can often be cured with surgery alone. MYCN amplification and PHOX2B mutation and LOH of 11q are all associated with neuroblastoma, not Wilms tumor. While PAX6 deletion is seen in patients with Wilms tumor who also have WAGR syndrome, it is not significant for prognosis.

(Section 24: Neoplastic Disorders; Part 3: Solid Tumors, Chapter 456, p 1646)

Answer 24-36. e

This child has opsoclonus-myoclonus-ataxia (OMA) syndrome, which is very rare, but seen in ~1% of children with neuroblastoma. Although the exact pathophysiology is unknown, it is thought to be a paraneoplastic syndrome caused by autoantibodies that develop against the tumor and cross-react with normal neurons. Unfortunately, these symptoms are likely to persist to some degree even with effective treatment of the tumor. Patients with neuroblastoma and OMA tend to have biologically favorable tumors and a good prognosis from an oncologic standpoint.

(Section 24: Neoplastic Disorders; Part 3: Solid Tumors, Chapter 457, p 1649)

Answer 24-37. a

Neuroblastoma is a complex disease, with many factors that appear to contribute to prognosis, including a number of genetic variables that can be detected in the tumor itself. DNA index is a measure of the number of chromosomes in a tumor cell. Normal cells are diploid, meaning that they have 2 copies of each chromosome. It is common for chromosomes to be lost (leading to "hypodiploidy") or gained (leading to "hyperdiploidy") in malignant cells. For neuroblastoma, hyperdiploidy is a favorable prognostic factor, up to a point. While near-triploid tumors, with 3 copies of most chromosomes, tend to correlate with more indolent tumor behavior, near-tetraploid tumors, with 4 copies of most chromosomes, tend to behave more aggressively. MYCN amplification, deletion of chromosome 1p, and extra copies of chromosome 17q are all associated with worse prognosis for patients with neuroblastoma.

(Section 24: Neoplastic Disorders; Part 3: Solid Tumors, Chapter 457, p 1650)

Answer 24-38. b

The use of 13-*cis*-retinoic acid to promote differentiation of neuroblastoma cells has been tested in a Phase III trial in the post-transplant setting and shown to produce superior event-free survival in patients with high-risk disease with acceptable toxicity, so it is now considered standard of care. A recent Phase III trial of immunotherapy (monoclonal chimeric mouse/human antibody ch14.18, which targets the neural GD2 cell-surface marker alternating with GM-CSF and IL-2), demonstrated improved event-free survival in children with high-risk disease, and is also likely to be incorporated into standard of care. All-*trans*-retinoic acid (ATRA) is used in the treatment of acute promyelocytic leukemia (APML) but not neuroblastoma. Allogeneic stem cell transplant has not been demonstrated to be superior to autologous stem cell transplant in neuroblastoma patients, and is of higher risk, so it is generally avoided. Currently, ^{131}I-MIBG therapy is used primarily in the experimental setting, although given the success of this therapy in early-phase trials, this may change in the next Children's Oncology Group trial.

(Section 24: Neoplastic Disorders; Part 3: Solid Tumors, Chapter 457, p 1651)

Answer 24-39. d

Hepatoblastoma and hepatocellular carcinoma are the 2 most common types of liver tumors found in children. Hepatoblastoma is typically seen in young children, with a mean age of onset of approximately 18 months, and the vast majority of cases occurring in children under the age of 5. Hepatocellular carcinoma is typically seen in older children. The strongest risk factor for developing hepatocellular carcinoma is a history of infection with hepatitis B or hepatitis C viruses. High rates of hepatocellular carcinoma exist in countries with widespread hepatitis infections, and hepatitis vaccination programs have been shown to significantly reduce the incidence of this tumor.

Undifferentiated embryonal sarcoma and cholangiocarcinoma are rare in the pediatric population. Hemangioendotheliomas are relatively common, but this benign tumor would be unlikely to result in weight loss and cachexia.

(Section 24: Neoplastic Disorders; Part 3: Solid Tumors, Chapter 458, pp 1651–1652)

Answer 24-40. c

Familial adenomatous polyposis (FAP) is an inherited cancer syndrome caused by mutations in the adenomatous polyposis coli (APC) gene. It is an autosomal dominant syndrome characterized by polyp growth in the colon throughout adolescence and adulthood. Without medical attention, these polyps frequently progress to colon cancer.

Interestingly, mutations in this gene are frequently seen in children with hepatoblastoma who have a family history of colon cancer, and it is recommended that children of FAP families be screened for hepatoblastoma and children with hepatoblastoma be screened for *APC* mutations.

GPC3 is the gene associated with Simpson–Golabie–Behmel. While patients with a mutation in GPC3 are at increased risk of hepatoblastoma and other tumors, including colon cancer, children with this mutation have macrosomia and coarse facial features in addition to other genetic defects. Mutations in ABCB11 cause progressive familial intrahepatic cholestasis, mutations in NOTCH2 are associated with Alagille syndrome, and mutations in FAH can cause hereditary tyrosinemia, all of which are associated with an increased risk of hepatocellular carcinoma but not hepatoblastoma.

(Section 24: Neoplastic Disorders; Part 3: Solid Tumors, Chapter 458, p 1652)

Answer 24-41. b

Children with hepatoblastoma whose tumors have pure fetal histology generally have an excellent outcome. In fact, if the tumor can be completely resected, adjuvant chemotherapy may be avoidable. By contrast, small cell undifferentiated histology and low alpha-fetoprotein levels are associated with a worse outcome. History of prematurity and hemihypertrophy are each associated with an increased risk of hepatoblastoma, but do not affect outcome.

(Section 24: Neoplastic Disorders; Part 3: Solid Tumors, Chapter 458, p 1653)

Answer 24-42. c

Dysgerminoma is a germinoma arising from the ovary; Seminoma is a germinoma arising from the testes. As described in the vignette, these tumors stain strongly for placental alkaline phosphatase. They are rarely found in prepubertal girls.

Mature teratomas are the most common histologic subtype of childhood germ cell tumors and are typically diagnosed by ultrasound given characteristic sonographic findings suggestive of hair, teeth, and fat. Yolk sac tumors are the most common malignant germ cell tumor of childhood. These tumors stain positive for AFP. Embryonal carcinomas are AFP negative but CD30 positive, and most commonly found in adolescent testicular tumors. Choriocarcinomas stain positive for B-HCG.

(Section 24: Neoplastic Disorders; Part 3: Solid Tumors, Chapter 459, pp 1654–1655)

Answer 24-43. d

While most sacral tumors in newborns are mature or immature teratomas, malignant yolk sac tumors can also occur in this location. Teratomas, even though technically benign, often contain small amounts of yolk sac tumor, and about 10% of patients under the age of 2 months with teratoma will have recurrence in the form of a malignant yolk sac tumor after resection of the original tumor. In this patient, the elevated AFP indicates that there are detectable quantities of malignant yolk sac elements, and the presence of abundant cells with Schiller–Duval bodies on biopsy suggests that yolk sac elements make up a large proportion, if not all, of the tumor. Yolk sac tumors should be treated with chemotherapy and resection. Resection may be scheduled either upfront or after chemotherapy reduction.

(Section 24: Neoplastic Disorders; Part 3: Solid Tumors, Chapter 459, p 1654)

Answer 24-44. c

This patient meets clinical criteria for neurofibromatosis type 1, which is caused by a mutation or deletion of the tumor suppressor gene *NF1*. Patients with neurofibromatosis type 1 are at increased risk of developing optic pathway gliomas, and should undergo regular thorough eye exams by an experienced ophthalmologist. MRI is not indicated unless the patient develops symptoms of an intracranial tumor, vision disturbances, or changes in his ophthalmologic exam. Cardiac and/or renal defects are not part of neurofibromatosis type 1.

(Section 24: Neoplastic Disorders; Part 3: Solid Tumors, Chapter 460, p 1657)

Answer 24-45. e

This presentation, exam, and imaging findings are classic for juvenile pilocytic astrocytoma. This low-grade glioma can occur anywhere in the brain, but is most often seen in the posterior fossa. It is always Grade 1, and dissemination is very rare so further staging workup is not indicated. As this tumor is typically cured by complete resection, chemotherapy and/or radiation therapy are reserved for cases in which complete resection is not possible due to tumor size or location.

(Section 24: Neoplastic Disorders; Part 3: Solid Tumors, Chapter 460, p 1658)

Answer 24-46. b

Deletion of *INI1* is virtually pathognomonic of an atypical teratoid/rhabdoid tumor (ATRT). This tumor typically presents in infants and other very young children, and can be located anywhere in the brain. ATRT is associated with a terrible prognosis, in part because it occurs in children too young to have their brains irradiated without intolerable consequences for their development. Complete surgical resection and multiagent chemotherapy provide the best chance for cure.

(Section 24: Neoplastic Disorders; Part 3: Solid Tumors, Chapter 460, p 1659)

Answer 24-47. a

The 4-year-old girl most likely had the sporadic, non-hereditary form of retinoblastoma since her malignancy developed as a toddler and she had unilateral disease. Children with the inherited version of the disease typically (though not always) develop disease during infancy and have bilateral tumors. Mutation of the *RB1* gene is highly penetrant, and since both of the girl's parents are healthy without eye tumors, it is unlikely that either of them carry the mutation. Therefore, the risk of retinoblastoma for their second child is likely to be about 1%. Regardless, genetic counseling and screening the second child for eye tumors during infancy (or testing for the sibling's RB1 mutation, if known) is indicated.

(Section 24: Neoplastic Disorders; Part 3: Solid Tumors, Chapter 461, p 1661)

Answer 24-48. d

The most effective therapy for Kaposiform hemangioendotheliomas (KHE) is complete surgical resection, although tumors may still recur. When lesions are large, complete surgical resection may not be possible. The tumors can be partially resected in combination with sclerosing or embolizing feeder blood vessels as a palliative measure, but typically medications such as steroids, interferon, or vincristine are attempted first to try to shrink the tumor. Radiation is reserved as a last resort, and is rarely effective.

(Section 24: Neoplastic Disorders; Part 3: Solid Tumors, Chapter 462, p 1663)

Answer 24-49. b

This child has widespread cutaneous Langerhans cell histiocytosis (LCH), and given the systemic symptoms of fever and weight loss, may have additional organ involvement. He requires a laboratory evaluation to screen for involvement of the bone marrow and liver, and a skeletal survey to look for bony lesions. The most common complication of LCH is diabetes insipidus (DI) due to involvement of the pituitary gland, and all children with suspected or confirmed LCH should be screened by history and urinalysis for DI.

A brain MRI is used to assess CNS involvement. Although a chest X-ray to screen for pulmonary involvement should be included as part of the initial diagnostic workup, the higher-radiation chest CT should be reserved only for patients with respiratory symptoms. Bone marrow biopsy is usually only performed if the CBC reveals abnormal blood counts.

(Section 24: Neoplastic Disorders; Part 4: Mononuclear Phagocytic System Disorders, Chapter 463, p 1665)

Answer 24-50. a

Currently, to make the diagnosis of hemophagocytic lymphohistiocytosis (HLH), a patient must meet 5 of 8 diagnostic criteria: (1) fever, (2) splenomegaly, (3) cytopenias of at least two lineages in the peripheral blood, (4) elevated triglycerides OR low fibrinogen, (5) evidence of hemophagocytosis in the tissue (eg, bone marrow, spleen, lymph nodes), (6) low or absent natural killer cell activity, (7) high ferritin level, and (8) elevated soluble IL-2 receptor levels. The patient in the vignette has a very high ferritin level and a low fibrinogen level, which combined with her fever and splenomegaly give her 4 of the 5 required criteria.

HLH can be acquired (usually in response to a viral infection or a malignancy), or caused by a germline genetic mutation. Increasingly, a molecular diagnosis can be made in the latter group of patients suspected of having HLH by sequencing the genes that encode perforin (*PRF1*), Munc13-4 (*UNC13D*), and syntaxin-11 (*STX11*), which are all involved in the cytolytic perforin granule pathway.

(Section 24: Neoplastic Disorders; Part 4: Mononuclear Phagocytic System Disorders, Chapter 463, p 1666)

CHAPTER 25 | Disorders of the Kidney and Urinary Tract

Kartik Pillutla and Erica Winnicki

25-1. Which of the statements regarding the epidemiology of acute renal failure is correct?

  a. Gastroenteritis is an uncommon cause of acute renal failure in Africa and Tropical Asia

  b. The incidence of hospital acquired acute renal failure in pediatric patients has steadily decreased in the last 2 decades

  c. Nephrotoxin use and congenital heart disease is now a common cause of acute renal failure in the United States

  d. The incidence of acute renal failure is less in children who are mechanically ventilated

  e. None of the above

25-2. A previously healthy 2-year-old boy is brought into the Emergency Department with a 3-day history of nonbilious and nonbloody vomiting and diarrhea. He has refused PO intake aside from occasional sips of juice and water. He has made little urine output in the last 12 hours. On physical exam, he is afebrile with a HR of 130. A blood pressure cannot be be taken. Laboratory results reveal a BUN of 60, creatinine of 1.7, and a bicarbonate level of 14. What is the most appropriate first step?

  a. Bladder catheterization

  b. Intravenous furosemide

  c. 20 mL/kg bolus of intravenous normal saline

  d. Obtaining a renal ultrasound

  e. Renal biopsy

25-3. A concerned parent calls you regarding a local outbreak of E. coli gastroenteritis traced to contaminated beef from a fast food restaurant. He has read on the internet that E. coli can be associated with HUS and wants to know more about the disease. Which of the following statements regarding HUS is correct?

  a. Platelet transfusions should be used sparingly in patients with HUS

  b. Atypical HUS remains far more common than diarrhea-associated HUS in the United States

  c. S. pneumoniae associated HUS has a more favorable prognosis than diarrhea-associated HUS

  d. Antibiotics should be given to patients who are positive for E. coli 0157:H7 to prevent HUS

  e. The anemia seen in HUS is due to insufficient bone marrow production of red blood cells

25-4. A previously healthy 5-year-old girl is brought to urgent care with bloody diarrhea, pallor, and fatigue. Her vital signs are notable for a HR of 130 with a blood pressure of 145/101. On physical exam, she is irritable with dry mucous membranes. Laboratory data is significant for a WBC of 17,000, hemoglobin of 8, platelet count of 65, BUN of 70, and creatinine of 3.2. Which of the following is the next best diagnostic step?

  a. Obtaining a peripheral blood smear, LDH, and reticulocyte count

  b. Calculating the fractional excretion of sodium (FeNa)

  c. Sending the stool for ova and parasites examination

  d. Renal ultrasound

  e. Renal biopsy

25-5. A 9-month-old male presents to clinic with feeding difficulties and change in growth curve percentile from the 50th% at 4 months of age to 10th% at present. On physical examination, he is noted to be irritable with a slightly sunken fontanelle. You obtain the following laboratory values: Na 141 mEq/L (normal: 135–145), K 2.1 mEq/L (normal: 3.5–5.0), Cl 97 mmol/L (normal: 98–108), HCO_3 11 mmol/L (normal: 22–30), BUN 5 mg/dL (normal: 6–22 mg/dL), Cr < 0.3 mg/dL (normal: 0.2–0.4), Ph 1.2 mg/dL (normal: 3.2–6.3), Mg 1.1 mEq/L (normal: 1.3–2.0). Urinalysis is notable for pH of 5 and the presence of glucose. Which of the following is the most likely underlying diagnosis in this patient?

  a. Acute gastroenteritis

  b. Bartter syndrome

  c. Liddle syndrome

  d. Cystinosis

  e. Lithium intoxication

25-6. A 7-year-old previously healthy boy presents with his parents with a complaint of swelling in his eyelids for the past 2 weeks. There is no eye discharge or pruritus. The swelling appears to be worse when he gets up in the morning. His parents report that he has otherwise been well, though he did have a runny nose, cough, and fever 2 weeks ago. On physical examination, he is afebrile and well appearing. His examination is only notable for bilateral periorbital swelling that is non-tender with minimal erythema. There is no scleral injection and his fundoscopic examination and visual acuity are normal. What is the most appropriate first step?

a. Urgent ophthalmology referral

b. Computerized tomography scan of the orbits

c. Prescription for an antihistamine

d. Urinalysis

e. Hospital admission for intravenous antibiotics

25-7. A 6-year-old previously healthy girl comes to your clinic today presenting with periorbital edema for the past 2 weeks. Initially her parents thought she was having allergies and have tried over the counter antihistamines with no improvement. They have observed that she has gained weight over the past 2 weeks and is not fitting into her clothes. Her weight today is 20 kg compared to 18 kg last month. On physical examination, she is afebrile with a heart rate of 112, respiratory rate of 22, oxygen saturation of 100% on room air, and a blood pressure of 92/64. Her examination is notable for non-tender periorbital edema and mild ascites. Her cardiovascular and lung examination are normal. You suspect nephrotic syndrome, and a urinalysis is significant for proteinuria. A urine protein to urine creatinine ratio is 6 mg/mg. What is the most appropriate next step?

a. Oral prednisone therapy for 6 weeks followed by a 6 week taper

b. Intravenous albumin infusion

c. Oral cyclophosphamide therapy for 6 weeks

d. Urgent nephrology consultation for renal biopsy

e. No medication is indicated at this time

25-8. Which of the following statements regarding focal segmental glomerulosclerosis (FSGS) is correct?

a. Oral corticosteroid therapy induces remission in the majority of patients with FSGS

b. FSGS can be idiopathic, inherited, or acquired from secondary causes

c. FSGS is a clinical diagnosis and a renal biopsy is not required

d. Steroid responsiveness is not a prognostic indicator in patients with FSGS

e. FSGS never recurs after a renal transplantation

25-9. An 11-year-old patient with newly diagnosed chronic kidney disease (CKD) secondary to renal hypoplasia is admitted to your service with an asthma exacerbation. Upon reviewing the child's medical history, you discover that her height is significantly below the third percentile for her age. What is the most appropriate next step in the management of her growth retardation?

a. Immediate start of growth hormone therapy

b. Correction of metabolic acidosis and hyponatremia if present

c. Endocrinology consultation

d. Measurement of serum GH and IGF-1 levels

e. Placement of gastrostomy tube

25-10. A 13-year-old previously healthy child presents with a 1-day history of gross hematuria, dysuria, and urinary urgency. A plain abdominal film demonstrates nephrolithiasis. He is started on IV hydration and soon after, he passes what he thinks is a stone and his symptoms resolve. What is the most appropriate next step?

a. Nonenhanced computed tomography (CT) scan of the abdomen and pelvis

b. Urological consultation for shock wave lithotripsy

c. Oral thiazide diuretic

d. Timed urine collection for calcium, oxalate, urate, citrate, and sodium

e. Calcium-restricted diet

25-11. An 8-year-old with a history of sickle cell nephropathy is admitted to the ER with a sickle cell pain crisis. Electrolytes reveal a potassium of 7.3 and an EKG demonstrates peaked T-waves. What is the most appropriate next step?

a. Intravenous calcium gluconate

b. Oral kayexelate

c. Echocardiography

d. Intravenous sodium bicarbonate

e. Intravenous furosemide

25-12. A 1-month-old presents to your clinic for well-child care. His parents note that a prenatal ultrasound showed a left multicystic dysplastic kidney. Since birth, he has been breastfeeding well and makes multiple wet diapers a day. What is the most appropriate next step?

a. Analysis for Wilms tumor 1 of (WT1) gene mutation

b. Urological consultation for an immediate nephrectomy

c. Sending of serum PTH

d. Renal ultrasound at 3 months of age

e. Oral amoxicillin antibiotic prophylaxis

25-13. As you take a round in the newborn nursery, you are notified regarding the birth of a full-term male infant with a prenatal diagnosis of agenesis of the right kidney. He has urine output and is well-appearing on exam. The parents would like to know more about renal agenesis. Which of the following statements regarding renal agenesis is correct?

  a. Patients with unilateral renal agenesis have similar renal outcomes as compared to patients without renal agenesis

  b. Patients with renal agenesis typically develop end-stage renal disease by young adulthood

  c. Hypertension and proteinuria can develop in patients with renal agenesis

  d. Patients with renal agenesis have an increased risk of developing Wilms tumor

  e. Patients with renal agenesis require antibiotic prophylaxis

25-14. Which of the following statements regarding renal dysplasia is correct?

  a. It may be discovered incidentally on antenatal ultrasound

  b. Unilateral renal dysplasia is associated with oligohydramnios

  c. A dysplastic kidney on ultrasound will have a loss of echogenicity

  d. Renal dysplasia is not associated with urological anomalies

  e. Patients with unilateral renal dysplasia usually present with renal failure

25-15. A 16-year-old previously healthy girl presents to your clinic for well-child care. A nurse alerts you that her blood pressure is 136/74 with a HR 83. She has no complaints today including no headaches, dizziness, or palpitations. Her father notes that both he and her mother developed hypertension at 42 and 45 years of age, respectively. Multiple family members have hypertension as well. On physical exam, she has a weight of 110 kg and a height of 174 cm. She is obese with a darkish discoloration behind her neck. The remainder of her physical exam is normal. What is the most appropriate next step?

  a. Immediate hospital admission for hypertension management

  b. Renal ultrasound

  c. Serum aldosterone and renin level

  d. Fasting glucose and lipid profile

  e. Renal angiography with renal vein sampling

25-16. A 5-year-old female had a urinalysis performed for evaluation during a febrile illness, which had negative leukocytes and negative nitrites, as well as a specific gravity of 1.025 and the presence of trace protein. A urine culture was sent, which was negative. The febrile illness resolved and was thought to be due to a viral syndrome. A few months later, during her well-child visit, a repeat urine dipstick test is performed, which is notable for 1+ urine protein. This result is followed by measurement of a spot urine protein-to-creatinine ratio, which is 0.4 mg/mg.

Which of the following is the most appropriate next step?

  a. Reassure her parents that this is a normal finding and that no further evaluation is required

  b. Have the child return to the clinic in 1–2 weeks for a repeat urinalysis with spot urine protein-to-creatinine ratio, preferably on an early morning urine sample

  c. Refer the child to a pediatric nephrologist for further evaluation

  d. Obtain serum creatinine concentration and serum complement levels

  e. Order an ultrasound to evaluate renal anatomy

25-17. The father of a 6-year-old girl brings his daughter in for evaluation of bed wetting. He states that she wets the bed approximately 3 nights per week and has never consistently remained dry throughout the night. A urinalysis is performed in the clinic and has a specific gravity of 1.020 and is negative for glucose, nitrates, or leukocyte esterase. Which of the following is appropriate advice to give to the patient's father?

  a. Counsel that nocturnal enuresis is unlikely to resolve without pharmacologic intervention

  b. Instruct him to restrict his daughter's intake of beverages prior to bedtime

  c. Advise him against obtaining a bed wetting alarm, as the alarms have not been shown to be effective

  d. Suggest that the child void frequently during the daytime

  e. Counsel him to punish his daughter by having her change her bed sheets alone after every accident

25-18. Which of the following statements regarding nephrolithiasis in children is correct?

  a. Struvite stones are the most common type of stone in the pediatric population

  b. Use of thiazide diuretics is a common cause of hypercalciuria

  c. Hypercalciuria in children is usually associated with hypercalcemia

  d. Sodium citrate should be given to prevent calcium containing stones

  e. Stones less than 5 mm in size will usually pass spontaneously

25-19. You are evaluating a 2-week-old former full-term male infant in the clinic. Review of his medical records reveals that he was prenatally diagnosed with left-sided renal agenesis. Which of the following is true regarding unilateral renal agenesis?

a. Microscopic hematuria is a frequent complication in persons with a solitary kidney

b. It is rare for unilateral renal agenesis to be associated with vesicoureteral reflux

c. An abdominal ultrasound should be performed to rule out an ectopic location of the second kidney

d. Renal agenesis is more common in females than in males

e. Unilateral renal agenesis is not a risk factor for hypertension

25-20. A 9-year-old male presents with his mother to your clinic with a chief complaint of gross hematuria. His mother noticed blood on his underwear when doing the laundry. When she questioned him about this finding, he stated that he has also seen bright red blood at the end of his urine streams on a few occasions. He denies any associated abdominal or flank pain, and denies discomfort with voiding. Examination shows a normal appearing, circumcised penis without evidence for trauma. You perform a urinalysis in clinic, which is negative for blood or protein. Which of the following is the most likely diagnosis?

a. Post-streptococcal glomerulonephritis

b. Nephrolithiasis

c. Urethrorrhagia

d. Acute cystitis

e. Bladder carcinoma

25-21. A 5-year-old female with CKD Stage 4 due to reflux nephropathy is hospitalized for supportive management of a respiratory infection. During that time, screening labs are sent. The labs are notable for a calcium of 8.1 (normal 8.7–10.1 mg/dL), phosphorus 5 (normal 2.8–6.2 mg/dL), Vit D 25, OH of 34 ng/mL (>30 ng/mL indicates sufficiency), and a PTH of 450 ng/L (normal range 12–65 ng/L). Which of the following would be the most appropriate treatment to initiate?

a. Cholecalciferol daily

b. Sevelamer three times daily with meals

c. Calcium carbonate three times daily with meals

d. Calcitriol 3 times weekly

e. Dietary restriction of phosphorus

25-22. A 3-year-old male with end-stage renal disease due to obstructive uropathy from posterior urethral valves presents for routine evaluation in the clinic. He is maintained on continuous cycling peritoneal dialysis. Review of his laboratory studies shows: Hgb 8.5 g/dL, hematocrit 26%, transferrin 210 mg/dL (normal: 130 – 275 mg/dL), percent saturation 31%, and reticulocyte count 0.5%. Review of his medications show that he is taking ferrous sulfate at a dose of 3 mg/kg BID. Which would be the most beneficial treatment for this patient?

a. Increase ferrous sulfate to 6 mg/kg/dose twice daily

b. Initiate treatment with epogen subcutaneously twice weekly

c. Give the patient a single dose of iron sucrose in clinic

d. Start folate supplementation

e. Transfuse the patient with 10 mL/kg of PRBCs

25-23. You are evaluating a 1-day-old term newborn female in the nursery. Review of her records indicates that prenatal ultrasounds were notable for dilation of the left renal pelvis. Which of the following is true in the diagnosis and management of this infant?

a. A renal and bladder ultrasound should be obtained immediately

b. A renal and bladder ultrasound should be obtained within the first few days of life

c. A renal and bladder ultrasound should be obtained at 2 weeks of life

d. The infants is unlikely to have normal function of the left kidney

e. Laparoscopic pyeloplasty is indicated for this infant

25-24. A 15-year-old male with CKD stage II secondary to lupus nephritis presents for evaluation of persistent hypertension. His blood pressures have been consistently above the 95th% for age, gender, and height. His vital signs in the clinic are as follows: T 36°C, Pulse 84, BP 138/86. His laboratory evaluation is notable for normal serum electrolytes, BUN of 14, serum creatinine concentration of 1.4 mg/dL, and urinalysis with a urine protein-to-creatinine ratio of 0.6 mg/mg. Which of the following would be the best initial antihypertensive agent in this patient?

a. Enalapril

b. Amlodipine

c. Minoxidil

d. Clonidine

e. Metoprolol

25-25. You have been following a 16-year-old female for routine care. At her last visit 1 month ago, you noted that her blood pressure was elevated. She has since had 2 repeat blood pressure measurements that confirm an elevation of systolic blood pressure between the 90th and 95th percentile for age, gender, and height. Her exam is notable for a BMI of 31. There is a family history of hypertension in the patient's father and mother, and a history of diabetes mellitus in the patient's paternal grandmother. Which of the following would be the most appropriate next step in management of this patient?

a. Initiate amlodipine for blood pressure control and see the patient back in clinic in 1 month

b. Obtain a renal ultrasound to evaluate for anatomical abnormality

c. Obtain thyroid function tests as exam is concerning for thyroid dysfunction

d. Obtain a CT angiogram to exclude renal artery stenosis

e. Advise dietary modifications and increase in physical activity and re-evaluate the patient in 6 months

25-26. A 2-year-old male patient with end stage renal disease who is peritoneal dialysis dependent presents to the emergency department with a 1-day history of abdominal pain, persistent emesis, and cloudy peritoneal fluid. On presentation, he has a fever of 38.9°C. A sample of dialysate fluid is obtained for cell count, Gram stain, and culture. Which of the following is true regarding the diagnosis and management of this patient?

a. The most likely causative organism is *Escherichia coli*

b. A peritoneal white blood cell count of 100/μL and 80% polymorphonuclear cells would be suggestive of peritonitis

c. The patient should be discharged home with vancomycin as empiric intraperitoneal antibiotic coverage

d. Intravenous antibiotic administration would be more appropriate than intraperitoneal antibiotic administration in this patient

e. Peritoneal dialysis is unlikely to be effective after an episode of peritonitis

25-27. Which of the following is correct regarding autosomal recessive polycystic kidney disease (ARPKD)?

a. Enlargement of fetal kidneys is evident on first-trimester ultrasound

b. Liver dysfunction from congenital hepatic fibrosis frequently develops prior to renal dysfunction

c. A negative renal ultrasound in both parents makes the diagnosis of ARPKD more likely than autosomal dominant polycystic kidney disease (ADPKD)

d. The majority of patient's with ARPKD will be diagnosed prenatally

e. ARPKD is more common than ADPKD

25-28. A 13-year-old previously healthy male presents to the emergency department with back pain that developed after a grueling cross-country race. In the emergency department, he is given a dose of Ketorolac for his pain. Serum chemistries are then performed, which are notable for a BUN of 49 and a serum creatinine concentration of 2.1 mg/dL. Which of the following is correct regarding this patient's kidney injury?

a. Urine sediment is likely to contain red blood cell casts

b. Urine specific gravity of >1020 would be consistent with an intrinsic renal etiology for acute kidney injury

c. Volume resuscitation should be avoided as this patient will likely be oliguric

d. A calculated fractional excretion of sodium <1% would be consistent with a prerenal etiology of acute kidney injury

e. Appropriate choice of intravenous fluids would be ½ NS with 20 mEq KCl/L and 1.5 times maintenance rate

25-29. For which of the following patient scenarios is acute hemodialysis most clearly indicated?

a. A 10-year-old male with oliguria and the following serum chemistries: Na 132, K 6.1, Cl 92, CO_2 17, BUN 50, SCr 3.1, Ca 8.9

b. A 13-year-old female with nonoliguric acute renal failure and a vancomycin trough of 90

c. A 9-year-old female with CKD stage IV and progressive fatigue and anorexia

d. A 15-year-old hypertensive male with anuric renal failure unresponsive to diuretic therapy with pulmonary edema on chest X-ray

e. A 4-year-old male with CKD stage V and refractory metabolic acidosis

25-30. A 6-year-old previously healthy male presents to the urgent care clinic with a 1-day history of hematuria. In the clinic, he is noted to be mildly hypertensive with periorbital edema. A urine sample obtained in clinic has a dark brown appearance. He denies any recent rash or joint pain, but does report a sore throat 2 weeks ago for which he did not seek care. Which of the following is most likely to be true in this patient?

  a. Antibiotic administration for pharyngitis would likely have prevented this disease

  b. Low serum C3 and normal serum C4 would be consistent with this disease

  c. Low serum C4 and normal serum C3 would be consistent with this disease

  d. If the patient were to have a renal biopsy, immunofluorescence would reveal mesangial deposits of IgA

  e. Abnormalities on urinalysis should resolve within 5–10 days

25-31. A 10-kg patient presents to the emergency room with a 1-week history of diarrhea. His mother reports that his urine output has decreased over the past 24 hours despite drinking a lot of fluids, and that he is having approximately 6 loose stools daily. His vital signs are normal but his exam shows sunken eyes. His serum chemistries show a sodium of 125 mEq/L. He is given 20 mL/kg of normal saline in the emergency room. What is his current estimated sodium deficit?

  a. 3 mEq

  b. 10 mEq

  c. 30 mEq

  d. 60 mEq

  e. 90 mEq

25-32. You are examining a 1-day-old male in the newborn nursery who was the product of in vitro fertilization. You notice that his urethral meatus is located on the distal portion of the penile shaft. Which of the following is true of this condition?

  a. The patient should be referred for urologic surgery immediately

  b. In vitro fertilization is not a risk factor for this condition

  c. The patient should be started on prophylactic antibiotics

  d. The patient should be not have a circumcision performed despite the parent's request

  e. An ultrasound of the kidneys and bladder should be obtained prior to discharge home

25-33. A 5-year-old with a history of acute lymphoblastic leukemia (ALL) is admitted to the intensive care unit with fever and respiratory distress. The patient soon requires intubation and is currently being mechanically ventilated. Serum chemistries, blood urea nitrogen, and creatinine are within normal limits. Which of the following is correct?

  a. Because this patient is receiving humidified air, his insensible losses are increased

  b. D5 ¼ NS is recommended, as this patient is at risk for developing hypernatremia

  c. Potassium containing intravenous fluids should be avoided in this patient

  d. His maintenance fluid requirement is less compared to a patient not receiving mechanical ventilation

  e. His plasma ADH level would be expected to be low

25-34. A newborn boy has not voided for 40 hours since birth. Examination reveals an alert infant with normal external genitalia, testes descended bilaterally, Tanner I. There is a firm abdominal mass. Ultrasound of the abdomen reveals a distended bladder with a "keyhole" appearance formed by a large bladder and a distended posterior urethra. Which of the following statements is true about this case?

  a. The ratio of males to females affected is 5 to 1

  b. Prognosis is worse if the child also has unilateral *vesicoureteral* reflux

  c. Immediate stabilization of the infant with bladder drainage is necessary

  d. The condition is caused by external compression of the urethra by aberrant vasculature

  e. Due to the insidious nature of the disease, prenatal ultrasound is an ineffective screening tool

25-35. A 3-year-old boy who weighs 16 kg is admitted for elective surgery and needs to be NPO overnight. What is the appropriate maintenance fluid and maintenance fluid rate?

  a. D5 ¼ NS @ 52 mL/hr

  b. D5W @ 52 mL/hr

  c. D5 ¼ NS @ 400 mL/hr

  d. D5W @ 400 mL/hr

  e. NS @ 20 cc/kg over 20 minutes

ANSWERS

Answer 25-1. c

Nephrotoxic medicines, congenital heart disease, renal ischemia, bone marrow transplantation, and sepsis have now overtaken hemolytic uremic syndrome (HUS) as the most common causes of acute renal failure in the developed world. In developing countries such as Africa and Asia, infections such as gastroenteritis leading to resultant hypovolemia and kidney injury are the most common causes for acute renal failure. The rates of hospital acquired acute renal failure in pediatrics have increased greatly in the last 2 decades. The risk of acute renal failure is even higher in patients who are mechanically ventilated or require vasoactive support.

(Section 25. Disorders of the Kidney and Urinary Tract. Chapter 471 Acute Renal Failure, p 1706)

Answer 25-2. c

Acute renal failure can be subdivided into 3 major categories: prerenal, intrinsic, and postrenal acute renal failure. Clinical examination is important to help distinguish the type of acute renal failure that is occurring. Tachycardia, vomiting, diarrhea and hypotension are evidence of intravascular volume depletion with resultant prerenal acute renal failure. As a result IV fluid resuscitation would be the most appropriate treatment. Bladder catheterization could be considered if postrenal acute renal failure from obstruction is highly suspected; however, there is no evidence for obstruction in this patient. Furosemide or other diuretic therapy would not correct the intravascular volume depletion that is the cause for the acute renal failure in this patient. A renal ultrasound could be considered to help distinguish acute renal failure from chronic renal failure but would not be the most appropriate first step in this patient. A renal biopsy is not indicated in cases of prerenal acute renal failure.

(Section 25. Disorders of the Kidney and Urinary Tract. Chapter 471 Acute Renal Failure, p 1710)

Answer 25-3. a

Diarrhea-associated HUS, most commonly the result of Shiga toxin producing *E. coli* O157:H7, is associated with the majority (near 70%) of all HUS cases in the United States and Europe. The Shiga toxin causes endothelial damage, which then results in the classic triad of renal failure, thrombocytopenia, and hemolytic anemia. The mainstay of management of patients with diarrhea associated HUS is supportive care, which has reduced mortality rates by 50%. This includes intravenous hydration. Dialysis should be performed if there is profound azotemia, electrolyte imbalances, oliguria, or fluid overload.

   As HUS results in a prothrombotic state with endothelial damage and resultant thrombotic microangiopathy, platelet transfusions are reserved for patients who are actively bleeding

or require an invasive procedure. There is no evidence that antibiotics prevent HUS in patients who have stool cultures positive for *E. coli* O157:H7. In fact, some studies show that receiving antibiotics may increase the risk of developing HUS. Patients with *S. pneumoniae* associated HUS have a worse prognosis compared to patients with diarrhea-associated HUS, with a mortality rate up to 12% in some studies. Atypical HUS is less commonly seen than diarrhea-associated HUS, accounting for 10% of all HUS cases.

(Section 25. Disorders of the Kidney and Urinary Tract. Chapter 472 Glomerular Diseases, p 1728)

Answer 25-4. a

HUS, caused by Shiga toxin producing *E. coli* O157:H7 is the most common cause of severe acute renal failure in young children. It is acquired usually through the consumption of undercooked beef or unpasteurized milk products. The bacteria produces Shiga toxin, which causes endothelial damage, resultant thrombotic microangiopathy, and the classic triad of renal failure, hemolytic anemia, and thrombocytopenia.

   In order to aid the diagnosis of HUS, hemolytic anemia should be confirmed. A peripheral blood smear would demonstrate schistocytes and helmet cells. An elevated LDH and reticulocyte count also confirms a hemolytic process. Fractional excretion of sodium (also known as a FeNa) helps distinguish pre-renal acute renal failure from intrinsic renal failure causes; however, it does not help diagnose HUS. An ova and parasite examination would not aid in the diagnosis of diarrhea associated HUS, which is caused by toxin-producing bacteria. A renal ultrasound would be helpful if obstruction or a structural anomaly is suspected but would not be helpful in diagnosing HUS. A renal biopsy is not necessary to diagnose HUS.

(Section 25. Disorders of the Kidney and Urinary Tract. Chapter 472 Glomerular Diseases, p 1728)

Answer 25-5. d

Cystinosis is the most common inherited cause of Fanconi syndrome in children. Fanconi syndrome usually presents in early childhood with failure to thrive, polydypsia, polyuria, and dehydration. Laboratory findings include metabolic acidosis secondary to impaired proximal tubule reabsorption of bicarbonate. A proximal tubular defect can be distinguished from a distal tubular defect in that, for proximal tubular disorders, the distal urinary acidification mechanism is still intact; thus, urine pH is classically maintained below 5.5. Additional findings in Fanconi syndrome include hypophosphatemia, hypokalemia, glucosuria, and amino aciduria secondary to impaired proximal tubular absorption.

   Acute gastroenteritis could account for bicarbonate losses and a metabolic acidosis, but would not be associated with the combination of hypokalemia, hypophosphatemia, hypomagnesemia, and glucosuria. Patients with Bartter syndrome present with a hypokalemic, hyperchloremic metabolic alkalosis. Patients with Liddle syndrome also present with hypokalemia and a metabolic alkalosis, as well as hypertension, due to augmented collecting tubule sodium transport. Patients with lithium intoxication present with a distal RTA, which would be characterized by inability to excrete urine with a pH of less than 5.5.

(Chapter 474: Renal Tubular Disorders. Section 25: Disorders of the Kidney and Urinary Tract, p 1733)

Answer 25-6. d

Minimal change nephrotic syndrome (MCNS) is seen in 2–7 per 100,000 children under the age of 16. Its pathophysiology is yet to be fully understood, but is thought to result from a circulating "nephrotic factor" that results in damage to the podocytes in the glomerulus. This results in an increase in the glomerular basement membrane permeability and the loss of protein in the urine. Proteinuria, hypoalbuminemia, and hypercholestermia are seen. Dependent edema is seen in patients with MCNS. For children, this is commonly seen in the eyelids, scrotum, and labia. Patients are often misdiagnosed as having an allergic conjunctivitis.

For this patient, a urinalysis to look for proteinuria is indicated to diagnose MCNS. Given the normal ophthalmologic examination, an ophthalmology referral and CT scan of the orbits are not appropriate. As the patient does not have evidence for an allergic conjunctivitis, an antihistamine is not required. The patient does not have clinical features consistent with an orbital cellulitis; thus, intravenous antibiotics are not indicated.

(Section 25. Disorders of the Kidney and Urinary Tract. Chapter 472 Glomerular Diseases, p 1723)

Answer 25-7. a

Nephrotic syndrome is characterized by proteinuria (defined as greater than 50 mg/kg/24 hr, 40 mg/m^2/hr, or a urine protein to creatinine ratio greater than 2 mg/mg), hypoalbuminemia (serum albumin less than 3 g/dL), and hypercholestermia. The loss of oncotic pressure results in dependent edema, which is commonly seen in the eyelids, scrotum, and labia in children. Ascites can also be seen in affected patients. MCNS is the most common type of nephrotic syndrome seen in children. Untreated, nephrotic syndrome can result in complications including peritonitis and thrombosis. Though spontaneous remission can occur, oral corticosteroid therapy can induce remission in up to 90% of patients and should be started if MCNS is suspected.

Oral prednisone therapy for 6 weeks followed by a 6-week taper is the most appropriate step for this patient. Intravenous albumin is reserved for patients with gross anasarca and should be used with caution as they can precipitate pulmonary edema in patients with nephrotic syndrome. Oral cyclophosphamide

is reserved for patients with MCNS who exhibit steroid dependency (eg, patients who relapse once their prednisone is discontinued or tapered to a low dose). As minimal change disease nephrotic syndrome is the likely diagnosis for this patient, a renal biopsy is not required prior to starting prednisone therapy.

(Section 25. Disorders of the Kidney and Urinary Tract. Chapter 472 Glomerular Diseases, p 1724)

Answer 25-8. b

FSGS is the second most common form of nephrotic syndrome in childhood, behind MCNS. Idiopathic FSGS is the most common variant, though inherited forms due to mutations in the slit diaphragm protein, podocin, can be seen. FSGS can also be acquired from secondary causes including hypertension and HIV. Unlike MCNS, it is characterized by a poor response to steroid therapy, with only 20–25% achieving remission on prolonged oral corticosteroid therapy. Patients with FSGS who achieve remission on corticosteroid therapy have a more favorable prognosis. Recurrence of FSGS in the transplanted kidney can be seen almost immediately and close monitoring is required. A renal biopsy is indicated when FSGS or other causes of steroid resistant nephrotic syndrome is suspected.

(Section 25. Disorders of the Kidney and Urinary Tract. Chapter 472 Glomerular Diseases, p 1725)

Answer 25-9. b

CKD is defined as an evidence of kidney damage or a glomerular filtration rate of less than 60 mL/min/1.73 m^2 for 3 months or longer. For children with CKD, medical complications include growth impairment. The cause of growth impairment is multifactorial and includes malnutrition, metabolic acidosis, electrolyte imbalances (such as hyponatremia), and renal osteodystrophy. In addition, though serum GH levels in children with CKD are often normal or elevated, they exhibit evidence of growth hormone resistance. Correction of any metabolic acidosis and hyponatremia is the initial step in management of growth impairment. In addition, if evidence of malnutrition is present, the addition of protein powders or supplemental renal formulas should be considered to increase caloric density. A gastrostomy tube can be considered in an infant or young child if they are unlikely to take in the required volume and calories by mouth. For the older child described in the vignette, the placement of a gastrostomy tube is not indicated. Growth hormone therapy can be considered in this child, but only after any electrolyte imbalances, malnutrition, and renal osteodystrophy is addressed. For this child, their growth impairment is likely related to their kidney disease thus an endocrinology consultation is not warranted at this time. Measurement of serum GH and IGF-1 levels is not indicated for this patient.

(Section 25. Disorders of the Kidney and Urinary Tract. Chapter 477 Chronic Kidney Disease, p 1750)

Answer 25-10. d

Nephrolithiasis is defined as the presence of stones in the kidney, whereas urolithiasis is defined as the presence of stones anywhere in the urinary tract. In North America, most stones present in the kidney. For children with stones and renal calculi, investigation is required to rule out metabolic risk factors. This includes a timed urine collection to rule out hypercaluria, hyperoxaluria, hyperuricosuria, and hypocitraturia. A high-sodium diet has been implicated as a risk factor for stone formation, so quantification of urinary sodium is helpful. Treatment and prevention of further stone formation includes adequate fluid intake and correction of any metabolic risk factors that are present. Stones less than 5 mm often pass spontaneously.

Since the patient described in the vignette has already passed the stone and his symptoms have resolved, further imaging such as a CT scan is not required. Similarly, shock wave lithotripsy is not indicated. Patients with hypercalciuria are often treated with a thiazide diuretic, but this should only be done after hypercalciuria is confirmed with a timed urine collection. There is no role for a calcium-restricted diet.

(Section 25. Disorders of the Kidney and Urinary Tract. Chapter 475 Urinary Tract Stone Diseases, p 1739)

Answer 25-11. a

Hyperkalemia can be a life-threatening emergency secondary to the electrocardiographic changes that it can induce. Untreated, dysrhythmias including ventricular tachycardia and ventricular fibrillation can occur. In cases of hyperkalemia where there is evidence of electrocardiographic changes, the first step of management is stabilization of the myocardium. This is achieved with intravenous calcium administration. For this patient, intravenous sodium bicarbonate therapy is useful in rapidly shifting potassium into the cell, but should be given after intravenous calcium is administered. Likewise, intravenous furosemide and oral kayexelate can be considered after the myocardium is stabilized. There is no indication for an echocardiogram in this patient.

(Section 25. Disorders of the Kidney and Urinary Tract. Chapter 466 Fluid, Electrolytes and Acid–Base Disorders, p 1684)

Answer 25-12. d

Multicystic dysplastic kidneys (MCKD) are a common cause of flank masses in infancy. On ultrasound they present as a large cystic nonuniform mass in the renal fossa. By definition, MCKD are nonfunctional. Previously, nephrectomies were commonly performed because of an association of MCKD with the development of Wilms tumor. However, the incidence of Wilms tumor in patients with MCKD is quite low and now observation and medical management is the mainstay of therapy. Serial ultrasounds, commonly performed every 3 months during the first year of life and every 6 months thereafter, are done to monitor for involution of the mass as

well as compensatory hypertrophy of the contralateral kidney. Though the contralateral kidney can have urological anomalies, antibiotic prophylaxis is not indicated unless a VCUG demonstrates significant reflux. WT1 gene mutation analysis is not indicated in patients that have a MCKD. Measurement of serum PTH is not indicated, as there is no evidence for renal osteodystrophy.

(Section 25. Disorders of the Kidney and Urinary Tract. Chapter 469 Renal Malformations, p 1700)

Answer 25-13. c

Renal agenesis is defined by the absence of a second kidney, either in the renal fossa or in an ectopic location. Ultrasound will show absence of the kidney with a contralateral kidney that appears hypertrophied. As long as the contralateral kidney is without anomalies and has appropriate compensatory hypertrophy, patients with renal agenesis have good long-term renal survival. However, recent studies have shown these patients are at risk for developing hypertension and proteinuria. There is no association between renal agenesis and Wilms tumor. Unilateral renal agenesis is associated with urological anomalies in the contralateral kidney; however, antibiotic prophylaxis is only indicated if the kidney has anomalies on a VCUG.

(Section 25. Disorders of the Kidney and Urinary Tract. Chapter 469 Renal Malformations, p 1699)

Answer 25-14. a

Unilateral renal dysplasia is usually discovered as an incidental finding on antenatal ultrasound. As long as the contralateral kidney has no anomalies, long-term renal survival is good, though there is a risk of developing hypertension and proteinuria in adulthood. On ultrasound, dysplastic kidneys appear more echogenic with a loss of corticomedullary differentiation. Cortical cysts will also be apparent. Bilateral renal dysplasia (as opposed to unilateral renal dysplasia) can result in oligohydramnios due to a loss of glomerular filtration. Such patients with bilateral dysplastic kidneys can present with renal failure along with other sequelae of oligohydramnios.

(Section 25. Disorders of the Kidney and Urinary Tract. Chapter 469 Renal Malformations, p 1699)

Answer 25-15. d

For children and adolescents, the etiologies of hypertension can be numerous. Good history taking can help establish the likely cause. For this adolescent patient, numerous risk factors for obesity-related hypertension are evident. A family history of adult-onset hypertension is also present. For this patient, who is obese with evidence of glucose intolerance, a fasting glucose and lipid profile would be useful. As she is asymptomatic with stage 1 systolic hypertension, she does not require admission for treatment of her hypertension. Instead, dietary and lifestyle modifications would be beneficial for this patient and is the recommendation by the National High Blood Pressure Education Group for initial management of patients with obesity-related hypertension. A renal ultrasound would be beneficial for preadolescents with hypertension, patients with diastolic hypertension, stage 2 hypertension, or abnormal screening studies. For this patient with obesity-related hypertension, it would provide little diagnostic value. Similarly, renal artery stenosis is unlikely in this patient and renal angiography with renal vein sampling is not indicated.

(Section 25. Disorders of the Kidney and Urinary Tract. Chapter 479 Systemic Hypertension, p 1763)

Answer 25-16. b

The child in the vignette has had two urine samples that are notable for the presence of protein. One of the samples showed trace protein in a concentrated urine sample, and it is unclear whether this actually represents abnormal urine protein excretion. A spot urine protein-to-creatinine ratio is a good screen for abnormal protein excretion, and in this case is abnormal with a ratio of >0.2 mg/mg. However, there are several reasons a child may have a transient increase in urine protein excretion, such as fever and exercise.

The most appropriate next step would be to repeat a urinalysis with a urine protein-to-creatinine ratio, as several urine samples should be examined to confirm the presence of proteinuria before performing more invasive evaluation for causes of proteinuria. An early morning urine sample is preferred to exclude orthostatic influences. It would not be appropriate to reassure the parents that the finding is normal given that the urine protein-to-creatinine ratio is abnormal for age. Obtaining serum studies and referral to a nephrologist would be appropriate after proteinuria is confirmed on several urine samples. Renal ultrasound would not be indicated without confirmation of the presence of proteinuria or other indicators of renal compromise.

(Chapter 467: Principles of Nephrology. Section 25. Disorders of the Kidney and Urinary Tract, p 1687)

Answer 25-17. b

Primary nocturnal enuresis is a common problem in children and most often is not associated with organic disease. Evaluation for possible organic causes should include a careful history as well as an early morning urinalysis is order to exclude a urinary concentrating defect, diabetes mellitus, or a urinary tract infection.

The patient in the vignette above has primary nocturnal enuresis with a normal urinalysis suggesting that organic causes are unlikely. Bed wetting is likely to resolve with time regardless of treatment approach, and while pharmacologic treatment may be useful, it may not be necessary. It would be appropriate to have the child decrease fluid intake prior to bedtime, as this would help to decrease urine production overnight. Bed-wetting alarms awaken the child during voids overnight, and have been shown to be effective with a cure rate

of 70%. Another approach would be to have the child increase bladder capacity by delaying voids as long as possible during the day. Nocturnal enuresis is not under the child's voluntary control, and punishment for accidents by having the child change her bed sheets would be inappropriate.

(Chapter 468: Kidney or Urinary Tract Disorders. Section 25: Disorders of the Kidney and Urinary Tract. p 1696)

Answer 25-18. e

Calcium phosphate and calcium oxalate stones are the most common types of stones, whereas struvite stones are more rare. Hypercalciuria is a common risk factor identified in children with nephrolithiasis. Hypercalcemia would predispose to hypercalciuria; however, most children with hypercalciuria are normocalcemic and the cause of hypercalciuria is often idiopathic. Thiazide diuretics increase distal tubular absorption of calcium and are used in the treatment of hypercalciuria. Citrate is beneficial in increasing the solubility of calcium salts; however, potassium citrate would be preferred to sodium citrate, as excess sodium increases hypercalciuria. Stones that are less than 5 mm in size on imaging are likely to pass spontaneously and are unlikely to require surgical intervention.

(Chapter 475: Urinary Tract Stone Diseases. Section 25: Disorders of the Kidney and Urinary Tract. p 1740)

Answer 25-19. c

An abdominal ultrasound should be performed to confirm the prenatal diagnosis of unilateral renal agenesis given the possibility that a second kidney may exist in an ectopic location, such as the pelvis.

Renal agenesis and dysplasia are approximately 1.5 times more common in males than in females. Persons with a solitary kidney are at risk for lower urinary tract anomalies, and vesicoureteral reflux may be found in 30% of cases. For this reason, further workup with a voiding cystourethrogram is appropriate in these individuals. Both hypertension and proteinuria may develop over time, and for this reason, persons with a solitary kidney should have their blood pressure regularly measured and urine samples sent for evaluation periodically. Microscopic hematuria is not an associated complication in persons with a solitary kidney.

(Chapter 469: Renal Malformations. Section 25: Disorders of the Kidney and Urinary Tract. p 1699)

Answer 25-20. c

Urethrorrhagia may occur in peripubertal males and presents with hematuria at the end of the urine stream after a grossly normal void. It may also present with blood in the underwear. It is an idiopathic, benign, and self-limited condition. Further evaluation should include a renal and bladder ultrasound to exclude an anatomic abnormality.

Glomerulonephritis would likely present with cola-colored or rust-colored urine. If glomerulonephritis was present, the urinalysis would confirm the presence of blood as well as red blood cell casts. Nephrolithiasis would be more likely to be accompanied by symptoms of flank pain or dysuria. Infection is unlikely given the negative urinalysis. Bladder carcinoma is rare; however, it would be prudent to have the bladder evaluated for pathology by ultrasound.

(Chapter 476: Urologic Abnormalities of the Genitourinary Tract. Section 25: Disorders of the Kidney and Urinary Tract, p 1744)

Answer 25-21. d

This patient with advanced CKD likely has deficient activation of cholecalciferol to the active form of 1,25-dihydrocholecalciferol in the kidney. As a result, calcium absorption is impaired, resulting in hypocalcemia. The fall in plasma calcium levels leads to an elevation of parathyroid hormone values, placing this patient at risk for renal bone disease with high bone turnover. Other factors that lead to metabolic bone disease in children with CKD include dietary vitamin D deficiency and retention of phosphate.

There are multiple potential interventions to decrease the risk for renal bone disease in patients with CKD. If dietary vitamin D is insufficient, this should be replaced to maintain normal serum levels of vitamin D 25, OH. If serum phosphate levels are elevated, this can be addressed with both dietary restriction and use of phosphorus binders (sevelamer or calcium carbonate with meals). In the case above, where the patient is vitamin D sufficient with a normal serum phosphate levels, neither cholecalciferol, further restriction of dietary phosphorus, or use of phosphorus levels is likely to be beneficial in decreasing PTH and thus bone turnover. The appropriate treatment is calcitriol (activated vitamin D) in order to improve calcium reabsorption and decrease PTH levels.

(Chapter 477: Chronic Kidney Disease. Section 25: Disorders of the Kidney and Urinary Tract, p 1752)

Answer 25-22. b

The most common cause of anemia in patients with CKD is deficiency of erythropoietin, which is normally produced by the peritubular interstitial cells of the kidney. Erythropoietin deficiency is evidenced in the patient by an inappropriately low reticulocyte count in the face of anemia and an iron-sufficient state. Erythropoietin stimulating agents are indicated in the treatment of anemia of CKD.

This patient is not iron deficient. Although he should continue to receive iron replacement to maintain normal serum levels of iron, neither increasing his dose of oral iron nor administering intravenous iron will be the most beneficial treatment. Folate deficiency is possible in this patient, but erythropoietin deficiency is more likely. A blood transfusion is not indicated in an otherwise asymptomatic patient with moderate anemia.

(Chapter 477: Chronic Kidney Disease. Section 25: Disorders of the Kidney and Urinary Tract, p 1752)

Answer 25-23. c

Dilation of the renal pelvis on prenatal ultrasound without accompanying dilatation of the ureter raises suspicion for ureteropelvic junction (UPJ) obstruction. A renal ultrasound should be obtained postnatally. However, if a renal ultrasound is obtained too soon after delivery it may underestimate the degree of obstruction because of low urine output in the first few days of life. Ideally, a renal ultrasound should be obtained between 1 to 4 weeks after delivery. Most infants with UPJ obstruction will have preserved function, although this is related to the degree of obstruction. Surgical intervention may be indicated, but not without additional information that includes the degree of obstruction and functional impairment.

(Chapter 476: Urologic Abnormalities of the Genitourinary Tract. Section 25: Disorders of the Kidney and Urinary Tract, p 1741)

Answer 25-24. a

Children with CKD are at increased risk for hypertension, and optimal control of blood pressure is indicated to slow the rate of deterioration of renal function. Proteinuria is an additional risk factor for progression of CKD. Angiotensin-converting enzyme (ACE) inhibitors are an ideal choice for hypertension management because they also reduce proteinuria. Side effects of ACE inhibitors include hyperkalemia and renal impairment, and serum electrolyte levels should be monitored closely after initiation of this medication.

Amlodipine (calcium channel blocker), metoprolol (beta-blocker), and clonidine (alpha-2-adrenergic receptor agonist) would be reasonable initial anti-hypertensive agents; however, they do not have the added benefit of reducing proteinuria. Minoxidil is a direct vasodilator that is reserved for refractory hypertension, and would not be appropriate as a first-line agent for the management of hypertension.

(Chapter 477: Chronic Kidney Disease. Section 25: Disorders of the Kidney and Urinary Tract, p 1766)

Answer 25-25. e

The adolescent patient described above has prehypertension, which is defined as an average systolic and/or diastolic blood pressure between the 90th and 95th percentiles for age, gender, and height. She is also obese, which is a risk factor for primary hypertension. At this time, the most appropriate management of this patient would be to encourage lifestyle modifications that would include dietary changes and an increase in physical activity. Weight reduction and exercise are likely to successfully reduce blood pressure in this patient.

Appropriate evaluation of this patient would include screening for the metabolic syndrome. She is unlikely to have a secondary cause for hypertension, and a diagnostic workup for secondary causes is unnecessary at this time. Further workup including an evaluation for target-organ damage should be considered if hypertension persists or worsens despite lifestyle changes. Similarly, initiation of an antihypertensive agent is not necessary at this time given the patient's prehypertensive state and likelihood to respond to lifestyle modification.

(Chapter 479: Systemic Hypertension. Section 25: Disorders of the Kidney and Urinary Tract, p 1762)

Answer 25-26. b

The patient above has signs and symptoms for peritonitis, which include cloudy peritoneal fluid, abdominal pain, and fever. Additional information that would be consistent with a diagnosis of peritonitis would be a peritoneal white blood cell count of $100/\mu L$ and greater than 50% polymorphonuclear cells.

Gram-positive organisms are the most common causative agents of peritonitis; however, empiric coverage should include broad-spectrum antibiotics for both gram-positive and gram-negative organisms. This patient should be admitted for initial management given the severity of his symptoms and persistent emesis; however, either an intraperitoneal or intravenous route for administration of antibiotics would be appropriate. Repeated episodes of peritonitis can lead to scarring of the peritoneal membrane and may make peritoneal dialysis less effective, but a single episode of peritonitis with early treatment is unlikely to result in scarring significant enough to make peritoneal dialysis ineffective.

(Section 25: Disorders of the Kidney and Urinary Tract. Chapter 478: Chronic Dialysis, p 1756)

Answer 25-27. c

ARPKD is associated with mutations on the PKHD1 gene and occurs in 1 in 6000 to 40,000 live births as compared to ADPKD, which occurs in 1:1000 of the general population. Diagnosis is most often made in the neonatal period, as enlargement of the kidneys may not occur until after 24–28 weeks of gestation and therefore may not be picked up by prenatal ultrasound. Congenital hepatic fibrosis is associated with ARPKD; however, generally renal failure develops prior to liver function abnormalities and portal hypertension. A negative renal ultrasound in the parents of a child with suspected ARPKD helps to distinguish the disease from early-onset ADPKD.

(Chapter 470: Cystic Diseases if the Kidney. Section 25: Disorders of the Kidney and Urinary Tract, p 1703)

Answer 25-28. d

This patient's history of volume depletion from his grueling cross-country race and renal vasoconstriction from administration of a nonsteroidal anti-inflammatory agent are consistent with a prerenal etiology for his acute kidney injury. Additional diagnostic features that would be consistent with a prerenal etiology would include a relatively bland urine sediment (eg, only granular or waxy casts, but no red blood cell casts), a urine specific gravity of >1020, and a fractional excretion of sodium that is <1%. Initial management of this patient should include prompt fluid resuscitation with normal

saline. Potassium-containing fluids should be avoided as GFR is decreased and tubular secretion of potassium may be impaired.

(Chapter 471: Acute Renal Failure. Section 25: Disorders of the Kidney and Urinary Tract, p 1707)

Answer 25-29. d

Acute hemodialysis is indicated in cases of fluid overload resulting in respiratory compromise that are unresponsive to diuretic therapy. Other indications for hemodialysis include severe electrolyte derangements such as hyperkalemia that cannot be managed with medical therapy, and symptomatic uremia. In response A, the patient may respond to correction of acidosis and diuretic therapy for management of hyperkalemia. In response B, vancomycin toxicity is not necessarily an indication for acute hemodialysis, and there are no other specified indications for acute hemodialysis. In responses C and E, the patients may require initiation of chronic renal replacement therapy to support normal growth and development; however, they do not have acute indications for hemodialysis.

(Chapter 471: Acute Renal Failure. Section 25: Disorders of the Kidney and Urinary Tract, p 1710)

Answer 25-30. b

The patient in the above scenario has a history and exam that are highly suggestive of acute poststreptococcal glomerulonephritis (APSGN). This is primarily a disease of school aged children and follows infection with specific strains of group A β-hemolytic streptococcus. Antibiotic treatment of GAS associated pharyngitis is indicated; however, it does not prevent development of acute glomerulonephritis.

Clinical features of APSGN include a low serum C3 and a normal serum C4 level. The serum C3 level generally returns to normal within 3 months after the initial presentation of glomerulonephritis. A biopsy is not necessary in order to confirm the diagnosis of ASPGN; however, if a biopsy were performed immunofluorescence would reveal subepithelial deposits of IgG and C3. Abnormalities on urinalysis such as microscopic hematuria may persist for up to 1 year after initial presentation with APSGN.

(Chapter 472: Glomerular Diseases. Section 25: Disorders of the Kidney and Urinary Tract, p 1714)

Answer 25-31. c

This child presents with hyponatremic dehydration due to diarrhea. Given that a normal serum sodium concentration is 135 mEQ/L, the patient's sodium deficit on presentation can be calculated as follows: [Total body water × (desired Na−current Na)] = 60 mEQ. However, the patient received 200 mL of normal saline in the emergency department, which contains approximately 30 mEQ of Na, so the child's current estimated sodium deficit is equivalent to 30 mEQ. Note that this represents his estimated deficit only, and does not reflect ongoing maintenance sodium needs and stool losses.

(Chapter 466: Fluid, Electrolyte, and Acid–Base Disorders. Section 25: Disorders of the Kidney and Urinary Tract, p 1680)

Answer 25-32. d

The infant described has hypospadias, which is the most common congenital abnormality of the penis. A circumcision should not be performed on this patient in the newborn nursery because the preputial tissues are often used during surgical repair. The patient should be referred to a urologist, and surgery is usually performed when the child is 6 or more months of age. Anomalies of the upper GU tract are not generally associated with hypospadias, and neither a renal ultrasound nor prophylactic antibiotics would be indicated in this patient. In vitro fertilization is a potential risk factor for hypospadias because of maternal exposure to higher levels of progesterone.

(Chapter 476: Urologic Abnormalities of the Genitourinary Tract. Section 25: Disorders of the Kidney and Urinary Tract, p 1745)

Answer 25-33. d

Maintenance fluid requirements are calculated taking into account a patient's urinary losses and insensible losses. Insensible losses are composed of the solute free water that evaporates from the lungs and the skin required to regulate the core body temperature. For healthy individuals, insensible losses can be estimated to be roughly one-third of the usual maintenance fluid requirements. For patients receiving mechanical ventilation, insensible fluid losses are less as they receive humidified air. As a result maintenance fluid requirements are decreased. The syndrome of inappropriate ADH hypersecretion (SIADH) can be seen in individuals receiving mechanical ventilation. As a result, this patient's plasma ADH level would be expected to be elevated. Given the risk of SIADH and hyponatremia, significantly hypotonic fluids

should be avoided. As this patient has normal renal function and does not have hyperkalemia, it would be safe to add potassium to the intravenous fluids.

(Chapter 466: Fluid, Electrolyte, and Acid–Base Disorders. Section 25: Disorders of the Kidney and Urinary Tract, p 1679)

Answer 25-34. c

The child has posterior urethral valve (PUV) syndrome, which is the most common cause of lower urinary tract obstruction in males. The disease only affects male infants with an incidence of 1 in 5000–8000 male births. The obstruction is due to a congenital pair of obstructing leaflets within the prostatic urethra. Bladder distention results from the blockage. The presence of unilateral *vesicoureteral* reflux damages the ipsilateral kidney, but "protects" the contralateral kidney. As a result, these children have a better long-term prognosis. With improvements in prenatal ultrasonography, most cases are now detected prenatally. If missed prenatally, the infant may present with delayed voiding, a distended bladder, poor urinary stream, or urosepsis and vomiting.

(Page 1743; Urologic Abnormalities of the Genitourinary Tract)

Answer 25-35. a

A general rule of thumb is 40 mL/hr for the first 10 kg of weight, 20 mL/hr for the next 10 kg of weight, and 10 mL/hr for each additional 10 kg of weight. Thus for a 16 kg child, the child would require 40 mL/hr (for the first 10 kg of weight) + 12 mL/hr (for the last 6 kg of weight) for a total of 52 mL/hr. The traditional maintenance fluid used is D5 ¼ NS, which contains 30 mmol/L of sodium and chloride and 50 g/L of dextrose, which for most patients contains enough sodium to account for maintenance needs. If the child is NPO, dextrose would be necessary to prevent ketosis and endogenous protein catabolism. D5W would not be appropriate due to the increased risk of hyponatremia. NS at 20 cc/kg is appropriate as a fluid bolus, but not for maintenance requirements.

(Fluid, Electrolyte and Acid–Base Disorders, p 1679)

CHAPTER 26 | Disorders of the Heart

Alaina K. Kipps and Laura A. Robertson

26-1. The order of events in mammalian heart development is:

a. The second heart field replaces the first heart field and develops into a tube—the tube loops to the right—neural crest cells migrate into the outflow tract—atrial and ventricular septation occurs

b. The first and second heart fields develop in a crescent shape—heart tube forms—tube loops to the right—neural crest cells migrate into the outflow tract—atrial and ventricular septation occurs

c. Heart fields develop in a crescent shape—neural crest cells migrate into the field—this block of cells loops to the right while forming a tube—atrial and ventricular septation

d. The first and second heart fields develop in a crescent shape—the heart tube forms—tube loops to the left—atrial and ventricular septation occurs

e. The first heart field develops into a tube—tube loops to the right—atrial and ventricular septation occurs—neural crest cells migrate into the outflow tract

26-2. You are taking a family history of a child with an atrial septal defect. Her mother also had an atrial septal defect that was closed with device-closure. Her grandfather also had an atrial septal defect and has a pacemaker due to complete heart block. What gene defect do you suspect may run in this family?

a. *NOTCH1*

b. *NKX2.5*

c. *NF1*

d. *TBX5*

e. *JAG1*

26-3. You are evaluating a newborn in the nursery for hypotonia, dysmorphic features (see photo), and a heart murmur. Based on these features, what is the most likely chromosome abnormality and heart defect?

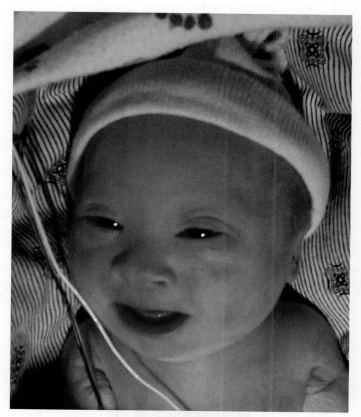

(Reproduced, with permission, from Rudolph CD, Rudolph AM, Lister GE, First LR, Gershon AA. *Rudolph's Pediatrics.* 22nd ed. New York: McGraw-Hill, 2011.)

a. Trisomy 13: Ventricular Septal Defect (VSD)

b. Trisomy 21: complete atrioventricular canal defect

c. Microdeletion 7q11: supravalvular aortic stenosis

d. Microdeletion 22q11: tetralogy of Fallot

e. Trisomy 18: VSD

26-4. A 12-year-old girl presents with lack of pubertal development, short stature, and broad chest. What are the appropriate next steps in evaluating this patient?

  a. Genetic testing of the genes involved in Noonan syndrome

  b. Genetic testing for Alagille syndrome

  c. Echocardiogram and blood pressure measurement in all four extremities

  d. MRI of the heart

  e. Reassurance that there are no cardiac issues in this condition

26-5. You are caring for a 2.2-kg term infant with cleft palate and a small chin. A fetal echocardiogram diagnosed truncus arteriosus, which was confirmed postnatally. There is a small or absent thymus on the echocardiogram. What is most likely underlying genetic abnormality?

  a. Deletion of 22q11.2

  b. *PTPN11* mutation in the RAS/MAP pathway

  c. *JAG 1* mutation

  d. A mutation in *NKX2.5*

  e. A deletion of 7q11

26-6. A 6-year-old who recently moved to your area is seen in your clinic with her mother for a well-child visit. On physical exam she has widely spaced eyes, a broad forehead, and low-set ears (see image below).

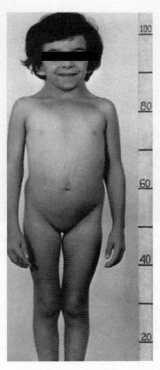

(Reproduced, with permission, from Rudolph CD, Rudolph AM, Lister GE, First LR, Gershon AA. *Rudolph's Pediatrics.* 22nd ed. New York: McGraw-Hill, 2011.)

She has a normal first and second heart sounds with a grade 3-4/6 systolic ejection murmur without any ejection clicks. You obtain an echocardiogram, which demonstrates asymmetric septal hypertrophy with no left ventricular outflow track gradient and a 40-mm peak gradient across her pulmonary valve. What is most likely underlying genetic abnormality?

  a. Deletion of 22q11.2

  b. *PTPN11* mutation in the RAS/MAP pathway

  c. *JAG 1* mutation

  d. A mutation in the beta myosin heavy gene 14q 11.2-3.

  e. A deletion of 7q11

26-7. Your gastroenterology colleagues request your help to evaluate a murmur in a 3-year-old with a history of jaundice and cholestasis. You note that he has a history of mild developmental delay and has unusual facial features (broad forehead, deep-set eyes, pointed chin). The chest X-ray shows a normal cardiac silhouette, but butterfly-shaped vertebrae. You hear normal S1 and S2, no valve clicks, and peripheral PS murmurs bilaterally. What gene defect should you test for?

  a. Deletion of 22q11.2

  b. *PTPN11* mutation in the RAS/MAP pathway

  c. *JAG 1* mutation

  d. A mutation in the beta myosin heavy gene 14q 11.2-3

  e. A deletion of 7q11

26-8. You are seeing a patient who was diagnosed with a ventricular septal defect at birth. The patient's mother is pregnant with her second child and wants to know if she should have a fetal echocardiogram. Which of the following is the most appropriate response?

  a. There are no maternal infections that would be an indication for fetal echocardiograph

  b. If a routine ultrasound shows an extracardiac abnormality, there is no indication for a formal cardiac evaluation

  c. The majority of positive referrals (pregnancies with fetal heart disease) come from known risk factors such as family history

  d. Prepregnancy maternal diseases are unlikely to be associated with congenital heart defects

  e. A family history of congenital heart disease, which includes any first-degree relative, is an indication for fetal echocardiograph

26-9. You are called to an emergent cesarean section delivery due to fetal bradycardia. The neonate is born at 29 weeks gestational age to a 32-year-old G1P 1 mother with no significant past medical history. The pregnancy was uncomplicated, and there were normal fetal heart tones noted on the prior routine obstetrician visits.

On the morning of delivery, the mother presented to her obstetrician and the fetus was found to have heart rate in 60s, prompting admission and urgent delivery. The baby is able to maintain spontaneous respirations, is warm and well perfused with good pulses, and is admitted to the NICU where this EKG was obtained:

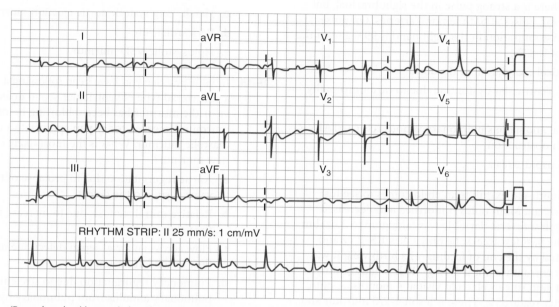

(Reproduced, with permission, from Hay WW, Levin MJ, Sondheimer JM, Deterding RR. *Current Diagnosis & Treatment: Pediatrics.* 21st ed. New York: McGraw-Hill, 2012.)

What does this EKG show and what is the best next work up for this kind of bradycardia?

a. This EKG is consistent with L-looped ventricles and associated complete heart block. Obtain echocardiogram to delineate cardiac anatomy and function

b. This EKG is consistent with sinus bradycardia. Begin workup for sepsis and start antibiotics

c. This EKG is consistent with first-degree atrioventricular block and a superior axis. Obtain echocardiogram to evaluate for endocardial cushion defect

d. This EKG is consistent with complete heart block. Send mother's blood for autoantibodies anti SSA-Ro and SSB-La to evaluate for neonatal lupus erythematosus and obtain an echocardiogram on the baby to evaluate for myocardial depression

e. This EKG is consistent with complete heart block. Send the neonate's blood for the NKX 2.5 mutation and obtain an echocardiogram to evaluate for associated atrial septal defect

26-10. A full-term baby girl is examined in the well-baby nursery and found to have an early systolic click and harsh 3/6 systolic ejection murmur, heard best at the second left intercostal space. S1 is normal, and S2 has normal physiologic split. She is comfortable with respiratory rate at 40 and heart rate 140. On pulse oximetry, she is desaturated at 82%. Several hours later, after transfer to the neonatal intensive care unit, her saturations are 73%. After prostaglandins are given, the saturation increases again to the low 80s. What is the most likely diagnosis?

a. Transposition of the great arteries

b. Critical Pulmonary stenosis (PS)

c. Tricuspid atresia

d. Truncus arteriousus with stenosis

e. Large VSD

26-11. You are seeing a newborn boy 10 days old. The birth was uncomplicated and he was discharged from the well-baby nursery at age 2 days. His mother notes that over the past day he has had "heavy breathing" and has a hard time breast-feeding. His vital signs are as follows: heart rate is 170, respiratory rate is 65 and labored, and it is difficult to obtain blood pressure in the leg. On exam there is a strong pulse in the right brachial, but very weak pulses at both femoral arteries. On pulse oximetry, saturation in the right hand is 99% and in the left foot is 82%.

   a. Critical coarctation of the aorta

   b. Left ventricular dysfuntion due to cardiomyopathy

   c. PS

   d. Total anomalous pulmonary venous return (TAPVR) with obstruction

   e. Tricuspid atresia

26-12. A 4-month-old ex-full term child comes to see his pediatrician. Mom notes rhinorrhea and decreased feeding last several days. He was taking up to 3 oz, but over the past few weeks, he only takes 1.5–2 oz and gets tired by the end of feeding. His birth weight was 3.3 kg; current weight is 5.1 kg. He has had minimal weight gain since well child visit at 4 months. A pulse oximeter reads 85%. There is a soft 1-2/6 murmur and widely split S2, which are new cardiac findings. A chest radiograph shows moderate cardiomegaly and mild pulmonary edema. What is the most likely cardiac lesion?

   a. Tetralogy of Fallot

   b. Total anomalous pulmonary venous return without obstruction

   c. Truncus arteriosus

   d. Transposition of the great arteries

   e. Ventricular septal defect

26-13. Which of the following forms of congenital heart lesions is most common?

   a. Truncus arteriosus

   b. Total anomalous pulmonary venous connection

   c. Transposition of the great arteries

   d. Hypoplastic left heart syndrome

   e. Aortic stenosis

26-14. You are called to examine a 2-day-old full-term infant with tachypnea (RR = 80), cyanosis, sinus tachycardia (HR = 170), hepatomegaly (5 cm below the costal margin), and a palpable spleen tip. He has a hyperdynamic precordium, normal S1, prominent S2, an S3, and bounding pulses but there are no precordial murmurs. CXR shows cardiomegaly, increased pulmonary vascular markings, and a dilated mediastinum. Auscultation for which of the following additional physical finding will help you identify the malformation causing cyanosis and congestive heart failure?

   a. Cranial bruit

   b. Continuous ductal shunt murmur

   c. Harsh, long systolic aortic ejection murmur

   d. Pericardial rub

   e. Holosystolic VSD murmur

26-15. In your practice you have been following a child with a subarterial type of ventricular septal defect. On past visits the murmur has been a blowing holosystolic murmur. However, today you appreciate a descrescendo diastolic murmur. What is the most likely cause for this new murmur?

   a. Aortic regurgitation due to prolapse of the aortic valve cusp into the defect

   b. Relative mitral stenosis due to increase flow across the valve

   c. Flow across an atrial septal defect due to increased flow in the left atrium

   d. Pulmonary regurgitation due to stretching of the pulmonary annulus from pulmonary hypertension

   e. Endocarditis of the tricuspid valve related to turbulence near the VSD has caused a left ventricle to right atrium shunt

26-16. You are seeing a 26-month-old who has been followed with the clinical diagnosis of a small VSD. At his recent examination he was noted to have a louder systolic murmur than at the past several visits. On examination today, he has a grade 4-5/6 systolic ejection-type murmur at the high to mid left sternal border and a grade 1/4 high-frequency diastolic decrescendo murmur at the lower left sternal border. There are no ejection clicks and the rest of the exam is normal.

His ECG shows right ventricular hypertrophy and an upright T-wave in V1. His echocardiogram demonstrated a small, perimembranous ventricular septal defect with aneurysmal closure, a fibrous subaortic ridge with an estimated peak left ventricular outflow A Doppler gradient of 20 mm Hg trivial to mild aortic regurgitation is seen. What other cardiac lesion would also likely be shown on this echocardiogram?

   a. Coarctation of the aorta

   b. Patent ductus arteriosus

   c. Valvar aortic stenosis

   d. Anomalous right ventricular muscle bundles

   e. Left superior vena cava to the coronary sinus

26-17. You are evaluating a 3-month-old boy in your office who you know to have tetralogy of Fallot. His mother informs you that the infant has had fever, diarrhea, and poor feeding in the last 24 hours. On physical examination, you note cyanosis of the extremities and perioral area, tachypnea, hyperpnea, and a heart rate of 180 beats per min. At the last visit you recall a harsh 3/6 systolic ejection murmur; today you do not hear a murmur.

Of the following, the MOST appropriate management strategy is to:

a. Administer antipyretics for fever

b. Reassure his mother because the murmur is gone

c. Order echocardiogram to evaluate the pulmonary valve

d. Encourage oral intake of fluids

e. Place him in the knee–chest position with oxygen

26-18. A 4-year-old comes for his well-child check up and to establish care in your clinic. On exam you auscultate an ejection click and a 3/6 harsh systolic murmur that increases with squatting. What is the most likely lesion and what is best treatment?

a. Congenital aortic stenosis; balloon valvoplasty

b. Subaortic stenosis due to hypertrophic cardiomyopathy; close observation

c. Bicuspid aortic valve and coarctation; coarctation repair

d. Pulmonary stenosis; balloon valvoplasty

e. Ventricular septal defect; surgical repair

26-19. A 7-month-old comes for a check-up due to "noisy breathing since birth." The mother notes it is worse now that the child is eating rice cereal and other baby foods. An echocardiogram is done and the arch vessel sequence is: left common carotid, right common carotid, right subclavian, and left subclavian arteries. There are patent vessels anterior to, to the right of, and posterior to the trachea but not to the left. There is a bulge in the proximal portion of the left subclavian artery. Which of the following is the best answer?

a. This may be a vascular ring but angiography is needed to confirm the diagnosis

b. This is a right arch with retroesophageal subclavian artery that does not form a true ring

c. This may be a vascular ring but the child needs a barium swallow to confirm the diagnosis

d. This is a vascular ring and the patient should have surgical division based on this imaging test alone

e. This is a left pulmonary artery sling, and the left pulmonary artery should be reimplanted surgically to relieve the symptoms

26-20. A 9-week-old infant presents with a dilated cardiomyopathy, ST segment changes on ECG, and Q waves in I and aVL. There is a holosystolic blowing murmur best heard at the apex. The ejection fraction is 20%. The right coronary artery appears dilated. The most likely cause of the cardiomyopathy is:

a. Anomalous left coronary artery from the pulmonary artery

b. Intramural left coronary artery from the right sinus

c. Left coronary artery ostium atresia

d. Myocarditis

e. Kawasaki disease

26-21. A 7-week-old, previously healthy infant comes to your office with a 2-week history of irritability while feeding, sweating, poor oral intake, and tachypnea. She is afebrile and has had no ill contacts. On exam, she is pale and ill-appearing. Her exam is notable for a respiratory rate of 60, without retractions, heart rate of 170, liver edge is 4 cm below the costal margin; she has an active precordium and a new pansystolic murmur at the apex. CXR shows increased cardiac silhouette and increased pulmonary vasculature. The ECG shows sinus tachycardia, increased LV forces, deep Q waves in leads I, aVL, and V4-6. There is ST elevation in V4-6. You can make the diagnosis before you stat page the ER and a cardiologist:

a. Glycogen storage disease

b. Pericarditis

c. Supraventricular tachycardia

d. Anomalous origin of the left coronary artery from the pulmonary artery

e. Endocardial fibroelastosis

26-22. A 6-year-old girl is admitted for appendectomy. After noting an irregular heart rate on preoperative examination, the nurse hands you this rhythm strip. What is the next most appropriate step?

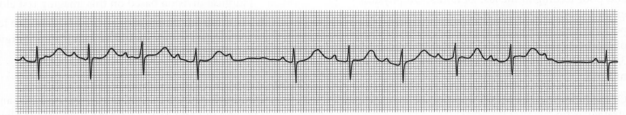

(Reproduced, with permission, from Rudolph CD, Rudolph AM, Lister GE, First LR, Gershon AA. *Rudolph's Pediatrics.* 22nd ed. New York: McGraw-Hill, 2011.)

a. Reassurance—this is sinus arrhythmia with a few escape beats.

b. Reassurance—this is second-degree Mobitz type I/ Wenckebach atrioventicular block, a normal variant

c. Consult cardiology—this is second-degree Mobitz type 2 atrioventicular block and could deteriorate to complete heart block

d. Consult cardiology—this is type 3/complete heart block and maybe very problematic for safe anesthesia

e. Check electrolytes—this is a junctional escape rhythm with a narrow QRS complex

26-23. A 13-year-old boy presents to the emergency room with palpitations and tachycardia. He has had two 20- to 30-minute episodes over the past week but he only told his mother about it this morning when he felt it for the third time after drinking a "redbull." He does not complain of chest pain or dizziness, and other vital signs are normal for age. Here is the rhythm strip:

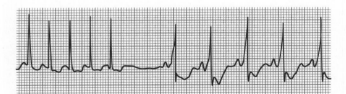

(Reproduced, with permission, from Rudolph CD, Rudolph AM, Lister GE, First LR, Gershon AA. *Rudolph's Pediatrics.* 22nd ed. New York: McGraw-Hill, 2011.)

The echocardiogram displays normal structure and function. What is the next most appropriate step in his evaluation and management?

a. Refer to cardiology clinic and discharge from ER with prescription for verapamil

b. Refer to cardiology clinic and discharge from ER with prescription for atenolol

c. Refer to cardiology clinic and discharge from ER with prescription for digoxin

d. Admit to the cardiology ward for close monitoring and an urgent electrophysiology test with ablation of the accessory pathway

e. Discharge from ER with instructions to cut back on caffeine intake and to follow up if the palpitations reoccur

26-24. You are evaluating a 15-year-old whose father recently drowned while swimming laps in a pool. Upon further inquiry, a couple of months ago, his father had had a fainting episode after running, but had attributed this to dehydration. Your patient admits that he has had some episodes of dizziness and palpitations during track practice, for which he took breaks, but he has never fainted or had any chest pain. He has a normal CXR and cardiovascular examination. What changes on his ECG would be most worrisome?

a. First-degree AV block (prolonged PR interval)

b. Premature atrial contractions

c. Prolonged QTc interval (>460 ms)

d. Sinus arrhythmia

e. Premature ventricular contractions

26-25. A 9-year-old boy with a history of syncope is found to have the following electrocardiogram show a prolonged QTc interval. What would be the most appropriate therapy?

a. Implant an intracardiac defibrillator

b. Initiate beta blocker therapy

c. Start digoxin

d. Start amiodarone

e. Implant a pacemaker

26-26. A 2-year-old patient with DiGeorge syndrome presents with hypocalcemia, seizure, and the following rhythm strip. Which of the following choices is the most likely cause of his erratic rhythm?

a. Ventricular fibrillation
b. Ventricular flutter
c. Atrial fibrillation
d. Movement artifact
e. Supraventricular tachycardia

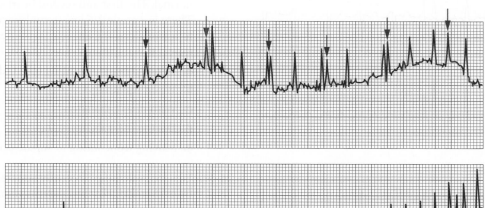

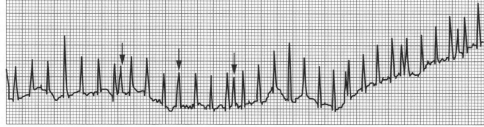

(Reproduced, with permission, from Fuster V, et al. *Hurst's The Heart*. 13th ed. New York: McGraw-Hill, 2011.)

26-27. A 14-year-old boy presents with a rash (see image below), some nonspecific joint pain, and the electrocardiogram shown below. What disease process will most appropriately explain these findings?

a. Rheumatic fever
b. Lyme disease
c. Myocarditis
d. Kawasaki disease
e. Juvenile rheumatoid arthritis

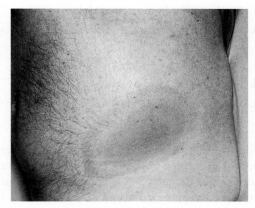

(Reproduced, with permission, from Weinberg S, Prose NS, Kristal L. *Color Atlas of Pediatric Dermatology*. 4th ed. New York: McGraw-Hill, 2007.)

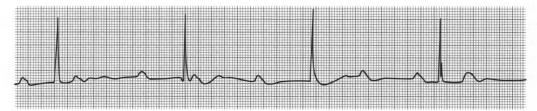

(Reproduced, with permission, from Rudolph CD, Rudolph AM, Lister GE, First LR, Gershon AA. *Rudolph's Pediatrics*. 22nd ed. New York: McGraw-Hill, 2011.)

26-28. A newborn develops tachycardia on day of life 1. She is feeding with good pulses and BP of 65/45 mm Hg. An ECG is obtained and shown here.

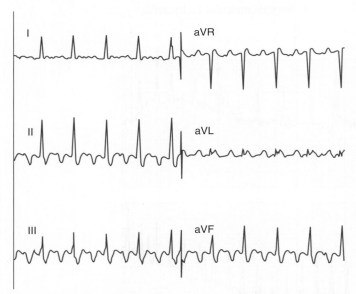

I   aVR

II   aVL

III   aVF

(Reproduced, with permission, from Rudolph CD, Rudolph AM, Lister GE, First LR, Gershon AA. *Rudolph's Pediatrics.* 22nd ed. New York: McGraw-Hill, 2011.)

Which of the following is the most appropriate therapy?

a. Discharge for home with a Holter monitor

b. IV adenosine to convert orthodromic reciprocating tachycardia

c. Atrial overdrive pacing for atrial flutter

d. Emergent DC cardioversion

e. Vagal maneuvers to convert AV node reentry tachycardia

26-29. You are evaluating a 4-year-old healthy girl at her annual health supervision visit. You note clear breath sounds, strong pulses, a quiet precordium, and a murmur. Your partner noted a murmur at last year's visit. Of the following, the finding MOST consistent with the diagnosis of a functional (innocent) murmur is:

a. A continuous "machinery" murmur under the left clavicle

b. A harsh systolic murmur at the right upper sternal border

c. A high-pitched systolic murmur in the back between the scapulae

d. A low-pitched, long, diastolic murmur at the left sternal border

e. A low-pitched, vibratory systolic murmur at the left sternal border

26-30. A 3-year-old healthy boy is referred for evaluation of a recently heard heart murmur. His peripheral pulses are normal. The first and second heart sounds are normal. There is a grade 2/6 low to mid frequency "vibratory" murmur along the left sternal border. One would expect this murmur to INCREASE in intensity:

a. When going from sitting to standing position

b. When squatting

c. With deep inhalation

d. During the Valsalva maneuver

e. Moving from sitting to supine position

26-31. You are evaluating a recently adopted 2-year-old from overseas. His new parents were told that he has a murmur. They noticed he loves to run around the house, but he often takes breaks squats down and breathes heavily. He has dark skin, but they wonder if he looks dusky when he runs. On examination, he has room air saturations of 80%, a right ventricular heave, and a harsh systolic ejection murmur at the LUSB that radiates to the lung fields. There is no hepatomegaly. Pulses are equal in all extremities. His upper and lower extremity blood pressures are normal for age. Which congenital cardiac lesion do you suspect?

a. Coarctation of the aorta

b. Patent ductus arteriosus

c. Tetralogy of fallot

d. Atrial septal defect

e. Ventricular septal defect

26-32. During a 10-year-old's well-child visit, you hear a loud first heart sound and a widely split second heart sound that does not vary with respiration. He has a RV lift and a soft systolic flow murmur at the LUSB. Pulses are normal. He is a good soccer player and has been healthy. What lesion is most likely to explain these findings?

a. Atrial septal defect

b. Ventricular septal defect

c. Coarctation of the aorta

d. Aortic stenosis

e. Pulmonic valve stenosis

26-33. A 16-year-old soccer player comes to the clinic complaining of left-sided chest pain for the past week. She has no history of chest trauma, fever, recent illness, palpitations, dizziness, or syncope. The pain is worse when she breathes deeply. Her cardiovascular and pulmonary examinations are normal. She has tenderness to palpation along the left sternal border. Of the following, the MOST likely diagnosis is:

a. Acute rheumatic fever

b. Costochondritis

c. Infective endocarditis

d. Myocarditis

e. Pericarditis

26-34. A 13-year-old altar boy comes to clinic with a history of multiple syncopal episodes during church services. He describes the episodes to you: after standing quietly for 5–10 minutes, he feels warm, his vision darkens from the periphery, he feels sweaty, and his heart races. He feels dizzy and loses consciousness. He has never injured himself during fainting episodes and returns to "normal" shortly afterwards. He drinks plenty of water every day. His mother recalls that she had similar episodes in adolescence. His physical examination in clinic is normal. His ECG shows normal axes, normal conduction, normal QRS and QT intervals for his age. What is the MOST LIKELY etiology of his syncope?

a. Long QT syndrome

b. Premature atrial contractions

c. Supraventricular tachycardia

d. Vasovagal syncope

e. Hypertrophic cardiomyopathy

26-35. A 6-year-old obese boy has a right-arm blood pressure of 145/60 and a left-arm blood pressure of 143/59 using an appropriately sized BP cuff. There is a family history of systemic hypertension. He has an aortic valve click on examination. You do not hear a murmur. He has good radial pulses, but you have difficulty identifying lower extremity pulses. His ECG has voltage criteria for left ventricular hypertrophy. What is the best next step?

a. Check a lower extremity blood pressure

b. Order a fasting lipid profile

c. Counsel him and his parents about exercise and diet. Schedule a return visit in a month.

d. Recommend portion control with a low-fat and low-salt diet.

e. Check chemistries with BUN and creatinine

26-36. Karen is a 13-year-old who was found to have hypertension at a school preathletic screening event. Her blood pressure in the right arm in your office is

152/96. Her heart rate is 75, her BMI is 23, and her exam was otherwise normal. Her past medical history is significant for a urinary tract infection at the age of 3. She also had a high fever and rash at age 5 that responded after treatment with amoxicillin. She has had normal growth and development. Her family history is notable for a father with hypertension. The most likely cause of her hypertension is:

a. Coarctation of the aorta

b. Renal artery stenosis

c. Post streptococcal glomerulonephritis

d. Atrophic pylonephritis

e. Pheochromocytoma

26-37. Of the following patients, who is at *highest* risk for bacterial endocarditis?

a. A child with tetralogy of Fallot with an aortopulmonary shunt

b. A toddler with transposition of the great arteries following an arterial switch operation at age 1 week

c. A child who had a cardiac transplant 4 years ago

d. An infant with unrepaired total anomalous pulmonary venous connection

e. A child with mild mitral stenosis

26-38. You are seeing a 4-year-old girl with tuberous sclerosis for the first time in your primary care practice. In addition to her seizure history, her mom mentions concern over a "heart tumor." For which of the following is this patient at highest risk

a. Hamartoma

b. Rhabdomyoma

c. Myxoma

d. Teratoma

e. Hemangioma

26-39. On a late night ER shift, you are asked to evaluate a 5-year-old who has had a rash and 5 days of persistent high fever (39–40 degrees) despite multiple doses of antipyretics. His parents are exasperated because he has been extremely irritable. You note that he has a bright red tongue, cracked red lips, conjunctivitis without eye discharge, and a diffuse erythematous rash. His joints are not tender or swollen, but his hands and feet are edematous. His palms and soles are erythematous. What is your diagnosis?

a. Kawasaki's disease

b. Streptococcal infection

c. Stevens–Johnson syndrome

d. Staph scaled skin syndrome

e. Rheumatic fever

26-40. You have recently diagnosed a 5-year-old boy with Kawasaki disease based on clinical exam and laboratory evaluation. He has had a fever for 5 days, has a bright red tongue, cracked red lips, conjunctivitis, a large cervical lymph node, and a diffuse erythematous rash. His ESR is 120. What would you do next to treat this patient?

   a. Perform a blood culture and start broad-spectrum antibiotics

   b. Admit tonight for intravenous immunoglobulin (IVIG) and high-dose aspirin. Order an echocardiogram for tomorrow

   c. Discharge from the ER with follow-up if fever persists another 48 hours

   d. Prescribe amoxicillin and follow up in primary care clinic tomorrow

   e. Perform a lumbar puncture and start broad-spectrum antibiotics due to concern for meningitis

26-41. Two weeks after having a nonspecific upper respiratory tract infection, a previously healthy 4-year-old boy is noted to have a respiratory rate of 40 breaths per min, a heart rate of 140 beats per min. His heart rate is occasionally irregular and a gallop rhythm is noted. A 1/6 blowing systolic murmur is heard at the apex. He has moderate hepatomegaly. Of the following, the MOST likely diagnosis is?

   a. Acute rheumatic fever

   b. Infective endocarditis

   c. Viral myocarditis

   d. Paroxysmal atrial tachycardia

   e. Pericarditis

26-42. A 6-year-old boy, with no previous cardiac history, is admitted to the PICU in congestive heart failure. Upon questioning his parents, he had a fever and culture-proven strep throat 3 weeks ago, but the family could not fill the antibiotic prescription. Your differential diagnosis includes ARF. Carditis is a major criterion. What other MAJOR criterion do you need to confirm to make this diagnosis?

   a. Arthritis

   b. Elevated erythrocyte sedimentation rate (ESR)

   c. Positive C-reactive protein (CRP)

   d. Anemia and elevated white blood count

   e. ECG changes of prolonged PR and/or QT intervals

26-43. You are seeing a 7-year-old boy with a documented antecedent strep infection, positive ASO, and evidence of carditis of echocardiography, how many MINOR criteria would you need to make the diagnosis of ARF?

   a. One

   b. Two

   c. Three

   d. Four.

   e. Five

26-44. A previously healthy 10-year-old girl has a 4-week history of low-grade fever, malaise, decreased appetite, weight loss, myalgia, and headaches. On examination, she has a new diastolic murmur, petechiae, and a palpable spleen tip. What is the most likely diagnosis?

   a. Infective endocarditis

   b. Tuberculosis

   c. Kawasaki's disease

   d. Rheumatic fever

   e. Scarlet fever

26-45. An otherwise healthy 14-year-old girl complains of chest pain that is particularly severe over the left precordium when she is lying supine. She has begun sleeping upright due to chest pain. She has had a mild viral respiratory infection and intermittent, low-grade fever (<38.5 degrees) for the past 2 weeks. Physical examination is remarkable only for mild jugular venous distention and distant heart sounds. The CXR shows a moderately enlarged cardiac silhouette, and the ECG shows diffusely decreased voltages throughout all leads. Of the following, the MOST likely diagnosis is?

   a. Acute rheumatic fever

   b. Costochondritis

   c. Infective endocarditis

   d. Myocarditis

   e. Pericarditis

26-46. You are called to evaluate a 15-year-old boy with a recently diagnosed systemic lupus erythematosis. He had a normal echocardiogram last month. Over the past week, he has had chest discomfort with inspiration, but now has shortness of breath and dyspnea on exertion. He is afebrile, tachycardic (130s), and ill-appearing with cold, clammy extremities. His ECG shows sinus tachycardia and diffusely decreased voltages. His CXR shows an enlarged cardiac silhouette, but no infiltrates, pulmonary edema or pleural effusions. What physical examination finding would help you make a diagnosis of tamponade at the bedside?

   a. Comparison of upper and lower extremity blood pressures

   b. Absent femoral pulses

   c. Conjunctival injection and strawberry tongue

   d. Splinter hemorrhages and Janeway lesion

   e. Blood pressure assessment with deep inspiration

26-47. You are in the ER evaluating a 4-year-old, who has had consistent well-child care and no significant prior medical history. She had a witnessed syncopal episode. She had been running on the playground and lost consciousness for <1 minute. Her mother thinks she "looked a bit blue" during the episode. There was no incontinence or seizure activity. On examination, she had a prominent left hemithorax and marked RV impulse. She has a regular rate and rhythm, normal S1 and a loud, single S2 that is palpable. There are no murmurs. Her abdominal examination is normal. She has full, equal pulses in all extremities and no blood pressure gradient between the arms and legs. There is no digital clubbing. Her room air saturations are 98%. CXR shows enlarged right ventricle and main pulmonary artery silhouettes. The ECG shows sinus rhythm, right axis deviation, and significantly increased RV voltages. What is your leading diagnosis based on the exam ECG and CXR?

   a. Tetralogy of Fallot with severe subvalvular outflow obstruction
   b. Severe pulmonary arterial hypertension
   c. Pulmonary valve stenosis
   d. Coarctation of the aorta
   e. Hypertrophic obstructive cardiomyopathy

26-48. Which of the following statements most accurately describes the normal maturation of change in the electrocardiogram during the first week of birth?

   a. A decrease of the right precordial R wave amplitude
   b. Regression of R/S ratio toward l in the right precordial leads
   c. A change in T wave polarity from positive to negative in the right precordial leads
   d. Loss of the right precordial Q wave
   e. A shift in the QRS frontal plane axis from greater than +135 degrees to less than +110 degrees

26-49. You are seeing a 12-year-old patient with Williams syndrome and known moderate supravalvar aortic stenosis. At echocardiogram today the pressure drop measured with spectral Doppler just above the aortic valve was 4.5 m/s. What is the gradient across the stenotic area?

   a. 91 mm Hg
   b. 18 mm Hg

   c. 45 mm Hg
   d. 20 mm Hg
   e. 81 mm Hg

26-50. Which of the following is a normal pulmonary vascular resistance (PVR) in children and adults (in Woods Units)?

   a. 1–3 Units/m^2
   b. 4–6 Units/m^2
   c. 7–10 Units/m^2
   d. 10–15 Units/m^2
   e. >15 Units/m^2

26-51. A cardiac catheterization was performed in room air (FiO$_2$ = 0.21) on a 6-month-old with a right arm BP = 70/40. Based on the catheterization data below, what congenital heart defect does this infant have?

Chamber	Saturation (%)	Pressure (mm Hg)
Superior Vena Cava	60	
Right Atrium	60	5
Left Atrium	99	8
Right Ventricle	85	70/5
Left Ventricle	85	70/8
Pulmonary Artery	85	10/5
Ascending Aorta	85	70/40
Descending Aorta	85	75/40

   a. Moderate membranous ventricular septal defect
   b. Tetralogy of fallot
   c. Large secundum atrial septal defect
   d. Aortic valve stenosis
   e. Coarctation of the aorta

26-52. A cardiac catheterization was performed in room air ($FiO_2 = 0.21$) on a 16-year-old with a right arm BP = 160/70. Based on the catheterization data below, what congenital heart defect does this adolescent have?

Chamber	Saturation (%)	Pressure (mm Hg)
Superior vena cava	75	
Right atrium	75	8
Left atrium	100	10
Right ventricle	75	25/8
Left ventricle	100	160/10
Pulmonary artery	75	10/5
Ascending aorta	100	160/70
Descending aorta	100	100/80

    a. Moderate membranous ventricular septal defect

    b. Tetralogy of Fallot

    c. Large secundum atrial septal defect

    d. Aortic valve stenosis

    e. Coarctation of the aorta

26-53. The mother of a 4-month-old is concerned because he is taking longer to finish feeds, sweats when he sucks, and breathes more quickly when he nurses. He has not gained much weight in the last month. He has little subcutaneous tissue, is tachypneic without retractions, has hepatomegaly, and diffusely diminished pulses. You hear a murmur on his examination. Which lesion is NOT likely to cause this clinical picture of failure to thrive and congestive heart failure?

    a. Large PDA

    b. Large VSD

    c. Truncus arteriosus

    d. Complete common AV canal

    e. Secundum atrial septal defect

26-54. You admit a patient with low cardiac output due to myocarditis, and decide to administer milrinone. How does this medication work?

    a. This medication is a calcium-sensitizing agent with inotropic and afterload reducing effects. It binds to troponin C and improves the efficiency of the contractile apparatus

    b. This medication acts by stimulating myocardial surface beta-adrenergic receptors, leading to increased adenylate cyclase and intracellular cyclic adenosine monophosphate

    c. This medication lowers filling pressures, systemic and pulmonary artery pressures, and systemic and pulmonary vascular resistances, while improving the cardiac index

    d. This medication is a sodium–potassium ATPase inhibitor with positive inotropy, negative chronotropy, and inhibition of neurohormonal activation

    e. This medication causes natriuresis, diuresis, vasodilatation, and increased renal blood flow, increased cardiac output and urine output

26-55. The following are cardiac lesions with single ventricle physiology EXCEPT:

    a. Pulmonary atresia with intact ventricular septum

    b. Hypoplastic left heart syndrome

    c. Tricuspid atresia with pulmonary stenosis

    d. Tetralogy of Fallot with pulmonary atresia and major aortopulmonary collaterals

    e. Tetralogy of Fallot with subpulmonary stenosis

26-56. A 4-day-old infant presents with decreased oral intake and decreased activity. Birth history was unremarkable and he was discharged home on day 2 of his life. Physical exam reveals a cool, mottled infant, with decreased pulses. No significant murmur is audible. Which is the most likely congenital heart defect?

    a. Tetralogy of Fallot

    b. Transposition of the great arteries

    c. Ebsteins anomaly

    d. Hypoplastic left heart syndrome

    e. Ventricular septal defect

26-57. A newborn born full term at a community hospital with Apgars of 8 and 8 is noted to be cyanotic at 9 hours of life. Oxygen is given by face-mask at 10 LPM, but pulse oximetry readings in the right hand remain in the low 70s. An umbilical arterial line is placed and the first blood gas shows pH 7.23, PCO_2 of 38, and PaO_2 of 33 mm Hg. Her lungs are clear and her breathing is unlabored with mild tachypnea and no retractions. She has full pulses at femoral and brachial areas and is well perfused. What intervention should be done while transport is arranged?

    a. Infusion of indomethacin

    b. Infusion of prostaglandin E1

    c. Bolus of digoxin

    d. Infusion of adenosine

    e. Bolus of saline

26-58. You are seeing a 14-year-old in the pediatrics clinic for a presports physical examination. Which of these patients may compete in school athletics without further cardiology evaluation?

  a. Unrepaired tetralogy of fallot

  b. Congenital atrio-ventricular block with transvenous pacemaker

  c. D-Transposition of the great arteries, status post arterial switch operation

  d. Moderate aortic valve stenosis

  e. Moderate pulmonary valve stenosis

26-59. Your 10-year-old patient with hypoplastic left heart syndrome has been stable for several years after his Fontan procedure. His family is considering a ski trip to Colorado and seeks your advice. Which of the following statements is most appropriate?

  a. Given his repair and Fontan physiology, he should have no problem at elevation

  b. The patient will not be able to tolerate the airline flight

  c. The patient will develop symptoms of respiratory distress and cyanosis within hours

  d. The patient may tolerate the high elevation but his exercise tolerance will be affected

  e. The patient should not travel above 500 feet

26-60. You are evaluating a 16-year-old boy for pre-participation sports screening. The boy states that his older brother was diagnosed with a seizure disorder and died suddenly during high school track practice. He also has a younger sister who has a history of syncope. Before approving him for sports participation, which of the following tests must be performed?

  a. MRI of the head

  b. Electrocardiography

  c. Electroencephalography

  d. 24-hour Holter monitor

  e. Tilt table test

26-61. The most common cause of sudden death during competitive exercise is?

  a. Postoperative congenital heart disease

  b. Hypertrophic cardiomyopathy

  c. Marfan syndrome

  d. Aortic valve stenosis

  e. Long QT syndrome

ANSWERS

Answer 26-1. b

Cardiogenesis involves a series of molecular and morphogenetic processes. The early cardiac progenitor cells arise from mesodermal cells that migrate from the primitive streak to the anterior portion of the embryo.

As illustrated in Figure 480-1, the first and second heart fields develop into a crescent shape in the anterior embryo. By the 3rd week, the heart tube forms from components of both heart fields. The heart tube loops to the right and neural crest cells then migrate into the outflow tract. Lastly there is atrial and ventricular septation to result in a four-chambered heart.

(Section 26: Disorders of the Cardiovascular System; Part 1: Principles of Cardiology, Chapter 480: pp 1770–1771)

Answer 26-2. b

Mutations in *NKX2.5* cause developmental atrial septal defects and progressively disrupt electrical conduction through the cardiac chambers and can result in complete heart block. Over time, the specialized muscle-derived conduction cells in the atrioventricular node are lost and replaced by fibrotic tissue, resulting in progressive defects in electrical conduction. This patient should be monitored in the long-term due to the strong family history of both ASD and conduction abnormalities.

NOTCH1 mutations in humans cause bicuspid aortic valves and later calcification. Neurofibromatosis is associated with thickened valves and is caused by mutation of the *NF1* gene. *TBX5* is associated with Holt–Oram syndrome. Although patients with the Holt–Oram syndrome can have ASDs, progressive conduction problems would be unexpected. *JAG 1*, a NOTCH ligand, can cause outflow tract defects associated with the autosomal-dominant disease, Alagille syndrome.

(Section 26: Disorders of the Cardiovascular System; Part 1: Principles of Cardiology, Chapter 480, pp 1773–1775)

Answer 26-3. b

This child's features are most consistent with Down syndrome, or trisomy 21. The prevalence of congenital heart defect (CHD) in this population is approximately 40%–50%. Complete atrioventricular septal defect (AVSD; also termed endocardial cushion defect, atrioventricular canal defect) accounts for 40% of all CHD in Down syndrome patients, and this figure increases to almost 60% when partial AVSD (primum atrial septal defect, inlet or canal-type ventricular septal defect) is included.

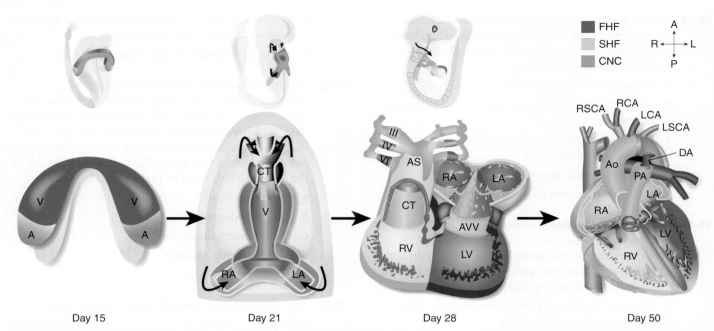

FIGURE 480-1. Mammalian heart development. Oblique views of whole embryos and frontal views of cardiac precursors during human cardiac development are shown. First panel: First heart field (FHF) cells form a crescent shape in the anterior embryo with second heart field (SHF) cells medial and anterior to the FHF. Second panel: SHF cells lie dorsal to the straight heart tube and begin to migrate (*arrows*) into the anterior and posterior ends of the tube to form the right ventricle (RV), conotruncus (CT), and part of the atria (A). Third panel: Following rightward looping of the heart tube, cardiac neural crest (CNC) cells also migrate (*arrow*) into the outflow tract from the neural folds to septate the outflow tract and pattern the bilaterally symmetric aortic arch artery arteries (III, IV, and VI). Fourth panel: Septation of the ventricles, atria, and atrioventricular valves (AVVs) results in the 4-chambered heart. V, ventricle; LV, left ventricle; LA, left atrium; RA, right atrium; AS, aortic sac; Ao, aorta; PA, pulmonary artery; RSCA, right subclavian artery; LSCA, left subclavian artery; RCA, right carotid artery; LCA, left carotid artery; DA, ductus arteriosus. (Reproduced, with permission, from Rudolph CD, Rudolph AM, Lister GE, First LR, Gershon AA. *Rudolph's Pediatrics.* 22nd ed. New York: McGraw-Hill, 2011.)

The American Academy of Pediatrics recommends routine echocardiographic screening of neonates with Down syndrome to facilitate early diagnosis of CHD and intervention because of the increased risk of pulmonary vascular disease in this population.

(Section 26: Disorders of the Cardiovascular System; Part 1: Principles of Cardiology, Chapter 481, p 1775)

Answer 26-4. c

The features presented here most likely represent those of Turner syndrome, or monosomy X. Approximately 25–30% of patients have associated congenital heart disease, predominately left-sided obstructive lesions. Coarctation of the aorta is present in 10–20% of patients; therefore, screening for coarctation is indicated at 5-year intervals. Unlike hypoplastic aortic arches, major intracardiac anomalies are not commonly found with isolated coarctation of the aorta; however, there is a high association of this lesion with Turner syndrome and with bicuspid aortic valve.

Genetic testing of the genes involved in Noonan syndrome would not be indicated unless Turner is ruled out. There can be overlap of the features between Noonan and Turner. Genetic testing for Alagille syndrome is not indicated. While an MRI

of the heart may be a more sensitive way to detect subtle coartcation, it is not indicated as the first-line test.

(Section 26: Disorders of the Cardiovascular System; Part 1: Principles of Cardiology, Chapter 481, p 1777)

Answer 26-5. a

The physical characteristics of the infant described in this vignette are classically associated with DiGeorge syndrome (22q11 microdeletion deletion syndrome). This includes neonatal hypocalcemia, micrognathia, thymic hypoplasia, Immunodeficiency, feeding and speech disorders, behavioral and psychiatric disorders, renal anomalies, and congenital heart disease. Approximately 75% of affected individuals have congenital heart disease, most commonly aortic arch anomalies including interrupted aortic arch, truncus arteriosus, and tetralogy of Fallot.

Due the incidence of 22q11 microdeletion syndrome (1 in 6000 live births), the American Heart Association and the American Academy of Pediatrics (AAP) have recently advocated fluorescence in situ hybridization (FISH) testing for the 22q11 deletion in all infants with the following cardiac lesions: type B interrupted arch, ventricular septal defect with aortic arch anomaly, truncus arteriosus, isolated aortic arch anomaly, and tetralogy of Fallot, especially when associated with either absent pulmonary valve, aortic arch or pulmonary artery anomalies, or aortopulmonary collaterals.

PTPN11 mutation in the RAS/MAP pathway is one of the genetic abnormalities associated with Noonan syndrome. A *JAG 1* mutation is seen in Alagile syndrome. Mutation in the beta myosin heavy gene 14q 11.2-3 is the genetic abnormality that is frequently seen in hypertrophic cardiomyopathy. A deletion of 7q11 is associated with William syndrome. None of these are associated with conotruncal cardiac abnormalities and cleft palate.

(Section 26: Disorders of the Cardiovascular System; Part 1: Principles of Cardiology, Chapter 481, p 1777)

Answer 26-6. b

The patient most likely has Noonan syndrome. Noonan syndrome is an autosomal dominant disorder which presents with hypertelorism, ptosis, epicanthal folds, low-set posteriorly rotated ears, short stature, and congenital heart defects. Congenital heart defects occurs in 80–90% of patients with Noonan syndrome, most often valvular pulmonic stenosis (PS) and hypertrophic cardiomyopathy. This patient's cardiac exam and echocardiogram are consistent with a dysplastic pulmonary valve and hypertrophic cardiomyopathy. *PTPN11* mutation in the RAS/MAP pathway is one of the genetic abnormalities associated with Noonan syndrome.

Deletion of 22q11 is the genetic anomaly seen with DiGeorge syndrome. A *JAG 1* mutation is seen in Alagille syndrome. Mutation in the beta myosin heavy gene 14q 11.2-3 is the genetic abnormality that is frequently seen in hypertrophic cardiomyopathy. Although the patient in this vignette shows evidence of hypertrophic cardiomyopathy, the physical exam consistent with a dysplastic pulmonary valve and the classic facial features are diagnostic of Noonan syndrome. A deletion of 7q11 is associated with Williams syndrome.

(Section 26: Disorders of the Cardiovascular System; Part 1: Principles of Cardiology, Chapter 481, p 1778)

Answer 26-7. c

The constellation of symptoms and facial features is most consistent with Alagille syndrome. Alagille syndrome is caused by mutations in *JAG1*, which encodes a cell surface protein that acts as a ligand in the NOTCH signaling pathway. Alagille syndrome is characterized by a paucity of bile ducts, cholestasis, and jaundice. Some patients need liver transplantation. Alagille patients have distinctive facial features and vertebral anomalies. The cardiac defects usually involve stenosis in the peripheral pulmonary arteries. Rare patients will have tetralogy of Fallot.

Deletion of 22q11.2 is the genetic abnormality with DiGeorge syndrome, which does not have associated hepatic disease or skeletal involvement. *PTPN11* mutation in the RAS/MAP pathway is one of the genetic abnormalities associated with Noonan syndrome. Noonan patients usually have

dysplastic pulmonary valves and can also develop hypertrophic cardiomyopathy. Skeletal and hepatic abnormalities are not associated with Noonan's. The genetic abnormality in the beta myosin heavy gene is frequently seen in hypertrophic cardiomyopathy. A defect in the elastin gene with deletion of 7q11 is the abnormality associated with Williams syndrome. It causes an arterial vasculopathy and can cause supravalvar aortic stenosis, supravalvar pulmonary stenosis, and branch pulmonary artery stenosis as well as aortic hypoplasia and renal artery stenosis.

(Section 26: Disorders of the Cardiovascular System; Part 1: Principles of Cardiology, Chapter 481, p 1779)

Answer 26-8. e

Fetal echocardiograms are used to evaluate structural, functional, and rhythm-related defects. A family history of congenital heart defects (CHD) in the fetus's mother, father, or siblings is an indication for fetal screening. Additionally, a family history of a syndrome associated with CHD is also an indication. Maternal indications include prepregnancy diseases such as diabetes, phenylketonuria, or autoimmune disorders. Fetal indications include suspected cardiac abnormalities on routine ultrasound, suspected extracardiac abnormalities, and abnormal fetal rhythms. Importantly, the majority of positive referrals come from low-risk population without known risk factors who were referred because of suspicion for CHD on routine ultrasound.

(Section 26: Disorders of the Cardiovascular System; Part 2: Approach to the Patient, Chapter 482, p 1782)

Answer 26-9. d

This EKG shows complete heart block with complete atrial (p-wave) and ventricular (QRS complex) dissociation. The ventricular rate is in the 60s, and although this is much slower than the typical neonatal heart rate, the child is compensating with larger stroke volume and has adequate cardiac output. The QRS complexes are narrow and normal, indicating that the escape focus generating the ventricular rhythm is high in the conducting system. The block often occurs in utero, and at times cesarean section is done due to concern for fetal distress inferred from the slow heart rate. The autoantibodies anti SSA-Ro and SSB-La are observed in maternal systemic lupus erythematosus or mixed connective tissue disease, but also occur in the absence of clinical autoimmune disease, a more common finding in mothers of affected fetuses just like in this vignette. It is important to evaluate the neonate's myocardial function as 15–20% of fetuses with maternal autoimmune-mediated atrioventricular block can develop more diffuse myocardial disease.

This EKG does not have the features of L-looped ventricles. Although complete heart block is associated with this form of congenital heart disease, it is much less common than neonatal lupus. Also, neonates with heart block and bradycardia in the 60s with congenital heart lesions are typically much more symptomatic than those with structurally normal hearts. Although the most common form of fetal bradycardia is sinus bradycardia, this EKG shows complete dissociation of p-waves from the QRS complexes and is not consistent with sinus bradycardia. Also, sinus bradycardia is typically associated with a gradual slowing of the fetal heart rate and rapid resolution. The EKG is not consistent with first-degree atrioventricular block (when there is prolongation of the PR interval, but otherwise preserved conduction) or a superior axis (with a frontal plane QRS axis of −90° to −180° (or 0° to +270°). Although complete heart block is associated with this genetic mutation, it is much less common than neonatal lupus. NKX2.5 is also associated with atrial septal defects, which can be difficult to diagnose on physical exam alone.

(Section 26: Disorders of the Cardiovascular System; Part 2: Approach to the Patient, Chapter 483, p 1786 & Chapter 485, p 1847)

Answer 26-10. b

This vignette describes a neonate with inadequate pulmonary blood flow. This may be due to an obstruction of the blood into the right ventricle, from the right ventricle, or ejection of the blood itself. This patient's exam and clinical course are most consistent with severe PS, which presents in the immediate postnatal period and can resemble pulmonary atresia with severe cyanosis and cardiac collapse as the ductus arterious closes. Once the ductus closes, pulmonary blood flow decreases substantially. In this patient, at the time of the first exam the ductus was still patent; several hours later it was more restrictive, and saturations improved with prostaglandins. While the ductus is patent, there is left to right flow across it, allowing more pulmonary blood flow. In infants with PS, there will be right ventricular hypertrophy and right axis deviation, the degree depending on the severity of the stenosis. Apart from the systolic ejection murmur, there is typically a loud variable ejection click. The electrocardiogram shows the right atrial hypertrophy with peaked P waves. The right precordial leads show tall R waves, and with severe stenosis, they may also show T-wave inversion and S–T segment depression.

Transposition of the great arteries does not present with cyanosis in the immediate newborn period. At birth, pulmonary vascular resistance falls rapidly, resulting in pulmonary blood flow 2 to 4 times that of systemic flow. This results in oxygen saturations in the high 80s to low 90s. Cyanosis may then progress gradually, over hours to days, or, as often happens, is first noticed when the newborn cries or is fed. With these events there is increased oxygen utilization and decreased pulmonary blood flow. Tricuspid atresia results in inadequate filling of the right ventricle and thus a hypoplastic right ventricle and does not generate a parasternal impulse. Although this defect would lead to inadequate pulmonary blood flow, in the case described above, the right ventricle ejects a reasonable amount of blood under high pressure, and thus there is a normal to increased parasternal impulse.

Truncus with mild stenosis of truncal valve would present with an ejection murmur. Oxygen saturations are typically between 85% and 90%; therefore, the infant rarely appears cyanotic. A ventricular septal defect results in a left to right shunt and does not cause cyanosis.

(Section 26: Disorders of the Cardiovascular System; Part 2: Approach to the Patient, Chapter 483, pp 1792–1795)

Answer 26-11. a

The child in this vignette most likely has a critical coarctation of the aorta. The coarctation usually occurs in the region of the aorta across from the ductus arterious, at the distal end of the aortic isthmus. Children will present with increasing respiratory distress; as the left heart outflow is obstructed, pulmonary venous pressures rise resulting in pulmonary edema. Workup should include pulses and upper and lower blood pressures. Systolic, not mean pressures, should be compared because blood flows through the aortic arch in systole.

Although patients with left ventricular dysfunction present with respiratory distress due to a similar mechanism as described above, normal radial pulses make ventricular dysfunction unlikely. An EKG of a patient with cardiomyopathy typically shows low voltages or ST segment changes. Both PS and tricuspid atresia present with decreased pulmonary blood flow. This physiology would not lead to differential saturations, differential pulses, or respiratory distress. TAPVR presents earlier than 10 days of life. The more proximal the obstruction, the earlier the onset of symptoms.

(Section 26: Disorders of the Cardiovascular System; Part 2: Approach to the Patient, Chapter 483, pp 1796–1803)

Answer 26-12. b

Total anomalous pulmonary venous return without obstruction often presents as failure to thrive because the respiratory distress is so subtle and these children often do not have a significant heart murmur on exam. These children are often diagnosed incidentally when a child presents with bronchiolitis, leading to a chest X-ray or pulse oximetry. Cardiac findings include a well-split second heart sound in the setting of markedly increased pulmonary blood flow. Cyanosis becomes more significant as congestive heart failure progresses.

In tetralogy of Fallot the murmur would have been heard earlier and be harsher at 4 months. CXR shows darker lung fields indicating decreased pulmonary blood flow. In truncus arteriosus there is no split S2 as there is only 1 semilunar valve and there is usually a systolic ejection click. Truncus commonly presents with tachypnea and modest desaturations. In transposition of the great arteries there is a single loud S2 since aorta is anterior. In VSD, there should not be desaturation or a widely split S2.

(Section 26: Disorders of the Cardiovascular System; Part 2: Approach to the Patient, Chapter 483, pp 1798–1803)

Answer 26-13. c

Transposition of the great arteries accounts for 5.2% of all congenital heart disease. Aortic stenosis accounts for 4%. Hypoplastic left-heart syndrome is 2.9%, while Truncus arteriosus and TAPVR each account for 1%.

(Section 26: Disorders of the Cardiovascular System; Part 2: Approach to the Patient, Chapter 484, p 1804 (Table 484-1))

Answer 26-14. a

A cranial bruit may be present in the vein of Galen malformation; this is a type of intracranial arteriovenous fistula. These AV fistulas usually produce immediate, severe hemodynamic changes in neonates. They involve vessels of large caliber and the left-to-right shunt is often large, causing severe congestive heart failure in the first days after birth. Clinically, they have continuous murmurs over either side of the skull and bounding carotid pulses and distended jugular veins. The superior vena cava is generally markedly dilated on chest radiograph, and there is significant right and left ventricular volume overload.

   A large ductal shunt and a large VSD will not cause congestive heart failure until the pulmonary vascular resistance drops in the first weeks of life. A pericardial rub caused by a pericardial effusion is not associated with congestive heart failure. Valvar aortic stenosis murmurs are not associated with severe congestive heart failure.

(Section 26: Disorders of the Cardiovascular System; Part 2: Approach to the Patient, Chapter 484, p 1807)

Answer 26-15. a

The murmur in the vignette is characteristic of aortic regurgitation: a high-pitched, early diastolic murmur that starts at the aortic component of the second heart sound. This occurs due to prolapse of the aortic valve cusp into the subpulmonic or doubly committed subarterial defects. With a ventricular septal defect adjacent to the aortic annulus, the support of the adjacent aortic cusp is weakened. The cusp tends to sag into the left ventricle, and the left-to-right shunt through the ventricular septal defect exerts force on the cusp through the defect. Repair of the defect may buttress the aortic cusp sufficiently to reduce the aortic regurgitation and prevent surgery on the aortic valve.

   The murmur described does not correlate with mitral stenosis or ASDs. Pulmonary regurgitation is not associated with VSDs. Infective endocarditis (IE) is a rare problem, even after spontaneous closure of the defect; however, this clinical vignette is not consistent with endocarditis.

(Section 26: Disorders of the Cardiovascular System; Part 2: Approach to the Patient, Chapter 484, pp 1807–1814)

Answer 26-16. d

There is a strong association of VSD, anomalous right ventricular muscle bundles, and subpulmonic stenosis. This is known as double-chambered right ventricle. This double-chambered right ventricle is caused by large, aberrant muscular bands that divide the right ventricular cavity into 2 separate chambers and obstruct flow through the subpulmonic infundibular area. This is usually associated with VSD. The result is increased right ventricular pressure, as indicated by the upright T wave in V1.

   Although VSD, subaortic stenosis, and coarctation of the aorta are frequently related, this is not the best answer based on the ECG and physical exam (with normal distal pulses). The physical exam does not suggest valvar aortic stenosis or a patent ductus ateriosus (PDA). A PDA in a toddler would most likely be heard as the classic machinery type continuous murmur. Left superior vena cava to the coronary sinus is not associated with VSD and subpulmonic stenosis.

(Section 26: Disorders of the Cardiovascular System; Part 2: Approach to the Patient, Chapter 484, p 1823)

Answer 26-17. e

Placing the patient in the knee–chest position with supplemental oxygen is one of the ways to help abort a Tet spell. Tet spells are hypercyanotic episodes with paroxysmal hyperpnea that occur spontaneously, after early morning feedings, prolonged crying, or fever. The attacks may last only a few moments and have no sequelae; they may cause obtundation, limpness, deep exhaustion, or sleep; rarely, they may end in unconsciousness, convulsions, or even death. Administering antipyretics or oral hydration is not correct as the patient's hypoxia is the most acute concern. The absence of murmur is not reassuring; it is one of the signs of a "Tet spell," and steps to correct the hypoxia are the most important. An echocardiogram would not help with management as the diagnosis has already been made.

(Section 26: Disorders of the Cardiovascular System; Part 2: Approach to the Patient, Chapter 484, p 1826)

Answer 26-18. a

The heart murmur described above is most consistent with aortic stenosis. This is a loud crescendo–decrescendo systolic murmur, often grade 4 to 5 in intensity and associated with a suprasternal notch thrill. Additionally, a prominent apical third sound is frequently heard. Balloon valvoplasty has become the treatment of choice (see Chapter 499 for more information about balloon valvoplasties).

   Although a bicuspid valve may also cause an ejection click, the coarctation would result in a blood pressure and pulse intensity differential not noted in the vignette. In subaortic stenosis due to hypertrophic cardiomyopathy, when the patient squats this increases venous return and causes left ventricular dilation, which results in a softer murmur. The murmur of PS is an ejection systolic murmur of the crescendo–decrescendo type best heard at the upper left sternal border, with radiation to the left infraclavicular area. A PS murmur does not change with squatting, although it does decrease with Valsalva. The murmur of a moderate-sized VSD would be holosystolic and blowing in character and should not appreciably change with Valsalva.

(Section 26: Disorders of the Cardiovascular System; Part 2: Approach to the Patient, Chapter 484, pp 1818–1826)

Answer 26-19. d

The vignette is most consistent with either a right aortic arch with aberrant left subclavian causing a ring or a double arch with an atretic left arch. Elective surgery should be done and there is no other imaging necessary. Infants with severe obstructions are very ill with vomiting, choking, and often dysphagia; often leading to feeding difficulties and poor weight gain. Wheezing and stridor, usually inspiratory, are often symptoms and made worse by feeding. These infants frequently will hyperextend their heads to reduce tracheal compression. The most common malformation is the double aortic arch, which can result from failure of absorption of any part of the embryonic fourth arches. The subclavian artery is not causing the patient's noisy breathing. The large proximal left subclavian bulge is known as a "diverticulum of Kommerell." This indicates that there is a ring with either a ligamentum arteriosum or an atretic left arch (or both). Although a left pulmonary artery sling can cause symptoms similar to those in the vignette, dysphagia is rare. The echocardiogram would show the left pulmonary artery arises from the right pulmonary artery and passes between the esophagus and trachea, compressing the trachea and the right main bronchus.

(Section 26: Disorders of the Cardiovascular System; Part 2: Approach to the Patient, Chapter 484, pp 1833–1834)

Answer 26-20. a

Patients with an anomalous left coronary artery arising from pulmonary artery (ALCAPA) present with myocardial failure from ischemia or even a myocardial infarct between 2 weeks and 6 months of age. Episodes of restlessness and crying, as if in pain, associated with pallor and sweating have been described in infants with this anomaly, but poor feeding, tachypnea, and respiratory symptoms related to left ventricular failure are more common. Other findings include severe cardiomegaly with mitral regurgitant murmurs, prominent third and fourth heart sounds, and ECG findings consistent with an anterolateral infarct pattern.

Although intramural left coronary artery from the right sinus can be associated with sudden death, especially after exercise, this does not present as cardiomyopathy in infancy. Left coronary artery ostium atresia is extremely rare and would not lead to the left to right shunt type steal that causes ischemia like in ALCAPA. Although ECG changes and poor ventricular function are common findings in myocarditis, the mitral regurgitation and specific ischemic changes on the EKG make ALCAPA more likely. Kawasaki can affect infants, and could explain the dilation of the right coronary artery; however, it is unusual to present this young with these ischemic findings without other preceding Kawasaki symptoms.

(Section 26: Disorders of the Cardiovascular System; Part 2: Approach to the Patient, Chapter 484, p 1834)

Answer 26-21. d

The ECG findings of ischemia and anterolateral infarct are consistent with anomalous origin of the left coronary artery from the pulmonary artery (ALCAPA). The infant's irritability and poor feeding are likely due to chest pain and ischemia. She has signs of left ventricular failure and a new mitral insufficiency murmur.

The ECG of a patient with glycogen storage disease shows diffusely increased voltages for both ventricles. The ECG in pericarditis shows diffusely diminished voltages due to the pericardial effusion. The ECG in supraventricular tachycardia shows a higher heart rate (220–300 bpm) and generally no visible P waves. In endocardial fibroelastosis, there generally are increased LV forces, but no deep Q waves.

(Section 26: Disorders of the Cardiovascular System; Part 2: Approach to the Patient, Chapter 485, p 1834)

Answer 26-22. b

This figure shows second-degree, Mobitz type I/Wenckebach atrioventricular block. The tracing shows 2 Wenckebach cycles with progressive lengthening of the P–R interval until the atrial beat is not conducted to the ventricles. The first atrial impulse of a group of beats is conducted normally, but the next atrial impulse reaches the AV node while it is still partly refractory and thus is conducted more slowly, giving a longer PR interval. The next atrial impulse arrives even earlier in the AV nodal refractory period, resulting in an even longer PR interval. Eventually the atrial impulse reaches the AV node in its absolute refractory period and is blocked so that no QRS complex follows. Mobitz type I second-degree AV block may occur in healthy people, particularly athletes with slow sinus rates. In this setting, it occurs at night and is caused by increased vagal tone. If it is asymptomatic in someone with no structural or functional heart disease, it does not require aggressive evaluation or treatment.

In contrast, Mobitz type II second-degree AV block occurs when a QRS complex drops out without prior lengthening of the PR intervals. It is less common, but more serious than type I second-degree AV block and is more likely to lead to complete AV block. It usually results from disease in the His–Purkinje system and always requires careful evaluation, therefore reassurance would be incorrect. Third-degree AV block occurs if no atrial beats are conducted so that the ventricles are driven by a junctional or ventricular focus, then there are normal P waves at one rate and QRS complexes at a slower rate, usually with no fixed relationship between P waves and QRS complexes. Phasic sinus arrhythmia is a normal variant in which the sinus rate varies; usually, but not always, the rate increases with inspiration and slows with expiration. During expiration the sinus rate may be sufficiently slowed to allow escape beats from an atrial or junctional pacemaker. An escape beat is recognized by its late appearance (R–R interval longer than normal) and evidence of an ectopic focus (abnormal P-wave axis and morphology for an atrial ectopic focus; no P wave, very short PR; or retrograde P wave for junctional focus). An escape rhythm is characterized by an ectopic rhythm that is slower than a normal sinus rhythm.

(Section 26: Disorders of the Cardiovascular System; Part 2: Approach to the Patient, Chapter 485, pp 1837–1847)

Answer 26-23. b

This patient has Wolff–Parkinson–White syndrome. The narrow complex, supraventricular tachycardia terminates suddenly to sinus rhythm, with pre-excitation evident following the termination. Note the short PR interval and the delta wave (slurred initial QRS deflection) at the beginning of each sinus rhythm QRS. It is important to document an echocardiogram, as WPW is associated with both Ebstein anomaly and hypertrophic cardiomyopathy. A beta-blocker, such as atenolol, is the treatment of choice to prevent recurrences of tachycardia. This child would also be referred for elective radiofrequency ablation as definitive treatment since he has been symptomatic with SVT due to the WPW. Radiofrequency ablation of the accessory pathway is the treatment of choice for patients with WPW syndrome, with >90% cure rate. However, this patient is mostly asymptomatic and it can be done on an elective basis.

The AV nodal blocking agents, including verapamil and digoxin are contraindicated in WPW due to the potential for enhancing anterograde conduction in the accessory pathway (see Table 485-1). Although caffeine can increase automaticity and may cause increased frequency of SVT due to a premature atrial or ventricular beat setting off the re-entrant circuit, cutting back will not always prevent further episodes. Additionally, any symptomatic child should be referred for definitive treatment with radiofrequency ablation.

(Section 26: Disorders of the Cardiovascular System; Part 2: Approach to the Patient, Chapter 485, pp 1839–1843)

Answer 26-24. c

This clinical history is concerning for a cardiac-cause for syncope (with his family history of sudden death and his exertional dizziness). A referral to a pediatric cardiologist is warranted.

Long QT syndrome is a cause of ventricular arrhythmias and sudden death and would be the most worrisome of these findings. All first-degree relatives of a child with a long QTc interval should be screened by a cardiologist. First-degree AV block, premature atrial contractions, sinus arrhythmia, and premature ventricular contractions can be seen in normal children.

(Section 26: Disorders of the Cardiovascular System; Part 2: Approach to the Patient, Chapter 485, p 1846)

Answer 26-25. b

Beta-blockers are the primary treatment for long QT syndrome. Beta blockers are useful for minimizing the

adrenergic stimulation that results in rapid changes in heart rate with dispersion of repolarization across the myocardium. The after depolarizations are thought to be the inciting events for torsades de pointes. Pacemaker or ICD may be needed in select cases when symptoms persist despite beta-blocker therapy; however, they are not a substitute for beta blockers, which remain the primary treatment for long QT syndrome.

(Section 26: Disorders of the Cardiovascular System; Part 2: Approach to the Patient, Chapter 485, p 1846)

Answer 26-26. d

Children with the DiGeorge syndrome and hypocalcemia are prone to having seizures from hypocalcemia. A rhythm strip during the seizure may have artifact that will appear as a supraventricular or ventricular tachycardia. Careful marching of the R waves will show an underlying sinus rhythm.

(Section 26: Disorders of the Cardiovascular System; Part 2: Approach to the Patient, Chapter 485)

Answer 26-27. b

The ECG and rash depicted above are consistent with Lyme disease. The incidence of cardiac involvement in Lyme disease has been estimated to be 8% and usually occurs within a few weeks of the onset of the illness. The most common feature of Lyme carditis is atrioventricular block, as shown here. The AV block usually resolves gradually with normalization of the PR interval in 1–2 weeks. Persistence of AV block requiring a pacemaker is unusual.

Although first-degree AV Block (P–R prolongations) can occur in acute rheumatic fever (ARF), the carditis generally does not involve the conduction system. Higher grade AV block is not seen. Typical ECG findings in pericarditis are of decreased voltages, but not of the AV block. Although Kawasaki disease may affect the coronary arteries, it does not affect AV conduction. Juvenile rheumatoid arthritis is not associated with AV block.

(Section 26: Disorders of the Cardiovascular System; Part 2: Approach to the Patient, Chapter 485, p 1837)

Answer 26-28. c

The rhythm strip shows a regular and rapid atrial rate with variable conduction and narrow QRS complexes, consistent with atrial flutter. Atrial flutter is characterized by rapid atrial rates of about 300 per minute in older children and adolescents and as high as 450–500 beats per minute in newborns. In the typical form, there is a sawtooth configuration of atrial waves best seen in leads II, III, and V1. It can sometimes occur transiently in otherwise normal newborn infants. Overdrive pacing with the use of an esophageal lead is an effective treatment. An alternative treatment is digoxin to increase the atrioventricular block and slow ventricular rate. After conversion, digoxin can be started to help prevent further episodes.

The patient should be treated before discharge. The patient described is stable and does not require emergent DC cardioversion. This vignette is not consistent with AV node reentry tachycardia or orthodromic reciprocating tachycardia. Vagal maneuvers and adenosine will not convert atrial flutter to sinus rhythm. They can, however, slow the ventricular rate so that the sawtooth pattern is more easily seen.

(Section 26: Disorders of the Cardiovascular System; Part 2: Approach to the Patient, Chapter 485, pp 1844–1845)

Answer 26-29. e

The classic functional murmur, Still's murmur, is a low-pitched, vibratory systolic murmur best heard between the left sternal border and apex. Typically this murmur decreases in intensity as the patient moves from supine to sitting position. These innocent murmurs are frequently heard after age 3 years, when the child is quietly cooperative with the physical exam.

A continuous "machinery" murmur under the left clavicle describes a patent ductus arteriosus. The harsh systolic ejection murmur of valvar aortic stenosis is best heard at the right upper sternal border and radiates to the carotid arteries in the neck. It often is associated with a suprasternal notch thrill. The murmur of an aortic coarctation is best heard in the interscapular area, which is closest to the aortic narrowing. Diastolic murmurs are always pathologic.

(Section 26: Disorders of the Cardiovascular System; Part 2: Approach to the Patient, Chapter 486, p 1848)

Answer 26-30. e

Functional (innocent) murmurs increase in intensity when the child moves from sitting to supine position. It is flow-dependent and should change in intensity during postural change, which increase venous return and preload to the heart. Moving from sitting to standing, deep inspiration, and the Valsalva maneuver decrease preload on the heart and therefore would cause the murmur to decrease in intensity. Squatting causes an increase in afterload, which will not change a functional murmur.

(Section 26: Disorders of the Cardiovascular System; Part 2: Approach to the Patient, Chapter 486, pp 1848–1849)

Answer 26-31. c

Given his examination and low baseline oxygen saturations, this child likely has tetralogy of Fallot: right ventricular outflow tract obstruction, pulmonary stenosis, and a VSD. This is the most common form of cyanotic heart disease. He is having hypercyanotic ("Tet") spells, which are caused by an acute reduction in pulmonary blood flow during exertion. Squatting increases the systemic vascular resistance, decreases the volume of right to left shunting across the

VSD, and thereby increases pulmonary blood flow. The PDA, ASD, and VSD likely would shunt from left to right and there for not be associated with cyanosis in a toddler. Normal blood pressures and pulses make coarctation unlikely in this cyanotic patient.

(Section 26: Disorders of the Cardiovascular System; Part 2: Approach to the Patient, Chapter 486, p 1849)

Answer 26-32. a

An ASD shunt increases the volume of flow across the pulmonic valve, causing the fixed split S2 and the flow murmur in the main pulmonary artery. Most children with an ASD are asymptomatic and the lesion is detected on routine examinations. There is minimal pressure difference between the atria, so the murmur is due to increased flow volume across the pulmonic valve.

Aortic stenosis, pulmonic valve stenosis, and VSD murmurs generally are detected early in infancy/childhood due to increased pressure gradients. The pulses and blood pressure are normal, so aortic coarctation is unlikely.

(Section 26: Disorders of the Cardiovascular System; Part 2: Approach to the Patient, Chapter 486, p 1849)

Answer 26-33. b

Reproducible chest wall tenderness at the costochondral border supports the diagnosis of costochondritis. Adolescents often develop nonspecific inflammation of the costochondral cartilage, which is relieved by nonsteroidal anti-inflammatory medications. Rheumatic fever, endocarditis, myocarditis, and pericarditis are all more likely to present with fever and other symptoms of infection. The pain associated with pericarditis is not associated with tenderness.

(Section 26: Disorders of the Cardiovascular System; Part 2: Approach to the Patient, Chapter 486, p 1850)

Answer 26-34. d

His description of the episodes, the normal exam, and ECG are characteristic of vasovagal syncope. It is a benign condition and can be avoided by increasing fluid and salt intake and by avoiding situations that promote venous blood pooling in the lower extremities, thereby reducing systemic venous return, that is, standing for prolonged periods of time. Once the patient faints, and thereby lies flat, the systemic venous return increases and the relative cerebral blood flow increases, thus re-establishing consciousness.

Long QT syndrome, hypertrophic cardiomyopathy, and supraventricular tachycardia have distinct ECG patterns. Premature atrial contractions are benign. Syncope episodes due to long QT syndrome are often associated with increased emotion or exercise.

(Section 26: Disorders of the Cardiovascular System; Part 2: Approach to the Patient, Chapter 486, pp 1851–1852)

Answer 26-35. a

Having documented elevated arm blood pressures with a proper-sized cuff, it is important to rule out an aortic coarctation. His distal pulses are difficult to feel. With an aortic click on exam, he likely has a bicuspid aortic valve; however, there no evidence of aortic stenosis on exam. There is LV hypertrophy on ECG. If his lower extremity blood pressure is lower than his arms, he is likely to have an aortic coarctation. He needs a cardiology evaluation and an echocardiogram.

Once a coarctation has been ruled out, then you should investigate other etiologies of systemic hypertension, including renal disease, familial hypercholesterolemia, and essential hypertension.

(Section 26: Disorders of the Cardiovascular System; Part 2: Approach to the Patient, Chapter 486, p 1852)

Answer 26-36. d

Atrophic pyelonephritis is the most likely cause for her hypertension. The key is the history of urinary tract infection. She likely had other asymptomatic episodes of UTI causing scar over time.

Coarctation is unlikely since her diastolic blood pressure is also high; most children with coarctation have isolated systolic hypertension. You would also expect an abnormal physical exam such as a murmur in the back and weak femoral pulses. Although renal artery stenosis could cause this degree of blood pressure elevation, you might expect to hear an abdominal bruit. Moreover, renal artery stenosis is an uncommon diagnosis. The history of high fever and rash may represent a streptococcal infection. However, an elevated blood pressure at age 13, 8 years after this episode, is more consistent with glomerular scarring rather than glomerulonephritis. Pheochromocytoma is unlikely since she is not tachycardic and does not have other historical features consistent with this diagnosis. Additionally, pheochromocytoma is a rare diagnosis.

(Section 26: Disorders of the Cardiovascular System; Part 2: Approach to the Patient, Chapter 486, p 1852 and see Section 25: Disorders of the Kidney and Urinary Tract, Ch 479: Systemic Hypertension, pp 1762–1763)

Answer 26-37. a

Patients with prosthetic material used during palliative or corrective surgery are at the highest risk for bacterial endocarditis. In the current 2007 AHA guidelines, patients with aorto-pulmonary shunts continue to be in the small subset of patients for whom antibiotic prophylaxis is recommended. The other patients in this vignette would not warrant prophylaxis unless they had a history of prior bacterial endocarditis (or if there is valve disease in the transplant patient). Prophylaxis would have been recommended for the child with transposition and transplant for the first 6 months following the operation. The child with unrepaired total anomalous pulmonary veins and the child with mitral stenosis have not had surgical or cardiac interventional procedures.

(Section 26: Disorders of the Cardiovascular System; Part 2: Approach to the Patient, Chapter 486, pp 1853–1854, Table 486-6)

Answer 26-38. b

Rhabdomyomas are the most common cardiac tumor of childhood and approximately half are associated with tuberous sclerosis. Most are asymptomatic and many regress; however, they may cause arrhythmias, heart block, or even death by obstructing blood flow. Mortality is highest among children less than 5 years old. Hamartomas are a type of fibroma that can occur in the ventricular wall. Myxomas are benign and usually arise from the atrial septum. Teratomas are rare and usually occur in infants at the base of the heart. Hemangiomas are usually in the atrial wall and spontaneously resolve. Any of these lesions may present with similar symptoms of arrhythmia or obstruction but are not associated with tuberous sclerosis.

(Section 26: Disorders of the Cardiovascular System; Part 3: Acquired Cardiovascular Disease, Chapter 487, p 1855)

Answer 26-39. a

This patient meets the clinical criteria for Kawasaki disease: The persistent high fever, conjunctival injection, changes in the extremities, red lips, and strawberry tongue are consistent with Kawasaki disease. Cervical lymphadenopathy (node >1.5 cm), is the 5th principal feature, excluding fever (see Table 488.1). To meet the classical definition, the patient must have at least 5 days of fever and 4 of the 5 principle features. His presentation is not as consistent with streptococcal infection, which usually presents with a pharyngeal exudate and without mucosal involvement. Children with Steven–Johnson syndrome and staphylococcal scaled skin syndrome typically have a more toxic appearance. Rheumatic fever classically has a history of joint swelling, pain, or erythema.

(Section 26: Disorders of the Cardiovascular System; Part 3: Acquired Cardiovascular Disease, Chapter 488, pp 1855–1857)

Answer 26-40. b

If the patient meets the clinical criteria for diagnosis of Kawasaki disease, the treatment of choice is intravenous immunoglobulin, as well as high-dose aspirin, to reduce inflammatory response and decrease the risk of coronary aneurysm formation. There is a limited window of time in which one can give IVIG to help prevent coronary aneurysm formation (<10 days after the onset of fever).

Blood cultures and antibiotics, or a lumbar puncture with antibiotics are appropriate if sepsis and meningitis are primary concerns, but he meets diagnostic criteria for Kawasaki disease and antibiotics have no role in its treatment. To discharge the patient and follow up the next day in clinic would delay diagnosis and treatment of the Kawasaki disease, and may increase the risk of coronary involvement.

(Section 26: Disorders of the Cardiovascular System; Part 3: Acquired Cardiovascular Disease, Chapter 488, p 1858)

Answer 26-41. c

This patient most likely has acute myocarditis. Its course ranges from very mild to fulminant, with death in a few days or weeks. Often there is a history of a recent upper respiratory tract infection, and viruses are usually the causative agents. Viral myocarditis is commonly associated with ventricular dysrhythmias and conduction abnormalities. The murmur is most likely from mitral regurgitation.

Although ARF can cause myocarditis, there are no other signs of the disease such as prior infection with streptococcus, arthritis, or rash. IE is unlikely in a previously healthy patient and he has not had persistent fevers or other signs of IE. Paroxysmal atrial tachycardia would not cause this degree of illness with hepatomegaly and would not explain the murmur or gallop. Pericarditis can follow a viral URI, but typically would cause chest pain and not cause a gallop.

(Section 26: Disorders of the Cardiovascular System; Part 3: Acquired Cardiovascular Disease, Chapter 489, p 1859)

Answer 26-42. a

To diagnose ARF a patient must have 2 major criteria or 1 major and 2 minor criteria. The 5 major criteria include: (1) migratory polyarthritis, (2) carditis, (3) subcutaneous nodules, (4) erythema marginatum, and (5) Syndenham's chorea. Minor criteria include: fever, arthralgia, increased ESR or CRP, leukocytosis, ECG changes showing features of heart block, evidence of streptococcal infection such as elevated DNAse or antisteptolysin O (ASO), or previous history of rheumatic fever. Rheumatic myocarditis can occur early in ARF and almost always causes mitral or aortic valve regurgitation.

(Section 26: Disorders of the Cardiovascular System; Part 3: Acquired Cardiovascular Disease, Chapter 489, p 1859 and Section 17: Infectious Diseases; Part 2: Infections of Oran Systems, Chapter 235, pp 941–944)

Answer 26-43. a

This patient has 1 major criterion of ARF, carditis. He also has 1 minor criterion, documented evidence of recent strep infection. To be diagnosed with ARF, he would need 1 additional minor criterion. This includes elevated ESR, positive CRP, anemia, and leukocytosis, ECG changes of PR and QT prolongation, and arthralgia.

(Section 26: Disorders of the Cardiovascular System; Part 3: Acquired Cardiovascular Disease, Chapter 489, p 1859 and Section 17: Infectious Diseases; Part 2: Infections of Oran Systems, Chapter 235, pp 941–944)

Answer 26-44. a

IE is an infection of the endocardium, typically involving the cardiac valves. The presentation of endocarditis can be variable. Presentation can be slow onset, or subacute, with intermittent fevers and few other symptoms. Other cases may present with fever, fulminant symptoms of heart failure, and embolic complications. IE can occur in children with or without underlying cardiac disease. The diagnosis is primarily dependent on clinical features (see Table 490-1 for Revised Duke Clinical Diagnostic Criteria). Importantly, identifying the causative organism through multiple blood cultures is imperative *before* starting an antibiotic. Treatment usually lasts for 4–6 weeks. Echocardiography is a secondary diagnostic modality; it can identify the valve involved and the potential risk of embolic events.

Tuberculosis can present with intermittent fevers and a pericardial friction rub, but generally does not directly involve the heart or the valves. Kawasaki disease has a 4- to 5-day course of high fever, irritability, conjunctivitis, and rash. Rheumatic fever can present with carditis; however, this presentation does not fit the major or minor criteria of ARF. Scarlet fever has a more self-limited course (<1 week) and is associated with pharyngitis and a rash.

(Section 26: Disorders of the Cardiovascular System; Part 3: Acquired Cardiovascular Disease, Chapter 490, p 1862)

Answer 26-45. e

Given this history, examination, and CXR, this patient most likely has acute pericarditis with a pericardial effusion. Symptoms of acute pericarditis include sharp precordial chest pain that is improved by sitting up, an intermittent pericardial friction rub, and fever. Pericardial effusions alone may have no symptoms, however can present as in this vignette, with muffled heart sounds, enlarged cardiac silhouette on chest X-ray, and low voltages on ECG. Importantly, pulsus paradoxus should be checked. She should have an echocardiogram to assess the size of the effusion. She may need pericardiocentesis to drain the effusion.

The patient in the vignette does not have an antecedent strep infection or other physical findings to support ARF. There is no chest wall tenderness consistent with costochondritis. IE is a possibility with the history of intermittent fevers, but the viral respiratory infection history and cardiomegaly on CXR make pericardial effusion more likely. Myocarditis is possible with the history of viral illness, but her need to sleep upright, dyspnea, ECG and CXR are more consistent with pericarditis.

(Section 26: Disorders of the Cardiovascular System; Part 3: Acquired Cardiovascular Disease, Chapter 491, pp 1863–1864)

Answer 26-46. e

Pulsus paradoxus is the single most important bedside test for tamponade. To measure pulsus paradoxus, blood pressure is measured with the patient breathing normally and then with deep inspiration. In tamponade, the systolic blood pressure with inspiration will be >10 mm Hg lower than the resting blood pressure. This is due to the inability of the right heart to fill during diastole when there is a constricting effusion. This effect profoundly compromises systemic cardiac output.

An upper extremity systolic blood pressure that is >15 mm Hg more than the lower extremity blood pressure and absent femoral pulses are signs of aortic coarctation. Nonpurulent conjunctival injection and strawberry tongue are seen in Kawasaki disease. Splinter hemorrhages and Janeway lesions are findings in IE.

(Section 26: Disorders of the Cardiovascular System; Part 3: Acquired Cardiovascular Disease, Chapter 491, p 1865)

Answer 26-47. b

Pulmonary arterial hypertension has multiple etiologies, but a common pathophysiology. The small pulmonary arteries (the lung does not have arterioles) are muscularized, which elevates the pulmonary vascular resistance and pulmonary arterial pressures. The right ventricle dilates and hypertrophies in response. During exercise, when the right heart is unable to maintain cardiac output through the hypertensive pulmonary vascular bed, syncope occurs. It is an ominous sign in late-stage pulmonary hypertension. Both tetralogy and pulmonary stenosis would have RV hypertrophy on ECG, but on examination patients with these cardiac defects should present with a murmur. Coarctation is unlikely given the normal pulses and blood pressures. Both coarctation and hypertrophic cardiomyopathy would have increased left ventricular voltages on ECG.

(Section 26: Disorders of the Cardiovascular System; Part 3: Acquired Cardiovascular Disease, Chapter 492, pp 1867–1868)

Answer 26-48. c

The mean T-vector undergoes rapid and marked changes after birth. By 24 hours after birth there is a positive T wave in V1; by about a week of life this T-wave should be down-going. The R-wave amplitude, R/S ratio, and QRS axes do not change appreciably in the first week, although by 3 months the normal QRS axis averages 65 with a range of 0–105 degrees. The right precordial Q-wave is abnormal at any age.

(Section 26: Disorders of the Cardiovascular System; Part 4: Diagnostic Tools in Heart Disease, Chapter 493, p 1871)

Answer 26-49. e

The quantitative assessment of flow events in the heart and great vessels is performed using spectral Doppler velocity measurement of flow velocities. In many situations, the blood velocity can be used to predict a pressure drop across the area of flow. Using the modified Bernoulli equation, the pressure drop is $4v^2$, where **v** is the velocity in meters per second. Thus, a peak jet velocity of 4.5 m/s predicts a peak pressure drop of 4×4.5^2, or 81 mm Hg. This gradient can be used to predict a chamber or vessel pressure or may be used to assess stenosis severity. A gradient of 81 mm Hg denotes severe left ventricular outflow tract obstruction and surgical correction would be warranted.

(Section 26: Disorders of the Cardiovascular System; Part 4: Diagnostic Tools in Heart Disease, Chapter 495, p 1882)

Answer 26-50. a

The normal pulmonary vascular resistance is <3 Units/m². Although high at birth, the PVR drops to adult levels by 4 weeks of age. If the patient has mild-moderate pulmonary vascular disease, the PVR will be in the 4–12 Units/m² range. Severe pulmonary vascular disease is characterized by high PVR (>15 Units). By testing the responsiveness of the pulmonary vasculature to vasodilators (oxygen, nitric oxide, and iloprost), cardiologists can assess the patient's suitability for various medications or lung transplant.

(Section 26: Disorders of the Cardiovascular System; Part 4: Diagnostic Tools in Heart Disease, Chapter 496, pp 1885–1886)

Answer 26-51. b

There is a 60 mm Hg pressure change between the right ventricle and pulmonary artery, indicating severe right ventricular outflow obstruction. There are equal pressures in the RV and LV due to the associated large VSD. As there is some right to left shunting at the VSD level, the saturation in the LV and Aorta are lower than normal. These data describe a child with tetralogy of Fallot.

A moderate VSD would cause mildly elevated RV and PA pressures, but would be expected to have only left to right shunting and no desaturation in the LV or Aorta. There is no shunting at the atrial level, as indicated by the fact that there is no increase in saturations from the SVC to the right atrium. The left atrial saturation is normal. There is no pressure gradient from the left ventricle to the ascending aorta, ruling out aortic valve stenosis. And there is no pressure gradient between the ascending and descending aorta, excluding coarctation of the aorta. The mildly increased descending aortic systolic pressure is normal. This elevation is caused by the standing wave effect of the blood rushing down the abdominal aorta.

(Section 26: Disorders of the Cardiovascular System; Part 4: Diagnostic Tools in Heart Disease, Chapter 496, p 1885)

Answer 26-52. e

There is a 60 mm Hg pressure gradient between the ascending and descending aorta, indicating the presence of a severe aortic coarctation.

A moderate VSD would cause mildly elevated RV and PA pressures, but would be expected to have only left to right shunting and no desaturation in the LV or Aorta. The data show normal pressures and saturations in the right ventricle and pulmonary artery, excluding RV outflow obstruction as in tetralogy of Fallot. There is no shunting at the atrial level, with no increase in saturations from the SVC to the right atrium. There is no pressure gradient from the left ventricle to the ascending aorta, ruling out aortic valve stenosis.

(Section 26: Disorders of the Cardiovascular System; Part 4: Diagnostic Tools in Heart Disease, Chapter 496, p 1885)

Answer 26-53. e

This patient is presenting with heart failure. Infants and young children present with poor feeding, failure to thrive, respiratory distress, diaphoresis, and pallor. Patients with a large PDA, large VSD, truncus arteriosus, and complete common AV canal all develop high pressure/high volume left to right shunts after the pulmonary vascular resistance drops. This subsequently causes an increase in pulmonary blood flow relative to systemic blood flow (increased Qp:Qs), which results in pulmonary over-circulation and symptoms of congestive heart failure symptoms. These patients may also have decreased systemic blood flow. Even large atrial septal defects will not cause such an increase in pulmonary blood flow and they seldom cause congestive heart failure at this age.

(Section 26: Disorders of the Cardiovascular System; Part 5: Management of Patients with Cardiovascular Disease, Chapter 497, pp 1888–1889)

Answer 26-54. c

Milrinone is a nonglycoside, noncatecholamine inotropic agent with additional vasodilatory and lusitropic properties. It inhibits phosphodiesterase type III, increasing intracellular cyclic adenosine monophosphate (AMP) and intracellular calcium, thus enhancing myocardial contractility. It also enhances diastolic relaxation of the myocardium by increasing the rate of reuptake of calcium after systole. It may also act synergistically with a beta-adrenergic agonist such as dopamine and has fewer side effects. Phosphodiesterase type III inhibitors have been used extensively in adults and more recently introduced to pediatric practice. Milrinone lowers filling pressures, systemic and pulmonary artery pressures, and systemic and pulmonary vascular resistances, while improving the cardiac index. Milrinone is usually initiated at 0.25 µ/kg/minute and can be titrated gradually to 1 µ/kg/minute based on the clinical response.

Levosimindan is a calcium-sensitizing agent with inotropic and afterload reducing effects. It binds to troponin C and improves the efficiency of the contractile apparatus. Catecholamines, either endogenous (eg, dopamine or epinephrine) or synthetic (eg, dobutamine), act by stimulating myocardial surface beta-adrenergic receptors, leading to increased adenylate cyclase and intracellular cyclic adenosine monophosphate (cAMP). Digoxin is a sodium–potassium ATPase inhibitor with positive inotropy, negative chronotropy, and inhibition of neurohormonal activation. Nisiritide causes natriuresis, diuresis, vasodilatation, and

increased renal blood flow, and increased cardiac output and urine output.

(Section 26: Disorders of the Cardiovascular System; Part 5: Management of Patients with Cardiovascular Disease, Chapter 497, pp 1889–1891)

Answer 26-55. e

Patients with single ventricle physiology have complete mixing of the pulmonary and systemic circulation. There is parallel circulation, instead of circulation in series; this creates an inefficient system where oxygenated blood may go to the lungs and deoxygenated blood may go to the systemic circulation. The balance between systemic and pulmonary blood flow depends on anatomic obstruction and resistance.

In patients with pulmonary atresia with an intact ventricular septum or tetralogy of Fallot with pulmonary atresia, the right ventricle cannot pump blood to the lungs, therefore pulmonary blood flow is dependent on the patent ductus arteriousus (PDA). Similar physiology occurs with tricuspid atresia. Despite the presence of the right ventricle, the physiology is a single-ventricle physiology. In the hypoplastic left heart syndrome, the left ventricle and left ventricular outflow tract are hypoplastic and therefore the right ventricle provides pulmonary blood flow and systemic blood flow through the PDA. In tetralogy of Fallot with subpulmonary stenosis, the pulmonary blood flow primarily is supplied by the right ventricle and does not depend on the balance of systemic and pulmonary vascular resistance.

(Section 26: Disorders of the Cardiovascular System; Part 5: Management of Patients with Cardiovascular Disease, Chapter 498, pp 1893–1896)

Answer 26-56. d

This infant is in cardiac shock and is presenting due to closure of the ductus arteriosus, which supports the systemic output. Most infants with hypoplastic left heart complex are acutely ill, with signs of congestive heart failure within the first days or weeks after birth. There are signs and symptoms of severe right-sided and left-sided heart failure: cyanosis of varying degree, and often a characteristic grayish pallor and poor peripheral pulses, which contrast with hyperdynamic cardiac pulsations. Murmurs are not prominent, but a short soft midsystolic murmur and middiastolic rumble may be present. The second heart sound is single, heard loudest at the upper left sternal border, and is accentuated until clinical deterioration with gross right heart failure is advanced.

Tetralogy of Fallot is not expected to cause cardiac shock and is most commonly associated with systolic ejection murmurs due to pulmonary stenosis and varying degrees of cyanosis without respiratory distress. Although transposition of the great arteries (TGA) also would likely not cause a murmur, the more typical presentation is a cyanotic infant without cardiac shock. If there is restriction to mixing, such as with restrictive atrial septal communication, the cyanosis can be profound. Ebsteins anomaly, when severe enough to cause symptoms in the neonate, typically is immediate in onset. Also, it would be very uncommon not to have some murmur such as a scratchy mid-diastolic murmur at the left sternal border and apex a widely split S2. And although large VSDs at 4 days of age would likely not cause a murmur, it would not cause cardiac shock.

(Section 26: Disorders of the Cardiovascular System; Part 5: Management of Patients with Cardiovascular Disease, Chapter 498, p 1894 (Figure 498-2) and Part 2: Approach to the Patient with Cardiovascular Disease, Chapter 484, pp 1830–1831)

Answer 26-57. b

This infant's presentation is very concerning for ductal-dependent cyanotic congenital heart disease, in this case pulmonary atresia with intact ventricular septum. She failed to increase saturations and had a low PaO_2 after oxygen was administered. To reopen and keep the ductus arteriosus patent, prostaglandin E1 should be given as soon as ductal-dependent heart disease is suspected. As this medication can cause hypoventilation, the transport team should be prepared to intubated and mechanically ventilate.

Indomethacin is used to promote closure of patent ductus arteriosus. Digoxin is not useful in this scenario. Adenosine is used to treat supraventricular tachycardia. This child has adequate perfusion and pulses and a saline bolus is not warranted.

(Section 26: Disorders of the Cardiovascular System; Part 5: Management of Patients with Cardiovascular Disease, Chapter 498, pp 1895–1897)

Answer 26-58. e

Mild-moderate pulmonary valve stenosis is very well tolerated. As long as the right ventricular pressures are less than one-half systemic and the right ventricular function is normal, patients should not have any restrictions. Patients who are dependent on pacemakers should not participate in school athletics. The pacemaker leads and generators are at risk for damage during contact sports. Tetralogy of Fallot patients should not compete in any sports until after they are repaired because of the risks of ventricular arrhythmias, hypercyanosis, and thromboembolic events associated with right to left shunting. D-transposition patients, who have had arterial switch repairs, have had their coronary arteries moved as part of the operation. They are potentially at risk for coronary ischemia and sudden death. They all should need exercise stress testing prior to approval for competitive sports. Additional sequelae that may affect their ability to participate are supravalvar PS or supravalvar aortic stenosis and dilation of the neoaortic root.

Asymptomatic patients with moderate aortic stenosis (defined as a catheterization gradient of 30–50 mm Hg or a mean gradient of 25–40 mm Hg on echocardiogram)

may participate in some sports, but they will need an echocardiogram/exercise testing prior to approval. Because all forms of subvalvar, valvar, and supravalvar aortic stenosis tend to progress with time, these patients will need serial follow up every 1–2 years with the possibility of a change in recommendations.

(Section 26: Disorders of the Cardiovascular System; Part 5: Management of Patients with Cardiovascular Disease, Chapter 500, pp 1904–1905 and eTable 500.1)

Answer 26-59. d

At higher altitudes the partial pressure of oxygen (PO_2) is reduced, which decreases the alveolar oxygen (PaO_2). In individuals with normal cardiopulmonary function, this only becomes significant at high elevation when the PO_2 is <60 mm Hg. This is due to the S-shaped oxygen dissociation curve. However, as the PaO_2 falls the pulmonary vascular resistance will increase due to hypoxia-induced vasoconstriction. In individuals with heart lesions that do not tolerate pulmonary vasoconstriction, such as single ventricles with Fontan circulation, this will cause cyanosis and respiratory distress. Most of these individuals are able to visit moderate elevations (5000–10,000 feet) or tolerate air travel. The longer they stay and the higher the elevation the more likely they are to develop symptoms. Even if they are not symptomatic at rest, their exercise tolerance will be affected. Ski trips should include contingency plans that allow the individual to return to a lower altitude quickly and supplemental oxygen can be helpful.

(Section 26: Disorders of the Cardiovascular System; Part 5: Management of Patients with Cardiovascular Disease, Chapter 500, p 1905)

Answer 26-60. b

According to the 2007 AHA guidelines for sports-screening, a positive family history includes sudden death, syncope, chest pain, arrhythmias, or heart disease. It is particularly likely in hypertrophic cardiomyopathy, right ventricular dysplasia, long QT syndrome, premature atherosclerosis, and Marfan syndrome. This patient has a very strong family history syncope and sudden death, and an EKG would help evaluate for long QT syndrome and hypertrophic cardiomyopathy.

A brain MRI and electroencephalography can be useful in diagnosing seizure disorders. This patient has no history of seizures and most likely his brother, with his history of exertion related sudden death, was having post-syncopal seizures and not primary seizures. A 24-hour Holter monitor would be useful in diagnosing an arrhythmia however, an EKG would be the first step in this workup. A tilt-table test is done to evaluate vasovagal causes of syncope.

(Section 26: Disorders of the Cardiovascular System; Part 5: Management of Patients with Cardiovascular Disease, Chapter 501, pp 1906–1907)

Answer 26-61. b

There are approximately 3000–5000 sudden death episodes per year in children and adolescents in the United States. The majority, approximately 40%–50% of sudden deaths, are caused by hypertrophic cardiomyopathy. Between 10% and 20% will be caused by coronary abnormalities—usually the left or right coronary artery arising from the wrong sinus origin or a single-coronary artery origin. The remaining 30% will be caused by such lesions as myocarditis, dilated cardiomyopathy including noncompaction, ion channelopathies (long QT) syndrome, Brugada syndrome, catecholaminergic polymorphic ventricular tachycardia (CPVT), arrhythmogenic right ventricular dysplasia (AVRD), Wolff–Parkinson–White (WPW) syndrome, previous Kawasaki disease with undiagnosed coronary involvement, commotio cordis, and connective tissue disorders with dilated aortic roots (eg, Marfan).

(Section 26: Disorders of the Cardiovascular System; Part 5: Management of Patients with Cardiovascular Disease, Chapter 501, p 1906)

CHAPTER 27 | Disorders of the Respiratory System

Amy G. Filbrun, Danielle M. Goetz, and Nanci Yuan

27-1. A 10-year-old girl presents with an inability to stop fidgeting for the past 6 months. Her mother states that both she and her teachers are complaining that the girl "cannot sit still." The nonrhythmic movement only occurs when she is awake. Her physical exam is unremarkable. The girl states that she feels as if "bugs are crawling up her legs," and she only feels better when she moves her legs as if trying to squash them.

What is the most likely diagnosis?

a. Essential tremor

b. Periodic limb movement disorder

c. Physiologic myoclonus

d. Restless leg syndrome

e. Tourette syndrome

27-2. A 6-year-old girl presents with a 8-month history of being unable to fall asleep at night. The mother reports that just as she starts to fall asleep, her daughter starts crying and rubbing her legs. The mother states that she also suffered from similar discomfort when she was pregnant. The mother's symptoms resolved after her doctor did a test and started her on daily pills. The mother cannot remember the name of the pills but recalls that they left a bad taste in her mouth.

What is the most likely test that the mother's doctor ordered?

a. TSH

b. Complete metabolic panel

c. CBC

d. Urinalysis

e. Serum copper level

27-3. A 7-year-old boy presents with an 8-month history of inconsolable screaming 3–4 times per week. The father states that after falling asleep his son will typically awaken 1–2 hours later screaming at the top of his lungs and sweating. He is inconsolable and terrified. He does not remember what happens the following morning. What do you tell his dad?

a. The child needs to be evaluated by a mental health professional

b. The child needs to be evaluated by neurologist

c. The symptoms are consistent with sleep terrors

d. The symptoms are consistent with nightmares

e. The symptoms are concerning for seizure disorder

27-4. A 16-year-old boy presents to clinic for excessive daytime sleepiness (EDS) for the past year. As per his mom, his teachers state that he is falling asleep in class. He feels a little better on the weekends but gets worse again during the school week. There is no history of snoring or mouth breathing. What is the most likely cause of EDS in this patient?

a. Alcohol abuse

b. Obstructive sleep apnea

c. Insufficient sleep

d. Narcolepsy

e. Anemia

27-5. A father brings his 13-year-old daughter in as she refuses to go to bed at 8 PM. Dad states that 8 PM had been her nightly bedtime since she was a toddler. She tells you that she just does not feel sleepy at 8 PM. What physiologic change during adolescents occurs which may be affecting her ability to fall asleep at 8 PM?

a. Phase advance

b. Phase delay

c. Growing pains

d. GERD

e. Menarche

27-6. A 28-month-old girl presents to your office for second opinion for persistent irritability. Her mom states that her previous pediatrician said she was fine. Her physical exam is normal. Her mom brings in laboratory tests (CBC, thyroid) which are normal. What screening tool may be helpful in determining the cause of her persistent irritability?

  a. BEARS

  b. DREAMS

  c. CAGE

  d. SALSA

  e. HEEADSSS

27-7. A 10-week-old former-32 week premature male infant comes to the clinic today. He was recently discharged from the neonatal intensive care unit and they are now establishing care at your practice. During the visit, the parents state that they are worried that since he was a premature infant that his lungs will not grow.

What do you tell them?

  a. The lungs stop growing at birth

  b. The lung tubes or conducting airways continue to grow in number after birth

  c. The lung sacs or alveoli continue to grow in number after birth

  d. The lung tubes and sacs continue to grow in number throughout life

  e. The lung tubes and sacs continue to remodel throughout life

27-8. A 2-week-old girl comes to clinic for observed pauses in her sleep. Her mom says that she now sleeps with her daughter sleeping on her stomach to make sure she is breathing.

What test would be most helpful is assessing her breathing pattern while she sleeps?

  a. CXR

  b. ABG

  c. EEG

  d. Polysomnogram

  e. Spirometry

27-9. An 8-year-old boy comes to clinic with complaint of persistent cough and wheeze with respiratory infections. His parents state that he has no problems when he is well. The parents state that he was given a "breathing medication" but that they do not know what it is for.

What test in your office clinic could be done to assess his lung function?

  a. CXR

  b. ABG

  c. Plethysmography

  d. Peak flow meter

  e. Spirometry

27-10. A 12-year-old boy with a history of mild-persistent asthma presents for his annual well-child visit. He is currently on a daily controller medication. His typical triggers include seasonal allergies, smoke exposure, and mold. He has been hospitalized three times, with the most recent hospitalization 2 years ago. Which of the following statements are correct regarding this patient's asthma control?

  a. For this patient, asthma control should be assessed at a visit at least every 6 months

  b. It is not possible to assess asthma control for this patient because he has already been started on a daily controller medication

  c. The patient's asthma control is optimal because he has had no hospitalizations or emergency department visits in the last year

  d. Asthma control describes the patient's intrinsic intensity of disease, while his asthma severity is based on the intensity of disease and the appropriateness of asthma management

  e. There are no validated questionnaires to help measure asthma control for children

27-11. A 2-year-old boy comes to the ED with sudden onset of cough and respiratory distress. His father was watching football on television and eating popcorn when he noted his son coughing on the floor. On exam you hear wheezing in the left lung.

What is the most appropriate study to order?

  a. CT scan of the chest

  b. Bronchoscopy

  c. CBC

  d. CXR

  e. Spirometry

27-12. A 13-year-old girl with a history of asthma presents for her annual well-child visit. She has mild, intermittent asthma. She has recently been seen by an allergist who has confirmed that she is sensitive to house dust mite allergen. House dust mite allergen seems to be a trigger for her asthma exacerbations.

Which of the following allergen avoidance strategies would be inappropriate for this patient?

a. Removal of wall-to-wall carpeting in the bedroom

b. Weekly washing all the sheets and bedding in hot water at a temperature greater than 130°F

c. Use of encasings for the child's bedroom mattresses

d. Use of encasings for the child's bedroom pillows

e. Use of a warm mist humidifier at night in the child's bedroom

27-13. A 1-month-old boy comes to the ED with stridor and respiratory distress. His parents state that he developed a runny nose and then a harsh barky cough. From the following choices, which would be the most appropriate test to order?

a. CT scan

b. Frontal and lateral neck X-rays

c. CXR

d. Ultrasound

e. CBC

27-14. A 4-year-old girl comes to the ED with sudden onset of wheezing. The patient's mother says she heard the wheezing right after the family opened up their holiday gifts. The patient's mother states that the girl's older brother received a set of toy cars with detachable wheels.

What is the most appropriate test to order?

a. Inspiratory and expiratory films

b. Decubitus films

c. Ultrasound

d. CT scan

e. MRI

27-15. A 16-year-old girl presents to the ED with sudden onset of chest pain. She just came back from a 16-hour flight from Europe. On exam you note that she is in a cast, as she broke her leg a week ago skiing.

What is the most appropriate test to order to rule out a pulmonary embolism?

a. Ultrasound of the lower extremities

b. CXR

c. CT angiography

d. Ventilation/perfusion scan

e. MRI

27-16. A 3-month-old infant is brought to your office by her parents for evaluation of "noisy breathing." The parents have noticed that as she has gotten more active, her breathing has become noisier. Her breathing is louder when she gets active or excited, and was much louder when she had a recent cold. Her breathing is quiet when she sleeps. They deny cough, fever, feeding intolerance, or cyanosis. On your exam, the baby is thriving, with normal vital signs and excellent growth. As she gets excited, you note inspiratory stridor and mild chest wall retractions.

Of the following, the most appropriate next step is to:

a. Order an X-ray of the neck looking for a steeple sign

b. Refer the child for surgical correction

c. Reassure the family that this will improve with time

d. Initiate therapy with bronchodilators

e. Order an upper GI series

27-17. Primary ciliary dyskinesia (PCD) is a rare condition. An appropriate index of suspicion in the primary care setting is important for timely referral, early diagnosis, and appropriate management of the condition. You are seeing a 2-year-old child in primary care clinic. Which of the following findings would most likely be present in a 2-year-old child with PCD that has not yet been diagnosed?

a. Prominent digital clubbing

b. Bronchiectasis

c. Situs inversus

d. Rhinosinusitis since birth

e. Nasal polyps

27-18. A 16-year-old girl who is a competitive cheerleader presents for evaluation of chest tightness and dyspnea during a cheerleading competition. She notices symptoms within a few minutes of activity. Upon further questioning, you learn that she feels she cannot catch her breath, and has more difficulty breathing in. She has felt lightheaded at times, and once thought she was going to faint. If she stops and rests, and takes a drink of water, she feels better in a few minutes, and can return to activity. She denies symptoms at other times, and has no sleep-related symptoms. She has a history of allergic rhinitis and eczema, but feels these have been well-controlled. Pulmonary function testing shows flattened inspiratory loops.

Which of the following diagnoses is most likely?

a. Exercise-induced asthma

b. Vocal cord dysfunction

c. Restrictive lung disease

d. Cystic fibrosis

e. GERD

27-19. Which of the following statements about tracheobronchomalacia (TBM) is correct?

    a. TBM is usually an isolated abnormality

    b. Chest X-ray and neck films are usually diagnostic

    c. Rigid bronchoscopy should be used for direct visualization of the airways

    d. TBM will generally improve by one year of age

    e. Chest physiotherapy can be helpful to clear retained secretions

27-20. A 4-year-old previously healthy boy presents with fever to 102.5°F, sore throat, irritability, and refusal to eat or drink. Symptoms began that morning and have progressed over the past few hours. You note the child to be ill appearing, leaning forward, and drooling. There are no ill contacts and the child has received all immunizations. You keep the child comfortable with his mother and immediately contact anesthesia and otolaryngology to assist with further management.

If neck films were ordered, the most likely finding would be:

    a. Thumbprint sign

    b. No acute abnormality

    c. Steeple sign

    d. Reverse spine sign

    e. Irregularity of the tracheal air column

27-21. The chest radiograph of a 12-hour-old full-term baby boy with respiratory distress shows a uniformly dense left upper lobe and a shift of the mediastinum from left to right. On repetition of the study at 72 hours of age, the left upper lobe is more lucent than the rest of the lung, but mediastinal shift persists.

Of the following, the most likely diagnosis is:

    a. Bronchogenic cyst

    b. Meconium aspiration syndrome

    c. Pulmonary sequestration

    d. Congenital large hyperlucent lobe

    e. Congenital cystic adenomatoid malformation

27-22. Which of the following statements is true regarding antenatal diagnosis of fetal lung lesions?

    a. If a fetal lesion demonstrates an aortic blood supply, pulmonary sequestration may be definitively diagnosed

    b. All abnormalities should be detectable on 2nd trimester scans

    c. Oligohydramnios is often associated with congenital cystic lesions and confers poorer prognosis

    d. All neonates with prenatally diagnosed with a fetal lung lesion require a chest computerized tomography (CT) scan prior to discharge

    e. Congenital thoracic malformations peak in size at 25 weeks, and then regress

27-23. You follow a baby diagnosed with PCD, who was found to have bilateral right lung (right isomerism). Parents are reluctant to provide routine immunizations, but are willing to provide those that you feel are most critical.

Which of the following vaccines do you recommend is most important for your patient to receive?

    a. MMR vaccine

    b. Hepatitis B vaccine

    c. Pneumococcal vaccine

    d. RSV prophylaxis

    e. DTaP vaccine

27-24. A 14-year-old boy followed in your practice comes in with his 3rd episode of pneumonia in the last 8 months. He was previously healthy with no symptoms between episodes. His symptoms started with nasal congestion, post nasal drainage, cough, and low-grade fever. On exam, you note a temperature of 38°C, respiratory rate of 16, oxygen saturation of 97% in RA. He does have cloudy nasal drainage. Lung exam reveals slightly coarse breath sounds bilaterally without focal wheezing or crackles. The remainder of exam is within normal limits. Chest X-ray reveals a round infiltrate in the same area in the left lower lobe as seen previously. You order a follow-up chest X-ray 6 weeks after treatment with antibiotics. Despite complete resolution of clinical symptoms, the same appearance is noted on repeat imaging. You suspect this may be a congenital anomaly.

Which of the following is most likely?

    a. Pulmonary arteriovenous malformation

    b. Pulmonary sequestration

    c. Bronchogenic cyst

    d. Tracheomalacia

    e. Congenital cystic adenomatoid malformation

27-25. You receive a call on a Saturday evening from the mother of one of your patients. Her 2-year-old son was found with an open bottle of lamp oil about 20 minutes ago. He is coughing a little, but seems to be fine otherwise.

You explain the following to the mother:

a. She should not worry. It is likely that the child did not actually ingest the fluid

b. She should try to induce emesis for gastric cleanout to reduce potential side effects

c. She should bring the child to your office the following Monday for a chest X-ray. It is too soon to see changes before then

d. She should bring the child to the Emergency Department for evaluation and observation as symptoms may worsen over the next several hours

e. She should watch for signs of central nervous system depression, which is the most common problem after hydrocarbon ingestion

27-26. Which of the following statements about swallowing dysfunction is correct?

a. The inflammatory response is characterized by eosinophilic infiltration

b. Acute-onset large-volume aspiration is a common complication

c. Neurologically intact children are more likely to have silent aspiration

d. The larynx must lower during the pharyngeal phase in order for a food bolus to pass into the esophagus

e. If left untreated, chronic dysphagia can lead to bronchiectasis as well as chronic hypoxia and dyspnea

27-27. A 3-year-old boy is brought in to your office by his mother with complaints of cough, wheeze, and low-grade fever. The child was well until the prior evening, when he developed sudden onset of cough after dinner. He came to find his mother when he was coughing, but she is unsure what he was doing just prior to that time. He has no signs of an upper respiratory infection, no history of prior wheeze, and has had no abdominal complaints. Upon further questioning, his older brother admits that they were playing a game, trying to catch peanuts in their mouths when the younger boy began coughing. You have a high suspicion of foreign body aspiration (FBA). You order a chest X-ray. The most likely finding is:

a. Unilateral hyperinflation of the right side

b. Right-sided bronchiectasis

c. Focal infiltrate in the left lower lobe

d. Left-sided atelectasis

e. Radiopaque foreign body in the trachea

27-28. Once a FBA has been diagnosed, the next step would be:

a. Upper GI series to be sure the foreign body is truly in the airways

b. Flexible bronchoscopy

c. Chest CT to confirm likely location of the foreign body

d. Rigid bronchoscopy

e. Reassure the family that a 10-day course of antibiotics should be all that is necessary

27-29. Which of the following statements about diagnostic tests for gastroesophageal reflux is true?

a. An upper GI series (or barium swallow study) is considered the gold standard for diagnosing gastroesophageal reflux

b. Bronchoscopy with bronchoalveolar lavage (BAL) can definitively diagnose gastroesophageal reflux

c. Multichannel intraluminal impedance with pH monitoring can detect both acid and nonacid reflux

d. 24-hour esophageal pH probe monitoring can determine aspiration

e. Gastroesophageal scintigraphy or "milk scan" has a high sensitivity for aspiration in children

27-30. Approximately 40% of children who wheeze before 3 years of age do not have episodes of wheezing after 6 years of age. These children are labeled "transient wheezers," as opposed to "persistent wheezers"

Which of the following characteristics is associated with transient wheezing of childhood rather than persistent wheezing?

a. Family history of asthma

b. Lack of exposure to daycare

c. Eczema

d. RSV infection in the first year of life

e. Maternal smoking during pregnancy

27-31. You are seeing a 14-year-old boy with exercise-induced bronchospasm (EIB). As you counsel him regarding his condition, which of the following factors can potentially increase the likelihood of an episode of EIB?

a. Recent use of a bronchodilator 10–20 minutes before exercise

b. Conserving energy by avoiding a warm-up period prior to exercise

c. Participation in sports associated with a warm, moist air environment (such as swimming) versus a cold-weather sport (eg, skiing, speed-skating)

d. Wearing a mask to cover the nose and mouth during exercise when the weather is cold

e. Exercising indoors during days with high pollen counts or high levels of pollution

27-32. A 7-year-old girl presents to your office for evaluation of chronic cough and wheeze. By history, you determine that triggers for her symptoms include: upper respiratory infections, weather change, exercise, and laughter. She was seen in the ED once and received an oral steroid burst and was sent home with bronchodilator therapy. She reports that anytime she is active, she will use bronchodilators often to relieve her symptoms. Her mother reports that the girl has nighttime cough at least once a week.

You diagnose her with asthma, and classify the severity as follows:

a. Exercise-induced bronchospasm

b. Mild intermittent asthma

c. Mild persistent asthma

d. Moderate persistent asthma

e. Severe persistent asthma

27-33. A 17-year-old girl is admitted to the pediatric intensive care unit in status asthmaticus. She is intubated, mechanically ventilated, and treated aggressively. However, her clinical condition deteriorates despite the best efforts of the intensive care team. Ultimately, her parents elect to withdraw medical care. Of the following, the risk factor most closely associated with fatal asthma is:

a. Caucasian race

b. Female gender

c. Sensitivity to pollen

d. Use of daily inhaled corticosteroids

e. Poor perception of symptoms

27-34. An 8-year-old obese boy comes to see you for follow-up of his asthma. His mother reports that he has been having more difficulties with flares, and that they note an increase in nighttime cough. He has not had symptoms of acute upper respiratory infection and has no fevers. His allergic symptoms seem to be controlled without nasal congestion, itching, or rhinorrhea. There is no abdominal pain, emesis, or heartburn. His mother describes a decline in his energy level, and he has been using more rescue medication recently, which does help some of his symptoms. They both report that he is taking his combination high-dose inhaled corticosteroid—long-acting bronchodilator well, with rare missed doses. He is also taking his leukotriene modifier every day.

Your next step in managing his asthma is to:

a. Order a chest X-ray to evaluate for pneumonia

b. Make no changes to the current regimen

c. Order a polysomnogram to evaluate for OSA

d. Order a methacholine challenge test to assess airway reactivity

e. Order a sinus CT to evaluate for acute sinusitis

27-35. A 15-year-old boy has recently transferred his care to your office. He and his parents report that he was recently diagnosed with exercise-induced asthma. He began noticing symptoms when he made the high school cross country team. Prior to this, he had not had difficulty with exercise. He has no history of prolonged upper respiratory infections or pneumonia. He denies frequent sinus infections or otitis media. He does have a history of peanut allergy, and carries an Epipen. He denies chronic rhinorrhea, sneezing, or other signs of environmental allergy. There is no history of eczema. He reports that he eats well, and denies abdominal discomfort, heartburn or emesis. Generally his symptoms begin within the first 5 minutes of exercise, and he feels a tightness in his throat and upper chest. He generally stops and rests for a few minutes and then can return to running again. He has tried an inhaler, but he felt it did not help as much as a brief rest.

The most definitive diagnostic test you can order is:

a. Upper GI series

b. Methacholine challenge

c. Spirometry

d. Flexible laryngoscopy

e. Nasal ciliary biopsy

27-36. A cohort of school-age children who were born prematurely and developed BPD undergo pulmonary function testing. The mean test values are compared with those of an appropriate control group who had been born at term.

When comparing the results for the two groups, the survivors of BPD would be more likely to exhibit:

a. No evidence of abnormality

b. Restrictive lung disease

c. Decreased chest wall compliance

d. Airways hyperresponsiveness

e. Oxygen desaturation on incremental exercise testing

27-37. A 5-month-old infant born at 26 weeks gestation presents to your office with chronic cough. The child has a history of bronchopulmonary dysplasia, and is being treated with oxygen at 0.5 LPM and diuretics. The parents report no associated upper respiratory symptoms, no fever, and no ill contacts. The cough is most commonly heard one to two hours after feeds or when the child is lying down. On exam, you note that the child has not been growing as well as she had previously. Oxygen saturation is 98% in 0.5 liters per minute (LPM) by nasal cannula, respiratory rate is 30 breaths per minute, and lungs are clear bilaterally with no increased work of breathing. Remainder of exam is within normal limits.

The most likely diagnosis in this case is:

a. Lower respiratory tract infection

b. Gastroesophageal reflux disease

c. Pulmonary edema

d. Tracheomalacia

e. Tracheoesophageal fistula

27-38. There has been increasing recognition of the effects of oxygen toxicity and barotrauma on the premature lung and the association with bronchopulmonary dysplasia (BPD). Despite changes in management and the development of new treatments, BPD still exists; however, this "classic" BPD has evolved into a "new" BPD.

Which of the following is most characteristic of the "new" bronchopulmonary dysplasia?

a. Reduced airways resistance

b. Ventilation–perfusion mismatch

c. Increased compliance of the respiratory system

d. Increased lung volumes

e. Cysts alternating with linear densities on X-ray

27-39. Which of the following statements is true regarding BPD?

a. The incidence of BPD has increased steadily over the past 2 decades

b. The risk of BPD decreases with increasing maternal age

c. The risk of BPD increases with lower birth weight

d. The risk of BPD is lower with younger maternal age

e. BPD is a disorder limited to premature children

27-40. A 5-month-old former 25-week preterm infant presents to your office for follow up of BPD. The child was discharged from the neonatal intensive care unit 5 days ago. You review the discharge summary, and learn that the infant weighed 850 g at birth, and required mechanical ventilation for the first 6 weeks of life. Complications included maternal chorioamnionitis and neonatal sepsis, intraventricular hemorrhage (grade 1), and poor growth. The child was discharged on oxygen at 0.5 LPM by nasal cannula. The parents report that the child has been well since discharge, without any increased respiratory symptoms. There is no cough or wheeze, and no cyanosis. The child has been feeding orally, and is on increased calorie formula to promote growth. Exam reveals normal oxygen saturation, tachypnea with mild retractions, and clear lungs.

Which of the following therapies is most appropriate to prescribe at this time?

a. Low-dose inhaled corticosteroids

b. Oral diuretics

c. Inhaled bronchodilator

d. Anti-reflux medications

e. Respiratory syncycial virus (RSV) prophylaxis

27-41. A 14-year-old boy with cystic fibrosis has a low-grade fever, sore throat, fatigue, and increased urinary frequency. Since his last visit 2 months ago, he has had a 4.0 kg weight loss, essentially unchanged findings on chest examination, and only minimally decreased pulmonary function (3% decrease in FEV1 and 8% decrease in FEF25-75). Which of the following is the most likely diagnosis?

a. Urinary tract infection

b. Diabetes mellitus

c. Distal intestinal obstruction syndrome

d. Pulmonary exacerbation

e. Allergic bronchopulmonary aspergillosis

27-42. Which of the following descriptions meet accepted criteria for the diagnosis of cystic fibrosis?

a. Positive newborn screen and sweat chloride value of 65 mEq/L with adequate sweat volume

b. Four-year-old with failure to thrive and steatorrhea and sweat chloride value of 45 meq/L with adequate sweat volume

c. Positive newborn screen that identifies 2 disease causing CF mutations on the state's newborn screen DNA testing

d. Positive newborn screen in an infant with a sibling with CF

e. Twelve-year-old with recurrent sinusitis and nasal polyps with one known CF mutation identified on DNA testing

27-43. A 12-year-old girl with cystic fibrosis returns to your office after a second course of an oral as well as inhaled antibiotics for a pulmonary exacerbation. She reports she has been doing extra airway clearance. She continues to have an increased cough. In addition, her lung function has not yet returned to her usual baseline. She has lost 1 pound since her last visit, and continues to have fatigue. The most appropriate next step is:

   a. Begin an appetite stimulant to improve appetite and encourage weight gain

   b. Begin treatment for allergic bronchopulmonary aspergillosis

   c. Admit her for initiation of IV antibiotics for a 2- to 3-week course

   d. Perform outpatient bronchoscopy to clear mucus and continue increased airway clearance

   e. Assume this is her new baseline and continue routine therapies

27-44. Which class of CFTR mutation is most commonly associated with pancreatic sufficiency and milder lung disease?

   a. Class I

   b. Class II

   c. Class IIa

   d. Class III

   e. Class IV

27-45. A 16-year-old football player with cystic fibrosis presents with complaints of diffuse crampy abdominal pain. Football season began 2 weeks ago, and he is practicing 3 days per week, with games on weekends. He reports that he has not had a regular formed bowel movement in the last 3 days. He has had some loose stool the morning of his appointment. He usually has 2 formed stools per day. He reports feeling well between pain episodes. He denies any blood or mucus in his stools. He denies vomiting, heartburn, or epigastric pain. He has been eating a bit less in the last day, but does not note worsening after eating.

The most likely diagnosis is:

   a. Gallstones

   b. Gastroesophageal reflux

   c. Intussusception

   d. Distal intestinal obstruction syndrome

   e. Fibrosing colonopathy

27-46. A patient is found to be homozygous for the PI Z mutation in the Alpha1-antitrysin (AAT) gene. Which of the following is true regarding the pathophysiology of this disorder in the lung?

   a. Decreased levels of AAT are able to decrease apoptosis in the lung

   b. Neutrophil elastase (NE) is the only substrate for the activity of AAT

   c. Inhibition of NE by AAT involves irreversible binding and translocation of NE from one pole of AAT to the other side

   d. Decreased levels of AAT allow for increased neutrophil elimination within the pulmonary capillaries which lie in close juxtaposition with interstitial elastin fibers

   e. AAT may be destructive to airway and alveolar epithelial and endothelial cells.

27-47. A 50-year-old man who has smoked since he was 18 years old presents to his primary care doctor with cough and difficulty breathing. These symptoms have been present for "years" but worsened over the past year. His spirometry shows obstruction with positive bronchodilator response. His chest radiograph shows hyperinflation; while chest CT scan demonstrates panacinar emphysema. What is the next step you would take to help diagnose this patient's condition?

   a. Obtain tuberculin skin testing

   b. Perform video assisted thoracoscopic lung biopsy

   c. Perform flexible bronchoscopy with BAL

   d. Obtain alpha-1 antitrypsin level and isoelectric focusing

   e. Obtain nasal potential difference

27-48. An 8-year-old boy's father is diagnosed with alpha1-antitrypsin deficiency. The boy does not have any evidence of liver or lung disease based on thorough testing, though he is also homozygous for the PiZ alpha1-antitrypsin gene. What is the most important piece of anticipatory guidance to give the family?

   a. Avoid all exposure to tobacco smoke, through the family and for the patient himself

   b. Start antibiotics at the first sign of cough

   c. Avoid going to school to prevent contracting any viral illnesses

   d. Start an exercise program to help avoid complications of the disease

   e. Start corticosteroids immediately for the first episode of wheezing

27-49. Which of the following statements is true regarding replacement therapy for alpha1-antitrypsin (AAT) deficiency lung disease?

a. IV infusion increases pulmonary function measures over a period of years

b. The primary endpoint for therapy is restoration of plasma levels of alpha1-antitrypsin (AAT)

c. Monthly replacement therapy is generally recommended

d. Aerosol therapy is regarded as equal to IV therapy in randomized controlled trials

e. After lung transplantation, replacement therapy for alpha1-antitrypsin is no longer necessary

27-50. A 15-year-old girl is found to have anemia, cough, and bibasilar infiltrates on chest radiograph. BAL is performed and confirms pulmonary hemorrhage. Video-assisted thoracoscopic lung biopsy is performed and there is evidence on pathology of small and medium vessel neutrophilic inflammation. Which of the following can be eliminated from the differential diagnosis?

a. Polygranulomatosis with angiitis (PGA)

b. Churg–Strauss syndrome

c. Microscopic polyangiitis

d. Polyarteritis nodosa

e. Takayasu arteritis

27-51. A 13-year-old girl presents with sinusitis and epistaxis. She is admitted to the hospital for nasal cautery and is found to have proteinuria and renal insufficiency with increasing creatinine levels. On further review of her history, she was found to have pneumonia 2 years ago, which was associated with microcytic anemia and bilateral pulmonary infiltrates. What is the most likely diagnosis?

a. Churg–Strauss syndrome

b. Polyarteritis nodosa

c. Behcet disease

d. Polygranulomatosis with angiitis (PGA)

e. Sarcoidosis

27-52. A 15-year-old boy with a history of epistaxis, proteinuria, and hemoptysis presents with hypoxemia, respiratory distress, and acute worsening hemoptysis. His vital signs include a respiratory rate of 45, heart rate of 120, blood pressure of 100/60, oxygen saturation of 88%, continued hemoptysis, and severe suprasternal and subcostal retractions. What is the most appropriate next step in treatment?

a. Administer IV corticosteroids

b. Intubate using 100% oxygen

c. Administer IV cyclophosphamide

d. Give a blood transfusion

e. Start chest compressions

27-53. A 9-year-old male presents to his pediatrician after a 6 month history of worsening cough and dyspnea, associated with limiting physical activity and weight loss. He has also had recurrent fevers and was diagnosed with pneumonia based on increased cough, hemoptysis, and bilateral pulmonary infiltrates on 2 occasions over the past 6 months. He was treated with inhaled corticosteroids and bronchodilators for asthma, but without any improvement in symptoms. Which of the following is the most appropriate next diagnostic test?

a. Ophthalmologic examination

b. Flexible bronchoscopy with BAL

c. CBC, ESR, and C-reactive protein

d. Double-stranded DNA antibody

e. Antineutrophil cytoplasmic antibodies (ANCAs)

27-54. A 12-year-old girl presents with hemoptysis. Her evaluation has thus far has included a complete blood count showing microcytic anemia, chest radiograph with bilateral opacities, and chest CT scan also with bilateral opacities and a right upper lobe cavitary lesion. Flexible bronchoscopy with BAL demonstrates the presence of hemosiderin macrophages and video assisted thoracoscopic lung biopsy demonstrates small to medium vessel vasculitis. What test would help confirm the diagnosis?

a. C-reactive protein

b. Angiotensin converting enzyme level

c. Antiribonucleoprotein antibody

d. Antiphospholipid antibody profile

e. Antineutrophil cytoplasmic antibodies

27-55. Which of the following statements is true about pulmonary surfactant?

a. Function includes increasing surface tension, thereby preventing alveolar collapse

b. It is composed primarily of proteins (90%) and also of lipids (10%)

c. It is secreted into alveoli by type I alveolar epithelial cells

d. Surfactant protein B deficiencies are reported to occur in 1 in 1000 births

e. Surfactant protein C deficiencies are associated with interstitial lung disease

27-56. A 1-year-old boy develops cough and increased work of breathing. He has a thorough evaluation including lung biopsy. This demonstrates well-preserved alveolar wall architecture, but filling of the alveoli with surfactant. The diagnosis in this case is most likely which of the following?

   a. ABCA3 dysfunction

   b. Surfactant protein B deficiency

   c. Surfactant protein C dysfunction

   d. NKTF-1 (thyroid transcription factor) dysfunction

   e. Granulocyte/macrophage-colony stimulating factor receptor α chain dysfunction

27-57. A 5-year-old girl develops cough and hypoxemia. She has a thorough evaluation including chest CT scan, which shows diffuse ground-glass opacities in both lungs. Which of the following diagnostic tests should be performed next?

   a. Thoracoscopic lung biopsy

   b. BAL for surfactant levels

   c. Genetic testing for lysinuric protein intolerance

   d. Genetic testing for ABCA-3 mutations

   e. Genetic testing for granulocyte/macrophage-colony stimulating factor receptor α chain mutations

27-58. A 5-year-old girl develops cough and hypoxemia. She has a thorough evaluation including chest CT scan which shows diffuse ground-glass opacities in both lungs. Genetic testing confirms the presence of two mutations in the ABCA-3 gene. What is the next step in treatment of this disorder?

   a. Surfactant administration

   b. Whole-lung lavage

   c. Supplemental oxygen

   d. Chronic systemic steroids

   e. Lung transplant

27-59. Which of the following clinical scenarios best describes a patient with autoimmune pulmonary alveolar proteinosis?

   a. A nonsmoking 39-year-old male who develops dyspnea and exercise intolerance

   b. A 12-month-old boy who develops shortness of breath over the first year of life

   c. A 3-year-old girl with acute myeloid leukemia who develops dyspnea

   d. A term infant with respiratory failure requiring emergent intubation

   e. A 12-year-old male with chronic cough and diffuse infiltrates

27-60. Which of the following is true regarding the pulmonary physiology of an infant?

   a. Compliance of the chest wall is less than in the adult

   b. Laryngeal braking helps maintain FRC

   c. As an infant ages, less of the diaphragm is in direct contact with the inner thoracic cavity

   d. The chest wall of an infant is less likely to collapse inward

   e. Prolonged expiration helps to maintain FRC

27-61. Which of the following muscles helps to increase the intrathoracic volume by a "bucket handle" mechanism?

   a. Scalenes

   b. Serratus anterior

   c. Diaphragm

   d. Sternocleidomastoids

   e. External intercostals

27-62. A 10-year-old boy is being evaluated for Duchenne muscular dystrophy. His spirometry suggests decreased forced vital capacity compared to the standards for his age and height. Which of the following abnormalities is most likely to be found on testing?

   a. Elevated total lung capacity

   b. Increased residual volume to total lung capacity ratio

   c. Increased maximum expiratory pressure

   d. Decreased end-tidal carbon dioxide

   e. Increased oxyhemoglobin saturation

27-63. A 16-year-old female athlete is being evaluated for exercise-induced asthma with an exercise test. During her run on the treadmill, which of the following is true regarding her pulmonary physiology?

   a. Contraction of the internal intercostal muscles may aid in expiration

   b. Contraction of the abdominal muscles may aid in inspiration

   c. Expiration is passive and dependent on the elastic recoil of the lung and chest wall

   d. Contraction of the sternocleidomastoids may aid in expiration

   e. Contraction of the serratus anterior may aid in expiration

27-64. A 4-month-old infant presents with choking when taking his bottles, tongue fasciculation, and profound hypotonia. Which of the following would you tell the parents?

a. Without assisted ventilation, median age of death is at 12 years

b. Their child will likely be able to sit but not to walk

c. The chest wall may increase in diameter over time due to weakness of the intercostal muscles

d. Tracheostomy is the only option for survival

e. Cough is impaired and use of an airway clearance device is recommended

27-65. A term newborn whose mother did not have prenatal care presents with short-limb dwarfism, small, narrow, bell-shaped rib cage with shortened ribs, hypoxemia, respiratory distress, and renal insufficiency. Which of the following is true regarding this patient and disorder?

a. It is inherited in an autosomal dominant fashion

b. It results in obstructive lung disease

c. Vertically expandable prosthetic titanium rib placement is a treatment option

d. Recurrent pneumonia is unlikely

e. It is known as achondroplasia

27-66. A 15-year-old girl with chronic cough productive of sputum and poor growth is found to have enlargement of the terminal segments of her fingers and toes. No other family members have this finding. Which of the following is true regarding this finding?

a. It is likely to be idiopathic and does not need further evaluation

b. The depth of the finger at the proximal nail fold is less than the depth of the distal interphalangeal joint

c. It is likely to be painful and recognized by the patient

d. The nail bed shows increased numbers of blood vessels and primitive fibroblasts

e. When this finding is present, Schamroth sign should disappear

27-67. A 10-month-old infant presents to her pediatrician's office with respiratory rate of 70 bpm, diffuse crackles on auscultation of all lung fields, as well as oxygen saturation of 88% on room air. Her symptoms continue for months and she does not respond to inhaled bronchodilators. She is kept on supplemental oxygen. Chest CT scan reveals ground glass opacities most prominent in the right middle lobe and lingula. Lung biopsy demonstrates normal lung histology, but

increased cells that stain positive for bombesin. Which of the following is correct regarding this diagnosis?

a. It most commonly occurs following adenovirus infection

b. Treatment with corticosteroids is usually effective

c. The most common cause in children is exposure to avian antigens

d. Supplemental oxygen may be required for a period of years

e. Lung transplantation is ultimately required for the majority of cases

27-68. A 3-year-old girl presents to the hospital with tachypnea, hypoxemia, and bilateral diffuse infiltrates on chest radiograph. She becomes more comfortable on 2 L nasal cannula oxygen and her respiratory rate is 30. The patient is found to be anemic.

What is the next step you would take in the management of this patient?

a. Request lung biopsy using video-assisted thoracoscopy

b. Perform bronchoscopy with BAL

c. Prescribe high-dose intravenous corticosteroids

d. Order high-resolution CT of the chest

e. Order genetic testing for mutations in surfactant proteins B and C

27-69. An 18-year-old male with cystic fibrosis underwent lung transplantation 1 year ago due to severe airway obstruction and progressive disease. He had been doing well but has noticed over the past 2 months that he has been more short of breath with exercise and is also coughing more. His spirometry suggests increased airway obstruction compared to baseline. High-resolution CT of the chest shows mosaic perfusion and central bronchiectasis. What recommendations would you give to the patient and his family regarding his most likely diagnosis?

a. Reassure the family that the symptoms are unlikely to be progressive and therefore no treatment is necessary

b. Explain to the family that steroids have been proven in multiple studies to prevent airway fibrosis

c. Counsel the family that anti-TNF has been used successfully for treatment and can be started immediately

d. Recommend bronchoscopy with BAL to help make a definitive diagnosis

e. Suggest treatment with systemic corticosteroids and consideration of lung biopsy if symptoms continue

27-70. A 4-year-old child with snoring is found to have OSA on a polysomnogram. Which of the following is true regarding the upper airway physiology in this patient?

 a. Decreased inspiratory effort results in collapse of the upper airway

 b. Impaired arousal responses to obstructive events result in obstructive alveolar hypoventilation

 c. Increased growth rate of lymphadenoid tissue compared to other upper airway structures contributes to upper airway obstruction

 d. Pharyngeal airway neuromotor responses are increased compared to normal children

 e. Hypoxia and hypercapnic ventilatory drive is impaired compared to normal children

27-71. An infant is found to have OSA. Which of the following is true regarding this condition in the first year of life?

 a. It is more common in females than in males

 b. The upper airway is most likely obstructing in the retroglossal region

 c. A child with trisomy 21 and laryngomalacia is at increased risk

 d. It is not commonly associated with hypoxemia

 e. The laryngeal chemoreflex is less likely playing a role compared to an older child

27-72. A full-term infant is born to a G1P0 mother without prenatal complications by vaginal delivery. The infant weighs 8 pounds and is vigorous at birth, but develops respiratory failure and cyanosis during sleep. Arterial blood gas reveals PCO_2 of 80 mm Hg. The infant is intubated and mechanically ventilated. After thorough evaluation in the neonatal intensive care unit, genetic testing reveals the presence of a heterozygous mutation in the paired-like homeobox 2B (PHOX2b) gene with a 20/27 polyalanine expansion, consistent with congenital central hypoventilation syndrome (CCHS)

What can you tell the parents regarding CCHS?

 a. It is inherited in an autosomal recessive fashion

 b. Their child is likely to outgrow the disorder as maturation of the autonomic nervous system occurs

 c. Hirschsprung disease is associated with this condition

 d. Their child's mutation is *not* the most common to cause this disorder

 e. Ventilation is most affected during REM sleep

27-73. A 12-month-old girl with normal birth history and normal development until 6 months of age is found to have developmental delay, loss of ability to babble, and flapping hand movements. The girl also develops breath-holding spells and rapid shallow-

breathing during sleep. These events do lead to oxygen desaturations during sleep. Which of the following is also consistent with this condition?

 a. Mutation in the gene encoding methyl-CpG-binding protein 2 (MeCP2)

 b. Absence of the paternally inherited genes on the proximal long arm of chromosome 15

 c. Autosomal dominant inheritance

 d. Cerebellar aplasia with thickened superior cerebellar peduncles ("molar tooth sign")

 e. Abnormal development and survival of unmyelinated sensory and autonomic neurons

27-74. An infant born at 33 weeks gestation to a mother without prenatal problems is admitted to the neonatal intensive care unit. After several hours of life the baby is found to have pauses in his breathing of 15- to 25-second duration associated with bradycardia (heart rate to the 60 bpm). The events occur 1 to 2 times per hour, and the infant does require stimulation by the nurse to stop the episodes. The infant has a temperature of 38°C, heart rate of 140, respiratory rate of 36–48, pulse oximetry of 99% on room air, and does not appear in distress in between these episodes. Arterial blood gas shows a normal pH, PCO_2, PO_2, and bicarbonate. Electrolytes and serum glucose are within normal limits. What is your next step in the management of this infant?

 a. Start caffeine citrate

 b. Start nasal continuous positive airway pressure (CPAP)

 c. Order a pH probe

 d. Order a head ultrasound

 e. Order a blood culture and complete blood count

27-75. A 6-year-old boy with normal growth and development is being evaluated by his pediatrician for OSA due to parental complaint that the boy snores loudly every night. Which of the following is true regarding assessment for OSA?

 a. The predictive value of clinical history is increased when the patient is referred to a sleep specialist, often obviating the need for a polysomnogram

 b. Diagnosis can be made with an overnight pulse oximetry study or with an overnight polysomnogram

 c. Less than 10% of children with OSA report excessive daytime sleepiness

 d. Transcutaneous carbon dioxide tension measurements are recommended in addition to end-tidal capnography

 e. Children are more likely to manifest electroencephalographic arousals following obstructive apneas

ANSWERS

Answer 27-1. d

Based on the history and physical examination this patient most likely has restless leg syndrome. Restless legs syndrome (RLS) is a clinical diagnosis characterized by uncomfortable leg sensations that usually occur *prior* to sleep onset. Periodic limb movement disorder (PLMD) is characterized by periodic limb movements *during* sleep, which are associated with symptoms of insomnia or excessive daytime sleepiness.

Both RLS and PLMD are common in adults, with a prevalence of up to 10%. Approximately one-third of adult patients report the onset of symptoms before the age of 20 years. Nonspecific symptoms, such as growing pain, restless sleep, and hyperactivity, may accompany RLS or PLMD. A family history of RLS and PLMD is common.

The etiology of RLS and PLMD is not known. Pregnancy, uremia, iron deficiency, and anemia are associated with increased risk of RLS and PLMD (secondary RLS). Treatment of RLS and PLMD includes avoidance of caffeine and sleep hygiene. There is currently no FDA-approved medication available to treat RLS and PLMD in children.

A tremor is defined as an involuntary oscillating movement with a fixed frequency. The most common cause of tremor in children is *essential (familial) tremor*, which transmitted in autosomal dominant trait. In this case, the child does not have a movement with fixed frequency. Myoclonus is characterized by sudden, brief, shock-like movements, which can be rhythmic or nonrhythmic, focal, multifocal, or generalized. Myoclonic movement can be activated by another movement or sensory stimulation. Physiologic myoclonus can occur as nocturnal myoclonus during sleep, or myoclonus induced by anxiety. Tourette syndrome is part of the spectrum of tic disorder. In this case, the child does not have a tic, which is an involuntary, sudden, rapid, repetitive, nonrhythmic, stereotyped movement.

(Section 27: Disorders of the Respiratory System, Chapter 509: Sleep Disorders, Page 1943. Section 29: Disorders of the Nervous System, Chapter 566: Movement Disorders, Tics, and Tourette Syndrome)

Answer 27-2. c

Based on the history and physical examination this patient most likely has RLS, which is a clinical diagnosis characterized by uncomfortable leg sensations that usually occur *prior* to sleep onset. Other nonspecific symptoms include growing pains, restless sleep, and hyperactivity. The prevalence of RLS is estimated to be approximately 2% in children 8–17 years of age.

Many children with RLS have low iron storage, as evidenced by low serum ferritin and/or iron. As iron deficiency and anemia are associated with RLS, it is important to screen for this condition. The mother's physician most likely ordered a CBC to screen for anemia and iron deficiency. Based on

the mother's history, she was most likely treated with iron supplementation.

Although the etiology of RLS is not known, studies suggest that genetic predisposition, dopamine dysfunction, and low iron stores are related to the pathophysiology of RLS. Thyroid disease, electrolyte anomalies, urinary tract disease, and copper metabolism have not been linked to RLS. As a result, it is unlikely that any of the other tests were previously ordered.

(Section 27: Disorders of the Respiratory System, Chapter 509: Sleep Disorders, Page 1943)

Answer 27-3. c

A sleep terror is a parasomnia characterized by night-time awakening in an agitated state from non-REM sleep. The events correspond to prominent slow-wave sleep. Sleep terrors are associated with intense autonomic nervous system manifestations such as dilated pupils, diaphoresis, tachypnea, and tachycardia. After the event, the child is not consolable, but returns to sleep after a few minutes. In the morning, the child has *no* recollection of the event. It is estimated that up to 6.5% of children experience night terrors, which are most common between 2 and 6 years of age. Sleep terrors can be precipitated by stress, sleep deprivation, anxiety, and environmental noises.

In contrast, a nightmare is a frightening dream that awakes a child. Nightmares occur during REM sleep. The child is consolable after the event and may also have a recollection of the event in the morning. While night terrors occur in younger children, nightmares are more common in school-age children and adolescents. The occurrence is normal and management is counseling and reassurance.

Night terrors and nightmares do not require referral to a mental health professional or a neurologist. There is no reported association with seizure disorders.

(Section 27: Disorders of the Respiratory System, Chapter 509: Sleep Disorders, Page 1944)

Answer 27-4. c

Although adolescents need 9 hours of sleep, most sleep only 7–7.5 hours each night, with irregular sleep patterns, as well. This "sleep debt" can lead to significant issues in adolescents, such as daytime sleepiness, as in this case. Other associated problems are changes in mood, memory, behavior, and decreased academic performance.

During puberty, there are physiologic changes and a shift in melatonin secretion and circadian sleep phase. These changes lead to a phase delay and a greater likelihood of later onset of sleep as well as a later wake-up time. In addition, changes in academic demands and social activities during adolescence increase the likelihood of sleep deprivation and sleeping longer during the weekend, which can make the phase delay worse.

Obstructive sleep apnea (OSA) is defined as partial or complete upper airway obstruction during sleep, resulting in disruption of normal gas exchange and sleep patterns. Although one of the symptoms of OSA is daytime sleepiness, other daytime symptoms include morning headaches, mouth breathing, difficulty in waking up, moodiness, nasal obstruction, and cognitive problems. Severe OSA is associated with cor pulmonale. The prevalence is 2%–3% of children. No other symptoms of OSA are present, which make OSA less likely in this case.

Narcolepsy is unlikely in this case due to the history, symptoms, and epidemiology of the condition. Although narcolepsy is also associated with excessive daytime sleepiness, it is also associated with cataplexy (sudden loss of muscle tone), hypnagogic hallucination, and sleep paralysis, which were not reported in this case. Normally, rapid eye movement (REM) sleep occurs after deep sleep; however, patients with narcolepsy enter REM sleep immediately in the sleep cycle. The prevalence of narcolepsy is approximately 1 in 1000 to 1 in 10,000 in the United States. The diagnosis of narcolepsy is based on clinical history and sleep study.

Although anemia can cause fatigue, the patient does not have any risk factors associated with anemia. A complete social history is always helpful; however, based on the information provided, there is no specific reason to suspect alcohol abuse in this case.

(Section 27: Disorders of the Respiratory System, Chapter 509: Sleep Disorders, Page 1948)

Answer 27-5. b

The major change in sleep patterns during adolescence is a shift in melatonin secretion and circadian sleep phase. These changes lead to phase delay with propensity to later onset of sleep and later wake-up time.

"Growing pains" most commonly occur between the ages of 3 and 12. Although the pain occurs intermittently during sleep, it is not directly associated with difficulty falling asleep at night. Similarly, although symptoms of gastroesophageal reflux disease (GERD) can be worse in a supine or prone position, GERD is not directly associated with difficulty falling asleep. Phase advance is not a standard term. Menarche is generally not a risk factor for sleep disturbances.

(Section 27: Disorders of the Respiratory System, Chapter 509: Sleep Disorders, Page 1948)

Answer 27-6. a

The BEARS (Bedtime, Excessive daytime sleepiness, Awakenings, Regularity, Snoring) instrument provides a comprehensive screening process for the common sleep disorders (eTable 509-1). The instrument can be used for children 2–18 years of age.

The CAGE questionnaire is used for alcoholism. HEEADSSS exam is a psychosocial interview tool to address adolescent health and risk behaviors. SALSA is a depression screening mneumonic (Sleep distrurbance, Anhedonia, Low Self-esteem, Appetite decreased). DREAMS is not a standard screening tool.

(Section 27: Disorders of the Respiratory System, Chapter 509: Sleep Disorders, Page 1948)

Answer 27-7. c

Lung development begins in embryonic life with outpouching of the tracheal primordium from foregut endoderm. There are

eTABLE 509-1. BEARS Sleep Screening Tool with Developmentally Appropriate Trigger Questions

	Toddler/Preschool (2–5 yr)	School-Aged (6–12 yr)	Adolescent (13–18 yr)
Bedtime problems	Does your child have any problems going to bed?	Does your child have any problems at bedtime? (P) Do you have any problems going to bed?(C)	Do you have any problems falling asleep at bedtime? (C)
Excessive daytime sleepiness	Does your child seem overtired or sleepy a lot during the day?	Does your child have difficulty waking in the morning, seem sleepy during the day, or take naps? (P) Do you feel tired a lot? (C)	Do you feel sleepy a lot during the day? In school? While driving? (C)
Awakenings during the night	Does your child wake up a lot at night?	Does your child seem to wake up a lot at night? Any sleepwalking or nightmares? (P) Do you wake up a lot at night? Have trouble getting back to sleep? (C)	Do you wake up a lot at night? Have trouble getting back to sleep? (C)
Regularity and duration of sleep	Does your child have a regular bedtime and wake time? What are they?	What time does your child go to bed and get up on school days? Weekends? Do you think he or she is getting enough sleep? (P)	What time do you usually go to bed on school nights? Weekends? How much sleep do you usually get? (C)
Snoring	Does your child snore a lot or have difficulty breathing at night?	Does your child have loud or nightly snoring or any breathing difficulties at night? (P)	Does your teenager snore loudly or nightly? (P)

4 characteristic periods, including the pseudoglandular period, the canalicular period, the terminal saccular period, and the alveolar period. Normal development of the lung during postnatal development in infancy and childhood is dominated by formation and differentiation of alveoli during the first years of life.

Time	Period	Description
Weeks 6–16 of gestation	Pseudoglandular period	All of the major lung elements, except alveoli have formed
Weeks 16–26 of gestation	Canalicular period	Lung becomes vascularized; bronchi enlarge. Respiration is possible towards the end of this phase
Weeks 26 to birth	Terminal saccular period	Specialized cells emerge in respiratory epithelium. Type I alveolar cells promote gas exchange occurs. Type II alveolar cells produce pulmonary surfactant, which allows expansion of saccules
Birth to 8 years of age	Alveolar Period	Saccules, alveolar ducts, and alveoli develop and increase in number

(Section 27: Disorders of the Respiratory System, Chapter 502: Lung Growth in Infancy and Childhood, Page 1909)

Answer 27-8. d

Assessing the function of the respiratory control centers is not straightforward. Polysomnography measures a wide variety of physiologic variables during sleep, including nasal and oral airflow, chest and abdominal wall motion, oxygen saturation (SpO_2), end-tidal (exhaled) pCO_2, and electrocardiogram. Sleep state is monitored by electroencephalogram (EEG), electrooculogram, and electromyogram. Abnormalities of respiratory drive (especially central apneas and periodic breathing) can be detected with this testing.

Spirometry is the measurement of pulmonary airflow during a maximally forced exhalation. CXR, ABG, and EEG would not be helpful for assessing breathing patterns.

(Section 27: Disorders of the Respiratory System, Chapter 503: Physiologic Basis of Pulmonary Function, Page 1913)

Answer 27-9. e

Spirometry is the measurement of airflow during a maximally forced exhalation. Many common pediatric lung diseases (asthma and cystic fibrosis) are obstructive in nature, and are characterized by reduced airflows, based on the shape of the flow-volume curve. Furthermore, in the smaller airways, minimal effort is needed to achieve a maximal flow rate. The tests are reproducible within subjects, making them useful for assessing response to treatment over time.

Peak flow meter readings are useful for characterizing large airway disease; however, there is less information about small airway obstruction. Plethysmography is useful for measuring airway resistance. CXR and an ABG are not directly useful for assessing lung function.

(Section 27: Disorders of the Respiratory System, Chapter 503: Physiologic Basis of Pulmonary Function, Page 1915)

Answer 27-10. a

According to the National Institutes of Health Expert Panel Report 3, even if a patient is in very good asthma control, it is important to assess asthma control every 6 months. Asthma control is the degree to which the manifestations of asthma (symptoms, impairments, and risk) are minimized and the goals of therapy are met. Asthma control can help guide decisions to maintain or adjust asthma therapy for this patient.

While asthma severity describes the patient's intrinsic intensity of disease, asthma control is based on the intensity of disease and the appropriateness of asthma management. Thus, it is possible that a patient with very severe asthma can still have well-controlled asthma. Likewise, a patient with very mild asthma can still have very poorly controlled asthma. Because asthma severity describes the intrinsic intensity of disease, it is not possible to assess asthma severity for this patient because he has already been started on a daily controller medication. However, it is possible to assess asthma control for this patient.

Asthma control is not only based on recent hospitalizations. Components of asthma control include the level of impairment (frequency of symptoms, nighttime awakenings, interference with normal activity, use of short-acting beta-agonists, FEV_1, and the results from validated questionnaires) and risk (exacerbations in the last year, loss of lung function, and treatment-related adverse events). There are several validated questionnaires that can be used to assess asthma control in children. These include the Childhood Asthma Control Test (C-ACT) for children 4–11 years of age, as well as the Asthma Therapy Assessment Questionnaire (ATAQ), Asthma Control Questionnaire (ACQ), and the Asthma Control Test (ACT) for children 12 years and older.

(Section 27: Disorders of the Respiratory System, Chapter 512: Asthma, Pages 1962–1973)

Answer 27-11. d

Plain radiographs of frontal and lateral views of the chest remain the mainstay of screening imaging for any child with a suspected abnormality within the chest. In this case, it would be the most appropriate initial study for suspected foreign body aspiration (FBA). Plain films may be normal with FBA, but certain findings may be present and strongly support the diagnosis in the context of this clinical history.

If the object causes lower airway obstruction and air trapping, local hyperinflation of the lung can be seen. Partial obstruction can lead to atelectasis. If the aspiration is more remote, later developments that can be seen include pneumonia, lung abscess, and bronchiectasis.

CT involves a much larger dose of ionizing radiation and this would not be the first study to pursue. Bronchoscopy may be appropriate upon further workup, but a CXR should be done prior to bronchoscopy. CBC and Spirometry have no utility in this scenario.

(Section 27: Disorders of the Respiratory System, Chapter 506: Tools for Diagnosis and Management of Respiratory Disease, Page 1925)

Answer 27-12. e

House dust mites (*Dermatophagoides pteronyssinus* and *Dermatophagoides farinae*) feed on human skin flakes which are shed onto and into mattresses, pillows, carpets, stuffed toys and upholstered furniture. House dust mites (HDM) also prefer a humid environment. As a result, the use of a warm mist humidifier at night could potentially improve the environment for HDM.

The feces of HDM contain allergens (Der p 1 and Der f 1) that can trigger asthma symptoms for some sensitized children. Removal of wall-to-wall carpeting in the bedroom, weekly washing all the sheets and bedding in hot water at a temperature greater than 130°F, and the use of encasings for the child's bedroom mattresses and pillows can all help eradicate HDM and exposure to HDM feces.

(Section 27: Disorders of the Respiratory System, Chapter 512: Asthma; Environmental Allergen Avoidance. Pages 1972–1973)

Answer 27-13. b

This child is presenting with stridor and barky cough shows signs of upper airway obstruction. In such cases, radiographs of the neck with frontal and lateral projections can be helpful in distinguishing whether the obstruction is due to an intrinsic or extrinsic mass, foreign body, or inflammation such as croup or epiglottitis. Masses that may be seen include abscesses, cysts, or abnormal vessels. Croup is classically associated with a "steeple sign" due to subglottic narrowing. Epiglottitis is associated with a "thumb sign" from an enlarged epiglottis.

CT scan or ultrasounds would not be appropriate first-line tests to order, but may be needed for further evaluation of neck masses causing obstruction. CXR would not be as helpful in this child with signs of upper airway obstruction. CBC would not be indicated.

(Section 27: Disorders of the Respiratory System, Chapter 506: Tools for Diagnosis and Management of Respiratory Disease, Page 1925)

Answer 27-14. b

This child's history is suspicious for FBA. Plain films may be normal with FBA, but certain findings may be present that strongly support the diagnosis. If children are old enough to cooperate with breath-holding, obtaining inspiratory and expiratory radiographs increases the sensitivity of identifying air trapping and local hyperinflation from foreign body obstruction.

Decubitus views of the chest do not require cooperation for inspiratory and expiratory breath-holding and are more useful for infants and young children. With FBA, the expected deflation of the dependent lung is not seen due to the foreign body causing air trapping. Ultrasound, CT scan, and MRI would not be the first-line tests in this scenario.

(Section 27: Disorders of the Respiratory System, Chapter 506: Tools for Diagnosis and Management of Respiratory Disease, Page 1925)

Answer 27-15. c

Computed tomography (CT) angiography to evaluate pulmonary embolism (PE) is faster and more sensitive than nuclear medicine ventilation/perfusion (V/Q) scanning.

When the probability of PE is high, CT angiography is the preferred method for confirming this diagnosis. When the probability of PE is low, D-dimer may be used to help rule out the diagnosis. Ultrasound of the lower extremity can support the diagnosis of PE if a deep vein thrombosis is found, but not rule out PE. CXR and MRI have are not used in the diagnosis of PE.

(Section 27: Disorders of the Respiratory System, Chapter 506: Tools for Diagnosis and Management of Respiratory Disease, Page 1926)

Answer 27-16. c

The symptoms are most consistent with laryngomalacia. Laryngomalacia commonly presents as stridor that worsens with activity and crying. It may improve when the infant is placed in the prone position. Diagnosis is usually based on the history and physical examination. The lack of fever or other signs of upper respiratory infection make croup less likely. In more severe cases, surgery (supraglottoplasty) may be necessary; however, this infant is thriving. Bronchodilators would more likely provide relief of wheezing, such as in asthma. GERD, has been linked to laryngomalacia, and the possibility of concurrent GERD should be considered if suggested by history.

(Section 27: Disorders of the Respiratory System, Chapter 510: Disorders Causing Airway Obstruction, Page 1949)

Answer 27-17. d

PCD is a rare condition with an estimated prevalence of 1 in 15,000–30,000. Nasal congestion is a nonspecific symptom of PCD that can occur in all individuals; however, in the child who has nasal congestion from birth, PCD should be considered. In PCD, the cilia demonstrate abnormal or no motility. As a result, there is stasis of secretions, which can lead to upper and lower respiratory tract infections.

Other factors that would alert the clinician to the diagnosis of PCD are chronic wet cough, wheeze, and particularly severe recurrent sinusitis and otitis media. Situs inversus is seen in one half of people with PCD. Bronchiectasis is generally a later finding. Digital clubbing and nasal polyposis, often seen in cystic fibrosis, are not often present in PCD.

(Section 27: Disorders of the Respiratory System, Chapter 510: Disorders Causing Airway Obstruction, Page 1955)

Answer 27-18. b

Vocal cord dysfunction (VCD), also known as paradoxical vocal fold motion, has gained recognition recently as a cause of upper airway obstruction as a result of paradoxical closure of the true vocal folds during inspiration. It is most commonly seen in females and it usually presents in early adolescence. VCD may be confused with a diagnosis of asthma, and patients are placed on unnecessary medications such as corticosteroids. Spirometry may reveal attenuation of inspiratory flow with flattened inspiratory loops, indicating extrathoracic airway obstruction. Reductions in expiratory flows, reduced FEV_1/FVC ratio, and air trapping, suggested by elevated RV/TLC, are consistent with intrathoracic airway obstruction commonly seen with asthma. Restrictive lung disease with reduced TLC would not be expected. GERD and asthma may be comorbidities associated with VCD.

(Section 27: Disorders of the Respiratory System, Chapter 510: Disorders Causing Airway Obstruction, Page 1950)

Answer 27-19. e

Secretions are often trapped by collapsible airways, and airway clearance devices can be used to facilitate removal of retained secretions in children with TBM. Most infants and children with TBM have an underlying or associated problem. Cardiovascular anomalies may occur in up to 60% of the cases, and half of infants with TBM have bronchopulmonary dysplasia (BPD) and/or GER. Because it does not "stent" open collapsible airways, flexible bronchoscopy is a better alternative to rigid bronchoscopy when evaluating TBM. Bronchoscopy not only identifies the area of TBM but can determine the etiology. Plain radiographs of the neck and chest are not helpful for evaluating TBM. Fluoroscopy of the neck and chest provides a cinegraphic view of the airway, allowing the observer to determine if there is dynamic collapse of the airway. TBM will improve by 2–3 years of age, although those with tracheoesophageal fistula may have significant problems into adult years.

(Section 27: Disorders of the Respiratory System, Chapter 510: Disorders Causing Airway Obstruction, Page 1954)

Answer 27-20. a

Acute epiglottitis can progress quickly to becoming a life-threatening emergency. Children affected are usually between 2 and 8 years old. It presents quite suddenly (over 6–24 hours)

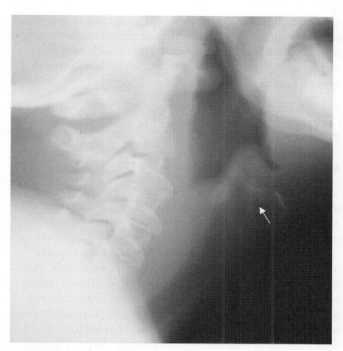

FIGURE 263-2. Lateral soft-tissue X-ray of the neck demonstrating thickening of aryepiglottic folds and thumbprint sign of epiglottis (arrow). (Reproduced, with permission, from Rudolph CD, Rudolph AM, Lister GE, First LR, Gershon AA. *Rudolph's Pediatrics.* 22nd ed. New York: McGraw-Hill, 2011.)

with high fever, irritability, throat pain, stridor, and what is known as a "hot potato" or muffled voice. Unlike croup, there is usually no preceding viral prodrome or cough. A "thumbprint sign," which describes a round and thickened epiglottis, can be seen on the X-ray (Figure 263-2).

In croup, a "steeple sign," which is the tapering of the subglottic airway, may be seen, but many patients will also have normal X-rays. Reverse curve of thoracic spine signifies an enlarged retropharyngeal space seen with retropharyngeal abscess. Irregularity of the tracheal air column (indicating sloughing of pseudomembranous material from the tracheal wall) is most consistent with bacterial tracheitis.

(Section 27: Disorders of the Respiratory System, Chapter 510: Disorders Causing Airway Obstruction, Page 1952)

Answer 27-21. d

Congenital large hyperlucent lobe (congenital lobar emphysema) is a rare condition that affects the left upper (42%), right middle (35%), right upper (21%), and lower lobes (2%). The affected lobe is overdistended and displaces adjacent structures. There is resulting respiratory distress from compression and collapse of the adjacent lung, ipsilateral depression of the diaphragm, and mediastinal shift.

Bronchogenic cysts are most often located near the carina, and are distinguished by cartilage in the wall. Chest X-ray in meconium aspiration syndrome generally shows patchy atelectasis and hyperinflation. Pulmonary sequestration occurs most often in the left lower lobe, and symptoms in neonates are uncommon. Congenital cystic adenomatoid malformations usually present as either larger (>2 cm) cysts or multiple smaller cysts. Rarely there is a fully adenomatous lesion that appears solid.

(Section 27: Disorders of the Respiratory System, Chapter 507: Congenital Disorders of the Lower Airways and Mediastinum, Page 1932)

Answer 27-22. e

The prognosis for a fetus with a congenital thoracic malformation is good as the lesions often regress in the 3rd trimester. Pulmonary sequestrations are not the only malformations with an aortic blood supply, as congenital cystic adenomatoid malformation may also have an aortic blood supply. While most abnormalities are detectable after 20 weeks, diaphragmatic hernia and pleural effusion may not be detected until later in the 3rd trimester. Congenital cystic lesions are often associated with hydrops or polyhydramnios, which may indicate poor prognosis, and has led to consideration of fetal interventions. While chest CT is the gold standard for congenital thoracic malformations, since many fetal lung lesions may regress prior to birth, chest X-ray is the recommended initial screening test, particularly for asymptomatic neonates.

(Section 27: Disorders of the Respiratory System, Chapter 507: Congenital Disorders of the Lower Airways and Mediastinum, Page 1931)

Answer 27-23. c

Nearly 80% of children with bilateral right lung have asplenia and are thus at risk of overwhelming pneumococcal sepsis. They are therefore particularly at risk from polysaccharide encapsulated bacteria, including pneumococcus, *Hemophilus influenza,* and meningococcus. Bilateral left lung is associated with polysplenia in nearly 80% of patients. Other associated abnormalities with both right and left isomerism include midline liver, malrotation of the gut, and cardiac abnormalities.

(Section 27: Disorders of the Respiratory System, Chapter 507: Congenital Disorders of the Lower Airways and Mediastinum, Page 1930)

Answer 27-24. b

Pulmonary sequestration is often diagnosed after adolescence and symptoms are uncommon in infants. Intralobar sequestration is more common than extralobar, and treatment is surgical excision. The vascular supply must be carefully delineated preoperatively.

Pulmonary arteriovenous malformation is characterized by dyspnea, cyanosis, and possibly hemoptysis, and clubbing is generally seen on exam. Bronchogenic cyst is most often located near the carina, and when infected will usually have an air fluid level. Tracheomalacia would present with wheeze and/

or stridor, and would not present with left lower lobe infiltrate. Congenital cystic adenomatoid malformations are generally multicystic abnormalities rather than a single round infiltrate.

(Section 27: Disorders of the Respiratory System, Chapter 507: Congenital Disorders of the Lower Airways and Mediastinum, Page 1931)

Answer 27-25. d

Hydrocarbon ingestion (lamp oil, solvents, paint remover, etc.) is a significant issue, especially in young children. Pneumonitis is the most common effect, but CNS depression, GI upset and cardiac problems may also be seen. The hydrocarbons with the highest potential of causing aspiration injury are those with low viscosity, low surface tension, and higher volatility. These characteristics allow for easier penetration of the hydrocarbon deep into the tracheobronchial tree and easier spread over a greater surface area.

There is a risk for secondary aspiration with emesis of material with hydrocarbons, so inducing emesis in these children should be avoided. It is important to observe children for at least 6–8 hours after a suspected aspiration, to follow serial chest radiographs, and to admit any child with respiratory symptoms or abnormal chest films for observation. Most children do recover without significant long-term sequelae.

(Section 27: Disorders of the Respiratory System, Chapter 511: Aspiration Syndromes, Page 1958)

Answer 27-26. e

Chronic aspiration from swallowing dysfunction leads to increased levels of interleukin-8 and tumor necrosis factor-alpha, and there is a significant neutrophilic migration to the site of aspiration with subsequent activation and sequestration of the neutrophils. Generally swallow dysfunction leads to chronic small-volume aspiration with typical symptoms including cough, wheeze, choking, and gagging that is temporally related to the intake of food.

Children with neuromuscular disorders are among those who are at higher risk for chronic aspiration, and those with neurologic compromise in particular are more likely to have silent aspiration of food. There are three phases of swallowing: the oral phase, pharyngeal phase, and the esophageal phase. During the pharyngeal phase, the larynx elevates and the glottis closes to prevent aspiration into the airway, and to allow relaxation of the upper esophageal sphincter so the bolus may pass into the esophagus. If left untreated, children can develop progressive irreversible lung disease that may progress to respiratory failure and death.

(Section 27: Disorders of the Respiratory System, Chapter 511: Aspiration Syndromes, Page 1959)

Answer 27-27. a

The most common location for FBA is a right sided bronchus. Therefore, unilateral hyperinflation may be seen. Inspiratory and expiratory films may be helpful to identify air trapping. Bronchiectasis would not develop this quickly, but can be a long-term sequela of untreated aspiration. Left-sided foreign body is less common, so X-ray findings on the left side would be less likely. Most foreign bodies are radiolucent, and peanuts would not be visible on chest X-ray.

(Section 27: Disorders of the Respiratory System, Chapter 511: Aspiration Syndromes, Page 1958)

Answer 27-28. d

Rigid bronchoscopy is the procedure of choice to remove foreign bodies. This allows for better control of the airway and maintains ventilation. Flexible bronchoscopy can be used, but the inability to maintain airway patency and ventilation makes it inferior to rigid bronchoscopy. It is unlikely that chest CT or Upper GI series will be helpful in the immediate management of a foreign body. The goal is to remove a foreign body, particularly in a child who is symptomatic. Therefore, a course of antibiotics is unlikely to be sufficient for resolution of symptoms long term.

(Section 27: Disorders of the Respiratory System, Chapter 511: Aspiration Syndromes, Page 1958)

Answer 27-29. c

Multichannel intraluminal impedance with pH monitoring has some advantages over standard pH probe monitoring. It can track the movement of a bolus along the length of the esophagus, and detects both acid and nonacid liquid boluses. It can tell how high in the esophagus a bolus goes, so is better able to detect pharyngeal level reflux. However, it is not yet widely available.

Standard 24-hour pH probe monitoring remains the gold standard for the diagnosis of gastroesophageal reflux, but does not differentiate acid from above (aspiration) versus below (reflux). Upper GI series can be used to diagnose reflux, but captures gastroesophageal reflux only if it happens to occur during the test. BAL can detect the presence of lipid in the lower airways, but cannot distinguish between gastroesophageal reflux and aspiration.

(Section 27: Disorders of the Respiratory System, Chapter 511: Aspiration Syndromes, Page 1959)

Answer 27-30. e

Transient wheezing, which generally resolves by school age, is associated with decreased lung function, maternal smoking during pregnancy, and exposure to other siblings or children at day care centers. This is in contrast to persistent wheezing, which is associated with RSV infection in the first year of life, family history of asthma or allergy, early allergic sensitization, and atopy.

(Section 27: Disorders of the Respiratory System, Chapter 512: Asthma, Page 1962)

Answer 27-31. b

Asthma should not limit physical activity. For patients with EIB, the airways are sensitive to changes in humidity and temperature. During exercise or vigorous physical activity, the body temperature increases and the respiratory rate increases quickly, leading to a loss of airway moisture. For some patients, these changes trigger bronchospasm.

Methods to address this issue include a gradual "warm-up" period prior to planned exercise or activity. In addition, the use of a bronchodilator prior to exercise can also help relax the airways. Sports in low humidity and cold conditions (eg, skiing, speed skating, etc.) are a greater risk for EIB compared to sports in more humid settings (eg, swimming, diving). It may be helpful to avoid exercise outdoors during high pollen counts or during days with high levels of pollution. Also, it may be helpful to wear a mask to cover the nose and mouth during exercise when the weather is cold.

(Section 27: Disorders of the Respiratory System, Chapter 512: Asthma, Pages 1962–1967)

Answer 27-32. d

According to the Expert Panel Report 3, this child would have moderate persistent asthma based on having nighttime symptoms at least once per week and likely daily symptoms given activity-related symptoms described (Figure 512-3).

Given her age, she would need to have nighttime symptoms every night to be classified as severe persistent asthma, or only 3–4 times per month to classify as mild persistent asthma. Spirometry would also be useful in classifying her asthma severity. She clearly has too many symptoms for her asthma to be considered mild intermittent. Keep in mind that an individual should be assigned to the most severe category in which any feature occurs.

(Section 27: Disorders of the Respiratory System, Chapter 512: Asthma, Page 1968)

Answer 27-33. b

Demographic factors linked to fatal asthma include: female, nonwhite and current smokers. Additional factors include those with poor adherence to the treatment plan, psychosocial factors such as stress, and socioeconomic factors. Additionally, people who report a sense of danger from there asthma are more at increased risk of asthma exacerbation or death. See Table 512-2 for additional factors associated with fatal asthma.

(Section 27: Disorders of the Respiratory System, Chapter 512: Asthma, Page 1969)

Answer 27-34. c

OSA and nocturnal asthma can present with similar symptoms. According to the National Guidelines Expert Panel Report 3, evaluation for OSA is recommended in patients with unstable, poorly controlled asthma, particularly those who are overweight or obese. Without daytime cough, fever, or acute respiratory symptoms, pneumonia or acute sinusitis

Classification of Asthma Severity in Children				
	Intermittent	Mild persistent	Moderate persistent	Severe
(Children 0–4 years of age)				
	Step 1	Step 2	Step 3/Step 4	Step 5/Step 6
Symptoms	≤2 d/w	>2 d/w, but not daily	Daily	Throughout the day
Nighttime symptoms	0	1–2 times per mo	3–4 times per mo	>1 times per w
Short-acting β₂-agonist use for symptom control	≤2 d/w	>2 d/w but not daily	Daily	Several times per day
Interference with normal activity	None	Minor limitation	Some limitation	Extremely limited
Exacerbations requiring oral systemic corticosteroids	0–1 y		≥2 in 6 months	
(Children ≥5 years of age)				
Symptoms	≤2 d/w	≤2 d/w but not daily	Daily	Throughout the day
Nighttime symptoms	≤2 times per mo	3–4 times per mo	>1 times per w but not nightly	Often 7 times per week
Short-acting β₂-agonist use for symptom control	≤2 d/w	>2 d/w but not daily	Daily	Several times per day
Interference with normal activity	None	Minor limitation	Some limitation	Extremely limited
Lung function	Normal FEV_1 between exacerbations FEV_1 >80% predicted FEV_1/FVC normal	FEV_1 ≥80% FEV_1/FVC normal	FEV_1 ≥60% but <80% predicted FEV_1/FVC reduced 5%	FEV_1 <60% predicted FEV_1/FVC reduced 5%
Exacerbations requiring oral systemic corticosteroids	0–1/year		≥2 /year	

Classification of severity of asthma by clinical features before treatment according to the guidelines for the diagnosis and management of asthma, highlights of the expert panel report 3.
An individual should be assigned to the most severe grade in which any feature occurs.
An individual's classification may change over time.
Patients at any level of severity can have mild, moderate, or severe exacerbations.
Key: FEV_1, Forced expiratory volume in 1 second; FVC, Forced vital capacity.

FIGURE 512-3. (Reproduced, with permission, from Rudolph CD, Rudolph AM, Lister GE, First LR, Gershon AA. *Rudolph's Pediatrics.* 22nd ed. New York: McGraw-Hill, 2011.)

are less likely. A methacholine challenge is unlikely to be helpful in this scenario, as it will likely be positive given the patient's history. Given the increase in asthma flares and use of rescue medications, continuing current care without further investigation is not optimal.

(Section 27: Disorders of the Respiratory System, Chapter 512: Asthma, Comorbid Conditions (only in online version))

Answer 27-35. d

This young man's symptoms are most consistent with VCD. It is most definitively diagnosed via flexible laryngoscopy with direct observation of paradoxical vocal cord movement. Spirometry can show flattened inspiratory loops, but it is not a definitive diagnostic test and is often highly variable. A methacholine challenge may be negative in the absence

TABLE 512-2. Predictors Associated with Increased Risk of Asthma Exacerbation or Death

Severe airflow obstruction, as detected by spirometry
Two or more emergency department visits or hospitalizations for asthma in the last year
History of intubation or intensive care unit admission, especially in the last 5 years
Patients report that they feel a sense of danger from their asthma
Demographics: female, nonwhite, and current smoking
Psychosocial factors: depression, increased stress, socioeconomic factors
Problems with adherence to treatment plan

of asthma, but that will not make the diagnosis of VCD. An upper GI series would likely show normal anatomy, and given the lack of abdominal symptoms, would not likely show frank reflux leading to the respiratory symptoms. However, GER can be a contributing factor to the development of VCD. A nasal ciliary biopsy would be used to diagnose ciliary dyskinesia, which is not consistent with this history.

(Section 27: Disorders of the Respiratory System, Chapter 512: Asthma, Page 1967)

Answer 27-36. d

Lung disease from BPD should improve over time. Although lung volumes and exercise capacity generally reach the normal range, there may be a persistence of airway hyperresponsiveness. Additionally, there may be evidence of impaired gas exchange. Survivors of BPD may use different ventilation strategies during exercise.

(Section 27: Disorders of the Respiratory System, Chapter 513: Bronchopulmonary Dysplasia, Page 1975)

Answer 27-37. b

GERD is one of the more common comorbidities and complications often associated with BPD. The history of increased cough after feeds and when lying down are suggestive of GER. This pattern is not typical of lower respiratory tract infection, which would likely have a more acute presentation with persistent cough and perhaps fever.

Pulmonary edema may be accompanied by edema and often with a change in vital signs with tachypnea as well. Tracheomalacia generally is worse with activity and better with sleep and when quiet. Tracheoesophageal fistula may also worsen with feeds, but would also be more likely to lead to difficulty during feeding due to aspiration. By this age, most tracheoesophageal fistulas, other than the H-type, would already have been diagnosed.

(Section 27: Disorders of the Respiratory System, Chapter 513: Bronchopulmonary Dysplasia, Page 1976)

Answer 27-38. b

BPD was first described by Northway in 1967. Premature infants with severe respiratory distress syndrome (RDS) who were treated with mechanical ventilation and oxygen supplementation developed a chronic lung disease. In this "classic" BPD, radiographs showed cysts alternating with strands of increased density, suggestive of injury and repair affecting both the parenchyma and the airways. Radiographs of "new" BPD evolve from clear lung fields to a hazy and diffuse pattern of opacification, then into evenly distributed coarse interstitial opacities.

This heterogeneous distribution of disease with regional differences in lung compliance and airway caliber, leads to ventilation–perfusion mismatch. The respiratory system compliance is reduced while airways resistance is elevated and persists beyond the newborn period. Overall lung volumes tend to be reduced, and radiographic findings in "new" BPD tend to demonstrate more evenly distributed interstitial opacities without cysts.

(Section 27: Disorders of the Respiratory System, Chapter 513: Bronchopulmonary Dysplasia, Page 1974)

Answer 27-39. c

The risk of BPD increases with lower birth weight or younger gestational age at birth. Other factors that increase the risk of BPD include factors associated with preterm birth, including:, lower socioeconomic status, African American descent, prenatal infection with *Ureaplasma ureolyticum*, and chorioamnionitis.

Although younger maternal age is associated with increased likelihood of BPD, advanced maternal age is also associated with increased likelihood of BPD. The incidence of BPD has decreased since the 1980s, but there is variation in reporting due to differences in how BPD is defined. While BPD is primarily a disorder of preterm infants, definitions have included infants with other early lung injuries such as from Group B streptococcus pneumonia, meconium aspiration syndrome, or ventilator-induced injury in term infants with pulmonary hypertension.

(Section 27: Disorders of the Respiratory System, Chapter 513: Bronchopulmonary Dysplasia, Page 1974)

Answer 27-40. e

RSV prophylaxis with palivizumab is routinely given to children under 2 years of age who have BPD and who require medical therapy in the 6 months prior to the onset of the RSV season. A significant reduction in hospitalizations for RSV has been demonstrated in this group.

Studies in the use of inhaled corticosteroids, diuretics, and bronchodilators are mixed in terms of efficacy. In older infants with BPD that has already developed, use of corticosteroids and bronchodilators has utility in those with asthma-like symptoms. Antireflux medications should be considered when gastroesophageal reflux is present, particularly in the setting of poor growth, but there is not enough information that suggests that such medications are indicated for this case.

(Section 27: Disorders of the Respiratory System, Chapter 513: Bronchopulmonary Dysplasia, Page 1976)

Answer 27-41. b

The constellation of features is most suggestive of CF-related diabetes mellitus. This complication becomes more common with age. Annual screening is recommended for early diagnosis and timely management. Insulin remains the only therapy at this time.

A pulmonary exacerbation or allergic bronchopulmonary aspergillosis would generally show a significant decline in lung function, with more respiratory symptoms. Distal intestinal obstruction syndrome (DIOS) generally presents with abdominal pain and change in bowel habits. Minimally decreased pulmonary function makes a pulmonary exacerbation less likely.

(Section 27: Disorders of the Respiratory System, Chapter 514: Cystic fibrosis, Page 1979)

Answer 27-42. a

The accepted criteria for the diagnosis of CF include are listed in Table 514-2. Diagnosis is based on a combination of clinical history and laboratory test results.

(Section 27: Disorders of the Respiratory System, Chapter 514: Cystic fibrosis, Page 1980)

Answer 27-43. c

This patient has evidence of ongoing pulmonary exacerbation that has not responded to outpatient antibiotics. In addition, the patient has continued to lose weight, and has fatigue, which may impair the ability to complete all the treatments necessary in the home. An IV antibiotic course is indicated in this scenario, and may be completed in the hospital, or in the home setting based on individual scenario.

TABLE 514-2. Diagnostic Criteria for Cystic Fibrosis[a]

Clinical History	Laboratory Evidence of Abnormal CFTR/CFTR Function
One or more characteristic phenotypic features (chronic obstructive pulmonary disease, exocrine pancreatic insufficiency, sweat salt loss syndrome, male infertility)	A positive sweat test chloride concentration >60 meq/L on a sample of at least 100 mg, obtained after maximal stimulation by pilocarpine iontophoresis
CF in a sibling or a positive newborn screen	Identification of two CFTR mutations known to cause CF
	Diagnostic nasal potential difference

[a]Diagnosis requires at least one from each column.

An appetite stimulant may be useful, but would not treat the pulmonary exacerbation, which is likely contributing to the weight loss. Allergic bronchopulmonary aspergillosis may be considered, but treatment should not be initiated until a diagnosis is confirmed. Bronchoscopy may be helpful, but generally in this situation, bronchoscopy without further treatment would not fully treat the exacerbation. It may be helpful in identifying other organisms to target with therapy. It would be early to make an assumption that this patient could not recover lung function, and aggressive treatment should be implemented before this conclusion is made.

(Section 27: Disorders of the Respiratory System, Chapter 514: Cystic fibrosis, Page 1982)

Answer 27-44. e

Class IV mutations are those of altered conductance, with CFTR that reaches the membrane but does not activate properly. These are commonly associated with pancreatic sufficiency. Delta F508 is the most common CFTR mutation, and is a class II mutation, a block in processing. A knowledge of the class of mutation involved is becoming more important as new drugs targeting specific classes are being developed.

(Section 27: Disorders of the Respiratory System, Chapter 514: Cystic fibrosis, Page 1978)

Answer 27-45. d

DIOS is often triggered in warmer months when patients become dehydrated more easily. The condition generally begins with constipation and progresses to obstruction if not treated promptly. Symptoms include crampy abdominal pain with decreased stooling, with or without emesis. It is usually treated with enemas followed by polyethylene glycol. Enzyme therapy should be reviewed and optimized.

The symptoms described are not classic for GERD or gallstones. Intussusception can present with similar symptoms, but may also include currant jelly stools, and is less common than DIOS. Fibrosing colonopathy is uncommon, and generally is seen when high doses of enzymes are being used. Fibrosing colonopathy generally presents with signs of obstruction and bloody stools.

(Section 27: Disorders of the Respiratory System, Chapter 514: Cystic fibrosis, Page 1985)

Answer 27-46. c

The patient is homozygous for a mutation that causes Alpha1-antitrysin deficiency.

The major role of AAT is to inhibit NE, the mechanism for which is correctly described in correct answer choice C. However AAT has many other substrates, including proteinase 3, cathepsins, and alpha-defensins (making choice B incorrect). Decreased levels of AAT as seen in Alpha1-antitrypsin deficiency lead to uncontrolled apoptosis in the lung, which could lead to lung damage, making choice A incorrect. In addition, in Alpha1-antitrypsin deficiency, decreased levels of AAT lead to neutrophil *accumulation*, and not elimination, making choice D incorrect. AAT appears to be cytoprotective by inhibition of enzyme activities, so it is not destructive to airway cells, making choice E incorrect.

(Section 27: Disorders of the Respiratory System; Chapter 516: Alpha-1 Antitrypsin Lung Disease, Page 1989)

Answer 27-47. d

Although some forms of alpha1-antitrypsin manifest during the neonatal period (eg, liver disease), the average age of diagnosis of alpha1-antitrypsin deficiency lung disease is 52 years of age. Based on the clinical vignette, the patient has chronic obstructive pulmonary disease and, with "panacinar emphysema" as demonstrated on chest CT scan, is likely to have alpha1-antitrypsin deficiency.

Tuberculin skin testing for tuberculosis, video-assisted thoracoscopic lung biopsy, flexible bronchoscopy with BAL, and nasal potential difference for cystic fibrosis are not likely to be helpful in making this patient's diagnosis. The patient should have a total plasma level of alpha1-antitrypsin drawn, as well as isoelectric focusing to verify the presence of an abnormal migration pattern or absence of the normal M band, or both.

(Section 27: Disorders of the Respiratory System; Chapter 516: Alpha-1 Antitrypsin Lung Disease, Page 1990)

Answer 27-48. a

The patient described above is at risk for development of complications of alpha1-antitrypsin deficiency. At his young age, he has not yet developed lung disease but he is at risk for this condition, especially if he has personal or second-hand exposure to environmental tobacco smoke. Therefore, choice A, avoidance of tobacco smoke, is the most important piece of anticipatory guidance to give the family.

Choices B through E are not practical and there is no evidence that using these measures will help *prevent* the development of alpha1-antitrypsin lung disease. In a patient who already has evidence of alpha1-antitrypsin lung disease (airway obstruction, chronic cough or other respiratory symptoms), Choices B (antibiotics) and E (corticosteroids), may be warranted.

(Section 27: Disorders of the Respiratory System; Chapter 516: Alpha-1 Antitrypsin Lung Disease, Page 1990)

Answer 27-49. b

Replacement therapy for alpha1-antitrypsin deficiency is recommended *weekly* by IV infusion rather than *aerosol*. However, it has been difficult to demonstrate improvement in pulmonary function over time with IV AAT, perhaps given the episodic nature of pulmonary symptoms, the variability in pulmonary function measurements and the slow rate of decline in lung function with the disease.

Choice B is correct because the primary endpoint of therapy and the key to avoiding progression of lung disease has been considered restoration of plasma levels of AAT above 11 micromoles. Finally, for those patients who receive lung transplantation, AAT levels are still insufficient and replacement therapy for AAT is still needed.

(Section 27: Disorders of the Respiratory System; Chapter 516: Alpha-1 Antitrypsin Lung Disease, Page 1990)

Answer 27-50. e

The girl described in the vignette has a small- to medium-vessel vasculitis with inflammation of these vessels on lung pathology. Choices A through D all fit into this category of small to medium-vessel vasculitis. Only Takayasu arteritis (Choice E) is incorrect, because this is a large-vessel vasculitis.

(Section 27: Disorders of the Respiratory System; Chapter 517: Pulmonary Vasculitis Syndromes, Page 1991)

Answer 27-51. d

The girl described in the vignette is most likely to have Wegener granulomatosis, based on the triad of involvement of upper respiratory tract with sinusitis and epistaxis, lower respiratory tract with history of pneumonia and likely pulmonary hemorrhage, as well as the kidney, with proteinuria and renal insufficiency.

Churg–Strauss syndrome is incorrect because it is more likely to be associated with asthma and eosinophilia, and is very rare in the pediatric population. Polyarteritis nodosa is not usually associated with upper respiratory findings, but instead may involve fever, weight loss, arthritis, skin lesions, and central nervous system disease. Behcet disease is a large-vessel vasculitis more likely associated with oral and genital ulcers and iritis rather than upper and lower respiratory and kidney findings. Sarcoidosis is a multisystem granulomatous disease, typically with multiple organ involvement, but respiratory symptoms are more likely to include cough and dyspnea rather than pulmonary hemorrhage.

(Section 27: Disorders of the Respiratory System; Chapter 517: Pulmonary Vasculitis Syndromes, Page 1991)

Answer 27-52. b

The patient described in the vignette has severe respiratory distress with continuing hemoptysis and his airway needs to be protected. Following basic cardiopulmonary resuscitation measures, attention to airway, breathing, and circulation should ensue before other interventions. Therefore, intubation is the correct next step in treatment. The patient may need a blood transfusion, but this would occur after initial assessment and stabilization. The patient does not yet require chest compressions as he has an adequate heart rate and blood pressure. The patient also likely has Wegener granulomatosis and may at some point require IV corticosteroids or IV cyclophosphamide as part of the chronic therapy, but these would not be the next step in acute management of his hemoptysis and respiratory distress.

(Section 27: Disorders of the Respiratory System; Chapter 517: Pulmonary Vasculitis Syndromes, Page 1993)

Answer 27-53. c

The child in the clinical vignette is suspected to have a pulmonary vasculitis syndrome. Although the approach to diagnosis varies depending on the clinical presentation, in this case the most appropriate next diagnostic test to obtain would be a complete blood cell count and differential, as this would help evaluate for anemia with the hemoglobin and hematocrit as well as for inflammation with the white blood cell count and platelet count. Next steps in evaluation may include all of the other choices provided, but initial evaluation with inflammatory markers may help to guide the differential diagnosis. Flexible bronchoscopy with BAL may be considered after chest radiograph or CT scan. Ophthalmologic evaluation may be considered to assess for uveitis, especially if there are eye symptoms or findings on physical examination. Double stranded DNA antibody testing is incorrect as this would usually be performed after a positive serum antinuclear antibody (ANA) test is positive. Choice E is incorrect as ANCA testing would also be considered, but a complete blood cell count would be warranted first.

(Section 27: Disorders of the Respiratory System; Chapter 517: Pulmonary Vasculitis Syndromes, Page 1992)

Answer 27-54. e

The most likely diagnoses for the patient in the vignette include polygranulomatosis with angiitis (PGA) and microscopic polyangiitis, both of which are antineutrophil cytoplasmic antibody (ANCA)-associated vasculitides. Therefore, the best answer is Choice E, antineutrophil cytoplasmic antibodies. C-reactive protein is likely to be elevated with pulmonary vasculitides but is not specific, so will not help confirm the diagnosis. Angiotensin converting enzyme level is incorrect as this would likely be elevated with sarcoidosis rather than with Wegener granulomatosis or microscopic polyangiitis, which are the 2 diagnoses under consideration based on the clinical vignette. Antiribonucleoprotein antibody is incorrect as this would be elevated in mixed connective tissue disease. Antiphospholipid antibody profile is incorrect as this would be ordered to give an assessment of autoimmune related thrombosis risk rather than confirm the diagnosis of either Wegener granulomatosis or microscopic polyangiitis.

(Section 27: Disorders of the Respiratory System; Chapter 517: Pulmonary Vasculitis Syndromes, Page 1992)

Answer 27-55. e

Surfactant protein C deficiencies are autosomal dominant or sporadic and are associated with interstitial lung disease. The function of pulmonary surfactant is to *reduce* surface tension, which prevents alveolar collapse. Surfactant is composed

primarily of lipids (90%) and also of proteins (10%). Surfactant is secreted by type II alveolar epithelial cells, not type I cells. Surfactant protein B deficiencies occur in an estimated 1 in 1 to 1.5 million births.

(Section 27: Disorders of the Respiratory System; Chapter 518: Pulmonary Alveolar Proteinosis, Page 1994)

Answer 27-56. e

Lung histopathology in primary alveolar proteinosis (PAP), which is caused by granulocyte/macrophage-colony stimulating factor receptor α chain dysfunction, is most consistent with that described in the vignette. Namely, there is preserved alveolar wall architecture but filling of the alveoli with surfactant. All of the other answer choices are incorrect as they are associated with surfactant metabolic dysfunction disorders whose pathological findings include fibrosis, alveolar wall thickening, and significant parenchymal lung distortion.

(Section 27: Disorders of the Respiratory System; Chapter 518: Pulmonary Alveolar Proteinosis, Page 1995)

Answer 27-57. d

The child described in the vignette is most likely to have ABCA-3 mutations leading to surfactant dysfunction, especially given the ground-glass appearance throughout both lungs on chest CT scan, as opposed to PAP, in which there are normal-appearing secondary pulmonary lobules adjacent to highly abnormal secondary lobules. Therefore, Choice D is correct, as genetic testing for surfactant mutations should be performed before lung biopsy since this is less invasive, as long as the patient is stable enough to do so.

BAL for surfactant levels is incorrect because this is performed on research basis only and is not routinely recommended for clinical decision-making. If genetic testing for surfactant mutations is negative, then genetic testing for lysinuric protein intolerance should be considered. Therefore Choice C is incorrect as ABCA-3 mutation testing should be performed first. Lung biopsy plays a more important role in diagnosing PAP, rather than genetic testing for granulocyte/macrophage-colony stimulating factor receptor α chain mutations. Based on the clinical and radiologic appearance, the patient described above is more likely to have ABCA-3 dysfunction rather than PAP.

(Section 27: Disorders of the Respiratory System; Chapter 518: Pulmonary Alveolar Proteinosis, Page 1995)

Answer 27-58. c

Treatment for pulmonary surfactant dysfunction disorders typically includes first supportive care, including oxygen supplementation and nutritional support. Therefore, treatment should begin with supplemental oxygen. Surfactant administration is incorrect because in older children surfactant administration does not result in improvement in clinical condition. Whole lung lavage is incorrect because this technique is technically challenging and of uncertain efficacy.

Chronic systemic steroids is incorrect because although the use of chronic steroids has been reported, there are no controlled studies supporting their clinical utility. Lung transplantation is incorrect because it should be considered in severe and progressive disease from ABCA3 mutations, but not before supportive care such as supplemental oxygen is given.

(Section 27: Disorders of the Respiratory System; Chapter 518: Pulmonary Alveolar Proteinosis, Page 1995)

Answer 27-59. a

Given the clinical scenarios described above, the one most likely to describe a patient with autoimmune pulmonary alveolar proteinosis is Choice A, an adult who was previously healthy.

Choice B is more likely to describe primary pulmonary alveolar proteinosis, where there is insidious onset of dyspnea in infancy, or one of the surfactant mutations. Choice C is incorrect as it describes a child who has risk for secondary pulmonary alveolar proteinosis. Choice D is incorrect as it is more likely to describe surfactant protein B deficiency or one of the surfactant deficiencies. Choice E is incorrect as it is more likely to describe surfactant protein C or ABCA3 deficiencies.

(Section 27: Disorders of the Respiratory System; Chapter 518: Pulmonary Alveolar Proteinosis, Page 1994)

Answer 27-60. b

Choice B is correct because laryngeal braking helps to maintain an adequate volume of air in the thorax, thus helping to maintain FRC. The chest wall of the newborn infant is actually very compliant much more so that the chest wall of an adult.

Due to the increased compliance of an infant's chest wall, there is an increased likelihood of collapse inward. As an infant ages, *more* of the diaphragm is actually in direct contact with the inner surface of the thoracic cavity. Choice E is incorrect because premature termination of the expiratory phase rather than prolonged expiration helps to maintain FRC.

(Section 27: Disorders of the Respiratory System; Chapter 519: Chest Wall and Respiratory Muscle Disorders, Page 1996)

Answer 27-61. d

Choice D is correct because the sternocleidomastoids help to lift the sternum and increase intrathoracic volume by a "bucket handle" mechanism. Choices A and B are incorrect because although the scalenes and serratus anterior are accessory muscles of inspiration, their mechanisms of action do not involve the "bucket handle" movement. Choice C is incorrect as the function of the diaphragm is to act like a piston and increase intrathoracic volume by displacing abdominal contents downward. Choice E is incorrect because the external intercostals act to the increase the anteroposterior diameter of the thorax.

(Section 27: Disorders of the Respiratory System; Chapter 519: Chest Wall and Respiratory Muscle Disorders, Page 1996)

Answer 27-62. b

Choice B is correct because with neuromuscular weakness as in Duchenne muscular dystrophy, there are decreases in lung volumes but increased residual volume to total lung capacity ratio (RV/TLC). The total lung capacity should be low, not elevated. The relationships of the different lung volume measurements are shown in Figure 503-3.

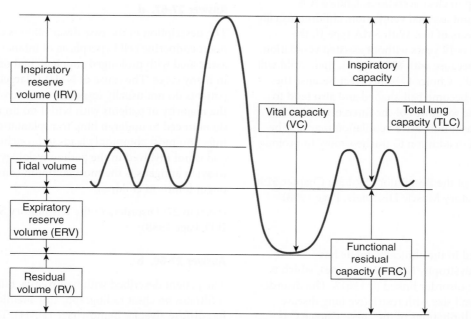

FIGURE 503-3. Fractional lung volume measurements. After measurement of FRC by dilution or plethysmography, and FVC and ERV by spirometry, RV (FRC-ERV), and TLC (RV + VC) are calculated arithmetically. FRC, functional residual capacity; FVC, forced vital capacity; ERV, expiratory reserve volume; RV, residual volume; TLC, total lung capacity; VC, vital capacity. (Reproduced, with permission, from Rudolph CD, Rudolph AM, Lister GE, First LR, Gershon AA. *Rudolph's Pediatrics.* 22nd ed. New York: McGraw-Hill, 2011.)

With neuromuscular weakness there should also be reduced muscle pressures, including maximum expiratory pressure. End-tidal carbon dioxide is more likely to be elevated, rather than decreased, in cases of neuromuscular weakness due to hypoventilation. Choice E is incorrect because these patients should have normal or low oxyhemoglobin saturations.

(Section 27: Disorders of the Respiratory System; Chapter 519: Chest Wall and Respiratory Muscle Disorders, Page 1997)

Answer 27-63. a

Choice A is correct because the internal intercostal muscles are accessory muscles of expiration which may be utilized during exercise. Contraction decreases the anteroposterior diameter of the thorax, aiding in expiration.

Choice B is incorrect because the abdominal muscles are also accessory muscles of expiration, not inspiration. Choice C is incorrect because expiration is passive only during normal tidal breathing, not during exercise, coughing, sneezing, or speaking. Choices D and E are incorrect because both the sternocleidomastoids and serratus anterior muscles are accessory muscles of inspiration rather than expiration.

(Section 27: Disorders of the Respiratory System; Chapter 519: Chest Wall and Respiratory Muscle Disorders, Page 1996)

Answer 27-64. e

The infant described in the vignette has spinal muscular atrophy (SMA) type I (Wernig–Hoffman disease) due to presentation as an infant with the above described clinical features. Choice E is correct as cough is expected to be impaired and the use of a cough assist device (mechanical in-exsufflator) will help to clear secretions. Choice A is incorrect because without assisted ventilation, children usually die within the first 2 years of life. With SMA type II, the median age of survival is 12 years without assisted ventilation. Choice B is incorrect because with SMA type I, their child will not be able to sit or walk. Choice C is incorrect because the chest wall may start to become bell-shaped and also tend to draw inward, due to the weakness of the intercostal muscles. Choice D is incorrect as noninvasive ventilation may also be presented as an option in addition to tracheostomy to prolong survival.

(Section 27: Disorders of the Respiratory System; Chapter 519: Chest Wall and Respiratory Muscle Disorders, Page 1998)

Answer 27-65. c

The newborn described in the clinical vignette has asphyxiating thoracic dystrophy (Jeune syndrome), which is an autosomal recessive disorder linked to 15q13. The disorder results in fixed chest wall size with restrictive lung disease due to the mechanical limitations of the chest. Choice C is correct because the vertically expandable prosthetic titanium rib placement has been used for treating children with thoracic dystrophy.

Choice D is incorrect, unfortunately, because in this patient recurrent pneumonia is likely given the restrictive lung disease and tendency for atelectasis. Choice E is incorrect as achondroplasia is an autosomal dominant condition associated with dwarfism but not with the characteristic features of the narrow bell-shaped chest with shortened ribs as described above for Jeune syndrome.

(Section 27: Disorders of the Respiratory System; Chapter 519: Chest Wall and Respiratory Muscle Disorders, Page 1997)

Answer 27-66. d

The girl described in the vignette has digital clubbing of the fingers and toes. Choice D is correct because clubbing is associated with increased caliber and number of blood vessels, as well as primitive fibroblasts and an increased number of lymphocytes and eosinophils.

Choice A is incorrect because in a girl with chronic productive cough and poor growth, clubbing is likely a sign of respiratory disease, such as bronchiectasis due to cystic fibrosis or other causes, chronic lung infection, or pulmonary abscess. Choice B is incorrect because with clubbing, the depth of the finger at the proximal nail fold exceeds the depth of the distal interphalangeal joint. Choice C is incorrect because clubbing is usual painless and *not* recognized by the patient. Choice E is incorrect because when clubbing is present, Schamroth sign is present; that is there is an obliteration of the normal rhombus that is seen when the dorsal surfaces of the right and left index finger are placed against each other.

(Section 27: Disorders of the Respiratory System; Chapter 505: Clinical Presentation of Respiratory Illness, Page 1923)

Answer 27-67. d

The description in the case description is consistent with neuroendocrine cell hyperplasia of infancy (NEHI), which is associated with prolonged supplemental oxygen requirement in many cases. The cause of NEHI is largely unknown, and patients do not usually respond to corticosteroids. Luckily, the majority of patients with NEHI do improve over time and do not need to undergo lung transplantation. Adenovirus infection most commonly leads to bronchiolitis obliterans (BO) and is not involved in the pathophysiology of NEHI. Exposure to avian antigens is the most common cause of hypersensitivity pneumonitis in children.

(Section 27: Disorders of the Respiratory System; Chapter 515: ILD, Page 1988)

Answer 27-68. b

The patient described with hypoxemia, bilateral diffuse infiltrates on chest radiograph, and anemia most likely has diffuse alveolar hemorrhage (DAH). The next step in management would be to confirm pulmonary hemorrhage by looking for hemosiderin-stained macrophages in the BAL fluid. Lung biopsy would be performed to look for pulmonary

Disorders of the Respiratory System

capillaritis, but due to the invasiveness of the procedure, one would perform BAL to confirm pulmonary hemorrhage first, then serologic tests to rule out immune-mediated lung disease, cardiac evaluation, followed by lung biopsy. High-dose intravenous corticosteroids are used for idiopathic pulmonary hemosiderosis and other causes of pulmonary hemorrhage, but are not indicated for immediate management unless the diffuse alveolar hemorrhage is life-threatening. High-resolution CT of the chest would not be performed next in the management of this patient as it may not provide much additional information and would expose the patient to unnecessary radiation. Surfactant protein B and C mutations cause surfactant dysfunction and can be associated with respiratory distress, but not characteristically with anemia in combination with infiltrates on chest radiograph.

(Section 27: Disorders of the Respiratory System; Chapter 515: ILD, Page 1987)

Answer 27-69. e

The patient described in the clinical vignette has BO following lung transplantation for cystic fibrosis. BO affects small- to medium-sized airways and causes obstruction during exhalation. Chronic rejection can manifest as BO. Median time to diagnosis of BO post-transplant is 16–20 months.

Lung biopsy may not be necessary for diagnosis if clinical signs and symptoms as well as radiography are consistent with the diagnosis. Still, treatment should begin with corticosteroids and consideration of lung biopsy should occur if there is no improvement with therapy. Unfortunately, BO following lung transplantation usually follows a progressive course, so treatment is indicated, thus eliminating Choice A. Although steroids are often given and have been somewhat helpful in the treatment of BO, the studies behind this practice are lacking. Anti-TNF has been used in BO related to bone marrow transplantation, but not related to lung transplantation. Lung biopsy would help confirm the diagnosis, but bronchoscopy with BAL would not in and of itself help make the diagnosis.

(Section 27: Disorders of the Respiratory System; Chapter 515: ILD, Page 1988)

Answer 27-70. b

Children with OSA do have impaired arousal responses to obstructive events. The upper airway behaves as a collapsible tube, therefore *increased* inspiratory effort (rather than decreased inspiratory effort as in Choice A) may only result in more collapse of the airway rather than increased flow. Choice C is incorrect as the growth rate of lymphadenoid tissue is proportional to other tissues within the upper airway in children aged 2–8 years, contrary to popular belief. Choice D is incorrect because pharyngeal airway neuromotor responses are impaired in children with OSA compared to normal children. Choice E is incorrect because hypoxic and hypercapnic ventilatory drive appears to be normal in children

with OSA; however, centrally mediated augmentation of upper airway neuromotor function is abnormal.

(Section 27: Disorders of the Respiratory System; Chapter 508: Disorders of Respiratory Control and Sleep Disordered Breathing, Page 1939)

Answer 27-71. c

OSA in infants is more common in children with chromosomal disorders such as trisomy 21 or with craniofacial abnormalities and any disease leading to upper airway inflammation, such as laryngomalacia. OSA is also more likely in premature infants and in males, which may be attributable to sex- related differences in anatomy or to a protective role of female hormones. Thus, OSA in infants is more common in males. Choice B is incorrect because MRI and manometry studies have shown that infants with clinically significant OSA are more likely to have upper airway obstruction in the retropalatal region (80%) compared with the retroglossal region (20%). Choice D is incorrect because OSA in infants is commonly associated with hypoxemia. This finding is likely due to the higher chest wall compliance in infants and the need for dynamically active maintenance of FRC. Therefore, in sleep when FRC is reduced, infants are more likely to desaturate, even in the absence of apnea. Choice E is incorrect because the laryngeal chemoreflex is more likely to play a role in an infant than in an older child as the reflex is reduced with maturation. The reflex is more prominent in premature infants as well, such that episodes of gastroesophageal reflux can lead to apnea and bradycardia.

(Section 27: Disorders of the Respiratory System; Chapter 508: Disorders of Respiratory Control and Sleep Disordered Breathing, Page 1940)

Answer 27-72. c

CCHS is inherited in autosomal dominant fashion, rather than in an autosomal recessive manner. There are also de novo mutations described. CCHS is a lifelong disorder and patients usually require up to 24 hours per day of assisted ventilation. Hirschsprung disease is found in 20% of CCHS patients, while autonomic neural crest tumors such as neuroblastoma are found in 5–10% of CCHS patients, making Choice C the correct answer. The most common mutations causing CCHS are those in the PHOX2B gene, which plays essential roles in the embryogenesis of the autonomic nervous system. Ventilation is actually most affected during quiet or NREM sleep, a time when autonomic control is most prominent.

(Section 27: Disorders of the Respiratory System; Chapter 508: Disorders of Respiratory Control and Sleep Disordered Breathing, Page 1935)

Answer 27-73. a

This question describes a young girl with Rett syndrome, who is likely to have abnormal cardiorespiratory patterns and can have hyperventilation, apnea, breath holding, and rapid shallow-breathing during wakefulness and sleep. This disorder is caused by a mutation in the MeCP2 gene as described in Choice A.

Choice B describes the microdeletion defect characteristic of Prader–Willi syndrome, a disorder that can lead to excessive daytime sleepiness or disturbances in circadian rhythms. Obesity and hypotonia may also lead to OSA in Prader–Willi syndrome. Choice C is incorrect as the inheritance for Rett syndrome is not autosomal dominant. The cerebellar abnormalities described in Choice D are associated with Joubert syndrome. The respiratory manifestations of Joubert syndrome include marked hyperpnea with severe alveolar hypoventilation. Finally, Choice E is incorrect as this describes familial dysautonomia (Riley–Day syndrome), in which abnormalities in the autonomic nervous system leads to inappropriate cardiovascular or catecholamine responses to physical stress, exercise or position change. Patients can have breath-holding episodes with emotional outbursts, as well as periodic breathing and central apnea during sleep.

(Section 27: Disorders of the Respiratory System; Chapter 508: Disorders of Respiratory Control and Sleep Disordered Breathing, Page 1937)

Answer 27-74. e

Based on the clinical information, the infant was born prematurely and may be more at risk for apnea of prematurity, which is defined as pauses in breathing of greater than 20 seconds or an apneic event of less than 20 seconds but associated with bradycardia or cyanosis. However, as the baby has a low grade temperature of 38 degrees in addition to the apneic pauses, it is prudent to rule out underlying sepsis or infection as a cause of apnea as in Choice E. Central nervous system problems should also be ruled out and a head ultrasound would be indicated after a thorough evaluation looking for infection. pH probe could be done to look for gastroesophageal reflux; however, infection and intracranial abnormalities would take precedence over this evaluation. In addition, there is no clear evidence that treating gsatroesophageal reflux, if present, will lead to a decrease in the frequency or severity of apnea of prematurity in preterm infants.

Treatment for apnea of prematurity with caffeine citrate should not be initiated until sepsis, seizure disorders and severe GERD have been ruled out, since caffeine can lower the seizure threshold and decrease muscle tone in the esophageal sphincter. Treatment of apnea of prematurity with CPAP may also be considered if apnea is frequent or severe; however, evaluation for other etiologies should be undertaken first as described above.

(Section 27: Disorders of the Respiratory System; Chapter 508: Disorders of Respiratory Control and Sleep Disordered Breathing, Page 1938)

Answer 27-75. d

The assessment of OSA involves clinical history and examination and then polysomnogram. Choice D is correct because in young children the measurement of transcutaneous carbon dioxide tension is recommended in addition to end-tidal capnography to increase the sensitivity of the test. This assessment is needed because in children, complete obstructive events are less likely due to the resistance of the pediatric upper airway to collapse. Therefore, the complete obstructive events are often replaced by prolonged periods of increased upper airway resistance leading to alveolar hypoventilation, which may be detected by transcutaneous carbon dioxide tension measurement. Choice A is incorrect as the clinical history, even when performed by a sleep medicine specialist, does not have high predictive accuracy for OSA. At this time, the gold standard for diagnosis is only the overnight polysomnogram, and not overnight pulse oximetry as in Choice B. Other methods for making the diagnosis are being evaluated such as video monitoring and overnight pulse oximetry. Choice C is incorrect because more children actually report excessive daytime sleepiness than initially thought; the numbers indicate 40–50% of children have this complaint. Finally, Choice E is incorrect because children are less likely to have electroencephalographic arousals following obstructive events and sleep architecture is more likely preserved in children.

(Section 27: Disorders of the Respiratory System; Chapter 508: Disorders of Respiratory Control and Sleep Disordered Breathing, Page 1941)

CHAPTER 28 | Endocrinology

Andrea K. Goldyn and Todd D. Nebesio

28-1. A 16-year-old boy presents to his primary care physician after noticing an asymmetric enlargement in his neck. On exam, neuromas were noted on his tongue and he has a marfanoid body habitus. Thyroidectomy revealed medullary thyroid cancer.

What is the most likely genetic cause of this child's disorder?

a. Gain of function in the *RET* proto-oncogene

b. Inactivating mutation in the *RET* proto-oncogene

c. Germline mutation in the *MEN1* gene

d. Mutation in the *PRKARIA* gene

e. Activating mutations of the G-protein subunit of adenyl cyclase system

28-2. A 12-year-old male is seen in clinic for a well-child visit. On exam, he has adult body odor, scant axillary hair, Tanner stage III pubic hair, and 8 mL testes bilaterally.

Which of the following statements about normal male puberty is correct?

a. The onset of puberty in males is defined as an increase in testicular volume to 8 mL

b. The serum concentration of prolactin increases in normal male puberty

c. The circulation of LH stimulates testosterone secretion by Leydig cells

d. The circulation of FSH stimulates spermatogenesis in Leydig cells

e. The circulation of inhibin stimulates FSH secretion

28-3. Which of the following scenarios depicts abnormal pubertal development?

a. A 14-year-old girl who grows 2 inches after menarche

b. A 14-year-old girl with Tanner stage I breast development

c. A 12-year-old boy with 3-mL testicles bilaterally

d. A 13-year-old girl with Tanner stage II breast development on the right and Tanner stage III breast development on the left

e. A 10-year-old girl who has achieved menarche

28-4. A 5-year-old female presents to clinic for concerns about breast development that began 1 year ago. On exam, she has Tanner stage III breasts, estrogenization of her vaginal mucosa, and Tanner stage II pubic hair. Since her last well-child visit, she has developed a seizure disorder. A bone age reveals that her skeletal age is closest to 8 years. A brain MRI revealed a pedunculated mass in the region of the posterior hypothalamus, which projects into the suprasellar cistern. What is the most likely diagnosis for this patient?

a. Optic glioma

b. Craniopharyngioma

c. Ependymoma

d. Astrocytoma

e. Hamartoma of the tuber cinereum

28-5. Which of the following is true in familial gonadotropin-independent sexual precocity?

a. Affected girls achieve menarche before age 7

b. Fertility is negatively affected in adulthood

c. Testicular enlargement is more pronounced than penile enlargement

d. Results from an activating mutation of the LH receptor

e. Elevated testosterone with elevated gonadotropin concentrations is common

28-6. A 5-year-old girl has had recent concerns of weight loss, restlessness, and difficulty going to sleep at night. Laboratory testing reveals that she is hyperthyroid. On exam, she has multiple jagged hyperpigmented macules on her truck that do not cross the mid-line. She also has Tanner stage II breast development. What is her most likely diagnosis?

  a. Peutz–Jeghers syndrome

  b. McCune–Albright syndrome

  c. Classic congenital adrenal hyperplasia

  d. Familial gonadotropin-independent puberty

  e. Granulosa cell tumor

28-7. Which of the following statements is true regarding premature thelarche?

  a. Small for gestational age is a risk factor

  b. Gonadotropin levels are in pubertal ranges

  c. Most cases are self-limited and benign

  d. Patients are at an increased risk for polycystic ovarian syndrome in adulthood

  e. Most case occur after the age of 4 years

28-8. A 16-month-old black male is seen in clinic for a well-child visit. On history, his mother states that he has not started to walk and was exclusively breast fed until 14 months. On physical exam, his anterior fontanelle is open, wrists appear thickened, and he is below the 3rd percentile for both length and weight.

  Which of the following laboratory results are most consistent with his diagnosis?

  a. Decreased calcium, increased phosphate, normal alkaline phosphatase, normal parathyroid hormone (PTH)

  b. Decreased calcium, decreased phosphate, increased alkaline phosphatase, increased PTH

  c. Increased calcium, decreased phosphate, decreased alkaline phosphatase, increased PTH

  d. Decreased calcium, decreased phosphate, decreased alkaline phosphatase, decreased PTH

  e. Increased calcium, increased phosphate, increased alkaline phosphatase, increased PTH

28-9. A 4-day-old infant presents for his first clinic visit after birth. The child was born full term to a healthy mother with no significant past medical history. The child was diagnosed with congenital hypothyroidism by the newborn screen. On exam, heart rate and blood pressure were normal and no goiter or neck masses were appreciated. What is the most common reason for congenital hypothyroidism in this child?

  a. Thyroid dysfunction due to prematurity

  b. Maternal antithyroid antibodies

  c. Ingestion of goitrogenic substances by the mother

  d. Inborn defects in thyroid hormone synthesis or action

  e. Defect in thyroid embryogenesis

28-10. Which statement is true regarding congenital hypothyroidism?

  a. Three to 5% of infants with the disorder are not detected on the newborn screen

  b. The incidence of congenital hypothyroidism is 1:400

  c. Preferred thyroid hormone preparation for therapy is triiodothyronine

  d. Physical growth and development are not normalized by early and adequate therapy

  e. The diagnosis is confirmed by serum measurements of thyroid-stimulating hormone (TSH) and T3

28-11. An 8-year-old boy presents to clinic for concerns about early pubertal development. On history, his father noted testicular and penile enlargement without pubic hair development in the past year along with intermittent fatigue. On exam, he has a slightly enlarged thyroid, delayed relaxation phase of his patellar reflexes, and his growth channel has fallen from the 50th to the 10th percentile on the height chart. A bone age is read as 4 years.

  Which laboratory value is most likely seen in this patient?

  a. Normal TSH of 1.0 mU/L

  b. Elevated free T4 of 7.0 ng/dL

  c. Elevated TSH of 600 mU/L

  d. Normal free T4 of 1.8 ng/dL

  e. Mildly elevated TSH 6.0 mU/L

28-12. A 9-year-old healthy girl presents for her yearly well child visit. On physical exam, her thyroid is full, smooth, symmetric, and easily palpable. Blood tests reveal that her TSH is mildly elevated at 9.634 mcU/mL and total T4 is normal at 6.5 mcg/dL.

  Which of the following is the best additional test to perform to confirm the diagnosis?

  a. MRI of the brain

  b. Thyroid ultrasound

  c. TSH receptor antibody

  d. Thyroid peroxidase antibody

  e. Total T3 level

28-13. A 14-year-old female presents to the clinic for the second time in 3 months for concerns about depression and declining school performance. She has been on an antidepressant for the past two months without improvement of her symptoms. On physical exam, her pulse rate was 144 beats per minute and blood pressure was 154/68. Proximal muscle weakness was detected on exam. Of the following hormones, which is most likely to be elevated?

a. Thyroid-stimulating hormone

b. Estradiol

c. LH

d. Thyroxine (T4)

e. Follicle-stimulating hormone (FSH)

28-14. A 17-year-old male was diagnosed with Graves disease 2 years ago and has been on antithyroid medication (methimazole) since diagnosis. What clinical prognostic sign is most likely to suggest remission of his Graves disease when antithyroid medication is discontinued?

a. Resolution of orbitopathy

b. Resolution of goiter

c. Resolution of widened pulse pressure

d. Resolution of muscle weakness

e. Maintenance of a normal body mass index (BMI)

28-15. Which statement is true regarding the metabolism and action of thyroid hormones?

a. T3 and reverse T3 (rT3) are produced at different rates

b. The thyroid gland is the sole source of T3

c. Deiodination is the main pathway of thyroid hormone metabolism

d. The concentration of T4 is 50 to 100 times less than that of T3

e. T4 is more potent than T3

28-16. Of the following conditions, which are associated with an increased prevalence of autoimmune thyroid disease and require periodic screening for hypothyroidism?

a. Type 1 diabetes, Turner syndrome, and Down syndrome

b. Turner syndrome, Prader–Willi syndrome, and McCune–Albright syndrome

c. Down syndrome, type 1 diabetes, and congenital adrenal hyperplasia (CAH)

d. Prader Willi syndrome, Down syndrome, and CAH

e. McCune–Albright syndrome, type 1 diabetes, and CAH

28-17. A 39-week gestation infant was born after an uneventful pregnancy. Following delivery, the infant has respiratory distress and is found to have truncus arteriosus. Further examination reveals a low calcium (6.0 mg/dL) and low PTH. What is this child's most likely diagnosis?

a. Williams syndrome

b. DiGeorge syndrome

c. Neonatal Graves disease

d. Beckwith–Wiedemann syndrome

e. Congenital hypothyroidism

28-18. An 11-year-old boy presents to clinic for concerns about short stature. He has been consistently growing at the 3rd percentile for the last 10 years. On exam, his weight is at the 75th percentile. He has a round face with a flattened nasal bridge. Brachydactyly and small cutaneous nodules are felt beneath the skin of his finger tips. Which of the following laboratory results are the most representative of this child's diagnosis?

a. Low PTH, low calcium, low phosphorous

b. Elevated PTH, elevated calcium, elevated phosphorous

c. Elevated PTH, low calcium, elevated phosphorous

d. Low PTH, elevated calcium, elevated phosphorous

e. Elevated PTH, elevated calcium, low phosphorous

28-19. A 10-year-old boy presents to an emergency room with fever and dehydration. During the evaluation, a basic metabolic panel is drawn and reveals a total calcium level of 11.3 mg/dL. After recovering from his illness, he has further testing for hypercalcemia, which reveals a total calcium of 11.4 mg/dL and hypocalciuria with a low calcium clearance/creatinine clearance of <0.01. Which of the following statements is most likely true about his diagnosis?

a. Treatment with aggressive hydration is indicated

b. Most patients with this disorder have symptoms of hypercalcemia

c. Vitamin D levels should be obtained before a definitive diagnosis is made

d. This disorder is inherited in an X-linked recessive pattern

e. This disorder is due to a mutation in the calcium-sensing receptor (CaSR)

28-20. Which of the following statements is true regarding hormone effects on the skeleton?

　a. Glucocorticoids accelerate osteoblast formation and enhance bone formation

　b. Thyroid hormone increases bone resorption through increasing the number of osteoclasts

　c. Estrogens and androgens suppress maturation of chondrocytes

　d. Growth hormone decreases the synthesis of type I collagen and bone-specific alkaline phosphatase

　e. Insulin-like growth factor-1 (IGF-1) decreases bone mineral content and density

28-21. An 11-year-old boy presents to clinic for a well-child exam. During the encounter, his family asks if his final adult height can be estimated. His biological mother is 166 cm tall and his father is 183 cm tall. What is his mean parental height?

　a. 174 cm

　b. 181 cm

　c. 168 cm

　d. 183 cm

　e. 178 cm

28-22. A 15-year-old male presents to clinic for concerns of lack of pubertal development. On exam, he has 3-mL testes bilaterally, which are not firm. Review of systems is significant for the inability to smell coffee brewing. FSH, LH, and testosterone levels are low. What is the child's most likely diagnosis?

　a. Klinefelter syndrome

　b. Noonan syndrome

　c. Prader–Willi syndrome

　d. Turner syndrome

　e. Kallman syndrome

28-23. Growth hormone has been approved by the U.S. Food and Drug Administration for the treatment of which disorders?

　a. Noonan syndrome, cystic fibrosis, Turner syndrome

　b. Cystic fibrosis, Down syndrome, Prader–Willi syndrome

　c. Turner syndrome, Prader–Willi syndrome, Down syndrome

　d. Idiopathic short stature (ISS), cystic fibrosis, Turner syndrome

　e. Prader–Willi syndrome, Noonan syndrome, ISS

28-24. Which of the following statements about childhood growth is true?

　a. Supine measurement of length should be used for children younger than 36 months

　b. Height velocity should be calculated using measurements taken at least 6 weeks apart

　c. Height growth occurs primarily as a continuous linear process

　d. Growth velocity during the first 2 years of life averages 15 cm per year

　e. A device with a flexible mounted arm should be used to obtain standing height measurements

28-25. A 6-year-old girl presents to clinic for concerns about short stature and a decline in her linear growth and growth velocity. Two years ago, her height plotted at the 25th percentile, and at today's clinic visit, her height is at less than the 3rd percentile for her age or at −3 standard deviations below the mean. Her weight is proportional to her height. Previous workup has included a normal female karyotype (46,XX). A bone age radiograph indicates that her skeletal maturity is 2 years delayed. Growth hormone deficiency is suspected.

What biochemical evaluation should be sent to screen for growth hormone deficiency?

　a. Growth hormone level

　b. Insulin-like growth factor-1 (IGF-1) and insulin-like growth factor binding protein-3 (IGFBP-3)

　c. Free T4 and TSH

　d. IgA level and tissue transglutaminase IgA antibody

　e. Complete blood cell count and erythrocyte sedimentation rate

28-26. A 16-year-old girl presents as a new patient for concerns of primary amenorrhea. On physical exam, she is tall for her family background. She has normal adult breast development and her vaginal mucosa appears pink, dull, and thick. Her physical exam is otherwise normal with the exception of minimal pubic hair and axillary hair. She is on no medications and her past medical history is unremarkable. Family history reveals that her younger sister presented in early infancy with an inguinal hernia. What test would be most helpful in establishing a diagnosis?

　a. Testosterone

　b. LH

　c. Follicle-stimulating hormone (FSH)

　d. Estradiol

　e. Karyotype

28-27. A 14-year-old girl has recently moved and presents for a well-child visit before she starts at her new school. She has always been one of the shortest children in her class. She has a B average in school, but she struggles in mathematics. Past medical history reveals that she has had frequent ear infections and has had bilateral myringotomy tubes placed as a young child. Her height is 134 cm, which is <3rd percentile or at –4 SDS. Findings on physical exam include a high arched palate, low set ears, ptosis, and multiple nevi. Breast development is Tanner stage II on the right and Tanner stage I on the left.

Besides a karyotype, what additional test will likely be elevated and suggestive of the diagnosis?

a. Thyroid-stimulating hormone (TSH)

b. Insulin-like growth factor 1 (IGF-1)

c. FSH

d. Estradiol

e. Tissue transglutaminase IgA antibody

28-28. Which of the following statements about Klinefelter syndrome is correct?

a. Klinefelter syndrome is a rare cause of primary gonadal failure

b. The most common karyotype found in individuals with Klinefelter syndrome is 47,XYY

c. Individuals with Klinefelter syndrome often have problems with deviant and criminal behavior

d. Gynecomastia commonly occurs in adolescent males with Klinefelter syndrome

e. Testosterone replacement in Klinefelter syndrome corrects the symptoms of androgen deficiency and reverses infertility

28-29. Which of the following is the most common cause of ambiguous genitalia in a newborn?

a. Turner syndrome

b. Congenital adrenal hyperplasia (CAH)

c. Noonan syndrome

d. 5-alpha reductase deficiency

e. Klinefelter syndrome

28-30. A 5-year-old boy presents with Tanner III pubic hair, oily skin, and acne. A bone age radiograph of his left hand and wrist is advanced at 9 years. There is concern that the child may have nonclassic congenital adrenal hyperplasia (CAH). Which of the following would be the best laboratory test to evaluate for CAH?

a. Cortisol

b. Testosterone

c. ACTH

d. 17-hydroxyprogesterone

e. DHEA-S

28-31. A 14-year-old girl presents to her primary care physician with increased fatigue, weakness, abdominal pain, and nausea. She has no significant past medical history. Growth and development have been normal and she is fully pubertal. Physical exam is remarkable for orthostatic hypotension and darkening of the creases on her hands. Which of the following is the most likely diagnosis?

a. Addison disease

b. Adrenoleukodystrophy

c. Salt-wasting congenital adrenal hyperplasia

d. Nonclassic congenital adrenal hyperplasia

e. Brain tumor with subsequent ACTH deficiency

28-32. Which of the following is the best initial test to screen for adrenal insufficiency?

a. Dexamethasone suppression test

b. 12-hour urine cortisol collection

c. Cortisol level drawn at 4 PM

d. ACTH level

e. Cortisol level drawn at 8 AM

28-33. Which of the following are the earliest and most commonly seen signs and symptoms in children with Cushing syndrome?

a. Hypertension and weight gain

b. Buffalo hump and striae

c. Weight gain and growth failure

d. Depression and acne

e. Headache and weight gain

28-34. Which of the following children has the highest likelihood of developing glucocorticoid withdrawal?

    a. A 5-year-old girl with a brain tumor was treated with 2 mg of dexamethasone every 6 hours for 6 weeks and then the medication was stopped

    b. A 8-year-old boy with asthma was treated with 2 mg/kg of prednisolone for 5 days and then the medication was stopped

    c. A 14-year-old boy with Crohn disease was treated with 60 mg of prednisone per day for a week and then the dose was gradually weaned over 2 months and then stopped

    d. A 6-year-old girl with asthma was treated with 2 mg/kg of prednisolone for 5 days and then the dose was weaned over another 5 days and then stopped

    e. A 12-year-old girl with a severe allergic skin reaction receives a 6-day methylprednisolone dose pack where she took 4 pills the first day and then the dose was decreased daily

28-35. A 12-year-old boy presents with a 3-week history of fatigue as well as increased thirst, increased urination, and 15-pound weight loss. On physical exam, his blood pressure is 115/82 and his pulse is 108 beats per minute. A complete blood cell count reveals a normal hemoglobin and hematocrit, but his white blood cell count is elevated at 25,000. A comprehensive metabolic profile reveals a sodium of 127 mEq/L, potassium of 5.9 mEq/L, chloride of 92 mEq/L, bicarbonate of 16 mEq/L, and glucose of 902 mg/dL. His venous pH is 7.32. Urinalysis shows > 1000 glucose and large ketones. Which of the following is the most likely explanation for this patient's hyponatremia?

    a. Hyperkalemia

    b. Hyperglycemia

    c. Leukocytosis

    d. Syndrome of inappropriate anti-diuretic hormone (SIADH)

    e. Acidosis

28-36. A previously healthy 10-year-old boy presents with a 2-day history of abdominal pain and vomiting. His mother thought that he had the flu since his older brother was recently diagnosed with a viral illness. On exam, he is afebrile but appears ill as he is tachypneic and tachycardic. Laboratory testing reveals a plasma glucose of 745 mg/dL. His bicarbonate level is 6 mEq/L and his venous pH is 7.10. A urinalysis is positive for glucose and large ketones. The most appropriate first step in this patient's management is which of the following?

    a. Start an insulin drip at 0.1 units per kg per hour

    b. Start maintenance IV fluids

    c. Bolus with insulin at 0.1 units/kg

    d. Bolus with normal saline at 20 mL/kg

    e. Administer bicarbonate

28-37. A 4-year-old girl is admitted to the hospital with DKA. Her weight is 20 kg. She received 2 L of IV fluids initially when she arrived in the Emergency Department 6 hours ago. She had been feeling better and was conversational, but now she is more somnolent and difficult to arouse. Her blood sugar is 214 mg/dL, and she is on an insulin drip and IV fluids at 2 times maintenance. Which of the following is the most appropriate step in the management of this patient?

    a. Order a stat head CT

    b. Administer bicarbonate

    c. Intubate and hyperventilate

    d. Administer mannitol

    e. Increase the IV fluid rate

28-38. A 5-year-old girl with known type 1 diabetes presents with a 2-day history of fever and diarrhea. She has not vomited and her mother has been monitoring blood sugars and checking for ketones in her urine. On exam, she appears to be well hydrated and the remainder of her exam is unremarkable. A urinalysis reveals positive glucose and moderate ketones. Additional laboratory studies show that her complete blood cell count is normal. Her electrolytes are unremarkable, including a bicarbonate of 23 mEq/L. The only abnormality is a serum blood glucose of 315 mg/dL. In addition to giving her extra insulin, what else would be recommended?

    a. Encourage sugar free fluid intake

    b. Admit to the hospital for observation

    c. Monitor her blood sugar twice a day

    d. Place an IV and give a 20 mL/kg bolus of normal saline

    e. Check her urine ketones twice a day

28-39. Which of the following scenarios has the highest likelihood for the development of ketones?

a. A 12-year-old male with type 1 diabetes goes to a birthday party and eats 2 pieces of cake and a bowl of ice cream. He does not give himself insulin to cover his food intake

b. A 16-year-old girl with type 1 diabetes spends the weekend at her grandmother's house. She received her long-acting insulin each day but only intermittently took her short-acting insulin

c. A 10-year-old girl with type 1 diabetes is on an insulin pump. She takes her pump off during a tennis match and then reattaches it an hour later

d. A 14 year-old girl with type 1 diabetes is playing in a soccer tournament and has 2 games today. She decides to decrease the amount of short-acting insulin she receives at breakfast and lunch

e. A 15-year-old male with type 1 diabetes is on an insulin pump. He changes his pump site at bedtime. When he wakes up 8 hours later, he discovers that his pump site has fallen off

28-40. A 12-year-old boy has type 1 diabetes diagnosed 4 years ago. He is on multiple daily injections and his recent hemoglobin A1c was 8.4%. His mother reports frustration in trying to gain better blood sugar control. She reviews his blood sugar records weekly and makes insulin dose adjustments based on the trends in his numbers. He checks his blood sugar 4–6 times a day, and he receives his insulin injections in his abdomen, upper arms, and thighs. On exam, there is evidence of blood sugar testing on several of his fingers. His exam is otherwise unremarkable with the exception of 2 small lumps on either side of his umbilicus consistent with lipohypertrophy. Which of the following recommendations would likely lead to improved blood sugar control and a lower hemoglobin A1c?

a. Switch to a different type of insulin

b. Rotate his insulin injection sites

c. Change to an insulin pump

d. Check his blood sugar more often

e. Refer him to a dermatologist

28-41. Which of the following is a true statement about type 2 diabetes?

a. Elevated insulin levels are commonly seen in obese adolescents and should initially be treated with metformin

b. DKA cannot occur in type 2 diabetics since β cells are still able to produce insulin

c. The average age at diagnosis of type 2 diabetes in children is 10 years old, which corresponds to the onset of puberty

d. Genetics plays a larger role in the development of type 2 diabetes than in type 1 diabetes in children

e. Type 2 diabetes is more commonly seen in non-Hispanic whites than in other ethnic groups in the United States

28-42. A 15-year-old obese African American girl has struggled with weight gain for many years. She presents with concerns of fatigue and lack of energy. Other review of systems is positive for increased thirst and urination over the past few weeks. Her weight is 120 kg and she has lost 5 kg in the last 2 months. On exam, she has darkening of the skin on the back and sides of her neck. She also has a vaginal yeast infection. A urinalysis reveals >1000 glucose and no ketones. Additional tests show that her plasma glucose is 256 mg/dL, bicarbonate is 26 mEq/mL, and her hemoglobin A1c is 9.5%.

Which of the following would be the most appropriate treatment?

a. Refer her to a diabetes specialist to start insulin injections

b. Refer her to a dietitian to start a calorie-restricted diet

c. Refer her to a diabetes specialist to start metformin

d. Refer her to a diabetes specialist to start a sulfonylurea

e. Admit her to the hospital for IV fluids and an insulin drip

28-43. Which of the following tests is the most helpful in differentiating between new-onset type 1 and type 2 diabetes?

a. Blood glucose

b. C-peptide

c. Hemoglobin A1c

d. Urine ketones

e. Glutamic acid decarboxylase antibody

28-44. A 2-year-old girl presents to the Emergency Department with decreased feeding, tachycardia, and lethargy. Her blood glucose is found to be low at 25 mg/dL. Her weight is 12 kg. She is admitted to the hospital for IV fluids and observation. A septic work-up is negative. She has no low blood sugars for the first 48 hours while she is on IV fluids of 0.45% NaCl with 5% dextrose at 20 mL per hour. As she has been stable, it is decided to wean her off IV fluids. However, as the IV fluid rate is decreased, her blood glucose drops. A critical sample is drawn during an episode of hypoglycemia, which shows a plasma glucose of 21 mg/dL, elevated growth hormone of 20 mcg/L, elevated cortisol of 38 mcg/dL, undetectable c-peptide, and elevated insulin level of 42 mcU/mL. Urine ketones are negative. What is the most likely reason for the child's hypoglycemia?

 a. Insulinoma

 b. Growth hormone deficiency

 c. Sulfonylurea ingestion

 d. Cortisol deficiency

 e. Exogenous insulin

28-45. A term 36-hour-old male infant is hypoglycemic in the nursery with a plasma blood glucose of 18 mg/dL. His birth weight was 7 pounds and 2 ounces. On exam, he has a midline cleft lip and palate as well as a micropenis with a stretched penile length of 1.8 cm and bilaterally descended testes. Which of the following is the most likely cause of his hypoglycemia?

 a. Congenital hyperinsulinism

 b. Growth hormone deficiency

 c. Small for gestational age

 d. Gonadotropin deficiency

 e. Beckwith–Wiedemann syndrome

28-46. A 4-day-old infant was born full term, and the pregnancy was complicated by the mother having eclampsia and hypertension. He has had problems with hypoglycemia and is on IV fluids with a GIR of 15 mg/kg/minute. During one episode of hypoglycemia, the serum blood glucose was 28 mg/dL. Glucagon was administered and the serum blood glucose rose to 65 mg/dL. Which of the following medications would be the initial drug of choice for this infant?

 a. Growth hormone

 b. Nifedipine

 c. Diazoxide

 d. Hydrocortisone

 e. Octreotide

28-47. A 4-year-old girl presents for her well-child visit in August. Her linear growth and development appear to be normal. The mother's primary concern is that her daughter has had increased thirst and urination over the summer. She was toilet trained when 3 years old, but over the past 2 months, she has needed to use pull-up diapers at night to prevent accidents. She wakes up every 2 hours during the night to drink and urinate. She carries a water bottle with her during the day, and her mother refills it at least 8 times throughout the day. Her mother has tried to restrict her water intake. However, when fluids have been restricted, she gets upset but calms down after she is allowed to drink. Which of the following details from the history is most concerning for a pathological condition?

 a. She was previously toilet trained during the night

 b. She carries a water bottle with her during the day

 c. She wakes up at night to drink and urinate

 d. She is drinking 8 or more bottles of water per day

 e. She gets upset when fluids are restricted

28-48. A 15-year-old girl presents to her physician's office with increased thirst and increased urination for the past 3 months. She drinks up to 8 L of water per day as she constantly feels thirsty and she urinates 10 times or more a day. Her height, weight, and vital signs are all normal. Her physical exam is unremarkable. Electrolyte panel shows a serum sodium of 135 mEq/L, potassium of 4.2 mEq/L, calcium of 9.3 mg/dL, and glucose of 89 mg/dL. Her TSH is normal at 1.35 mU/mL. Urinalysis reveals a specific gravity of 1.002 and no glucosuria. She is admitted to the hospital for a water deprivation test. After 12 hours, her sodium is 137 mEq/L, serum osmolaltity is 286 mosm/kg, and her urine specific gravity is 1.025. Which of the following is the most likely diagnosis?

 a. SIADH

 b. Compulsive water drinking

 c. Nephrogenic diabetes insipidus

 d. Central diabetes insipidus

 e. Cerebral salt wasting

28-49. A 13-year-old boy is a restrained back seat passenger in a motor vehicle accident 2 days ago. He sustained an injury to his brain and is on a ventilator. For the first 24 hours after the accident, his urine output was 3 mL/kg/hour. His urine output has subsequently decreased. Laboratory studies now reveal that his serum sodium is 129 mEq/L, serum osmolality is 281 mosm/kg, and urine sodium is 40 mEq/L. Which of the following would be the most appropriate management at this time?

a. Decrease the IV fluid rate

b. Start oral salt supplementation

c. Bolus with furosemide

d. Start a vasopressin drip

e. Bolus with hypertonic (3%) saline

28-50. A 16-year-old male is an unrestrained front seat passenger in a motor vehicle accident. He has suffered extensive trauma to his body. Head imaging reveals that he has significant disruption of the pituitary stalk. Of the following hormones, which would most likely be expected to be elevated?

a. Growth hormone

b. Prolactin

c. IGF-1

d. Free T4

e. Testosterone

ANSWERS

Answer 28-1. a

With the patient's history of medullary thyroid cancer combined with neuromas on his tongue and marfanoid body habitus, the patient most likely has Multiple Endocrine Neoplasia 2b (MEN2b). MEN 2 syndromes, which are inherited in an autosomal dominant pattern, are caused by a gain of function mutation in the *RET* proto-oncogene, not an inactivating mutation of the gene. MEN1, which encodes the tumor suppressor gene MENIN, is mutated in Multiple Endocrine Neoplasia 1 (MEN1). The parathyroid glands, pituitary gland, and pancreatic islet cells are most often affected in MEN1. The most common endocrine abnormality in MEN1 involves hypercalcemia due to hyperparathyroidism. Pancreatic tumors, including gastrinomas and insulinomas, are the second most common endocrine problem in MEN1. Pituitary tumors occur in over 40% of MEN 1 patients—prolactinomas are the most common followed by tumors secreting growth hormone and ACTH. The PRKARIA gene is responsible for Carney complex, which involves pituitary-independent Cushing syndrome along with an association of heart myxomas and lentigines. Activating mutations of the G-protein alpha subunit are associated with McCune–Albright syndrome, which presents with autonomous endocrine function, fibrous dysplasia, and/or café au lait macules.

(Pages 2059–2060: Section 28, Chapter 537: Endocrine Neoplasia Syndromes; Page 2080: Section 28, Chapter 541: Abnormal Pubertal Development)

Answer 28-2. c

Normal male pubertal development occurs between the ages of 9 and 14 years with the average age being approximately 11.5 years (see Figure 540-1). In males, the testicular Leydig cells produce testosterone as a result of stimulation of receptors by circulating luteinizing hormone (LH). The onset of central male puberty is defined as an increase in testicular volume greater than or equal to 4 mL. This is followed by penile enlargement, pubic hair development, and lastly a linear growth spurt.

The serum concentration of prolactin increases in normal female puberty, but it does not change in normal male puberty. The circulation of FSH stimulates spermatogenesis by attaching to the FSH receptors of seminiferous tubules. Inhibin, which is produced by the testicular Sertoli cells, suppresses FSH secretion in normal male puberty.

(Pages 2074–2076: Section 28, Chapter 540: Normal Pubertal Development)

Answer 28-3. b

Breast development is the first sign of central puberty in girls and testicular enlargement (greater than or equal to 4 mL in volume) is the first sign of central puberty in boys. Puberty is delayed if a girl has not entered puberty by age 13 and delayed in a boy if he has not entered puberty by age 14. Following menarche, girls grow approximately 2 to 7 cm (or 0.8 inches to 2.8 inches). Breast development may begin unilaterally, and asymmetric breast growth is not uncommon. The average age of menarche is approximately 12.5 years in girls. Menarche occurs about 2 years after the onset of breast development. Although there is controversy surrounding when puberty is precocious, most agree that puberty that begins before the age of 8 years in girls and before the age of 9 years in boys is early.

(Pages 2074–2076: Section 28, Chapter 540: Normal Pubertal Development)

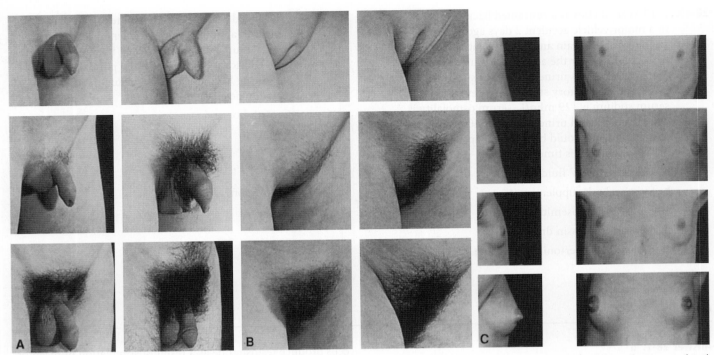

FIGURE 540-1. **(A)** Genital development and pubic hair growth among boys. Stage G1 (*upper left*), prepubertal. Stage G2 (*upper right*), enlargement of testis to more than 2.5 cm, appearance of scrotal reddening, and increase in rugations. Stage G3, increase in length or 4 cm volume and, to a lesser extent, breadth of penis with further growth of testis. Stage G4, further increase in size of penis and testes and darkening of scrotal skin. Stages G5 and G6 (*lower panels*), adult genitalia. Stage P1 (*upper panels*), preadolescent, no pubic hair. Stage P2 (*middle left*), sparse growth of slightly pigmented, slightly curved pubic hair mainly at the base of the penis. Stage P3 (*middle right*), thicker curlier hair spread laterally. Stage P4 (*lower left*), adult-type hair that does not yet spread to medial thighs. Stage P5 (*lower right*), adult-type hair spread to medial thighs. **(B)** Appearance of pubic and labial hair among girls. Stage PH1 (*upper left*), prepubertal, no pubic hair. Stage PH2 (*upper right, middle left*), sparse growth of long, straight, or slightly curly minimally pigmented hair, mainly on labia. Stage PH3 (*middle right*), considerably darker and coarser hair spreading over mons pubis. Stage PH4 (*lower left*), thick adult-type hair that does not yet spread to the medial surface of the thighs. Stage PH5 (*lower right*), hair is adult type and is distributed in the classic inverse triangle. **(C)** Breast development. Stage B1 (*upper panels*), prepubertal, elevation of the papilla only. Stage B2, breast buds visible or palpable with enlargement of the areola. Stage B3, further enlargement of the breast and areola with no separation of their contours (not shown). Stage B4, projection of areola and papilla to form a secondary mound over the rest of the breast. Stage B5 (*lower panel*), mature breast with projection of papilla only. (Reproduced, with permission, from Rudolph CD, Rudolph AM, Lister GE, First LR, Gershon AA. *Rudolph's Pediatrics.* 22nd ed. New York: McGraw-Hill, 2011.)

Answer 28-4. e

The patient has evidence of central precocious puberty with breast and pubic hair development, estrogenization of her vaginal mucosa, and advanced skeletal maturation. The patient in the scenario mostly likely has a hamartoma of the tuber cinereum, which is associated with gelastic seizures, precocious puberty, and a characteristic appearance of the hamartoma on brain imaging. On MRI, the hamartoma appears as a pedunculated or sessile mass attached to the posterior hypothalamus. The hamartoma is nonmalignant and may have GnRH-synthesizing neurons.

An optic glioma, craniopharyngioma, ependymoma, or astrocytoma can cause central precocious puberty, but they are not classically associated with seizures and the described characteristic appearance on MRI.

(Page 2078: Section 28, Chapter 541: Abnormal Pubertal Development)

Answer 28-5. d

Familial gonadotropin-independent sexual precocity (or "testotoxicosis") is caused by an activating mutation of the LH receptor. Due to this mutation, which is inherited in an autosomal dominant pattern, testosterone is constantly produced. This disorder manifests clinically only in males. Fertility is normal in adulthood. Boys with this condition have minimal enlargement of the testes because the Leydig cells are predominantly stimulated and not the seminiferous tubules. Therefore, penile enlargement, pubic hair, growth acceleration, and acne are seen, but testicular volume is disproportionately small. Biochemical testing reveals elevated testosterone levels with low gonadotropin concentrations.

(Page 2079: Section 28, Chapter 541: Abnormal Pubertal Development)

Answer 28-6. b

This child has precocious puberty, hyperthyroidism, and café au lait spots. This clinical presentation is most consistent with McCune–Albright syndrome. The classic triad of McCune–Albright syndrome is polyostotic fibrous dysplasia, irregular or jagged bordered café au lait macules, and autonomous endocrine function. The most common endocrinopathy is GnRH-independent precocious puberty followed by hyperthyroidism. However, all 3 entities of the classic triad do not need to be apparent to make the diagnosis of McCune–Albright syndrome. Activating mutations of the stimulatory G-protein of the adenyl cyclase system are responsible for the autonomous activity in endocrine glands. Cushing syndrome, acromegaly, and hyperparathyroidism can also occur.

Peutz–Jeghers syndrome presents with nasal polyps, hyperpigmentation of the lips, and macules on the buccal mucosa. This autosomal dominant condition can also present with gynecomastia and precocious puberty with Sertoli cell tumors in boys and ovarian cysts in girls. Classic congenital adrenal hyperplasia (CAH) is an autosomal recessive disorder most commonly due to 21-hydroxylase deficiency and presents at birth with ambiguous genitalia in females. Boys with classic CAH may present in infancy with a salt-wasting crisis but they do not have ambiguous or abnormal genitalia. Familial gonadotropin-independent puberty is a disorder seen only in males and is caused by an activating mutation of the LH receptor. Affected males present with signs of virilization and penile enlargement with only a small and disproportionate increase in testicular volume. Granulosa cell tumors are a rare functional neoplasm, which can manifest as gonadotropin-independent premature puberty. Peutz–Jeghers syndrome, CAH, familial gonadotropin-independent puberty, and granulosa cell tumors are not associated with cafe-au-lait macules or hyperthyroidism.

(Pages 2079–2080: Section 28, Chapter 541: Abnormal Pubertal Development)

Answer 28-7. c

Premature thelarche is usually best managed with reassurance as it is a benign, self-limited condition that is considered a normal variant in development. Girls most often present with premature thelarche before 2 years of age and almost always before 4 years of age. The majority of cases regress within 6 months of onset, but breast tissue can persist. In girls with premature thelarche, no other signs of pubertal development are present. There is no nipple or areolar complex development. Girls with premature thelarche have normal linear growth and normal skeletal maturation. The differential diagnosis of breast development in young girls includes exogenous estrogen exposure, estrogen-secreting tumor, McCune–Albright syndrome, or central precocious puberty.

In premature thelarche, gonadotropin levels are in the prepubertal range. Small for gestational age is a risk factor for premature adrenarche (not thelarche). Some girls with premature adrenarche are at an increased risk for polycystic ovary syndrome and insulin resistance as adults.

(Page 2082: Section 28, Chapter 541: Abnormal Pubertal Development)

Answer 28-8. b

This child has rickets, which is most likely due to decreased vitamin D intake. Breast milk is deficient in vitamin D and recommendations state that breastfeeding mothers should take 1000 IU of vitamin D daily while their infant should receive 400 IU of vitamin D per day. Individuals with darkly pigmented skin are at an increased risk for vitamin D deficiency. As the child in this case is black and was exclusively breast fed, he is at high risk for vitamin D deficiency. In children with rickets, delayed closure of fontanelles can be seen along with short stature, poor weight gain, and delayed walking. Common findings on radiographs include cupping and fraying of the metaphyses of the long bones and demineralization. In mild vitamin D deficient rickets, laboratory abnormalities are more subtle and calcium, phosphate, and parathyroid levels may be normal with an increased alkaline phosphatase (Table 543-2). In more severe cases, calcium and phosphate are low with a notable increase in alkaline phosphatase and PTH.

(Pages 2098–2100: Section 28, Chapter 543: Disorders of Bone Formation)

Answer 28-9. e

The most common reason for congenital hypothyroidism is a defect in thyroid embryogenesis with more than 95% of cases being idiopathic or sporadic. The prevalence of congenital hypothyroidism is approximately 1 in 4000 newborns. The remaining answers are also reasons for congenital hypothyroidism (Table 527-1), but they are less likely in this case.

The child is not premature, and therefore, dysfunction due to prematurity would be unlikely. Premature infants may have an immature hypothalamic–pituitary–thyroid axis and are predisposed to thyroid dysfunction. The child's mother is healthy and has no history of thyroid disease, which makes the transplacental acquisition of maternal TSH receptor blocking antibodies unlikely. Ingestion of a goitrogenic substance, such as iodines or sulfonamides, by the mother was not given in the history but could cause hypothyroidism and a neonatal goiter. Thyroid dyshormonogenesis can occur from a variety of enzymatic defects, including organification and thyroid iodide transport defects. However, cases of thyroid dyshormonogenesis are less common than defects in thyroid embryogenesis. Infants with thyroid dyshormonogenesis have a normal-appearing thyroid gland in the normal location on ultrasound, and they may have a goiter on exam.

(Pages 2031–2035: Section 28, Chapter 527: Hypothyroidism in the Infant)

TABLE 543-2. Laboratory Data in Rickets of Different Causes

Type	Calcium	Phosphate	Alkaline Phosphatase	Calcidiol	Calcitriol	Parathyroid Hormone
Calcium deficiency	↓↓	↓	↑↑	N	↑	↑
Phosphate deficiency	N, ↑	↓↓	↑↑	N	↑	N, ↓
Vitamin D deficiency						
Mild	N, ↓	N, ↓	↑	↓	N	N
Moderate	N, ↓	↓	↑↑	↓	↓, N, ↑	↑
Severe	↓	↓	↑↑	↓↓	↓	↑↑
Loss-of-function *CYP2R1* (25-hydroxylase)	↓	↓	↑	N	N, ↓	N
Loss-of-function *CYP27B1* (25OHD-1α-hydroxylase)	↓↓	↓↓	↑↑↑	N	↓↓↓	↑↑↑
Loss-of-function *VDR* (Resistance to calcitriol)	↓↓	↓↓	↑↑↑	N	↓↓↓	↑↑↑
Loss-of-function *PHEX* (X-linked hypophosphatemic rickets)	N	↓↓	↑	N	N, ↓	N

N, normal; ↓, low; ↑, high.

Modified with permission from Root AW, Diamond FB Jr. Disorders of bone mineral metabolism in the newborn, infant, child, and adolescent. In: Sperling MA, ed. *Pediatric Endocrinology*. 3rd ed. Philadelphia, PA: Saunders/Elsevier; 2008:686–769. (*Italics* indicate genes.)

Answer 28-10. a

Methods of thyroid testing in newborn screening programs vary from state to state, but screening is commonly conducted with either thyroid-stimulating hormone (TSH) only or a combination of TSH and thyroxine (T4). The majority of infants with congenital hypothyroidism have primary thyroid disease and an elevated TSH. Approximately 15% of infants with congenital hypothyroidism can have a normal T4 level. Although newborn screening detects the great majority of affected infants, 3–5% of infants with congenital hypothyroidism are not detected by newborn screening. The incidence of congenital hypothyroidism is approximately 1 in 4000 newborns. Preferred thyroid hormone replacement therapy is T4, and the goal is to start thyroid hormone replacement no later than 2 weeks of life as thyroid hormone is critically important for normal brain growth and development. Physical growth and development are usually normalized with timely and adequate therapy along with close monitoring of thyroid function tests. Confirmation of the diagnosis of congenital hypothyroidism is made by measuring serum TSH and T4 (Figure 527-1).

(Pages 2031–2036: Section 28, Chapter 527: Hypothyroidism in the Infant)

Answer 28-11. c

This child has severe hypothyroidism evidenced by an extremely high thyroid-stimulating hormone (TSH) value (Table 526-1), sexual precocity (pubertal signs before age 9), delayed bone age, goiter, and delayed relaxation of deep tendon reflexes. Pseudoprecocious puberty due to severe hypothyroidism can occur in both boys and girls. Boys exhibit penile and testicular enlargement with lack of androgen-mediated body hair, while girls can present with menstruation and breast development. These findings occur due to high levels of TSH cross-reacting with FSH receptors, as both have identical alpha subunits. Galactorrhea can also occur due to increased thyrotropin-releasing hormone (TRH) production from the hypothalamus, which stimulates both TSH and prolactin from the pituitary gland. The bone age delay reflects the duration of the hypothyroidism. Once a child receives treatment, the signs and symptoms of pseudoprecocious puberty regress.

Normal thyroid function levels are not linked to precocious puberty. A markedly elevated free T4 value (with an accompanying low TSH value) would suggest hyperthyroidism. Unlike this patient, the bone age would not be markedly delayed and the patient would be hyper-reflexive if he was hyperthyroid. A mildly elevated TSH of 6.0 mU/L would not explain this clinical scenario.

(Pages 2037–2038: Section 28,Chapter 528: Acquired Hypothyroidism; Page 2080: Section 28, Chapter 541: Abnormal Pubertal Development)

Answer 28-12. d

Hashimoto thyroiditis is the most common cause of goiter and hypothyroidism in a 9-year-old child. It an autoimmune condition and is more common in females than in males. The onset of Hashimoto thyroiditis is usually insidious, and some children may have no signs or symptoms of hypothyroidism.

Most children with Hashimoto thyroiditis and autoimmune hypothyroidism have detectable levels of circulating antithyroid antibodies, which are markers of inflammation in the thyroid gland. An antithyroid peroxidase (TPO) antibody is more often detected compared to an antithyroglobulin antibody.

A goiter and elevated TSH level establishes that the disease originates in the thyroid gland. An MRI of the brain with specific emphasis on the hypothalamus and pituitary gland would only be necessary in cases of central (not primary) hypothyroidism. An enlarged thyroid on physical exam would not be present in cases of central hypothyroidism. A thyroid ultrasound would be helpful if there was thyroid asymmetry or a nodule present. However, in this case, the patient has a thyroid gland that is enlarged but smooth and symmetric. A TSH receptor antibody (TRAb) and total T3 would be helpful in the evaluation of hyperthyroidism and Graves disease.

(Pages 2037–2038: Section 528: Acquired Hypothyroidism)

Answer 28-13. d

This child has hyperthyroidism, which is most commonly due to Graves disease. Other causes of hyperthyroidism in children include Hashimoto thyrotoxicosis (or Hashitoxicosis), hyperfunctioning thyroid nodule, or ingestion of thyroid hormone. Classically, the diagnosis of hyperthyroidism is confirmed with a low or suppressed TSH level, elevated T4 and/or free T4, and an elevated T3. TSH receptor antibody (TRAb), which is also called a thyroid-stimulating immunoglobulin (TSI), is positive in Graves disease. Clinical features of hyperthyroidism include muscle weakness, behavioral problems, frequent or loose stools, declining school performance, and emotional lability. Cardiovascular signs of hyperthyroidism include a widened pulse pressure, tachycardia, and exercise intolerance. Weight loss in conjunction with an increased appetite is also common.

Estradiol, LH, and FSH are hormones that are important in pubertal development but are not associated with hyperthyroidism.

(Pages 2039–2040: Section 28, Chapter 529: Hyperthyroidism)

Answer 28-14. b

The incidence of Graves disease sharply increases as children approach adolescence. Graves disease is 6–8 times more common in girls than in boys. Treatment options include thyroidectomy, radioactive iodine ablation, and antithyroid drugs. In this scenario, the patient is taking methimazole, which inhibits the oxidation of iodine and blocks the production of thyroid hormones. Side effects of methimazole include rash, arthralgia, and agranulocytopenia. Due to the risk of agranulocytopenia, it is recommended that patients have a complete blood count checked during times of illness to document their white blood cell count. If it is suppressed, the patient should stop methimazole. Drug therapy is typically continued for 1–2 years before a trial off is recommended.

The best clinical prognostic sign for determining if the patient has gone into remission is the size of the thyroid gland. Most patients with a persistent goiter will relapse when the medication is discontinued.

Orbitopathy, widened pulse pressure, muscle weakness, and weight loss are all clinical features of Graves disease. Other clinical signs include emotional lability, tremor, fatigability, and rapid tendon reflex relaxation. However, the resolution of these signs does not suggest that the patient has gone into remission.

(Pages 2039–2040: Section 28, Chapter 529: Hyperthyroidism)

Answer 28-15. c

Thyroid hormone metabolism is mediated by iodothyronine monodeiodinase (MDI) enzymes (Figure 526-3). T4 is progressively deiodinated by MDI-1, MDI-2, and MDI-3. In the first step of thyroid hormone metabolism, T4 is deiodinated to either active T3 or to inactive reverse T3 (rT3). Normally, T3 and rT3 are produced at the same rate, although rT3 is produced in greater quantity in sick euthyroid syndrome. T4 is produced only by the thyroid gland while T3 is produced by the thyroid gland and in other tissues, including the liver, brain, and placenta. T4 is deiodinated in these peripheral tissues to T3. The concentration of T4 is 50–100 times greater than that of T3, but T3 is more potent than T4. As T3 is the active and biologically relevant hormone, it binds with greater affinity to nuclear receptors in comparison to T4.

(Pages 2028–2030: Section 28, Chapter 526: The Thyroid)

Answer 28-16. a

Disorders associated with autoimmune hypothyroidism include type 1 diabetes, Turner syndrome, and Down syndrome. In children with type 1 diabetes, it is estimated that about 30% have detectable thyroid autoantibodies (thyroid peroxidase (TPO) or antithyroglobulin) and about 10% have an elevated TSH. In Turner syndrome, up to 30% of adults may become hypothyroid and as many as 50% have detectable thyroid autoantibodies. Periodic screening for thyroid disease is recommended in children with type 1 diabetes as well as in girls with Turner syndrome. In Down syndrome, autoimmune thyroid disease is more common than in the general population. Besides the newborn screen, thyroid studies should be checked at 6 months of life and then yearly thereafter.

CAH is not associated with an increased prevalence of autoimmune thyroid disease. Greater than 95% of CAH cases are caused by an autosomal recessive deficiency of 21 alpha-hydroxylase (mutations of CYP21A2 gene). Prader–Willi syndrome is not associated with autoimmune hypothyroidism. Endocrine issues associated with Prader–Willi syndrome include hypogonadism, type 2 diabetes, and central hypothyroidism. Growth hormone deficiency and adrenal insufficiency have also been linked to Prader–Willi syndrome. Prader–Willi syndrome is the most common cause of syndromic obesity. In McCune–Albright syndrome, defined as the classic triad of gonadotropin-independent precocious puberty, fibrous dysplasia, and café au lait macules, there is no association with hypothyroidism. However, the mutation associated with this disorder can cause continued stimulation of endocrine function, leading to hyperthyroidism, Cushing syndrome, and/or growth hormone excess.

(Page 2038: Section 28, Chapter 528: Acquired Hypothyroidism)

Answer 28-17. b

This child has DiGeorge syndrome as evidenced by the conotruncal defect of the heart and hypocalcemia due to hypoparathyroidism. The classic presentation for this syndrome includes conotruncal heart defect (such as tetralogy of Fallot, truncus ateriosus, aberrant right subclavian artery, and interrupted or right aortic arch), hypoplastic thymus, and hypocalcemia secondary to hypoparathyroidism. The hypoparathyroidism is not due to an autoimmune process, but secondary to defects in the development of the 3rd and 4th pharyngeal pouches, which causes parathyroid gland dysgenesis. Incidence ranges from 1:4000 to 1:10,000 births with approximately 70% having isolated hypoparathyroidism. Partial or complete absence of the thymus can result in an increased frequency of viral and fungal infections due to impaired cell-mediated immunity and defects in T lymphocyte function. The most common genetic cause of sporadic DiGeorge syndrome is a microdeletion in chromosome 22q11.2.

Williams syndrome is associated with idiopathic hypercalcemia, which is self-limited and not related to increased PTH secretion. Neither neonatal Graves disease, congenital hypothyroidism, nor Beckwith–Wiedemann syndrome is associated with hypocalcemia or hypoparathyroidism.

(Page 2089: Section 28, Chapter 542: Calcium, Phosphorous, and Magnesium Metabolism)

Answer 28-18. c

This child has Albright hereditary osteodystrophy and pseudohypoparathyroidism type IA (PHP-IA). Clinically, these children are short and often obese. Short stature may not be apparent in childhood but is nearly universal as adults. Typically, they have developmental delay, round face, subcutaneous calcifications, brachydactyly, and flattened nasal bridge. Lab abnormalities include hypocalcemia, hyperphosphatemia, and elevated PTH. This disorder is characterized by its lack of response to PTH and is inherited in an autosomal dominant pattern. Inactivating mutations in *GNAS* cause resistance to PTH and other hormones, such as TSH. When exogenous PTH is administered to these patients, it does not improve the hypocalcemia or hyperphosphatemia.

(Page 2090: Section 28, Chapter 542: Calcium, Phosphorous, and Magnesium Metabolism)

Answer 28-19. e

This child has hereditary hypocalciuric hypercalcemia type 1 (HHC1), which is also known as familial hypocalciuric hypercalcemia (FHH). This benign disorder is characterized by asymptomatic hypercalcemia (11–12 mg/dL) with hypocalciuria (calcium/creatinine clearance ratio <0.01). This condition is autosomal dominant and is usually discovered incidentally. Due to a heterozygous loss-of-function defect in the CaSR, documentation of mild hypercalcemia with hypocalciuria in 1 parent solidifies the diagnosis.

No treatment is indicated in this disorder and patients are asymptomatic. They do not have typical symptoms of hypercalcemia, such as polyuria, fatigue, anorexia, irritability, hypertension, behavioral changes, constipation, or seizures. Vitamin D levels are not necessary as definitive diagnosis is made through parental testing since it is inherited in an autosomal dominant fashion.

(Page 2093: Section 28, Chapter 542: Calcium, Phosphorous, and Magnesium Metabolism)

Answer 28-20. b

Various hormones and growth factors have profound effects on the growing skeleton, especially during childhood. Sixty percent of the total body bone mineral content is accrued during puberty. Thyroid hormone increases bone resorption as well as bone remodeling. Hyperthyroidism results in a generalized net loss of bone. Glucocorticoids suppress osteoblast formation and accelerate osteoblast death, which leads to impaired bone formation. Glucocorticoid excess can also disrupt GH/IGF-1 action as well as alter vitamin D and calcium metabolism. Estrogen and testosterone increase during puberty and promote the proliferation and maturation of chrondrocytes. These pubertal hormones promote long bone growth and are necessary for bone mineral accrual. Growth hormone increases osteoblast proliferation, which leads to increased synthesis of bone-specific alkaline phosphatase, IGF-I, and type I collagen. IGF-I increases both bone mineral content and bone mineral density.

(Pages 2097–2098: Section 28, Chapter 543: Disorders of Bone Formation)

Answer 28-21. b

Most children establish a pattern of growth by about 2–3 years old, and they do not deviate from this growth channel until puberty. Genetic potential is a significant factor in a child's growth, and the mean parental height (also termed midparental or target height) should be considered when evaluating a child's growth pattern. Mean parental height is calculated for boys by averaging parental height and adding 6.5 cm. For girls, mean parental height is calculated by averaging parental heights and subtracting 6.5 cm. Two standard deviations for the calculated mean parental height is approximately 10 cm. Final adult height typically falls within 2 inches above or below the mean parental height.

(Page 2013: Section 28, Chapter 522: Growth and Growth Impairment)

Answer 28-22. e

This patient has Kallman syndrome based on his clinical findings of hyposmia (or anosmia) and hypogonadotropic hypogonadism based on his pubertal exam and laboratory studies. Although he is 15 years old, this patient has no evidence of central puberty as evidenced by his small testicular volume. In Kallman syndrome, GnRH neurons do no migrate correctly from the olfactory placode to the hypothalamus and the olfactory bulbs do not develop, which results in hypogonadotropic hypogonadism and hyposmia/anosmia. As there is a deficiency of GnRH (from the hypothalamus), this leads to a deficiency of LH and FSH (from the pituitary gland) and central puberty does not proceed normally. Kallman syndrome occurs more commonly in males.

Klinefelter syndrome affects males, and the most common karyotype is 47,XXY. Gonadotropin levels are elevated at the time of normal pubertal development and it is not associated with hyposmia. Noonan syndrome, which is an autosomal dominant disorder, is often associated with short stature and cardiac defects. Delayed puberty and cryptorchidism can be seen in Noonan syndrome, and it is not associated with hyposmia. Hypogonadism frequently occurs in Prader–Willi syndrome and is characterized by hypothalamic dysfunction (low LH) along with primary gonadal dysfunction (high FSH). Many boys also have cryptorchidism. Hyposmia is not associated with Prader Willi syndrome. Turner syndrome is seen only in females and many have primary gonadal failure, illustrated by an increased FSH level. Turner syndrome is not associated with hyposmia.

(Page 2083: Section 28, Chapter 541: Abnormal Pubertal Development)

Answer 28-23. e

The US Food and Drug Administration has approved the use of growth hormone in the treatment of various disorders in children, including growth hormone deficiency, Turner syndrome, chronic renal insufficiency, children born with intrauterine growth restriction (or small for gestational age) who do not have catch-up growth by the age of 2 years, Prader–Willi syndrome with growth failure, Noonan syndrome, and ISS. Children with ISS are defined as those with a height that is more than −2.25 standard deviations below the mean for sex and age, and epiphyses are not closed. Growth hormone is approved in children with ISS who have a growth rate that is unlikely to attain a final adult height within the normal range, which is at least 63 inches (160 cm) for boys and 59 inches (150 cm) for girls.

Although children with Down syndrome are typically short, growth hormone is not approved for this syndrome. Research suggests that growth hormone therapy may improve lung function and have other positive benefits in cystic fibrosis, but it is considered experimental and has not been approved in the treatment of children with cystic fibrosis.

(Page 2021: Section 28, Chapter 523: Endocrine Abnormalities Causing Growth Impairment)

Answer 28-24. d

A child's growth pattern is an important indicator of their overall general health. Therefore, height measurements need to be accurately obtained and plotted on appropriate growth charts at each clinic visit. During the first 2 years of life, growth velocity averages 15 cm per year and decreases to an average of 6 cm per year later in childhood. During the pubertal growth spurt, peak growth velocity is between 7 and 11 cm per year. Because boys usually begin and complete puberty later than girls and thus stop growing later, this leads to a 13 cm final height difference between males and females (see Figure 2-2).

Supine length measurements should be used for children younger than 2 years, and standing height measurements are recommended thereafter. To calculate an accurate height velocity, two measurements of height should be made at least 4 months apart, although measurements taken 9–12 months apart minimize error. Typically, growth occurs as periodic bursts followed by times of growth arrest; in some children, growth may occur as a continuous process. Devices with a flexible arm mount are often inaccurate as the measurement arm does not always remain in a perpendicular plane. Wall-mounted devices are more accurate, and when taking an upright height measurement, the child should be standing with heels together with the thoracic spine, buttocks, and heals touching the measuring device.

(Pages 2012–2013: Section 28, Chapter 522: Growth and Growth Impairment)

Answer 28-25. b

A diagnostic evaluation for growth failure should be pursued in a child whose height percentile differs largely from that of their midparental height, in a child who is falling from their growth channel, or in a child whose height is more than 3 standard deviations below the mean height for age. Pathological causes of poor growth and short stature include various endocrinopathies, including growth hormone deficiency, thyroid hormone deficiency, and glucocorticoid excess.

IGF-1 and IGFBP-3 are the screening laboratory tests of choice in the evaluation of growth hormone deficiency. IGF-1 and IGFBP-3 are proteins made by the liver and are growth hormone dependent. Growth hormone levels can be measured during provocative stimulation testing to evaluate for growth hormone deficiency (Figure 522-1). However, random growth hormone levels should not be drawn as a screen for growth hormone deficiency since growth hormone is secreted in a pulsatile manner.

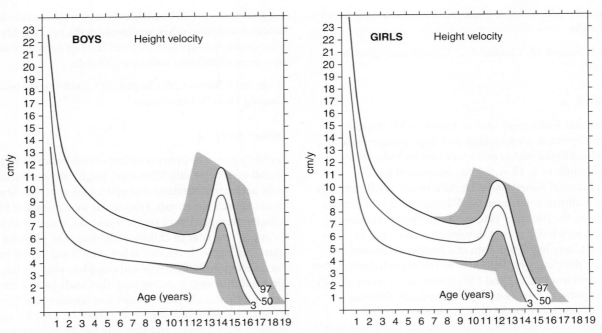

FIGURE 2-2. Ranges of linear growth velocities in males and females. (Reproduced, with permission, from Kappy MS, Allen DB, Geffner ME. *Pediatric Practice: Endocrinology.* New York: McGraw-Hill, 2010.)

The rest of the choices are various screening tests that may be done during the evaluation of a child with growth failure and short stature (Table 522-3). Thyroid function testing (free T4 and TSH) should be drawn to screen for hypothyroidism. Children with celiac disease can sometimes present with no gastrointestinal symptoms (eg, diarrhea, constipation, or abdominal pain) but only with poor growth and short stature. A tissue transglutaminase IgA antibody should be obtained to screen for celiac disease. A sedimentation rate and complete blood cell count are useful to screen for anemia and inflammatory bowel disease. The patient has already had a normal female karyotype, which rules out the diagnosis of Turner syndrome.

(Pages 2014–2015: Section 28, Chapter 522: Growth and Growth Impairment)

Answer 28-26. e

Based on the family history and physical exam, the patient most likely has complete androgen insensitivity syndrome. Females with this condition have a mutation in the androgen receptor. Therefore, testosterone levels are elevated but affected individuals lack physical signs of androgen exposure, such as acne, oily skin, pubic hair, and axillary hair. Testosterone is aromatized to estrogen, which results in normal breast development. This patient has signs of estrogen exposure but not androgen exposure. The karyotype in individuals with complete androgen insensitivity is 46,XY. Patients with complete androgen insensitivity syndrome are phenotypically female and identify themselves as female. Amenorrhea occurs due to lack of a uterus, which does not develop due to production of anti-Müllerian hormone (AMH) from the intra-abdominal testicles.

Infants with complete androgen insensitivity syndrome may present with an inguinal hernia. As it is X-linked, her younger sister may also have this condition. Individuals with partial androgen insensitivity have a wide clinical phenotype with variable degrees of masculinization.

Testosterone and estradiol levels would be at normal pubertal levels. LH and FSH are helpful in evaluating for primary versus secondary gonadal problems (elevated in primary gonadal dysfunction and low in secondary causes). However, a karyotype would be the most helpful test in this clinical scenario.

(Page 2067: Section 28, Chapter 539: Disorders of Sexual Development (DSD))

Answer 28-27. c

Based on the history and physical exam, the patient has Turner syndrome, which occurs in about 1 in 2000 females. Short stature is universal in this condition, and more than 90% of girls require hormone replacement to initiate and progress through puberty due to gonadal dysgenesis. The description of the patient includes many classic features of Turner syndrome (Figure 539-3). Girls with Turner syndrome are prone to recurrent otitis media as well as conductive and sensorineural hearing loss. The mean IQ of girls with Turner syndrome is normal, but they often have difficulties in mathematics, multitasking, and social interactions. As the patient is 14 years old and only has Tanner stage II breast development on one side, it is likely that she has primary ovarian failure.

Girls with Turner syndrome are at risk for the development of autoimmune conditions, such as hypothyroidism and celiac disease. However, a TSH and tissue transglutaminase

IgA antibody may be elevated but would be a less likely reason for delayed pubertal development. An IGF-1 level is an important test to screen for growth hormone deficiency. However, children with Turner syndrome are not growth hormone deficient but are short due to loss of the SHOX gene on the distal short arm of the X chromosome. Estradiol produced by the ovaries may be normal or low in cases of ovarian dysfunction. However, an FSH level is a more sensitive indicator of ovarian function. An elevated FSH level due to gonadal dysgenesis is frequently seen in girls with Turner syndrome before the age of 4 years and after the age of 10 years.

(Pages 2068–2069: Section 28, Chapter 539: Disorders of Sexual Development (DSD))

Answer 28-28. d

Klinefelter syndrome is the most common cause of primary gonadal failure in males, occurring in about 1 in 500 to 1 in 1000 males. The most common karyotype is 47,XXY. Affected individuals usually enter puberty at a normal age but are not able to progress through and complete puberty.

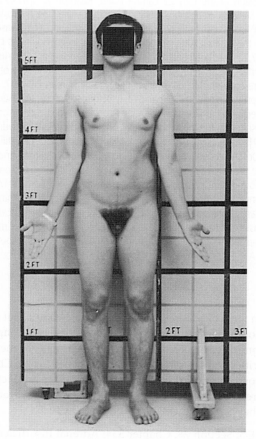

Klinefelter syndrome in a 20-year-old man. Note relatively increased lower/upper body segment ratio, gynecomastia, small penis, and sparse body hair with a female pubic hair pattern. (Reproduced, with permission, from Gardner DG, Shoback D, eds. *Greenspan's Basic & Clinical Endocrinology*. 9th ed. New York: McGraw-Hill, 2011.)

On physical exam, pubic hair development will be normal but the testes are firm and usually no larger than 6 mL. During puberty, gynecomastia commonly occurs in about 90% of patients with Klinefelter syndrome. They may have learning and behavioral problems, but there is a wide clinical spectrum. They are similar to other men with hypogonadism in regards to job status, social adjustment, and criminal behavior. Due to dysgenesis and fibrosis of the seminiferous tubules, infertility occurs. Testosterone replacement results in increased strength, masculinity, and secondary sexual characteristics, but it does not reverse the infertility. By isolating sperm from the testis and using intracytoplasmic sperm injection (ICSI), fertility can be successful.

(Page 2070: Section 28, Chapter 539: Disorders of Sexual Development (DSD))

Answer 28-29. b

CAH due to 21-hydroxylase deficiency accounts for at least half of all cases of ambiguous genitalia in newborns. Male infants appear normal, but females have varying degrees of virilization due to in utero androgen exposure. The appearance of the external genitalia in a girl with 21-hydroxylase deficiency may be indistinguishable from a normal male with the exception of non-palpable gonads.

Newborns with Turner, Noonan, and Klinefelter syndromes do not have ambiguous genitalia. Individuals with 5-alpha reductase may have ambiguous genitalia but this condition is much less common than CAH.

(Page 2063: Section 28, Chapter 539: Disorders of Sexual Development (DSD))

Answer 28-30. d

The best screening test to evaluate for CAH is 17-hydroxyprogesterone. The most common cause of CAH is 21-hydroxylase (p450c21) deficiency. Due to deficiencies in this enzyme, 17-hydroxyprogesterone is not able to be converted to 11-deoxycortisol (Figure 531-1).

Testosterone is a less sensitive screening marker of CAH as it may be elevated in other conditions, and it is also produced by the testes. Cortisol may be low and ACTH may be elevated in CAH, but neither are sensitive or specific screening tests to evaluate for CAH. DHEA-S is a good screening test for adrenal activation, but like the other tests, it is not a sensitive or specific test to screen for CAH. DHEA-S levels may be slightly elevated in children with premature adrenarche, and the DHEA-S level corresponds to the Tanner stage of pubertal development. Markedly elevated levels of DHEA-S would be concerning for an adrenal tumor or cancer.

(Page 2050: Section 28, Chapter 533: Genetic Lesions in Steroidogenesis)

Answer 28-31. a

The patient is exhibiting many signs and symptoms of adrenal insufficiency (Table 534-1).

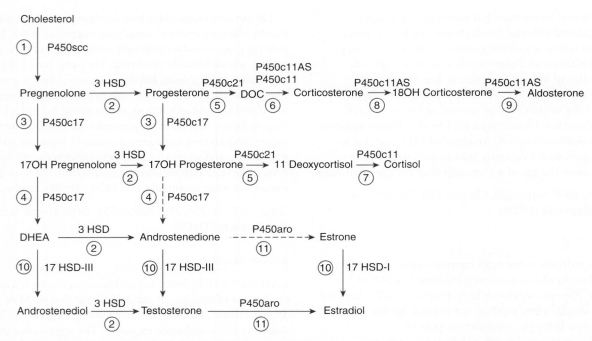

FIGURE 531-1. Principal pathways of human adrenal steroid hormone synthesis. Other quantitatively and physiologically minor steroids are also produced. The names of the enzymes are shown by each reaction, and the traditional names of the enzymatic activities correspond to the *circled numbers*. Reaction 1: Mitochondrial cytochrome P450scc mediates 20α-hydroxylation, 22-hydroxylation, and scission of the C20–22 carbon bond. Reaction 2: 3βHSD mediates 3β-hydroxysteroid dehydrogenase and isomerase activities, converting Δ5 steroids to Δ4 steroids. Reaction 3: P450c17 catalyzes the 17α-hydroxylation of pregnenolone to 17OH-pregnenolone and of progesterone to 17OH-progesterone. Because P450c17 has both 17 α hydroxylase activity and 17,20-lyase activity, it is the branch point in steroid hormone synthesis. Neither activity of P450c17 is present in the adrenal zona glomerulosa; hence, pregnenolone is converted to mineralocorticoids. In the zona fasciculata, the 17 α hydroxylase activity is present, but 17,20-lyase activity is not; hence, pregnenolone is converted to glucocorticoids. In the zona reticularis, both activities are present so that pregnenolone is converted to sex steroids. Reaction 4: The 17,20-lyase activity of P450c17 converts 17OH-pregnenolone to DHEA; only insignificant amounts of 17OH-progesterone are converted to δ4 androstenedione by human P450c17, although this reaction occurs in other species. Reaction 5: P450c21 catalyzes the 21-hydroxylation of progesterone to DOC and of 17OH-progesterone to 11-deoxycortisol. 21-Hydroxylase deficiency causes more than 90% of all cases of congenital adrenal hyperplasia.[37–39] Reaction 6: DOC is converted to corticosterone by the 11-hydroxylase activity of P450c11AS in the zona glomerulosa and by P450c11β in the zona fasciculata. Reaction 7: 11-Deoxycortisol undergoes 11β-hydroxylation by P450c11β to produce cortisol in the zona fasciculata. Patients with disorders in P450c11β have classical 11b hydroxylase deficiency, but can still produce aldosterone. Reactions 8 and 9: The 18-hydroxylase and 18-methyl oxidase activities of P450c11AS convert corticosterone to 18OH-corticosterone and aldosterone, respectively, in the zona glomerulosa. Patients with disorders in P450c11AS have rare forms of aldosterone deficiency (so-called corticosterone methyl oxidase deficiency), while retaining the ability to produce cortisol. Reactions 10 and 11 are found principally in the testes and ovaries. Reaction 10: 17βHSD-III converts DHEA to androstenediol and androstenedione to testosterone, while 17βHSD-I converts estrone to estradiol. Reaction 11: Testosterone may be converted to estradiol and androstenedione may be converted to estrone by P450aro. Aromatase expression in extraglandular tissues, especially fat, can convert adrenal androgens to estrogens. Aromatase in the epiphyses of growing bone converts testosterone to estradiol; the tall stature, delayed epiphyseal maturation and osteopenia of males with aromatase deficiency, and their rapid reversal with estrogen replacement, indicate that estrogen, not androgen, is responsible for epiphyseal maturation in males. (Reproduced, with permission, from Rudolph CD, Rudolph AM, Lister GE, First LR, Gershon AA. *Rudolph's Pediatrics.* 22nd ed. New York: McGraw-Hill, 2011.)

The most common cause of adrenal insufficiency (Table 534-2.) at her age is autoimmune adrenalitis or Addison disease. In primary adrenal insufficiency, low levels of cortisol stimulate the pituitary gland to secrete ACTH, which subsequently leads to increased melanocyte-stimulating hormone (MSH) causing hyperpigmentation in the creases of the hands, buccal mucosa, knuckles, knees, and old scars.

The most common form of adrenoleukodystrophy is X-linked, and therefore, the disease occurs in males. Adrenal insufficiency occurs due to buildup and deposition of very-long chain fatty acids in the adrenal glands, which also occurs in the brain, leading to progressive central nervous system impairment. Salt-wasting congenital adrenal insufficiency is the most

common form of adrenal insufficiency in newborns, but it would not manifest at this age. Girls with nonclassic congenital adrenal insufficiency present with hirsutism, acne, or menstrual irregularities and not symptoms of cortisol deficiency. Children with secondary adrenal insufficiency lack ACTH production. Therefore, signs and symptoms of cortisol deficiency would be present but hyperpigmentation would not be seen.

(Page 2053: Section 28, Chapter 534: Adrenal Insufficiency)

Answer 28-32. e

Plasma concentrations of cortisol and ACTH are highest in the morning and lowest in the evening. ACTH levels peak around

TABLE 534-1. Signs and Symptoms of Adrenal Insufficiency

Features Shared by Acute and Chronic Insufficiency
Anorexia
Apathy and confusion
Dehydration
Fatigue
Hyperkalemia
Hypoglycemia
Hyponatremia
Hypovolemia and tachycardia
Nausea and vomiting
Postural hypotension
Prolonged neonatal jaundice
Salt craving
Weakness
Features of Acute Insufficiency (Adrenal Crisis)
Abdominal pain
Fever
Features of Chronic Insufficiency (Addison Disease)
Decreased pubic and axillary hair
Diarrhea
Hyperpigmentation
Low-voltage electrocardiogram
Small heart on X-ray
Weight loss

4–6 AM leading to a subsequent cortisol peak at about 8 AM. Therefore, a cortisol level drawn at 8 AM (not 4 PM) is the best choice as an initial screen for adrenal insufficiency. An ACTH level by itself is not helpful. If an ACTH level is elevated and cortisol is low, then this is highly suggestive of primary adrenal insufficiency. Due to the diurnal and episodic nature of ACTH and cortisol secretion, a 12-hour urine collection for cortisol would be inaccurate. A 24-hour urinary free cortisol collection as well as a dexamethasone suppression tests are used to evaluate for cortisol excess or Cushing syndrome.

(Page 2045, 2046, and 2053: Section 28, Chapter 531: The Adrenal Cortex; Chapter 532: Evaluation of Adrenal Function; Chapter 534: Adrenal Insufficiency)

Answer 28-33. c

The two most common early signs and symptoms of Cushing syndrome in children are weight gain and growth failure (Figure 535-1). The classic "cushingoid appearance" of cortisol

excess described in adults of striae, moon facies, plethora, buffalo hump/fat pad, hypertension, and muscle weakness often takes several years to manifest in children. Most children who are overweight are tall, as weight is a very strong driver of linear growth in childhood. Hormone causes of linear growth failure include cortisol excess, growth hormone deficiency, and profound hypothyroidism.

(Page 2055: Section 28, Chapter 535: Adrenal Excess

Answer 28-34. a

It is difficult to predict who may have problems with suppression of the hypothalamic–pituitary–adrenal (HPA) axis after glucocorticoid therapy. Some individuals are able to recover their HPA axis quickly after receiving high doses of glucocorticoids over short or long periods of time whereas others may take several weeks or months to recover. Steroid withdrawal symptoms include lethargy, fatigue, nausea, and anorexia. When glucocorticoids have been used for less than 10 days, therapy can typically be discontinued without concern for withdrawal symptoms. However, for the 5-year-old girl with a brain tumor who was treated with dexamethasone for 6 weeks, she will likely have withdrawal symptoms if the glucocorticoid is abruptly stopped without a gradual wean. Furthermore, dexamethasone is a very potent, long-acting glucocorticoid compared to other steroids (Table 536-1).

(Page 2058: Section 28, Chapter 536: Glucocorticoid Therapy and Withdrawal)

Answer 28-35. b

The patient has classic signs and symptoms of new-onset diabetes mellitus, including decreased energy, polydipsia, polyuria, and weight loss. The patient is not in diabetic ketoacidosis (DKA), which is defined by a venous pH less than 7.3 or a serum bicarbonate concentration less than 15 mEq/L. Hyperglycemia causes a factitious hyponatremia. The corrected sodium can be estimated by adding 1.6 mEq to the measured value for each 100 mg/dL of blood glucose above normal. With the patient's blood sugar of 902 mg/dL, this is 8 times higher than a normal blood sugar of 100 mg/dL. Therefore, $8 \times 1.6 = 12.8$. If this value is added to the measured sodium of 127, the corrected sodium is normal at 140 mEq/L.

Hyperkalemia is commonly seen in new-onset diabetes and results from hydrogen ions moving intracellularly and displacing potassium to the extracellular space. The hyperkalemia will improve with hydration, insulin, and correction of the acidosis. An elevated white blood cell count is commonly seen as a stress reaction and positively correlates with the degree of illness. Patients with SIADH will have decreased urine output and not increased urination.

(Page 2110: Section 28, Chapter 544: Diabetes Mellitus)

Answer 28-36. d

The patient has new-onset diabetes and is presenting with diabetic ketoacidosis (DKA). The goals of treatment of DKA

TABLE 536-1. Potency of Various Therapeutic Steroids (Set Relative to the Potency of Cortisol)

Steroid	Anti-Inflammatory Glucocorticoid Effect	Growth-Retarding Glucocortcoid Effect	Salt-Retaining Mineralocorticoid Effect	Plasma Half-life (min)	Biological Half-life (hr)
Cortisol (hydrocortisone)	1.0	1.0	1.0	80–120	8
Cortisone acetate (oral)	0.8	0.8	0.8	80–120	8
Cortisone acetate (IM)	0.8	1.3	0.8		18
Prednisone	4	5	0.25	200	16–36
Prednisolone	4		0.25	120–300	16–36
Methyl prednisolone	5	7.5	0.4		
Betamethasone	25		0	130–330	
Triamcinolone	5		0		
Dexamethasone	30	80	0	150–300	36–54
9α-fluorocortisone	15		200		
DOC acetate	0		20		
Aldosterone	0.3		200–1000		

are to restore perfusion, arrest ketone production, replace electrolyte losses, and avoid complications. The first line of treatment is to restore perfusion by giving NaCl (0.9%) at 20 mL/kg in the first 1 to 2 hours. After the initial fluid bolus, IV fluids should be given based on a rehydration plan accounting for the degree of dehydration and maintenance fluid requirement. Insulin should be started as an insulin drip at 0.1 units/kg/hr as a continuous infusion only after the initial fluid expansion is completed. A bolus of insulin is unnecessary and should be avoided as this could precipitously drop the serum blood sugar as well as increase the risk of cerebral edema. Bicarbonate is not indicated in this clinical scenario and would increase the potential risk for complications.

(Pages 2110–2112: Section 28, Chapter 544: Diabetes Mellitus)

Answer 28-37. d

A serious and potentially life-threatening complication of DKA is cerebral edema. As this patient is less than 5-years-old and received a large volume of fluids upon presentation (100 mL/kg), she is at high risk for cerebral edema. Cerebral edema typically occurs 4–12 hours after starting treatment, but it can occur later or even before treatment has started. Many if not all patients with DKA have some degree of cerebral edema, but most are asymptomatic. Case reports have shown some benefit with mannitol. Close monitoring and rapid recognition of cerebral edema may result in positive outcomes.

Treatment and clinical decision making should not be delayed for the results of a head CT. Bicarbonate is not indicated and would increase the likelihood of cerebral edema. Intubation is not necessary unless respiratory compromise

is present. Hyperventilation has been associated with poor outcomes in patients with cerebral edema. Besides mannitol, other early intervention measures include reduction in the IV fluid rate and elevation of the head of the bed.

(Page 2109: Section 28, Chapter 544: Diabetes Mellitus)

Answer 28-38. a

Although her blood sugar is elevated at 315 mg/dL, she is not in DKA as her bicarbonate level is normal. As she is not vomiting, she can drink oral sugar-free fluids to hydrate and eliminate the ketones. Supplemental insulin will help her to stop making ketones.

If she was not able to drink or was actively vomiting, then IV fluids or admission to the hospital may be necessary. Children with diabetes should check their blood sugar at least four times per day, specifically before breakfast, lunch, supper, and bedtime. Blood sugar testing should be performed more frequently during an illness. When a child with diabetes is ill, ketones should be checked with each void.

(Page 2115: Section 28 – Chapter 544: Diabetes Mellitus)

Answer 28-39. e

DKA occurs when there is a critical net effective deficit of insulin in the body (Figure 544-2). Without insulin, counter-regulatory hormones rise, adipocytes release free fatty acids, and hepatic fatty acid oxidation increases, resulting in ketone body production. Insulin pumps only deliver short-acting insulin and there is no long-acting or background insulin present to suppress ketone production. If a patient with diabetes is without insulin for several hours, ketones will be present in the blood and urine. If this is not recognized quickly, ketone bodies will rise and DKA may occur.

Children with diabetes cannot eat themselves into DKA. For the patient in choices A and B, their blood sugar will be elevated, but they will not develop ketones as long as they have received their long-acting insulin. For the patient in choice C, ketones should not develop if she is off her pump for only 1 hour. Blood sugar is affected by insulin, food, and activity. For the patient in choice D, it is appropriate for her to take less insulin to compensate for the increased physical activity. This decrease in insulin will lower her risk of hypoglycemia and should not result in ketone production. Increased physical activity can be countered by either decreasing the insulin dose or increasing carbohydrate consumption.

(Page 2108: Section 28, Chapter 544: Diabetes Mellitus)

Answer 28-40. b

Lipohypertrophy is due to repeated insulin injections in the same area of the skin. If insulin is injected into areas of lipohypertophy, absorption of insulin becomes erratic and unpredictable, which leads to inconsistent and difficult to regulate blood sugars. Although the patient noted that he is using his abdomen, arms, and legs for insulin injections, he is likely predominantly using just both sides of his abdomen. Lipohypertrophy can be avoided by rotating insulin injection sites and using all available areas, such as the upper arms, thighs, abdomen, hips, and buttocks. The best recommendation for this patient is to rotate his insulin injection sites and avoid the hypertrophied areas until it resolves. Rotation of injection sites will allow for more reliable and predictable insulin absorption.

Switching to a different type of insulin or changing to a pump would not be helpful as all insulin can cause lipohypertrophy due to repeated injections in the same area. The patient is already checking his blood sugar at least 4–6 times a day, which is appropriate. Referral to a dermatologist is not necessary. Rare skin findings in a diabetic patient that might be seen by a dermatologist include necrobiosis lipoidica diabeticorum.

(Page 2116: Section 28, Chapter 544: Diabetes Mellitus)

Answer 28-41. d

Genetics plays an important role in the risk and development of type 2 diabetes. Siblings of affected individuals with type 2 diabetes have a 3.5 times higher risk of developing diabetes than the general population. In studies of monozygotic twins, there is a concordance of almost 100% for type 2 diabetes compared to only about 30% for type 1 diabetes. Obese individuals commonly have elevated insulin levels, but metformin is not always necessary, especially if the patient does not have diabetes. Lifestyle modification, specifically decreased caloric intake and regular exercise, is the first step to improve hyperinsulinism, insulin resistance, and obesity.

DKA is more commonly seen in type 1 diabetes but it can also occur in type 2 diabetes due to severe insulin deficiency and β cell dysfunction from prolonged elevated blood sugar levels. The average age of diagnosis of type 2 diabetes corresponds to the peak of adolescent growth and development, which occurs later than 10 years. Type 2 diabetes is most commonly seen in Native Americans, Asians, African-Americans, and Hispanics.

(Page 2120: Section 28, Chapter 544: Diabetes Mellitus)

Answer 28-42. a

The patient has new-onset diabetes based on her symptoms and elevated random plasma glucose. The diagnostic criteria for diabetes includes symptoms of diabetes and a casual plasma glucose ≥200 mg/dL; fasting plasma glucose ≥126 mg/dL; 2-hour plasma glucose ≥200 mg/dL during an oral glucose tolerance test; or a hemoglobin A1c ≥6.5%. If the patient is asymptomatic, then the test needs to be repeated on a second day to confirm the diagnosis. It is sometimes difficult to determine if a patient has type 1 or type 2 diabetes, as obesity is increasing in all populations in the United States. As she has a history of obesity, is from a high-risk ethnic population, and has signs of insulin resistance (acanthosis nigricans), she most likely has type 2 diabetes. Regardless of whether she has type 1 or type 2 diabetes, she should be started on insulin injections due to her markedly elevated hemoglobin A1c value of 9.5%. Due to glucose toxicity and β cell dysfunction, neither metformin nor a sulfonylurea alone would be effective at this time. The patient does not have ketones in her urine and her bicarbonate level is normal; therefore, she does not have DKA and does not need to be started on IV fluids or an insulin drip. Referral to a dietitian would be helpful, but this is not the best initial management to improve her blood sugar control.

(Page 2124: Section 28, Chapter 544: Diabetes Mellitus)

Answer 28-43. e

Type 1 diabetes involves autoimmune destruction of β cells, and diabetic autoantibodies can be assayed as a reflection of β cell damage. Insulin antibodies, islet cell antibodies, and glutamic acid decarboxylase antibodies are commonly present in type 1 diabetes. Diabetic autoantibodies are uncommon in type 2 diabetes (Table 544-4). Blood glucose and hemoglobin A1c will both be elevated in new-onset diabetes, and therefore, are not helpful in differentiating the type of diabetes. Due to glucose toxicity to β cells in type 2 diabetes and β cell injury in type 1 diabetes, C-peptide and insulin levels may be low in both conditions at diagnosis. Ketones are a reflection of insulin deficiency and can be present in both conditions as well.

(Page 2106: Section 28, Chapter 544: Diabetes Mellitus)

Answer 28-44. e

The laboratory results in the critical sample are consistent with exogenous insulin administration (or factitious hyperinsulinism). The growth hormone and cortisol levels

TABLE 544-4. Differentiating Type 1 from Type 2 Diabetes in Children and Adolescents

	Type I Diabetes	Type 2 Diabetes	Comment
Demographics			
Family history	3–5%	74–10%	Extensive family history suggests type 2; type 2 affects minorities disproportionately
Age or pubertal status	Variable	> 10 or pubertal[a]	Type 1 can occur at any age; only 10% of type 2 children are younger than 10 or prepubertal
Gender	F = M	F > M	Some gender difference in type 2 may reflect differences in use of medical care
Presentation			
Asymptomatic	Rare	Common	Type 2 often detected incidentally on routine physical exam
Symptom duration	Days or weeks	Weeks or months	Predominant symptoms are polyuria, polydipsia, polyphagia, and nocturia
Weight loss	Common	Common	Type 2 children lose more pounds; type 1 usually lose greater percentage of body weight
Hyperglycemic hyperosmolar state[b]	Very rare	Occurs	Type 2 can develop severe/fatal dehydration, electrolyte disturbance
Physical Findings			
Body mass index at diagosis	≤75th Percentile	≥85th Percentile	Those with body mass index in 75th to 85th percentile often present greatest diagnostic challenge
Acanthosis	No	Common	Useful marker in hyperglycemic child
Biochemistry at Diagnosis			
Hyperglycemia	Variable	Varable	Degree of hyperglycemia at diagnosis is not useful in delineating diabetes type
Ketosis and ketonuria	Common	Common	Not useful for diagnosis of diabetes type
Acidosis	Common	Moderately common	Not useful for diagnosis of diabetes type
Other Markers			
HbA₁	Elevated	Elevated	Not useful for diagnosis of diabetes type
Insulin or C-peptide/Serum	Low (may be normal early)	Normal–high	Hyperinsulinism reflects insulin resistance. Low levels may be found in type 2 at diagnosis, repeat 3 to 6 months after diagnosis may be elevated
Autoimmune markers	Common	Uncommon	Includes anti-islet cell and antiglutamic acid carboxylase antibodies; absence does not rule out type 1

[a]Occasionally in 8- to 10-year-old group and as young as 4 years.
[b]Hyperglycemic hyperosmolar state.

are appropriately elevated in the setting of hypoglycemia. Patients with sulfonylurea ingestion or an insulinoma would have a detectable c-peptide level since the hypoglycemia results from endogenous insulin release. Prior to decreasing the IV fluid rate, her glucose infusion rate (GIR) was only 1.4 mg/kg/min [(5 × 20 × 0.167) divided by 12 = 1.4 mg/kg/min]. The normal GIR in healthy infants and young children is approximately 6 mg/kg/min. Therefore, her GIR was not

elevated before the hypoglycemic events. Children with congenital hyperinsulinism require much higher GIRs to maintain normal blood sugar levels. As the child is only 2 years old, it is likely that a caregiver is giving her exogenous insulin. A careful history of whom in the family has access to insulin and syringes should be solicited.

(Page 2129: Section 28, Chapter 545: Endocrine Cause of Hypoglycemia)

Answer 28-45. b

This child likely has growth hormone deficiency. On exam, he has midline abnormalities, including a cleft lip, cleft palate, as well as a micropenis. Children with a cleft lip and palate have a much higher incidence of growth hormone deficiency than children who do not have a cleft lip or palate. In the first few months of life, growth hormone is essential for maintenance of normal blood sugar and it does not become important for linear growth until about 9 months.

Congenital hyperinsulinism is the most common cause of persistent hypoglycemia in the newborn. Infants with congenital hyperinsulinism are often born large for gestational age. Perinatal stress-induced hyperinsulinism, which occurs in about 10% of small-for-gestational-age infants, is a transient state that can last for a few days or up to a few months or more of life. However, in this case, the infant has an appropriate for gestational age birth weight. Gonadotropins may be deficient in children with midline abnormalities and a micropenis, but this would not be responsible for hypoglycemia. Other pituitary hormone deficiencies that can cause hypoglycemia include ACTH deficiency, which results in cortisol deficiency. Infants with Beckwith–Wiedemann syndrome can have hypoglycemia from transient hyperinsulinism, but they do not have a cleft lip, cleft palate, or micropenis.

(Page 2129: Section 28, Chapter 545: Endocrine Cause of Hypoglycemia)

Answer 28-46. c

With the infant's history of hypoglycemia and maternal history of eclampsia and hypertension, the infant most likely has a transient form of hyperinsulinism due to perinatal stress. Infants with GIRs of greater than 10 mg/kg/minute likely have either hyperinsulinism or hypopituitarism. In hyperinsulinism, glycogenolysis is suppressed and glycogen stores are inappropriately not depleted in the setting of hypoglycemia. In this patient, a rise in the plasma glucose of greater than 30 mg/dL after the administration of glucagon indicates inappropriate stores of glycogen at the time of hypoglycemia and is diagnostic of hyperinsulinism. Diazoxide inhibits insulin secretion by activating the opening of the K_{ATP} channel in the β cell (Figure 545-3) and is the initial treatment of choice in infants with hyperinsulinism. Adverse effects include fluid retention and hypertrichosis. Octreotide is a long-acting analog of somatostatin that inhibits insulin release from β cells, but this medication is used only if diazoxide is ineffective. Nifedipine is a calcium channel blocker that has been used in infants with hyperinsulinism but is generally not effective. Growth hormone and hydrocortisone would be indicated if the child has hypopituitarism.

(Page 2126: Section 28, Chapter 545: Endocrine Cause of Hypoglycemia)

Answer 28-47. c

The most concerning symptom is that the child is waking up from sleep to drink and urinate. Psychogenic polydipsia is a behavioral problem that leads to compulsive water drinking. Behavioral problems of increased drinking manifest during the day time when the child is awake but not during the night. Normal children can have primary polydipsia where they drink large volumes of fluid during the day leading to volume overload and increased urination. Young children may use drinking as a way to get their parent's attention, and they will be upset if the fluids are restricted. However, waking up at night to drink and urinate points to a more pathologic condition, such as diabetes insipidus or diabetes mellitus.

(Page 2025: Section 28, Chapter 525: Primary Disturbances in Water Homeostasis)

Answer 28-48. b

The differential diagnosis of polyuria and polydipsia includes diabetes melltitus, diabetes insipidus, psychogenic, hypercalcemia, hypokalemia, and hyperthyroidism. Initial screening labs were unremarkable except for a low urine specific gravity. After a water deprivation test, the patient was able to appropriately concentrate her urine and her serum sodium and osmolality were normal. These labs are most consistent with psychogenic polydipsia or compulsive water drinking.

The syndrome of inappropriate anti-diuretic hormone (SIADH) would present with decreased urine output and hyponatremia. After a prolonged fast, patients with either nephrogenic or central diabetes insipidus would have hypernatremia, hyperosmolality, and an inability to concentrate their urine. Patients with cerebral salt wasting have increased urine output and hyponatremia.

(Page 2025: Section 28, Chapter 525: Primary Disturbances in Water Homeostasis)

Answer 28-49. a

The patient is currently in the second phase of the triphasic response, which commonly occurs after neurosurgery or trauma. The first phase is a transient diabetes insipidus state due to loss of regulation of vasopressin release after neuronal damage. This phase can last for 12 hours or up to several days. The second phase is due to uncontrolled vasopressin release by dying neurons that produce vasopressin, which creates the syndrome of inappropriate anti-diuretic hormone (SIADH). This phase can last for a couple of days or up to a couple of weeks. The third phase is due to complete vasopressin deficiency from neuronal death, which results in permanent diabetes insipidus. SIADH is best treated with fluid restriction. Therefore, the best initial management in this patient is to decrease the IV fluid rate.

Furosemide and hypertonic saline are not part of the initial management of SIADH, and they are only indicated if the patient is neurologically symptomatic (eg, seizures) and serum sodium is less than 120 mEq/L. A vasopressin drip would be indicated in a patient with diabetes insipidus and not SIADH. Oral salt supplementation is used in patients with cerebral salt wasting and not SIADH. Cerebral salt wasting and SIADH are sometimes difficult to differentiate as both have hyponatremia. However, in cerebral salt wasting, urine output is increased and urine sodium is more elevated (>100–150 mEq/L) than in SIADH.

(Page 2025 and 2028: Section 28, Chapter 525: Primary Disturbances in Water Homeostasis)

Answer 28-50. b

Unlike other pituitary hormones, prolactin secretion is tonically inhibited by dopamine. With any disruption in the pituitary stalk, prolactin levels will be elevated. The pituitary is connected by a stalk to the hypothalamus (Figure 521-2). Disruption of the stalk results in a decrease in communication between the hypothalamus and pituitary gland. Therefore, growth hormone will be decreased leading to decreased IGF-1 production; TSH will be decreased leading to decreased free T4 production; and LH will be decreased leading to decreased testosterone production. Cortisol may initially be increased due to stress and illness, but it may also be decreased from ACTH deficiency.

(Page 2012: Section 28, Chapter 521: Disorders of the Anterior Pituitary Gland)

CHAPTER 29 | Neurology

Amy A. Gelfand and Kendall B. Nash

29-1. An 8-year-old girl with juvenile inflammatory arthritis presents with headache 2 weeks after completing a prolonged course of corticosteroids for an arthritis flare. While on corticosteroids, she gained 15 lb and her BMI is now 29 kg/m². Her headache began 1 week ago and is dull in quality, diffuse in location, and constant. It is worse at night and has started to wake her up from sleep. In the last 2 days, she has also developed diplopia. On examination, she has Cushingoid facies. Neurologic examination is significant for bilateral papilledema and a right sixth nerve palsy. MRI of the brain, including MR venogram, is normal. Opening pressure on lumbar puncture is 30 cm H_2O, and CSF composition is normal.

Which medication would be most appropriate for her treatment?

a. Propranolol

b. Acetazolamide

c. Ibuprofen

d. Cyproheptadine

e. Sumatriptan

29-2. A 6-year-old boy complains of episodic severe headaches for the past 6 months. The headaches occur once every 2 weeks and last for 2 hours. He says it hurts "all over" his head, and feels like something is going "boom boom" in his head. His mother notes that he pulls the covers over his head and he asks her to turn off the lights when he has a headache. There are no cranial autonomic symptoms (eg, lacrimation) with the headaches. The mother experiences severe headaches every month before her period that are associated with nausea and vomiting. The child's neurologic examination is normal. What is his diagnosis?

a. Tension-type headaches

b. Idiopathic intracranial hypertension

c. Migraine

d. Cluster headache

e. Seizure

29-3. Which of the following would be the most appropriate migraine preventive medication for a sexually active adolescent girl?

a. Sumatriptan

b. Divalproex sodium

c. Clonidine

d. Propranolol

e. Levetiracetam

29-4. A 10-year-old girl has migraine headaches once every 2 weeks. Her head pain is severe in intensity and there is significant associated nausea and vomiting. Her parents have tried giving her ibuprofen; however, she usually vomits the medication within minutes of taking it. Her parents ask if there is anything else she could try for these headaches. Which of the following would be the most appropriate treatment to recommend?

a. Sumatriptan nasal spray.

b. Continue to use ibuprofen.

c. Ondansetron oral dissolving tablet.

d. Oxygen at 12 L/min.

e. Amitriptyline.

29-5. A 3-day-old term neonate presents to the emergency department because of tachypnea and poor feeding. He was born to a 25-year-old G1P1 mother by normal spontaneous vaginal delivery after an uncomplicated pregnancy. Apgar scores were 8 and 9. His examinations in the nursery were normal and he was discharged to home on day of life 2 latching well and taking colostrum, although his mother's milk had not yet come in. In triage, he is noted to have a respiratory rate of 72. His eyes are closed and he is sluggishly reactive to painful stimuli. Emergent CT of the head rules out intracranial hemorrhage but suggests diffuse cerebral edema. Which laboratory test is most likely to reveal the reason for his encephalopathy?

a. Blood glucose

b. Ammonia

c. Venous blood gas

d. Urine toxicology screen

e. Sodium

29-6. A term neonate develops recurrent focal motor seizures at 12 hours of life. The seizures were first noted by the mother while she was breast-feeding. She reports the infant's left arm began to jerk rhythmically and then the left side of his face began to jerk as well. This lasted for 1 minute before self-resolving. The infant was brought to the nursery where he had a second event, identical to the first. Review of his history revealed that he was born to a 28-year-old G1P1 mother by vaginal delivery. Labor was complicated by a prolonged second stage; however, his fetal heart tracing remained reassuring and he was delivered spontaneously with Apgar scores of 8 and 9. The infant was vigorous at delivery. His neurologic examination at the time of the evaluation was normal. A bedside head ultrasound was performed and intracranial hemorrhage ruled out. Electrolytes were normal. A lumbar puncture was performed and cell counts and chemistries were normal. What is the most likely diagnosis?

a. Viral meningitis

b. Nonepileptic seizures

c. Nonaccidental trauma

d. Hypoxic-ischemic injury

e. Arterial ischemic stroke

29-7. A 3-year-old boy presents with hypotonia and gross motor delay. He can pull to stand, but is not yet walking. He was born at term. His mother recalls decreased fetal movements in utero. The neonatal period was complicated by feeding difficulty. On examination, he has a high-arched palate and a narrow face. There is facial diplegia and his mouth tends to hang open. His speech is nasal in quality and dysarthric. Muscle bulk is diminished throughout, and he is hypotonic. He has proximal weakness in a limb-girdle distribution. The weakness is not fatiguable. Sensation is normal. Deep tendon reflexes are present. What is the localization of his neurologic condition?

a. Upper motor neuron disease

b. Neuromuscular junction

c. Muscle

d. Lower motor neuron disease

e. Peripheral nerve

29-8. A 9-month-old baby girl is evaluated for profound global developmental delay. Examination is notable for coarsened facial features, a gibbous deformity of the thoracolumbar spine, and hepatomegaly. Neurologic examination reveals hypotonia and positional plagiocephaly. Laboratory analysis reveals low β-galactosidase activity.

Which of the following would be most likely on ophthalmologic examination?

a. Cherry-red spot

b. Optic nerve hypoplasia

c. Coloboma

d. Uveitis

e. Congenital cataract

29-9. A 12-year-old boy presents to the emergency room complaining of a severe headache that involves only the right side of his face. He has been having this type of headache on and off for 2 days. The headaches occur twice a day and last for 1 hour each time. There is associated right-sided conjunctival injection, lacrimation, and nasal rhinorrhea during the attacks. His mother notes that he had a similar bout of headaches 6 months ago that lasted for 3 weeks. Of the following, which would be the best first-line therapy?

a. Ketoralac IM

b. Prochlorperazine IV

c. Oxygen via non-rebreather

d. Topiramate

e. Sodium valproate IV

29-10. A baby boy was born at term to a 34-year-old G3P2 mother. Pregnancy was complicated by borderline gestational diabetes. Delivery was complicated by shoulder dystocia, although the infant was ultimately able to be delivered vaginally. Apgars were 8 and 9. Birth weight was 4700 g. In the delivery room, the pediatrics team noted the infant was not moving his left arm. Closer examination in the nursery several hours later revealed a left-sided Horner syndrome. What is the most likely reason for his inability to move the left arm?

a. Pain secondary to clavicular fracture

b. Brachial plexus palsy

c. Postictal Todd paralysis

d. Neonatal stroke

e. In utero drug exposure

29-11. A 12-year-old boy presents to the emergency department complaining of an acute-onset, severe, holocephalic headache that began 12 hours ago. There was no antecedent head trauma. He vomited once at headache onset. He reports this is the worst headache of his life. He is afebrile and neurologic examination is normal; however, he has some neck stiffness. A CT scan is negative for intracranial hemorrhage. What is the next most appropriate step in his care?

a. Reassurance that his headache is benign, and ibuprofen for pain.

b. Lumbar puncture to evaluate for xanthochromia.

c. MRI scan to rule out ischemic stroke.

d. EEG to evaluate for seizure.

e. Start antibiotics for presumed meningitis.

29-12. A 7-year-old comes to see you for "funny movements" for the past 6 weeks. His mother has noticed that at times he wiggles his nose or clears his throat repetitively. These behaviors occur several times per day. She is always able to get his attention during these movements, and he is not sleepy afterwards. The patient says he tries not to make the movements in class as some of the kids make fun of him. After a few minutes of suppressing the behaviors, he finds it difficult not to do them. His neurologic examination is normal. Which of the following is the most appropriate next step in his care?

a. Obtain an EEG.

b. Order an MRI of the brain.

c. Send a serum ceruloplasmin level.

d. Reassurance and counseling.

e. Lumbar puncture.

29-13. A 13-year-old girl with acute migraine is treated in the emergency department with intravenous fluids and prochlorperazine. She develops a dystonic reaction. What is the most appropriate treatment?

a. Diphenhydramine

b. Chlorperazine

c. Phenytoin

d. Acetaminophen

e. Observation

29-14. An 8-year-old boy comes in with 2 days of left-sided facial weakness. He awoke with it in the morning and it has been stable since. He reports that things sound louder than usual and his taste on the left side of his tongue seems abnormal. On examination, the left side of his face moves significantly less than the right. The forehead is involved. The remainder of his neurologic examination is normal. What is the localization of his facial weakness?

a. Cortex

b. Muscle

c. Seventh nerve

d. Eighth nerve

e. Midbrain

29-15. A 15-year-old boy comes to the office complaining of headache for 1 day. The day prior he had played in a football game and banged his helmet against another player's during a tackle. He did not lose consciousness, however felt "dazed" immediately following the event and had to sit out for the rest of the game. The headache began within an hour of the event. He also reports trouble concentrating, and sensitivity to light and sound. Neurologic examination is normal. Neuropsychological testing indicates he is currently performing below his preseason baseline. He asks if he can go to football practice later that afternoon. What would be the most appropriate counseling?

a. He can warm up with the team, but should not participate in any tackling drills.

b. He can play, but if his headache starts to get worse, he should sit out.

c. He should stay home for now on cognitive and physical rest until symptoms resolve.

d. He should focus on schoolwork, and only return to football once he can concentrate on academics again.

e. He can practice as long as his headache improves with ibuprofen.

29-16. A 2-month-old baby boy comes into the emergency department after having a focal convulsive seizure at home. The parents state that he rolled off the changing table and hit his head. On examination, he is lethargic and difficult to arouse. An emergent head CT shows a left-sided subdural hemorrhage with an overlying skull fracture. What other testing is indicated to evaluate this child?

a. Seizure protocol brain MRI

b. Skeletal survey

c. Lumbar puncture

d. Vascular imaging of the intracranial vessels

e. Serum electrolytes

29-17. A term infant is born by emergency cesarean section for fetal distress. Intraoperatively the obstetricians suspect that a placental abruption has caused the fetal distress. Labor had been uneventful until the fetal heart rate dropped suddenly.

At delivery, the infant has low tone, a poor suck, and an absent Moro reflex. Apgar scores were 1 and 4 at 1 and 5 minutes, respectively. He is treated with therapeutic hypothermia for presumed hypoxic-ischemic injury. At 18 hours of life he develops seizures, which are controlled with phenobarbital and stop after 24 hours. His neurologic examination remains mildly abnormal after the cooling is completed; however, he is opening his eyes and beginning to breast-feed. His EEG background is normalized by 48 hours of life. An MRI scan suggests moderate brain injury. Which of the following is the most accurate way to counsel the family?

a. Therapeutic hypothermia prevented any permanent neurologic injury, and the child will definitely develop normally.

b. The baby now has epilepsy and will need antiseizure medication for at least 2 years.

c. The baby is at risk for both motor and cognitive disabilities, and needs close monitoring.

d. An elective C-section could have prevented the child's injury.

e. The child is neurologically devastated, and will never learn to walk, talk, or feed himself.

29-18. A 9-year-old girl with a history of severe birth asphyxia with resultant quadriplegic cerebral palsy comes to clinic. Her mother reports that the child's legs are so stiff that the physical therapists are having difficulty doing range of motion exercises with her. On examination, she has severe spasticity in all extremities, particularly the legs. She appears uncomfortable when the examiner tries to range her lower extremities, and she has contractures at the ankles. What medication might be helpful in treating her spasticity?

a. Baclofen

b. Chlorpromazine

c. Phenobarbital

d. Valproic acid

e. Venlafaxine

29-19. A 3-year-old girl comes to urgent care because since she woke up that morning she has been "clumsy" and "has been falling much more than usual." She has not vomited. On examination, she is afebrile and well appearing. There is horizontal nystagmus on end-gaze bilaterally. When she reaches for a toy, her accuracy is poor bilaterally. Her gait is wide-based and she tends to veer to the side and prefers to walk along the hallway wall to help her balance. Her mother notes that about 10 days earlier she had a febrile illness with vomiting and diarrhea. What is the most likely diagnosis?

a. Posterior fossa mass

b. Hydrocephalus

c. Acute cerebellar ataxia

d. Seizure

e. Guillain-Barré syndrome

29-20. A 6-year-old boy presents to the emergency room with fever and altered mental status. On examination, there is nuchal rigidity. On neurologic examination, he is somnolent and pupils are dilated and slow to react to light. The treating physician is concerned for bacterial meningitis. Which of the following correctly describes the optimal timing of when antibiotics should be started?

a. After the CT scan is done

b. Without any delay

c. Once the lumbar puncture has been performed

d. When the lab calls with the STAT Gram stain results

e. After the hearing test

29-21. A 12-year-old girl tells you her neurologist started her on a preventive medication for migraine. She can't remember the name of the medication, but complains that since starting it she is having more difficulty concentrating at school and is having word-finding difficulties. Which medication was she most likely started on?

a. Propranolol

b. Topiramate

c. Valproate

d. Amitriptyline

e. Gabapentin

29-22. A 16-year-old girl complains of left eye pain and visual blurring in the left eye. Her acuity in that eye is 20/100 compared with 20/20 in the right eye. When the examiner shows her a red object, she states it appears "less red" on the left compared with the right. The fundoscopic examination is normal and there are no eye movement abnormalities. The remainder of her neurologic examination is normal. What is the neuroanatomic localization of her visual disturbance?

a. Optic nerve

b. Optic chiasm

c. Lateral geniculate nucleus

d. Visual cortex

e. Not localizable (ie, conversion disorder)

29-23. A 21-month-old girl is brought to the pediatrician's office for several days of unusual eye movements. Her mother notes that she also has not been sleeping well for the last couple of weeks. On examination, she has random, conjugate, chaotic eye movements. She is somewhat dysmetric on reaching for objects bilaterally. There are no abnormal jerking movements. What condition should she be promptly investigated for?

a. Ovarian teratoma

b. Limbic encephalitis

c. Neurotransmitter disorder

d. Neuroblastoma

e. Landau-Kleffner syndrome

29-24. A term infant is noted to be hypoglycemic in the first few hours of life. Labor and delivery were uneventful and the mother did not have diabetes. The hypoglycemia corrects with intravenous dextrose, but the infant requires continuous intravenous dextrose to maintain a normal glucose. The physician notes that the infant's pupils do not react to light and he does not attend to visual stimuli. However, he responds well to sound and is interested in feeding. An ophthalmologist examines the infant and notes optic nerve hypoplasia bilaterally. The remainder of his neurologic examination is normal. What is most likely to be seen on brain MRI?

a. Agenesis of the corpus callosum

b. Absence of the septum pellucidum

c. Stenosis of the cerebral aqueduct

d. Cerebellar-pontine hypoplasia

e. Evidence of hypoxic-ischemic injury

29-25. You have been referred a new 7-year-old patient to your clinic. She has a history of neurofibromatosis type 1 (NF1). What screening examination should young children with NF1 have annually?

a. Ophthalmologic examination

b. Brain MRI

c. Hearing tests

d. Cardiac echo

e. Wood's lamp examination

29-26. A 2-year-old little boy presents because the mother is concerned that he is having seizures. She describes that when he gets frustrated or upset, he will cry, and then turn purple in the face and lose consciousness. He has a few seconds of jerking movements after losing consciousness. He regains consciousness immediately and does not seem sleepy afterwards. He never has a spell without first becoming upset and crying. What is the most likely diagnosis?

a. Epilepsy

b. Child abuse

c. Gastroesophageal reflux

d. Cardiac arrhythmia

e. Breath-holding spell

29-27. A 9-month-old infant has episodes of torticollis every 3 weeks that last between 20 and 30 minutes. He typically does not want to feed during these periods and sometimes looks pale. He is also not as playful as he usually is. Between episodes he returns completely to his normal self. His neurologic examination is normal and he has achieved normal developmental milestones. What condition might he develop later in childhood?

a. Epilepsy

b. Depression

c. Migraine

d. Breath-holding spells

e. Anxiety

29-28. A 12-year-old girl presents complaining of fatigue for the last few weeks. She notes that while she feels normal in the morning, as the day goes on she gets more tired. She cannot exercise as much as she used to. In the evenings, she sometimes gets double vision while watching TV, and needs to rest while eating dinner or she notes that she starts to drool. On examination, she has mild ptosis bilaterally at baseline, although it is more noticeable on the right. On sustained upgaze testing, the ptosis becomes more prominent and she complains of diplopia. What is the localization for her symptoms?

a. Muscle

b. Nerve

c. Neuromuscular junction

d. Pons

e. Spinal cord

29-29. A 2-week-old baby boy comes into urgent care for seizures. He has been feeding poorly with minimal weight gain. On examination, his skin feels lax and his hair is kinky and lightly pigmented compared with his skin. He has a pectus excavatum. His visual tracking is poor. His prenatal course was unremarkable and he had a normal newborn screen.

What is his most likely diagnosis?

a. Phenylketonuria

b. Menkes disease

c. Biotinidase deficiency

d. Urea cycle defect

e. GM1 gangliosidosis

29-30. You are asked to see a child with Fabry disease. He has bouts of painful crises that often involve "burning" or "piercing" pains that originate in the hands and feet. What medication can be used to treat the pain crises that often occur in Fabry disease?

a. Carbamazepine

b. Baclofen

c. Propranolol

d. Diphenhydramine

e. Prochlorperazine

29-31. A 7-year-old boy began to have trouble with attention and hyperactivity both at school and at home several months ago. His parents bring him to clinic after he complains of difficulty seeing for several weeks, and then has a generalized convulsion. Examination shows poor visual attention and mild spasticity in the legs. An MRI of the brain shows abnormalities of the parieto-occipital white matter. Plasma levels of very-long-chain fatty acids are elevated.

What is the most likely diagnosis?

a. Aicardi-Goutières syndrome

b. X-linked adrenoleukodystrophy

c. Attention deficit-hyperactivity disorder

d. Neuronal ceroid lipofuscinosis

e. Juvenile-onset Alexander disease

29-32. The port wine stain characteristic of Sturge-Weber syndrome is most commonly found:

a. In an upper motor neuron seventh nerve pattern

b. In a lower motor neuron seventh nerve pattern

c. In the first division of the trigeminal nerve, bilaterally

d. In the first division of the trigeminal nerve, unilaterally

e. In the distribution of the greater occipital nerve

29-33. A 2-day-old, former full-term neonate has seizures that are difficult to control. Her mother reports that in utero the baby had significantly more "hiccups" than her other children did. On examination, the infant is encephalopathic and hypotonic. Labor and delivery were uneventful and the infant had Apgar scores of 8 and 9. What test or intervention would be most useful in identifying the etiology for her seizures?

a. Brain MRI

b. EEG

c. Lumbar puncture

d. EMG

e. Response to therapeutic hypothermia

29-34. A 3-year-old boy has been having headaches that wake him up from sleep for the last week. He has vomited several times. He says he sees "2 doctors" when he looks at you. On examination, he has end-gaze horizontal nystagmus bilaterally and gait ataxia. He cannot bury his sclera on the left. He is unable to tolerate a funduscopic examination. What is the most likely etiology for his headaches?

a. Migraine

b. Tension-type headache

c. Idiopathic intracranial hypertension

d. Cerebral aneurysm

e. Posterior fossa mass

29-35. Which cranial nerve is most likely to be affected by Lyme disease?

  a. Optic nerve

  b. Oculomotor nerve

  c. Trigeminal nerve

  d. Facial nerve

  e. Hypoglossal nerve

29-36. A 12-year-old girl is being evaluated for possible seizures. She has a seizure about once a week. Typically they occur when she is in a stressful situation or frightened. Her eyes roll up and she has asynchronous jerking movements of all extremities and pelvic thrusting for about 15 minutes. A routine EEG is normal; however, no events were captured. What is the next best step in her management?

  a. Start an antiepileptic medication.

  b. Benzodiazepines as needed.

  c. Referral for behavioral therapy.

  d. The parents should ignore the events.

  e. Admit for video EEG monitoring.

29-37. A 10-year-old boy presents with 10 hours of progressive bilateral lower extremity weakness and urinary retention. He is awake and alert. Cranial nerve function is normal. What is the neuroanatomic localization of his symptoms?

  a. Brain stem

  b. Spinal cord

  c. Lumbosacral plexus, bilateral

  d. Brain

  e. Neuromuscular junction

29-38. A neonate is being loaded on phenobarbital for seizures. What is the most likely side effect the neonatology team should be prepared for?

  a. Hyponatremia

  b. Respiratory suppression

  c. Anaphylaxis

  d. Hypertension

  e. Dystonic reaction

29-39. A 15-month-old girl presents to the emergency department after a reported generalized convulsion at home that lasted 60 seconds. A rectal temperature on arrival is 39.5°C. She is well appearing and back to her baseline with a normal neurologic examination. She is an otherwise healthy and normally developing girl. Mom had a febrile seizure when she was 2 years old. What are the clinical features that would increase this child's risk of future epilepsy?

  a. Family history of febrile seizures in a first-degree relative

  b. Age of fist febrile seizure <18 months

  c. Level of temperature at first seizure

  d. Complex febrile seizure (focal, prolonged, or repeated)

  e. Duration of illness before seizure

29-40. A 6-month-old normally developing boy presents to pediatric urgent care for episodes of brief arm jerks for the past 5 days. The movements occur in clusters on awakening. The parents report he is quiet during the arm jerks, which last only a few seconds, but he cries after each jerk. His examination is normal.

You develop a broad differential diagnosis that includes several potential diagnoses including benign myoclonic epilepsy of infancy, infantile spasms, and focal seizures. In planning your workup, which of the following neurologic diagnoses requires an electroencephalogram to confirm the diagnosis?

  a. Benign myoclonic epilepsy of infancy

  b. Benign sleep myoclonus

  c. Infantile spasms

  d. Focal seizures

  e. Tonic seizures

29-41. A healthy 7-year-old girl presents to your clinic with her mother, who claims she has noticed that her daughter has been "spacing out" many times a day over the past month. On further questioning, mom reports that these episodes last about 10 seconds, during which she is unresponsive with a behavioral arrest. Her teachers have also reported similar episodes at school. The patient endorses feeling that she "loses time" sometimes and was recently hit on the head with a soccer ball during one of these episodes. Her examination is normal.

Based on the most likely diagnosis, what is the best next step?

  a. Obtain blood work, including CBC and LFTs.

  b. Schedule a referral to a neurologist and an EEG.

  c. Obtain a brain MRI.

  d. Ask the patient's mother to keep an event diary and schedule follow-up in 1 month.

  e. Schedule a referral to a psychiatrist.

29-42. Which of the following antiepileptic drugs is most likely to cause an allergic skin reaction?

    a. Levetiracetam

    b. Topiramate

    c. Valproic acid

    d. Lamotrigine

    e. Zonisamide

29-43. You are taking care of a 5-year-old boy who has had recurrent seizures and was recently diagnosed as having idiopathic epilepsy. What is the most common form of idiopathic epilepsy in children?

    a. Childhood absence epilepsy

    b. Juvenile myoclonic epilepsy

    c. Benign epilepsy with centrotemporal spikes (BECTS)

    d. Childhood occipital epilepsy, Gastaut type

    e. Benign occipital epilepsy, Panayiotopoulos syndrome

29-44. A 13-year-old girl with a history of generalized tonic–clonic seizures arrives to the emergency department by ambulance after having a convulsion lasting 5 minutes at home. She is sleepy but arousable on arrival without any focal neurologic findings. Vital signs are normal. There is no history of illness or trauma. She takes lamotrigine for seizure control.

As part of her diagnostic evaluation, what test would be most important in this situation?

    a. Head CT scan

    b. EEG

    c. Lamotrigine level

    d. CBC and LTs

    e. Lumbar puncture

29-45. A 6-month-old with developmental regression and a 1-month history of seizures is seen for a follow-up visit in your clinic. The cause of her developmental regression and new-onset seizures is unknown. Imaging and laboratory tests have not yet been performed.

The local neurologist's first available clinic appointment is in 4 weeks.

In the interim, which of the following antiepileptic medications should *not* be started in this child?

    a. Phenobarbital

    b. Valproic acid (VPA)

    c. Topiramate

    d. Levetiracetam

    e. Zonisamide

29-46. A 12-year-old boy presents to the emergency room after having an episode of unresponsiveness with shaking of all extremities lasting 2 minutes. The event occurred during wakefulness and was witnessed by his mother. When the paramedics arrived, he was sleepy but arousable. His serum glucose was 100.

When he arrives to the ER by ambulance, he is well appearing with normal vital signs, and is alert with a normal neurologic examination.

What is the most appropriate course of action?

    a. Admission to the hospital for observation.

    b. Perform a lumbar puncture to exclude meningitis.

    c. Diagnose the patient with epilepsy.

    d. Contact the PMD to coordinate an outpatient referral to a neurologist.

    e. Start an antiepileptic medication.

29-47. An 8-month-old boy with unexplained developmental delay who recently moved to the area presents in urgent care for worsening spells over the past month. These spells are described as "jackknife" movements in which there is a quick head drop with flexion at the waist and lower extremities. These episodes have been occurring over the past 3 weeks with increasing frequency, and they tend to cluster on waking up. On examination, he is hypotonic and 5 hypomelanotic macules are noted.

What is the patient's most likely underlying diagnosis?

    a. Tuberous sclerosis complex (TSC)

    b. Severe myoclonic epilepsy in infancy (Dravet syndrome)

    c. Benign myoclonic epilepsy in infancy

    d. Ohtahara syndrome

    e. Hydrocephalus

29-48. A 2-year-old girl presents to your clinic for a routine checkup. She is meeting her developmental milestones, has a normal examination, and does not have any medical problems. Her mother is concerned about her history of febrile seizures, which includes 4 simple febrile seizures over the past 12 months, and asks you if her risk of future epilepsy is increased due to the number of febrile seizures.

How will you counsel this patient?

a. If she continues to have frequent febrile seizures past age 2 years, then her risk will increase.

b. The number of seizures does not predict risk of future epilepsy, but her age of onset (before 18 months) does increase her risk.

c. The number of simple febrile seizures does not correlate with risk of future epilepsy.

d. If she has 1 more simple febrile seizure, then her risk of epilepsy increases.

e. Her risk is already 15% of developing future epilepsy.

29-49. What percentage of children with new-onset epilepsy will eventually be able to discontinue medication and remain seizure-free?

a. 10%

b. 30%

c. 50%

d. 70%

e. 90%

29-50. You are taking care of a 4-year-old girl who has had several generalized tonic–clonic (GTC) seizures over the past 6 weeks. She has no significant past medical history. You decide to refer her to a neurologist in hopes of pursuing a formal diagnosis.

Which if the following is the most important reason for accurate identification of an epilepsy syndrome?

a. It may avoid the need to obtain an EEG and hospitalization.

b. It may avoid the need to check antiepileptic drug levels and drug interactions.

c. It may prompt genetic testing for future pregnancies and screening of siblings.

d. It may help with prognosis and choice of antiepileptic therapy.

e. It can determine if prenatal and environmental exposures were associated with symptoms.

29-51. A 4-month-old infant is seen in the office for a new patient visit. The patient's mother reports that her daughter had "seizures" involving clonic movements starting at 5 days of life and remitting at 1 month of life spontaneously. Brain MRI and metabolic studies at the time of seizure onset were normal. Her examination and developmental are normal. There is no family history of seizures. What is the most likely diagnosis?

a. Infantile spasms

b. Early myoclonic epilepsy (EME)

c. Benign neonatal convulsions

d. Benign familial neonatal convulsions

e. Nonketotic hyperglycinemia

29-52. A 9-month-old with a history of seizures is admitted to the pediatric ICU for status epilepticus. The infant has had seizures since several days of life and the etiology is unclear.

In addition to traditional antiepileptic medications, which of the following therapies should be considered in an infant with unexplained intractable epilepsy?

a. Folic acid

b. Pyridoxine (vitamin B_6)

c. Vitamin D

d. Glucose

e. Cobalamin (vitamin B_{12})

29-53. A 6-month-old infant presents to the emergency room after a brief convulsion at home in the setting of fever for 3 days. In the emergency room, his temperature is 40.0°C, his anterior fontanelle is bulging and firm, pupils are equal and responsive to light bilaterally, and he moves all extremities equally to stimulation. What is the most important initial intervention?

a. Antibiotics

b. Neuroimaging

c. Antiepileptic medication

d. EEG

e. Lumbar puncture

29-54. A 2-year-old boy presents to your clinic for a well-child visit. You notice that his head circumference plots above the 90th percentile. Which of the following conditions is *not* associated with macrocephaly?

a. Hydrocephalus

b. Sotos syndrome

c. Tay-Sachs disease

d. Hypoxic-ischemic encephalopathy

e. Canavan disease

29-55. You are evaluating an otherwise healthy and normally developing 6-month-old with stable macrocephaly. Which part of the history is most helpful in making the diagnosis?

a. Birth history

b. Family history of seizures

c. Parental head circumference scores

d. Pregnancy history

e. Immunization status

29-56. A 10-year-old girl with a history of transient left-sided weakness due to a partial transverse myelitis now presents to urgent care with a 3-day history of worsening blurry vision of her right eye. On examination, her right eye demonstrates decreased visual acuity (20/200) and papillitis. The rest of her neurologic examination is normal. Lumbar puncture reveals normal cell count and normal glucose and protein. Brain MRI shows right optic nerve enhancement and several T2 hyperintense lesions in the periventricular white matter. What is the most likely diagnosis?

a. Acute disseminated encephalomyelitis (ADEM)

b. Clinically isolated syndrome

c. Increased intracranial pressure

d. Focal arterial ischemic stroke

e. Multiple sclerosis

29-57. A 12-year-old girl with a history of transverse myelitis now presents to urgent care with a 2-day history of worsening blurry vision of her right eye. On examination, her right eye demonstrates decreased visual acuity and papillitis. What is the best acute treatment for this patient?

a. Antibiotics

b. Plasmapheresis

c. High-dose methylprednisolone

d. Oral steroids

e. Cytoxan

29-58. A 10-year-old boy presents with altered mental status and lower extremity weakness. Based on neuroimaging, he is diagnosed with acute disseminated encephalomyelitis (ADEM). What percentage of children who present with ADEM will have only 1 event without recurrence?

a. 10%

b. 20%

c. 40%

d. 60%

e. 80%

29-59. An 8-year-old previously healthy boy develops subacute onset of bilateral leg weakness with bowel and bladder incontinence over 3 days. On examination in the emergency room, he has bilateral leg weakness, increased lower extremity deep tendon reflexes, and absent anal wink reflex. Emergent spinal MRI is indicated to exclude which of the following diagnoses?

a. Multiple sclerosis

b. Guillain-Barré syndrome

c. Acute arterial ischemic stroke

d. Spinal epidural hematoma

e. Transverse myelitis

29-60. A 12-year-old girl with recent diagnosis of multiple sclerosis presents to your clinic with complaints of blurry vision. Which of the following symptoms or signs would support a diagnosis of optic neuritis?

a. Proptosis

b. Color vision deficit

c. Inability to abduct the affected eye

d. Foreign body sensation

e. Eyelid swelling

29-61. A 15-year-old girl has a history of multiple episodes of transient neurologic symptoms with associated T2 hyperintense white matter lesions suggestive of multiple sclerosis. Which of the following diagnostic tests offers further support of a diagnosis of multiple sclerosis?

a. Low serum vitamin D level

b. Elevated ESR

c. Presence of 2 or more oligoclonal bands in the CSF but not in the serum

d. Presence of 2 or more oligoclonal bands in the CSF and in the serum

e. Elevated vitamin B_{12}

29-62. A 3-month-old infant is brought to the pediatrician for evaluation of excessive startle response to tactile stimulation and developmental regression over the past month. On examination, there is mild hepatosplenomegaly. He does not make good eye contact, does not vocalize, and has axial hypotonia with appendicular hypertonia and increased reflexes. Ophthalmologic examination performed earlier that day showed a macular cherry-red spot. What is the enzyme deficiency in this disease?

a. β-Hexosaminidase α-subunit

b. β-Hexosaminidase β-subunit

c. Ornithine transcarbamylase

d. Acid α-glucosidase

e. α-Galactosidase A

29-63. Which statement is correct regarding diagnostic tests in Tay-Sachs and Sandhoff diseases?

   a. Tay-Sachs is associated with hexosaminidase A deficiency in white blood cells, while Sandhoff disease is associated with hexosaminidase A and B deficiency.

   b. Tay-Sachs is associated with hexosaminidase B deficiency in white blood cells, while Sandhoff disease is associated with hexosaminidase A and B deficiency.

   c. Tay-Sachs is associated with hexosaminidase A and B deficiency in white blood cells, while Sandhoff disease is associated with hexosaminidase A deficiency.

   d. Tay-Sachs is associated with hexosaminidase A and B deficiency in white blood cells, while Sandhoff disease is associated with hexosaminidase B deficiency.

   e. Tay-Sachs is associated with hexosaminidase A deficiency in white blood cells, while Sandhoff disease is associated with hexosaminidase B deficiency.

29-64. Gaucher disease displays which type of inheritance pattern?

   a. Autosomal dominant

   b. X-linked recessive

   c. X-linked dominant

   d. Autosomal recessive

   e. Mitochondrial

29-65. A 2-year-old boy has a history of myoclonic seizures since 9 months of life, slowly progressive ataxia, acquired microcephaly, and recent-onset visual decline. His ophthalmologic examination reveals macular degeneration, retinal degeneration, and optic atrophy. EEG displays epileptiform discharges in response to low-frequency photic stimulation. What is the most likely diagnosis?

   a. Dravet syndrome

   b. Infantile spasms

   c. Neuronal ceroid lipofuscinosis (NCL)

   d. Lennox-Gastaut syndrome

   e. Ohtahara syndrome

29-66. What clinical characteristic can be seen in all of the following metabolic disorders: sialidosis type I, Gaucher, Sandhoff, and Neimann-Pick type A?

   a. Hepatosplenomegaly

   b. Cherry-red spot

   c. Hyperpigmented skin lesions

   d. Cognitive impairment

   e. Early death

29-67. You are seeing a 7-year-old boy with new-onset attention deficit-hyperactivity disorder, cognitive decline, visual changes, and elevated very-long-chain fatty acids (VLCFA). Which is the most accurate prognosis for this patient?

   a. Stabilization of symptoms within next 2 years

   b. Recovery of symptoms within next 2 years

   c. Slow worsening of symptoms within next 10 years

   d. Significant neurologic impairment and often death within the next 2 years

   e. Normalization of VLCFA within next 2 years

29-68. In a child diagnosed with X-linked leukodystrophy, what is an important initial assessment?

   a. ACTH

   b. Vitamin B_{12}

   c. Platelets

   d. ESR

   e. Bicarbonate

29-69. A 4-month-old girl presents with extreme irritability and developmental regression. On examination, there is diffusely increased tone. CSF evaluation reveals increased protein. MRI showed extensive T2 hyperintense lesions involving the brain stem and centrum semiovale, and T2 hypointensity of the bilateral thalami. Which laboratory test is diagnostic of this disorder?

   a. Undetectable galactocerebrosidase level

   b. Elevated galactocerebrosidase level

   c. Elevated very-long-chain fatty acids (VLCFA)

   d. Absence of arylsulfatase A activity

   e. Duplication of PLP1

29-70. You see a 6-month-old infant with Pelizaeus-Merzbacher disease (PMD) in your office for routine checkup. What feature of this disease is incorrect?

   a. X-linked recessive inheritance pattern.

   b. Typical clinical presentation occurs in boys and girls with equal frequency.

   c. The majority of PMD cases can be linked to abnormalities in the proteolipid protein 1 (PLP1) gene on chromosome Xq22.

   d. In the connatal and classic forms of PMD, nystagmus is one of the defining clinical features.

   e. Treatment is supportive.

29-71. West syndrome refers to the triad including which features?

   a. Abnormal neuroimaging, abnormal development, infantile spasms

   b. Abnormal development, microcephaly, infantile spasms

   c. Abnormal development, hypsarrhythmia, infantile spasms

   d. Normal development, hypsarrhythmia, infantile spasms

   e. Abnormal neuroimaging, hypsarrhythmia, infantile spasms

29-72. The ketogenic diet would be a reasonable option relatively early in the course of all of the following epilepsies except which one?

   a. Dravet syndrome

   b. Lennox-Gastaut syndrome

   c. Doose syndrome

   d. Benign rolandic epilepsy

   e. Infantile spasms

29-73. A 17-year-old otherwise healthy boy presents to the emergency room 1 hour after experiencing sudden-onset right face and arm weakness along with expressive and receptive aphasia as witnessed and reported by his mother. There were no preceding symptoms. His examination reveals right-sided hemiparesis and global aphasia. What is the first diagnosis to exclude?

   a. Migraine

   b. Conversion disorder

   c. Seizure

   d. Multiple sclerosis

   e. Childhood stroke

29-74. A 5-year-old girl with acute bacterial meningitis is comatose in the intensive care unit with an intracranial pressure (ICP) monitor, which shows raised ICP. What measure would help lower the ICP acutely?

   a. Administer mannitol.

   b. Change the dose of antibiotics.

   c. Hypoventilation.

   d. Perform a neuroimaging study.

   e. Put the patient in Trendelenburg position.

29-75. A 2-month-old girl with developmental delay, new-onset infantile spasms, and chorioretinal lacunae received a brain MRI. What is the most likely finding?

   a. Normal

   b. Hypoplastic cerebellum

   c. Astrocytoma

   d. Focal stroke

   e. Absent corpus callosum, partial or complete

ANSWERS

Answer 29-1. B

Idiopathic intracranial hypertension (IIH), previously known as pseudotumor cerebri, is characterized by elevated intracranial pressure in the absence of any structural cause or CSF abnormality. The underlying cause is not well understood. Before puberty, girls and boys are equally likely to be affected. After puberty, there is a female predominance. Recent use of certain medications, including corticosteroids, has been associated with IIH. Being overweight is also associated, and weight loss is an important component of long-term management in overweight patients.

Elevated intracranial pressure should be suspected in a patient who complains of a headache that is worse when laying flat; the patient may describe this as worse when they lay down to go to sleep, or that the headache is waking them up from sleep. A fundoscopic examination is essential to evaluate for papilledema, which is swelling of the optic nerve head due to increased pressure. However, early on this finding can be absent. Neuroimaging, including venous imaging, is necessary to rule out other causes of elevated intracranial pressure such as an intracranial mass or venous sinus thrombosis. Following neuroimaging, lumbar puncture with measurement of opening pressure should be performed with the patient in the lateral decubitus position with the legs extended. IIH can be vision threatening and close monitoring of visual function is needed.

Carbonic anhydrase inhibitors, such as acetazolamide, are first-line therapies as they decrease CSF production. Propranolol and cyproheptadine are used as migraine preventives in children; ibuprofen and sumatriptan are acute therapies for migraine.

(Page 2177, Section 29: Disorders of the Nervous System, Chapter 553: Hydrocephalus and Pseudotumor Cerebri)

Answer 29-2. c

Primary headache disorders are relatively common in pediatrics. This child meets diagnostic criteria for migraine. Migraineurs typically describe a pounding or pulsating quality to their head pain; children may describe this as "booming" like their heartbeat. Pediatric migraine can be shorter in duration than adult migraine, with a minimum duration of 1 hour. In addition, symptoms such as photophobia (light sensitivity) and phonophobia (sound sensitivity) can be inferred from the child's behavior, such as pulling the covers over their head. There is usually a family history of migraine, although it is not uncommon for the family member to think it is "normal" to get frequent headaches. Interviewing family members directly about the features of their headaches can be helpful.

Tension-type headaches are not accompanied by migrainous features such as photophobia or nausea. Idiopathic intracranial hypertension is characterized by head pain that is worse when lying flat, whereas migraineurs typically prefer to lay down when they have severe headache. Cluster headache is a rare headache disorder that is characterized by unilateral headache associated with at least 1 cranial autonomic symptom (eg, ptosis, conjunctival injection, nasal congestion). While headache can occur postictally, isolated ictal headache would be quite rare.

(Page 2217, Section 29: Disorders of the Nervous System, Chapter 565: Migraine and Headache Disorders)

Answer 29-3. d

The β-blocker propranolol is effective for migraine prophylaxis in adults and there is some supportive evidence in the pediatric population as well. Divalproex sodium is also efficacious; however, it is teratogenic and so less optimal in sexually active individuals unless reliable contraception is being used. Sumatriptan is an acute migraine medication and is not appropriate for preventive use. Clonidine and levetiracetam are not effective as migraine preventive agents.

(Page 2218, Section 29: Disorders of the Nervous System, Chapter 565: Migraine and Headache Disorders)

Answer 29-4. a

Sumatriptan nasal spray has been well studied in children for the treatment of acute migraine in children as young as age 6. It is an appropriate choice in children who have severe head pain, particularly those who have difficulty taking oral medication due to nausea and vomiting. Triptans are migraine-specific therapies that treat head pain as well as associated migraine symptoms such as photophobia, phonophobia, nausea, and vomiting. Her attack frequency is low enough that using sumatriptan would not be expected to lead to medication overuse headache.

Ibuprofen is an excellent first-line agent for many children with acute migraine. However, in this patient's case she cannot tolerate it due to emesis. Ondansetron oral dissolving tablets could be used to treat the nausea, but will have no impact on the headache. Oxygen therapy can be useful in cluster headache, another headache disorder, but is not a proven therapy for migraine. Amitriptyline is a preventive migraine agent and not useful in the acute setting.

(Page 2218, Section 29: Disorders of the Nervous System, Chapter 565: Migraine and Headache Disorders)

Answer 29-5. b

This is a classic presentation of a hyperammonemic neonate. While neonatal hyperammonemia can be due to fatty acid oxidation disorders or disorders of amino acid metabolism, the most common cause is a urea cycle defect. There are 6 enzymes in the urea cycle, and a defect in any one of them can lead to hyperammonemia. A neonatal presentation in a male infant would be most suggestive of ornithine transcarbamylase (OTC) deficiency, the only enzyme that has an X-linked inheritance. Breastfed infants with OTC deficiency are asymptomatic until the mother's milk comes in, which is typically on day of life 3, particularly in a primiparous mother. Often the infants have already gone home before they become symptomatic. While some urea cycle defects can be tested for with routine newborn screening, not all can be detected. Furthermore, results of newborn screening tests usually are not completed by the time infants with OTC deficiency present, requiring clinicians to have a high index of suspicion.

Ammonia levels are often elevated at presentation. Urgent diagnosis is critical as significant prolonged hyperammonemia leads to cerebral edema, neurologic damage, and, potentially, death. Hemodialysis should be rapidly initiated and ammonia-scavenging medications provided. The infant should be transferred to a center that is experienced in the management of inborn errors of metabolism. Hyperammonemia is often accompanied by a respiratory alkalosis. This can be detected via arterial blood gas; a venous sample will not be as helpful.

Methamphetamine or cocaine ingestion, via mother's milk, would only cause an acute encephalopathy by causing an intracranial bleed, and hemorrhage was ruled out by imaging. Hypoglycemia and hyponatremia would not cause tachypnea, and while cerebral edema can result from hyponatremia, breastfed infants are at lower risk for this than formula-fed infants as formula can be prepared incorrectly.

(Page 583, Section 11: Inherited Disorders of Metabolism, Chapter 145: Urea Cycle and Related Disorders)

Answer 29-6. e

Recurrent focal motor seizures in a neonate are often due to arterial ischemic stroke. Perinatal stroke is significantly more common than previously appreciated. It is usually not possible to pinpoint the exact timing of stroke onset, but it is generally thought to be at or near the time of birth. Neonates do not typically present with a hemiparesis after an ischemic stroke, as an older child or an adult would. Instead, recurrent focal motor seizures in day 1 or 2 of life are the most typical presentation. Some infants with perinatal stroke will be asymptomatic in the nursery and then present later in infancy with an early hand preference (eg, being left-handed or right-handed).

Hypoxic-ischemic injury is a common cause of seizures in the neonatal period; however, there is usually a history of fetal distress in labor and the infant is not neurologically normal at birth. Electrolyte disturbance is a treatable cause of focal motor seizures and should be ruled out. CNS infection can be evaluated for with CSF examination. Head ultrasound is significantly more sensitive for intracerebral hemorrhage than for ischemic stroke; MRI is preferred for evaluating for ischemic stroke. Nonaccidental trauma, while always a possibility, is less common in the neonatal period, and would usually present with encephalopathy due to axonal shear injury. Nonepileptic seizures, a type of somatization disorder, do occur in children, however not in infancy.

(Page 2166, Section 29: Disorders of the Nervous System, Chapter 552: Stroke and Cerebrovascular Disease)

Answer 29-7. c

This child has a congenital myopathy. There are several different forms of congenital myopathies, each with a different pathologic change in muscle on histology. Typical clinical features include feeding or respiratory difficulty in the neonatal period and a high-arched palate at birth. However, the diagnosis may not be made until the child presents with delayed motor milestones. Neurologic examination findings that suggest a muscle localization include diminished bulk, hypotonia, and proximal greater than distal weakness.

Upper motor neuron injury presents with hypertonia (spasticity), hyperreflexia, and distal greater than proximal weakness. Weakness in neuromuscular junction disease is fluctuating and fatiguable. The bulbar musculature is not commonly involved in peripheral nerve disease. More typical features would be sensory abnormalities and diminished or absent reflexes (depending on severity). Lower motor neuron disease that presents in the neonatal period would be spinal muscular atrophy (SMA), which is typically progressive and entirely spares the cranial nerves.

(Page 2241, Section 29: Disorders of the Nervous System, Chapter 572: Myopathies)

Answer 29-8. a

This infant has GM1 gangliosidosis, an inborn error of metabolism due to β-galactosidase deficiency. Buildup of GM1 ganglioside in neurons leads to progressive neurologic dysfunction, and buildup of metabolites in the bone, liver, and soft tissues of the face leads to bony malformations, organomegaly, and coarsened facial features. Metabolites also build up in the retina nerve fiber layer; however, the macula is spared because the nerve fiber layer is thinned in this region. This leads to the macula appearing as a bright "cherry-red spot" compared with the surrounding retina.

Optic nerve hypoplasia is a congenital anomaly that can be seen in other neurodevelopmental disorders, for example, septo-optic dysplasia. Congenital cataracts are seen in certain metabolic and genetic disorders such as trisomy 21. They are important to diagnose early, as there is a critical period to early vision development. Uveitis is seen in inflammatory autoimmune disorders such as multiple sclerosis.

(Page 633, Section 11: Inherited Disorders of Metabolism, Chapter 160: Mucopolysaccharidosis, Glycoproteinosis, and Mucolipidosis)

Answer 29-9. c

This child suffers from a cluster headache, a primary headache disorder. Cluster headache pain is severe in intensity, lateralized, and associated with at least 1 cranial autonomic symptom. Examples of cranial autonomic symptoms include conjunctival injection, lacrimation, periorbital edema, and nasal congestion or rhinorrhea. The cranial autonomic symptoms lateralize to the side of the headache. High-flow oxygen via non-rebreather mask for 20 minutes is an effective acute therapy in some patients.

Both prochlorperazine (a dopamine receptor antagonist) and ketorolac (an NSAID) are used in the acute treatment of migraine in children in the emergency room setting, with prochlorperazine being superior. Topiramate is migraine preventive medication. Sodium valproate is also a preventive migraine medication, although there are several small studies suggesting some efficacy of an IV load of sodium valproate in the treatment of acute migraine.

(Page 2216, Section 29: Disorders of the Nervous System, Chapter 565: Migraine and Headache Disorders)

Answer 29-10. b

This baby has brachial plexus injury, most likely due to birth injury. Shoulder dystocia and macrosomia are risk factors for brachial plexus injury. In this infant, the accompanying Horner syndrome helps with the localization as the sympathetic chain runs close to the brachial plexus and its involvement signals this is a severe, proximal injury that will not spontaneously recover. Physical findings of Horner syndrome include ptosis and miosis, which is a smaller pupil on the affected side. The pupillary asymmetry is most easily appreciated in a darkened room as the other pupil will dilate. Anhydrosis, or decreased facial sweating on that side, can be part of Horner syndrome, but is difficult to appreciate in a neonate. Infants with severe brachial plexus injury at birth should be referred for evaluation for possible surgical reconstruction of the plexus within the first few months of life.

A clavicular fracture can occur during a difficult delivery and may cause pain and lead to asymmetric arm movement; however, it is unlikely to cause compete absence of movement in the arm. Neonates with stroke do not present with a hemiparesis at birth. In utero drug exposure can lead to perinatal stroke, but these infants do not manifest a hemiparesis in the nursery. Postictal Todd paralysis is unlikely, as the flaccid limb was noted immediately in the delivery room, so the child would have had to be seizing immediately prior to delivery. It also would not account for the Horner syndrome.

(Page 2233, Section 29: Disorders of the Nervous System, Chapter 570: Peripheral Nerve Disorders and Anterior Horn Cell Diseases)

Answer 29-11. b

Acute-onset severe headache is concerning for aneurysmal subarachnoid hemorrhage. While CT scan is generally highly sensitive for acute intracranial blood, a small bleed can be missed, particularly if several hours have passed since headache onset. When subarachnoid hemorrhage is suspected, a negative CT scan should be followed up by a lumbar puncture to evaluate for xanthochromia in CSF. Xanthochromia is the pigment seen after blood has begun to break down; its presence distinguishes a subarachnoid hemorrhage from a traumatic lumbar puncture. In this patient, his neck stiffness suggests meningeal irritation, which can be from subarachnoid blood.

While a CT scan is not as sensitive as MRI for ischemic stroke, isolated acute headache with no other neurologic symptoms or examination findings would be unusual for stroke. Similarly, isolated, severe, ongoing headache is not suggestive of seizure. An afebrile patient with normal mental status would be relatively unlikely to have an infectious meningitis; however, lumbar puncture should be performed if there is a clinical suspicion for CNS infection. A benign headache disorder, such as migraine, is a diagnosis of exclusion and should not be made until the evaluation for secondary causes of headache has been completed.

(Page 2172, Section 29: Disorders of the Nervous System, Chapter 552: Stroke and Cerebrovascular Disease)

Answer 29-12. d

Motor and vocal tics commonly present in this age group. Boys are more likely to be affected. Patients with tics describe being able to suppress the movements for a few minutes, but the urge to perform them mounts, and when they do them, they typically feel a sense of relief. It is possible to have motor tics, vocal tics, or both. Tic disorders are generally benign, although if the tics cause significant social distress, they can be treated with medication. Tourette disorder is diagnosed when both motor and vocal tics are present and have been going on for at least 1 year.

The fact that there is no impairment of consciousness and no postictal state makes these unlikely to be seizures. In addition, the movements themselves are more characteristic of tics than absence seizures. There are no neuroimaging findings associated with tic disorders, and imaging is not necessary unless there is a question as to the diagnosis. Low ceruloplasmin levels testing can help to diagnose Wilson disease, an inherited condition of copper accumulation that often manifests as a movement disorder. However, the abnormal movements are usually dystonia or chorea rather than tics. There are also neuropsychiatric symptoms that frequently accompany the movement disorder. Examination of cerebrospinal fluid would be indicated if there was a question of an inflammatory etiology for a movement disorder, for example, anti-NMDA receptor encephalitis. However, these patients characteristically have abnormal mental status, and sometimes seizures and cardiovascular instability.

(Page 2221, Section 29: Disorders of the Nervous System, Chapter 566: Movement Disorders, Tics, and Tourette Syndrome)

Answer 29-13. a

Prochlorperazine (Compazine) is a commonly used acute migraine therapy in children in the emergency department setting. It is a dopamine receptor antagonist and therefore can cause movement-related side effects, most commonly dystonic reactions or akathisia (a sense of needing to move). Diphenhydramine is typically effective in relieving this side effect. Observation is an option; however, the dystonic reaction is typically uncomfortable and so treatment is generally preferred.

Chlorperazine is another dopamine receptor antagonist used to treat migraine, and would be expected to worsen the dystonic reaction. Acetaminophen may help with discomfort, but would not treat the underlying abnormality. Phenytoin is a seizure medication and would not be expected to have an effect.

(Page 460, Section 8: The Acutely Ill Infant and Child, Chapter 120: Toxic Ingestions and Exposures)

Answer 29-14. c

This child has a Bell's palsy. This results from an abnormality of the seventh cranial nerve on the affected side. Many cases are idiopathic, although some cases are associated with infections such as Lyme disease or HSV. Early treatment (within 72 hours of onset) with corticosteroids improves recovery. Some patients with Bell's palsy experience hyperacusis due to weakness of the stapedius muscle, an inner ear muscle that is innervated by the seventh nerve and responsible for dampening sound intensity. The seventh nerve also provides taste sensation to the anterior two thirds of the tongue; hence, many patients with Bell's palsy report abnormal taste on the affected side.

The involvement of the forehead denotes a lower motor neuron (peripheral) cause of facial weakness; facial weakness from a central cause (cortex) would spare the forehead, as there is bilateral cortical innervation to the forehead. The seventh nerve is in the pons, which is below the midbrain in the brain stem. A lesion of the eighth cranial nerve would be expected to cause diminished hearing.

(Page 2233, Section 29: Disorders of the Nervous System, Chapter 570: Peripheral Nerve Disorders and Anterior Horn Cell Disease)

Answer 29-15. c

This young athlete has suffered a concussion, sometimes referred to as mild traumatic brain injury. The majority of concussions are not associated with loss of consciousness. Typically postconcussive symptoms take 7 to 10 days to resolve, although a longer recovery course is possible. Both cognitive and physical rest are recommended while recovering from a concussion. This means that both schoolwork and athletics should be put on hold. Once he is symptom-free, he can then return to his usual activities in a graded fashion, ensuring that he remains symptom-free with each increase in activity. Returning to play before he has fully recovered from the concussion puts him at risk for second-impact syndrome, a potentially fatal consequence that can result from suffering a second concussion before the first has resolved. While ibuprofen or other medications may help his headache, he should not return to athletics until he is symptom-free without medications.

(Page 2160, Section 29: Disorders of the Nervous System, Chapter 551: Trauma to the Nervous System)

Answer 29-16. b

The clinical story is concerning for nonaccidental head trauma. Two-month-old infants do not have the gross motor control to roll over; hence, the parents' story is questionable. A skeletal survey to look for bone fractures is indicated, as is an ophthalmologic examination to look for retinal hemorrhages. The seizure was provoked by trauma and intracranial blood; hence, investigations for other seizure etiologies such as CNS infection, electrolyte disturbance, or focal brain anomaly are not indicated. Similarly, there is no indication to pursue a vascular anomaly in this infant as the etiology of the subdural hemorrhage was clearly trauma.

(Page 2162, Section 29: Disorders of the Nervous System, Chapter 551: Trauma to the Nervous System)

Answer 29-17. c

This infant suffered perinatal birth asphyxia and as a result was encephalopathic at delivery. He was appropriately treated with therapeutic hypothermia and his acute symptomatic seizures were appropriately managed. He does not have epilepsy, although he is at some risk for it. This infant's neurologic examination, EEG background, and brain MRI suggest moderate brain injury. Certainly normal development cannot be assured; however, it would be equally inappropriate to suggest to the family that the child's developmental prospects are dire. He is at risk for both motor and cognitive disabilities, and will need close monitoring during early childhood, with early referral for therapies if developmental concerns arise. Elective C-section does not eliminate the risk of birth asphyxia and carries higher risks of maternal morbidity and mortality than vaginal delivery.

(Page 2178, Section 29: Disorders of the Nervous System, Chapter 554: Cerebral Palsy and Static Encephalopathies)

Answer 29-18. a

CNS damage can lead to an imbalance between the afferent excitatory and descending inhibitory pathways, which is associated with muscle hypertonia and involves γ-aminobutyric acid (GABA).

Baclofen can be useful in the treatment of spasticity. It is a derivative of GABA and an agonist for GABA receptors. It can be given orally, or in more severe cases through a continuous intrathecal pump. Some degree of spasticity can actually be helpful in some individuals in making transfers

easier or helping with ambulation, so treating spasticity is an individualized decision that often depends on factors such as discomfort, or the inability to participate fully in therapies.

Chlorpromazine is a dopamine-receptor antagonist that does not treat spasticity, and can cause dystonic reactions. Phenobarbital is an antiepileptic and may indirectly mildly lower tone; however, it is not typically used for that purpose. Valproic acid is an antiepileptic, and venlafaxine is a serotonin–norepinephrine reuptake inhibitor.

(Page 2181, Section 29: Disorders of the Nervous System, Chapter 554: Cerebral Palsy and Static Encephalopathies)

Answer 29-19. c

Acute cerebellar ataxia is an infectious or postinfectious process that typically affects preschool aged children. The course of the illness is typically monophasic. For those in the postinfectious category, there is often a history of a recent febrile or GI illness. It is important to rule out more serious causes of new ataxia in young children, such as a posterior fossa mass or a cerebellar hemorrhage, with brain MRI. However, most children with cerebellar hemorrhage are not well appearing and the onset of ataxia is quite acute.

Ataxia from a posterior fossa mass is usually more insidious in onset, unless there has been bleeding into the mass. Hydrocephalus can cause gait disturbance; however, it would not explain the nystagmus or limb ataxia. Young children with Guillain-Barré syndrome are sometimes initially mistaken as being ataxic when they have a lower extremity weakness from ascending paralysis. As a result, in this age group it is important for the clinician to always question whether what they are calling acute-onset ataxia could actually be weakness. However, in this child the nystagmus and limb dysmetria are prominent and make a muscle weakness less likely.

(Page 2182, Section 29: Disorders of the Nervous System, Chapter 555: Infections of the Central Nervous System)

Answer 29-20. b

This clinical situation is concerning for bacterial meningitis. His neurologic examination suggests elevated ICP given his lethargy and slowly reactive pupils. When there is concern for high ICP, a CT scan should be performed before performing a lumbar puncture as there is the potential to precipitate herniation through the foramen magnum. If necessary, lumbar puncture can even be put off even longer until the patient is stable. However, empiric antibiotic coverage at meningitic doses should be started without delay. Concerns about being able to identify the specific organism do not justify a delay in treatment. It may still be possible to identify the infectious organism through blood or urine culture, and if necessary an empiric course of antibiotics can be completed based on the most likely etiologic agents.

(Page 2183, Section 29: Disorders of the Nervous System, Chapter 555: Infections of the Central Nervous System)

Answer 29-21. b

All of these medications can be used for migraine prevention. Some of the more frequent side effects of topiramate are cognitive slowing and word-finding difficulties. Propranolol can decrease exercise tolerance. Valproate is teratogenic and can cause weight gain. Amitriptyline can cause fatigue and dry mouth. Gabapentin can also cause fatigue.

(Page 2211, Section 29: Disorders of the Nervous System, Chapter 562: Epilepsy Treatment: Antiepileptic Drug Therapy)

Answer 29-22. a

This girl has an optic neuritis, a disorder of the optic nerve that can be inflammatory or infectious in etiology. Typical symptoms include diminished visual acuity and red desaturation. The optic nerve is anterior to the optic chiasm, where inputs from both eyes cross, so all visual information in the optic nerve is coming from a single eye. Once the optic chiasm is reached, visual information is crossing, so manifestations will be apparent in both eyes. This holds true for the lateral geniculate nucleus in the thalamus and the visual cortex as well. Her symptoms can easily be localized within the nervous system, making conversion disorder unlikely.

(Page 2194, Section 29: Disorders of the Nervous System, Chapter 556: Immune and Inflammatory-mediated Central Nervous System Disorders)

Answer 29-23. d

This child has opsoclonus-myoclonus-ataxia syndrome. About half of children with this condition have a detectable neuroblastoma, so an abdominal ultrasound and urine catecholamines should be promptly performed. Not all patients will have all 3 of these neurologic symptoms, and it is possible for 1 symptom to precede the others.

Ovarian teratomas can be associated with the NMDA receptor antibody syndrome, which is typically characterized by seizures, autonomic instability, and mental status or behavioral changes. Limbic encephalitis also typically presents with seizures and behavioral or mental status changes. A neurotransmitter disorder can present with abnormal eye movements and a movement disorder; however, this patient's age and the potential for an oncologic process make neuroblastoma the first consideration to investigate. Landau-Kleffner syndrome is characterized by language regression and electrical status epilepticus of sleep.

(Page 2197, Section 29: Disorders of the Nervous System, Chapter 556: Immune and Inflammatory-mediated Central Nervous System Disorders)

Answer 29-24. b

This infant has septo-optic dysplasia (also known as de Morsier syndrome), a condition characterized by absence of the septum pellucidum, optic nerve hypoplasia, and abnormalities of the hypothalamic–pituitary axis with resultant endocrine dysfunction. Symptoms of septo-optic dysplasia are variable, but may include unilateral or bilateral blindness, nystagmus, hypotonia, pituitary hypoplasia, inability to develop a stress response, developmental delay, and seizures.

The corpus callosum is the white matter tract that connects the 2 hemispheres of the brain. Agenesis of the corpus callosum, either partial or complete, is the result of abnormal prosencephalic development and is sometimes seen in children with developmental delay. Stenosis of the cerebral aqueduct can be seen in X-linked hydrocephalus. There are several types of cerebellar-pontine hypoplasia; infants may be notably weak in the neonatal period. This infant's delivery was not concerning for birth asphyxia, and other than his visual impairment he has a normal neurologic examination with no evidence of encephalopathy.

(Page 2151, Section 29: Disorders of the Nervous System, Chapter 548: Cranial Development Abnormalities)

Answer 29-25. a

Children with NF1 are at increased risk for optic pathway gliomas; therefore, annual ophthalmologic screening examinations are recommended for those 10 years of age or younger.

Screening neuroimaging is not recommended, and should only be done to evaluate neurologic symptoms. Vestibular schwannomas are associated with neurofibromatosis type 2, not NF1. Patients with NF1 should have blood pressure checked annually as they are at risk for hypertension; however, annual cardiac echo in the absence of symptoms is not necessary. While revisiting the skin examination annually in a patient with known or suspected NF1 may help satisfy diagnostic criteria and track the number of neurofibromas, a Wood's lamp examination is not necessary. Wood's lamp examination is useful in detecting the hypopigmented lesions sometimes seen in tuberous sclerosis, so-called ash leaf macules, which can be difficult to see in light-skinned individuals.

(Page 2269, Section 29: Disorders of the Nervous System, Chapter 578: Phakomatoses)

Answer 29-26. e

This child's history is characteristic for breath-holding spells. Typically breath-holding spells occur in young children and are triggered by being frightened or upset. The child will cry and then hold their breath in expiration and turn either pale or cyanotic. Loss of consciousness is possible and convulsive movements are relatively common. EEG during the spell shows no electrographic seizure.

Children with epilepsy typically do not have a reliable trigger for their seizures, except in the rare case of reflex epilepsies. While it is important to have a low index of suspicion for child abuse, nothing about this child's story is developmentally or medically inconsistent or concerning for abuse. Reflux can cause crying or accompany crying, but does not typically lead to loss of consciousness. A cardiac arrhythmia is possible, for example, due to long QT syndrome; however, the age of the patient and the clinical presentation are quite classic for breath-holding spells.

(Page 2223, Section 29: Disorders of the Nervous System, Chapter 567: Other Paroxysmal Disorders)

Answer 29-27. c

Benign paroxysmal torticollis of infancy is an episodic disorder characterized by bouts of torticollis that can last from minutes to hours or even several days. In between bouts children are completely normal. Typically the disorder remits by age 3; however, there is an association with the development of migraine later in life. Many of these infants also have a family history of migraine. There is no known association with mood disorders, seizures, or breath-holding spells.

(Page 2223, Section 29: Disorders of the Nervous System, Chapter 567: Other Paroxysmal Disorders)

Answer 29-28. c

This girl has myasthenia gravis, an autoimmune disorder that affects the neuromuscular junction. Diurnal variation is common, with patients feeling relatively well in the morning but becoming more symptomatic as the day goes on. Rest can often improve symptoms, while exercise and sustained muscle use, as with prolonged upgaze, brings out the weakness. Predominance of ocular and bulbar symptoms is common in myasthenia gravis.

Weakness from a muscle cause typically does not have such marked diurnal fluctuation. There are no sensory symptoms to suggest sensory nerve involvement, and motor involvement at the nerve level is not fluctuating. Ptosis in myasthenia is due to weakness of the levator palpebrae; the nucleus innervating them is in the midbrain and not the pons. While careful testing late in the day would likely reveal some weakness in the proximal extremities and neck flexors, the ocular and bulbar symptoms exclude a spinal cord localization.

(Page 2236, Section 29: Disorders of the Nervous System, Chapter 571: Diseases of the Neuromuscular Junction)

Answer 29-29. b

This baby's presentation is consistent with Menkes disease, a disorder of copper transport due to mutation in the X-linked gene *ATP7A* that results in copper deficiency and dysfunction of copper-dependent enzymes. Infants present within the first few weeks or months of life with systemic signs and evidence of neurologic dysfunction. Retinal degeneration leads to poor visual function. Connective tissue dysfunction leads to lax skin, and the hair is typically twisted and lightly pigmented. The prognosis is poor.

Phenylketonuria is detected on the newborn screening tests in all states. Biotinidase deficiency and urea cycle defects can present in early infancy; however, the hair findings would not

be characteristic. GM1 gangliosidosis is a storage disease and presents with coarsened facial features, hepatosplenomegaly, and thoracolumbar kyphoscoliosis. There is often hypotonia and developmental delay.

(Page 674, Section 11: Inherited Disorders of Metabolism, Chapter 169: Disorders of Metal Metabolism)

Answer 29-30. a

Fabry disease is an X-linked lysosomal disorder that results in accumulation of glycosphingolipids throughout the body. It is caused by a deficiency of the enzyme α-galactosidase A. The incidence is estimated to be 1 in 55,000 male births. It is probably underdiagnosed as individuals with milder phenotypes may go undiagnosed. Patients may also complain of numbness and paresthesias of the hands and feet (acroparesthesia).

Another classic manifestation of the disease is bouts of painful crises that often involve burning or lancinating (ie, cutting or piercing) pains that originate in the hands and feet. Carbamazepine and gabapentin can be useful therapeutically.

Baclofen is a treatment for spasticity. Propranolol is used as an antihypertensive or migraine preventive. Diphenhydramine is an antihistamine and useful in treating dystonic reactions that sometimes arise from use of dopamine receptor antagonists such as prochlorperazine.

(Page 2252, Section 29: Disorders of the Nervous System, Chapter 574: Lysosomal Storage Disorders)

Answer 29-31. b

The cerebral form of X-linked adrenoleukodystrophy is most common and boys typically present between 4 and 8 years of age. New behavioral disturbances, often concerning for attention deficit-hyperactivity disorder, are often the first symptom. However, other symptoms such as visual impairment and seizures rapidly follow. Corticospinal tract signs typically come later. Brain MRI most typically shows white matter changes in parieto-occipital cortex, involving visual cortex. The condition is caused by a mutation in the gene that codes for the adrenoleukodystrophy protein, which plays a role in β-oxidation of very-long-chain fatty acids. Disruption in this protein's function leads to accumulation of very-long-chain fatty acids.

Aicardi-Goutières syndrome is a leukoencephalopathy that presents in infancy. Neuronal ceroid lipofuscinosis is a group of disorders characterized by neuronal dysfunction due to accumulation of autofluorescent material in the lysosomes. The juvenile form can present at a similar age and is also characterized by visual and behavioral problems; however, there is no male predominance and the typical imaging and lab findings are different. Juvenile-onset Alexander disease is another leukoencephalopathy that can present in this age group; however, the presenting symptoms are spasticity and bulbar dysfunction.

(Page 2257, Section 29: Disorders of the Nervous System, Chapter 576: Leukoencephalopathies)

Answer 29-32. d

Sturge-Weber syndrome is a sporadic disorder characterized by seizures and a port wine stain skin lesion. The port wine stain is unilateral and most often involves the first division of the trigeminal nerve, although lower divisions can also be involved.

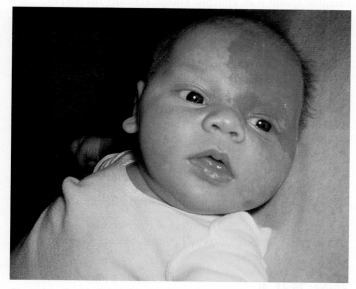

(Reproduced, with permission, from Weinberg S, Prose NS, Kristal L. *Color Atlas of Pediatric Dermatology*. 4th ed. New York: McGraw-Hill, 2007.)

The seventh cranial nerve, the facial nerve, innervates the muscles of facial expression. The forehead receives bilateral innervation and so an upper motor neuron lesion, such as a stroke, will result in unilateral facial weakness that spares the forehead. Lower motor neuron facial weakness, such as that from a Bell's palsy, involves the forehead. The greater occipital nerves provide sensation over the back of the head, with innervation from the upper cervical cord.

(Page 2270, Section 29: Disorders of the Nervous System, Chapter 578: Phakomatoses)

Answer 29-33. c

Glycine encephalopathy classically presents in the neonatal period with difficult to control seizures in an encephalopathic infant. Some infants will have experienced seizures in utero, which the mother may report as frequent "hiccups." A high CSF to plasma glycine ratio, and therefore lumbar puncture with measurement of serum and CSF glycine, is essential in making the diagnosis.

A glycine peak may be seen on magnetic resonance spectroscopy, but brain imaging is the not the typical way of making the diagnosis. EEG will show frequent seizures, but will not be specific to etiology. EMG is used to evaluate for peripheral nerve, neuromuscular junction, or muscle

pathology. Neonates who have experienced hypoxic-ischemic brain injury at birth may suffer seizures and benefit from therapeutic hypothermia; however, this infant had an uncomplicated delivery with good Apgar scores and no evidence of birth asphyxia.

(Page 572, Section 11: Inherited Disorders of Metabolism, Chapter 139: Disorders of the Glycine, Serine, and Proline Metabolism)

Answer 29-34. e

His clinical picture is concerning for increased intracranial pressure in that the headaches wake him from sleep and he has apparent diplopia from a left sixth nerve palsy. In addition, he has nystagmus and ataxia, which suggest a cerebellar localization. He may have papilledema, but it can be difficult to get a good funduscopic examination in young children. Taken together, this clinical situation is concerning for a posterior fossa mass.

Children with a primary headache disorder such as migraine or tension-type headache should have a normal neurologic examination. Idiopathic intracranial hypertension is rare in this age group and does not have cerebellar examination findings. Cerebral aneurysms typically do not cause pain unless they rupture and cause subarachnoid hemorrhage with a "thunderclap-onset" headache.

(Page 2146, Section 29: Disorders of the Nervous System, Chapter 547: Clinical Approach to Neurologic Disease)

Answer 29-35. d

Neurologic complications of Lyme disease include cranial nerve palsies and meningitis. The facial nerve is most likely to be affected, and Lyme disease is an important consideration in evaluating a child with a Bell's palsy. Early treatment (within 72 hours of onset) with corticosteroids improves recovery. Some patients with Bell's palsy experience hyperacusis due to weakness of the stapedius muscle, an inner ear muscle that is innervated by the seventh nerve and responsible for dampening sound intensity. The seventh nerve also provides taste sensation to the anterior two thirds of the tongue; hence, many patients with Bell's palsy report abnormal taste on the affected side.

(Page 1046, Section 17: Infectious Diseases, Chapter 267: Lyme Disease)

Answer 29-36. e

This girl's events could be nonepileptic seizures, a form of conversion disorder. The asynchronous jerking of the limbs and pelvic thrusting are common manifestations of nonepileptic seizures in teenaged girls. However, many patients with nonepileptic seizures also have epilepsy, so an admission for video EEG monitoring to capture events is essential in clarifying the diagnosis. It will also afford an opportunity for private discussions with the adolescent about whether there is any concern for abuse. Starting a medication typically should be delayed until the diagnosis is clear, particularly as the goal of the admission is to record events. If the diagnosis is ultimately shown to be nonepileptic seizures, then referral for behavioral therapy would be recommended.

(Page 2223, Section 29: Disorders of the Nervous System, Chapter 567: Other Paroxysmal Disorders)

Answer 29-37. b

Bowel or bladder symptoms, along with lower extremity weakness, point to the spinal cord as the localization. His clinical picture is that of a transverse myelitis, for which there are a number of infectious and inflammatory etiologies.

Hydrocephalus can cause bladder and gait dysfunction; however, with onset over just a few hours, if he were developing rapid hydrocephalus, his mental status would likely be abnormal. Absence of cranial nerve involvement rules out a brain stem localization. Neuromuscular junction pathology usually causes fluctuating weakness and bulbar involvement is common. Bilateral lumbosacral involvement would not explain the bladder involvement.

(Page 2192, Section 29: Disorders of the Nervous System, Chapter 556: Immune and Inflammatory-mediated Central Nervous System Syndromes)

Answer 29-38. b

Multiple loading doses of phenobarbital can sometimes be required to control neonatal seizures. Respiratory suppression is not uncommon and infants may need respiratory support, particularly with escalating doses.

Phenobarbital-induced electrolyte disturbances are not expected. Allergic reactions are rare. Dystonic reactions are associated with dopamine receptor antagonists, not barbiturates.

(Page 2211, Section 29: Disorders of the Nervous System, Chapter 562: Epilepsy Treatment: Antiepileptic Drug Therapy)

Answer 29-39. d

Several studies have shown that the factors that define a complex febrile seizure are risk factors for subsequent epilepsy after a first febrile seizure. These factors include a focal seizure, prolonged seizure, and repeated seizures within a single febrile illness. Developmental delay or abnormal neurologic examination is also associated with an increased risk of future epilepsy.

Children with a history of febrile seizures with no risk factors for epilepsy have a 2% chance of developing epilepsy. A single risk factor increases the risk of epilepsy to 5%, and 2 or more risk factors increase the risk to 15%. Even so, the majority of all children with febrile seizures will not develop epilepsy.

The other choices listed above are risk factors for having a recurrent febrile seizure after a first febrile seizure. Positive family history and younger age of first febrile seizure are most predictive, but low temperature and shorter duration of illness at first seizure are also risk factors.

(Page 2205, Section 29: Disorders of the Nervous System, Chapter 559: Febrile Seizures)

Answer 29-40. c

Infantile spasm is an epileptic encephalopathy marked by epileptic spasms and an EEG pattern called hypsarrhythmia. The spasms are brief seizures characterized by a sudden contraction of the axial muscles, resulting in either flexion or extension of the neck or upper and/or lower extremities. The EEG shows a characteristic pattern in between the seizures (the "interictal" EEG) called hypsarrhythmia, and while not all infants with spasms will have this pattern, the vast majority do. Therefore, the diagnosis is confirmed with an EEG. The prompt diagnosis of infantile spasms is important because the developmental outcome may be improved with earlier treatment. Accurate diagnosis is important because traditional first-line antiepileptic drugs are generally ineffective in this disorder and rather vigabatrin or steroids offer greater success.

(Page 2200, Section 29: Disorders of the Nervous System, Chapter 557: Epidemiology of Epilepsy, Seizure Classification, Epilepsy Syndromes)

Answer 29-41. b

The patient's age and clinical description of her spells are most consistent with childhood absence epilepsy (CAE), and therefore she should be evaluated by a neurologist as soon as possible given her presumed frequent seizures. The EEG shows a typical pattern of 3 Hz generalized spike and wave during the absence seizures, which are easily provoked by hyperventilation. CAE is an age-related idiopathic generalized epilepsy that occurs in otherwise normal children, more frequently in girls, with a strong genetic predisposition. Remission usually occurs before the age of 12 years, but infrequent generalized tonic–clonic seizures may develop in adolescence.

Brain imaging is normal and therefore unnecessary in children with CAE. Similarly, laboratory evaluations are also normal and not required for diagnosis. Since this is a typical story for absence seizures and they are occurring many times per day, planning to see the patient back in a month is inappropriate. Neurologic diagnoses should be excluded prior to concluding that these symptoms are a psychiatric or behavioral issue.

(Page 2201, Section 29: Disorders of the Nervous System, Chapter 557: Epidemiology of Epilepsy, Seizure Classification, Epilepsy Syndromes)

Answer 29-42. d

The overall risk of a skin reaction with lamotrigine is approximately 5%. Phenytoin and carbamazepine also carry roughly similar risk of an allergic skin reaction. The risk of an AED skin reaction is increased if there is a history of prior AED skin reaction.

The other choices have reported rates of rash that are less than 1%.

(Page 2211, Section 29: Disorders of the Nervous System, Chapter 562: Epilepsy Treatment: Antiepileptic Therapy)

Answer 29-43. c

BECTS is the most common form of idiopathic epilepsy in children, accounting for up to nearly 25% of epilepsies in children less than 16 years of age. It is characterized by childhood onset of partial motor seizures occurring mostly but not exclusively during sleep, a genetic predisposition, absence of neurologic impairment, and a characteristic EEG with centrotemporal spikes.

Except for benign occipital epilepsy (Gastaut type), the other epilepsy syndromes listed are still quite common, with Panayiotopoulos syndrome occurring most often in younger children (3-6 years of age) and juvenile myoclonic epilepsy occurring in older children (12-18 years of age).

(Page 2201, Section 29: Disorders of the Nervous System, Chapter 557: Epidemiology of Epilepsy, Seizure Classification, Epilepsy Syndromes)

Answer 29-44. c

It is important to check a lamotrigine level to determine if the patient is taking the medication, as this will affect the management plan going forward. Nonadherence is a significant problem with patients with epilepsy.

The patient has known epilepsy without recent trauma, and has a nonfocal neurologic examination, and therefore a head CT scan is unnecessary. An EEG is also unnecessary, as the patient has known epilepsy and is waking up (therefore low risk of ongoing subclinical seizures). CBC, LFTs, and a lumbar puncture are also unnecessary in this patient who is otherwise well appearing without recent fevers or infection.

(Page 2209, Section 29: Disorders of the Nervous System, Chapter 562: Epilepsy Treatment: Antiepileptic Drug Therapy)

Answer 29-45. b

The risk of VPA-associated fatal hepatotoxicity is highest in young children, with the risk reaching 1 in 600 in children under 2 years of age receiving VPA as polytherapy. In addition to age and polytherapy, developmental delay and coincident metabolic disorders are also risk factors. For this reason VPA should not be started in any child with abnormal neurodevelopment of unknown cause prior to performing basic laboratory studies to screen for a metabolic disorder. VPA is a branched medium-chain fatty acid known to inhibit mitochondrial β-oxidation, and therefore particular attention to excluding an underlying mitochondrial disorder

is important. The other antiepileptic drugs listed are often used in young children.

(Page 2209, Section 29: Disorders of the Nervous System, Chapter 562: Epilepsy Treatment: Antiepileptic Drug Therapy)

Answer 29-46. d

After a first-time afebrile seizure, a child should be evaluated by a neurologist. As in this case, if a child quickly returns to baseline and the history and examination are not concerning for an acute medical or neurologic process, then the evaluation can be done as an outpatient.

Given the child is otherwise well and has a normal neurologic examination in the emergency room, an admission to the hospital and lumbar puncture are unnecessary. Epilepsy is defined by 2 or more unprovoked seizures, and therefore this patient does not have epilepsy. His risk of recurrence is 20% to 60%, depending on the results of his EEG, which can be done as an outpatient. Given this relatively low risk of recurrence, the standard of care is to wait to start a daily antiepileptic medication until the second seizure.

(Page 2206, Section 29: Disorders of the Nervous System, Chapter 560: Evaluation of New Onset Seizures)

Answer 29-47. a

This infant has infantile spasms in the setting of developmental delay and hypomelanotic macules, or ash leaf spots, which raises high suspicion for TSC. TSC is a multisystem genetic disorder that causes hamartomatous lesions of all organs, but primarily affects skin, central nervous system, eye, kidney, heart, and lung. It is a clinical diagnosis based on major and minor criteria. Cortical tubers are common in patients with TSC, occurring in up to 95% of patients. Infantile spasms develop in approximately one third of individuals with TSC.

The other options are epilepsy syndromes with early onset, but none have the characteristic ash leaf spots, and Ohtahara presents with seizures during the first few weeks of life.

(Page 2203, Section 29: Disorders of the Nervous System, Chapter 558: Etiologies of Epilepsies)

Answer 29-48. c

Children with simple febrile seizures have a 2% chance of developing subsequent epilepsy (compared with the 1% prevalence of epilepsy in children). The number of febrile seizures does not increase this risk. Complex febrile seizures and abnormal neurodevelopment or an abnormal neurologic examination increase the risk of future epilepsy.

The other options are incorrect. Earlier age of onset (<18 months) increases the risk of recurrent febrile seizures, not epilepsy. The risk of developing subsequent epilepsy in a child with 2 or more risk factors (eg, focal febrile seizures and abnormal neurodevelopment) is up to 15%.

(Page 2205, Section 29: Disorders of the Nervous System, Chapter 559: Febrile Seizures)

Answer 29-49. c

About 50% of all children with new-onset epilepsy will ultimately outgrow their epilepsy and no longer require medication. Response to medication is a positive predictor, with about 65% of children who are seizure-free for 2 years on medication remaining seizure-free after weaning medication.

(Page 2208, Section 29: Disorders of the Nervous System, Chapter 562: Epilepsy Treatment: Antiepileptic Drug Therapy)

Answer 29-50. d

A key part of the diagnostic evaluation in all children with a first-time seizure or epilepsy is an EEG. In fact, an EEG is required to diagnose many epilepsy syndromes. The EEG should never be deferred, as it can identify abnormalities that place an individual at risk of recurrent seizures and it can help confirm epilepsy syndromes. The need to check antiepileptic drug levels is not based on the underlying etiology of the epilepsy. It is important to correctly identify epilepsy syndromes, as some idiopathic epilepsy syndromes of childhood such as childhood absence epilepsy and benign rolandic epilepsy are not associated with structural brain disorders and therefore neuroimaging is not necessary. Prognosis is greatly impacted by the epilepsy syndrome. Lastly, seizures may respond better to particular medications depending on the syndrome.

(Page 2200, Section 29: Disorders of the Nervous System, Chapter 557: Epidemiology of Epilepsy, Seizure Classification, Epilepsy Syndromes)

Answer 29-51. c

Benign neonatal convulsions, also known as fifth-day fits, are marked by seizure onset between 4 and 6 days of life in otherwise healthy newborns. Diagnostic evaluation for an underlying cause is negative. The seizures remit by 2 months of life. The diagnosis is made retrospectively, after the seizures remit and development remains normal.

Infantile spasms present around 6 months of age and are generally associated with poor developmental outcomes. Similarly, EME is associated with poor developmental outcomes, and the early-onset myoclonic seizures tend to be refractory to treatment. Metabolic disorders, such as nonketotic hyperglycinemia, are the most common underlying cause. Benign familial neonatal convulsions also present in the first several days of life in a healthy newborn and are associated with favorable prognosis, but there is a family history of seizures during the newborn period. This syndrome is associated with mutations in the potassium channel gene KCNQ2/KCNQ3.

(Page 2200, Section 29: Disorders of the Nervous System, Chapter 557: Epidemiology of Epilepsy, Seizure Classification, Epilepsy Syndromes)

Answer 29-52. b

Pyridoxine-dependent (vitamin B_6–dependent) epilepsy is a rare metabolic disorder manifesting as unexplained medically refractory seizures usually in the neonatal period that rapidly respond to pyridoxine. The underlying genetic abnormality is a deficiency in α-aminoadipic semialdehyde dehydrogenase (antiquitin). Importantly, folinic acid–dependent seizures have been found to be allelic with pyridoxine dependency, and therefore a trial of folinic acid should also be considered. The other choices do not abort intractable seizures.

(Page 543, Section 11: Inherited Disorders of Metabolism, Chapter 134: Principles of Inborn Errors of Metabolism)

Answer 29-53. a

It is crucial to start antibiotics immediately in any child with a clinical picture concerning for meningitis or meningoencephalitis to minimize mortality and morbidity. All of the other therapies or diagnostic evaluations are important but should never delay antibiotics. Concerns about being able to identify the specific organism do not justify a delay in treatment. It may still be possible to identify the infectious organism through blood or urine culture, and if necessary an empiric course of antibiotics can be completed based on the most likely etiologic agents.

(Page 915, Section 17: Infectious Diseases, Chapter 231: Bacterial Infections of the Central Nervous System)

Answer 29-54. d

Hypoxic-ischemic encephalopathy results in either normocephaly or microcephaly, if the injury was significant enough to cause poor brain growth. The other choices are all associated with increased head size due to pressure (hydrocephalus), disorders of somatic size (Sotos syndrome), and metabolic disorders (Tay-Sachs, Canavan diseases).

(Page 2156, Section 29: Disorders of the Nervous System, Chapter 550: Macrocephaly and Microcephaly)

Answer 29-55. c

Increased head size with an autosomal dominant inheritance pattern, known as familial macrocephaly, is the most common type of anatomic macrocephaly.

The other choices would not contribute to making the diagnosis in this case of a normally developing child with a normal neurologic examination. It is important to establish the diagnosis to avoid unnecessary testing.

(Page 2156, Section 29: Disorders of the Nervous System, Chapter 550: Macrocephaly and Microcephaly)

Answer 29-56. e

Multiple sclerosis is a chronic demyelinating disorder affecting the brain and spinal cord. The diagnosis is suspected clinically and confirmed radiographically. The first demyelinating attack of the central nervous system is termed a clinically isolated syndrome.

ADEM is typically monophasic and presents with encephalopathy and multifocal symptoms, with MRI showing demyelinating lesions affecting the brain and sometimes spinal cord. Increased intracranial pressure can present with bilateral papilledema rather than unilateral papillitis. Focal ischemic arterial stroke presents with an acute-onset neurologic deficit rather than subacute onset, and imaging shows an infarct in an arterial vascular territory.

(Page 2195, Section 29: Disorders of the Nervous System, Chapter 556: Immune- and Inflammatory-mediated Central Nervous System Disorders)

Answer 29-57. c

The first-line therapy for an acute demyelinating CNS attack is a course of high-dose intravenous steroids. While it does not appear that this treatment alters long-term disability, it does hasten functional recovery.

Oral steroids are not recommended as initial treatment. As second-line therapy, plasmapheresis is also used. Cytoxan can be considered, but due to the adverse side effect profile is reserved for cases in which other treatments have failed. With lack of systemic symptoms, antibiotics are not indicated in this case.

(Page 2193, Section 29: Disorders of the Nervous System, Chapter 556: Immune- and Inflammatory-mediated Central Nervous System Disorders)

Answer 29-58. e

About 80% of children who present with ADEM will only have a single event. The remaining 20% of children will have a recurrent event, usually within the first 3 months. Those who have a recurrence after 3 months of the initial event can be classified as recurrent ADEM (if the symptoms are the same as the initial event) or multiphasic ADEM (if the symptoms are different). Even if there is clear encephalopathy with the recurrence in multiphasic ADEM, the classification of this group remains controversial. Overall, about 10% of children who are initially diagnosed with ADEM will go on to be diagnosed with multiple sclerosis.

(Page 2191, Section 29: Disorders of the Nervous System, Chapter 556: Immune- and Inflammatory-mediated Central Nervous System Disorders)

Answer 29-59. d

Emergent neuroimaging is indicated in this case to exclude a compressive spinal lesion, such as an epidural hematoma or abscess, which would require an emergent neurosurgical procedure to prevent severe neurologic disability. While an acute stroke does require emergent neuroimaging, this child has been symptomatic for 3 days and therefore acute therapy would not be indicated, and furthermore the clinical history of subacute-onset weakness is not consistent with acute stroke. This clinical picture is consistent with transverse myelitis and therefore urgent neuroimaging should be obtained, but establishing the diagnosis and starting high-dose steroids will

not significantly alter final outcome. This is the first clinical event, excluding a diagnosis of multiple sclerosis. Guillain-Barré could also present with these symptoms, although the reflexes would be decreased or absent.

(Page 2193, Section 29: Disorders of the Nervous System, Chapter 556: Immune- and Inflammatory-mediated Central Nervous System Disorders)

Answer 29-60. b

Color vision deficit can be seen in optic neuritis. The major presenting symptom of optic neuritis is vision loss, which typically affects central visual field more than periphery. In children, vision loss is usually severe with acuity of 20/200 or worse. Bilateral involvement occurs in about 50% of patients.

The inability to abduct the affected eye, which implies a cranial nerve VI palsy, would not be seen in isolated optic neuritis, which involves cranial nerve II exclusively. Proptosis, foreign body sensation, and eyelid swelling would also not be expected with optic neuritis.

(Page 2194, Section 29: Disorders of the Nervous System, Chapter 556: Immune- and Inflammatory-mediated Central Nervous System Disorders)

Answer 29-61. c

Oligoclonal band testing involves a comparison of immunoglobulin patterns in the CSF to the serum. The presence of bands in the CSF but not the serum indicates abnormal synthesis of immunoglobulin in the CSF, and the presence of 2 or more of such bands is considered a positive result and supports the diagnosis of MS.

The presence of bands both in the CSF and in the serum is suggestive of a systemic process, rather than an isolated CNS process. Low serum vitamin D level at first demyelinating event is associated with a higher risk for future development of multiple sclerosis. Elevated ESR is a marker of systemic inflammation and would point against multiple sclerosis. Vitamin B_{12} level is not known to play a role in multiple sclerosis.

(Page 2195, Section 29: Disorders of the Nervous System, Chapter 556: Immune- and Inflammatory-mediated Central Nervous System Disorders)

Answer 29-62. b

β-Hexosaminidase β-subunit deficiency causes Sandhoff disease, which differs clinically from β-hexosaminidase α-subunit deficiency (Tay-Sachs) only by the occasional presence of hepatosplenomegaly. The age of onset, duration, neurologic symptoms, and ophthalmologic signs in patients with Sandhoff disease are otherwise identical to Tay-Sachs disease. Symptoms can include excessive startle response, motor delay and loss of motor skills, loss of verbal skills, and loss of awareness of environment. Physical findings common to both disorders include macular cherry-red spot and macrocephaly.

Affected children can also develop seizures. Choices C, D, and E are other enzymes involved in metabolic disorders (urea cycle disorder, Pompe disease, and Fabry disease).

(Page 2251, Section 29: Disorders of the Nervous System, Chapter 574: Lysosomal Storage Disorders)

Answer 29-63. a

The clinical presentations of Tay-Sachs and Sandhoff diseases are often indistinguishable, and therefore the diagnosis is confirmed with evaluation of hexosaminidase A and B in the white blood cells, with both being deficient in Sandhoff disease and only A in Tay-Sachs. The age of onset, duration, neurologic symptoms, and ophthalmologic signs in patients with Sandhoff disease are identical to those in patients with Tay-Sachs disease with the exception of occasional mild hepatosplenomegaly in Sandhoff disease. Symptoms can include excessive startle response, motor delay and loss of motor skills, loss of verbal skills, and loss of awareness of environment. Physical findings common to both disorders include macular cherry-red spot and macrocephaly. Affected children can also develop seizures.

(Page 2251, Section 29: Disorders of the Nervous System, Chapter 574: Lysosomal Storage Disorders)

Answer 29-64. d

Gaucher disease is an autosomal recessive disorder that results from deficiency of the lysosomal enzyme glucocerebrosidase and is inherited in an autosomal recessive pattern. This leads to accumulation of glycolipid in the macrophage–monocyte system throughout the body. Three major clinical types are determined by presence or absence of CNS involvement: Type 1, nonneuronopathic; Type 2, infantile onset, acute neuronopathic; Type 3, chronic neuronopathic.

(Page 2253, Section 29: Disorders of the Nervous System, Chapter 574: Lysosomal Storage Disorders)

Answer 29-65. c

NCLs are a group of progressive hereditary neurodegenerative disorders characterized by the accumulation of an autofluorescent material rich in lipid, protein, and carbohydrate in the lysosomes. Although all tissues have this accumulation, only neurons are affected. NCLs are characterized by progressive neurodegeneration, with cognitive and motor dysfunction, seizures, and vision loss. Progressive visual decline is a hallmark of NCL, and usually occurs as the initial symptom in juvenile-onset NCL. The other choices, while associated with seizures and developmental delay or regression, are not associated with progressive visual loss.

(Page 2254, Section 29: Disorders of the Nervous System, Chapter 574: Lysosomal Storage Disorders)

Answer 29-66. b

Cherry-red macula can be seen in all of these disorders. Hepatosplenomegaly is not seen in sialidosis type I.

Hyperpigmented skin lesions, or café au lait spots, are not seen in any of these disorders. Sialidosis type I is not associated with cognitive decline or premature death.

(Pages 2251-2253, Section 29: Disorders of the Nervous System, Chapter 574: Lysosomal Storage Disorders)

Answer 29-67. d

X-linked adrenoleukodystrophy (cerebral form) is marked by onset of ADHD symptoms in a previously healthy childhood-age boy, followed by progressive cognitive decline, visual abnormalities, ataxia, and spasticity. The diagnosis is confirmed with elevated VLCFA in the serum. Prognosis is poor, with mean time from onset to a vegetative state of approximately 2 years.

(Page 2257, Chapter 576: Leukoencephalopathies)

Answer 29-68. a

The majority of symptomatic boys with X-linked ALD (cerebral form) have abnormal adrenal function, and therefore adrenal assessment through plasma ACTH level or cortical response in an ACTH stimulation test is important. The other choices do not have abnormal values in X-linked ALD.

(Page 2257, Chapter 576: Leukoencephalopathies)

Answer 29-69. a

This clinical presentation is suggestive of Krabbe disease, which is a leukodystrophy due to a mutation of the GALC gene on chromosome 14q31 encoding the lysosomal enzyme galactocerebrosidase. The mutation results in an undetectable or extremely low activity level, not an elevated level. Choices C, D, and E are abnormalities found in other leukodystrophies.

(Page 2261, Chapter 576: Leukoencephalopathies)

Answer 29-70. b

PMD is inherited in an X-linked autosomal recessive pattern, with males being affected and females being carriers who are either mildly affected or asymptomatic. PLP1 gene abnormalities are identified in the majority of cases (80%-95%). Children presenting with the early onset forms (connatal and classic) have abnormal eye movements (nystagmus) and hypotonia early in the course and then develop progressive spasticity, ataxia, and cognitive impairment. SPG2 presents at an older age, typically between 2 and 5 years, with lower extremity spasticity and bladder dysfunction, although nystagmus can be seen in some of these cases as well. At this time there is no treatment other than supportive care.

(Page 2264, Chapter 576: Leukoencephalopathies)

Answer 29-71. c

West syndrome refers to the triad of infantile spasms, which is a specific type of seizure occurring on average at 6 months of age, an interictal EEG pattern called "hypsarrhythmia," and abnormal development. There are many causes of West syndrome, and not all have abnormal neuroimaging studies or microcephaly. A minority of children do have normal development following infantile spasms, but the majority have neurologic impairment.

(Pages 2198-2201, Chapter 557: Epidemiology of Epilepsy, Seizure Classification, Epilepsy Syndromes)

Answer 29-72. d

Studies have shown that the ketogenic diet can be quite effective for seizure control in some epileptic encephalopathies such as those listed in choices A, B, C, and E. The ketogenic diet requires significant parental dedication and can be very difficult to administer effectively, and therefore is typically reserved for severe epilepsies that do not respond to typical antiseizure medications. Benign rolandic epilepsy is an age-dependent epilepsy associated with spontaneous seizure cessation and normal developmental outcomes and medication is rarely necessary. Therefore, the ketogenic diet would not be an optimal therapeutic choice.

(Page 2213, Chapter 562: Epilepsy Treatment)

Answer 29-73. e

Conversion order is a diagnosis of exclusion and should never be diagnosed prior to excluding other treatable neurologic conditions. Unlike the sudden onset of maximum neurologic deficit in this case, demyelinating episodes such as those in multiple sclerosis evolve in severity over the course of the attack. Migraine can present with transient unilateral weakness, but there are no typical migrainous features to suggest this diagnosis and it also is a diagnosis of exclusion. Seizure itself is typically not associated with unilateral weakness but postictal hemiparesis is common and suggests a focal seizure onset.

Childhood stroke is the most likely diagnosis in this case, and it is the first diagnosis to exclude because emergent therapies (such as clot removal called embolectomy) may be an option in the first several hours following the stroke.

(Pages 2167-2174, Chapter 552: Stroke and Cerebrovascular Disease)

Answer 29-74. a

As an osmotic diuretic, mannitol increases water and sodium excretion and therefore decreases extracellular fluid volume, which then lowers ICP. Hypoventilation raises ICP by causing cerebral vasodilatation and increased cerebral blood volume, whereas hyperventilation lowers ICP by causing cerebral vasoconstriction and decreased cerebral blood volume. Putting the patient in Trendelenburg position with the head below the feet will increase cerebral blood volume and therefore raise ICP. The dosing of antibiotics and neuroimaging studies do not change the patient's ICP.

(Page 421, Chapter 111: Management of Cerebral Edema; Pages 2167-2174, Chapter 552: Stroke and Cerebrovascular Disease)

Answer 29-75. e

This patient has Aicardi syndrome, which is an X-linked dominant disorder with lethality but no gene or region on the X chromosome has been identified. The classic triad consists of chorioretinal lacunae identified on ophthalmologic examination, infantile spasms, and a dysplastic corpus callosum. The brain MRI is never normal. Hypoplastic cerebellum is not a feature of this disorder, although other cerebral malformations such as polymicrogyria can been seen. Astrocytomas and strokes are not associated with this syndrome.

(Page 2151, Chapter 548: Cranial Developmental Abnormalities)

CHAPTER 30 | Disorders of the Eyes

Lance M. Siegel and Tina Rutar

30-1. A 6-year-old girl is running in the department store and gets her eyelid torn by a coat hanger. On examination, you notice the lower lid is torn irregularly around 3 mm from where it inserts into the medial aspect near the nose. The globe itself is not involved. Which of the following structures are of concern for damage?

   a. The medial canthal ligament, canaliculi, and puncta

   b. The cornea, iris, and limbus

   c. The lacrimal gland and lateral limbus

   d. The lateral canthal ligament and orbicularis muscles

   e. Ciliary body and retina

30-2. A 10-year-old boy is struck in the eye by a baseball while trying to field a line drive. Vision is 20/20 in each eye. There is no afferent pupillary defect. The eyelids are very swollen, the conjunctiva is red and boggy, and there is mild limitation of extraocular movements in all fields of gaze. The eye appears intact. A CT of the orbits is ordered. The CT is most likely to show which of the following?

   a. A displaced tripod fracture involving the lateral orbital wall

   b. A trapdoor fracture of the orbital floor

   c. A blowout fracture of the orbital floor

   d. Traumatic optic neuropathy

   e. An orbital roof fracture

30-3. Mom brings in a healthy 4-year-old into the office for a well-child check. The child is developmentally normal, but refuses to speak. What would be the most appropriate initial way to try and estimate visual acuity for this patient?

   a. Pattern visual evoked potential with multiple check sizes.

   b. MRI of the optic pathways.

   c. Wait to check the vision next year.

   d. Use a lap card so the patient can point to responses.

   e. Refer the patient to the local pediatric ophthalmologist.

30-4. A 3-year-old male is struck in the eye by a toy thrown by a classmate. The child is very photophobic and tearing. Your examination reveals a normal pupil, conjunctival injection, and a deep and quiet anterior chamber without hyphema. No foreign body is seen and the eye appears intact. The next step in assessing this child is to:

   a. Order an orbital CT scan to rule out a foreign body embedded in the fornix.

   b. Refer to ophthalmology for occult iritis.

   c. Refer to psychiatry for malingering.

   d. Use fluorescein and a cobalt blue filter to look for a corneal abrasion.

   e. Begin copious irrigation with water or isotonic saline for 30 minutes.

30-5. A 16-year-old is working on a farm and gets a large amount of unknown liquid splashed into the eyes. He immediately experiences burning pain and decreased vision. Which of the following is true?

   a. Highly alkaline (basic) chemical burns to the eyes have more severe ocular outcomes than acid chemical burns.

   b. The eyes should be patched immediately and the patient transported to the nearest emergency room.

   c. The eye should be neutralized by pouring in copious antibiotic eye drops.

   d. Activated charcoal should be put into the eyes.

   e. Fluorescein staining should be done, before any other treatment, to define the extent of damage.

30-6. A 4-year-old boy was running when he impaled his eye on the branch of a bush. The parents put ice over his swollen eyelid and brought him into the emergency room. The examination reveals upper eyelid edema and ecchymosis. The child cries when you attempt to manipulate the eyelid and refuses to cooperate with visual acuity testing. When he spontaneously opens the eye, you can visualize subconjunctival hemorrhage, with brown tissue within the hemorrhage, and a poorly reactive pupil. The next best step in management is:

  a. After sedating the child, remove the suspected brown foreign body so that it can be sent for culture.

  b. Administer topical anesthetic and antibiotic eye drops.

  c. Patch the eye with a sterile eye pad.

  d. Cover the eye with a metal shield.

  e. Copiously irrigate the eye with sterile saline.

30-7. A 15-year-old boy is hit with a paintball in the eye; the pupil is cat-eye shaped with some brown material coming from the iris and poking out through the junction of the cornea and sclera. There is a layer of blood in the anterior chamber. The lens looks cloudy. Your concern is for:

  a. Corneal abrasion

  b. Blowout fracture of the orbital floor

  c. Ruptured globe/hyphema

  d. Foreign body reaction

  e. Chemical burn reaction

30-8. A concerned mom calls your office stating that her developmentally normal 12-year-old child has failed the school vision test in both eyes. Your office records document that the patient has always had normal vision and normal eye examinations in the past. The most likely cause of the failed vision test is:

  a. Ptosis

  b. Traumatic cataract

  c. Myopia

  d. Hereditary retinal dystrophy

  e. Amblyopia

30-9. An 8-year-old boy comes into your office having undergone amblyopia therapy with the local pediatric ophthalmologist. Your office examination shows the vision having improved with glasses and patching treatment from 20/400 to 20/25 in the affected left eye. Your advice to the patient should be:

  a. Continue the regimen of full-time glasses wear and taper off of patching while monitoring the vision regularly.

  b. Use glasses PRN (as desired), as the vision is now adequate in both eyes.

  c. Stop the patching since the patient is too old for patching now.

  d. Refer the child for refractive surgery.

  e. Patch the better-seeing right eye full time and see the patient in follow-up 6 months later.

30-10. A 7-month-old infant presents to your office with the following examination (see Figure 586-1):

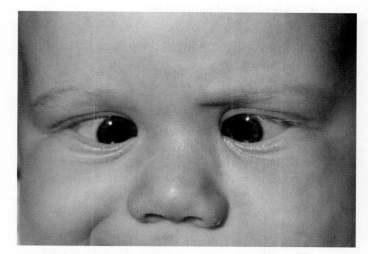

FIGURE 586-1. (Reproduced, with permission, from Rudolph CD, Rudolph AM, Lister GE, First LR, Gershon AA. *Rudolph's Pediatrics.* 22nd ed. New York: McGraw-Hill, 2011.)

Your best advice to the family is:

  a. Tell the family to wait for approximately 6 to 12 months to see if the esotropia spontaneously resolves.

  b. Do vision therapy until the child is 2 years old.

  c. Alternate patch the eyes until the child is old enough for surgery.

  d. Referral for surgery to optimize the best prognosis for binocular vision.

  e. Reassure the family that this is pseudoesotropia.

30-11. A 14-month-old infant is brought to your office because the mother has noted crossing of the eyes. On examination, the light reflex is centered in the pupils, there is no movement on the alternate cover test, and the patient has full eye movements. The most likely diagnosis is:

a. Fourth nerve palsy

b. Acute sixth nerve palsy

c. Intermittent exotropia

d. Accommodative esotropia

e. Pseudostrabismus

30-12. A 2-month-old child presents with a history of falling off the bed. The child is lethargic, and a head CT shows bilateral subdural hemorrhages. A skeletal survey has been requested, and social work has been consulted. Additional assessment should include:

a. A visual evoked potential test

b. A fundoscopic examination

c. Hemoglobin electrophoresis to rule out coagulopathy

d. Antinuclear antibody test to screen for lupus vasculitis

e. Blood culture to rule out infection

30-13. A 2-week-old full-term and otherwise healthy infant is brought into the emergency room due to unilateral eyelid swelling and conjunctival injection, with mucopurulent discharge. The baby is breast-feeding well. She is well appearing, and her vital signs and physical examination are otherwise normal. The mother received prenatal care; however, HIV, *gonococcus*, and *Chlamydia* status were not tested. She delivered the baby by C-section due to failure to progress. What would be the next best step in management?

a. Gram stain, Giemsa stain, bacterial culture of the conjunctival discharge, and scraping of the conjunctiva for chlamydial culture or PCR.

b. Treat with oral erythromycin.

c. Perform a CBC with differential and blood culture.

d. Treat with oral erythromycin, intravenous ceftriaxone, and intravenous acyclovir.

e. Perform a CBC with differential and blood culture, liver function tests, and lumbar puncture.

30-14. A 16-year-old high school student spent the entire night working in the computer lab while wearing her contact lenses. Although her vision is normal, she has bilateral conjunctival injection with crusting of the lashes bilaterally. The most likely diagnosis is:

a. Dry eyes from sleeping with eyes open

b. Bacterial conjunctivitis

c. Chlamydial conjunctivitis

d. Parinaud oculoglandular syndrome

e. Contact lens overwear

30-15. A 7-year-old child has spent the majority of the summer afternoons swimming in the community pool. He develops a bright red eye with scant discharge; the eye is irritated and has a sandpaper feeling to it. Two days later, the other eye becomes involved. The conjunctival injection lasts for 3 weeks. The most likely diagnosis is:

a. Viral conjunctivitis, likely adenoviral

b. Bacterial conjunctivitis, likely streptococcal

c. Corneal abrasion

d. Foreign body in the eye

e. Chemical reaction to chlorine

30-16. A 5-year-old female complains of a swollen right knee and left ankle, and mildly decreased vision. The ophthalmologist detects an iritis in both eyes with posterior synechiae (adhesions between iris and lens) and a cataract in 1 eye. The most likely diagnosis is:

a. Sarcoidosis

b. Leukemic infiltrate

c. Enthesitis-related spondyloarthropathy

d. Systemic lupus erythematosus (SLE)

e. ANA+ juvenile idiopathic arthritis (JIA)

30-17. A 6-year-old African American male presents to your office with a history of eczema and asthma. Which of the following are most consistent with allergic vernal conjunctivitis?

a. Mucopurulent discharge, adenopathy, and matted eyelashes

b. Vesicles on the eyelid with unilateral conjunctivitis

c. Lower eyelid follicles and preauricular lymphadenopathy

d. Gelatinous elevations along the limbus and cobblestones on the palpebral conjunctiva

e. Unilateral conjunctival injection with profuse tearing

30-18. A 15-month-old male comes into your office with the parental complaint of "lazy eyes," unchanged since birth. Further history reveals that he has droopy eyelids bilaterally. The physical examination of the child is otherwise normal, including neurological reflexes and tone. The child is not walking and has a large chin-up position while sitting. Other than bilateral ptosis of the lids, the eye examination, including ocular motility and pupils, is completely normal. The most likely diagnosis is:

a. Horner syndrome

b. Third nerve palsy

c. Myasthenia gravis

d. Muscular dystrophy

e. Congenital ptosis

30-19. A 3-year-old male, who was developing normally, now presents with a 3-week history of losing his balance, vomiting intermittently, and waking up at night from a headache. The examination reveals a new-onset ptosis, with mild unilateral third and fourth nerve palsies that were not there on your prior examination. Your plan and concern should be:

a. Antibiotics and bed rest for presumed mastoiditis

b. IVIG and aspirin for presumed Kawasaki disease

c. Lumbar puncture and supportive care for presumed viral meningitis

d. Brain MRI and hospital admission for presumed brain tumor

e. Observation for migraine headache

30-20. A 1-year-old child presents with a firm 0.5 cm mass on the upper eye lid. The lesion was not present at birth and developed only a week prior. The most likely diagnosis is:

a. Chalazion

b. Hemangioma

c. Epiblepheron

d. Molluscum

e. Dacryocele

30-21. A 14-month-old presents with persistent tearing and recurrent conjunctivitis. There is no mass palpable in the location of the lacrimal sac, but massaging the lacrimal sac expresses copious mucoid discharge. The cause of this chronic condition is:

a. Herpes simplex virus conjunctivitis

b. Varicella zoster conjunctivitis

c. Congenital glaucoma

d. Nasolacrimal duct obstruction (NLDO)

e. Congenital dacryocele

30-22. A 2-month-old full-term infant is noted to have a decreased red reflex bilaterally. The pupils are normal, the conjunctiva is not inflamed, and something white can be seen in the center of both pupils. There is a family history of cataracts in the mom and the maternal aunt at a young age.

The most likely diagnosis is:

a. Retinoblastoma

b. Retinal detachment

c. Coats disease

d. Bilateral congenital cataracts

e. Corneal scarring

30-23. A newborn baby girl born at term weighing 2100 g is noted to have blueberry-type skin lesions, mild icterus, and a large spleen on palpation. The eye examination is grossly normal, but brain imaging shows periventricular calcifications. The most likely diagnosis is:

a. Herpes simplex virus

b. Cytomegalovirus

c. Rubella

d. Lymphocytic choriomeningitis virus

e. Toxoplasmosis

30-24. A 4-year-old ex-premature female who had laser treatment for retinopathy of prematurity (ROP) has come into your office. The best prospective management would include discussion with her parents about the following:

a. Myopia, strabismus, and late retinal detachments

b. Cataracts, glaucoma, and dermoids

c. Coloboma and iris transillumination defects

d. Ptosis and absent color vision

e. Marcus Gunn jaw winking and blepharospasm

30-25. Which of the following criteria are used to determine laser treatment for retinopathy of prematurity?

a. Zone of disease, stage of disease, and gestational age

b. Zone of disease, stage of disease, and the presence of plus disease

c. Stage of disease only

d. Presence of plus disease and gestational age

e. Mature retina

30-26. An ex–24-week twin with birth weight of 530 g who is now 27 weeks has had bowel surgery for necrotizing enterocolitis, been treated for *E. coli* sepsis and meningitis, received 3 packed red blood cell transfusions for anemia, and required an oscillator for mechanical ventilation. The ophthalmologist should examine the baby for retinopathy of prematurity:

   a. As soon as possible

   b. At corrected gestational age of 31 weeks

   c. At corrected gestational age of 34 weeks

   d. At term (corrected gestational age of 40 weeks)

   e. At the time of discharge from the neonatal intensive care unit

30-27. An otherwise healthy newborn baby girl is noted to have very large bright red reflexes. On further examination, the neonatologist notes an absence of iris in both eyes, and thus no pupillary response. There is no family history of eye disease or of nystagmus. What systemic testing will be necessary in the future?

   a. Brain MRI

   b. Renal ultrasonography

   c. Skeletal survey

   d. Upper GI series

   e. Chest x-ray

30-28. A 15-year-old male reports slowly worsening vision and glasses do not seem to help. His vision is worse at night. The patient has had severe hearing loss since birth. Two other relatives have a history of vision loss in their teens and hearing loss since birth. The most likely diagnosis is:

   a. Horner syndrome

   b. Usher syndrome

   c. Stargardt disease

   d. Nystagmus

   e. Congenital rubella

30-29. A 16-year-old female presents with blurred vision. Her history is significant for 10-lb weight gain and the use of retinoic acid for acne. Examination reveals a mild sixth nerve paresis in a moderately obese female. Examination of the optic discs shows edema. The most likely diagnosis is:

   a. Sagittal sinus thrombosis

   b. Idiopathic intracranial hypertension

   c. West Nile virus meningitis

   d. Bacterial meningitis

   e. Brain tumor

30-30. A 17-year-old female complains of decreased vision in 1 eye for the past 2 weeks. The event was preceded by a viral illness. The ophthalmologist measures visual acuity of 20/30 in the involved eye, and notes decreased color vision, an afferent pupillary defect, and a normal optic disc appearance. An MRI with flair sequence shows 6 areas of periventricular white matter plaques. The most likely cause of the decreased vision is:

   a. Compressive lesion of the optic nerve

   b. Macular edema

   c. Optic neuritis

   d. Traumatic optic neuropathy

   e. Leber hereditary optic neuropathy

30-31. to 30-45.   Match the ophthalmologic findings on the left side (#31-45) with the condition most associated with it on the right side.

Ophthalmic Findings	Associated Conditions
30-31. Lisch nodules, optic nerve gliomas	a. Type I diabetes mellitus
30-32. Iris neovascularization; episodic and recurrent myopia	b. Mucopolysaccharidosis
30-33. Chorioretinal colobomas	c. Stickler syndrome
30-34. Corneal clouding, optic atrophy	d. Wilson disease
30-35. Cherry-red spot	e. Down syndrome
30-36. Glaucoma; choroidal hemangioma	f. Tuberous sclerosis
30-37. Optically empty vitreous; high myopia; retinal detachment	g. Sturge-Weber syndrome
30-38. Iris transillumination defects; foveal hypoplasia; nystagmus	h. CHARGE association
30-39. Limbal dermoid; abduction deficit	i. Neurofibromatosis type 1
30-40. Lens subluxation; myopia	j. Riley-Day syndrome
30-41. Dry eye, absent corneal sensation	k. Marfan syndrome
30-42. Retinal astrocytomas	l. Goldenhar syndrome
30-43. Shallow orbits; hypertelorism; strabismus; exposure keratopathy	m. Tay-Sachs disease
30-44. Brushfield spots; nasolacrimal duct obstruction; snowflake cataract	n. Oculocutaneous albinism
30-45. Kayser-Fleischer ring	o. Crouzon syndrome

ANSWERS

Answer 30-1. a

The medial canthal ligament, canaliculi, and puncta are the structures near where the eyelid joins the nasal bridge. In case of trauma that occurs around the eye or eyelids, the eye should be checked for injury first. This process may include checking for corneal abrasion (with fluorescein and cobalt filter), and ruling out ruptured globe. Examine the patient for an irregular iris (eg, cat-eye pupil), and examine the anterior chamber for a hyphema. The vignette, however, states that the globe is not involved. Answer B, which includes parts of the anterior segment of the eye, is thus incorrect, as is choice E, which includes parts of the posterior segment of the eye. Answers C and D are also incorrect as the lacrimal gland is above the lateral canthal ligament and on the lateral side, *not* the medial side where the injury took place. See Figure 579-2 for a schematic of the nasolacrimal tear drainage system.

(Page 2275, Section 30: Disorders of the Eyes, Part 1: General Principles, Chapter 579; Page 2286, Part 2: Disorders of the Eye, Chapter 583)

Answer 30-2. c

The red and boggy conjunctiva and diffuse limitation of extraocular motility indicate diffuse edema and/or hemorrhage within the orbit. An orbital blowout fracture frequently accompanies these findings. This is also consistent with the mechanism of injury. This type of orbital fracture does not need to be urgently repaired. Indications for future repair may include enophthalmos (sinking in of the eye, the opposite of proptosis or exophthalmos) or residual strabismus (misalignment of the eyes).

A displaced tripod fracture of the lateral orbital wall is a fracture usually found with severe blunt force trauma, for example, a high-speed motor vehicle accident. A trapdoor fracture of the orbital floor is a condition that needs to be recognized urgently. In these cases the mechanism is often similar to this event; the floor of the orbit breaks open; however, the bone is flexible and snaps back into place trapping a portion of the inferior rectus muscle within the maxillary sinus. The eye has minimal injection (thus, this fracture type is referred to as a white-eyed blowout); the CT scan is often subtle with only a small "crack" in the orbital floor and sometimes tissue visualized below it within the maxillary sinus (see eFigures 583-11 and 583-12). The examination, however, is pathognomonic; the patient usually cannot look up (or down), and the pain is out of proportion to the injury, usually with severe nausea and vomiting with any attempted

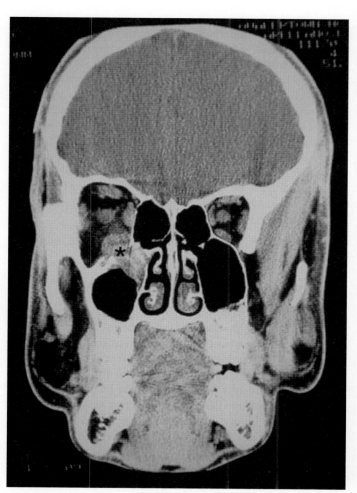

eFIGURE 583-11. CT scan showing blowout fracture with entrapment of inferior rectus muscle and orbital fat (*). (Reproduced, with permission, from Rudolph CD, Rudolph AM, Lister GE, First LR, Gershon AA. *Rudolph's Pediatrics*. 22nd ed. New York: McGraw-Hill, 2011.)

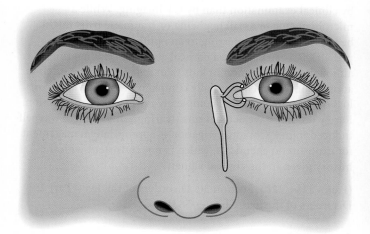

FIGURE 579-2. Schematic showing the position of the nasolacrimal duct system. (Reproduced, with permission, from Rudolph CD, Rudolph AM, Lister GE, First LR, Gershon AA. *Rudolph's Pediatrics*. 22nd ed. New York: McGraw-Hill, 2011.)

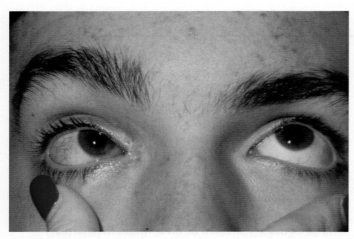

eFIGURE 583-12. Inferior orbital blowout fracture showing limited upgaze on the right from entrapment of inferior rectus muscle. (Reproduced, with permission, from Rudolph CD, Rudolph AM, Lister GE, First LR, Gershon AA. *Rudolph's Pediatrics.* 22nd ed. New York: McGraw-Hill, 2011.)

upgaze. Failure to undergo surgical release of the muscle within 1 to 2 days results in irreversible damage to the muscle and permanent inability to move the eye up or down. Because of the quiet-looking eye and minimal CT findings, these patients may be mistakenly sent home from the ER without surgical intervention. A traumatic optic neuropathy is ruled out by the normal visual acuity and absence of afferent pupillary defect. It is usually due to more traumatic injury—such as a closed head injury; direct blunt impact to the globe is not required. An orbital roof fracture is more common in early childhood, often from impact along the brow from a fall. There is usually a prominent hematoma of the upper lid.

(Pages 2275-2278, Section 30: Disorders of the Eyes, Part 1: General Principles, Chapter 580; Page 2288, Part 2: Disorders of the Eye, Chapter 583)

Answer 30-3. d

Children may be shy, may not want to talk, or may not want to say something wrong; pointing helps ease the fear. Developmentally, 3-year-old children can match letters, such as in the HOTV test, even if they cannot read the letters aloud. Some of the picture charts and symbols are difficult—many children have difficulty with the "tumbling E test." Having the lap card with the same items as the eye chart makes screening much easier; children can match what they see with the letters on the card. (Be careful to watch for "cheating.") Although assessing vision in children can be difficult, it is critically important. Light perception and fixation on the caregiver's face is present at birth or shortly thereafter. Babies can fix and follow an object held in the examiner's hands by approximately 3 months. Formal visual acuity testing begins at age 3 years but is possible in some 2-year-old children. Children aged 3 years and older should have a quantitative assessment of vision.

Patients should be referred according to the following visual acuity guidelines:

Three to 4 years of age: acuity of 20/50 or worse, or a 2 or greater line difference between the 2 eyes

Five years of age: visual acuity of 20/40 or worse, or a 2 or greater line difference between the 2 eyes

Six years of age: visual acuity of 20/30 or worse, or a 2 or greater line difference between the 2 eyes

Referral to an ophthalmologist is indicated if the patient has failed a vision screening test, or if there are developmental problems that preclude assessment of vision (such as Down syndrome, autism).

Pattern visual evoked potential testing with multiple check sizes can be used to estimate vision in a nonverbal child, but it is not routine. MRI is not appropriate, as most visual disorders affecting young children (amblyopia, strabismus) have no imaging findings detected by brain MRI. Brain MRI may be done if the pupillary responses are abnormal, or if other factors suggest a central nervous system disorder (ie, new-onset nystagmus, cranial nerve abnormalities, or other neurological signs). Waiting until the following year is not acceptable; delaying the vision assessment by 1 year could result in inadequate treatment of age-sensitive visual disorders, such as amblyopia.

(Pages 2276-2277, Section 30: Disorders of the Eyes, Part 1: General Principles; Chapter 580)

Answer 30-4. d

Once a ruptured globe has been ruled out, assessment of unilateral red eye after trauma requires a fluorescein stain. If an abrasion is noted, prescribe antibiotic eye drops or ointment to be administered 4 times daily, ± a cycloplegic agent. Do not patch the eye.

The mechanism of injury does not warrant CT scanning. In addition, a forniceal foreign body would be better detected by clinical examination than by CT imaging. While a microhyphema or small hyphema or traumatic iritis might be present, prior to referring to an ophthalmologist, the pediatrician can rule out a corneal abrasion. Malingering, although more common in kids than realized, occurs often in adolescent/teens. They usually complain of loss of vision, or loss of visual field, with a completely normal eye examination. Rarely do they have actual signs (tearing), unless there was self-induced injury. Copious irrigation is appropriate management for exposure to chemicals, which is not consistent with the history given in the clinical vignette.

(Pages 2284-2285, Section 30: Disorders of the Eyes, Part 2: Disorders of the Eye, Chapter 583)

Answer 30-5. a

Immediate and copious irrigation with saline (or water) is critical when any unknown chemical gets into the eye. The irrigation will help remove the chemical and/or any

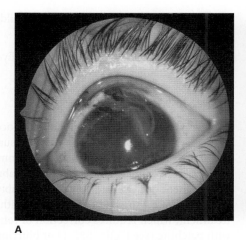 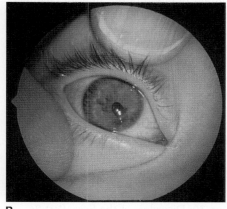

FIGURE 583-3. **(A)** Full-thickness laceration of cornea and sclera with iris and choroid extrusion into the wound. Note pupil moved upward in direction of the wound. **(B)** Pupil moved downward in direction of inferior corneal laceration with iris plugging the wound. (Reproduced, with permission, from Rudolph CD, Rudolph AM, Lister GE, First LR, Gershon AA. *Rudolph's Pediatrics.* 22nd ed. New York: McGraw-Hill, 2011.)

precipitates, and will neutralize the ocular surface. Highly alkaline substances (lye, cement, oven cleaner) cause severe and often irreversible damages immediately. In contrast, acids cause ocular proteins to precipitate, and while they can cause severe damage, the protein precipitation limits the depth of penetration of the chemical into the eye.

The eyes should not be patched, but rather irrigated immediately at the scene of the accident with transport to the emergency room as soon as possible. There are no "chemicals or antibiotics" to administer into the eye. Moreover, the liquid used for irrigation should be administered in large volumes, not in drops. Fluorescein staining is useful in characterizing corneal abrasions but is not indicated in the initial management of chemical burns.

(Page 2285, Section 30: Disorders of the Eyes, Part 2: Disorders of the Eye, Chapter 583)

Answer 30-6. d

This scenario describing a penetrating injury through the sclera and cornea is suspicious for a ruptured globe. Whenever there is violation of the cornea or the sclera, the uveal tissue of the eye (the iris or choroid) attempts to seal the wound. This tissue typically has a dark brown color (see Figure 583-3). Placement of a shield over the surface of the globe will protect the globe from additional manipulation. An ophthalmologist should be consulted emergently. The child should be kept calm in the interim to avoid Valsalva maneuver. The child should not eat or drink in anticipation of requiring general anesthesia for further globe examination and subsequent repair.

The "brown tissue" may represent intraocular contents; therefore, any attempt to remove this would be incorrect (Figure 583-4). It is not safe to administer any topical ophthalmic drops to a patient with suspected globe rupture as not all eye drops are safe if they enter the eye. Patching the eye may result in further extrusion of intraocular contents

due to pressure applied by the patch onto the surface of the globe. Irrigation could cause additional injury to the ruptured globe.

(Pages 2286-2287, Section 30: Disorders of the Eyes, Part 2: Disorders of the Eye, Chapter 583)

Answer 30-7. c

Globe rupture can occur due to sharp/penetrating trauma to the eye (eg, a pencil), blunt trauma to the eye (eg, a high-velocity paintball), or explosion (eg, fireworks injury). Sharp/penetrating trauma has a better prognosis than the other 2 mechanisms of globe violation. Half of all paintball injuries to the eye cause severe loss of vision or loss of the eye.

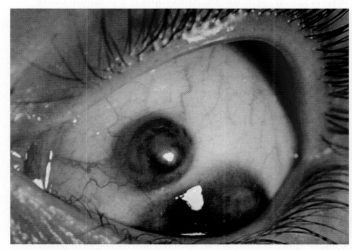

FIGURE 583-4. Eye is looking down, revealing superior scleral perforation with plugging of wound by choroidal tissue. (Reproduced, with permission, from Rudolph CD, Rudolph AM, Lister GE, First LR, Gershon AA. *Rudolph's Pediatrics.* 22nd ed. New York: McGraw-Hill, 2011.)

The examination findings of blood in the anterior chamber, irregular iris protruding through the limbus, and traumatic cataract are not seen with corneal abrasions or chemical burns. A paintball is insufficient in size to cause both globe rupture and blowout of the orbital floor. Most blunt trauma resulting in both globe rupture and orbital fractures results from larger objects, such as a fist or a baseball. A foreign body can cause inflammation or infection of the ocular surface, if embedded in the cornea or conjunctiva, or intraocular inflammation or infection, if located within the globe. However, the mechanism of injury does not suggest an intraocular foreign body, and the associated ophthalmic findings are classic for globe rupture.

(Pages 2286-2288, Section 30: Disorders of the Eyes, Part 2: Disorders of the Eye, Chapter 583)

Answer 30-8. c

Myopia, or nearsightedness, is common in early teens (see figure below). It is more likely to be diagnosed in patients with a positive family history, in certain ethnic groups, and in patients who are avid readers. Prolonged accommodation due to focused near-work is thought to influence the growth of the eye and is associated with myopia.

Ptosis can cause visual loss from occlusion or an induced refractive error due to astigmatism by the pressure of the droopy lid. Ptosis is rarely progressive; thus, if the examination in the office was previously normal, the possibility of developing bilateral ptosis at 12 years of age is unlikely. The patient's vision test was abnormal in both eyes, and it would be highly unusual to have bilateral traumatic cataracts. Hereditary retinal dystrophy is possible but would not be the most likely explanation. Retinal dystrophies have a progressive nature in which the vision does not improve with glasses, and often have symptoms such as photophobia, night blindness, or a decrease in peripheral vision. They are associated with several genetic syndromes. Amblyopia is a common cause of unilateral, and rarely bilateral, decreased vision in young children, but would not be expected to develop after the

age of approximately 7 or 8 years in a child with previously normal eye examinations.

(Page 2290, Section 30: Disorders of the Eyes, Part 2: Disorders of the Eye, Chapter 584)

Answer 30-9. a

Amblyopia is defined as "monocular (or occasionally binocular) vision loss due to impaired visual development in the brain." Strabismus (ie, ocular misalignment), refractive error, or congenital cataract may lead to abnormal visual development of 1 eye and subsequent amblyopia.

In spite of having had good success with amblyopia treatment, which requires correction of refractive error along with patching (see Figure 585-1) or blurring the better-seeing eye (eg, with atropine), amblyopia can recur when the treatment is discontinued or tapered too rapidly. On the cessation of amblyopia therapy, up to 50% may regress and lose gained vision if under the age of 8 to 10 years. Continued use of glasses and a gradual decrease of amblyopia therapy are recommended. Of note, modest success with amblyopia treatment has been shown to work up to the age of 12 years, and perhaps even up to the age of 17 years.

Using the glasses on an as-needed basis, or discontinuing patching, may cause amblyopia to recur. Additionally, it may decrease the patient's binocular vision. Refractive surgery (Lasik) is not approved for children, in part because their eyes are still growing, and refractive error changes over time. Refractive surgery is occasionally used in children with certain subtypes of amblyopia due to asymmetric or high refractive errors, especially if there is no possibility of compliance with spectacles or contact lenses due to neurobehavioral disorders. While patching full time may occasionally be used in the treatment of severe amblyopia, the mild degree of amblyopia now and the long length of follow-up make this an unacceptable choice. Typical follow-up for full-time patching is 1 week for every year of life.

(Pages 2291-2292, Section 30: Disorders of the Eyes, Part 2: Disorders of the Eye, Chapter 585)

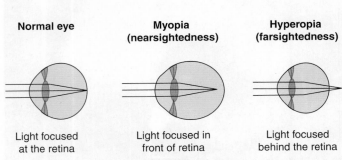

Refractive errors. In a normal eye, light rays converge and focus on the retina. In a myopic (nearsighted) eye, the light rays converge in front of the retina; in a hyperopic eye, they converge behind the retina. (Reproduced, with permission, from Lueder GT. *Pediatric Practice: Ophthalmology.* New York: McGraw-Hill, 2011.)

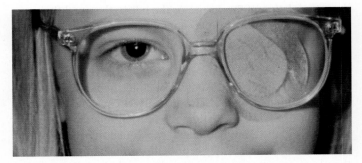

FIGURE 585-1. Note that the patch is on the skin and not on the glasses. The patch is on the child's healthy, nonamblyopic left eye. Amblyopia is present in the right eye. (Reproduced, with permission, from Rudolph CD, Rudolph AM, Lister GE, First LR, Gershon AA. *Rudolph's Pediatrics.* 22nd ed. New York: McGraw-Hill, 2011.)

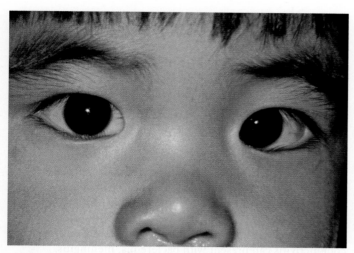

FIGURE 586-3. Pseudoesotropia. Note that the Hirschberg light reflex is symmetric in the pupil of both eyes. Even though the eyes look grossly esotropic, they are actually aligned. (Reproduced, with permission, from Rudolph CD, Rudolph AM, Lister GE, First LR, Gershon AA. *Rudolph's Pediatrics.* 22nd ed. New York: McGraw-Hill, 2011.)

Answer 30-10. d

This child has primary infantile esotropia. This usually develops in the first few weeks to months of life, and there is often a family history. Multiple large studies have showed that constant large-angle esotropia that is still present at age 2 to 4 months is unlikely to resolve without treatment. In a center with access to pediatric anesthesia, surgery for infantile esotropia is generally performed as soon as the ophthalmologist is satisfied with his or her ability to obtain accurate measurements of the degree of ocular misalignment. Prolonged delays, and especially delays beyond the age of 2 years, will decrease the possibility of binocular vision development, and may increase the risk of amblyopia.

There is no evidence for vision therapy being effective in treating infantile esotropia. Alternate patching of the eyes until the time of surgery is a rarely prescribed treatment; the theory behind this treatment is maintaining the capability of the primary visual cortex to respond to binocularly driven inputs, and to ensure that the child does not develop amblyopia in either eye. However, alternate patching is not used to delay surgery, and there is no particular age at which the child becomes "old enough for surgery." Psuedoesotropia is often due to prominent epicanthal folds creating the optical illusion of the esotropia. The Hirschberg light reflex test is normal as seen in Figure 586-3.

(Pages 2294-2295, Section 30: Disorders of the Eyes, Part 2: Disorders of the Eye, Chapter 586)

Answer 30-11. e

Pseudostrabismus or pseudoesotropia is noted when the patient has broad epicanthal folds and the skin is prominent over the medial canthus, covering an increased amount of the sclera nasally, which makes the eyes appear crossed. This is also seen in children with wide nasal bridges. Alternatively, parents may believe an eye is crossed if they look at the child from the side, or take a photograph of the child from the side, and see an unequal amount of nasal sclera showing. A symmetric corneal light reflex and alternate cover test showing no movement of the eyes make true strabismus extremely unlikely. If the pediatrician is unsure of the examination findings, or if the patient has risk factors for true esotropia, such as a family history of esotropia or was born more than 2 months prematurely, the patient can be further evaluated by the pediatric ophthalmologist.

A fourth nerve palsy presents with a head tilt, or a hypertropia. This will be elicited by alternate cover testing. Both accommodative esotropia and acute sixth nerve palsy would present with true esotropia, which would be detected by a decentered corneal light reflex in 1 eye, and outward shift of the eyes on alternate cover testing, limited abduction of 1 eye, and frequently a face turn opposite the direction of abduction deficit. The most common causes of acquired sixth nerve palsy in a child are head trauma and postviral inflammation, although it can also be seen with elevated intracranial pressure, a mass lesion anywhere along the course of the sixth nerve, meningitis, intracranial hypotension, and Gradenigo syndrome (mastoiditis extending to the petrous bone). The best assessment for accommodative esotropia is with the child fixating on a small target near the examiner, such as a sticker or small toy with fine details. Accommodative esotropia is usually treated by glasses and often presents after 2 years of age. This is in contrast to infantile esotropia that is treated by surgery and is evident before 1 year of age. Intermittent exotropia can be detected when the child fixates at a distant object, and the examiner performs an alternate cover test, noting inward shift of the eyes. The history is typically of intermittent outward drift of 1 or either eye, noted primarily when the child is sick or tired, and is often more noticeable on distant gaze.

(Pages 2293-2296, Section 30: Disorders of the Eyes, Part 2: Disorders of the Eye, Chapter 586)

Answer 30-12. b

The examination finding of subdural hemorrhages with a history of a short fall in a 2-year-old child is suspicious for nonaccidental trauma (NAT), specifically shaken baby syndrome. Evaluation for retinal hemorrhages is an important part of the NAT workup. Half of NAT victims die, and of those who survive, half are neurologically devastated. Bleeding in the brain is thought to be due to shearing forces of the brain against the skull. Retinal hemorrhages are common in patients with repetitive acceleration/deceleration forces applied to the head, such as occur with shaking of an infant. One postulated mechanism for retinal hemorrhages is due to shearing forceps exerted by attachments of the jelly-like vitreous onto the retinal vessels. Hemorrhages that extend to the ora serrata (the most peripheral retina), and hemorrhages affecting multiple layers (preretinal, intraretinal, subretinal), are more common with

NAT than other conditions causing retinal hemorrhages. Retinoschisis is a splitting of the retina, and in NAT, it occurs in the macula, with hemorrhage layered between the splits in the macula. Hemorrhagic macular schisis in young children is quite specific for NAT, although it has also been rarely reported in fatal motor vehicle crashes and severe accidental crush injuries of the head.

The visual evoked potential is a test used to estimate visual function by stimulating the retina with patterns and lights, while recording electrical activity from the visual cortex. This test would not be used in the acute setting, or without knowledge about the patient's retinal examination. Coagulopathies and lupus vasculitis are on the differential diagnosis for retinal hemorrhages, although they present with a different set of systemic problems. The presence or absence of retinal hemorrhages has not yet been determined for this particular patient. Hemoglobin electrophoresis would not be the appropriate laboratory test to screen for a coagulopathy potentially associated with bilateral subdural hemorrhages. Although sepsis may present as lethargy in 2 months, given the concern for NAT, ophthalmologic examination is the most appropriate answer.

(Pages 2298-2199, Section 30: Disorders of the Eyes, Part 2: Disorders of the Eye, Chapter 587)

Answer 30-13. a

The clinical description is that of ophthalmia neonatorum, or neonatal conjunctivitis, which by definition occurs within the first month of life. In order to rule out chlamydial conjunctivitis and gonococcal conjunctivitis, Gram stain, Giemsa stain, and bacterial cultures of the conjunctival discharge are the most appropriate initial workup. Chlamydial conjunctivitis presents between 5 and 25 days from birth. If left untreated, pneumonitis may develop in 20% to 40% of affected children. It can be visualized on Giemsa stain as intracellular inclusions within epithelial cells, or cultured or detected by PCR using scrapings of actual conjunctival epithelial cells, not merely conjunctival discharge. *Gonococcus* can be detected as gram-negative diplococci on Gram stain or by culture using modified Thayer-Martin medium. Importantly, the differential for neonatal conjunctivitis includes chemical conjunctivitis, which typically presents bilaterally and begins within 48 hours after instillation of prophylactic agent into the eyes; this was most common when silver nitrate was used for prophylaxis. In addition to chlamydial conjunctivitis and gonococcal conjunctivitis, other bacterial conjunctivitides (such as *Staphylococcus aureus*, *Streptococcus pneumoniae*, *Streptococcus viridans*, *Enterococcus* spp., and *Haemophilus* spp.) should be considered, as well as herpetic keratoconjunctivitis. Bacterial conjunctivitis not due to *Chlamydia* or *gonococcus* is the most common cause of ophthalmia neonatorum in countries where women receive prenatal care and thus have a lower prevalence of peripartum chlamydial and gonococcal infections. Many nonchlamydial and nongonococcal conjunctivitides resolve on their own without treatment, but administration of a broad-spectrum topical antibiotic is prudent and hastens recovery.

Although chlamydial conjunctivitis is on the differential diagnosis, in the absence of clinical signs of pneumonia, oral erythromycin treatment does not need to be instituted until chlamydial infection is confirmed by laboratory testing. If chlamydial conjunctivitis is confirmed, the infant should be treated with oral erythromycin for 14 days and monitored for development of pneumonia. As the child is afebrile and otherwise asymptomatic, a septic workup and evaluation for HSV is not warranted at this time. Of note, herpetic keratoconjunctivitis can present in the setting of viremia, meningoencephalitis, and hepatitis. Herpetic keratoconjunctivitis can present late because not all infections are due to exposure to HSV at the time of delivery. Neonates can also be exposed secondarily via contact with caregivers who have oral HSV lesions or herpetic whitlow. Gonococcal conjunctivitis can present with bacteremia, meningitis, and septic arthritis. It usually presents within the first 5 days of life and appears aggressive, with copious purulent discharge. In the presence of conjunctivitis and a Gram stain showing gram-negative diplococci or a maternal history of untreated gonococcal infection, the baby should be treated with intravenous ceftriaxone. An ill-appearing neonate with conjunctivitis should receive oral erythromycin, intravenous ceftriaxone, and intravenous acyclovir while awaiting results of the diagnostic workup.

(Pages 2300-2301, Section 30: Disorders of the Eyes, Part 2: Disorders of the Eye, Chapter 588; also see Page 910, Section 17: Infectious Disease, Part 1: Principles of Infectious Disease, Chapter 230)

Answer 30-14. e

Contact lenses should not be worn overnight, as they impair normal oxygen diffusion to the cornea and can irritate the ocular surface. In addition, although all contact lens wearers are at increased risk of microbial keratitis, those who wear their contact lenses overnight or for multiple days in a row are especially at risk. The patient in this clinical scenario probably does not have bilateral microbial keratitis, but irritant conjunctivitis and drying of the corneal epithelium caused by contact lens overwear.

Dry eyes from sleeping with eyes open, known as lagophthalmos, develop in patients with eyelid disorders, such as cranial nerve 7 palsies. Bacterial conjunctivitis is a common cause of bilateral conjunctival injection, although it is more common in younger children than in teenagers. In addition to conjunctival injection, the patient will have purulent discharge. Treatment for bacterial conjunctivitis is use of a broad-spectrum antibiotic drop, and good hygiene. Chlamydial conjunctivitis in a teenager or child does not occur acutely. It causes unilateral or bilateral conjunctival injection with a follicular reaction and scant discharge, and it lasts for weeks. It should prompt a query into possible sexual abuse. Parinaud oculoglandular syndrome, which is associated with *Bartonella henselae* infection, or cat scratch disease, presents with unilateral conjunctivitis, large follicles in the lower lid conjunctiva, and ipsilateral preauricular lymphadenopathy.

(Pages 2300-2303, Section 30: Disorders of the Eyes, Part 2: Disorders of the Eye, Chapter 588)

Answer 30-15. a

Viral conjunctivitis often starts in 1 eye and then spreads to the second, less severely affected, eye several days later, with conjunctivitis lasting from a few days to 1 month. Adenoviral epidemic keratoconjunctivitis can also involve the cornea, and it lasts for many weeks. This conjunctivitis is treated with artificial tear drops for comfort, and by following precautions to prevent spread to other individuals: strict hand washing and not sharing towels or linens. Occasionally, an ophthalmologist treats corneal involvement due to adenoviral conjunctivitis with topical steroids. Topical steroid eye drops should not be prescribed by the pediatrician. Bacterial conjunctivitis usually has more purulent discharge; *Streptococcus pneumoniae* is a common pathogen. A corneal abrasion and foreign body would be unilateral, not spread to the other eye, and associated with tearing and with photophobia. Corneal abrasions typically heal within a few days. A chemical reaction to chlorine could cause similar symptoms; however, it would have bilateral simultaneous onset, usually cause a lesser degree of irritation, and would improve during the course of a day.

(Pages 2300-2304, Section 30: Disorders of the Eyes, Part 2: Disorders of the Eye, Chapter 588)

Answer 30-16. e

Among the subtypes of JIA, oligoarticular, polyarticular, or systemic, the highest risk of ophthalmic involvement occurs in young girls affected by ANA-positive oligoarticular JIA. This is typically characterized by chronic iritis causing complications such as corneal opacification, glaucoma, cataract, and macular edema. Importantly, JIA uveitis may be asymptomatic; therefore, regular screening is essential to management.

A leukemic infiltrate can also cause bilateral iritis, but the additional clinical history does not support the diagnosis. The clinical symptoms are not consistent with sarcoidosis, which presents most often with cough or shortness of breath. Sarcoidosis, while rare in children, is more common in African Americans, and can be further investigated with laboratory studies consisting of angiotensin-converting enzyme and lysozyme, chest x-ray, or CT showing hilar lymphadenopathy and biopsy of involved tissues showing noncaseating granulomas. Enthesitis-related spondyloarthropathy is more common in boys, is associated with HLA B27, and presents with sacroiliitis and enthesitis, most often of the Achilles tendon. It can present with anterior uveitis; however, the associated findings in this vignette make this diagnosis less likely. SLE almost never causes iritis; when it affects the eye, it typically causes a retinal vasculitis.

(Page 2302, Section 30: Disorders of the Eyes, Part 2: Disorders of the Eye, Chapter 588; also see Section 15: Rheumatology, Chapters 201, 202, 204, 209)

Answer 30-17. d

Vernal keratoconjunctivitis is a severe form of allergic conjunctivitis that occurs primarily in boys with an atopic history. It causes severe itching of the eyes, and is most bothersome in the spring and summer months. Ocular findings include large, flattened "cobblestone" papillae on the tarsal conjunctivae, white gelatinous elevations along the limbus (the junction of the sclera and cornea), and corneal ulceration (see figures below).

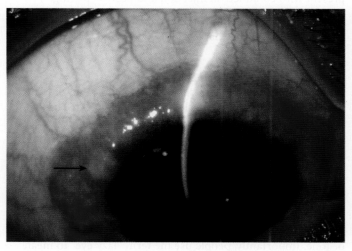

Limbal vernal conjunctivitis. Note gelatinous thickening of conjunctiva at corneal limbus, with white-centered nodules (Horner-Trantas dots) (arrow). (Reproduced, with permission, from Lueder GT. *Pediatric Practice: Ophthalmology.* New York: McGraw-Hill, 2011.)

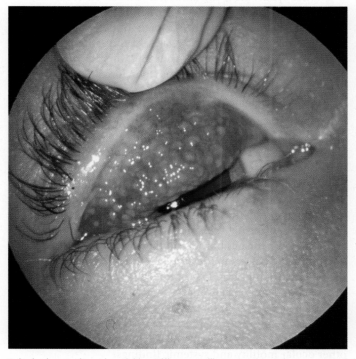

Palpebral vernal conjunctivitis. Diffuse papillary reaction of upper tarsal conjunctiva. (Reproduced, with permission, from Lueder GT. *Pediatric Practice: Ophthalmology.* New York: McGraw-Hill, 2011.)

Mucopurulent discharge, adenopathy, and matted eyelashes are signs of bacterial conjunctivitis.

Vesicles on the eyelid with unilateral conjunctivitis are indicative of a herpetic infection of the eyelid and conjunctiva. Herpes often initially presents unilaterally as eyelid vesicles. Recurrent infections are common even months to years later, often occurring after illness or prolonged sunlight exposure. Lower eyelid follicles and preauricular lymphadenopathy are associated with viral conjunctivitis. Corneal abrasions will present with conjunctival injection and profuse tearing.

(Pages 2303-2304, Section 30: Disorders of the Eyes, Part 2: Disorders of the Eye, Chapter 588)

Answer 30-18. e

Bilateral congenital ptosis results from abnormal development of the levator palpebrae muscle in the upper eyelid. These patients have absent eyelid creases, virtually no ability to elevate the eyelid without engaging the frontalis muscle of the forehead, and (when severe) chin-up head postures. The patient has mildly delayed walking due to having to maintain a chin-up posture to see from under his ptotic eyelids. The problem has been present since birth, is stable, and is not associated with other physical examination findings, such as weakness, or abnormalities in muscle bulk or tone. Importantly, people use the term "lazy eye" to mean different things; additional history may reveal the parent is reporting ptosis, exotropia, esotropia, nystagmus or roving eye movements, or poor vision in 1 or both eyes. Treatment for congenital ptosis requires surgical repair.

Horner syndrome is the unilateral association of miosis, mild ptosis, and anhidrosis. It is not severe enough to cause a chin-up head posture, as the sympathetically innervated muscle of the upper eyelid is a relatively unimportant elevator of the eyelid. Bilateral Horner syndrome would be unusual. It is essential to rule out neuroblastoma; therefore, the workup for Horner syndrome requires urine studies for homovanillic acid (HVA) and vanillyl mandelic acid (VMA) and imaging studies along the sympathetic nerve chain. Third nerve palsy would present with ocular motility abnormalities in addition to ptosis. If the third nerve palsy is complete, the pupil would also be dilated on the ipsilateral side. Again, bilateral third nerve palsy is unusual. Third nerve palsy requires neuroimaging due to very high incidence of tumor or brain pathology. Myasthenia gravis rarely presents as ptosis since birth. However, it can occur due to placental transmission of antiacetylcholine antibodies in neonates born to mothers with the disease, or due to genetic defects in the acetylcholine receptor. However, the presence of ptosis and no other ocular or systemic findings in a 15-month-old male would be highly atypical. Acquired myasthenia gravis in children can present with ptosis or abnormal eye movements. Muscular dystrophies, including mitochondrial myopathies, are usually progressive and have other ocular motility and systemic findings.

(Pages 2305-2306, Section 30: Disorders of the Eyes, Part 2: Disorders of the Eye, Chapter 589)

Answer 30-19. d

Multiple cranial nerve palsies, vomiting, and headaches severe enough to awaken the child suggest a CNS mass lesion. Immediate neuroimaging is essential.

Mastoiditis would present with redness and swelling behind the ear, fever, headache, and decreased hearing, but not multiple cranial nerve palsies. Kawasaki disease presents with swollen palms and soles, a strawberry tongue, adenopathy, conjunctivitis, and 5 days or longer of high fever, none of which are present in this patient. The management includes coronary artery imaging and treatment with IVIG and aspirin. Viral meningitis might present with headaches and multiple cranial nerve palsies, but would likely also have fever and more systemic findings. Migraines often are associated with an aura, photophobia and phonophobia, and visual phenomena. However, multiple cranial nerve palsies would be unusual. Initial treatment includes avoiding migraine triggers and NSAIDs. A headache that wakes a child at night and is associated with recurrent vomiting suggests increased intracranial pressure until proven otherwise.

(Page 2305, Section 30: Disorders of the Eyes, Part 2: Disorders of the Eye, Chapter 589; also see Section 24: Neoplastic Disorders, Part 3: Solid Tumors, Chapter 460)

Answer 30-20. a

Both chalazia and hordeola are commonly referred to as "styes." A chalazion is a nodule secondary to chronic inflammation due to a blocked gland in the eyelid tarsus and presents as a firm, occasionally painful mass in the eyelid. Hordeola are similar blocked glands that are often erythematous and inflamed. Most lesions will resolve on own over many months. Treatment consists of hot compresses, for weeks to months. The lesions will often get bigger and redder initially with heat as the hardened oil liquefies and passes into the surrounding tissue. Over weeks the lesion will resolve. Hand washing, hygiene of the lid margins (with lid scrubs/baby shampoo), and possibly diet with less saturated fats will decrease the incidence of the chalazia. Lesions can resolve faster with surgical drainage by an ophthalmologist, or, rarely, with intralesional steroid injection. Because these measures require general anesthesia for young children, chalazia and hordeola in children are generally treated conservatively.

Hemangiomas usually present around birth, as reddish purple fleshy lesions. Most grow during the first year, and then spontaneously resolve over the subsequent 5 years. Treatment historically has been reserved for vision-compromising lesions and was primarily with steroids, local and systemic. Newer treatment options include systemic propranolol and topical β-blocker eye drops.

Epiblepheron is lid inversion usually of the lower lid due to overriding orbicularis muscles. The incidence is more common in Asians and Hispanics. As the face grows, the lids often evert spontaneously. In severe cases of corneal damage, eyelid surgery can be performed. Molluscum typically presents with multiple smaller, firm, umbilicated lesions. They may cause

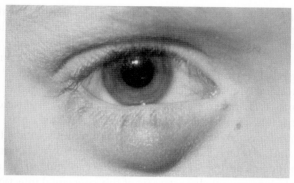

A

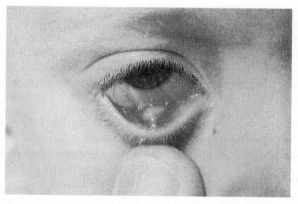

B

Chalazion. (**A**) Right lower lid, external view. (**B**) Right lower lid conjunctival surface. (Reproduced, with permission, from Hay WW, Levin MJ, Deterding RR, et al. *Current Diagnosis & Treatment: Pediatrics.* 21st ed. New York: McGraw-Hill, 2012.)

a reactive conjunctivitis if near the lid margin. A dacryocele is a mucocele overlying the lacrimal sac due to nasolacrimal obstruction. This is a bluish mass that typically presents within days of birth below the medial canthal ligament.

(Pages 2306-2308, Section 30: Disorders of the Eyes, Part 2: Disorders of the Eye, Chapter 589)

Answer 30-21. d

NLDO is present in 20% of neonates, but approximately 95% resolve without treatment by the age of 1 year. While massaging the lacrimal sac can help keep mucoid discharge from accumulating in the nasolacrimal drainage system, the true effect of massage is unknown. Lid hygiene and prophylactic antibiotic ointment to prevent or treat conjunctival infections may be helpful. If the tearing and discharge do not resolve by 1 year of age, most pediatric ophthalmologists would recommend probing the nasolacrimal system since the likelihood of spontaneous resolution in subsequent months/years wanes.

Herpes simplex virus infection often presents around the eye as a vesicular dermatitis. There is often a history

of cold sores in a caregiver. The first infection typically involves only the eyelids. Recurrent/reactivated herpes simplex virus infections can present with conjunctivitis or keratitis, characterized by multiple episodes of conjunctival injection and/or corneal dendrites. Varicella zoster in the V1 distribution can mimic a primary periocular herpes simplex virus infection. This can occur even if the patient has had the vaccine for varicella. Varicella zoster may be associated with corneal infiltrates and iritis even weeks after the skin manifestations. When a child has had either herpes simplex virus or recurrent varicella zoster virus affecting the eyelid, and the ipsilateral eye becomes red, they should see an ophthalmologist urgently. The ophthalmologist will examine the cornea for dendrites and other types of corneal infiltrates with fluorescein, and will assess the anterior chamber for evidence of iritis. Congenital glaucoma can be differentiated from NLDO by severe photophobia, absence of discharge, and clouding and enlargement of the cornea. Tearing is common in both conditions; thus, congenital glaucoma is important to consider on the differential diagnosis of tearing in a neonate. A congenital dacryocele usually presents within days of birth as a bluish mass below the medial canthal ligament. This cyst extends into the nose and can cause respiratory compromise in children who are obligate nasal breathers. While dacryoceles can sometimes be ruptured and resolved with massage, those that do not resolve with massage require probing with marsupialization and removal of the cyst in the nose below the inferior turbinate since they can become infected. Up to 30% of dacryoceles are bilateral and can cause respiratory compromise or interfere with feeding.

(Pages 2307-2308, Section 30: Disorders of the Eyes, Part 2: Disorders of the Eye, Chapter 589)

Answer 30-22. d

This child has leukocoria, which presents as a white pupil or absent red reflex. The differential diagnosis of leukocoria in an infant is broad and includes cataract, retinoblastoma, retinal detachment, Coats disease, and toxoplasmosis and *Toxocara* infections (see Figure 15-23). Autosomal dominant cataracts are the most common cause of cataracts in infants, and they occur in the absence of other systemic findings. Given this child's family history, bilateral congenital cataract is the most likely diagnosis. If there is no family history of cataracts occurring at an early age in the mother or father, the patient may receive a workup for metabolic causes of cataracts, such as galactosemia or Lowe syndrome, for TORCH infections, and for chromosomal disorders, such as Down syndrome.

Retinoblastoma is less likely given the family history. Despite the fact that retinoblastoma is not suspected in this case, the ophthalmologist would examine the posterior segment of the eye with ultrasonography to rule out a mass or retinal detachment prior to performing cataract surgery. Retinal detachment in infants can occur due to retinopathy of prematurity, retinal dysplasias, such as familial exudative vitreoretinopathy or Norrie disease, incontinentia pigmenti, Stickler syndrome, and trauma. Coats disease is a disorder

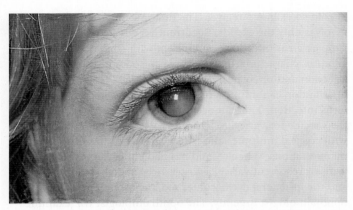

FIGURE 15-23. Cataract causing leukocoria. (Reproduced, with permission, from Hay WW, Levin MJ, Deterding RR, et al. *Current Diagnosis & Treatment: Pediatrics.* 21st ed. New York: McGraw-Hill, 2012.)

characterized by telangiectasias of retinal blood vessels, and it most commonly affects boys. It is most often unilateral with a mean age of diagnosis of 8 years. When severe, it can cause exudative retinal detachment. This diagnosis is not supported by the family history, the bilateral presentation, and the patient's young age. Corneal scarring can be bilateral and cause absence of the red reflex due to corneal opacification. However, the examiner should note that the level of the opacification is at the cornea, not at the lens or posterior to the lens. Opacification at the level of the cornea prevents the examiner from having a clear view of the iris, and when severe, a pupillary examination is not possible.

(Pages 2310-2312, Section 30: Disorders of the Eyes, Part 2: Disorders of the Eye, Chapter 590)

Answer 30-23. b

Many of the TORCH infections can present with eye pathology at birth. CMV infection is the most common congenital infection. Although most children are asymptomatic, some have severe sequelae and intrauterine growth retardation. As described in this vignette, findings associated with congenital CMV infection include hepatosplenomegaly, scleral icterus and jaundice due to hyperbilirubinemia, and periventricular calcifications within the brain. CMV retinitis can also occur, which may appear as grossly normal on examination. Diagnosis is made through urine CMV antigen testing. Treatment is with intravenous ganciclovir, and the prognosis is poor.

Herpes simplex virus infection in the neonate can manifest as disseminated disease, central nervous system disease, or skin/eye/mucous membrane (SEM) disease. Skin vesicles, rather than purpuric blueberry-type skin lesions, are common but need not be present with any of the 3 presentation types. Ocular findings can include keratoconjunctivitis and iritis. HSV infection in the neonate is treated with intravenous acyclovir. Congenital rubella infections have become very rare in parts of the world with effective rubella vaccination

campaigns. Congenital rubella results in intrauterine growth restriction, congenital heart disease, and ocular manifestations such as cataracts, microphthalmos, congenital glaucoma, and later-onset retinopathy. Purpuric lesions may occur, but congenital cerebral calcifications in general do not occur. Congenital lymphocytic choriomeningitis infection in the neonate is characterized by seizures, intracranial calcifications, hydrocephalus, and microcephaly or macrocephaly. Ophthalmic manifestations include chorioretinitis, cataracts, and optic atrophy. There may be a maternal history of contact with rodents during pregnancy. Splenomegaly and purpuric skin lesions are not characteristic of this congenital infection. Congenital toxoplasmosis infection results from maternal exposure to *Toxoplasma* cysts in undercooked meats or in cat excrement. Systemic findings in the neonate include hepatosplenomegaly, intracranial calcifications, hydrocephalus, and microcephaly or macrocephaly; however, blueberry-type skin lesions are not common. A common ophthalmic finding is the presence of bilateral chorioretinal scars, most often in the maculae.

(Page 2312, Section 30: Disorders of the Eyes, Part 2: Disorders of the Eye, Chapter 590; also see Section 17: Infectious Diseases, Part 1: Principles of Infectious Disease, Chapter 230)

Answer 30-24. a

In the United States, babies born with birth weight less than 1500 g or with gestational age 30 weeks or less undergo screening examinations for ROP. Only a small percentage of patients actually require laser treatment for ROP, and these babies have an average birth weight of 800 g. Laser helps prevent many of the immediate complications of progressive ROP, such as retinal detachment; however, babies treated for ROP with laser are still at risk of late complications. Myopia is common in more than 50% of these infants. Strabismus has been reported in approximately 25% of all infants born before gestational age of 32 weeks. (The normal incidence of strabismus in the population is approximately 3%-5%.) Late retinal detachments, which can occur in the teenage years, have also been reported.

Although cataracts and glaucoma are possible from sequelae of both laser and ROP, they generally present earlier, and dermoids have no association with ROP. Orbital dermoid cysts are embryological cysts containing remnants of epidermal tissue. They usually arise in utero at the sites where orbital bone suture fusion occurs (see Figure 589-4). Colobomas are due to incomplete formation of the eye embryologically; they present as a keyhole iris, with the defect pointing inferonasally, or as inferonasal defects of the optic nerve, retina, and choroid. Colobomas have no specific relation to ROP, although children with syndromes associated with colobomas may be more likely to be born prematurely than those without. Iris transillumination, ptosis, color blindness, Marcus Gunn jaw winking, and blepharospasm are not associated with ROP. Iris transillumination defects are most commonly associated with albinism in children. Five percent to 10% of all males have red-green color deficiency. Marcus Gunn jaw winking is a rare phenomenon in which the upper eyelid, normally innervated by branches of cranial nerve III, is instead innervated by misdirected branches of cranial nerve V, such that eyelid movement occurs with movement of the jaw. Blepharospasm, or periodic involuntary forceful closure of the eyelid, is rare in children. Blepharospasm cannot be willfully stopped by the child.

(Pages 2313-2318, Section 30: Disorders of the Eyes, Part 2: Disorders of the Eye, Chapter 591)

Answer 30-25. b

The current guidelines for ROP laser treatment incorporate zone of disease, stage of disease, and the presence of plus disease. Zone (I, II, or III) refers to the location of ROP relative to the optic disc; the lower the zone, the closer the disease is to the optic disc and thus to the macula, with greater risk of affecting central vision (see Figure 591-1).

The stage of disease (1-5) refers to the presence of specific findings at the border between vascular and avascular retina, or for stages 4 and 5, the extent of retinal detachment. Plus disease refers to vascular dilation and tortuosity around the optic disc; plus disease is the single most important factor determining the need for ROP treatment. The number of involved clock hours is no longer a treatment criterion, although it is still documented by the treating ophthalmologist to monitor the patient's progress.

Based on Early Treatment for Retinopathy of Prematurity guidelines from a large randomized multicenter clinical trial, ROP laser treatment is administered for:

- Zone I, any stage with plus disease
- Zone I, stage 3 whether or not plus disease is present
- Zone II, stage 2 or 3 with plus disease

Answer choices A and D are incorrect because gestational age is not a criterion for ROP treatment, although it is a criterion for determining whether the baby undergoes ROP

screening. Answer choice C is incorrect because stage of disease alone is not enough to guide treatment (with the exception of stages 4 and 5, which means a retinal detachment is present, and the baby may be treated with incisional intraocular surgery rather than with laser surgery alone). Retinal vascular maturity means that the retina has completely vascularized and ROP can no longer develop. ROP screening can be discontinued.

(Pages 2313-2316, Section 30: Disorders of the Eyes, Part 2: Disorders of the Eye, Chapter 591)

Answer 30-26. b

ROP requiring treatment typically develops between 36 and 39 weeks' corrected gestational age. Thus, current guidelines call for screening of at-risk neonates at corrected gestational age of 31 weeks or 4 weeks after birth, whichever is later. The highest-risk infants, those born at 27 weeks' gestational age or earlier, are examined at 31 weeks, and those born at 28 weeks' gestational age and older are examined at 32 weeks or later. This screening protocol attempts to minimize unnecessary examinations yet detect treatment-requiring ROP early enough.

At 27 weeks, this baby is too young to begin screening. The vitreous is likely still opacified, the retina is very immature, and the baby is too young to have developed ROP. The other answer choices are too late.

(Page 2315, Section 30: Disorders of the Eyes, Part 2: Disorders of the Eye, Chapter 592)

Answer 30-27. b

The clinical description is that of sporadic aniridia. Aniridia is technically a misnomer, as there is a residual stump of iris tissue present, but it is difficult to visualize without specialized equipment. Other ophthalmic features of aniridia include foveal hypoplasia, a deficiency of stem cells that repopulate

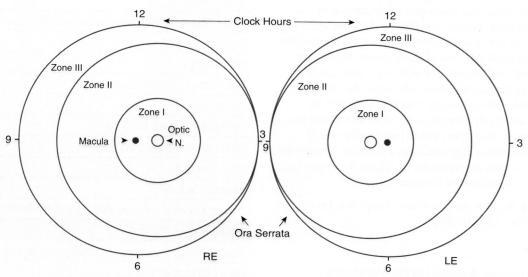

FIGURE 591-1. Zone system used to define location of ROP. (Reproduced, with permission, from Rudolph CD, Rudolph AM, Lister GE, First LR, Gershon AA. *Rudolph's Pediatrics.* 22nd ed. New York: McGraw-Hill, 2011.)

the corneal epithelium, cataracts, glaucoma, and nystagmus that develops within a few months of life. Two thirds of cases of aniridia are inherited in an AD fashion and not associated with systemic disease. A history of aniridia and nystagmus due to bilateral poor vision in the mother or father would be reassuring. When aniridia is sporadic, there is a high risk of deletion of the short of chromosome 11, which carries not only the gene for aniridia (PAX6) but also the Wilms tumor gene (WT1). These patients must be periodically screened for Wilms tumor with renal ultrasonography during childhood. WAGR syndrome refers to Wilms tumor, aniridia, genitourinary malformations, and mental retardation. The other answer choices would not detect the life-threatening renal tumor.

(Page 2317, Section 30: Disorders of the Eyes, Part 2: Disorders of the Eye, Chapter 592)

Answer 30-28. b

The most common cause of hereditary retinal dystrophy and hearing loss is Usher syndrome. These patients have retinitis pigmentosa, which manifests itself as nyctalopia (night blindness) and constriction of the peripheral visual field. In later stages, central vision also becomes affected. Depending on the age of onset of sensorineural hearing loss, the child may or may not have normal speech development. Usher syndrome is one of many diseases associated with retinitis pigmentosa (see Table 592-3).

Horner syndrome is the association of miosis, mild ptosis, and anhidrosis. The patient may also exhibit asymmetric flushing of the upper face. When congenital, iris heterochromia is also present. Horner syndrome occurs due to injury or mass lesions along the sympathetic tract. Although most cases are idiopathic, there are many known causes of Horner syndrome, including birth trauma, CNS disorders, upper thoracic surgeries, carotid artery dissection, and neuroblastoma. In infants and young children with acquired Horner syndrome, it is important to rule out neuroblastoma involving the sympathetic chain. Stargardt disease is a macular dystrophy characterized by decreased central vision. Because the disease does not affect the peripheral retina, in which rod photoreceptors predominate, the disease is not associated with loss of night vision. Nystagmus is a rapid back-and-forth movement of the eyes that can be due to disorders of the eye, the visual pathways, the vestibular system, and central nervous system disorders unrelated to vision. Although retinal dystrophies with onset at a young age can cause nystagmus, nystagmus would not develop due to slowly progressive retinitis pigmentosa in a teenager. Congenital rubella syndrome is also characterized by retinal dystrophy and hearing loss, but it would not be hereditary.

(Pages 2323-2324, Section 30: Disorders of the Eyes, Part 2: Disorders of the Eye, Chapter 592)

Answer 30-29. b

The signs and symptoms described in this vignette are consistent with "idiopathic" intracranial hypertension, also known as pseudotumor cerebrii. Specific risk factors

TABLE 592-3. Systemic Disease Associations With Retinitis Pigmentosa

Autosomal Dominant
Alagille syndrome (arteriohepatic dysplasia)
Charcot-Marie-Tooth disease
Flynn-Aird syndrome
Oculodentodigital dysplasia syndrome
Olivopontocerebellar atrophy
Paget disease
Pierre Robin syndrome
Steinert disease (myotonic dystrophy)
Stickler syndrome
Waardenburg syndrome
Wagner disease

Autosomal Recessive
Albers-Schönberg disease (osteoporosis)
Alström disease
Bardet-Biedl syndrome
Bassen-Kornzweig disease (abetalipoproteinemia)
Batten disease
Cockayne syndrome
Friedreich ataxia
Grönblad-Strandberg syndrome
Hallgren syndrome
Homocystinuria
Hurler syndrome (MPS 1-H)
Jeune syndrome
Juvenile Paget disease (hyperostosis corticalis deformans juvenilis)
Kearns-Sayre syndrome
Mannosidosis
Marinesco-Sjögren syndrome
Refsum disease
Sanfilippo syndrome (MPS III)
Scheie syndrome (MPS 1-S)
Usher syndrome
Wolfram syndrome
Zellweger syndrome (cerebrohepatorenal syndrome)

X-linked
Bloch-Sulzberger syndrome (incontinentia pigmenti)
Hunter syndrome (MPS II)
Pelizaeus-Merzbacher disease

include weight gain and obesity in postpubertal patients, the use of tetracycline, retinoic acid, growth hormone, some chemotherapeutics, or withdrawal of steroids. Optic disc swelling and a sixth nerve paresis are characteristic. This disorder is more common in postpubertal females. The diagnosis is confirmed by ruling out intracranial pathology and finding high intracranial pressure on a lumbar puncture once neuroimaging has ruled out an intracranial mass lesion. Fundoscopic examination reveals papilledema. Treatment consists of removal of the offending agent (in this case, retinoic acid) and weight loss. Even modest weight loss can be quite helpful in resolving symptoms and signs. Pharmacological treatment consists of oral acetazolamide, furosemide, and rarely steroids. Recalcitrant cases, or cases with impending vision loss, may require optic nerve sheath fenestration or lumboperitoneal shunting.

Venous sinus thrombosis is an underrecognized cause of "idiopathic" intracranial hypertension, and can be diagnosed on magnetic resonance venography, but it is not the most likely cause in this overweight female taking retinoic acid. Meningitis is usually associated with fevers and meningismus. A brain tumor could cause all of the findings in the vignette but would likely have other associated neurological signs and symptoms, and it is not the most likely diagnosis. Regardless, neuroimaging should be performed prior to lumbar puncture to rule out a mass lesion.

(Page 2329, Section 30: Disorders of the Eyes, Part 2: Disorders of the Eye, Chapter 593)

Answer 30-30. c

Optic neuritis is a demyelinating inflammatory condition of the optic nerve, which can develop after a viral infection (usually 1-2 weeks) or vaccination for viral disease. It is associated with multiple sclerosis (MS), Guillain-Barré syndrome, and syphilis. Findings in optic neuritis include decreased visual acuity, decreased color vision, decreased peripheral vision, an afferent pupillary defect, and an optic disc appearance that can be entirely normal during the initial weeks of the event. If the optic neuritis becomes chronic or recurrent, it can lead to optic atrophy (a pale disc appearance) over the course of many weeks. Optic neuritis occasionally affects the anterior portion of the optic nerve itself, resulting in optic disc hyperemia and edema; however, more often, it affects the posterior portions of the optic nerve, which cannot be seen on fundoscopic examination. Optic neuritis is less commonly associated with MS in children, compared with adults; however, given this patient's MRI finding and postpubertal age, it is the likely etiology.

A compressive lesion of the optic nerve, such as a pituitary adenoma, would be noted on MRI and would not have the associated periventricular white matter changes. Macular edema, without coexisting optic nerve inflammation, would not cause a decrease in color vision or an afferent pupillary defect. Macular edema is rare in children. Some causes include neuroretinitis (exudates accumulate in the macula in a star-shaped pattern; most often associated with *Bartonella henselae*

infection), pars planitis (an idiopathic type of uveitis affecting predominantly boys in the early teens that causes inflammation just behind the iris), and chronic juvenile idiopathic arthritis. There is no history of severe orbital or head trauma. Leber hereditary optic neuropathy affects boys almost exclusively and is due to a mitochondrial DNA defect. It does not have associated central nervous system findings. It usually presents in a teenage boy as visual loss in 1 eye progressing over weeks to months, and then involving the other eye.

(Page 2329, Section 30: Disorders of the Eyes, Part 2: Disorders of the Eye, Chapter 593)

Answer 30-31. i

Neurofibromatosis type I is an autosomal dominant disorder, but 50% of cases are due to new mutations. Most affected individuals develop Lisch nodules (benign hamartomas) of the iris by 8 years of age, but these are rarely seen in very young children. Optic nerve gliomas occur in less than 10% and are often present in the first few years of life. Two of 7 major diagnostic criteria establish the diagnosis:

1. Six or more café au lait macules over 5 mm in greatest diameter in prepubertal individuals and over 15 mm in greatest diameter in postpubertal individuals
2. Two or more neurofibromas of any type or 1 plexiform neurofibroma
3. Freckling in the axillary or inguinal regions (Crowe sign)
4. Optic glioma
5. Two or more Lisch nodules (iris hamartomas)
6. A distinctive osseous lesion such as sphenoid dysplasia or thinning of long bone cortex with or without pseudoarthrosis
7. A first-degree relative (parent, sibling, or offspring) with NF1 by the above criteria

(Section 30: Disorders of the Eyes, Part 2: Disorders of the Eye, Chapter 590, Table 590-4)

Answer 30-32. a

The severity of ocular manifestations of diabetes depends on the number of years with the disease and blood sugar control. Neovascularization of the iris, and the optic disc and retina, occurs when there is chronic retinal ischemia leading to vascular endothelial growth factor secretion, and it is a late sign, rarely occurring before 10 years with type 1 diabetes. Hyperglycemia can cause the lens to swell, leading to a myopic shift. Controlling blood sugar and thus decreasing the Hgb A1c will stop or slow progression of diabetic changes in the eye.

(Section 30: Disorders of the Eyes, Part 2: Disorders of the Eye, Chapter 590, Table 590-5)

Answer 30-33. h

The acronym CHARGE stands for: *c*olobomas of the eye, *h*eart defects, *a*tresia (choanal), *r*etardation of growth and development, *g*enital anomalies, and *e*ar anomalies.

Ocular colobomas occur because of abnormal closure of the embryonic fissure during ocular development. They are inferonasal in location and can affect the optic disc, choroid/retina, ciliary body, and iris.

(Page 2327, Section 30: Disorders of the Eyes, Part 2: Disorders of the Eye, Chapter 593; also see Section 12: Clinical Genetics and Dysmorphology, Part 3: Birth Defects, Malformations, and Syndromes, Chapter 176)

Answer 30-34. b

Mucopolysaccharidoses are lysosomal storage disorders due to abnormalities in the metabolic breakdown of glycosaminoglycans. Glycosaminoglycans can accumulate in the cornea and in the optic nerve, causing progressive corneal opacification and optic atrophy.

(Section 30: Disorders of the Eyes, Part 2: Disorders of the Eye, Chapter 590, Table 590-1)

Answer 30-35. m

Tay-Sachs disease is an autosomal recessive disorder with higher prevalence among Eastern European Ashkenazi Jews. It occurs due to insufficient activity of the β-hexosaminidase A enzyme, causing accumulation of ganglioside GM2 in the retina and the brain. The reason for formation of the cherry-red spot is that the central fovea lacks ganglion cells, whereas the perifoveal area is rich in ganglion cells. Ganglioside accumulates in the perifoveal ganglion cells, rendering them slightly opaque, and allowing the natural reddish/brownish color of the central fovea to appear most prominent. The accumulation of ganglioside in the retinal ganglion cells also causes optic atrophy, as the optic nerve is essentially the axonal extension of the ganglion cell bodies. Babies with Tay-Sachs disease progressively become blind.

(Section 29: Disorders of the Nervous System, Part 7: Developmental Delay and Regression, Chapter 574, Figure 574-1)

Answer 30-36. g

The association of a port wine stain, ipsilateral glaucoma, and seizure disorder with cerebral vascular malformation and calcification is termed Sturge-Weber syndrome. Children with port wine stain, including those with no central nervous system disease, should be monitored for development of glaucoma. Often, the conjunctiva of the eye ipsilateral to the port wine stain has a pink hue due to elevation of episcleral venous pressure. If the eye develops significant glaucoma, the eye grows and appears large and has a myopic refractive error compared with the contralateral eye. Choroidal hemangiomas are also associated with port wine stain and Sturge-Weber syndrome.

(Section 30: Disorders of the Eyes, Part 2: Disorders of the Eye, Chapter 590, Table 590-5)

Answer 30-37. c

Stickler syndrome is a hereditary autosomal dominant disorder due to a type 2 collagen defect. Affected individuals have a flattened midface, a high arched palate or frank clefting of the palate, micrognathia, hearing deficits, joint hypermobility, and various ocular findings. They are typically myopic at birth and develop a progressive degeneration of the vitreous that, along with retinal abnormalities, places them at high risk for retinal detachments.

(Page 2325, Section 30: Disorders of the Eyes, Part 2: Disorders of the Eye, Chapter 592)

Answer 30-38. n

These patients with albinism have lightly pigmented skin and hair, and blue irides. The irides have transillumination defects, best appreciated at the slit lamp. Because the patients' foveas are hypoplastic, visual acuity is decreased, and the patients have bilateral jerk or pendular nystagmus. Some patients have ocular albinism, without the involvement of the skin and hair; they also have iris transillumination defects and nystagmus on account of foveal hypoplasia.

(Section 30: Disorders of the Eyes, Part 2: Disorders of the Eye, Chapter 590, Table 590-4)

Answer 30-39. l

Goldenhar, also known as oculo-auriculo-vertebral, syndrome is characterized by dermoids, preauricular appendages, and vertebral anomalies. Patients with Goldenhar syndrome may also have hemifacial microsomia, and defects of the heart, kidneys, and central nervous system. Dermoids can occur anywhere on the surface of the eye, although they are most common inferotemporally straddling the junction between the sclera and cornea (the limbus), and they can also occur within the orbit. Duane syndrome, which results from congenital cranial misinnervation of the lateral rectus muscle by cranial nerve III instead of cranial nerve VI, can also coexist with Goldenhar syndrome. Most patients with Duane syndrome exhibit a deficit in abduction that mimics a congenital CNVI palsy.

(Section 30: Disorders of the Eyes, Part 2: Disorders of the Eye, Chapter 592, Table 592-2; also see Section 12: Clinical Genetics and Dysmorphology, Part 3: Birth Defects, Malformations, and Syndromes, Chapter 177)

Answer 30-40. k

Marfan syndrome occurs due to mutations in the fibrillin-1 gene. Skeletal abnormalities include tall stature, long fingers, chest wall deformities, and scoliosis; cardiac defects include aortic root dilation and mitral valve prolapse; ophthalmic abnormalities include lens subluxation and myopia. The lens subluxation occurs because fibrillin is a component of the zonules, which are thin fibers that attach the lens to the ciliary body. Loss or elongation of the zonules causes the lens to shift from a position centered with respect to the pupil.

(Section 30: Disorders of the Eyes, Part 2: Disorders of the Eye, Chapter 590, Table 590-5)

Answer 30-41. j

Riley-Day syndrome is also called familial dysautonomia. It has higher prevalence among Eastern European Ashkenazi Jews. Due to autonomous nervous system dysfunction, these patients have temperature instability, lability in blood pressure, abnormal sweating, and abnormal tear production, leading to dryness of the eye. They also have decreased taste, decreased pain perception, and corneal anesthesia. The combination of poor tear production and poor corneal sensation puts them at risk for progressive corneal ulceration and opacification.

(Page 2308, Section 30: Disorders of the Eyes, Part 2: Disorders of the Eye, Chapter 589)

Answer 30-42. f

Tuberous sclerosis is an autosomal dominant disorder due to mutations in either tuberin or hamartin. Patients typically have a seizure disorder associated with cortical tubers and subependymal nodules or astrocytomas. Skin manifestations include ash leaf spots, facial angiofibromas ("adenoma sebaceum"), periungual fibromas, and shagreen patches. They can also develop cardiac rhabdomyomas or rhabdomyosarcomas and renal benign and malignant angiomyolipomas. The primary ophthalmic feature is that of retinal hamartomas called astrocytomas, which rarely affect vision.

(Section 30: Disorders of the Eyes, Part 2: Disorders of the Eye, Chapter 592, Table 592-2)

Answer 30-43. o

Crouzon syndrome is one of the more common craniosynostosis syndromes, in which premature closure of the cranial sutures results in an abnormal shape of the skull and the orbits. Patients with Crouzon syndrome also have midface hypoplasia. The orbits are shallow, causing proptosis. When severe, there can be inadequate eyelid closure, resulting in corneal exposure, also known as exposure keratopathy, or spontaneous luxation of the globe forward and between the eyelids. Patients can develop optic nerve atrophy from elevated intracranial pressure or tight optic canals, and strabismus is common due to unusual locations/positions of the extraocular muscles.

(Section 12: Clinical Genetics and Dysmorphology, Part 3: Birth Defects, Malformations, and Syndromes, Chapter 177, Table 177-1)

Answer 30-44. e

Down syndrome, or trisomy 21, has many ophthalmic manifestations. The characteristic ocular appearance with narrow palpebral fissures, epicanthal folds, and almond-shaped eyes is by itself of no visual significance. Blepharitis and nasolacrimal duct obstruction are common in Down syndrome and can cause tearing and discharge. Brushfield spots are whitish spots occurring in the peripheral iris, have no visual significance, and can be seen in patients with blue irides in addition to Down syndrome patients. Down's patients can develop snowflake cataracts; they are occasionally visually significant. Patients with trisomy 21 also have a high incidence of refractive errors (requiring spectacle correction) and strabismus.

(Section 30: Disorders of the Eyes, Part 2: Disorders of the Eye, Chapter 590, Table 590-4)

Answer 30-45. d

Wilson disease is a rare disorder of copper transport, resulting in neurological deficits and liver disease. Deposition of the copper occurs in the peripheral cornea at the level of Descemet membrane, resulting in a golden brown ring in the peripheral cornea. This is best evaluated by slit lamp examination.

(Section 30: Disorders of the Eyes, Part 2: Disorders of the Eye, Chapter 590, Table 590-1)

INDEX

Note: Page numbers followed with '*f*' and '*t*' represents figures and tables respectively.

617